REVIEW OF ORTHOPAEDICS

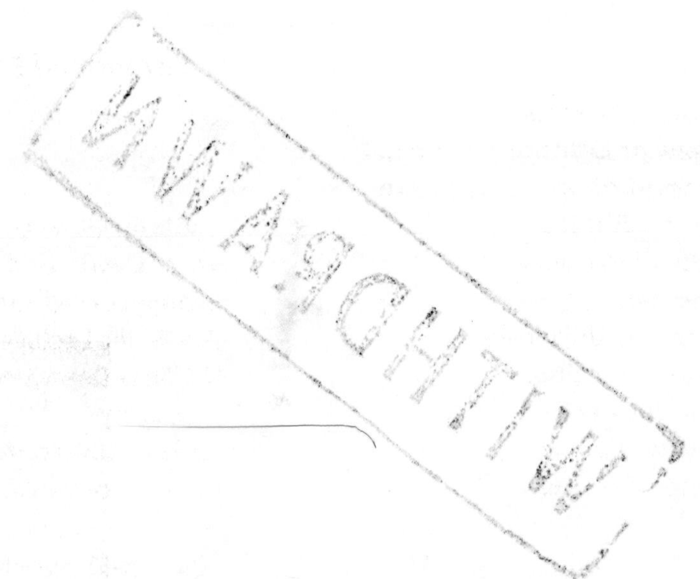

REVIEW OF ORTHOPAEDICS

Sixth Edition

Mark D. Miller, MD
S. Ward Casscells Professor
Department of Orthopaedic Surgery;
Head, Division of Sports Medicine
University of Virginia
Charlottesville, Virginia;
Team Physician
James Madison University
Harrisonburg, Virginia;
Founder and Director
Miller Review Course
Westminster, Colorado

Stephen R. Thompson, MD, MEd, FRCSC
Orthopaedic Sport Medicine Fellow
Fowler Kennedy Sport Medicine Clinic
University of Western Ontario
London, Ontario, Canada

Jennifer A. Hart, MPAS, PA-C
Physician Assistant
Department of Orthopaedic Surgery
University of Virginia
Charlottesville, Virginia

International Editors

Tom Cosker FRCS (Tr & Orth) MSc (Tr Surg)
Clinical Fellow and Academic Lecturer
Royal Devon and Exeter Hospital
Exeter, United Kingdom;
Academic Lecturer
Nuffield Department of Orthopaedic Surgery
Oxford, United Kingdom
Course Convenor, Miller UK Review Course

Sherief Elsayed, MB BCh, MRCS (Eng)
Orthopaedic Surgeon
Queens Medical Centre
Nottingham, United Kingdom
Course Convenor, Miller UK Review Course

ELSEVIER
SAUNDERS

ELSEVIER
SAUNDERS
An imprint of Elsevier, Inc.

1600 John F. Kennedy Blvd.
Ste 1800
Philadelphia, PA 19103-2899

REVIEW OF ORTHOPAEDICS ISBN: 978-1-4377-2024-2

Notices

Knowledge and best practice in this field are constantly changing. As new research and experience broaden our understanding, changes in research methods, professional practices, or medical treatment may become necessary.

Practitioners and researchers must always rely on their own experience and knowledge in evaluating and using any information, methods, compounds, or experiments described herein. In using such information or methods, they should be mindful of their own safety and the safety of others, including parties for whom they have a professional responsibility.

With respect to any drug or pharmaceutical products identified, readers are advised to check the most current information provided (i) on procedures featured or (ii) by the manufacturer of each product to be administered to verify the recommended dose or formula, the method and duration of administration, and contraindications. It is the responsibility of practitioners, relying on their own experience and knowledge of their patients, to make diagnoses, to determine dosages and the best treatment for each individual patient, and to take all appropriate safety precautions.

To the fullest extent of the law, neither the Publisher nor the authors, contributors, or editors assume any liability for any injury and/or damage to persons or property as a matter of products liability, negligence or otherwise, or from any use or operation of any methods, products, instructions, or ideas contained in the material herein.

Previous editions copyrighted 2008, 2004, 2000, 1996, 1992.

Library of Congress Cataloging-in-Publication Data
Review of orthopaedics / [edited by] Mark D. Miller, Stephen R. Thompson, Jennifer Hart ; international editors, Tom Cosker, Sherief Elsayed.—6th ed.
p. ; cm.
Includes bibliographical references and index.
ISBN 978-1-4377-2024-2 (hardcover : alk. paper)
I. Miller, Mark D.
[DNLM: 1. Musculoskeletal Diseases—Outlines. 2 Orthopedic Procedures—Outlines. WE 18.2]
616.7—dc23
2012006956

Executive Content Strategist: Delores Meloni
Content Developer: Joan Ryan
Publishing Services Manager: Anne Altepeter
Senior Project Manager: Cheryl A. Abbott
Senior Book Designer: Ellen Zanolle

Printed in the United States of America.

Last digit is the print number: 9 8 7 6 5 4 3 2 1

To my better 3/4, Ann, who has encouraged me to focus on my calling while calling me on my focus

MARK D. MILLER

For Shannon, who has my unending gratitude for her support, patience, and love

STEPHEN R. THOMPSON

For Joe, Drew, Julia, and Jordyn, who not only tolerated but supported the hours spent at the dining room table with constant, excited chatter about this NEW book. And for Mark Miller, who like all great mentors has taught me everything that I know about orthopaedics, but not necessarily everything that he knows

JENNIFER A. HART

CONTRIBUTORS

Clark C. Baumbusch, MD
Resident Physician
Department of Orthopaedic Surgery
Georgetown University Hospital
Washington, DC
SPINE

Mark R. Brinker, MD
Director, Acute and Reconstructive Trauma
Fondren Orthopedic Group
Texas Orthopedic Hospital
Houston, Texas;
Clinical Professor
Department of Orthopaedic Surgery
Tulane University School of Medicine
New Orleans, Louisiana;
Clinical Professor
Department of Orthopaedic Surgery
Baylor College of Medicine
Houston, Texas
BASIC SCIENCES

Lance M. Brunton, MD
Assistant Professor
Department of Orthopaedic Surgery
University of Pittsburgh Medical Center
Pittsburgh, Pennsylvania
HAND, UPPER EXTREMITY, AND MICROVASCULAR SURGERY

A. Bobby Chhabra, MD
Charles J. Frankel Professor and Vice Chair
Department of Orthopaedic Surgery
Professor of Plastic Surgery
Co-Director UVA Hand Center
University of Virginia
Charlottesville, Virginia
HAND, UPPER EXTREMITY, AND MICROVASCULAR SURGERY

Marc M. DeHart, MD
Clinical Assistant Professor
Department of Orthopaedics and Rehabilitation
University of Texas Medical Branch at Galveston;
Clinical Assistant Professor
Department of Surgery
Texas A&M Health Science Center, College of Medicine
Round Rock, Texas
PRINCIPLES OF PRACTICE

Deborah A. Frassica, MD
Associate Professor
Department of Pathology and Orthopaedic Surgery
The Johns Hopkins University
Baltimore, Maryland
ORTHOPAEDIC PATHOLOGY

Frank J. Frassica, MD
Professor of Orthopaedic Surgery and Oncology
Chair of Orthopaedic Surgery
Department of Orthopaedic Surgery
The Johns Hopkins University
Baltimore, Maryland
ORTHOPAEDIC PATHOLOGY

Frank A. Gottschalk, MD
Professor
Department of Orthopaedic Surgery
University of Texas Southwestern Medical Center at Dallas
Dallas, Texas
REHABILITATION: GAIT, AMPUTATIONS, PROSTHESES, ORTHOSES, AND NEUROLOGIC INJURY

Jennifer A. Hart, MPAS, PA-C
Physician Assistant
Department of Orthopaedic Surgery
University of Virginia
Charlottesville, Virginia
SPORTS MEDICINE

Joseph M. Hart, PhD, ATC
Assistant Professor
Department of Human Services/Kinesiology
Department of Orthopaedic Surgery
University of Virginia
Charlottesville, Virginia
RESEARCH DESIGN AND BIOSTATISTICS

Todd A. Irwin, MD
Assistant Professor
Division of Foot and Ankle Surgery
Department of Orthopaedic Surgery
University of Michigan
Ann Arbor, Michigan
DISORDERS OF THE FOOT AND ANKLE

Anish R. Kadakia, MD
Assistant Professor and Chief
Division of Foot and Ankle Surgery
Department of Orthopaedic Surgery
University of Michigan
Ann Arbor, Michigan
DISORDERS OF THE FOOT AND ANKLE

William C. Lauerman, MD
Professor of Orthopaedic Surgery
Chief
Division of Spine Surgery
Georgetown University Hospital
Washington, DC
SPINE

Edward F. McCarthy, MD
Professor
Departments of Pathology and Orthopaedic Surgery
The Johns Hopkins University
Baltimore, Maryland
ORTHOPAEDIC PATHOLOGY

Edward J. McPherson, MD, FACS, Lifetime Distinguished Fellow FACGS
Director and Founder
Los Angeles Orthopedic Institute
Los Angeles, California
ADULT RECONSTRUCTION

Todd A. Milbrandt, MD, MS
Program Director and Associate Professor
University of Kentucky
Shriners Hospital for Children
Lexington, Kentucky
PEDIATRIC ORTHOPAEDICS

Matthew D. Milewski, MD
Orthopaedic Sports Medicine Fellow
University of Virginia
Charlottesville, Virginia;
Pediatric Orthopaedic Fellow
Children's Hospital, Los Angeles
Los Angeles, California
SPORTS MEDICINE
TRAUMA

Mark D. Miller, MD
S. Ward Casscells Professor
Department of Orthopaedic Surgery;
Head, Division of Sports Medicine
University of Virginia
Charlottesville, Virginia;
Team Physician
James Madison University
Harrisonburg, Virginia;
Founder and Director
Miller Review Course
Westminster, Colorado
SPORTS MEDICINE

Daniel P. O'Connor, PhD
Associate Professor
Department of Health and Human Performance
University of Houston
Houston, Texas
BASIC SCIENCES

Matthew R. Schmitz, MD
Assistant Professor
Department of Orthopaedic Surgery and Rehabilitation
San Antonio Military Medical Center
San Antonio, Texas
ANATOMY

Franklin D. Shuler, MD, PhD
Director, Orthopaedic Research
Medical Director, Geriatric Fracture Program
Associate Professor, Orthopaedic Traumatology
Associate Residency Program Director
Joan C. Edwards School of Medicine
Department of Orthopaedic Surgery
Marshall University
Huntington, West Virginia
ANATOMY

James P. Stannard, MD
Chairman and Professor
Department of Orthopaedic Surgery
University of Missouri, Columbia;
Medical Director
Missouri Orthopaedic Institute
University of Missouri Health System
Columbia, Missouri
TRAUMA

Daniel J. Sucato, MD, MS
Chief of Staff
Department of Orthopaedic Surgery
Texas Scottish Rite Hospital for Children;
Professor
University of Texas Southwestern Medical Center
Dallas, Texas
PEDIATRIC ORTHOPAEDICS

Stephen R. Thompson, MD, MEd, FRCSC
Orthopaedic Sport Medicine Fellow
Fowler Kennedy Sport Medicine Clinic
University of Western Ontario
London, Ontario, Canada
TRAUMA

David B. Weiss, MD
Associate Professor
Head, Division of Orthopaedic Trauma
Department of Orthopaedic Surgery
University of Virginia
Charlottesville, Virginia
TRAUMA

PREFACE

We are proud to introduce the sixth edition of the orthopaedic best seller, ***Review of Orthopaedics.*** Although we are not sure how one substantiates this claim, this edition is perhaps the most revised edition of a textbook in the history of orthopaedic surgery, if not all of medicine! In response to our first-ever competitive text, we have radically updated and revised every chapter in this popular book. We started with the format, abandoning the cumbersome strict outline, and instead adapting an easier-to-follow bullet style. In addition, we added Testable Concepts to help with in-training and board preparation. We then focused on content and painstakingly updated each chapter, paying close attention to reader feedback from previous editions of this work. We added many additional figures, focusing on "composite figures" originally introduced in the first edition of this text and would like to recognize and thank the outstanding team of medical illustrators who brought our vision for this portion of the text to life. Their work on this text has transformed fragments of ideas into beautiful illustrations that aid readers even more than the written word (after all, a [good] picture is worth more than a thousand of them!). Lastly, the addition of color to the majority of the figures provides a visual enhancement to render content and procedures more detailed and understandable. The accompanying website includes the fully searchable text, all references linked to PubMed, questions and answers, and a supplemental image collection.

After five editions of a textbook, it is helpful to invite some fresh new talent to the mix. Dr. Stephen Thompson, who began as a "volunteer" and ended up as an associate editor, played a major role in breathing new life into the book. Jennifer Hart, as always, was also invaluable as an associate editor and collaborator. In addition, we gratefully acknowledge and appreciate the tremendous efforts of the chapter authors in revising this edition. The reader will note the addition of several new authors and co-authors, all of whom played a vital role in our major overhaul of the text. Finally, we are deeply indebted to the editors and staff at Elsevier, Dolores Meloni, Virginia Wilson, Joan Ryan, and their team for their insight, guidance, and contributions to this edition. ***So … what's new about Review 6? Everything!***

The writer does the most, who gives the reader the most knowledge and takes from him the least time.

C.C. Colton, *Lacon*, Preface
[From the preface for the first edition, 1992]

(Note: **Bold text** indicates material that is particularly important or has appeared on previous examinations. The *highlighter icon* indicates figures or tables that contain highly testable content.)

Mark D. Miller
Stephen R. Thompson
Jennifer A. Hart

CONTENTS

REVIEW OF ORTHOPAEDICS

Chapter 1

BASIC SCIENCES

Mark R. Brinker and Daniel P. O'Connor

CONTENTS

SECTION 1 BONE

I. HISTOLOGIC FEATURES OF BONE

A. Types (Figure 1-1; Table 1-1)

1. Normal bone: lamellar, either cortical or cancellous
2. Immature and pathologic bone: woven; more random, more osteocytes, increased turnover, weaker
   - Lamellar bone is stress oriented; woven bone is not.
3. Cortical (compact) bone
   - Constitutes 80% of the skeleton
   - Consists of tightly packed osteons or haversian systems
     - Connected by Haversian (or Volkmann's) canals
     - Contains arterioles, venules, capillaries, nerves, possibly lymphatic channels
   - Interstitial lamellae: between osteons
     - Fibrils connect lamellae but do not cross cement lines.
     - Cement lines define the outer border of an osteon.
       - Bone resorption has stopped, and new bone formation has begun.
   - Nutrition provided by intraosseous circulation
     - Canals and canaliculi (cell processes of osteocytes)
   - Characterized by slow turnover rate, higher Young's modulus of elasticity, more stiffness
4. Cancellous bone (spongy or trabecular bone)
   - Less dense, more remodeling according to lines of stress (Wolff's law)
   - Characterized by high turnover rate, smaller Young's modulus, more elasticity

B. Cellular biology (Figure 1-2)

1. **Osteoblasts**
   - Form bone by generating organic, nonmineralized matrix
     - Appear as cuboid cells aligned in layers along immature osteoid
   - Derived from undifferentiated mesenchymal stem cells
     - Have more endoplasmic reticulum, Golgi apparatus, and mitochondria than do other cells (for synthesis and secretion of matrix)

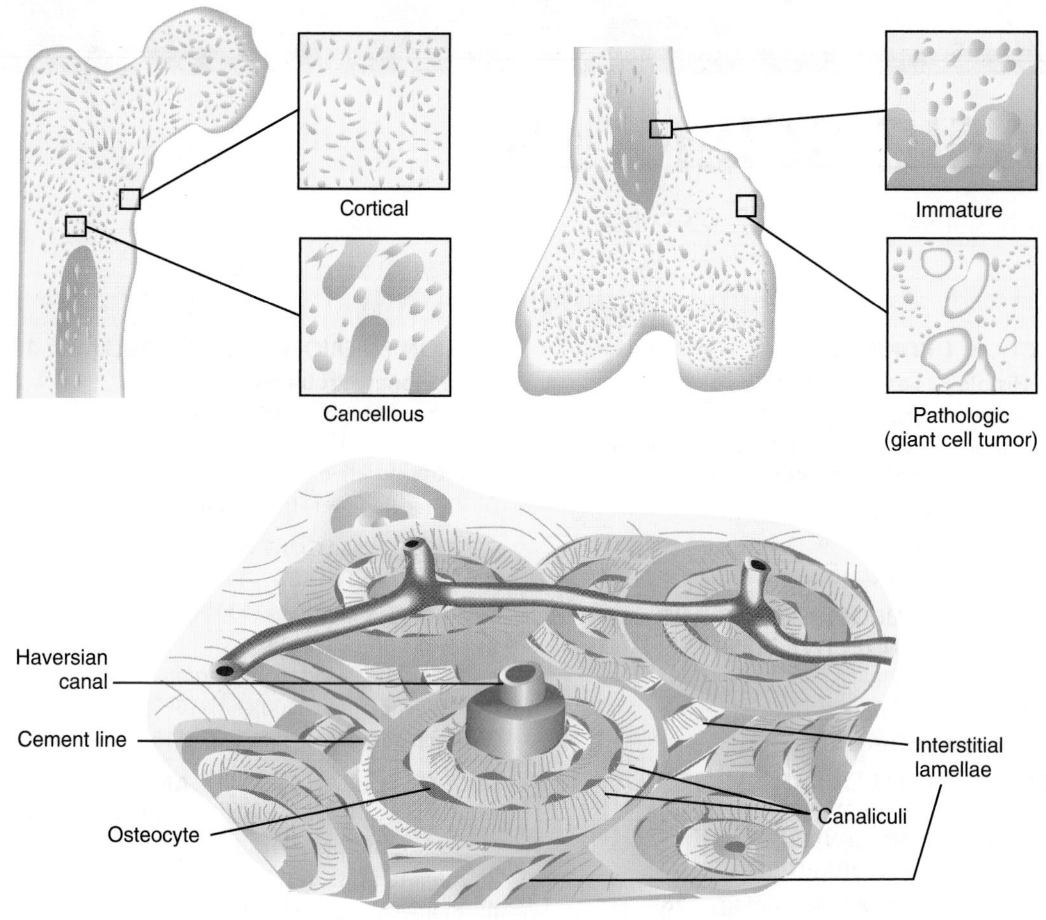

Figure 1-1 Types of bone. *Cortical* bone consists of tightly packed osteons. *Cancellous* bone consists of a meshwork of trabeculae. In *immature* bone, unmineralized osteoid lines the immature trabeculae. *Pathologic* bone is characterized by atypical osteoblasts and architectural disorganization. (Colorized from Brinker MR, Miller MD: *Fundamentals of orthopaedics,* Philadelphia, 1999, WB Saunders, p 2.)

    - **RUNX2 is a multifunctional transcription factor that directs mesenchymal cells to the osteoblast lineage.**
- Bone surfaces lined by more differentiated, metabolically active cells
- "Entrapped cells": less active cells in "resting regions"; maintain the ionic milieu of bone
    - Disruption of the active-lining cell layer activates entrapped cells
- Osteoblast differentiation in vivo effected by the following:
    - Interleukins
    - Platelet-derived growth factor (PDGF)
    - Insulin-derived growth factor (IDGF)
- **Receptor-effector interactions in osteoblasts** (Table 1-2)
- Osteoblasts produce the following:
    - Alkaline phosphatase
    - **Osteocalcin**
    - Type I collagen
    - Bone sialoprotein
    - Receptor activator of nuclear factor κB (NF-κB) ligand (RANKL)

Table 1-1 Types of Bone

Microscopic Appearance	Subtypes	Characteristics	Examples
Lamellar	Cortical	Structure is oriented along lines of stress Strong	Femoral shaft
	Cancellous	More elastic than cortical bone	Distal femoral metaphysis
Woven	Immature	Not stress-oriented	Embryonic skeleton Fracture callus
	Pathologic	Random organization Increased turnover Weak Flexible	Osteogenic sarcoma Fibrous dysplasia

Modified from Brinker MR, Miller MD: *Fundamentals of orthopaedics,* Philadelphia, 1999, WB Saunders, p 1.

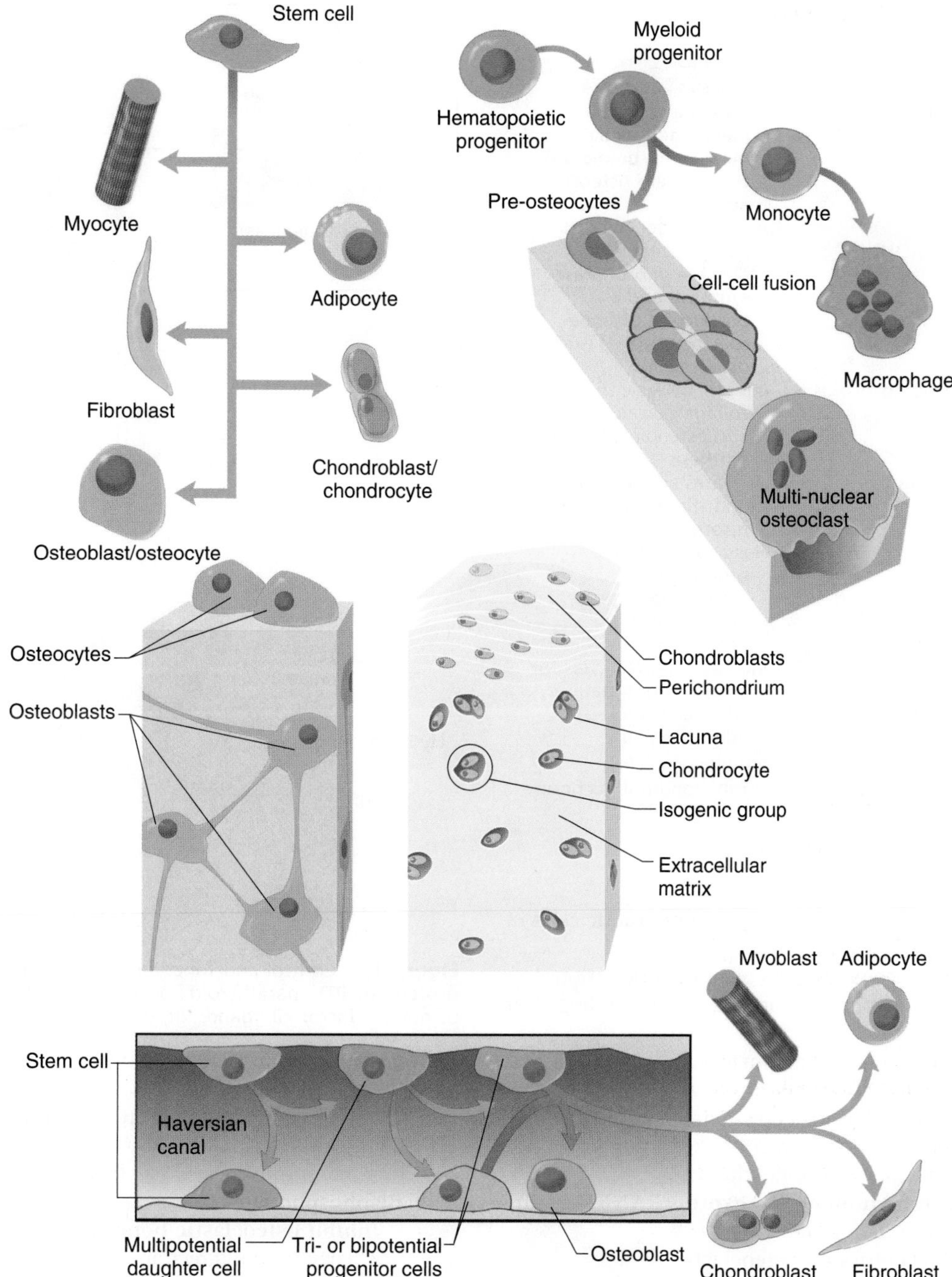

Figure 1-2 Cellular origins of bone and cartilage cells.

- Osteoblast activity stimulated by intermittent (pulsatile) exposure to parathyroid hormone (PTH)
- Osteoblast activity inhibited by tumor necrosis factor-α (TNF-α)
- Certain antiseptics toxic to cultured osteoblasts:
  - Hydrogen peroxide
  - Povidone-iodine (Betadine)
  - Bacitracin (believed to be less toxic)

2. **Osteocytes** (see Figure 1-1)
   - Maintain bone
   - Constitute 90% of the cells in the mature skeleton
     - Former osteoblasts surrounded by newly formed matrix
   - High nucleus/cytoplasm ratio
   - Long interconnecting cytoplasmic processes projecting through the canaliculi
   - Less active in matrix production than are osteoblasts
   - Important for control of extracellular calcium and phosphorus concentration
   - Directly stimulated by calcitonin, inhibited by PTH
3. **Osteoclasts**
   - Resorb bone
     - This activity occurs both normally and in certain conditions, including multiple myeloma and metastatic bone disease.
   - Multinucleated, irregular giant cells

Table 1-2 Bone Cell Types, Receptor Types, and Effects

Cell Type	Receptor	Effect
Osteoblast	PTH	**Releases a secondary messenger (exact mechanism unknown) to stimulate osteoclastic activity** Activates adenylyl cyclase
	1,25(OH)$_2$ vitamin D$_3$	Stimulates matrix and alkaline phosphatase synthesis and production of bone-specific proteins (such as osteocalcin)
	Glucocorticoids	Inhibits DNA synthesis, collagen production, and osteoblast protein synthesis
	Prostaglandins	Activates adenylyl cyclase and stimulates bone resorption
	Estrogen	Has anabolic (bone production) and anticatabolic (prevents bone resorption) properties Increases mRNA levels for alkaline phosphatase Inhibits activation of adenylyl cyclase
Osteoclast	Calcitonin	Inhibits osteoclast function (inhibits bone resorption)

mRNA, messenger RNA; PTH, parathyroid hormone.

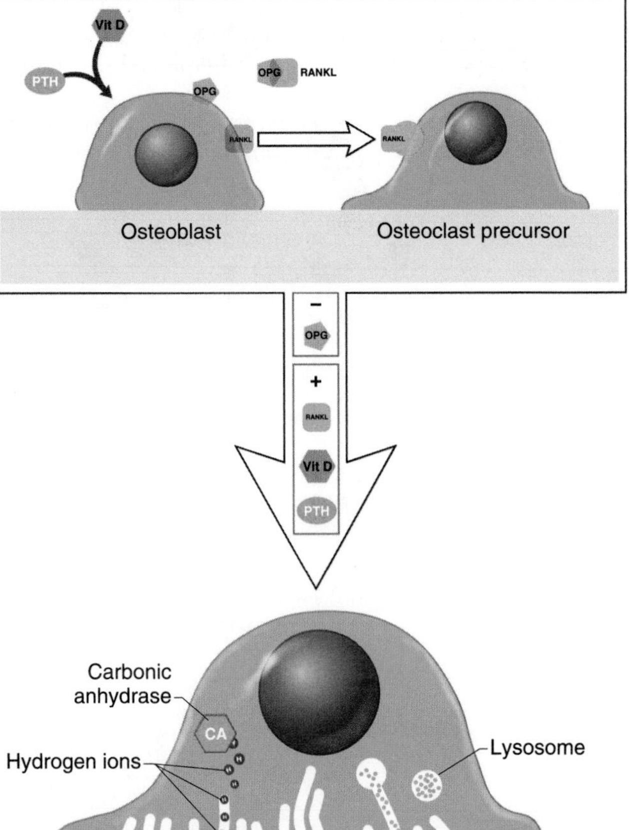

Figure 1-3 Control and function of the osteoclast. OPG, osteoprotegerin; PTH, parathyroid hormone; RANKL, receptor activator of nuclear factor κB ligand; Vit, vitamin.

- **These cells are derived from hematopoietic cells in macrophage lineage.**
- Monocyte progenitors form giant cells by fusion.

- Possess a ruffled ("brush") border and surrounding clear zone
  - Border consists of plasma membrane enfoldings that increase surface area for resorption.
- Bone resorption occurs in depressions: Howship's lacunae
  - Formation and resorption are linked ("coupled").
  - Resorption occurs more rapidly.
- **Osteoblasts (and tumor cells) express RANKL** (Figure 1-3), which acts as follows:
  - **Binds to receptors on osteoclasts**
  - **Stimulates differentiation into mature osteoclasts**
  - **Increases bone resorption**
  - **Inhibited by osteoprotegerin binding to RANKL**
- Synthesize tartrate-resistant acid phosphate
- **Bind to bone surfaces through cell attachment (anchoring) proteins**
  - Integrins, specifically $\alpha_v\beta_3$ or vitronectin receptor
  - Effectively seal the space below the osteoclast
- Produce hydrogen ions through carbonic anhydrase
  - Lower pH
  - Increase solubility of hydroxyapatite crystals
  - **Organic matrix then removed by proteolytic digestion through activity of the lysosomal enzyme cathepsin K**
- Have specific receptors for calcitonin
  - Calcitonin inhibits osteoclastic resorption.
- Interleukin-1 (IL-1)
  - Potent stimulator of osteoclast differentiation and bone resorption
  - Found in membranes surrounding loose total joint implants
  - In contrast, interleukin-10 suppresses osteoclasts
- **Bisphosphonates**
  - **Inhibit osteoclastic bone resorption.**
    - They have a direct anabolic effect on bone.
  - Categorized into two classes on the basis of presence or absence of a nitrogen side group
    - **Nitrogen-containing bisphosphonates are up to 1000-fold more potent in their antiresorptive activity.**
  - Nitrogen-containing bisphosphonates
    - Zoledronic acid (Zometa) and alendronate (Fosamax) are examples.
    - **They inhibit protein prenylation within the mevalonate pathway, blocking farnesyl pyrophosphate synthase.**
    - **This results in a loss of guanosine triphosphatase (GTPase) formation, which is needed for ruffled border formation and cell survival.**
  - Non–nitrogen-containing bisphosphonates
    - Metabolized into a nonfunctional adenosine triphosphate (ATP) analog, inducing apoptosis

- Decreases skeletal events in multiple myeloma
- **Associated with osteonecrosis of the jaw**
- **Orthopaedic implications of bisphosphonate use:**
  - Spine
    - **Reduced rate of spinal fusion in animal model; withholding bisphosphonate is recommended after surgery**
  - Hip and knee
    - Safe for use in cementless hip arthroplasty and cemented knee arthroplasty
    - May decrease rate of acetabular component subsidence
  - Fracture healing
    - No good data to recommend for or against use

4. **Osteoprogenitor cells**
   - Originate from mesenchymal stem cells
   - Become osteoblasts under conditions of low strain and increased oxygen tension
   - Become cartilage under conditions of intermediate strain and low oxygen tension
   - Become fibrous tissue under conditions of high strain
   - Line Haversian canals, endosteum, and periosteum
     - Awaiting the stimulus to differentiate
5. Lining cells
   - Narrow, flattened, "resting" osteoblasts that form an envelope around bone

C. **Matrix (Table 1-3)**

1. Organic components: 40% of the dry weight of bone
   - Collagen (90% of organic component)

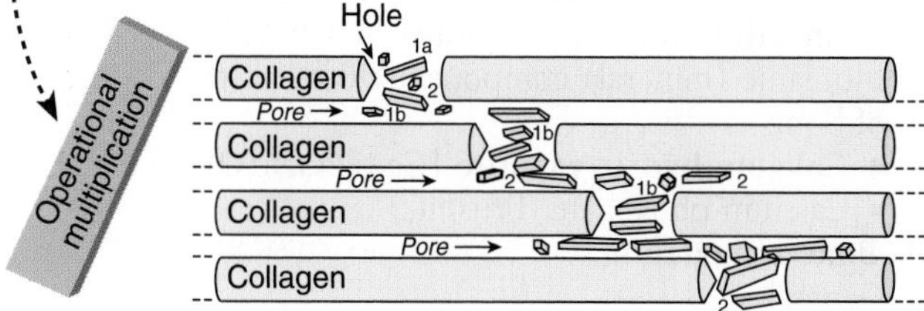

Progressively increasing mineral mass due to:
1. Increased number of new mineral phase particles (nucleation)
a. Heterogeneous nucleation by matrix in collagen holes (and pores)
b. Secondary crystal–induced nucleation in holes and pores
2. Initial growth of particles to ~400 Å × 15-30 Å × 50-75 Å
Hole
Collagen
Pore
Collagen
Pore
Collagen
Pore
Collagen
Operational multiplication

Figure 1-4 Biologic considerations of mineral accretion: heterogeneity within a collagen fibril. (From Simon SR [editor]: *Orthopaedic basic science*, Rosemont, Ill, 1994, American Academy of Orthopaedic Surgeons, p 139.)

- **Collagen is primarily type I (mnemonic: "bone" contains the word "one").**
- Hole zones (gaps) exist within the collagen fibril between the ends of molecules.
- Pores exist between the sides of parallel molecules.
- Mineral deposition (calcification) occurs within the hole zones and pores (Figure 1-4).
- Cross-linking decreases collagen solubility and increases its tensile strength.

- Proteoglycans
- Matrix proteins (noncollagenous)

Table 1-3 Components of Bone Matrix

Type of Matrix	Function	Composition	Types	Notes
Organic Matrix				
Collagen	Provides tensile strength	Primarily type I collagen		Constitutes 90% of organic matrix Structure: triple helix of one α_2 and two α_1 chains, quarter-staggered to produce a fibril
Proteoglycans	Partly responsible for compressive strength	Glycosaminoglycan-protein complexes		Inhibit mineralization
Matrix proteins (noncollagenous)	Promote mineralization and bone formation		Osteocalcin (bone γ-carboxyglutamic acid–containing protein)	Attracts osteoclasts; direct regulation of bone density; most abundant noncollagenous matrix protein (10%-20% of total)
			Osteonectin (SPARC)	Secreted by platelets and osteoblasts; postulated to have a role in regulating calcium or organizing mineral in matrix
			Osteopontin	Cell-binding protein, similar to an integrin
Growth factors and cytokines	Aid in bone cell differentiation, activation, growth, and turnover		TGF-β IGF IL-1, IL-6 BMPs	Present in small amounts in bone matrix
Inorganic Matrix				
Calcium hydroxyapatite [$Ca_{10}(PO_4)_6(OH)_2$]	Provides compressive strength			Most of the inorganic matrix; primary mineralization in collagen gaps (holes and pores), secondary mineralization on periphery
Osteocalcium phosphate (brushite)				Makes up the remaining inorganic matrix

BMP, bone morphogenetic proteins; IGF, insulin-like growth factor; IL, interleukin; SPARC, secreted protein, acidic, rich in cysteine; TGF-β, transforming growth factor-β.

- **Osteocalcin: most abundant noncollagenous protein in bone**
  - Inhibited by PTH and stimulated by 1,25-dihydroxyvitamin D_3
  - Can be measured in the serum or urine as a marker of bone turnover
- Growth factors and cytokines

2. Inorganic (mineral) components: 60% of the dry weight of bone
   - **Calcium hydroxyapatite [$Ca_{10}(PO_4)_6(OH)_2$]**
   - Calcium phosphate (brushite)

D. Bone remodeling

1. General
   - Cortical and cancellous bone is continuously remodeled throughout life by osteoclastic and osteoblastic activity (Figure 1-5).
   - **Wolff's law:** Remodeling occurs in response to mechanical stress.
     - Increasing mechanical stress increases bone gain.
     - Removing external mechanical stress increases bone loss, which is reversible (to varying degrees) on remobilization.
   - Piezoelectric remodeling occurs in response to electrical charge.
     - The compression side of bone is electronegative, stimulating osteoblasts (formation).
     - The tension side of bone is electropositive, stimulating osteoclasts (resorption).
   - **Hueter-Volkmann law:** Remodeling occurs in small packets of cells known as basic multicellular units (BMUs).
     - Such remodeling is modulated by hormones and cytokines.
     - **Compressive forces inhibit growth; tension stimulates it.**
     - This law suggests that mechanical factors influence longitudinal growth, bone remodeling, and fracture repair.
       - May play a role in scoliosis and Blount's disease
2. Cortical bone remodeling
   - Osteoclastic tunneling (cutting cones; Figure 1-6)
     - Followed by layering of osteoblasts and successive deposition of layers of lamellae
   - The head of the cutting cone is made up of osteoclasts.
   - Behind the osteoclast front are capillaries.
     - Followed by the laying down of osteoid by osteoblasts
3. Cancellous bone remodeling
   - Osteoclastic resorption occurs, and then osteoblasts lay down new bone.

E. Bone circulation

1. Anatomy
   - Bone receives 5% to 10% of the cardiac output.
     - Bones with a tenuous blood supply include the scaphoid, talus, femoral head, and odontoid.

BONE REMODELING

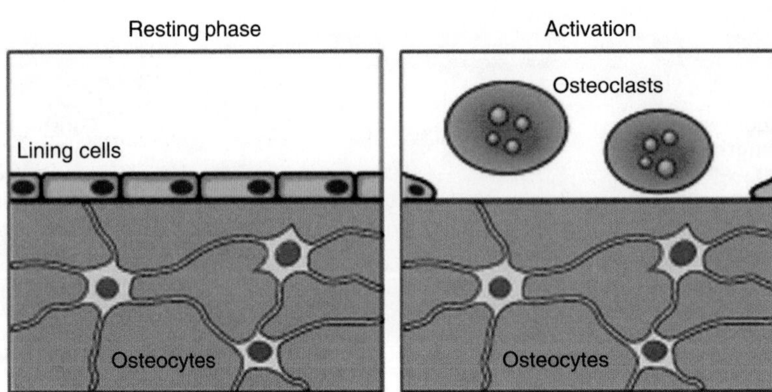

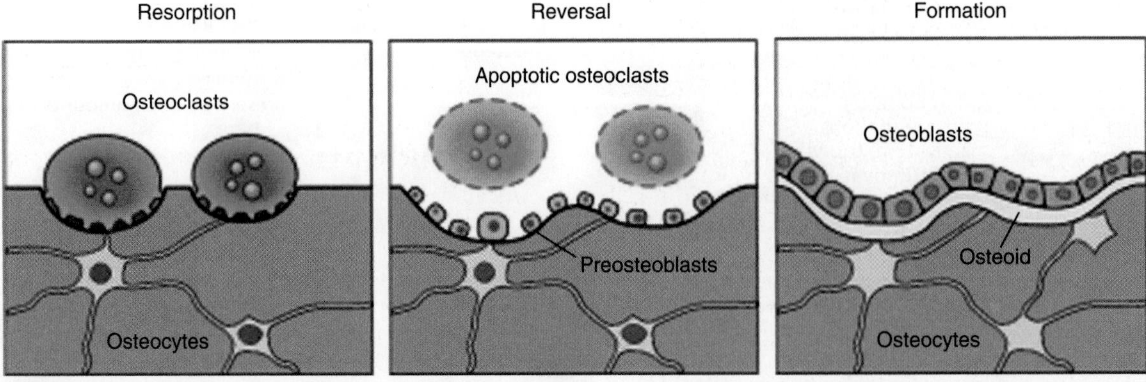

Figure 1-5 Bone remodeling. Osteoclasts dissolve the mineral from the bone matrix. Osteoblasts produce new bone, or osteoid, that fills in the resorption pit. Some of the osteoblasts are left within the bone matrix as osteocytes. (From Firestein GS, et al, editors: *Kelley's textbook of rheumatology,* ed 8, Philadelphia, 2008, WB Saunders.)

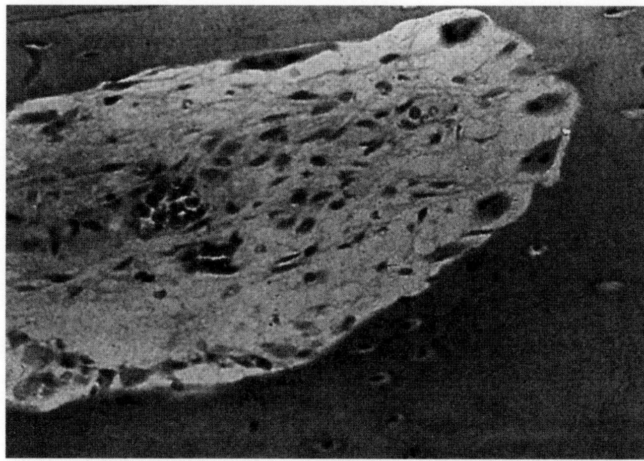

Figure 1-6 Mechanism of cortical bone remodeling via cutting cones. (From Simon SR, editor: *Orthopaedic basic science,* Rosemont, Ill, 1994, American Academy of Orthopaedic Surgeons, p 142.)

- Long bones receive blood from three sources (systems):
  - Nutrient artery system
    - Nutrient arteries branch from systemic arteries, enter the diaphyseal cortex through the nutrient foramen, enter the medullary canal, and branch into ascending and descending arteries (Figure 1-7).
    - Further branching into arterioles in the endosteal cortex enables blood supply to at least the inner two thirds of the mature diaphyseal cortex via the Haversian system (Figures 1-8 and 1-9).
    - The blood pressure in the nutrient artery system is high.
  - Metaphyseal-epiphyseal system
    - This system arises from the periarticular vascular plexus (e.g., geniculate arteries).
  - Periosteal system
    - This system consists mostly of capillaries that supply the outer third (at most) of the mature diaphyseal cortex.
    - The blood pressure in the periosteal system is low.

2. Physiologic features
   - Direction of flow (Figure 1-10)

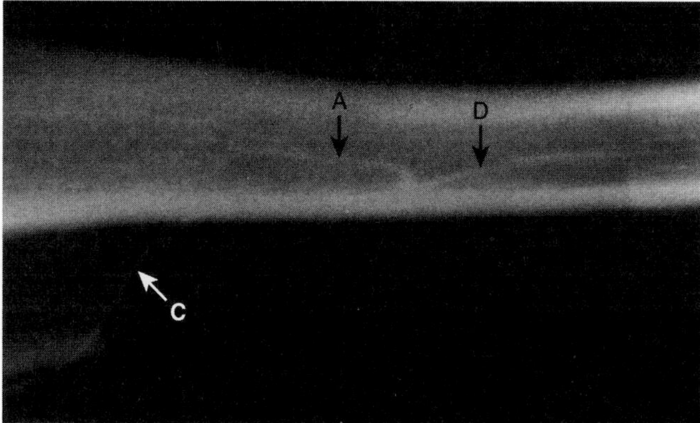

Figure 1-7 Intraoperative arteriogram (canine tibia) demonstrating ascending (A) and descending (D) branches of the nutrient artery. C, Cannula. (From Brinker MR, et al: Pharmacological regulation of the circulation of bone, *J Bone Joint Surg Am* 72:964-975, 1990.)

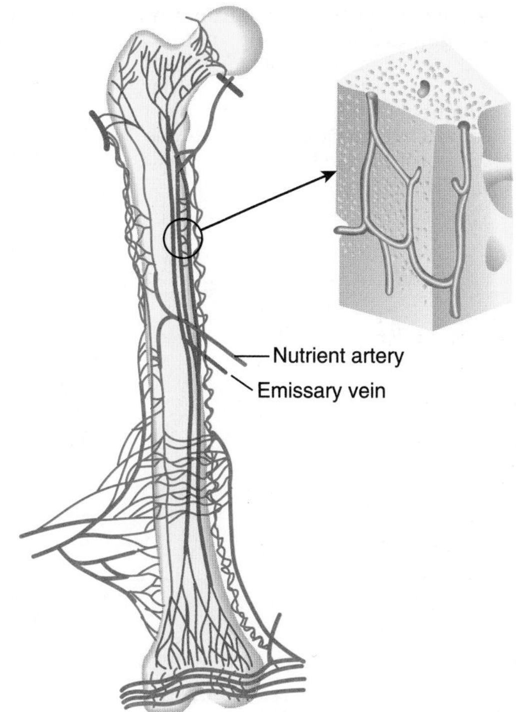

Figure 1-8 Blood supply to bone. (Colorized from Brinker MR, Miller MD: *Fundamentals of orthopaedics,* Philadelphia, 1999, WB Saunders, p 4.)

  - Arterial flow in mature bone is centrifugal (inside to outside), which is the net effect of the high-pressure nutrient artery system and the low-pressure periosteal system.
  - When fracture disrupts the nutrient artery system, the periosteal system pressure predominates, and blood flow is centripetal (outside to inside).
  - Flow in immature, developing bone is centripetal because the highly vascularized periosteal system is the predominant component.
  - Venous flow in mature bone is centripetal.
    - Cortical capillaries drain to venous sinusoids, which drain to the emissary venous system.
- Fluid compartments of bone
  - Extravascular: 65%
  - Haversian: 6%
  - Lacunar: 6%
  - Red blood cells (RBCs): 3%
  - Other: 20%
- Physiologic states
  - Hypoxia, hypercapnia, and sympathectomy increase flow.

3. **Fracture healing**
   - **Bone blood flow** is the major determinant of how well a fracture heals.
     - Delivers nutrients to the injury site
   - Initial response is a decrease in bone blood flow after vascular disruption at the fracture site.
   - Within hours to days, bone blood flow increases (as part of the regional acceleratory phenomenon), peaks at approximately 2 weeks, and returns to normal in 3 to 5 months.
   - Unreamed intramedullary nails preserve endosteal blood supply.

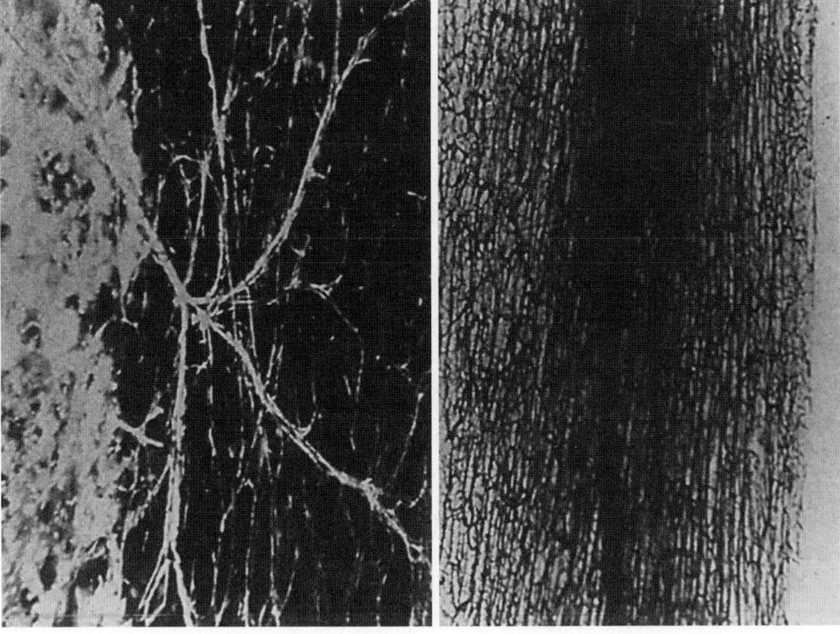

Figure 1-9 Vasculature of cortical bone at different magnifications showing nutrient artery branching in cortical bone *(left)* and the extent of the arterioles and Haversian system throughout the cortex *(right)*. (From Simon SR, editor: *Orthopaedic basic science,* Rosemont, Ill, 1994, American Academy of Orthopaedic Surgeons, p 131.)

- Reaming devascularizes the inner 50% to 80% of the cortex and delays revascularization of endosteal blood supply.
- Loose-fitting nails spare cortical perfusion and allow more rapid reperfusion than do canal-filling nails.

4. Regulation of bone blood flow
   - Influenced by metabolic, humoral, and autonomic inputs
   - Arterial system: great potential for vasoconstriction (from the resting state), less potential for vasodilation
   - Vessels within bone: have several vasoactive receptors (β-adrenergic, muscarinic, thromboxane/prostaglandin)

F. Tissues surrounding bone

1. Periosteum
   - This connective tissue membrane covers bone.
   - It is more highly developed in children.
   - The inner periosteum, or cambium, is loose and vascular and contains cells capable of becoming osteoblasts.
     - These cells enlarge the diameter of bone during growth and form periosteal callus during fracture healing.
   - The outer (fibrous) periosteum is less cellular and is contiguous with joint capsules.
2. Bone marrow
   - Source of progenitor cells; controls inner diameter of bone
     - Red marrow
       - Hematopoietic (40% water, 40% fat, 20% protein)
       - Slowly changes to yellow marrow with age, first in appendicular skeleton and later in axial skeleton
     - Yellow marrow
       - Inactive (15% water, 80% fat, 5% protein)

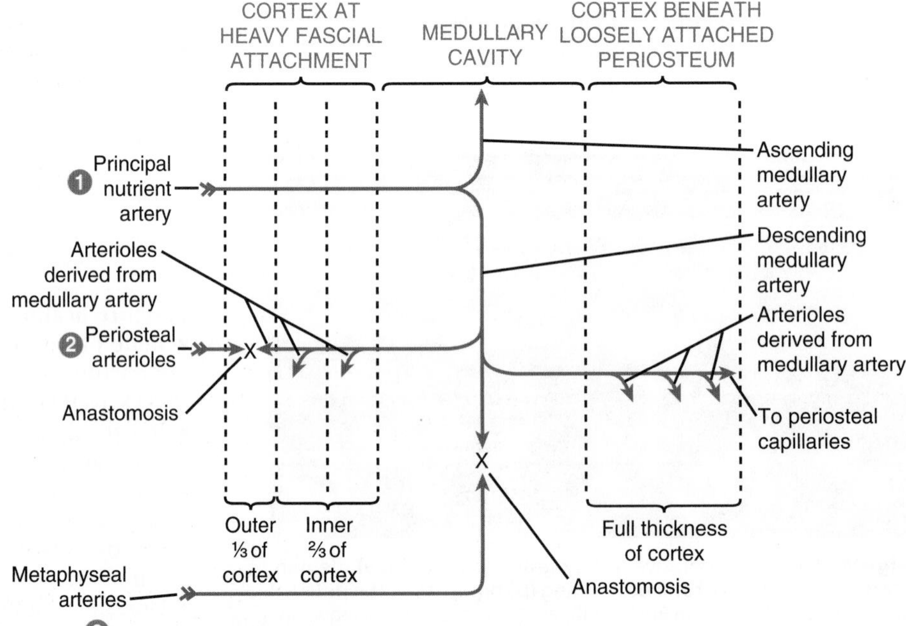

Figure 1-10 Major components of the afferent vascular system of long bone. Components *1, 2,* and *3* constitute the total nutrient supply to the diaphysis. *Arrows* indicate the direction of blood flow. (From Rhinelander FW: Circulation in bone. In Bourne G, editor: *The biochemistry and physiology of bone,* ed 2, vol 2, Orlando, Fla, 1972, Academic Press, pp 1-77.)

G. Types of bone formation (Table 1-4)

1. Enchondral bone formation and mineralization
   - General
     - Undifferentiated cells secrete the cartilaginous matrix and differentiate into chondrocytes.
     - The matrix mineralizes and is invaded by vascular buds that bring osteoprogenitor cells.
     - Osteoclasts resorb calcified cartilage, and osteoblasts form bone.
     - **Bone replaces the cartilage model;** cartilage is not converted to bone.
     - Examples of enchondral bone formation:
       - Embryonic formation of long bones
       - Longitudinal growth (physis)
       - **Fracture callus**
       - Bone formed with demineralized bone matrix
   - Embryonic formation of long bones (Figures 1-11 and 1-12)
     - These bones are formed from the mesenchymal anlage, at 6 weeks of gestation.
     - Vascular buds invade the mesenchymal model, bringing osteoprogenitor cells that differentiate into osteoblasts and form the primary ossification centers at 8 weeks.
       - Differentiation stimulated, in part, by binding of WNT protein to the LRP5 or LRP6 receptor.
     - The cartilage model increases in size through appositional (width) and interstitial (length) growth.
     - The marrow forms by resorption of the central cartilage anlage by invasion of myeloid precursor cells that are brought in by the capillary buds.
     - Secondary ossification centers develop at the bone ends, forming the epiphyseal centers (growth plates) responsible for longitudinal growth.
     - Arterial supply is rich during development, with an epiphyseal artery (terminates in the proliferative zone), metaphyseal arteries, nutrient arteries, and perichondrial arteries (Figure 1-13).
   - **Physis**
     - Two growth plates exist in immature long bones: (1) horizontal (the physis) and (2) spherical (growth of the epiphysis).
       - The spherical plate is less organized than the horizontal plate.
     - The perichondrial artery is the major source of nutrition of the growth plate.
     - Acromegaly and spondyloepiphyseal dysplasia affect the physis; multiple epiphyseal dysplasia affects the epiphysis.
     - Delineation of physeal cartilage zones is based on growth (see Figure 1-13) and function (Figures 1-14 and 1-15).
       - Reserve zone: Cells store lipids, glycogen, and proteoglycan aggregates; decreased oxygen tension occurs in this zone.
         - Lysosomal storage diseases (e.g., Gaucher's disease) can affect this zone.
       - Proliferative zone: Growth is longitudinal, with stacking of chondrocytes (the top cell is the dividing "mother" cell), cellular proliferation, and matrix production; increased oxygen tension and increased proteoglycans inhibit calcification.
         - **Achondroplasia causes defects in this zone** (see Figure 1-15).
         - **Growth hormone exerts its effect in the proliferative zone.**
       - **Hypertrophic zone:** This area is sometimes divided into three zones: maturation, degeneration, and provisional calcification.
         - Normal matrix mineralization occurs in the lower hypertrophic zone: chondrocytes increase five times in size, accumulate calcium in their mitochondria, die, and release calcium from matrix vesicles.
         - Chondrocyte maturation is regulated by systemic hormones and local growth factors (PTH-related peptide inhibits chondrocyte maturation; Indian hedgehog is produced by chondrocytes and regulates the expression of PTH-related peptide).
         - Osteoblasts migrate from sinusoidal vessels and use cartilage as a scaffolding for bone formation.
           - Low oxygen tension and decreased proteoglycan aggregates aid in this process.
         - This zone widens in rickets (see Figure 1-15), with little or no provisional calcification.

Table 1-4 Types of Bone Formation

Type of Ossification	Mechanism	Examples of Normal Mechanisms	Examples of Diseases with Abnormal Ossification
Enchondral	Bone replaces a cartilage model	Embryonic formation of long bones Longitudinal growth (physis) Fracture callus Bone formed with the use of demineralized bone matrix	Achondroplasia
Intramembranous	Aggregates of undifferentiated mesenchymal cells differentiate into osteoblasts, which form bone	Embryonic flat bone formation Bone formation during distraction osteogenesis Blastema bone	Cleidocranial dysostosis
Appositional	Osteoblasts lay down new bone on existing bone	Periosteal bone enlargement (width) The bone formation phase of bone remodeling	Paget's disease Infantile hyperostosis (Caffey's disease) Melorheostosis

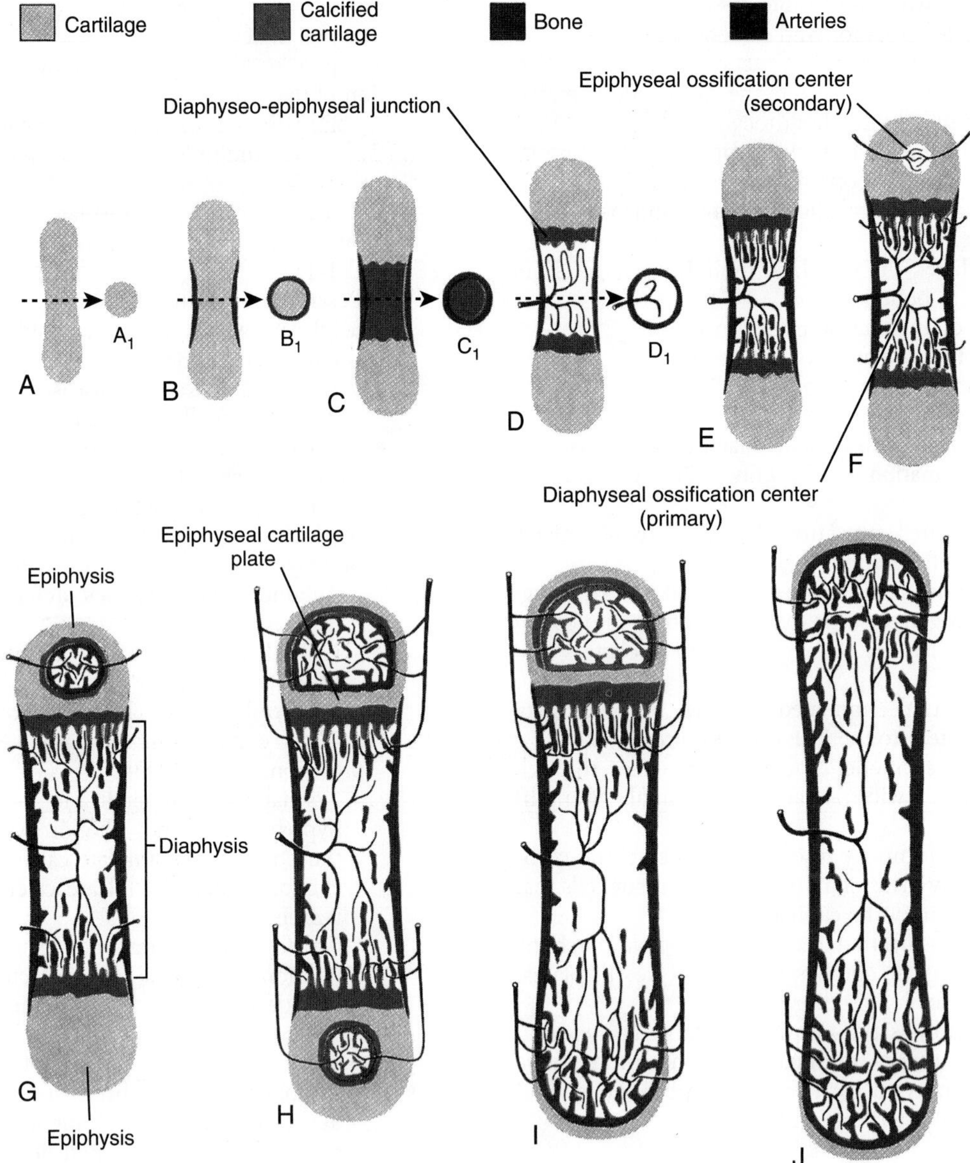

Figure 1-11 Enchondral ossification of long bones. Note that phases *F* through *J* often occur after birth. (From Moore KL: *The developing human,* Philadelphia, 1982, WB Saunders, p 346.)

  - Enchondromas originate here.
  - Mucopolysaccharide diseases (see Figure 1-15) affect this zone, leading to chondrocyte degeneration.
  - **Physeal fractures probably traverse several zones, depending on the type of loading** (Figure 1-16).
  - Slipped capital femoral epiphysis (SCFE) believed to occur here (through metaphyseal spongiosa with renal failure).
- Metaphysis
  - This is adjacent to the physis and expands with skeletal growth.
  - Osteoblasts from osteoprogenitor cells align on cartilage bars produced by physeal expansion.
  - Primary spongiosa (calcified cartilage bars) mineralizes to form woven bone and remodels to form secondary spongiosa and a "cutback zone" at the metaphysis.
  - Cortical bone forms as physeal (enchondral), and intramembranous bone remodels in response to stress along the periphery of the growing long bone.
- Periphery of the physis
  - Groove of Ranvier: supplies chondrocytes to the periphery for lateral growth (width)
  - Perichondrial ring of La Croix: dense fibrous tissue, primary membrane anchoring the periphery of the physis
- Mineralization
  - Collagen hole zones are seeded with calcium hydroxyapatite crystals through branching and accretion (crystal growth).
- Hormones and growth factors (Figure 1-17; Table 1-5)

2. **Intramembranous ossification**
   - This occurs without a cartilage model.

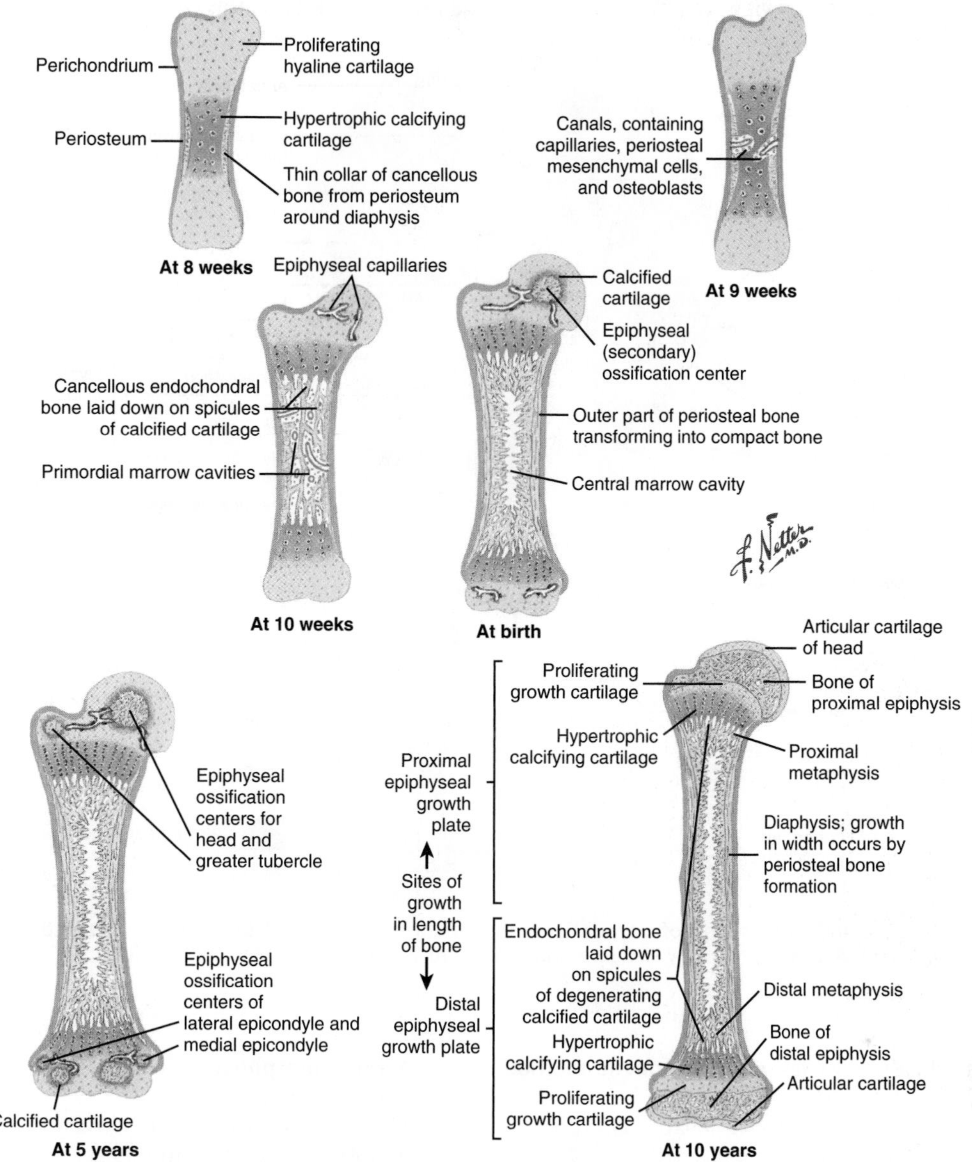

Figure 1-12 **Development of a typical long bone: formation of the growth plate and secondary centers of ossification.** (From Netter FH: *CIBA collection of medical illustrations,* vol 8: *Musculoskeletal system,* part I: *Anatomy, physiology and developmental disorders,* Basel, Switzerland, 1987, CIBA, p 136.)

- Undifferentiated mesenchymal cells aggregate into layers (or membranes), differentiate into osteoblasts, and deposit an organic matrix that mineralizes.
- Examples:
  - Embryonic flat bone formation
  - Bone formation during distraction osteogenesis
  - Blastema bone (in young children with amputations)

3. **Appositional ossification**
   - Osteoblasts align on the existing bone surface and lay down new bone.
   - Examples:
     - Periosteal bone enlargement (width)
     - Bone formation phase of bone remodeling

II. BONE INJURY AND REPAIR

A. Fracture repair (Table 1-6)

1. A Continuum: **inflammation** to **repair** (soft callus followed by hard callus) ending in **remodeling**
2. **Blood supply (bone blood flow): the most important factor**
3. Stages of fracture repair
   - Inflammation
     - Bleeding creates a hematoma, which provides hematopoietic cells capable of secreting growth factors.
     - Subsequently, fibroblasts, mesenchymal cells, and osteoprogenitor cells form granulation tissue around the fracture ends.
     - Osteoblasts from surrounding osteogenic precursor cells and fibroblasts proliferate.
   - Repair
     - Primary callus response within 2 weeks.
     - **For bone ends not in continuity, bridging (soft) callus occurs.**
       - Soft callus is later replaced through enchondral ossification by woven bone (hard callus).
       - Medullary callus supplements the bridging callus, forming more slowly and later (Figure 1-18).

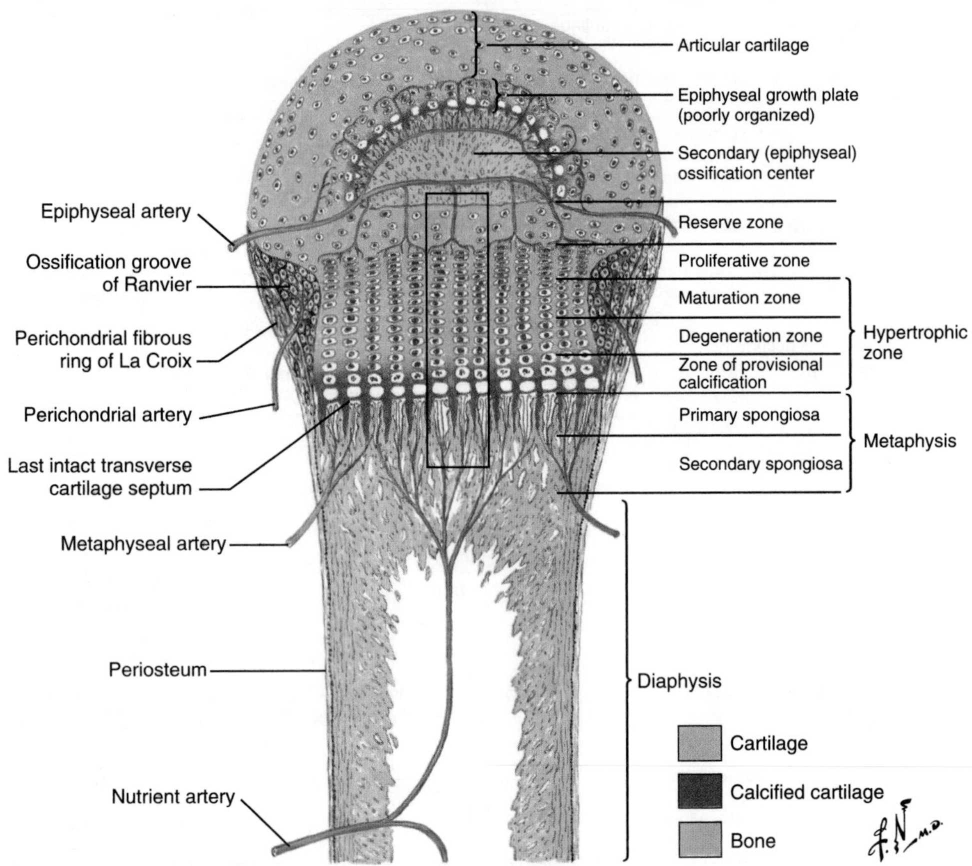

Figure 1-13 **Structure and blood supply of a typical growth plate.** (From Netter FH: *CIBA collection of medical illustrations,* vol 8: *Musculoskeletal system*, part I: *Anatomy, physiology and developmental disorders,* Basel, Switzerland, 1987, CIBA, p 166.)

- □ **Fracture healing varies with treatment method** (Table 1-7).
  - ▪ In unstable fracture, type II collagen is expressed early, followed by type I collagen.
  - ▪ Amount of callus is inversely proportional to the extent of immobilization.
- □ Progenitor cell differentiation:
  - ▪ High strain promotes development of fibrous tissue.
  - ▪ Low strain and high oxygen tension promote development of woven bone.
  - ▪ Intermediate strain and low oxygen tension promote development of cartilage.
- ▪ Remodeling
  - □ Remodeling begins in middle of repair phase and continues long after clinically healing (up to 7 years).
  - □ This process allows the bone to assume its normal configuration and shape according to stress exposure (Wolff's law).
  - □ Throughout, woven bone is replaced with lamellar bone.
  - □ Fracture healing is complete when the marrow space is repopulated.

4. Biochemistry of fracture healing (Table 1-8)
5. Growth factors of bone (Table 1-9)
   - ▪ **Bone morphogenetic protein (BMP)–2: acute open tibial fractures**
   - ▪ **BMP-3: no osteogenic activity**
   - ▪ **BMP-7: tibial nonunions**
6. Endocrine effects on fracture healing (Table 1-10)
7. Head injury
   - ▪ Can increase the osteogenic response to fracture
8. Nicotine (smoking)
   - ▪ Increases time to fracture healing
   - ▪ Increases nonunion risk (particularly in the tibia)
   - ▪ Decreases fracture callus strength
   - ▪ Increases pseudarthrosis risk after lumbar fusion up to 500%
9. Nonsteroidal anti-inflammatory drugs (NSAIDs)
   - ▪ These drugs have adverse effects on fracture healing and healing of lumbar spinal fusions.
   - ▪ **Cyclooxygenase-2 (COX-2) activity is required for normal enchondral ossification during fracture healing.**
10. **Quinolone antibiotics**
    - ▪ **Are toxic to chondrocytes and inhibit fracture healing**
11. Ultrasonography and fracture healing
    - ▪ **Low-intensity pulsed** ultrasonography accelerates fracture healing and increases the mechanical strength of callus.

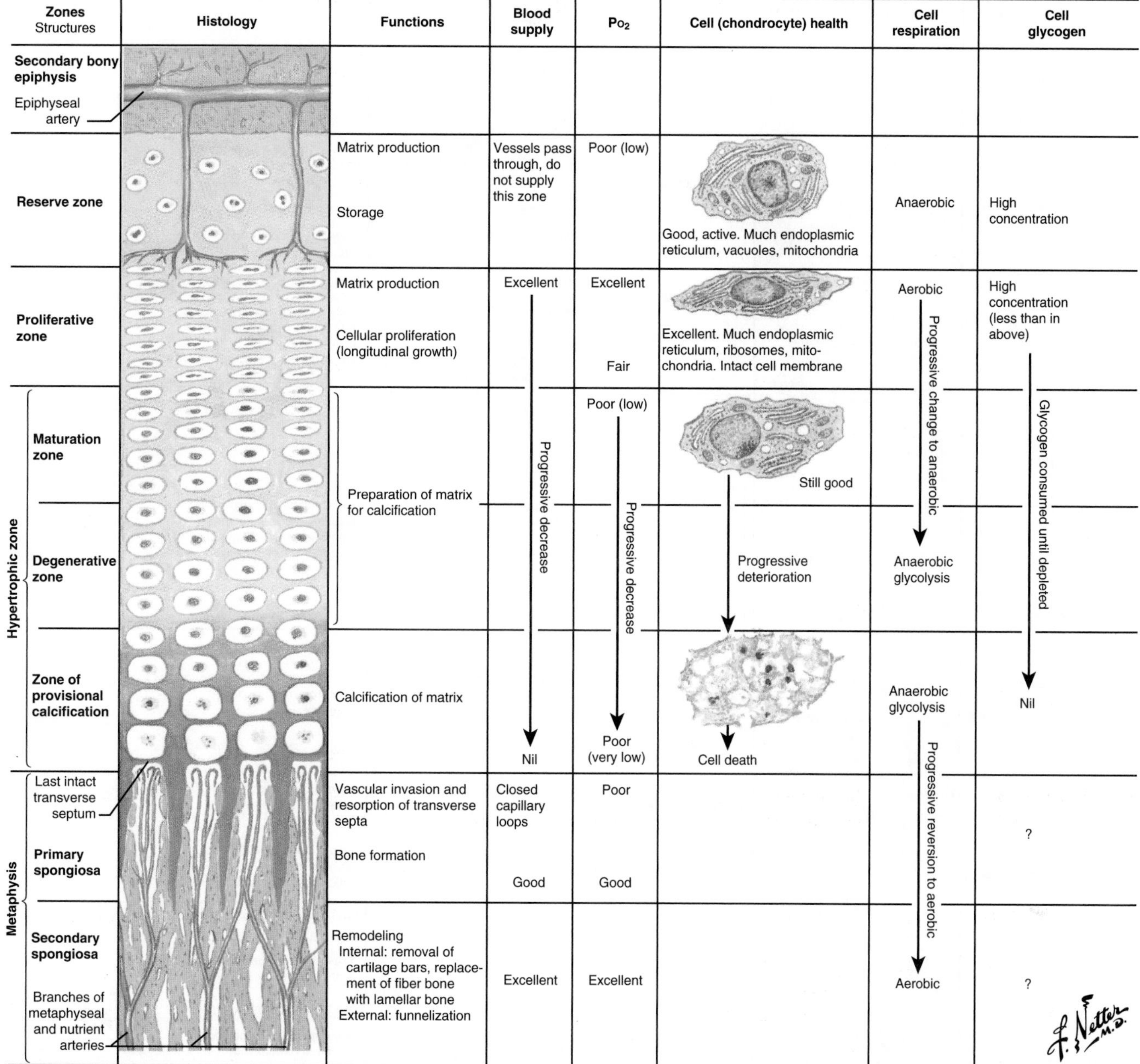

Figure 1-14 **Zone structure, function, and physiologic features of the growth plate.** (From Netter FH: *CIBA collection of medical illustrations,* vol 8: *Musculoskeletal system*, part I: *Anatomy, physiology and developmental disorders,* Basel, Switzerland, 1987, CIBA, p 164.)

- **A cellular response to the mechanical energy of ultrasonography has been postulated.**

12. Effect of radiation on bone
    - High-dose irradiation causes long-term changes within the haversian system and decreases cellularity.
13. Diet and fracture healing
    - Protein malnutrition results in negative effects in fracture healing:
        - Decreased periosteal and external callus
        - Decreased callus strength and stiffness
        - Increased fibrous tissue within callus
    - **In experimental models, oral supplementation with essential amino acids improves bone mineral density in fracture callus.**
14. Electricity and fracture healing
    - Definitions
        - Stress-generated potentials
            - Piezoelectric effect: Tissue charges are displaced secondary to mechanical forces.
            - Streaming potentials: These occur when electrically charged fluid is forced over a cell membrane that has a fixed charge.
        - Transmembrane potentials: generated by cellular metabolism
    - Types of electrical stimulation
        - Direct current (DC): stimulates an inflammatory-like response, resulting in decreased oxygen concentrations and increase in tissue pH (stage I)

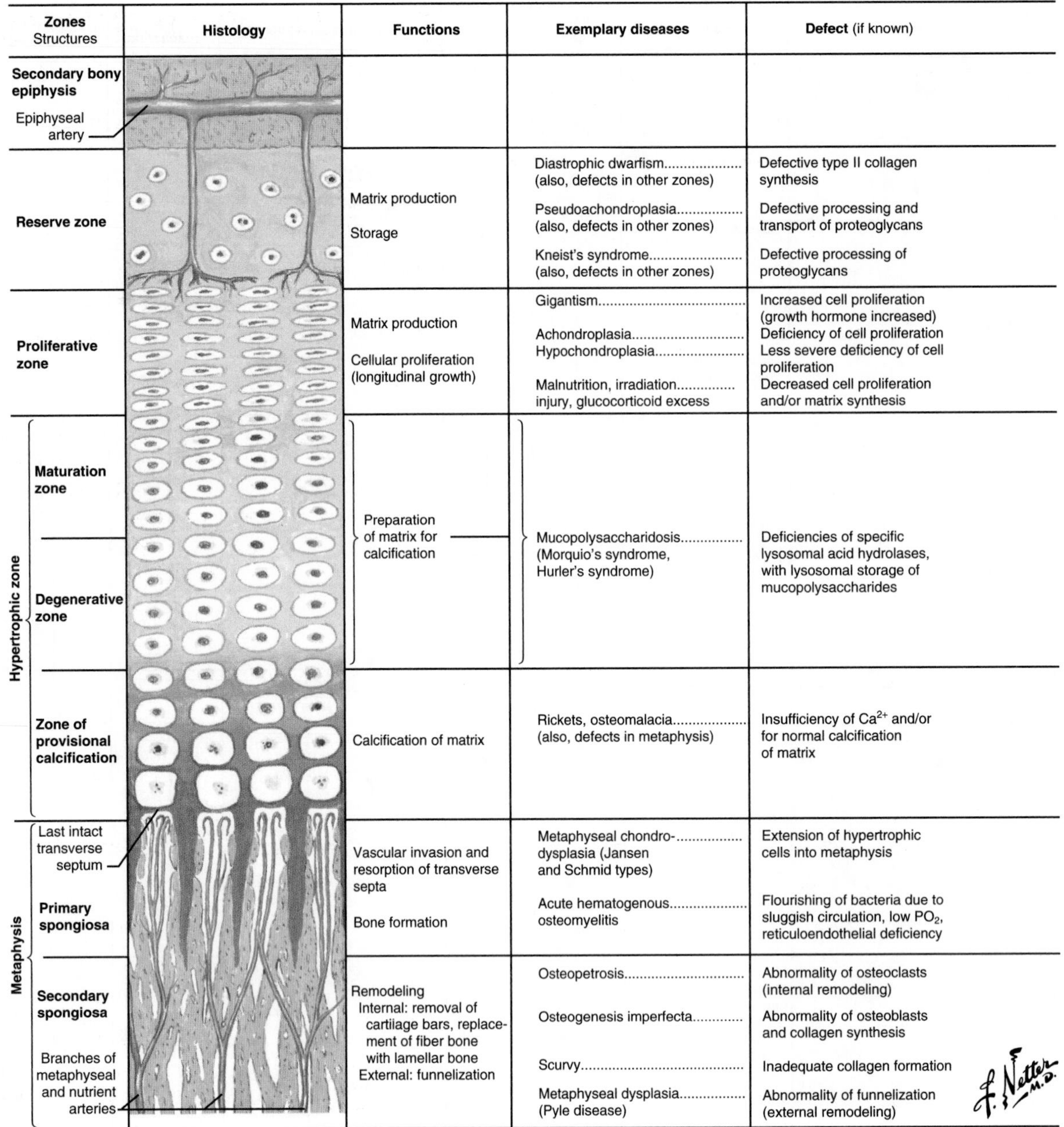

Zones
Structures
Histology
Functions
Exemplary diseases
Defect (if known)
Secondary bony epiphysis
Epiphyseal artery
Reserve zone
Matrix production
Storage
Diastrophic dwarfism
(also, defects in other zones)
Defective type II collagen synthesis
Pseudoachondroplasia
(also, defects in other zones)
Defective processing and transport of proteoglycans
Kneist's syndrome
(also, defects in other zones)
Defective processing of proteoglycans
Proliferative zone
Matrix production
Cellular proliferation (longitudinal growth)
Gigantism
Increased cell proliferation (growth hormone increased)
Achondroplasia
Deficiency of cell proliferation
Hypochondroplasia
Less severe deficiency of cell proliferation
Malnutrition, irradiation injury, glucocorticoid excess
Decreased cell proliferation and/or matrix synthesis
Hypertrophic zone
Maturation zone
Degenerative zone
Preparation of matrix for calcification
Mucopolysaccharidosis
(Morquio's syndrome, Hurler's syndrome)
Deficiencies of specific lysosomal acid hydrolases, with lysosomal storage of mucopolysaccharides
Zone of provisional calcification
Calcification of matrix
Rickets, osteomalacia
(also, defects in metaphysis)
Insufficiency of Ca2+ and/or for normal calcification of matrix
Metaphysis
Last intact transverse septum
Primary spongiosa
Vascular invasion and resorption of transverse septa
Bone formation
Metaphyseal chondrodysplasia (Jansen and Schmid types)
Extension of hypertrophic cells into metaphysis
Acute hematogenous osteomyelitis
Flourishing of bacteria due to sluggish circulation, low PO2, reticuloendothelial deficiency
Secondary spongiosa
Branches of metaphyseal and nutrient arteries
Remodeling
Internal: removal of cartilage bars, replacement of fiber bone with lamellar bone
External: funnelization
Osteopetrosis
Abnormality of osteoclasts (internal remodeling)
Osteogenesis imperfecta
Abnormality of osteoblasts and collagen synthesis
Scurvy
Inadequate collagen formation
Metaphyseal dysplasia (Pyle disease)
Abnormality of funnelization (external remodeling)
F. Netter M.D.

Figure 1-15 Zone structure and pathologic defects of cellular metabolism. (From Netter FH: *CIBA collection of medical illustrations,* vol 8: *Musculoskeletal system,* part I: *Anatomy, physiology and developmental disorders,* Basel, Switzerland, 1987, CIBA, p 165.)

- Alternating current (AC): "capacity coupled generators"; affects cyclic adenosine monophosphate (cAMP) synthesis, collagen synthesis, and calcification during the repair stage
- Pulsed electromagnetic fields (PEMFs): initiate calcification of fibrocartilage (but not fibrous tissue)

15. Pathologic fracture
    - In bone weakened by tumor, infection, or metabolic bone disease
    - Risk factors: pain, anatomic location, and pattern of bony destruction (scoring system of Mirels)
    - Risk for such fractures: highest in subtrochanteric femur

B. Bone grafting (Table 1-11)

1. Graft properties
    - **Osteoconductive matrix:** acts as a scaffold or framework for bone growth
    - **Osteoinductive factors:** growth factors (BMP) that stimulate bone formation
    - **Osteogenic cells:** primitive mesenchymal cells, osteoblasts, and osteocytes
    - **Structural integrity**
2. Overview
    - Autografts (from same person) or allografts (from another person)
    - Cancellous bone: for grafting nonunions or cavitary defects; remodels quickly and incorporates through the

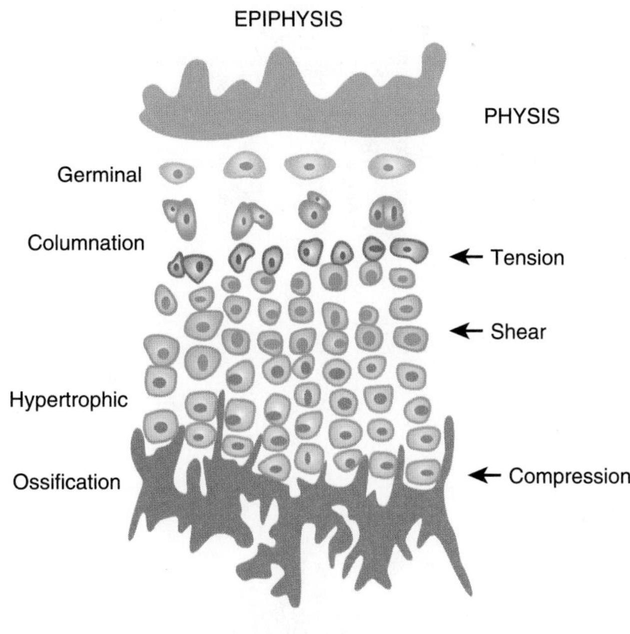

Figure 1-16 Histologic zone of failure varies with the type of loading applied to a specimen. (From Moen CT, Pelker RR: Biomechanical and histological correlations in growth plate failure, *J Pediatr Orthop* 4:180-184, 1984.)

laying down of new bone on old trabeculae ("creeping substitution")
- Cortical bone: slower to turn over; used for structural defects
- Osteoarticular (osteochondral) allograft used for tumor surgery
  - Immunogenic (cartilage is vulnerable to inflammatory mediators of immune response)
  - Articular cartilage preserved with glycerol or dimethyl sulfoxide (DMSO)
  - Cryogenically preserved grafts (leave few viable chondrocytes)
  - Tissue-matched (syngeneic) osteochondral grafts (produce minimal immunogenic effects and incorporate well)
- Vascularized bone grafts
  - Although technically difficult to implant, allow more rapid union and cell preservation; best for irradiated tissues or large tissue defects (morbidity may occur at donor site [e.g., fibula])
  - Nonvascular bone grafts are more common

3. **Allograft bone**
   - Fresh: increased immunogenicity
   - Fresh-frozen: less immunogenic than fresh; BMP preserved

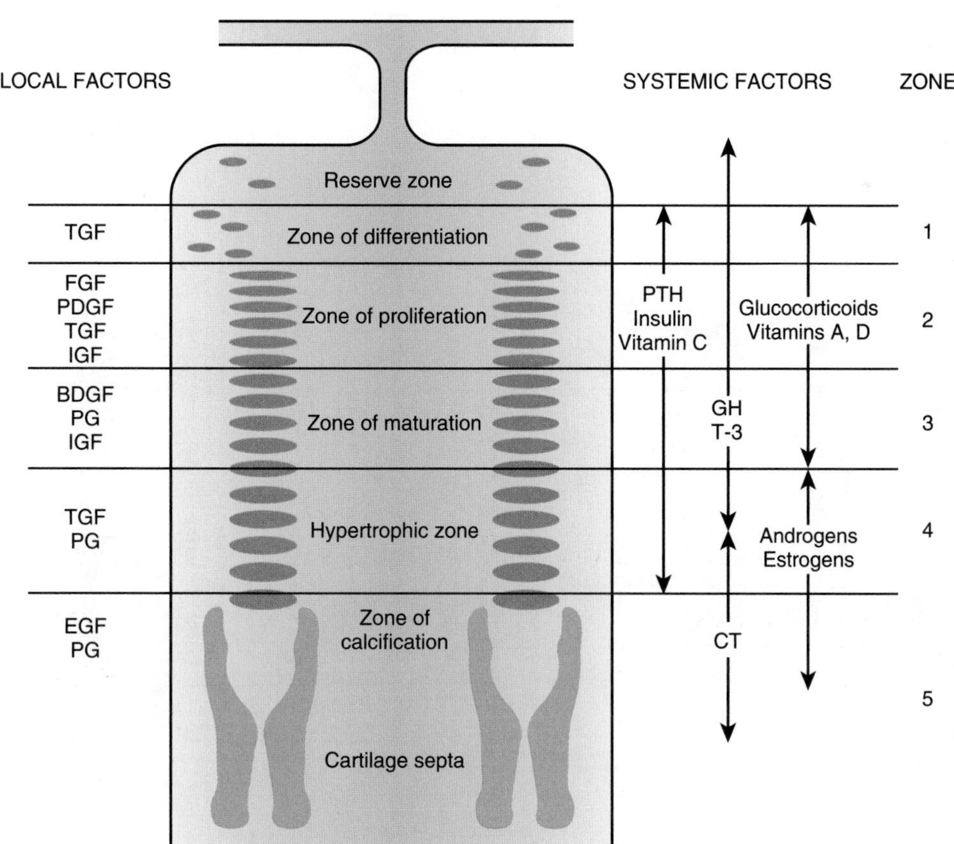

Figure 1-17 Growth plate demonstrating the proposed sites of action of hormones, growth factors, and vitamins. BDGF, bone-derived growth factor; CT, calcitonin; EGF, epidermal growth factor; FGF, fibroblast growth factor; GH, growth hormone; IGF, insulin-like growth factor; PDGF, platelet-derived growth factor; PG, proteoglycan; PTH, parathyroid hormone; T-3, triiodothyronine; TGF, transforming growth factor. (From Simon SR, editor: *Orthopaedic basic science,* Rosemont, Ill, 1994, American Academy of Orthopaedic Surgeons, p 197.)

Table 1-5 Effects of Hormones and Growth Factors on the Growth Plate

Biologic Effect of Hormone/Factor	Systemic/Local Derivation	Proliferation	Macromolecule Biosynthesis	Maturation Degradation	Matrix Calcification	Zone Primarily Affected
Thyroid hormone	Systemic (thyroid)	+ (T3 with IGF-I)	0	+ (T3 alone)	0	Proliferative zone and upper hypertrophic zone
Parathyroid	Systemic (parathyroid)	+	++ (Proteoglycan)	0	0	Entire growth plate
Calcitonin	Systemic (thyroid)	0	0	+	+	Hypertrophic zone and metaphysis
Excess corticosteroids	Systemic (adrenal glands)	–	–	–	0	Entire growth plate
Growth hormone	Systemic (pituitary)	+ (Through IGF-I locally)	+ (Slight)	0	0	Proliferative zone
Somatomedins	Systemic local paracrine (liver, chondrocytes)	+	+ (Slight)	0	0	Proliferative zone
Insulin	Systemic (pancreas)	+ (Through IGF-I receptor)	0	0	0	Proliferative zone
1,25(OH)$_2$-vitamin D$_3$	Systemic (liver, kidney)	0	0	+ Indirect effect serum Ca and PO		Hypertrophic zone
24,25(OH)$_2$D$_3$	Systemic (liver, kidney)	+	+ (Collagen II)	0	0	Proliferative zone and hypertrophic zone
Vitamin A	Systemic (diet)	0	0	–	0	Hypertrophic zone
Vitamin C	Systemic (diet)	0	+ (Collagen)	0	+ (Matrix vesicles)	Proliferative zone and hypertrophic zone
EGF	Local paracrine (endothelial cells)	+	– (Collagen)	0	0	Metaphysis
FGF	Local paracrine (endothelial cells)	+	0	0	0	Proliferative zone
PDGF	Local paracrine (platelets)	+	+ (Noncollagenous proteins)	0	0	Proliferative zone
TGF-β	Local paracrine (platelets, chondrocytes)	±	±	0	0	Proliferative zone and hypertrophic zone
BDGF	Local paracrine (bone matrix)	0	+ (Collagen)	0	0	Upper hypertrophic zone
IL-1	Local paracrine (inflammatory cells, synoviocytes)	0	–	++ (Activates tissue metalloproteinases)	0	Entire growth plate
Prostaglandin	Local autocrine	±	+ (Proteoglycan) – (Collagen and alkaline phosphatase)	0	Bone resorption with osteoclasts	Hypertrophic zone and metaphysis

From Simon SR, editor: *Orthopaedic basic science,* ed 2, Rosemont, Ill, 1994, American Academy of Orthopaedic Surgeons, p 196.

+, Increase stimulation; 0, no known effect; –, inhibitory; ±, depending on the local hormonal milieu.

BDGF, bone-derived growth factor; EGF, epidermal growth factor; FGF, fibroblast growth factor; IGF-I, insulin-like growth factor I; IL-1, interleukin-1; PDGF, platelet-derived growth factor; T3, triiodothyronine; TGF-β, transforming growth factor-β.

Table 1-6 Biologic and Mechanical Factors Influencing Fracture Healing

Biologic Factors	Mechanical Factors
Patient age Comorbid medical conditions Functional level Nutritional status Nerve function Vascular injury Hormones Growth factors Health of the soft tissue envelope Sterility (in open fractures) Cigarette smoke Local pathologic conditions Level of energy imparted Type of bone affected Extent of bone loss	Soft tissue attachments to bone Stability (extent of immobilization) Anatomic location Level of energy imparted Extent of bone loss

- Freeze-dried (lyophilized "croutons"): loses structural integrity and depletes BMP, is least immunogenic, is purely osteoconductive, has lowest risk of viral transmission
- Bone matrix gelatin (a digested source of BMP): demineralized bone matrix is osteoconductive and osteoinductive
- Antigenicity
  - Allograft bone possesses a spectrum of potential antigens, primarily from cell surface glycoproteins.
  - Classes I and II cellular antigens in allograft are recognized by T lymphocytes in the host.
  - Primary mechanism of rejection is cellular, as opposed to humoral.
    - Incorporation is related to cellularity and major histocompatibility complex (MHC) incompatibility.
  - Cellular components that contribute to antigenicity are marrow origin, endothelium, and retinacular activating cells.
    - Marrow cells incite the greatest immunogenic response.
  - Extracellular matrix components that contribute to antigenicity are as follows:
    - Type I collagen (organic matrix): stimulates cell-mediated and humoral responses
    - Noncollagenous matrix (proteoglycans, osteopontin, osteocalcin, other glycoproteins)
  - Hydroxyapatite does not elicit immune response.

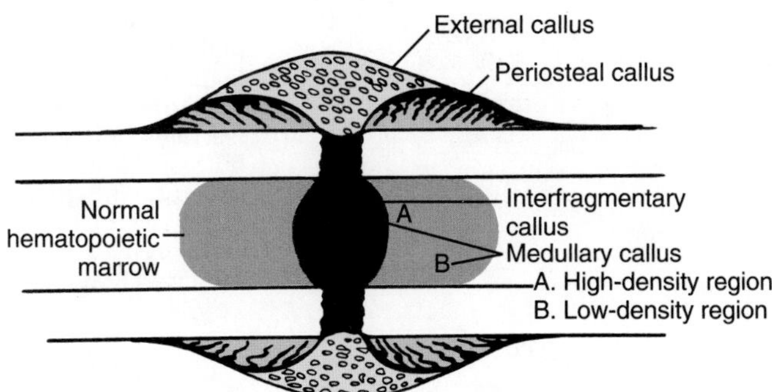

Figure 1-18 Histologic features of typical fracture healing. (From Brighton CT, Hunt RM: Early histological and ultrastructural changes in medullary fracture callus, *J Bone Joint Surg Am* 73:832-847, 1991.)

Table 1-7 Type of Fracture Healing Based on Type of Stabilization

Type of Stabilization	Predominant Type of Healing
Cast (closed treatment)	**Periosteal bridging callus and interfragmentary enchondral ossification**
Compression plate	Primary cortical healing (cutting cone–type or Haversian remodeling)
Intramedullary nail	Early: periosteal bridging callus; enchondral ossification Late: medullary callus and intramembranous ossification
External fixator	Dependent on extent of rigidity: Less rigid: periosteal bridging callus; enchondral ossification More rigid: primary cortical healing; intramembranous ossification
Inadequate immobilization with adequate blood supply	Hypertrophic nonunion (failed enchondral ossification); type II collagen predominates
Inadequate immobilization without adequate blood supply	**Atrophic nonunion**
Inadequate reduction with displacement at the fracture site	Oligotrophic nonunion

4. Five Stages of graft healing (Urist) (Table 1-12)
   - Factors influencing incorporation (Figure 1-19)
5. Specific bone graft types
   - **Cortical bone grafts**
     - Slower incorporation: remodels existing haversian systems through resorption (weakens the graft) and then deposits new bone (restores strength)
     - Resorption confined to osteon borders; interstitial lamellae are preserved
     - **Used for structural defects**
     - Of massive grafts, 25% eventually sustain insufficiency fracture
   - **Cancellous grafts**
     - These grafts revascularize and incorporate quickly.
     - Osteoblasts lay down new bone on old trabeculae, which are later remodeled ("creeping substitution").
   - **Synthetic bone grafts:** calcium, silicon, or aluminum

Table 1-8 Biochemical Steps of Fracture Healing

Step	Collagen Type
Mesenchymal	I, II, III, V
Chondroid	II, IX
Chondroid-osteoid	I, II, X
Osteogenic	I

Table 1-9 Growth Factors of Bone

Growth Factor	Action	Notes
Bone morphogenetic protein (BMP)	Osteoinductive; stimulates bone formation Induces metaplasia of mesenchymal cells into osteoblasts	Target cells of BMP are the undifferentiated perivascular mesenchymal cells; signal through serine-threonine kinase receptors Intracellular molecules called SMADs serve as signaling mediators for BMPs
Transforming growth factor-β (TGF-β)	Induces mesenchymal cells to produce type II collagen and proteoglycans Induces osteoblasts to synthesize collagen	Found in fracture hematomas; believed to regulate cartilage and bone formation in fracture callus; signal through serine/threonine kinase receptors Coating porous implants with TGF-β enhances bone ingrowth
Insulin-like growth factor II (IGF-II)	Stimulates type I collagen, cellular proliferation, cartilage matrix synthesis, and bone formation	Signal through tyrosine kinase receptors
Platelet-derived growth factor (PDGF)	Attracts inflammatory cells to the fracture site (chemotactic)	Released from platelets; signal through tyrosine kinase receptors

Table 1-10 Endocrine Effects on Fracture Healing

Hormone	Effect	Mechanism
Cortisone	–	Decreased callus proliferation
Calcitonin	+?	Unknown
TH, PTH	+	Bone remodeling
Growth hormone	+	Increased callus volume

PTH, parathyroid hormone; TH, thyroid hormone.

- Calcium phosphate–based grafts: capable of osseoconduction and osseointegration
  - Biodegrade very slowly
  - Highest compressive strength of any graft material
  - Many prepared as ceramics (heated apatite crystals fuse into crystals [sintered])
    - Tricalcium phosphate
    - Hydroxyapatite; purified bovine dermal fibrillar collagen plus ceramic hydroxyapatite granules and tricalcium phosphate granules
- Calcium sulfate: osteoconductive
  - Rapidly resorbed
- Calcium carbonate (chemically unaltered marine coral): resorbed and replaced by bone (osteoconductive)
- Coralline hydroxyapatite: calcium carbonate skeleton is converted to calcium phosphate through a thermoexchange process
- Silicate-based incorporate silicon as silicate (silicon dioxide); bioactive glasses and glass-ionomer cement
- Aluminum oxide: alumina ceramic bonds to bone in response to stress and strain between implant and bone

Table 1-11 Types of Bone Grafts and Bone Graft Properties

	PROPERTIES				
Graft	Osteoconduction	Osteoinduction	Osteogenic Cells	Structural Integrity	Other Properties
Autograft					
Cancellous	Excellent	Good	Excellent	Poor	Rapid incorporation
Cortical	Fair	Fair	Fair	Excellent	Slow incorporation
Allograft	Fair	Fair	None	Good	Fresh has the highest immunogenicity Freeze-dried is the least immunogenic but has the least structural integrity (weakest) Fresh-frozen preserves BMP
Ceramics	Fair	None	None	Fair	
Demineralized bone matrix	Fair	Good	None	Poor	
Bone marrow	Poor	Poor	Good	Poor	

Modified from Brinker MR, Miller MD: *Fundamentals of orthopaedics,* Philadelphia, 1999, WB Saunders, p 7.
BMP, bone morphogenetic protein.

Table 1-12 Stages of Graft Healing

Stage	Activity
1: Inflammation	Chemotaxis stimulated by necrotic debris
2: Osteoblast differentiation	From precursors
3: Osteoinduction	Osteoblast and osteoclast function
4: Osteoconduction	New bone forming over scaffold
5: Remodeling	Process continues for years

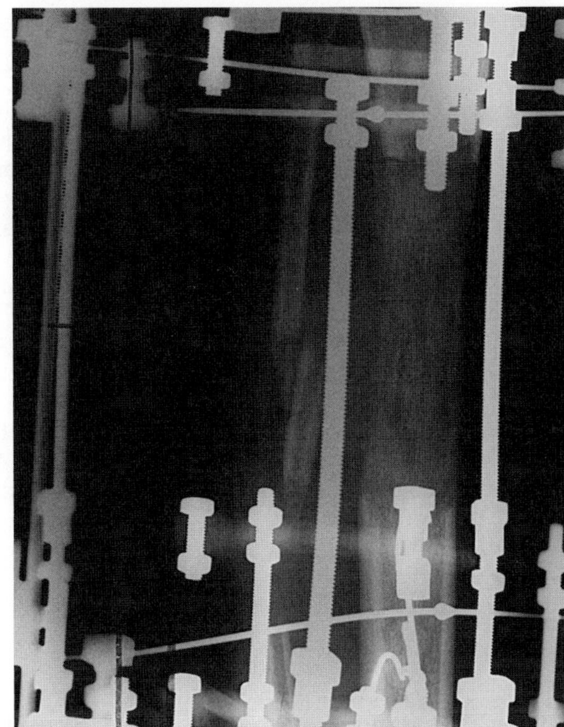

Figure 1-20 Anteroposterior radiograph of the proximal tibia in a patient who underwent bone transport for a large distal tibial segmental defect. Early regeneration of distraction osteogenesis is apparent; bone formation occurred through intramembranous ossification.

C. Distraction osteogenesis (Figure 1-20)

1. Definition: distraction-stimulated formation of bone
2. Clinical applications:
   - Limb lengthening
   - Hypertrophic nonunions
   - Deformity correction (via differential lengthening)
   - Segmental bone loss (via bone transport)
3. Biologic features:
   - Under optimal stability, intramembranous ossification occurs.
   - Under instability, bone forms through enchondral ossification.
     - Pseudarthrosis may occur under extreme instability.
   - Three histologic phases:
     - Latency phase (5 to 7 days)
     - Distraction phase (1 mm per day [approximately 1 inch per month])
     - Consolidation phase (typically twice as long as the distraction phase)
4. Optimal conditions during distraction osteogenesis:
   - Low-energy corticotomy/osteotomy
   - Minimal soft tissue stripping at the corticotomy site (preserves blood supply)
   - Stable external fixation and elimination of torsion, shear, and bending moments
   - Latency period (no lengthening) 5 to 7 days
   - Distraction: 0.25 mm three or four times per day (0.75 to 1.0 mm per day)
   - Neutral fixation interval (no distraction) during consolidation
   - Normal physiologic use of the extremity, including weight bearing

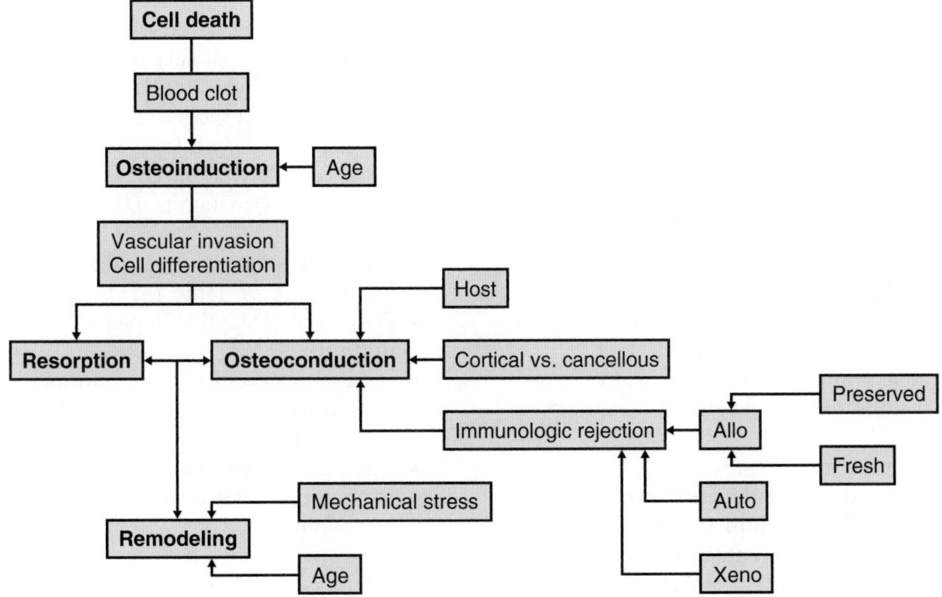

Figure 1-19 Major factors influencing bone graft incorporation. Allo, allograft; Auto, autograft; Xeno, xenograft. (From Simon SR, editor: *Orthopaedic basic science*, Rosemont, Ill, 1994, American Academy of Orthopaedic Surgeons, p 284.)

D. Heterotopic ossification

1. Ectopic bone forms in soft tissues.
   - Most commonly in response to injury or surgical dissection
   - Myositis ossificans: heterotopic ossification in muscle
2. Traumatic brain injury increases risk of heterotopic ossification.
   - Recurrence after resection is likely if neurologic compromise is severe.
   - The timing of surgery for heterotopic ossification after traumatic brain injury is important:
     - Time since injury (3 to 6 months)
     - Evidence of bone maturation on radiographs (sharp demarcation, trabecular pattern)
3. Heterotopic ossification may be resected after total hip arthroplasty (THA).
   - Resection should be delayed for 6 months or longer after THA.
   - Adjuvant radiation therapy may prevent recurrence of heterotopic ossification.
     - Optimal therapy: single postoperative dose of 600 to 700 rad
     - Prevents proliferation and differentiation of primordial mesenchymal cells into osteoprogenitor cells
4. Preoperative radiation (600 to 800 rad) may be used in treatment.
   - Helps prevent heterotopic ossification after THA in patients at high risk for this development.
   - Incidence of heterotopic ossification after THA among patients with Paget's disease is approximately 50%.
5. When oral bisphosphonate therapy is discontinued, heterotopic ossification may occur.
   - Oral bisphosphonate inhibits mineralization.
   - However, it does not prevent formation of osteoid matrix.

III. CONDITIONS OF BONE MINERALIZATION, BONE MINERAL DENSITY, AND BONE VIABILITY

A. Normal bone metabolism

1. **Calcium**
   - Important in muscle and nerve function, clotting, and many other areas
   - >99% of the body's calcium is stored in bones.
     - Plasma calcium is about equally free and bound (usually to albumin).
     - Approximately 400 mg of calcium is released from bone daily.
   - Absorbed in the duodenum by active transport
     - Requires ATP and calcium-binding protein
     - Regulated by 1,25$(OH)_2$-vitamin D_3
   - Absorbed in the jejunum by passive diffusion
   - The kidney reabsorbs 98% of calcium (60% in the proximal tubule).
     - Calcium may be excreted in stool.
   - **The primary homeostatic regulators of serum calcium are PTH and 1,25$(OH)_2$-vitamin D_3**
   - **Dietary requirement of elemental calcium:**
     - Approximately 600 mg/day for children
     - **Approximately 1300 mg/day for adolescents and young adults (ages 10 to 25 years)**
     - 750 mg/day for adults (ages 25 to 65 years)
     - 1500 mg/day for pregnant women
     - 2000 mg/day for lactating women
     - 1500 mg/day for postmenopausal women and for patients with a healing fracture in a long bone
   - Calcium balance is usually positive in the first three decades of life and negative after the fourth decade
2. **Phosphate**
   - A key component of bone mineral
     - Approximately 85% of the body's phosphate stores are in bone.
     - Plasma phosphate is mostly unbound.
   - Also important in enzyme systems and molecular interactions
     - It is a metabolite and buffer.
   - Dietary intake of phosphate is usually adequate.
     - Daily requirement is 1000 to 1500 mg.
   - Reabsorbed by the kidney (proximal tubule)
     - Phosphate may be excreted in urine.
3. **Parathyroid hormone**
   - PTH is an 84–amino acid peptide.
     - It is synthesized in and secreted from the chief cells of the (four) parathyroid glands.
     - The N-terminal fragment 1-34 is the active portion.
     - **Teriparatide, the synthetic form of recombinant human PTH, contains this active sequence.**
   - **The effect of PTH is mediated by the cAMP second-messenger mechanism.**
   - PTH helps regulate plasma calcium.
     - Decreased calcium levels in the extracellular fluid stimulate β_2 receptors to release PTH, which acts at the intestines, kidneys, and bones (Table 1-13).
   - PTH directly activates osteoblasts.
   - PTH modulates renal phosphate filtration.
   - PTH may accentuate bone loss in elderly persons.
   - PTH-related protein and its receptor have been implicated in metaphyseal dysplasia.
4. **Vitamin D**
   - Naturally occurring steroid
     - Activated by ultraviolet radiation from sunlight or utilized from dietary intake (Figure 1-21)
   - Hydroxylated to 25(OH)-vitamin D_3 in the liver and hydroxylated a second time in the kidney to one of the following:
     - 1,25$(OH)_2$-vitamin D_3, the active hormone
     - 24,25$(OH)_2$-vitamin D_3, the inactive form (Figure 1-22)
   - 1,25$(OH)_2$-vitamin D_3 works at the intestines, kidneys, and bones (see Table 1-13).
   - Phenytoin (Dilantin) impair metabolism of vitamin D.
5. **Calcitonin**
   - A 32–amino acid peptide hormone
     - Produced by clear cells in the parafollicles of the thyroid gland
   - Has a limited role in calcium regulation (see Table 1-13)
   - Increased extracellular calcium levels cause secretion of calcitonin
     - Controlled by a β_2 receptor
   - Inhibits osteoclastic bone resorption
     - Osteoclasts have calcitonin receptors.
     - Calcitonin decreases osteoclast number and activity.

Table 1-13 Regulation of Calcium and Phosphate Metabolism

Parameter	PTH (Peptide)	$1,25(OH)_2D$ (Steroid)	Calcitonin (Peptide)
Origin	Chief cells of parathyroid glands	Proximal tubule of kidney	Parafollicular cells of thyroid gland
Factors stimulating production	Decreased serum Ca^{2+}	Elevated PTH level Decreased serum Ca^{2+} level Decreased serum P_i	Elevated serum Ca^{2+} level
Factors inhibiting production	Elevated serum Ca^{2+} Elevated $1,25(OH)_2D$	Decreased PTH Elevated serum Ca^{2+} Elevated serum P_i	Decreased serum Ca^{2+}
Effect on end-organs for hormone action			
Intestine	No direct effect Acts indirectly on bowel by stimulating production of $1,25(OH)_2D$ in kidney	Strongly stimulates intestinal absorption of Ca^{2+} and P_i	?
Kidney	Stimulates 25(OH)D 1α-hydroxylase in mitochondria of proximal tubular cells to convert 25(OH)D to $1,25(OH)_2D$ Increases fractional resorption of filtered Ca^{2+} Promotes urinary excretion of P_i	?	?
Bone	Stimulates osteoclastic resorption of bone Stimulates recruitment of preosteoclasts	Strongly stimulates osteoclastic resorption of bone	Inhibits osteoclastic resorption of bone ? Role in normal human physiology
Net effect on Ca^{2+} and P_i concentrations in extracellular fluid and serum	Increased serum Ca^{2+} level Decreased serum P_i level	Increased serum Ca^{2+} level Increased serum P_i level	Decreased serum Ca^{2+} level (transient)

Adapted from Netter FH: *CIBA collection of medical illustrations,* vol 8: *Musculoskeletal system*, part I: *Anatomy, physiology and developmental disorders,* Basel, Switzerland, 1987, CIBA, p 179.

$1,25(OH)_2D$, 1,25-dihydroxyvitamin D; 25(OH)D, 25-hydroxyvitamin D; P_i, inorganic phosphate; PTH, parathyroid hormone.

- Decreases serum calcium level
- May also have a role in fracture healing and in reducing vertebral compression fractures in high-turnover osteoporosis

6. Other hormones affecting bone metabolism
   - **Estrogen**
     - Estrogen prevents bone loss by inhibiting bone resorption.
       - Decrease in urinary pyridinoline cross-links
     - Because bone formation and resorption are coupled, estrogen therapy also decreases bone formation.
     - Supplementation is helpful in postmenopausal women only if started within 5 to 10 years after onset of menopause.
       - Risk of endometrial cancer is reduced when estrogen therapy is combined with cyclic progestin therapy.
     - Certain regimens of hormone replacement therapy may increase risk of heart disease and breast cancer.
       - Other postmenopausal pharmacologic interventions (alendronate, raloxifene) should be strongly considered.
   - Corticosteroids
     - Increase bone loss
       - Decrease gut absorption of calcium by decreasing binding proteins
       - Decrease bone formation (cancellous more than cortical) by inhibiting collagen synthesis and osteoblast productivity
       - Do not affect mineralization
     - Alternate-day therapy may reduce the effects
   - Thyroid hormones
     - Affect bone resorption more than bone formation
       - Large (thyroid-suppressive) doses of thyroxine can lead to osteoporosis.
     - Regulates skeletal growth at the physis
       - Stimulates chondrocyte growth, type X collagen synthesis, and alkaline phosphatase activity
   - Growth hormone
     - Causes positive calcium balance
       - Increases gut absorption of calcium more than it increases urinary excretion
     - Insulin and somatomedins participate in this effect
   - Growth factors
     - Transforming growth factor β (TGF-β), PDGF, monokines, and lymphokines have roles in bone and cartilage repair.
7. Interactions
   - Calcium and phosphate metabolism
     - Affected by an elaborate interplay of hormones and the levels of the metabolites themselves
   - Feedback mechanisms: important in the regulation of plasma levels of calcium and phosphate

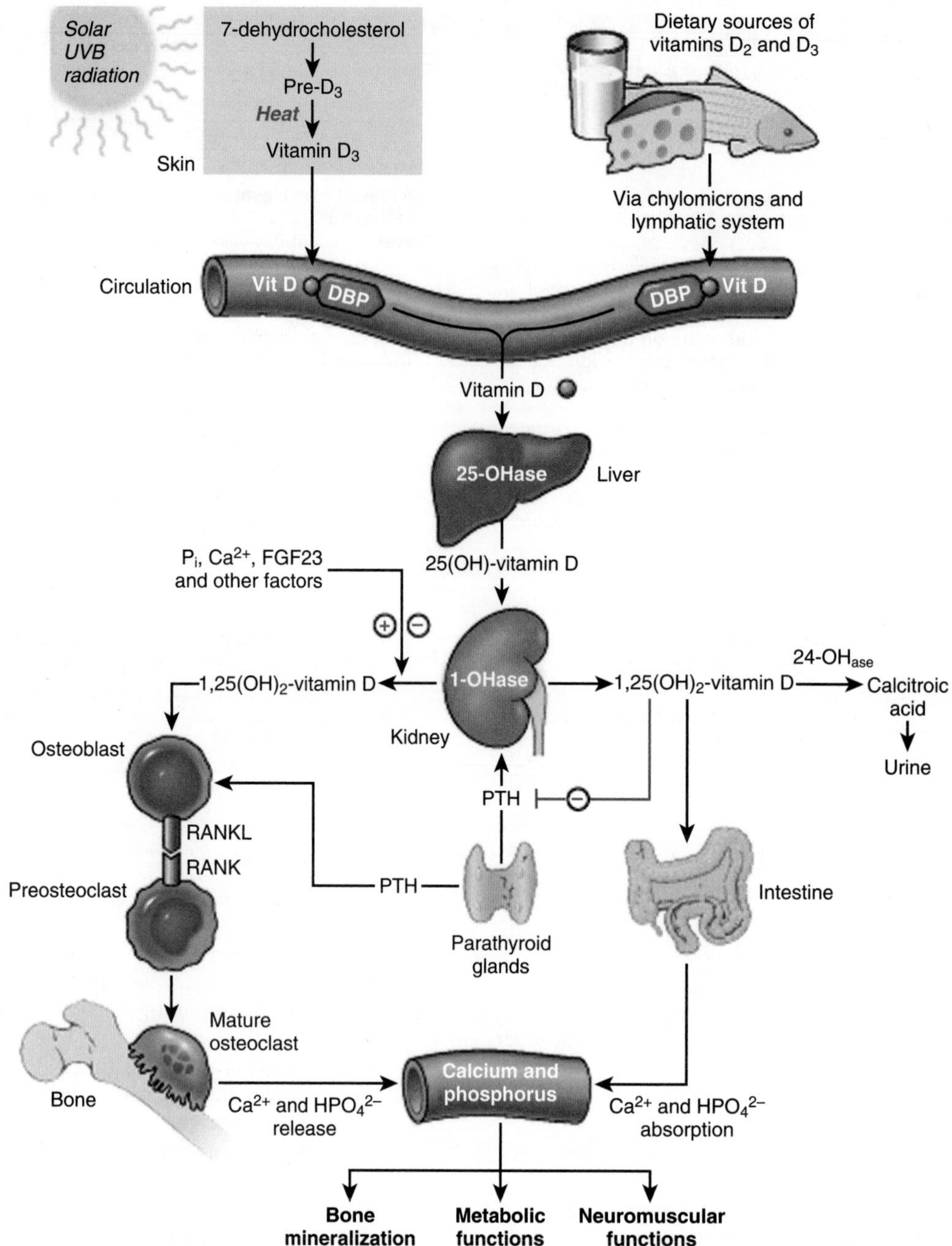

Figure 1-21 Vitamin D metabolism. $1,25(OH)_2D$, 1,25-dihydroxyvitamin D; 25(OH)D, 25-hydroxyvitamin D; DBP, vitamin D–binding protein; FGF23, fibroblast growth factor 23; OH_{ase}, 1α-hydroxylase; P_i, inorganic phosphate; PTH, parathyroid hormone; UVB, ultraviolet B. (From Kumar V, et al, editors: *Robbins and Cotran pathologic basis of disease,* Philadelphia, 2010, WB Saunders.)

8. Bone aging
   - Peak bone mass
     - Believed to occur between 16 and 25 years of age
     - Higher in men and in African Americans
   - After peak, bone loss occurs at a rate of 0.3% to 0.5% per year
     - Rate of bone loss is 2% to 3% per year in untreated women during the sixth through tenth years after menopause.
     - **Affects trabecular more than cortical bone**
       - Increase in trabecular rods results in increased anisotropy.
       - Cortical bone becomes thinner, and intracortical porosities increase.
       - Cortical bone becomes more brittle, less strong, and less stiff.
     - **Long bones have increased inner and outer diameter.**
9. Bone loss
   - Occurs at the onset of menopause, when both bone formation and resorption are accelerated

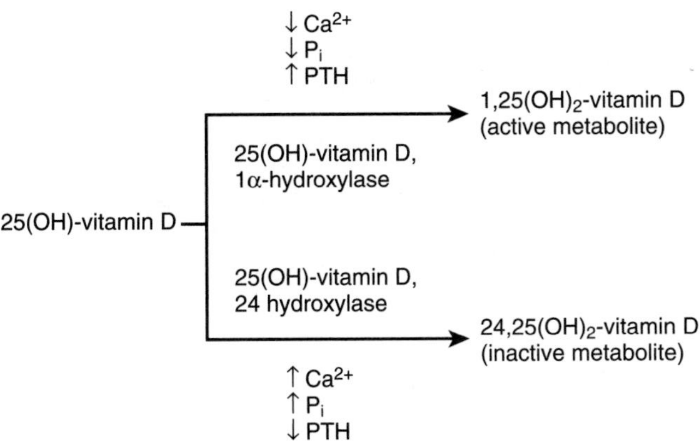

Figure 1-22 Vitamin D metabolism in the renal tubular cell. P_i, inorganic phosphate; PTH, parathyroid hormone. (From Simon SR [editor]: *Orthopaedic basic science,* Rosemont, Ill, 1994, American Academy of Orthopaedic Surgeons, p 165.)

- □ A net negative change in calcium balance: menopause decreases intestinal absorption and increases urinary excretion of calcium
- Both **urinary hydroxyproline and pyridinoline cross-links** are elevated when bone resorption occurs.
- **Serum alkaline phosphatase** level is elevated when bone formation is increased.
- Estrogen therapy is recommended for patients at high risk for osteoporosis.
  - □ Decreases urinary pyridinoline (decreased bone resorption)
  - □ Decreases serum alkaline phosphatase (decreased bone formation)
  - □ Increases bone density of the femoral neck, reducing the rate of hip fracture

B. Conditions of bone mineralization (Tables 1-14 through 1-16)

1. **Hypercalcemia**
   - Can manifest in a number of ways:
     - □ Polyuria
     - □ Polydipsia
     - □ Kidney stones
     - □ Excessive bony resorption with or without fibrotic tissue replacement (osteitis fibrosa cystica)
     - □ Central nervous system (CNS) effects (confusion, stupor, weakness)
     - □ Gastrointestinal effects (constipation)
   - Can also cause anorexia, nausea, vomiting, dehydration, and muscle weakness
   - Primary hyperparathyroidism
     - □ Overproduction of PTH, usually a result of a parathyroid adenoma
       - Generally affects only one parathyroid gland
     - □ Reflected in a net increase in plasma calcium and a decrease in plasma phosphate (as a result of enhanced urinary excretion)

Text continued on p. 28

Table 1-14 Overview of Clinical and Radiographic Aspects of Metabolic Bone Diseases

Disease	Cause	Clinical Findings	Radiographic Findings
Hypercalcemia			
Hyperparathyroidism	PTH overproduction: adenoma	Kidney stone, hyperreflexia	Osteopenia, osteitis fibrosa cystica
Familial syndromes	PTH overproduction: MEN/renal	Endocrine and renal abnormalities	Osteopenia
Hypocalcemia			
Hypoparathyroidism	PTH underproduction: idiopathic	Neuromuscular irritability, cataracts	Calcified basal ganglia
PHP/Albright's syndrome	PTH receptor abnormality	Short MC/MT, obesity	Brachydactyly, exostosis
Renal osteodystrophy	CRF: ↓ phosphate excretion	Renal abnormalities	"Rugger jersey" spine
Rickets (osteomalacia)			
Vitamin D–deficiency rickets	↓ Vitamin D diet; malabsorption	Bone deformities, hypotonia	"Rachitic rosary," wide growth plates, fractures
Vitamin D–dependent (types I and II) rickets	See Table 1-15	Total baldness	Poor mineralization
Vitamin D–resistant (hypophosphatemic) rickets	↓ Renal tubular phosphate resorption	Bone deformities, hypotonia	Poor mineralization
Hypophosphatasia	↓ Alkaline phosphatase	Bone deformities, hypotonia	Poor mineralization
Osteopenia			
Osteoporosis	↓ Estrogen: ↓ bone mass	Kyphosis, fractures	Compression vertebral fractures, hip fractures
Scurvy	Vitamin C deficiency: defective collagen	Fatigue, bleeding, effusions	Thin cortices, corner sign
Osteodensity			
Paget's disease	Osteoclastic abnormality: ↑ bone turnover	Deformities, pain, CHF, fractures	Coarse trabeculae, "picture frame" vertebrae
Osteopetrosis	Osteoclastic abnormality: unclear	Hepatosplenomegaly, anemia	Bone within bone

↓, Decreased; ↑, increased; CHF, congestive heart failure; CRF, chronic renal failure; MC, metacarpal; MEN, multiple endocrine neoplasia, MT, metatarsal; PHP, pseudohypoparathyroidism; PTH, parathyroid hormone.

Table 1-15 Laboratory Findings and Clinical Data Regarding Patients with Various Metabolic Bone Diseases

Disorder	CHANGES IN LEVEL OR CONCENTRATION: Serum Ca	Serum Phos	Alk Phos	PTH	25(OH)-Vitamin D	$1,25(OH)_2$-Vitamin D	Urinary Calcium	Other Findings or Possible Findings	Treatment	Comments
Primary hyperparathyroidism	↑	None or ↓	None or ↑	↑	None	None or ↑	↑	Active turnover observed on bone biopsy with peritrabecular fibrosis Brown tumors	Surgical excision of parathyroid edema Treat hypercalcemia (see text)	Most commonly caused by parathyroid adenoma Because PTH stimulates conversion of the inactive form to the active form [$1,25(OH)_2$-vitamin D] in the kidney, ↑ production of PTH leads to ↑ levels of $1,25(OH)_2$-vitamin D
Malignancy with bony metastases	↑	None or ↑	None or ↑	None or ↓	None	None or ↓	↑	Destructive lesions in bone	Treat cancer and hypercalcemia (see text)	↑ Calcium levels may lead to ↓ PTH production through feedback mechanism ↓ $1,25(OH)_2$-vitamin D levels result from to ↓ PTH (responsible for conversion of inactive to active form of vitamin D in the kidney) Patients with multiple myeloma display abnormal urinary and serum protein electrophoresis
Hyperthyroidism	↑	None	None	None or ↓	None	None	↑	↑ Free thyroxin index ↓ Thyroid-stimulating hormone Tachycardia, tremors	Treat hyperthyroidism	↑ Calcium levels caused by ↑ bone turnover (hypermetabolic state)
Vitamin D intoxication	↑	None or ↑	None or ↑	None or ↓	↑↑↑	None	↑		Normalize vitamin D intake and levels	History of excessive vitamin D intake Dietary vitamin D is converted to 25(OH)-vitamin D in the liver; very high concentrations of 25(OH)-vitamin D cross-react with intestinal vitamin D receptors to ↑ resorption of calcium and cause hypercalcemia
Hypoparathyroidism	↓	↑	None	↓	None	↓	↓	Basal ganglia calcification Hypocalcemic findings	Calcium and vitamin D supplementation	↓ PTH production most commonly follows surgical ablation of the thyroid (with the parathyroid) gland ↓ PTH leads to ↓ serum calcium and ↑ serum phosphate (as result of ↓ urinary excretion of phosphate) Because PTH stimulates conversion from the inactive to the active form of vitamin D (in the kidney), $1,25(OH)_2$-vitamin D is also ↓

Pseudohypoparathyroidism	↓	↑	None	None or ↑	None	↓	↓	Hypocalcemic findings	Calcium and vitamin D supplementation	PTH has no effect on the target cells (in the kidney, bone, and intestine) because of a PTH receptor abnormality Leads to a ↓ in the active form of vitamin D Therefore, serum calcium levels are ↓ as result of (1) lack of effect of PTH on bone and (2) ↓ levels of $1,25(OH)_2$-vitamin D
Renal osteodystrophy (high-turnover bone disease resulting from renal disease [secondary hyperparathyroidism])	↓ or none	↑↑↑	↑	↑↑↑	None	↓	—	Findings of secondary hyperparathyroidism: "rugger jersey" spine Osteitis fibrosa Amyloidosis	1. Correct underlying renal abnormality 2. Maintain normal serum phosphorous and calcium 3. Dietary phosphate restriction 4. Phosphate-binding antacid (calcium carbonate) 5. Administration of the active form of vitamin D: $1,25(OH)_2$-vitamin D (calcitriol)	↓ Renal phosphorus excretion leads to hyperphosphatemia Phosphorus retention leads to ↓ serum calcium and ↑↑↑ PTH (which can lead to secondary hyperparathyroidism) Elevated BUN and creatinine levels Associated with long-term hemodialysis
Renal osteodystrophy (low-turnover bone disease due to renal disease [aluminum toxicity])	↑ or none	None or ↑	↑	None or mildly elevated	None	↓	—	"Rugger jersey" spine Osteitis fibrosa Amyloidosis Osteomalacia may be observed	Treat the urinary obstruction or kidney disease	PTH levels may be suppressed because of (1) frequent episodes of hypercalcemia and (2) direct inhibitory effect of aluminum on PTH No secondary hyperparathyroidism is present Elevated BUN and creatinine levels Associated with long-term hemodialysis
Nutritional rickets: vitamin D deficiency	↓ or none	↓	↑	↑	↓	↓	↓	Osteomalacia, hypotonia Muscle weakness, tetany Bowing deformities of the long bones Rachitic rosary	Oral vitamin D (1500-5000 IU/day)	With ↓ vitamin D intake, intestinal calcium and phosphate absorption is reduced, leading to hypocalcemia ↓ Serum calcium stimulates ↑ PTH (secondary hyperparathyroidism), which leads to bone resorption and ↑ serum calcium (toward or to normal levels) Sources of vitamin D include sunlight, fish-liver foods, and fortified milk
Nutritional rickets: calcium deficiency	↓ or none	↓	↑	↑	None	↑ or none	↓	Clinical findings similar to those for vitamin D deficiency	Oral calcium (700 mg/day)	Hypocalcemia leads to secondary hyperparathyroidism. ↑ PTH leads to enhanced renal conversion of 25(OH)-vitamin D to $1,25(OH)_2$-vitamin D

↓, Decreased; ↑, increased; Alk, alkaline; BUN, blood urea nitrogen; Phos, phosphatase; PTH, parathyroid hormone.

Continued

Table 1-15 Laboratory Findings and Clinical Data Regarding Patients with Various Metabolic Bone Diseases—cont'd

Disorder	CHANGES IN LEVEL OR CONCENTRATION							Other Findings or Possible Findings	Treatment	Comments
	Serum Ca	Serum Phos	Alk Phos	PTH	25(OH)-Vitamin D	$1,25(OH)_2$-Vitamin D	Urinary Calcium			
Nutritional rickets: phosphate deficiency	None	↓	↑	None	None	↑↑↑	None	No changes of secondary hyperparathyroidism are observed	Oral supplementation of phosphate	Neither secondary hyperparathyroidism nor vitamin D deficiency is present ↓ Serum phosphate leads to ↑ renal production of $1,25(OH)_2$-vitamin D
Hereditary vitamin D–dependent rickets type I ("pseudo–vitamin D deficiency")	↓	↓	↑	↑	None or ↑	↓↓↓	↓	Osteomalacia Clinical findings similar to (but more severe than) those of nutritional rickets caused by vitamin D deficiency	Oral physiologic doses (1-2 μg/day) of $1,25(OH)_2$-vitamin D	There is a defect in renal 25(OH)-vitamin D 1α-hydroxylase. This enzymatic defect inhibits conversion from the inactive form [25(OH)-vitamin D] to the active form [$1,25(OH)_2$-vitamin D] of vitamin D in the kidney
Hereditary vitamin D–dependent rickets type II ["hereditary resistance to $1,25(OH)_2$-vitamin D"]	↓	↓	↑	↑	None or ↑	↑↑↑	↓	Osteomalacia Alopecia Clinical findings similar to (but more severe than) nutritional rickets caused by vitamin D deficiency	Long-term (3-6 months) daily administration of high-dose vitamin D analogue [$1,25(OH)_2$-vitamin D or (OH)-vitamin D 1α-hydroxylase] plus 3 g/day of elemental calcium	There is an intracellular receptor defect for $1,25(OH)_2$-vitamin D Patients with this disorder have the highest $1,25(OH)_2$-vitamin D levels observed in humans; this ↑↑↑ level of $1,25(OH)_2$-vitamin D distinguishes hereditary vitamin D–dependent rickets type II from type I, in which the level of $1,25(OH)_2$-vitamin D is ↓↓↓
Hypophosphatemic rickets (also known as vitamin D–resistant rickets and "phosphate diabetes"; Albright's syndrome is an example of a hypophosphatemic syndrome)	None	↓↓↓	↑	None	None	None	None or ↑	Osteomalacia No changes of secondary hyperparathyroidism Classic triad: 1. Hypophosphatemia 2. Lower limb deformities 3. Stunted growth rate	Oral administration of elemental phosphate (1-3 g/day) plus high-dose vitamin D (20,000-70,000 IU/day) Vitamin D administration is needed to counterbalance the hypocalcemic effect of phosphate administration, which otherwise could lead to severe secondary hyperparathyroidism	There is an inborn error in phosphate transport (probably located in the proximal nephron); this leads to failure of reabsorption of phosphate in the kidney and "spilling" of phosphate (phosphate diabetes) in the urine Although the absolute levels of $1,25(OH)_2$-vitamin D are normal, they are inappropriately low with regard to the degree of phosphaturia; production of $1,25(OH)_2$-vitamin D is normally stimulated by ↓ serum phosphorous (see Table 1-13) This is the most commonly encountered form of rickets
Hypophosphatasia	↑	↑	↓↓↓	None	None	None		Osteomalacia Early loss of teeth	There is no established medical therapy	There is an inborn error in the tissue-nonspecific (kidney, bone, liver) isoenzyme of alkaline phosphatase Elevated urinary phosphoethanolamine is diagnostic

↓, Decreased; ↑, increased; Alk, alkaline; BUN, blood urea nitrogen; Phos, phosphatase; PTH, parathyroid hormone.

Table 1-16 Differential Diagnosis of the Metabolic Bone Diseases, Based on Blood Chemistry Findings

CALCIUM LEVEL			PHOSPHORUS LEVEL		
Increased	**Decreased**	**Normal**	**Increased**	**Decreased**	**Normal**
Primary hyperparathyroidism Hyperthyroidism Vitamin D intoxication Malignancy without bony metastasis Malignancy with bony metastasis Multiple myeloma Lymphoma Sarcoidosis Milk-alkali syndrome Severe generalized immobilization Multiple endocrine neoplasias Addison's disease Steroid administration Peptic ulcer disease Hypophosphatasia Primary hyperparathyroidism Pseudohypoparathyroidism Renal osteodystrophy Nutritional rickets: vitamin D deficiency Nutritional rickets: calcium deficiency Hereditary vitamin D–dependent rickets (types I and II)	Hypoparathyroidism Pseudohypoparathyroidism Renal osteodystrophy (high-turnover bone disease) Nutritional rickets: vitamin D deficiency Nutritional rickets: calcium deficiency Hereditary vitamin D–dependent rickets (types I and II) Malignancy with bony metastasis Malignancy without bony metastasis Multiple myeloma Lymphoma Hyperthyroidism Vitamin D intoxication Hypoparathyroidism Sarcoidosis Milk-alkali syndrome Severe generalized immobilization	Osteoporosis Pseudohypoparathyroidism Nutritional rickets: vitamin D deficiency Nutritional rickets: calcium deficiency Nutritional rickets: phosphate deficiency Hypophosphatemic rickets Osteoporosis Malignancy with bony metastasis Multiple myeloma Lymphoma Vitamin D intoxication Pseudohypoparathyroidism Renal osteodystrophy (only low-turnover bone disease) Nutritional rickets: phosphate deficiency Hypophosphatemic rickets Hypophosphatasia Sarcoidosis Hyperthyroidism Milk-alkali syndrome Severe generalized immobilization	Malignancy with bony metastasis Multiple myeloma Lymphoma Vitamin D intoxication Hypoparathyroidism Pseudohypoparathyroidism Renal osteodystrophy Hypophosphatasia Sarcoidosis Milk-alkali syndrome Severe generalized immobilization Primary hyperparathyroidism Nutritional rickets: calcium deficiency Nutritional rickets: phosphate deficiency Hereditary vitamin D–dependent rickets type II Sarcoidosis	Primary hyperparathyroidism Malignancy without bony metastasis Nutritional rickets: vitamin D deficiency Nutritional rickets: calcium deficiency Nutritional rickets: phosphate deficiency Hereditary vitamin D–dependent rickets (types I and II) Hypophosphatemic rickets Malignancy with bony metastasis Malignancy without bony metastasis Multiple myeloma Lymphoma Hypoparathyroidism Pseudohypoparathyroidism Renal osteodystrophy Nutritional rickets: vitamin D deficiency Hereditary vitamin D–dependent rickets type I	Osteoporosis Primary hyperparathyroidism Malignancy with bony metastasis Multiple myeloma Lymphoma Hyperthyroidism Vitamin D intoxication Renal osteodystrophy (only low-turnover bone disease) Sarcoidosis Milk-alkali syndrome Severe generalized immobilization Osteoporosis Primary hyperparathyroidism Malignancy with bony metastasis Multiple myeloma Lymphoma Hyperthyroidism Vitamin D intoxication Nutritional rickets: calcium deficiency Hypophosphatemic rickets Hypophosphatasia

- Increased osteoclastic resorption and failure of repair attempts (poor mineralization as a result of low phosphate level)
- Diagnosis
  - Signs and symptoms of hypercalcemia
  - Characteristic laboratory results
    - Increased serum calcium, PTH, urinary phosphate
    - Decreased serum phosphate
- Bony changes
  - Osteopenia
  - Osteitis fibrosa cystica (fibrous replacement of marrow)
  - "Brown tumors" (Figure 1-23): increased giant cells, extravasation of RBCs, hemosiderin staining, fibrous tissue hemosiderin
  - Chondrocalcinosis
- Radiographs
  - Deformed, osteopenic bones
  - Fractures
  - "Shaggy" trabeculae
  - Radiolucent areas (phalanges, distal clavicle, skull)
  - **Destructive metaphyseal lesions**
  - Calcification of the soft tissues
- Histologic changes
  - Osteoblasts and osteoclasts active on both sides of the trabeculae (as in Paget's disease)
  - Areas of destruction
  - Wide osteoid seams
- Surgical parathyroidectomy is curative.

- Other causes of hypercalcemia
  - Familial syndromes
    - Pituitary adenomas associated with multiple endocrine neoplasia (MEN) types I and II
    - Familial hypocalciuric hypercalcemia
      - Poor renal clearance of calcium
  - Other disorders
    - **Malignancy** (most common)
      - Can be life-threatening, commonly associated with muscle weakness
      - Initial treatment should include hydration with normal saline (reverses dehydration).
      - Can occur in the absence of extensive bone metastasis
      - Most commonly results from the release of systemic growth factors and cytokines that stimulate osteoclastic bone resorption at bony sites not involved in the tumor process
    - PTH-related protein secretion (lung carcinoma)
    - Lytic bone metastases and lesions (such as multiple myeloma)
    - Hyperthyroidism
    - Vitamin D intoxication
    - Prolonged immobilization
    - Addison's disease
    - Steroid administration
    - Peptic ulcer disease (milk-alkali syndrome)
    - Kidney disease
    - Sarcoidosis
    - Hypophosphatasia
  - Treatment of hypercalcemia
    - Hydration (saline diuresis)
    - Loop diuretics
    - Dialysis (for severe cases)
    - Mobilization (prevents further bone resorption)
    - Specific drugs (bisphosphonates, mithramycin, calcitonin, and gallium nitrate)

2. Hypocalcemia (Figure 1-24)
   - Low plasma calcium
   - Results from low levels of PTH or vitamin D_3
   - Neuromuscular irritability (tetany, seizures, Chvostek's sign), cataracts, fungal nail infections, electrocardiographic (ECG) changes (prolonged QT interval), and other signs and symptoms
   - Hypoparathyroidism
     - Decreased PTH level causes decrease in plasma calcium level and increase in plasma phosphate level.
       - Urinary excretion not enhanced because of the lack of PTH

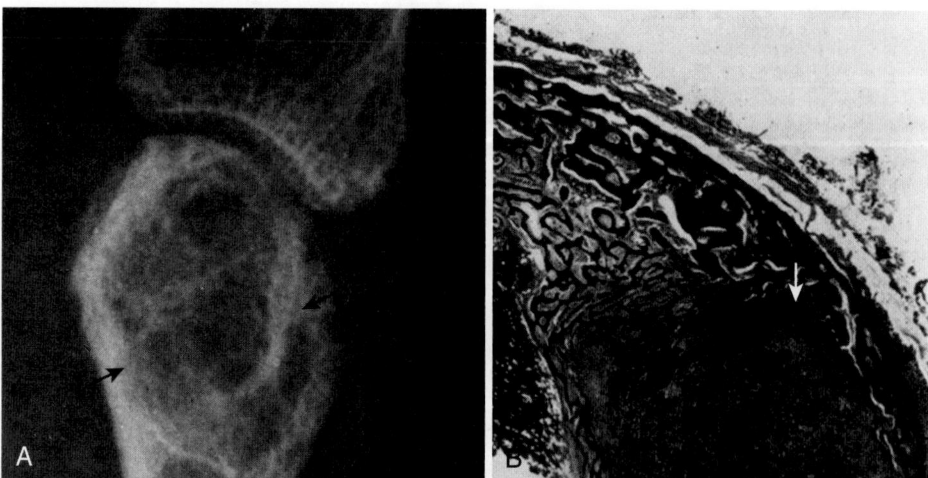

Figure 1-23 Radiograph **(A)** and photomicrograph **(B)** showing delineation of brown tumor *(arrows)* of hyperparathyroidism. (From Resnick D, Kransdorf MJ, editors: *Bone and joint imaging,* ed 3, Philadelphia, 2005, WB Saunders, p 608.)

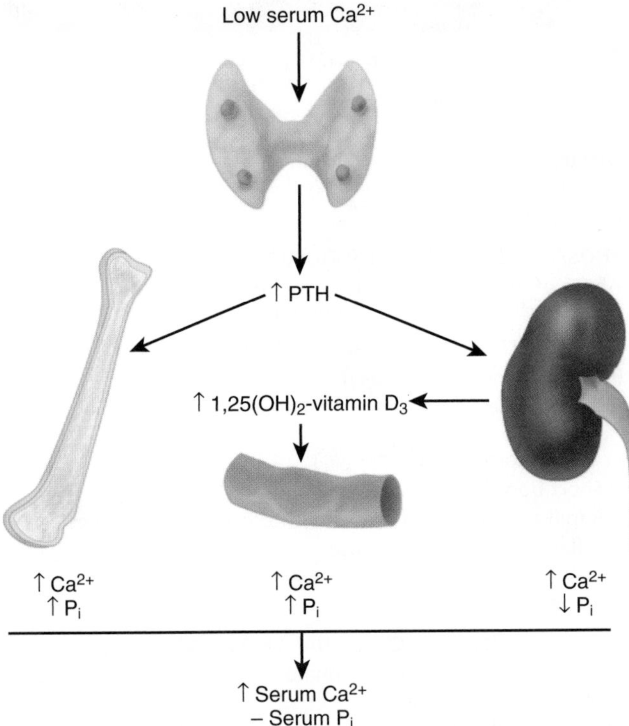

Figure 1-24 Body's reaction to hypocalcemia, with the consequent resorption of bone. When calcium level falls, parathyroid hormone (PTH) is secreted, which releases calcium and inorganic phosphate (P_i) from bone. PTH increases renal reabsorption of calcium while inhibiting phosphate reabsorption. These actions, in combination, restore calcium concentration. If hypocalcemia persists, PTH stimulates renal production of 1,25$(OH)_2$-vitamin D_3, which increases intestinal calcium absorption. (From Goldman L, Ausiello D, editors: *Cecil medicine,* ed 23, Philadelphia, 2008, WB Saunders–Elsevier.)

- Common findings:
  - Fungal nail infections
  - Hair loss
  - Blotchy skin (pigment loss; vitiligo)
- Skull radiographs may show basal ganglia calcification.
- Iatrogenic hypoparathyroidism most commonly follows thyroidectomy.

- Pseudohypoparathyroidism (PHP)
  - A rare genetic disorder
    - This disorder is caused by lack of effect of PTH on the target cells.
  - PTH is normal or high.
    - PTH action is blocked by an abnormality at the receptor, by the cAMP system, or by a lack of required cofactors (e.g., Mg^{2+}).
  - Albright's hereditary osteodystrophy, a form of PHP
    - Short first, fourth, and fifth metacarpals and metatarsals
    - Brachydactyly
    - Exostoses
    - Obesity
    - Diminished intelligence
  - Pseudo-pseudohypoparathyroidism (pseudo-PHP)
    - Normocalcemic disorder that is phenotypically similar to PHP
    - However, response to PTH is normal
- Renal osteodystrophy (Figure 1-25)
  - A spectrum of bone mineral metabolism disorders in chronic renal disease
    - Renal disease impairs excretion and compromises mineral homeostasis.
    - This process leads to abnormalities in bone mineral metabolism.
  - High-turnover renal bone disease
    - Chronically elevated serum PTH level leads to **secondary hyperparathyroidism** (hyperplasia of the chief cells of the parathyroid gland).
    - **Factors contributing to sustained, increased PTH, and secondary hyperparathyroidism include the following:**
      - **Diminished renal phosphorus excretion; phosphorus retention promotes PTH secretion by three mechanisms:**
        - **Hyperphosphatemia lowers serum calcium, stimulating PTH.**
        - **Phosphorus impairs renal 1α-hydroxylase activity, impairing production of 1,25$(OH)_2$-vitamin D_3.**
        - **Phosphorus retention may directly increase the synthesis of PTH.**
      - Hypocalcemia

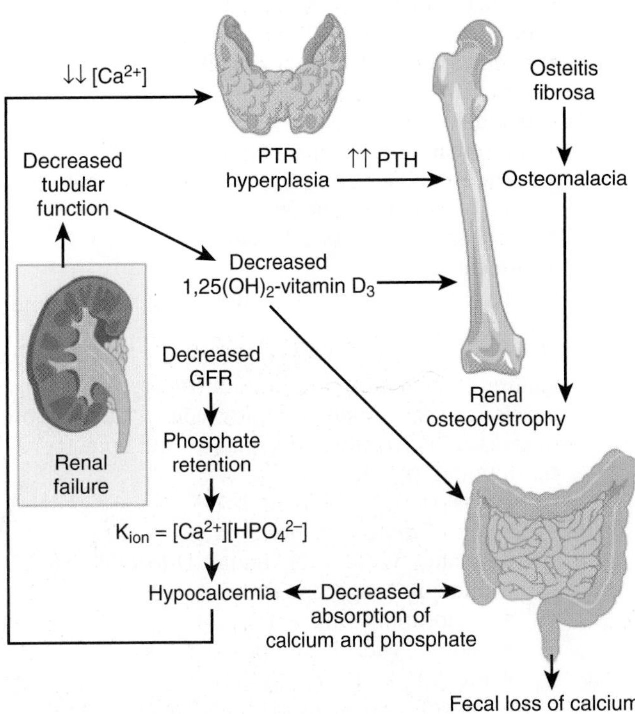

Figure 1-25 Pathogenesis of bony changes in renal osteodystrophy. GFR, glomerular filtration rate; PTR, proximal tubule reabsorption. (From McPherson RA, Pincus MR, editors: *Henry's clinical diagnosis and management by laboratory methods,* ed 21, Philadelphia, 2007, WB Saunders–Elsevier.)

- Impaired renal calcitriol [1,25(OH)$_2$-vitamin D$_3$]
- Alterations in the control of PTH gene transcription secretion
- Skeletal resistance to the actions of PTH

- Low-turnover renal bone disease (adynamic lesion of bone and osteomalacia)
  - Secondary hyperparathyroidism is not characteristic with this condition.
    - Serum PTH level is normal or mildly elevated.
  - Bone formation and turnover are reduced.
  - Excess deposition of aluminum into bone (aluminum toxicity) negatively affects bone mineral metabolism.
    - Impairs differentiation of precursor cells to osteoblasts
    - Impairs proliferation of osteoblasts
    - Impairs PTH release from the parathyroid gland
    - Disrupts the mineralization process
    - Adynamic lesion: accounts for the majority of cases of low-turnover bone disease in patients with chronic renal failure
    - Osteomalacia: defects in mineralization of newly formed bone
- Radiographs may demonstrate a "rugger jersey" spine (vertebral bodies appear to have increased density in the upper and lower zones, in a striated appearance), like that in childhood osteopetrosis, and soft tissue calcification
- β_2-microglobulin may accumulate with chronic dialysis, leading to amyloidosis
  - Amyloidosis may be associated with carpal tunnel syndrome, arthropathy, and pathologic fractures.
  - In amyloidosis, Congo red stain causes material to turn pink.
- Laboratory test results:
  - Abnormal glomerular filtration rate (GFR)
  - Increased alkaline phosphatase, blood urea nitrogen (BUN), and creatinine levels
  - Decreased venous bicarbonate level
- Treatment:
  - Directed at relieving the urologic obstruction or kidney disease

- **Rickets** (osteomalacia in adults; Box 1-1)
  - Failure of mineralization, leading to changes in the physis in the zone of provisional calcification (increased width and disorientation) and bone (cortical thinning, bowing)
  - Nutritional rickets (see Table 1-15)
    - Vitamin D–deficiency rickets
      - Rare after addition of vitamin D to milk, except in the following populations:
        - Asian immigrants
        - Patients with dietary peculiarities
        - Premature infants
        - Patients with malabsorption (celiac sprue)
        - Patients receiving chronic parenteral nutrition
      - Decreased intestinal absorption of calcium and phosphate leads to secondary hyperparathyroidism
      - **Laboratory studies**

Box 1-1

Causes of Rickets and Osteomalacia

NUTRITIONAL DEFICIENCY

Vitamin D deficiency

Dietary chelators (rare) of calcium

Phytates

Oxalates (spinach)

PHOSPHORUS DEFICIENCY (UNUSUAL)

Abuse of antacids (which contain aluminum), leading to severe dietary phosphate binding

GASTROINTESTINAL ABSORPTION DEFECTS

Postgastrectomy (rare today)

Biliary disease (interference with absorption of fat-soluble vitamin D)

Enteric absorption defects

- Short-bowel syndrome
- Rapid-transit (gluten-sensitive enteropathy) syndromes
- Inflammatory bowel disease
  - Crohn's disease
  - Celiac disease

RENAL TUBULAR DEFECTS (RENAL PHOSPHATE LEAK)

X-linked dominant hypophosphatemic vitamin D–resistant rickets or osteomalacia

Classic Albright's syndrome or Fanconi's syndrome type I

Fanconi's syndrome type II

Phosphaturia and glycosuria

Fanconi's syndrome type III

Phosphaturia, glycosuria, aminoaciduria

Vitamin D–dependent rickets (or osteomalacia) type I (a genetic or acquired deficiency of renal tubular 25-hydroxyvitamin D 1α hydroxylase enzyme that prevents conversion of 25-hydroxyvitamin D to the active polar metabolite 1,25-dihydroxyvitamin D)

Vitamin D–dependent rickets (or osteomalacia) type II (which represents enteric end-organ insensitivity to 1,25-dihydroxyvitamin D and is probably caused by an abnormality in the 1,25-dihydroxyvitamin D nuclear receptor)

Renal tubular acidosis

- Acquired: associated with many systemic diseases
- Genetic
  - Debre–De Toni–Fanconi syndrome
  - Lignac-Fanconi syndrome (cystinosis)
  - Lowe's syndrome

RENAL OSTEODYSTROPHY: MISCELLANEOUS CAUSES

Soft tissue tumors secreting putative factors

- Fibrous dysplasia
- Neurofibromatosis
- Other soft tissue and vascular mesenchymal tumors

Anticonvulsant medication (induction of the hepatic P450 microsomal enzyme system by some anticonvulsants—e.g., phenytoin, phenobarbital, and primidone [Mysoline]—causes increased degradation of vitamin D metabolites)

Heavy metal intoxication

Hypophosphatasia

High-dose diphosphonates

Sodium fluoride

Adapted from Simon SR, editor: *Orthopaedic basic science*, ed 2, Rosemont, Ill, 1994, American Academy of Orthopaedic Surgeons, p 169.

- **Low-normal calcium level** (maintained by high PTH level)
- **Low phosphate level** (excreted because of the effect of PTH)
- **Increased alkaline phosphatase level**
- **Low vitamin D level**
- **Increased PTH level**
  - Increased bone absorption
- Examination
  - Enlargement of the costochondral junction ("rachitic rosary")
  - Bowing of the knees
  - Muscle hypotonia
  - Dental disease
  - Pathologic fractures (Looser's zones: pseudofracture on the compression side of bone)
  - Milkman's fracture (Figure 1-26)
  - Waddling gait
- Radiographic
  - **Physeal widening and cupping**
  - Coxa vara
  - "Codfish" vertebrae
  - Retarded bone growth (defect in the hypertrophic zone, widened osteoid seams)
- In affected children, height is commonly below the fifth percentile for age.
- Treatment with vitamin D (5000 IU daily) resolves most deformities.
- Calcium-deficiency rickets (Figure 1-27)
- Phosphate-deficiency rickets
- Hereditary vitamin D–dependent rickets
  - Rare disorders with features similar to vitamin D deficiency (nutritional) rickets, except that symptoms may be worse and patients may have total baldness
    - **Type I: Defect in renal 25(OH)-vitamin D 1α-hydroxylase, inhibiting conversion of inactive vitamin D to its active form**
      - Autosomal recessive inheritance
      - Gene on chromosome 12q14
    - **Type II:** Defect in an intracellular receptor for 1,25$(OH)_2$-vitamin D_3
- Familial hypophosphatemic rickets (vitamin D–resistant rickets or "phosphate diabetes")
  - Most commonly encountered form of rickets
  - X-linked dominant inheritance
    - Impaired renal tubular reabsorption of phosphate
  - Normal GFR with an impaired vitamin D_3 response
  - Treatment:
    - Phosphate replacement (1-3 g daily)
    - High-dose vitamin D_3
- Hypophosphatasia (Figure 1-28)
  - Autosomal recessive
  - Error in the tissue-nonspecific isoenzyme of alkaline phosphatase
    - Leads to low levels of alkaline phosphatase, required for synthesis of inorganic phosphate and important in bone matrix formation
  - Features are similar to those of rickets.
  - Increased urinary phosphoethanolamine is diagnostic.
  - Treatment may include phosphate therapy.

3. Conditions of bone mineral density
   - Bone mass is regulated by relative rates of deposition and withdrawal (Figure 1-29).
   - **Osteoporosis**
     - Age-related **decrease in bone mass**
       - Usually associated with estrogen loss in postmenopausal women (Figure 1-30)
     - A quantitative, not qualitative, defect
       - Mineralization remains normal.
     - **World Health Organization's definition**
       - **Lumbar (L2 to L4) density is 2.5 or more standard deviations less than mean peak bone mass of a healthy 25-year-old (T-score).**
       - **Osteopenia: Bone density is 1.0 to 2.5 standard deviations less than the mean peak bone mass of a healthy 25-year-old.**
     - Responsible for more than 1 million fractures/year
       - Fractures of the vertebral body are most common.
       - History of osteoporotic vertebral compression fractures are strongly predictive of subsequent vertebral fracture.
         - After initial vertebral fracture, the risk for a second vertebral fracture is 20%.
       - Vertebral compression fracture is associated with increased mortality rate.
         - The incidence of vertebral compression fractures is higher among men than among women.
     - Lifetime risk of fracture in white women after 50 years of age: 75%
       - The risk for hip fracture is 15% to 20%.
     - **Risk factors** (Box 1-2):

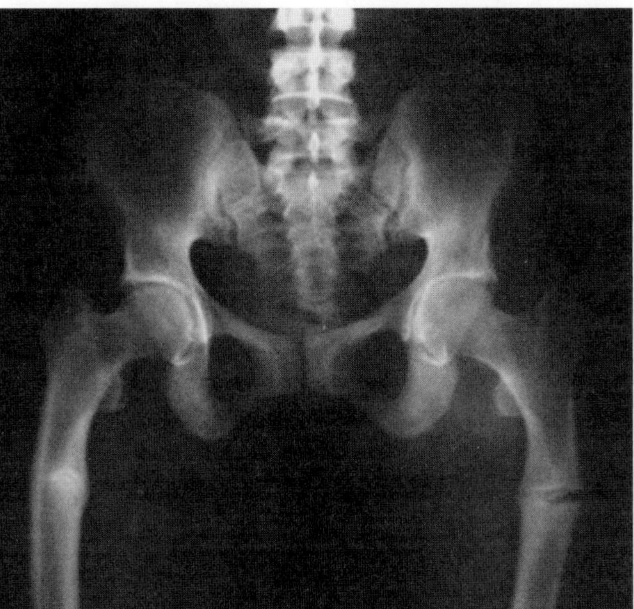

Figure 1-26 Pseudofracture in both femurs in an adult patient with X-linked hypophosphatemic osteomalacia. (From Adam A, Dixon AK: *Grainger & Allison's diagnostic radiology: a textbook of medical imaging,* ed 5, Philadelphia, 2008, Elsevier–Churchill Livingstone.)

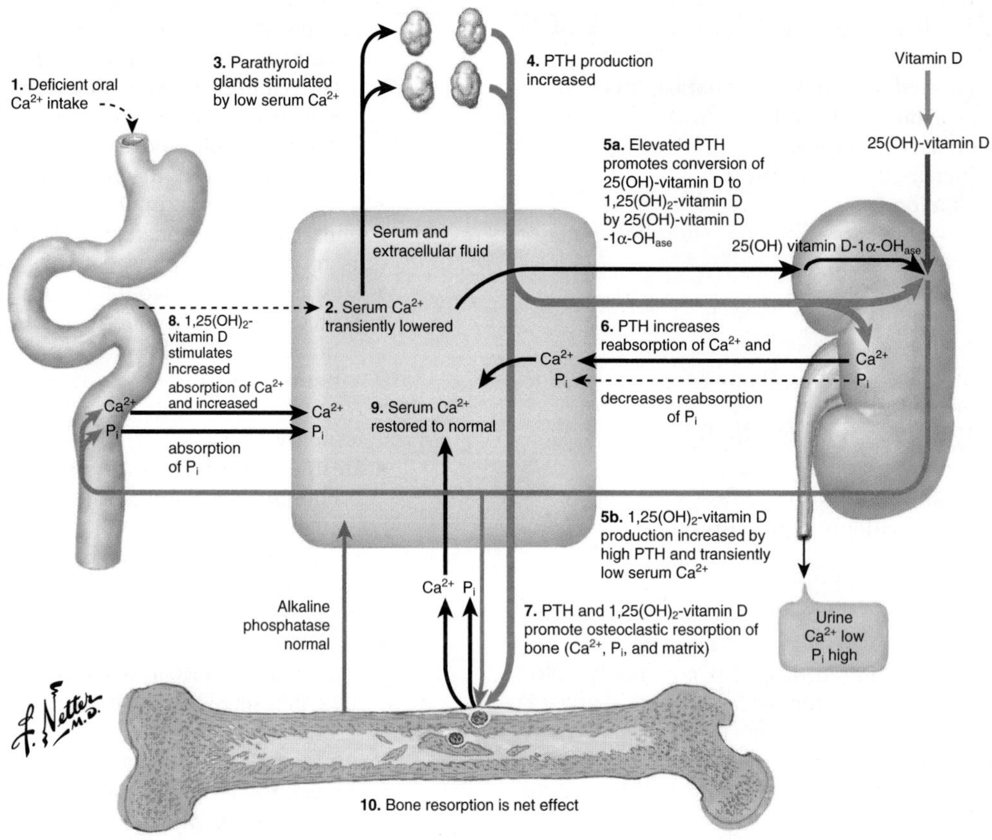

Figure 1-27 Nutritional calcium deficiency. 1,25(OH)$_2$D, 1,25(OH)$_2$-vitamin D; 25(H)D, 25(OH)-vitamin D; OH$_{ase}$, hydroxylase; P$_i$, inorganic phosphate; PTH, parathyroid hormone. (From Netter FH: *CIBA collection of medical illustrations,* vol 8: *Musculoskeletal system*, part I: *Anatomy, physiology and developmental disorders,* Basel, Switzerland, 1987, CIBA, p 184.)

- Cancellous bone is most affected.
- **Clinical features:**
  - Kyphosis and vertebral fractures
    - Compression fractures of T11 to L1 that create an anterior wedge-shaped defect or a centrally depressed "codfish" vertebra
  - Hip fractures
  - Distal radius fractures
- **Type I osteoporosis (postmenopausal)**
  - Primarily affects trabecular bone
  - Vertebral and distal radius fractures are common
- Type II osteoporosis (age-related)
  - In patients older than 75 years
  - Affects both trabecular and cortical bone
  - Related to poor calcium absorption
  - Hip and pelvic fractures are common
- Laboratory studies
  - Obtained to rule out secondary causes of low bone mass
    - Vitamin D deficiency, hyperthyroidism, hyperparathyroidism, Cushing's syndrome, hematologic disorders, malignancy
  - **Complete blood cell count; measurements of serum calcium, phosphorus, 25(OH)-vitamin D, alkaline phosphatase, liver enzymes, creatinine, and total protein and albumin levels; and measurement of 24-hour urinary calcium excretion**
  - Results of these studies are usually unremarkable in osteoporosis.
- Plain radiographs not helpful unless bone loss exceeds 30%
- Special studies
  - Single-photon (appendicular) absorptiometry
  - Double-photon (axial) absorptiometry
  - Quantitative computed tomography (CT)
  - Dual-energy x-ray absorptiometry (DEXA)
    - **Most accurate with less radiation**
- Biopsy
  - After tetracycline labeling
  - To evaluate the severity of osteoporosis and to identify osteomalacia
- Histologic changes:
  - Thinning trabeculae
  - Decreased osteon size
  - Enlarged haversian and marrow spaces
- **Treatment** (Figure 1-31):
  - Physical activity
  - **Calcium supplements**

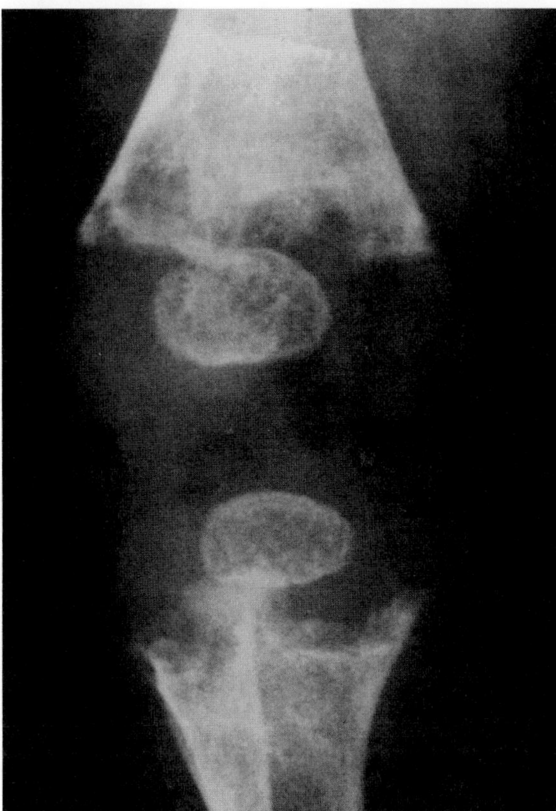

Figure 1-28 Hypophosphatasia. **Deossification is present adjacent to the growth plates. Characteristic radiolucent areas extend from the growth plates into the metaphysis.** (From Resnick D, Kransdorf MJ, editors: *Bone and joint imaging,* ed 3, Philadelphia, 2005, Saunders, p 574.)

  - **1000 to 1500 mg plus 400 to 800 IU of vitamin D per day**
  - More effective in type II (age-related) osteoporosis
- Fluoride
  - Inhibits bone resorption
  - However, bone is more brittle.
- Bisphosphonates: bind to bone resorption surfaces and inhibit osteoclastic membrane ruffling without destroying the cells
- Other drugs, such as intramuscular calcitonin, may be helpful.
  - Expensive
  - May cause hypersensitivity reactions
- Efficacy of bone augmentation with PTH, growth factors, prostaglandin inhibitors, and other therapies remains to be determined.
- Prophylaxis for patients at risk for osteoporosis:
  - Diet with adequate calcium intake
  - Weight-bearing exercise program
  - Estrogen therapy evaluation at menopause
- Idiopathic transient osteoporosis of the hip
  - Uncommon; diagnosis of exclusion
  - Most common during the third trimester of pregnancy in women but can occur in men
  - Groin pain, limited range of motion (ROM), and localized osteopenia without a history of trauma
    - Treatment: analgesics and limited weight bearing
    - Generally self-limiting and tends to resolve spontaneously after 6 to 8 months
      - This feature distinguishes idiopathic transient osteoporosis from osteonecrosis, which has progressive symptoms and does not resolve spontaneously
    - Stress fractures may occur.
  - Bone loss related to spinal cord injury
    - Bone mineral loss occurs throughout the skeleton (except the skull) for approximately 16 months
      - Levels off when bone mass reaches two thirds of the original value
    - High risk of fracture
    - Bone loss greatest in the lower extremities
- Osteomalacia
  - Qualitative defect
    - **Defect of mineralization** results in a large amount of unmineralized osteoid.
  - Causes:
    - Vitamin D–deficient diet
    - Gastrointestinal disorders
    - Renal osteodystrophy
    - Certain drugs
      - Aluminum-containing phosphate-binding antacids; aluminum deposition in bone prevents mineralization
      - Phenytoin (Dilantin)
    - Alcoholism
  - Radiographic findings:
    - Looser's zones (microscopic stress fractures)
    - Other fractures
    - Biconcave vertebral bodies
    - Trefoil pelvis
  - Biopsy (transiliac); required for diagnosis
    - Widened osteoid seams are histologic findings.
  - Femoral neck fractures are common
  - Treatment: usually includes large doses of vitamin D
  - Osteoporosis and osteomalacia are compared in Figure 1-32.
- Scurvy
  - Vitamin C (ascorbic acid) deficiency
  - Produces a decrease in chondroitin sulfate synthesis
    - Leads to defective collagen growth and repair
    - Also leads to impaired intracellular hydroxylation of collagen peptides
  - Clinical features:
    - Fatigue
    - Gum bleeding
    - Ecchymosis
    - Joint effusions
    - Iron deficiency
  - Radiographic findings:
    - May include thin cortices and trabeculae and metaphyseal clefts (corner sign)
  - Laboratory studies: normal results
  - Histologic features:
    - Primary trabeculae replaced with granulation tissue
    - Areas of hemorrhage
    - **Widening of the zone of provisional calcification in the physis**
  - Greatest effect on bone formation in the metaphysis

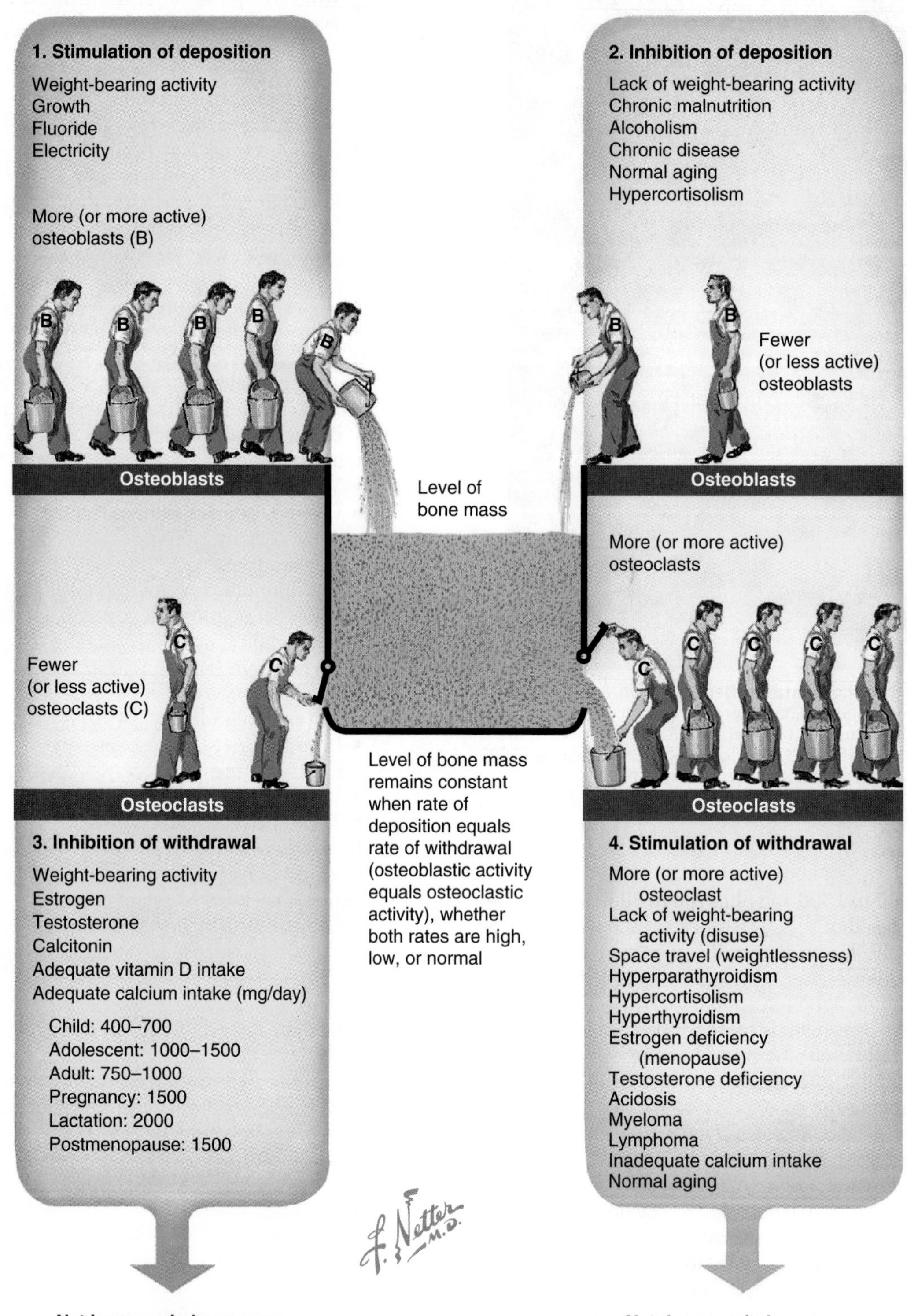

Figure 1-29 Four mechanisms of bone mass regulation. (From Netter FH: *CIBA collection of medical illustrations,* vol 8: *Musculoskeletal system,* part I: *Anatomy, physiology and developmental disorders,* Basel, Switzerland, 1987, CIBA, p 181.)

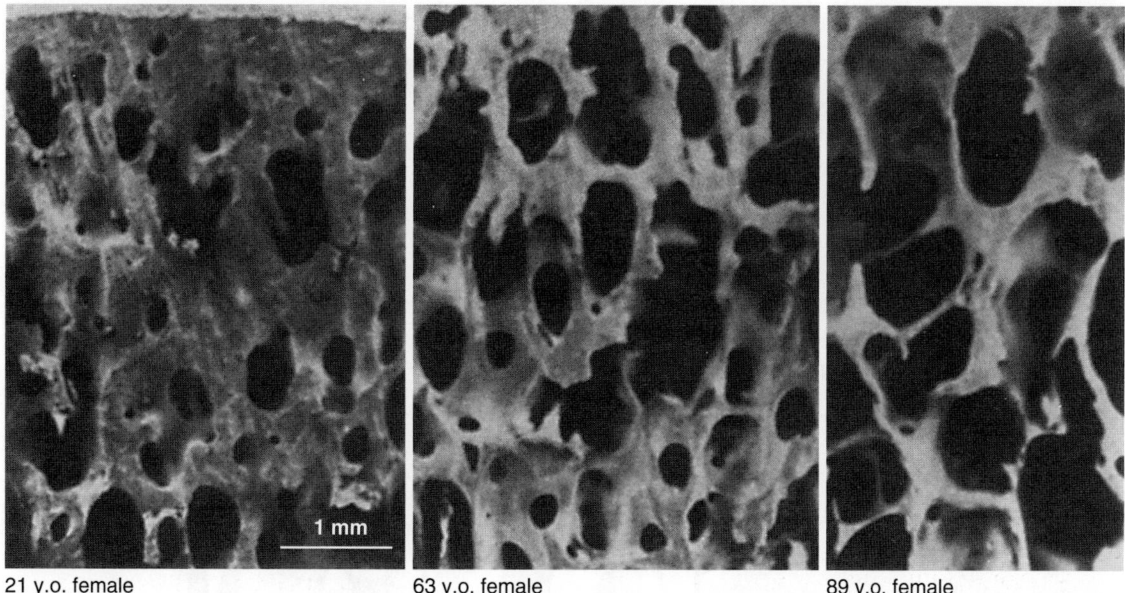

Figure 1-30 Age-related changes in density and architecture of human trabecular bone from the lumbar spine.

- Marrow packing disorders
  - Myeloma, leukemia, and other such disorders can cause osteopenia.
- Osteogenesis imperfecta
  - Caused by abnormal collagen synthesis
    - Failure of normal collagen cross-linking **as a result of glycine substitutions in procollagen.**
  - **Caused primarily by a mutation in genes responsible for metabolism and synthesis of type I collagen**
  - Increased bone turnover
- **Lead poisoning**
  - **Results in short stature and reduced bone density**
  - **Lead alters the chondrocyte response to PTH-related protein and to TGF-β.**

4. Increased osteodensity
   - Osteopetrosis (marble bone disease)
     - *Osteopetrosis* is the term for a group of bone disorders.
     - It is characterized by increased sclerosis and obliteration of the medullary canal as a result of decreased osteoclast (and chondroclast) function: failure of bone resorption. Osteoclast numbers may be increased, decreased, or normal.
     - It may result from an abnormality of the immune system (thymic defect).
     - Osteoclasts lack the normal ruffled border and clear zone.
     - Marrow spaces fill with necrotic calcified cartilage.
       - The cartilage may be trapped within the osteoid.

Box 1-2

Risk Factors for the Development of Osteoporosis

- White race, female gender, northern European descent (fair skin and hair)
- Sedentary lifestyle
- Thinness
- Smoking
- Heavy drinking
- Phenytoin (impairs vitamin D metabolism)
- Diet low in calcium and vitamin D
- History of breastfeeding
- Positive family history of osteoporosis
- Premature menopause

From Keaveney TM, Hayes WC: Mechanical properties of cortical and trabecular bone, *Bone,* 7:285-344, 1993.

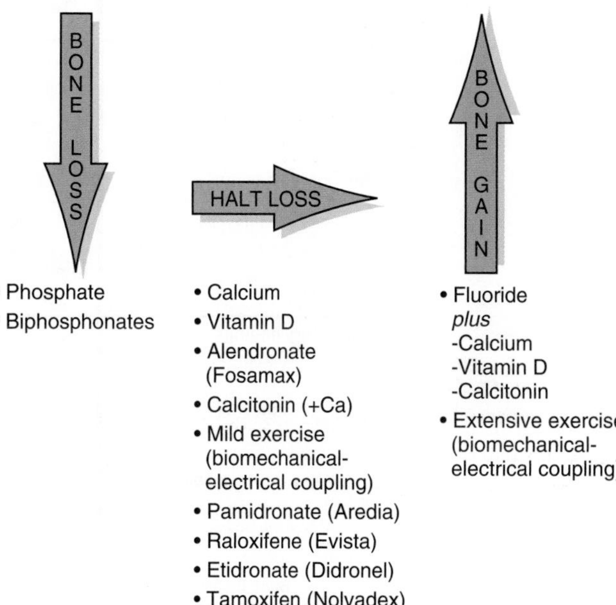

Figure 1-31 Treatment options for osteoporosis. (Adapted from Simon SR, editor: Orthopaedic basic science, Rosemont, Ill, 1994, American Academy of Orthopaedic Surgeons, p 174.)

Comparison of Osteoporosis and Osteomalacia

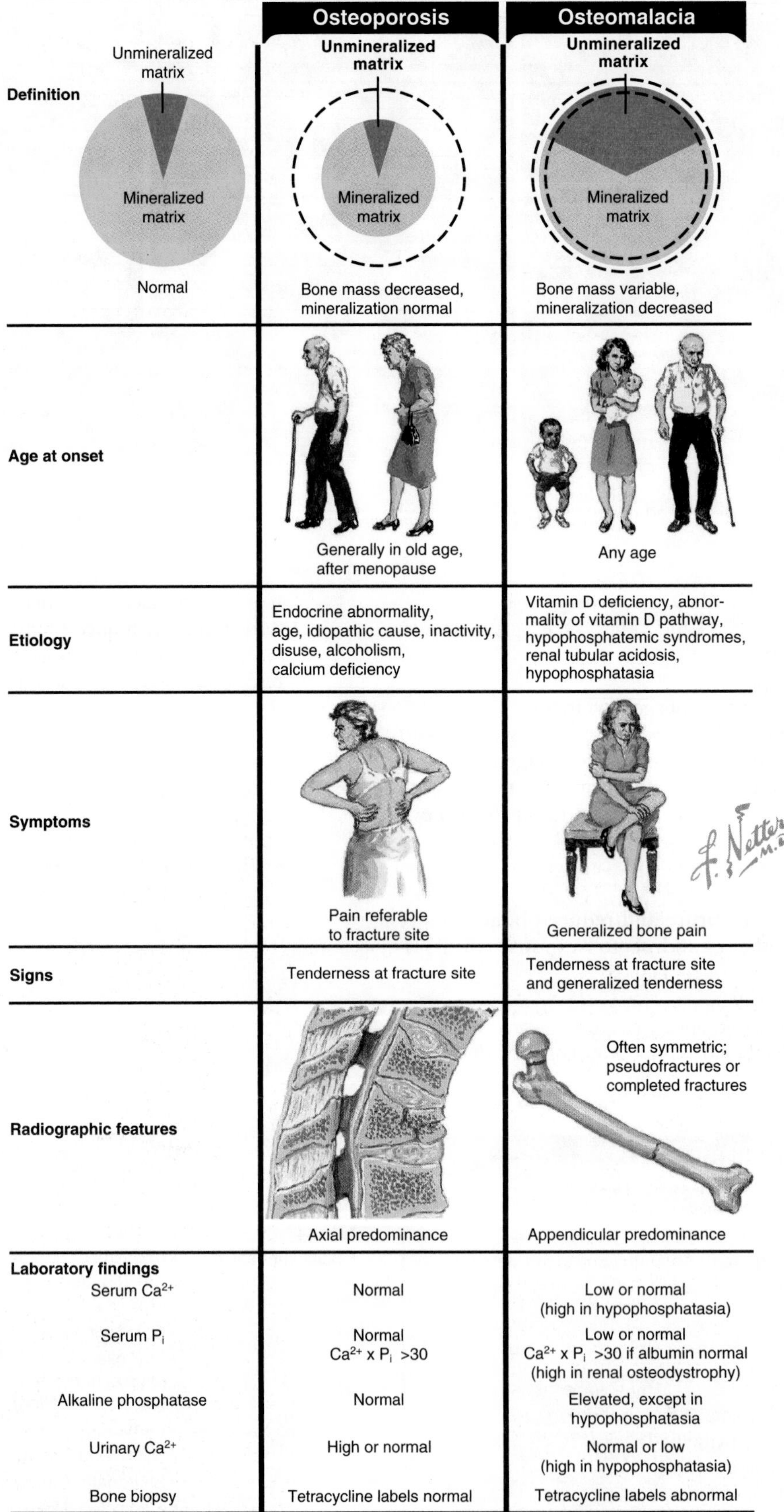

	Osteoporosis	Osteomalacia
Definition (Normal: Unmineralized matrix / Mineralized matrix)	Unmineralized matrix / Mineralized matrix Bone mass decreased, mineralization normal	Unmineralized matrix / Mineralized matrix Bone mass variable, mineralization decreased
Age at onset	Generally in old age, after menopause	Any age
Etiology	Endocrine abnormality, age, idiopathic cause, inactivity, disuse, alcoholism, calcium deficiency	Vitamin D deficiency, abnormality of vitamin D pathway, hypophosphatemic syndromes, renal tubular acidosis, hypophosphatasia
Symptoms	Pain referable to fracture site	Generalized bone pain
Signs	Tenderness at fracture site	Tenderness at fracture site and generalized tenderness
Radiographic features	Axial predominance	Often symmetric; pseudofractures or completed fractures Appendicular predominance
Laboratory findings		
Serum Ca^{2+}	Normal	Low or normal (high in hypophosphatasia)
Serum P_i	Normal $Ca^{2+} \times P_i > 30$	Low or normal $Ca^{2+} \times P_i > 30$ if albumin normal (high in renal osteodystrophy)
Alkaline phosphatase	Normal	Elevated, except in hypophosphatasia
Urinary Ca^{2+}	High or normal	Normal or low (high in hypophosphatasia)
Bone biopsy	Tetracycline labels normal	Tetracycline labels abnormal

Figure 1-32 Comparison of osteoporosis and osteomalacia. (From Netter FH: *CIBA collection of medical illustrations,* vol 8: *Musculoskeletal system*, part I: *Anatomy, physiology and developmental disorders,* Basel, Switzerland, 1987, CIBA, p 228.)

    - Empty lacunae and plugging of haversian canals are also observed.
  - One of these disorders is infantile autosomal recessive ("malignant") osteopetrosis.
    - Most severe form
    - "Bone within a bone" appearance on radiographs
    - Hepatosplenomegaly
    - Aplastic anemia
    - Can lead to death during infancy
    - Bone marrow transplantation (e.g., osteoclast precursors) can be lifesaving during childhood
    - High doses of calcitriol with or without steroids may also be helpful
  - **Another disorder is autosomal dominant "tarda" (benign) osteopetrosis (Albers-Schönberg disease).**
    - Generalized osteosclerosis, including the typical "rugger jersey" spine
    - Usually without other anomalies (Figures 1-33 and 1-34)
  - Pathologic fractures are common (brittle bone).
- Osteopoikilosis ("spotted bone disease")
  - Islands of deep cortical bone appear within the medullary cavity and the cancellous bone of the long bones.
    - Especially in the hands and feet
  - These areas are usually asymptomatic.
  - This disease is accompanied by no known incidence of malignant degeneration.

5. **Paget's disease**
- Elevated serum alkaline phosphatase and urinary hydroxyproline levels
- **Virus-like inclusion bodies in osteoclasts**
- Both decreased and increased osteodensity may be present.
  - Depends on phase of disease
  - Active phase
    - Lytic phase: intense osteoclastic bone resorption
    - Mixed phase
    - Sclerotic phase: osteoblastic bone formation
  - Inactive phase

D. Conditions of bone viability

1. **Osteonecrosis**
- Death of bony tissue from causes other than infection
  - Usually adjacent to a joint surface
- Caused by loss of blood supply as a result of trauma or another event (e.g., slipped capital femoral epiphysis)
- Idiopathic osteonecrosis of the femoral head and Legg-Calvé-Perthes disease may occur in patients with coagulation abnormalities
  - Deficiency of antithrombin factors protein C and protein S
  - Increased levels of lipoprotein (a)
- Commonly affects the hip joint
  - Leads to collapse and flattening of the femoral head, most frequently the anterolateral region
- **Associated with the following conditions:**
  - Steroid and heavy alcohol use
  - Blood dyscrasias (e.g., sickle cell disease)

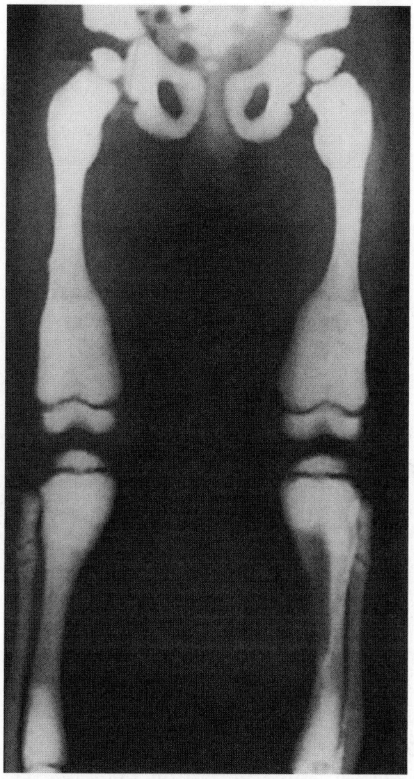

Figure 1-33 Typical "marble bone" appearance of osteopetrosis. (From Tachdjian MO: *Pediatric orthopaedics,* ed 2, Philadelphia, 1990, WB Saunders, p 795.)

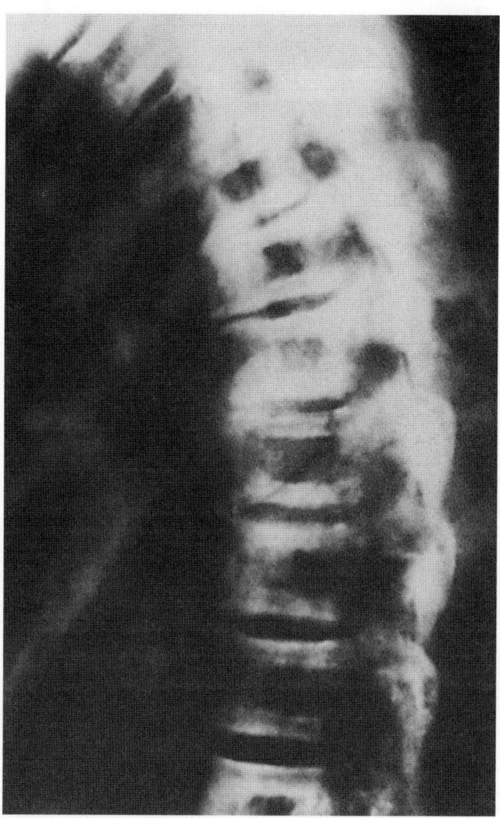

Figure 1-34 Typical "rugger jersey" spine observed in osteopetrosis. (From Tachdjian MO: *Pediatric orthopaedics,* ed 2, Philadelphia, 1990, WB Saunders, p 797.)

- Dysbarism (Caisson's disease)
- Excessive radiation therapy
- Gaucher's disease

- **Cause**
  - Theories vary (Figure 1-35).
  - Osteonecrosis may be related to enlargement of space-occupying marrow fat cells, which lead to ischemia of adjacent tissues
  - Vascular insults and other factors may also be significant.
  - Idiopathic (or spontaneous) osteonecrosis is diagnosed when no other cause can be identified.
    - Chandler's disease: osteonecrosis of the femoral head in adults
    - Medial femoral condyle osteonecrosis: most common in women older than 60 years
  - Idiopathic, alcohol, and dysbaric forms of osteonecrosis are associated with multiple insults.
  - These may be secondary to a hemoglobinopathy (e.g., sickle cell disease) or marrow disorder (e.g., hemochromatosis).

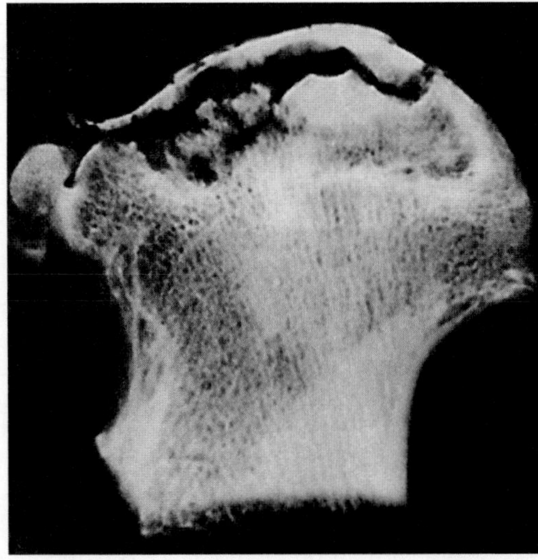

Figure 1-36 **Fine-grain micrograph demonstrating space between the articular surface and subchondral bone: "crescent sign" of osteonecrosis.** (From Steinberg ME: *The hip and its disorders,* Philadelphia, 1991, WB Saunders, p 630.)

  - Cyclosporine has reduced the incidence of osteonecrosis of the femoral head among renal transplant recipients.
- Pathologic changes
  - Grossly necrotic bone, fibrous tissue, and subchondral collapse may be observed (Figures 1-36 and 1-37).
  - Histologic findings:
    - Early changes (14 to 21 days) involve autolysis of osteocytes and necrotic marrow.

Hyperlipidemia
A Fatty liver
B Destabilization/coalescence of endogenous plasma lipoproteins
C Disruption of depot or marrow fat
Fat embolism Stage 0
Phase I Mechanical: Intraosseous vascular occlusion
Lipase
Phase II Chemical: Free fatty acids increased → Prostaglandins increased
Phase III Thrombotic: Focal intravascular coagulation → Platelet aggregation → Fibrin thrombosis
Osteonecrosis Stage 1

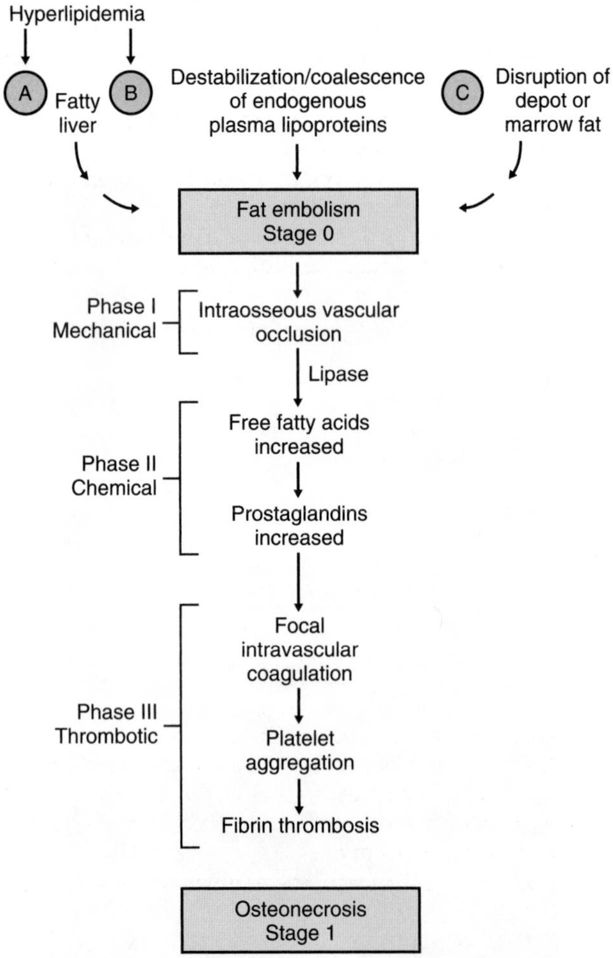

Figure 1-35 **Possible mechanisms by which intraosseous fat embolism leads to focal intravascular coagulation and osteonecrosis.** (From Jones JP Jr: Fat embolism and osteonecrosis, *Orthop Clin North Am* 16:595-633, 1985.)

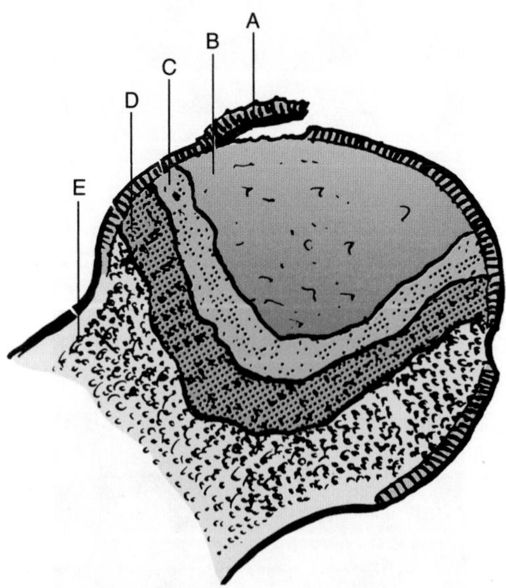

Figure 1-37 **Pathologic features of avascular necrosis. Illustration of articular cartilage *(A)*, necrotic bone *(B)*, reactive fibrous tissue *(C)*, hypertrophic bone *(D)*, and normal trabeculae *(E)*.** (From Steinberg ME: *The hip and its disorders,* Philadelphia, 1991, WB Saunders, p 630.)

- These are followed by inflammation with invasion of buds of primitive mesenchymal tissue and capillaries.
- Later, newly woven bone is laid down on top of dead trabecular bone.
- This is followed by resorption of dead trabeculae and remodeling through "creeping substitution."
- The bone is weakest during resorption and remodeling.
  - Collapse (crescent sign on radiographs) and fragmentation can occur.
- Evaluation
  - A careful history (to discern risk factors) and physical examination (e.g., to discern decreased ROM, limp) should precede additional studies.
  - Other joints (especially the contralateral hip) should be evaluated to identify the disease process early.
    - The process is bilateral in the hip in 50% of cases of idiopathic osteonecrosis and up to 80% of cases of steroid-induced osteonecrosis.
  - MRI and bone scanning are helpful for early diagnosis.
    - **MRI: earliest study to yield positive results; highest sensitivity and specificity**
  - Femoral head pressure measurement is possible but invasive.
    - Pressure higher than 30 mm Hg or increased more than 10 mm Hg with injection of 5 mL saline (stress test) is considered abnormal.
    - Values vary widely from one investigation to another.
- Treatment
  - Arthroplasty of the hip is associated with increased loosening.
  - Nontraumatic osteonecrosis of the distal femoral condyle and proximal humerus may improve spontaneously without surgery.

Table 1-17 Common Types of Osteochondrosis

Disorder	Site	Age (Yr)
Van Neck's disease	Ischiopubic synchondrosis	4-11
Legg-Calvé-Perthes disease	Femoral head	4-8
Osgood-Schlatter disease	Tibial tuberosity	11-15
Sinding-Larsen-Johansson syndrome	Inferior patella	10-14
Blount's disease (in infants)	Proximal tibial epiphysis	1-3
Blount's disease (in adolescents)	Proximal tibial epiphysis	8-15
Sever's disease	Calcaneus	9-11
Köhler's disease	Tarsal navicular	3-7
Freiberg's infarction	Metatarsal head	13-18
Scheuermann's disease	Discovertebral junction	13-17
Panner's disease	Capitellum of humerus	5-10
Thiemann's disease	Phalanges of hand	11-19
Kienböck's disease	Carpal lunate	20-40

  - The precise role of core decompression remains unresolved.
    - Results are best when core decompression is performed in early hip disease (Ficat stage I).

2. Osteochondrosis (Table 1-17)
   - This condition can occur at traction apophyses in children.
   - It may or may not be associated with trauma, joint capsule inflammation, vascular insult, or secondary thrombosis.
   - The pathologic process is similar to that of osteonecrosis in the adult.

SECTION 2 JOINTS

I. ARTICULAR TISSUES

A. Cartilage

1. Types
   - Growth plate (physeal) cartilage
   - Fibrocartilage at tendon and ligament insertion into bone (and healing articular cartilage)
   - Elastic cartilage in tissues such as the those of the trachea
   - Fibroelastic cartilage, which make up menisci
   - **Articular cartilage**, the focus of this section, which is critical in joint function
2. Articular cartilage: decreases friction and distributes loads
3. Classically described as avascular, aneural, and alymphatic
   - **Chondrocyte metabolism modulated primarily through mechanical stimulation**
   - Receives nutrients and oxygen from synovial fluid via diffusion
4. Ph of cartilage: 7.4
   - Changes in pH can disrupt cartilage structure.
5. Unlike mature articular cartilage, immature articular cartilage has a stem cell population
6. Rabbit autologous osteochondral progenitor cells can be isolated from bone marrow and grown in vitro
   - Apparently without losing the ability to differentiate into cartilage or bone
   - May be clinically useful for repairing articular cartilage defects (and subchondral bone)
   - Results of rabbit studies also suggest that TGF-β can induce chondrogenesis in periosteal explants cultured in agarose gel.
7. Articular cartilage composition
   - Water (65% to 80% of wet weight)

- ▫ Shifts in and out of cartilage to allow deformation of surface in response to stress
- ▫ Distribution: 65% of wet weight in deep zone, 80% at surface
- ▫ Increases in osteoarthritis (Table 1-18)
  - Increased permeability
  - Decreased strength
  - Decreased Young's modulus (*E*)
- ▫ Also responsible for nutrition and lubrication

- **Collagen** (10% to 20% of wet weight; more than 50% of dry weight) (Figure 1-38; Table 1-19)
  - ▫ Glycine, proline, hydroxyproline, and hydrogen bonding: responsible for collagen's unique characteristics
    - Hydroxyproline is unique to collagen; it can be measured in the urine to assess bone turnover.
  - ▫ Type II collagen
    - 95% of collagen content in articular cartilage
    - Provides cartilaginous framework and tensile strength
    - Very stable, with a half-life of approximately 25 years
  - ▫ Small amounts of types IV, V, VI, IX, X, and XI collagen
    - Collagen type VI: a minor component of normal articular cartilage but increases significantly in early stages of osteoarthritis
    - **Collagen type X**
      - ▫ Produced by hypertrophic chondrocytes during enchondral ossification:
        - Growth plate
        - Fracture callus
        - Heterotopic ossification formation
        - Calcifying cartilaginous tumors
      - ▫ Is associated with calcification of cartilage
      - ▫ A genetic defect in type X collagen is responsible for Schmid's metaphyseal chondrodysplasia (affects the hypertrophic physeal zone).
    - Collagen type XI: an adhesive that holds the collagen lattice together
- **Proteoglycans** (10% to 15% of wet weight) (Figure 1-39)
  - ▫ Have a half-life of 3 months
  - ▫ Provide structural properties, chiefly compressive and elastic strength

Table 1-19 Types of Collagen

Type	Location
I	Bone Tendon Meniscus Annulus of intervertebral disc Skin
II	Articular cartilage Nucleus pulposus of intervertebral disc
III	Skin Blood vessels
IV	Basement membrane (basal lamina)
V	Articular cartilage (in small amounts)
VI	Articular cartilage (in small amounts)*
VII	Basement membrane (epithelial)
VIII	Basement membrane (epithelial)
IX	Articular cartilage (in small amounts)
X	Hypertrophic cartilage†
XI	Articular cartilage (in small amounts) (acts as an adhesive)
XII	Tendon
XIII	Endothelial cells

*Tethers the chondrocyte to its pericellular matrix.
†Associated with calcification of cartilage (matrix mineralization).

Table 1-18 Biochemical Changes of Articular Cartilage

Parameter	Effect of Aging	Effect of Osteoarthritis
Water content (hydration; permeability)	↓	↑
Collagen	Content remains relatively unchanged	Becomes disorderly (breakdown of matrix framework) Content ↓ in severe osteoarthritis Relative concentration ↑ (because of loss of proteoglycans) Collagen type VI content ↑
Proteoglycan content (concentration)	↓ (Also, the length of the protein core and glycosaminoglycan chains decreases)	↓
Proteoglycan synthesis		↑
Proteoglycan degradation	↓	↑↑↑
Chondroitin sulfate concentration (includes both chondroitin-4- and -6-sulfate)	↓	↑
Chondroitin-4-sulfate concentration	↓	↑
Keratin sulfate concentration	↑	↓
Chondrocyte size	↑	
Chondrocyte number	↓	
Modulus of elasticity	↑	↓

↓, Decreased; ↑, increased.

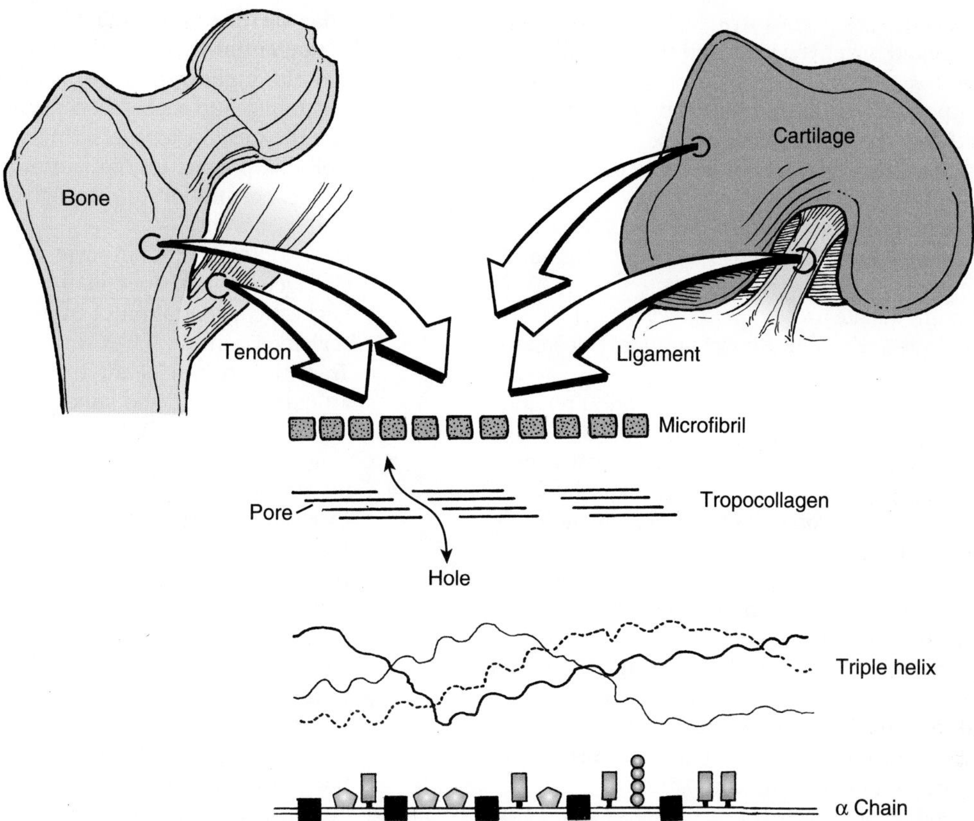

Figure 1-38 Microstructure of collagen. Collagen is composed of microfibrils that are quarter-staggered arrangements of tropocollagen. Note hole and pore regions for mineral deposition (for calcification). Tropocollagen in turn is made up of a triple helix of α chains of polypeptides. (From Brinker MR, Miller MD: *Fundamentals of orthopaedics,* Philadelphia, 1999, WB Saunders, p 3.)

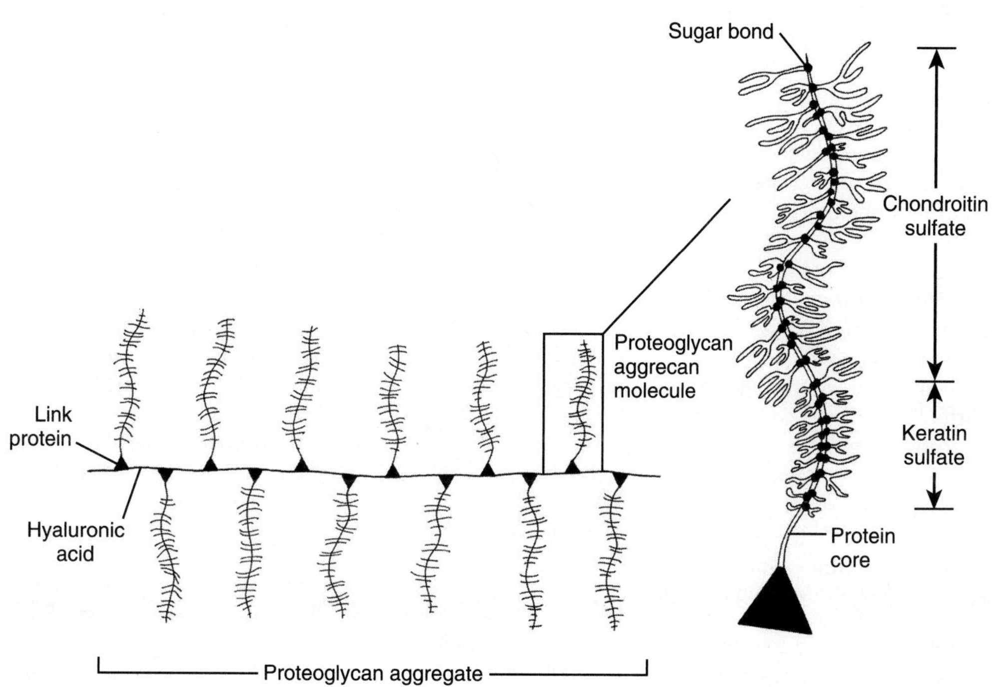

Figure 1-39 Proteoglycan aggregate and aggrecan molecule. (From Brinker MR, Miller MD: *Fundamentals of orthopaedics,* Philadelphia, 1999, WB Saunders, p 9.)

- Produce cartilage's porous structure
- Trap and hold water (regulate and retain fluid in the matrix)
- Protein polysaccharides produced by chondrocytes, secreted into the extracellular matrix
  - Composed of subunits known as **glycosaminoglycans** (disaccharide polymers)
  - Glycosaminoglycans include two subtypes:
    - Chondroitin sulfate (most prevalent glycosaminoglycan in cartilage)
    - Keratin sulfate
  - Chondroitin-4-sulfate concentration decreases with age.
  - Chondroitin-6-sulfate concentration remains essentially constant.
  - Keratin sulfate concentration increases with age.
- Glycosaminoglycans link to a protein core by sugar bonds to form a **proteoglycan aggrecan** molecule (see Figure 1-39).
- **Link proteins** stabilize these aggrecan molecules to hyaluronic acid to form a proteoglycan aggregate.

- **Chondrocytes (5% of wet weight)**
  - **Chondrocytes are derived from mesenchymal precursors; the SOX9 transcriptional factor is considered the "master switch."**
  - Chondrocytes are active in protein synthesis.
  - They possess a double effusion barrier.
  - They produce collagen, proteoglycans, and some enzymes.
    - Enzymes include the **metalloproteinases** (breakdown cartilage matrix) and **tissue inhibitor of metalloproteinases** (TIMPs).
  - Chondrocytes are least active in the calcified zone.
  - Deeper cartilage zone chondrocytes have two characteristics:
    - Decreased rough endoplasmic reticulum
    - Increased intraplasmic filaments (degenerative products)
  - Chondroblasts, derived from undifferentiated mesenchymal cells (stimulated by motion), are later trapped in lacunae to become chondrocytes.
- Other matrix components:
  - Adhesives
    - Noncollagenous proteins, such as fibronectin, chondronectin, and anchorin CII
      - Fibronectin may be associated with osteoarthritis.
    - Involved in interactions between chondrocytes and fibrils
  - Lipids: unknown function

8. **Articular cartilage layers** (Table 1-20; Figure 1-40).
   - **The tangential-superficial zone**
     - **Has the highest concentration of collagen fibers**
     - Right angles to each other, parallel to joint surface
     - Has the greatest tensile stiffness
     - Collagen parallel to joint surface
     - Low concentration of proteoglycans
   - The deeper zones
     - Have increased chondrocyte volume
     - Collagen fibers perpendicular to joint surface
     - Highest concentration of proteoglycans
   - The calcified zone
     - Transition region of intermediate stiffness between articular cartilage and subchondral bone
9. Articular cartilage metabolism
   - Collagen synthesis (Figure 1-41)
   - Collagen catabolism
     - Exact mechanisms are unknown.
     - Proposed enzymatic processes involve metalloproteinase collagenase cleaving to the triple helix.
     - Mechanical factors may play a role.
   - Proteoglycan synthesis (Figure 1-42)
     - Begins with proteoglycan gene expression and transcription of messenger RNA
     - Concludes with proteoglycan aggregate formation in the extracellular matrix
   - Proteoglycan catabolism (Figure 1-43)
10. Articular cartilage growth factors
    - Regulate cartilage synthesis; may have a role in osteoarthritis
    - PDGF
      - May affect healing of cartilage lacerations (and perhaps osteoarthritis)
    - TGF-β
      - Stimulates proteoglycan synthesis
      - Suppresses synthesis of type II collagen
      - Stimulates formation of plasminogen activator inhibitor-1 and TIMP
        - Prevents degradative action of plasmin and stromelysin
    - Fibroblast growth factor (basic) (b-FGF)
      - Stimulates DNA synthesis in adult articular chondrocytes
      - May affect cartilage repair
    - Insulin-like growth factor-I (IGF-I)
      - Previously known as *somatomedin C*
      - Stimulates DNA and cartilage matrix synthesis in adult articular cartilage
      - Stimulates immature cartilage of the growth plate

Table 1-20 Articular Cartilage Layers

Layer	Width (μm)	Characteristic	Orientation	Function
Gliding zone (superficial)	40	↓ Metabolic activity	Tangential	Opposes shear
Transitional zone (middle)	500	↑ Metabolic activity	Oblique	Opposes compression
Radial zone (deep)	1000	↑ Collagen size	Vertical	Opposes compression
Tidemark	5	Undulating barrier	Tangential	Opposes shear
Calcified zone	300	Hydroxyapatite crystals		As an anchor

↑, Increased; ↓, decreased.

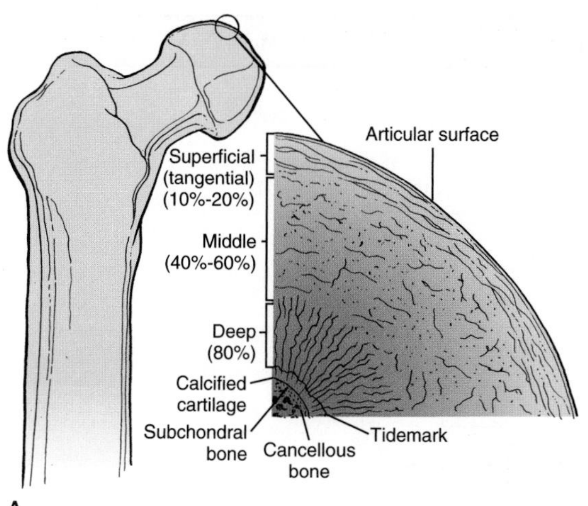

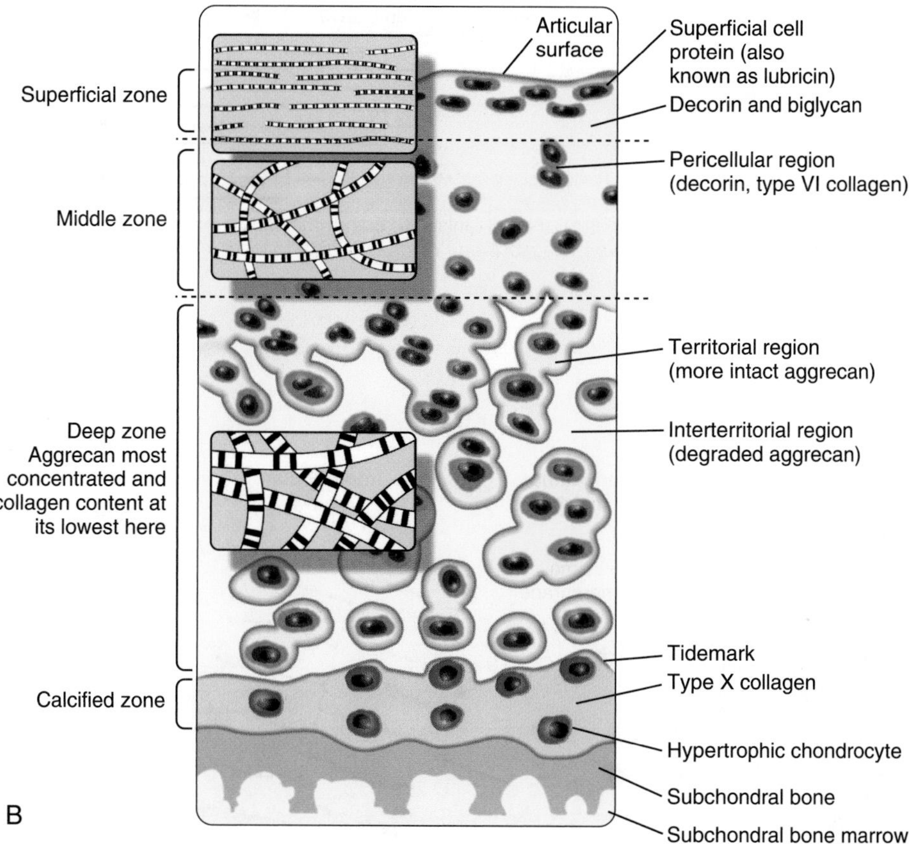

Figure 1-40 **A,** Articular cartilage layers. **B,** The structure of human adult articular cartilage, showing the zones of cellular distribution and the pericellular, territorial, and interterritorial regions of matrix organization. *Insets* show the relative diameters and orientations of collagen fibrils in the different zones. The positions of the tidemark and subchondral bone and other special features of matrix composition are also noted. (**A** from Brinker MR, Miller MD: *Fundamentals of orthopaedics,* Philadelphia, 1999, WB Saunders, p 9. **B** from Firestein B: *Kelley's textbook of rheumatology,* ed 8, Philadelphia, 2008, WB Saunders.)

11. Lubrication and wear mechanisms of articular cartilage (Figures 1-44 through 1-46)
    - The coefficient of friction for human joints varies from 0.002 to 0.04.
        - Factors decreasing articular cartilage coefficient of friction:
            - Fluid film formation
            - Elastic deformation of articular cartilage
            - Synovial fluid
            - Efflux of fluid from the cartilage
        - Factor increasing the coefficient of friction: fibrillation
    - Specific types of lubrication (see Figures 1-44 and 1-45)
        - **Elastohydrodynamic lubrication**
            - Predominant mechanism during dynamic joint function
            - Elastic deformation of articular surfaces and thin films of joint lubricants separate the surfaces.
            - The coefficient of friction is primarily a function of lubricant properties, not the surfaces.
            - Coefficient of friction is generally low.
        - **Boundary lubrication** (slippery surfaces)
            - Bearing surface is largely nondeformable.

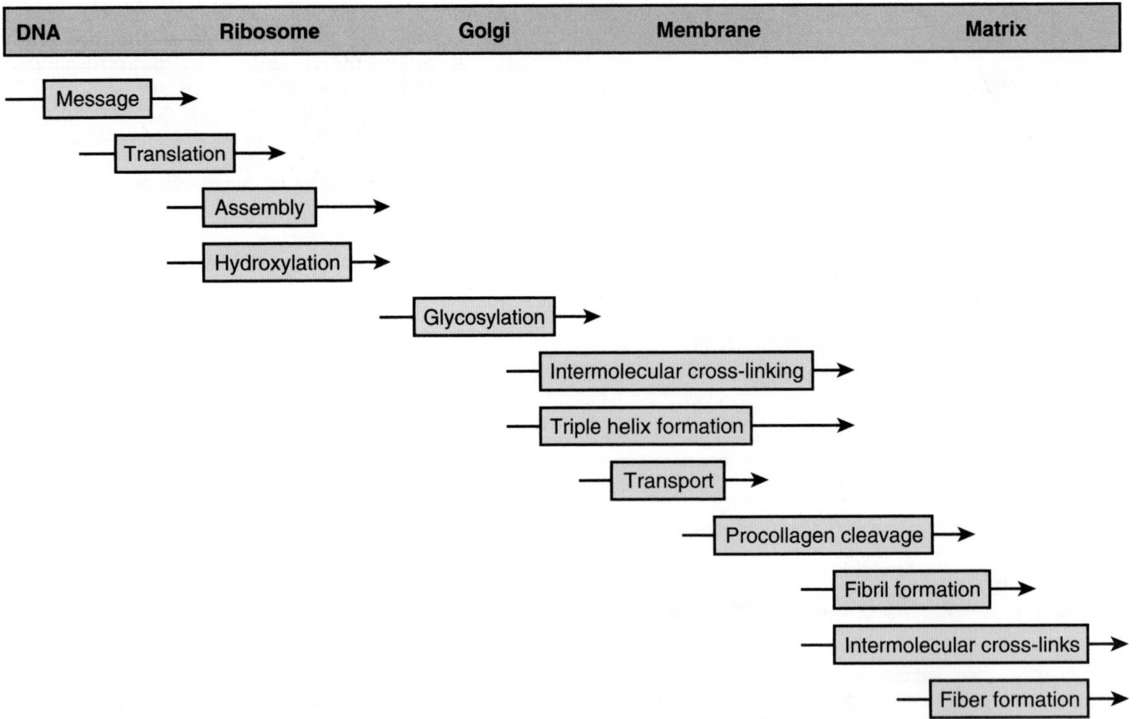

Figure 1-41 Collagen synthesis is accomplished at various intracellular sites. (From Mankin HJ, Brandt KD: Biochemistry and metabolism of articular cartilage in osteoarthritis. In Moskowitz RW, et al, editors: *Osteoarthritis: diagnosis and medical/surgical management,* ed 2, Philadelphia, 1992, WB Saunders, p 124.)

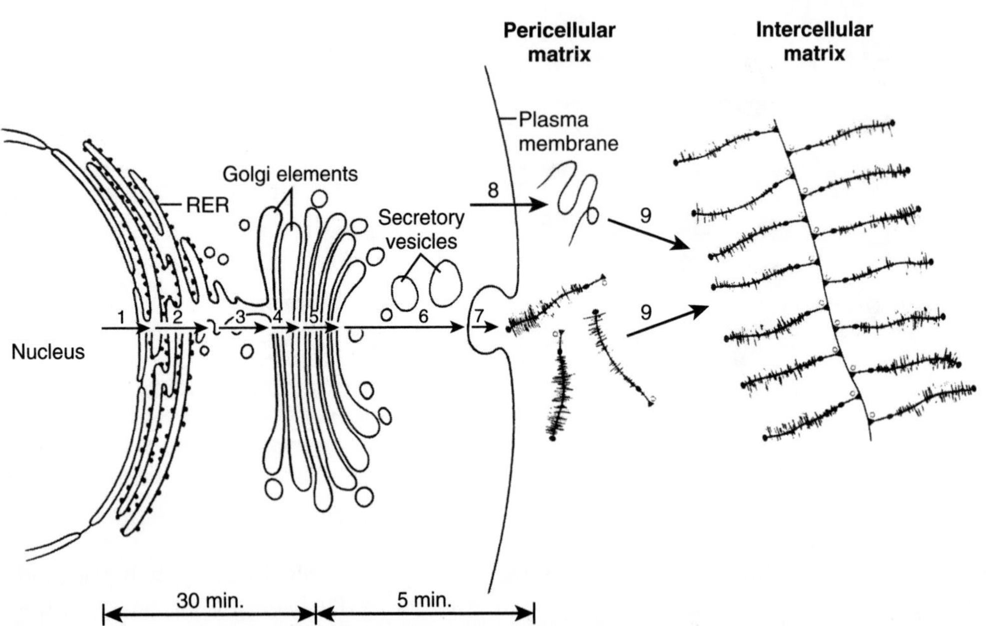

Figure 1-42 Synthesis and secretion of proteoglycan aggrecan molecules and link protein by a chondrocyte. *1,* Transcription of aggrecan and link protein genes to messenger RNA. *2,* Translation of messenger RNA to form protein core. *3,* Transportation. *4* and *5, cis*-Golgi and medial *trans*-Golgi compartments, respectively, where glycosaminoglycan chains are added to the protein core. *6,* Transportation to the secretory vesicles. *7,* Release into the extracellular matrix. *8* and *9,* Hyaluronate from the plasma membrane binds with the aggrecan and link proteins to form aggregates in the extracellular matrix. RER, rough endoplasmic reticulum. (From Simon SR, editor: *Orthopaedic basic science,* Rosemont, Ill, 1994, American Academy of Orthopaedic Surgeons, p 13.)

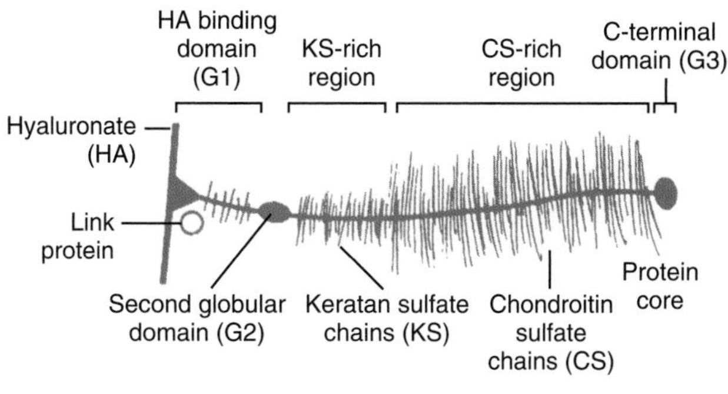

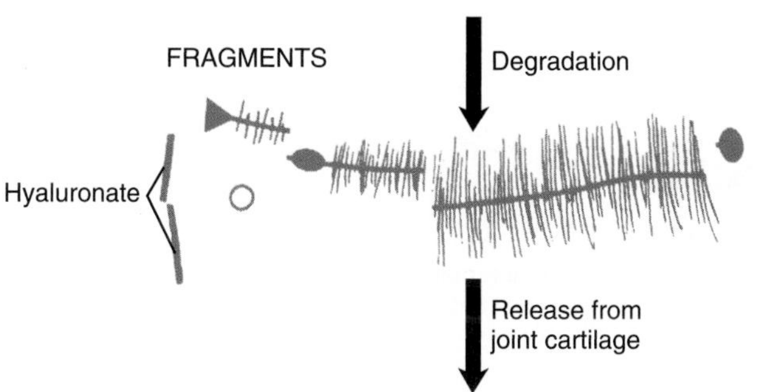

Figure 1-43 **Proteoglycan degradation in articular cartilage. Cleavage of the G1 and G2 domains renders the fragments nonaggregating.** (Modified from Simon SR, editor: *Orthopaedic basic science,* Rosemont, Ill, 1994, American Academy of Orthopaedic Surgeons, p 14.)

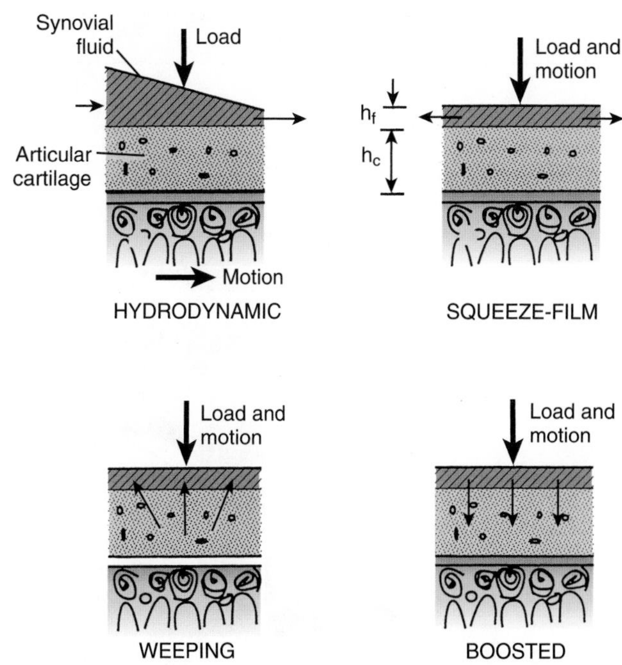

Figure 1-45 **Models of fluid film lubrication of articular cartilage.** (From Mow VC, Soslowsky LJ: Friction, lubrication, and wear of diarthrodial joints. In Mow VC, Hayes WC, editors: *Basic orthopaedic biomechanics,* New York, 1991, Raven Press, pp 245-292.)

- Lubricant only partially separates the surfaces.
- Superficial zone protein (**lubricin**) appears to have a role in boundary lubrication.

□ **Boosted lubrication** (fluid entrapment)
- Concentration of lubricating fluid in pools trapped by regions of bearing surfaces that are making contact
- The coefficient of friction is generally higher than with elastohydrodynamic lubrication.

□ Hydrodynamic lubrication
- Fluid separates the surfaces when one of the surfaces is sliding on the other.

□ Weeping lubrication
- Fluid shifts out of articular cartilage in response to load, separating the surfaces by hydrostatic pressure.

- **Articular cartilage aging** (Figure 1-47; see Table 1-18)
  - □ Chondrocytes become larger, acquire increased lysosomal enzymes, and no longer reproduce.

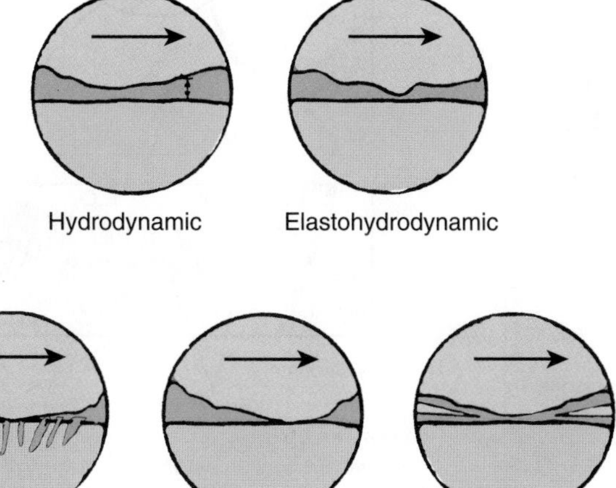

Figure 1-44 Types of lubrication of articular cartilage. (From Simon SR, editor: *Orthopaedic basic science,* Rosemont, Ill, 1994, American Academy of Orthopaedic Surgeons, p 465.)

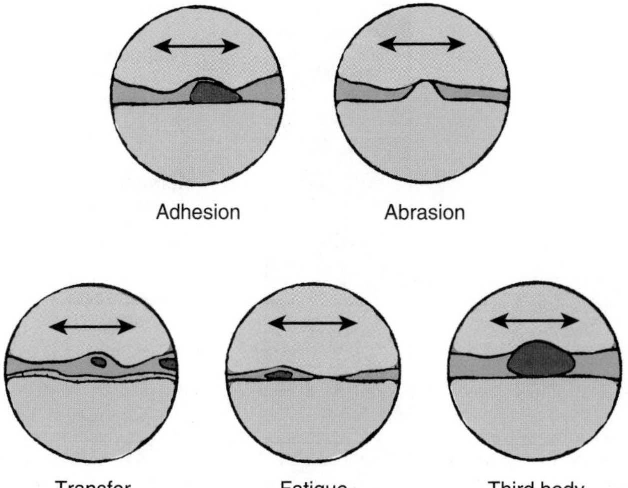

Figure 1-46 **Wear mechanisms of articular cartilage.** (From Simon SR, editor: *Orthopaedic basic science,* Rosemont, Ill, 1994, American Academy of Orthopaedic Surgeons, p 466.)

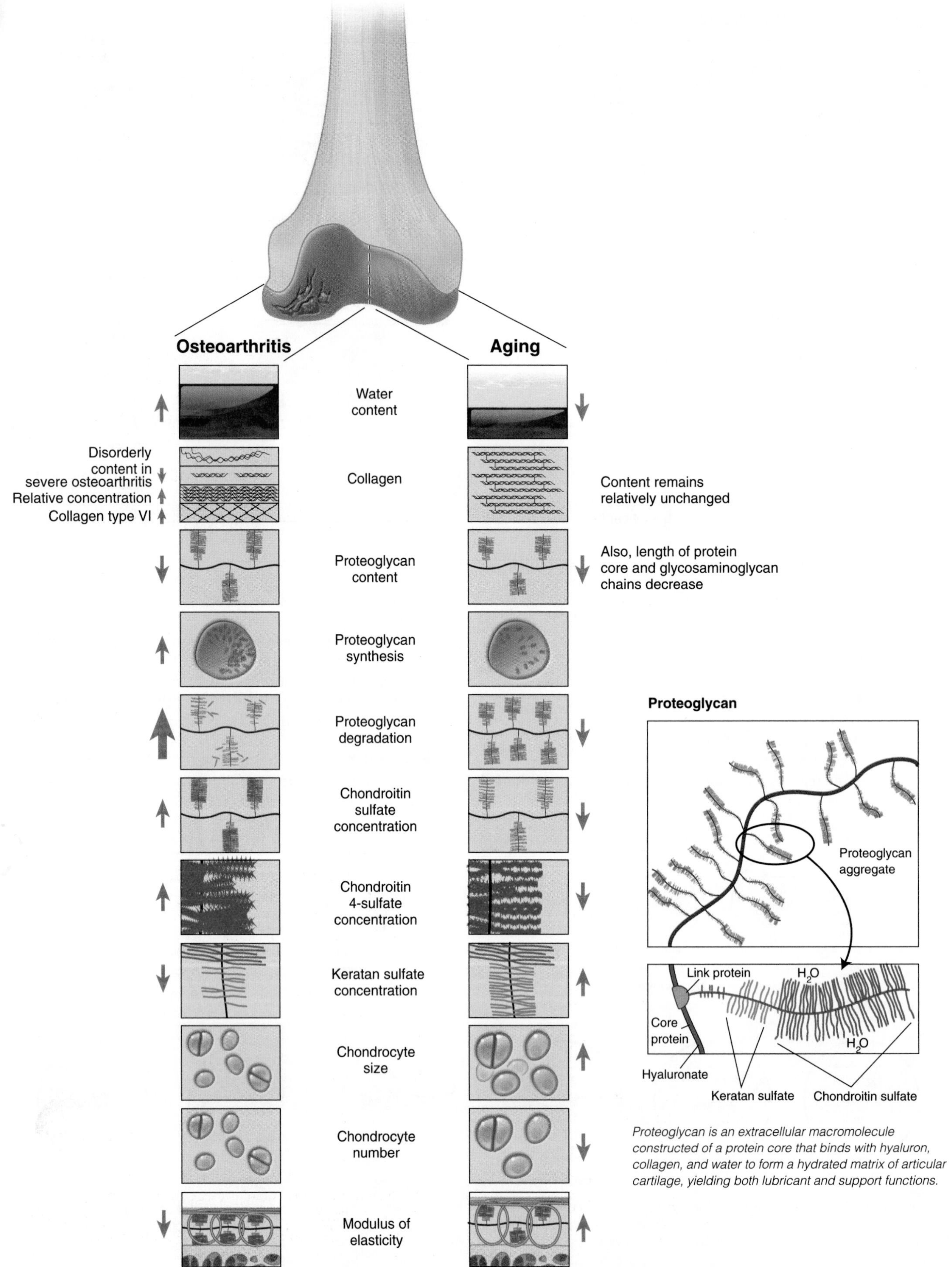

Figure 1-47 Articular cartilage changes in osteoarthritis and aging.

- Cartilage becomes relatively hypocellular.
- With aging, cartilage increases in stiffness and decreases in solubility.
- Cartilage proteoglycans decrease in mass and size (decreased length of the chondroitin sulfate chains) and change in concentrations (decreased chondroitin sulfate and increased keratin sulfate).
- Protein content increases, and water content decreases.
  - These changes decrease elasticity.
- In a normal joint, weight-bearing exercise increases proteoglycan content and thickens the cartilage.
  - However, moderate joint impact (without a fracture) decreases proteoglycan concentration and increases hydration.
- Glucosamine and chondroitin supplementation appears to slow degradation.
- **In osteoarthritis, the water content is increased, proteoglycan content is decreased, keratin sulfate concentration is decreased, and proteoglycan degradation is significantly increased.**

12. **Articular cartilage healing**
    - Damage above the tidemark:
      - Limited to the chondrocytes (type 1 injury) or articular cartilage surface (type 2 injury)
      - Have a poor potential for healing because cartilage is avascular
    - Lacerations extending below the tidemark:
      - Penetrate the underlying subchondral bone (type 3 injuries)
      - Cause an inflammatory response
      - May heal with fibrocartilage
        - Fibrocartilage is not as durable as hyaline cartilage.
        - The fibrocartilage is produced by undifferentiated marrow mesenchymal stem cells.
        - These stem cells differentiate into cells capable of producing fibrocartilage.
        - This is the theory behind abrasion chondroplasty.
      - An abundance of type I collagen is typical 1 year after injury.
    - Blunt trauma may induce cartilage changes similar to those observed with osteoarthritis.
    - Continuous passive motion is believed to benefit cartilage healing.
    - Joint immobilization leads to atrophy or cartilage degeneration.
      - In animal models, 4 weeks of joint immobilization decreases the proteoglycan/collagen ratio.
      - This ratio returns to normal after 8 weeks of joint mobilization.
    - Joint instability initially decreases the proteoglycan/collagen ratio (at 4 weeks).
      - Later (12 weeks), the ratio of proteoglycan to collagen is elevated, and hydration is increased.
      - Instability markedly decreases hyaluronan, whereas disuse does not.

B. Synovium

1. Vascularized connective tissue that lacks a basement membrane
2. Mediates nutrient exchange between blood and joint (synovial) fluid
3. Cell types
   - Type A: important in phagocytosis
   - Type B (fibroblast-like cells): produce synovial fluid
   - Other undifferentiated cells: have a reparative role
   - A third type of cell, type C, may exist as an intermediate cell type.
4. **Synovial fluid**
   - Hyaluronic acid, lubricin, proteinase, collagenases, and prostaglandins
   - An ultrafiltrate (dialysate) of blood plasma added to fluid produced by the synovial membrane
   - Contains no RBCs, clotting factors, or hemoglobin
   - Lubricates articular cartilage and provides nourishment through diffusion
   - Exhibits nonnewtonian flow characteristics
     - The viscosity coefficient μ is not a constant; the fluid is not linearly viscous.
     - Viscosity increases as the shear rate decreases.
   - Lubricin is the key lubricating glycoprotein component.
   - **Hyaluronan** molecules in the knee become entangled and behave like an elastic solid during high-strain activities (running, jumping).
5. Histologic finding: chronic inflammation of the synovium
   - Causes accumulation of lymphocytes
   - Leads to hyperplasia of the intimal lining
   - Neutrophils are absent

C. Meniscus

1. Deepens the articular surface of various synovial joints
   - The meniscus broadens the contact area and distributes load.
   - These joints include acromioclavicular, sternoclavicular, glenohumeral, hip, and knee joints.
   - The meniscus of the knee is the focus of this section.
2. More elastic and less permeable than articular cartilage
3. Transmits 50% of force across the knee in extension, up to 90% in deep flexion
4. Three years after total meniscectomy of the knee, 20% of patients have significant arthritic lesions and 70% have radiographic changes.
   - All patients experience arthrosis after 20 years.
   - The severity of degenerative changes is proportional to the amount of meniscus excised.
5. Anatomy (knee meniscus)
   - Triangular semilunar structure
   - Peripheral border attached to the joint capsule
   - Shape of medial meniscus: semicircular; shape of lateral meniscus: circular
6. Histologic findings
   - **Fibroelastic cartilage** (Figure 1-48)
   - An interlacing network of collagen fibers (90% type I)
   - Proteoglycans, glycoproteins, and cellular elements (Box 1-3)
7. Innervation and blood supply (knee meniscus)
   - Peripheral two thirds are innervated by types I and II nerve endings.
     - The concentration of mechanoreceptors is highest in the posterior horns.
     - Few fibers are found in the meniscal body.
   - **Blood supply is from the geniculate arteries.**
     - Vessels branch circumferentially to form a plexus supplying the **peripheral 25% of the meniscus.**

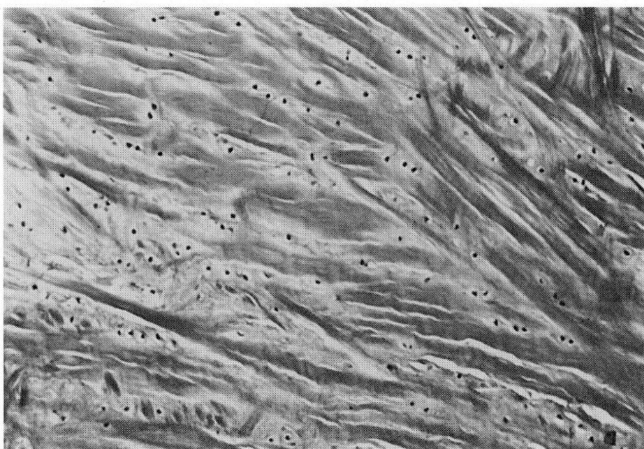

Figure 1-48 Histologic appearance of menisci.

- The remaining meniscus receives nutrition through diffusion.
- Tears in the peripheral, vascularized region ("red zone") can heal by means of fibrovascular scar formation.
  - More central tears in the avascular region ("white zone") cannot.
  - The fibrochondrocyte is responsible for meniscal healing.
  - **Peripheral acute meniscal tears with a rim width larger than 4 mm have the best healing characteristics.**

Box 1-3

Histologic Features of Meniscus

EXTRACELLULAR MATRIX

Collagen

- Types
  - Primarily type I collagen (55%-65% of dry weight)
  - Also types II, III, V, and VI (5%-10% of dry weight)
- Layers
  - Superficial layer: meshlike fibers oriented primarily radially
  - Surface layer (deep to superficial layer): irregularly aligned collagen bundles
  - Middle layer (deep): parallel circumferential fibers

Elastin (0.6% of dry weight)

Proteoglycans } 13% of dry weight
Glycoproteins }

Adhesive glycoproteins (fibronectin, thrombospondin)

CELLULAR COMPONENTS

Function

- Synthesize and maintain extracellular matrix
- Anaerobic metabolism (few mitochondria)

Components: chondrocytes and fibroblasts (fibrochondrocytes)

- Fusiform cells
  - Found in superficial layer
  - Resemble fibroblasts and chondrocytes
  - Found in lacunae
  - Contain abundant endoplasmic reticulum and Golgi cells
- Ovoid cells
  - Found in surface and middle layer
  - Contain abundant endoplasmic reticulum and Golgi cells

II. ARTHROSES

A. Groups (Table 1-21)

B. Joint fluid analysis (Table 1-22)

1. Noninflammatory arthritides
   - White blood cell (WBC) count: 200/mm^3, of which 25% are polymorphonuclear neutrophils (PMNs)
   - Equal serum values of glucose and protein
   - Normal viscosity (high)
   - Straw color
   - Firm mucin clot
2. Inflammatory arthritides
   - WBC count: 2000/mm^3 to 75,000/mm^3, of which up to 50% are PMNs
   - Moderately decreased glucose level (25 mg/dL lower than serum glucose level)
   - Low viscosity
   - Yellow-green
   - Friable mucin clot
   - Synovial fluid complement decreased in rheumatoid arthritis (RA), normal in ankylosing spondylitis
3. Infectious arthritides
   - WBC count: more than 80,000/mm^3, of which more than 75% are PMNs
   - Positive Gram stain (also positive cultures later)
   - Low glucose level (25 mg/dL lower than serum glucose level)
   - Opaque fluid
   - Increased synovial lactate

C. Noninflammatory arthritides

1. **Osteoarthritis** (degenerative joint disease; see Table 1-21)
   - **Most common form** of arthritis
   - Causes
     - Inflammation, overload, or decreased matrix production
     - Osteoarthritic cartilage:
       - **Increased water content** (in contrast with decreased water content with aging; see Table 1-18)
       - **Alterations in proteoglycans** (decreased content, shorter chains, increased chondroitin/keratin sulfate ratio)
       - **Collagen abnormalities** (disrupted by collagenase)
       - **Binding of proteoglycans to hyaluronic acid** (caused by proteolytic enzymes from increased prostaglandin E levels and decreased numbers of link proteins)
     - Cathepsins B and D levels and **metalloproteinases** (collagenase, gelatinase, stromelysin) increase.
       - IL-1 enhances enzyme synthesis and may have a catabolic effect leading to cartilage degeneration.
       - Glycosaminoglycans and polysulfuric acid may have a protective effect.
     - Articular cartilage degradation involves an enzymatic cascade (Figure 1-49).
     - Cartilage degeneration is prompted by shear stress.
       - Excessive stress and inadequate chondrocyte response
       - Prevented by normal compressive forces
     - Genetic predisposition may be important in osteoarthritis.
     - Rapidly destructive osteoarthritis
       - This type occurs most commonly in the hip.

Table 1-21 Comparison of Common Arthritides

Arthritis	Age Group Affected	Incidence by Sex	Symmetry	Joints	Physical Examination	Laboratory Tests	Radiographic Findings	Systemic Manifestations	Treatment
Noninflammatory									
Osteoarthritis	Elderly	M > F	Asymmetric	Hip, knee, CMC	↓ ROM, crepitus	Nonspecific	Asymmetric narrowing, eburnation, cysts, osteophytes	None	NSAIDs, arthrodesis, osteotomy, TJA
Neuropathic	Elderly	M > F	Asymmetric	Foot, ankle, lower extremity	Effusion, unstable	For underlying disease	Destruction/ heterotopic bone	None	Brace; TJA contraindicated
Acute rheumatic fever	Children	M = F	Asymmetric	Migratory; large joints	Red, tender joint; rash	ASO titer	Usually normal	Erythema marginatum nodules, carditis	Symptomatic
Ochronosis	Adults	M = F	Asymmetric	Large joints/ spine	↓ ROM, locking	Urine homogentisic acid	Destruction, disc calcification	Spondylosis	Supportive
Inflammatory									
Rheumatoid	Young adults	F > M	Symmetric	Hands, feet	Ulnar deviation, claw toes	ESR, CRP, RF	Symmetric narrow, periarticular resorption	Pericardial and pulmonary disease	Pyramid treatment for synovitis, reconstructive surgery
Systemic lupus erythematosus	Young adults	F > M	Symmetric	PIP joint, MCP joint, knee	Red, swollen joint; rash	ANA	Less destruction	Cardiac, renal, pancytopenia	Drug therapy as for rheumatoid arthritis
Juvenile rheumatoid arthritis	Children	F > M	Symmetric	Knee, multiple	Swollen joint, normal color	RF/ANA	Juxta-articular late, osteopenia	Iridocyclitis, rash	ASA; 75% remission
Relapsing polychondritis	Elderly	M = F	Symmetric	All joints	Eye, ear involved	ESR	Normal	Otic, cardiac	Supportive, dapsone?
Spondyloarthropathies									
Ankylosing spondylitis	Young adults	M > F	Symmetric	Sacroiliac, spine, hip	Rigid spine, "chin on chest"	ESR, alkaline phosphatase, CPK, HLA-B27	Sacroiliac arthritis, bamboo spine	Uveitis	Physical therapy, NSAID, osteotomy
Reiter's syndrome	Young adults	M > F	Asymmetric	Weight-bearing	Urethral discharge, conjunctivitis	ESR, WBC count, HLA-B27	MT head erosion, periostitis	Urethritis, conjunctivitis, ulcer	Physical therapy, NSAID, sulfa?
Psoriatic	Young adults	M = F	Asymmetric	DIP joint, small joints	Rash, sausage digit, pitting	ESR, HLA-B27	DIP joint: pencil-in-cup deformity	Rash, conjunctivitis	Drug therapy as for rheumatoid arthritis
Enteropathic	Young adults	M > F	Asymmetric	Weight-bearing	Synovitis, gastrointestinal manifestations	ESR, HLA-B27	Normal	Erythema nodosum, pyoderma	Treatment for bowel disease, symptomatic therapy

Continued

Table 1-21 Comparison of Common Arthritides—cont'd

Arthritis	Age Group Affected	Incidence by Sex	Symmetry	Joints	Physical Examination	Laboratory Tests	Radiographic Findings	Systemic Manifestations	Treatment
Crystal Deposition Disease									
Gout	Young	M > F	Asymmetric	Great toe, lower extremity	Tophi, red, swollen	Uric acid: Birefringent crystals	Soft tissue swelling, erosions	Tophi, renal stones	Colchicine, indomethacin
Chondrocalcinosis	Elderly	M = F	Asymmetric	Knee, lower extremity	Acute swelling	Birefringent rhombus-shaped crystals	Articular fibrocartilage calcified	Ochronosis, hyperparathyroidism, hypothyroidism	Symptomatic therapy; avoid surgery
Infectious									
Pyogenic	All	M = F	Asymmetric	Any joint	Red, hot, swollen	WBC count, ESR, bacterial cultures	Joint narrowing (late)	Fever, chills, infection	I&D, intravenous antibiotics
Tuberculous	Elderly	M > F	Asymmetric	Spine, lower extremity	Indolent, swelling	PPD, AFB, cultures	Both sides, cysts	Lung, multiorgan	Antibiotics ± I&D
Lyme disease	Young	M = F	Asymmetric	Any joint	Acute effusion	Culture, ELISA	Usually normal	ECM rash, neurologic, cardiac	Penicillin, tetracycline
Fungal	All	M > F	Asymmetric	Any joint	Indolent	Special studies/ cultures	Minimal changes	Immunocompromised	5-flucytosine, amphotericin
Hemorrhagic									
Hemophilia	Young	M	Asymmetric	Knee, upper extremity (elbow, shoulder)	↓ ROM, swelling	PTT, factor VIII	Squared-off patella	Soft tissue bleeding	Support, synovectomy, TJA
Sickle cell disease	Young	M = F	Asymmetric	Hip, any bone	Pain, ↓ ROM	Sickle preparation	Osteonecrosis	Infarcts, osteonecrosis	Supportive and symptomatic therapy
Pigmented villonodular synovitis	Young	M = F	Asymmetric	Knee, lower extremity	Pain, synovitis	Aspirate, biopsy	Juxtacortical erosion	None	Surgical excision

AFB, acid-fast bacilli; ANA, antinuclear antibody; ASA, acetylsalicylic acid; ASO, antistreptolysin O; CMC, carpometacarpal; CPK, creatine phosphokinase; CRP, C-reactive protein; DIP, distal interphalangeal; ECM, erythema chronicum migrans; ELISA, enzyme-linked immunosorbent assay; ESR, erythrocyte sedimentation rate; HLA, human leukocyte antigen; I&D, incision and drainage; MCP, metacarpophalangeal; MT, metatarsal; NSAID, nonsteroidal anti-inflammatory drug; PIP, proximal interphalangeal; PPD, purified protein derivative; PTT, partial thromboplastin time; RF, rheumatoid factor; ↓ ROM, decreased range of motion; TJA, total joint arthroplasty; WBC, white blood cell.

Table 1-22 Joint Fluid Analysis

Types of Arthritis	White Blood Cells	Polymorphonuclear Leukocytes	Other Characteristics
Noninflammatory	200/mm^3	25%	Joint aspirate levels of glucose and protein are equal to serum values
Inflammatory	2000/mm^3 to 75,000/mm^3	50%	↓ Joint aspirate glucose level
Infectious	>80,000/mm^3	>75%	Thick, cloudy fluid Positive Gram stain Positive cultures ↓ Joint aspirate glucose level, ↑ joint aspirate protein level

Modified from Brinker MR, Miller MD: *Fundamentals of orthopaedics,* Philadelphia, 1999, WB Saunders, p 26.

- It may mimic septic arthritis, RA, seronegative arthritis, neuropathic arthritis, or osteonecrosis.
- The femoral head may be so flat as to appear sheared off.

- General characteristics
  - Can be primary (intrinsic defect) or secondary (trauma, infection, congenital condition)
  - Begins with deterioration and loss of the weight-bearing surface
  - Followed by osteophyte development and osteochondral junction breakdown
  - Later, cartilage disintegration and subchondral microfractures expose the bony surface.
  - Radiographic findings:
    - Subchondral cysts (secondary to microfracture, may contain amorphous gelatinous material)
    - Osteophytes
    - Joint space narrowing
    - Eburnation of bone
    - Best shown on tomograms or CT scans
  - Microscopic changes (Figures 1-50 and 1-51)
    - Loss of superficial chondrocytes
    - **Chondrocyte cloning** (more than 1 chondrocyte per lacuna)
    - Replication and breakdown of the tidemark
    - Fissuring
    - Cartilage destruction with eburnation of subchondral "pagetoid" bone
  - The most common joint affected: the knee
  - Physical examination
    - Decreased ROM
    - Crepitus
    - Knee: asymmetric involvement
    - Hand: distal interphalangeal (DIP), proximal interphalangeal (PIP), and carpometacarpal joints
    - Hip: superolateral involvement
- Treatment
  - Supportive measures (e.g., activity modification, use of a cane), including NSAIDs
  - Surgical procedures
    - These range from arthroscopic débridement to total joint arthroplasty (TJA).

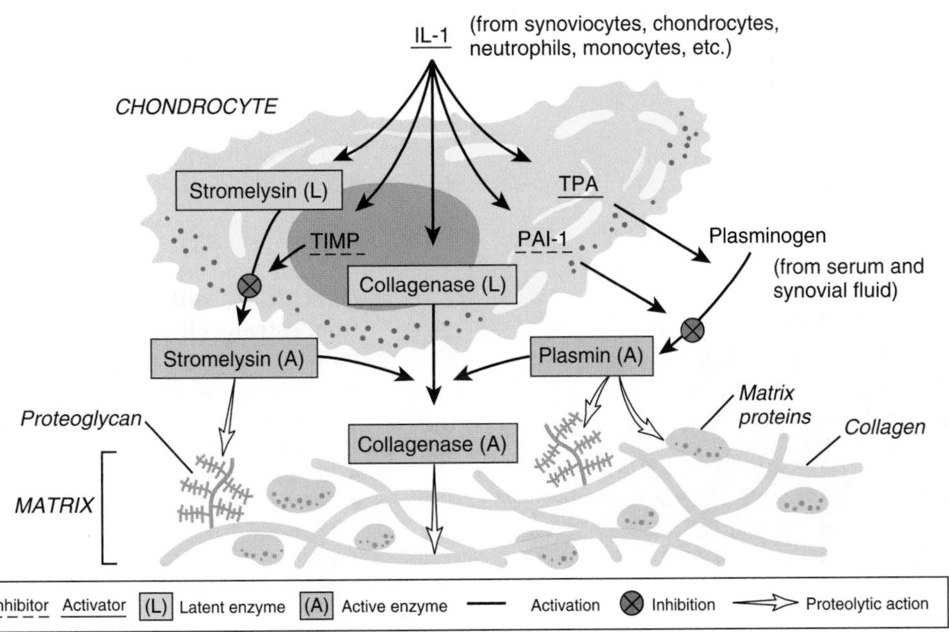

Figure 1-49 Enzyme cascade of interleukin-1–stimulated degradation of articular cartilage. (From Simon SR, editor: *Orthopaedic basic science,* Rosemont, Ill, 1994, American Academy of Orthopaedic Surgeons, p 40.)

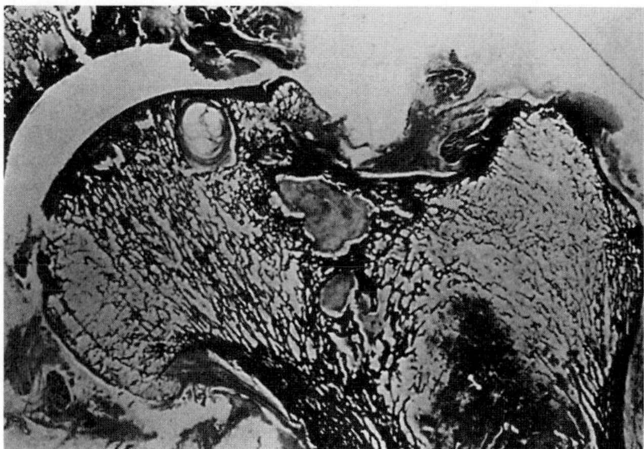

Figure 1-50 **Macrosection of an osteoarthritic human femoral head, demonstrating subarticular cysts, sclerotic bone formation, and an inferior femoral head osteophyte.** (From Simon SR, editor: *Orthopaedic basic science,* Rosemont, Ill, 1994, American Academy of Orthopaedic Surgeons, p 35.)

2. **Neuropathic arthropathy (Charcot joint disease) (Figure 1-52; see Table 1-21)**
   - An extreme form of osteoarthritis caused by disturbed sensory innervation
   - **Causes**
     - Diabetes
       - Most common overall cause
       - Charcot joint disease develops in 1% of patients with diabetic neuropathy
       - Foot and ankle most commonly involved
       - **Other anatomic sites possible, including knee and hip**
     - Tabes dorsalis (syphilitic myelopathy; lower extremity)
     - **Syringomyelia**
       - This is the most common cause of upper-extremity neuropathic arthropathy (shoulder and elbow).
       - Charcot joint disease develops in 25% of patients with syringomyelia; 80% of cases involve the upper extremity.
     - Hansen's disease
       - Second most common cause of upper extremity neuropathic arthropathy
     - Myelomeningocele: ankle and foot
     - Congenital insensitivity to pain: ankle and foot
     - Other neurologic problems (such as spinal cord injury)
   - Diagnosis
     - Typically in older patient with unstable, painless, swollen joint
       - May manifest with hemarthrosis
     - Radiographic findings:
       - Advanced (severe) destructive changes on both sides of the joint
       - Scattered "chunks" of bone embedded in fibrous tissue
       - Joint distension by fluid
       - Heterotopic ossification
     - **Difficult to differentiate Charcot's arthropathy from osteomyelitis with physical examination and radiographs**
       - Symptoms of both: swelling, warmth, erythema, minimal pain, and a variable WBC count and erythrocyte sedimentation rate (ESR)
       - Both entities common in diabetic patients
       - Technetium bone scan: may look "hot" (positive) for both diseases
       - Indium leukocyte scan: "hot" (positive) for osteomyelitis, "cold" (negative) for Charcot's arthropathy
   - Treatment
     - Limitation of activity and appropriate bracing or casting

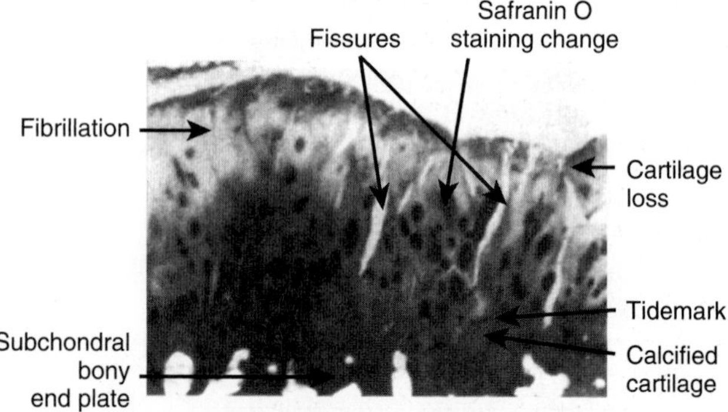

Figure 1-51 **Low-power micrograph of an osteoarthritic process, demonstrating fibrillation, fissures, and cartilage loss.** (From Simon SR, editor: *Orthopaedic basic science,* Rosemont, Ill, 1994, American Academy of Orthopaedic Surgeons, p 34.)

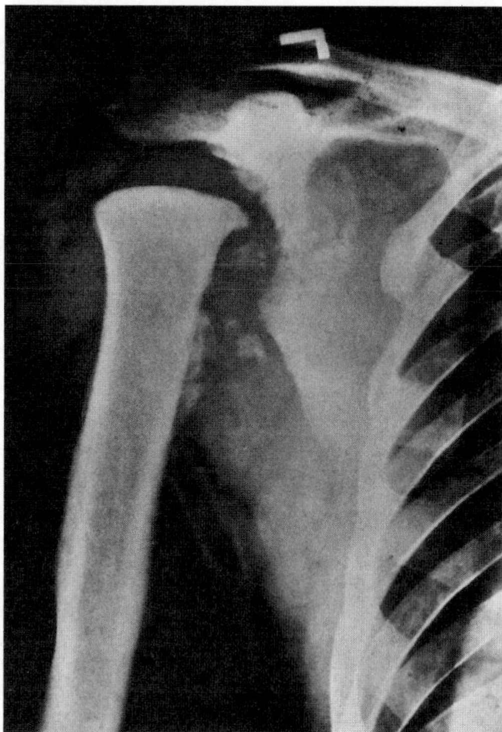

Figure 1-52 **Anteroposterior radiograph of a shoulder in which severe destructive changes characteristic of neuropathic arthropathy are evident.** (From Weissman BNW, Sledge CB: *Orthopedic radiology,* Philadelphia, 1986, WB Saunders, p 238.)

- Skin temperature of the involved side that is similar to that of the uninvolved side is the best indicator for discontinuing a total contact cast.
  - □ Charcot joint disease: usually a contraindication for TJA and the use of other orthopaedic hardware

3. Acute rheumatic fever (see Table 1-21)
   - This was formerly the most common cause of childhood arthritis.
     - □ Rare since the advent of antibiotics
   - Arthritis and arthralgias can follow untreated group A β-hemolytic streptococcal infections.
   - The onset of red, tender, extremely painful joint effusions is acute.
   - Systemic manifestations include the following:
     - □ Carditis
     - □ Erythema marginatum (painless macules with red margins, usually on the abdomen but never on the face)
     - □ Subcutaneous nodules (extensor surfaces of the upper extremities)
     - □ Chorea
   - Arthritis is migratory and typically involves multiple large joints.
   - Diagnosis is established if Jones criteria are fulfilled:
     - □ Preceding streptococcal infection with two of the following major criteria:
       - Carditis, polyarthritis, chorea, erythema marginatum, subcutaneous nodules
     - □ Or with one major criterion and two of the following minor criteria:
       - Fever, arthralgia, prior rheumatic fever, elevated ESR, prolonged PR interval on ECG study
   - Antistreptolysin O titers are elevated in 80% of affected patients.
   - Treatment includes penicillin and salicylates.
4. Ochronosis (see Table 1-21)
   - Degenerative arthritis resulting from **alkaptonuria**
     - □ A rare inborn defect of the homogentisic acid oxidase enzyme system (tyrosine and phenylalanine catabolism)
   - **Excess homogentisic acid** deposited in the joints
     - □ It then polymerizes (turns black), which leads to early degenerative changes.
     - □ It can also be deposited in other tissues, such as the heart valves.
   - Affected patients may also present with black urine
   - Ochronotic spondylitis (Figure 1-53):
     - □ Usually occurs during the fourth decade of life
     - □ Includes progressive degenerative changes, disc space narrowing, and calcification (Table 1-23)
5. Secondary pulmonary hypertrophic osteoarthropathy
   - A clinical diagnosis
   - Involves a lung tumor mass, joint pain and stiffness, periostitis of the long bones, and clubbing of the fingers

D. Inflammatory arthritides

1. Radiographic findings: generally evidence of destruction on both sides of a joint
2. Laboratory findings: sometimes confusing (Tables 1-24 and 1-25)
3. **Rheumatoid arthritis** (see Table 1-21)
   - The most common inflammatory arthritis
     - □ Affects 3% of women and 1% of men
   - Diagnostic criteria of the American Rheumatism Association:

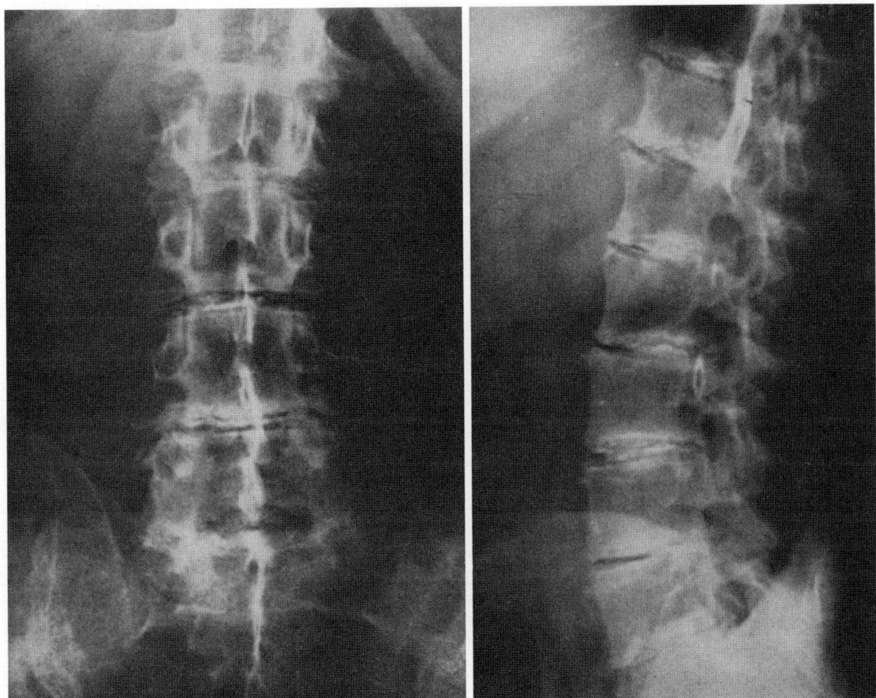

Figure 1-53 Ochronosis. Irregular calcification and narrowing of the intervertebral discs are present. Radiolucent streaks, evident anteriorly between the vertebral bodies, are not uncommon. Slipping of the vertebral bodies is typically minimal. (Courtesy of Samuel Fisher, MD.)

Table 1-23 Comparative Bony Changes of the Spine in the Arthritides

Disorder	Bony Change	Radiographic Appearance
Ochronosis	Syndesmophytes (ossification of the annulus fibrosis of the intervertebral disc)	Vertical syndesmophytes extending from the body of one vertebra to the adjacent vertebra
Ankylosing spondylitis	Syndesmophytes	Similar to those of ochronosis
Reiter's syndrome and psoriatic spondylitis	Ossification of the connective tissues adjacent to the spine	Area of ossification is separated from the margin of the vertebral body, that of the intervertebral disc, or both
Disseminated idiopathic skeletal hyperostosis	Ossification of the connective tissues adjacent to the spine, the anterior longitudinal ligament, and the intervertebral disc	Undulating osseous extension along the anterior portion of the spine

Table 1-24 Commonly Confused Laboratory Findings in Inflammatory Arthritic Conditions

Finding	Conditions in Which Finding May Be Positive	Conditions in Which Finding Is Usually Negative
Rheumatoid factor	Rheumatoid arthritis Sjögren's syndrome Sarcoid Systemic lupus erythematosus	Ankylosing spondylitis Gout Psoriatic arthritis Reiter's syndrome
Positivity for HLA-B27*	Ankylosing spondylitis Reiter's syndrome Psoriatic arthritis Enteropathic arthritis	
Antinuclear antibody (ANA)	Systemic lupus erythematosus Sjögren's syndrome Scleroderma	

Modified from Brinker MR, Miller MD: *Fundamentals of orthopaedics,* Philadelphia, 1999, WB Saunders, p 27.
*Approximately 6% of all white people are HLA-B27 positive.

Table 1-25 Associations between HLA Alleles and Susceptibility to Some Rheumatic Diseases

Disease	HLA Marker	Frequency (%) in Patients (Whites)	Frequency (%) in Controls (Whites)	Relative Risk
Ankylosing spondylitis	B27	90	9	87
Reiter's syndrome	B27	79	9	37
Psoriatic arthritis	B27	48	9	10
Inflammatory bowel disease with spondylitis	B27	52	9	10
Adult rheumatoid arthritis	DR4	70	30	6
Polyarticular juvenile rheumatoid arthritis	DR4	75	30	7
Pauciarticular juvenile rheumatoid arthritis	DR8	30	5	5
	DR5	50	20	4.5
	DR2.1	55	20	4
Systemic lupus erythematosus	DR2	46	22	3.5
	DR3	50	25	3
Sjögren's syndrome	DR3	70	25	6

Adapted from Nepom BS, Nepom GT: Immunogenetics and the rheumatic diseases. In McCarty DJ, Koopman WJ, editors: *Arthritis and allied conditions: a textbook of rheumatology,* ed 12, Philadelphia, 1993, Lea & Febiger.
HLA, human leukocyte antigen.

- Morning stiffness
- Swelling
- Nodules
- Positive laboratory test results
- Radiographic findings
- Causes
  - Unclear; probably related to a cell-mediated immune response (T cell):
    - Incites an inflammatory response
    - Response is initially against soft tissues
    - Response is later against cartilage (chondrolysis) and bone (periarticular bone resorption)
  - Mononuclear cells: the primary cellular mediators of tissue destruction in RA
  - May be associated with an infectious cause or a human leukocyte antigen (HLA) locus **(HLA-DR4 and HLA-DW4)**
  - Lymphokines, cytokines (particularly IL-1 and TNF-α), and other inflammatory mediators: initiate a destructive cascade that leads to joint destruction
    - **TNF-α** increases chondrocyte secretion of matrix metalloproteinases, which degrades the cartilage extracellular matrix.
  - In RA, cartilage is sensitive to PMN degradation and IL-1 effects (phospholipase A_2, prostaglandin E_2, and plasminogen activators)
  - **Class II molecules:** involved in antigen–T lymphocyte interaction
- General characteristics
  - Insidious onset, morning stiffness, and polyarthritis
  - Hands (ulnar deviation and subluxation of the metacarpophalangeal [MCP] joints) and feet (metatarsophalangeal joints, claw toes, and hallux valgus) affected early
    - Also common in the knees, elbows, shoulders, ankles, and cervical spine
  - **Subcutaneous nodules**
    - Observed in 20% of RA patients during their lifetime
  - Synovium and soft tissues affected first
    - Joints significantly involved only later
  - Early in the disease process, the RA-inflamed synovium shows a proliferation of blood vessels
  - **Late synovial changes**
    - **Hyperplastic cells**
    - **Intimal hyperplasia**
    - **Increased blood vessels**
    - **Abundant lymphocytes and rare neutrophils**
  - Pannus ingrowth denudes articular cartilage and leads to chondrocyte death
    - **There are almost no lymphocytes in pannus, however.**
  - Laboratory findings
    - **ESR and C-reactive protein level are elevated.**
    - Rheumatoid factor (RF) titer is positive in approximately 80% of affected patients.
    - **RF autoantibodies are directed against the crystallizable fragment (Fc) portion of immunoglobulin G (IgG). RF is most commonly immunoglobulin M (IgM) but can be any immunoglobulin type.**
  - Joint fluid assays can also demonstrate RF, decreased complement levels, and other helpful information.
  - **Systemic manifestations**
    - Rheumatoid vasculitis
    - Pericarditis
    - Pulmonary disease (pleurisy, nodules, fibrosis)
  - Popliteal cysts in rheumatoid patients (confirmed by ultrasonography), which can mimic thrombophlebitis
  - Felty's syndrome
    - RA with splenomegaly and leukopenia
  - Still's disease
    - Acute-onset juvenile RA (JRA) with fever, rash, and splenomegaly
  - Sjögren's syndrome
    - An autoimmune exocrinopathy often associated with RA.
    - **Decreased salivary and lacrimal gland secretion** (keratoconjunctivitis sicca complex) and lymphoid proliferation
- Radiographic characteristics (Figure 1-54):
  - Periarticular erosions and osteopenia

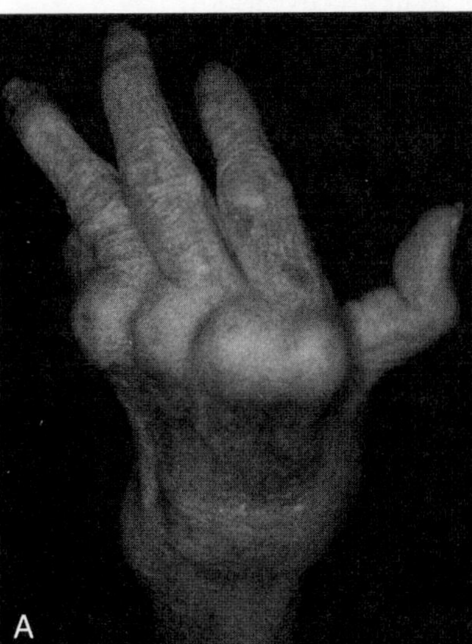

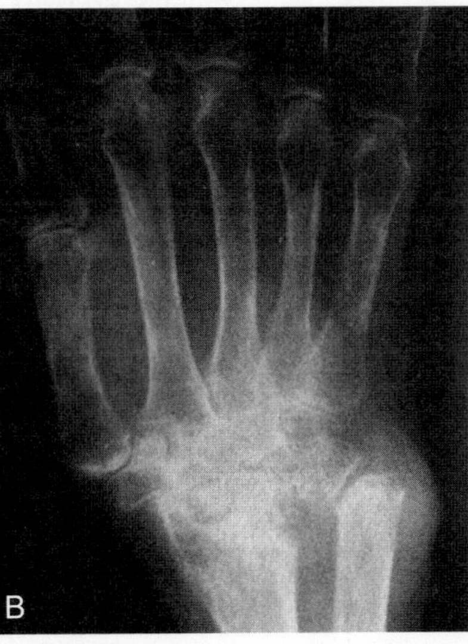

Figure 1-54 Rheumatoid arthritis. **A,** Clinical photograph of the hand of a patient with advanced rheumatoid arthritis. Note ulnar drift of the metacarpophalangeal (MCP) joints, caused by the ulnar shift of the extensor tendons, dislocations of the MCP joints, and thumb deformities. **B,** Anteroposterior radiograph of the hand and wrist of a patient with rheumatoid arthritis. Note severe erosive destruction of the distal radioulnar joint and diffuse osteopenia. (From Bogumil GP: The hand. In Wiesel SW, Delahay JN, editors: *Essentials of orthopaedic surgery,* ed 2, Philadelphia, 1997, WB Saunders, p 263.)

    - All three knee compartments may show osteoporosis and erosions.
  - Protrusio acetabuli
    - Medial displacement of the acetabulum beyond the radiographic teardrop with medial migration of the femoral head into the pelvis
    - Common in RA, as well as in ankylosing spondylitis, Paget's disease, metabolic bone diseases, Marfan's syndrome, Otto's pelvis, and other conditions
- **Treatment**
  - Goals:
    - Control synovitis and pain
    - Maintain joint function
    - Prevent deformities
  - A multidisciplinary approach involving therapeutic drugs, physical therapy, and sometimes surgery is necessary
  - The "pyramid" approach to RA drug therapy
    - Begins with NSAIDs
    - Slowly progresses to antimalarials, remittent agents (methotrexate, sulfasalazine, gold, and penicillamine), steroids, and cytotoxic drugs
    - May include experimental drugs
      - **Doxycycline has shown early promise in reducing inflammation in RA.**
  - The pyramid approach has been challenged in favor of **disease-modifying antirheumatic drugs (DMARDs).**
    - These drugs are intended to address underlying causes for the disease (e.g., autoimmune response) rather than only the effects (e.g., inflammation).
    - They include methotrexate, azathioprine, and anakinra (an IL-1 inhibitor).
    - **Most new DMARDs, such as infliximab and etanercept, target TNF-α.**
      - These drugs should be discontinued before elective surgery, to decrease risk of infection.
  - Surgery
    - Synovectomy, only if aggressive drug therapy fails
    - Soft tissue realignments
      - Usually not favored because deformity progresses
    - Various reconstructive procedures
      - Risk of infection after TJA is increased
  - If performed early, chemical and radiation synovectomy can be successful.
  - **Operative synovectomy** (open or arthroscopic) in the knee
    - Decreases pain and swelling associated with the synovitis
    - Does not prevent radiographic progression or the need for future total knee arthroplasty (TKA)
    - Does not improve joint ROM
  - After all forms of synovectomy, the synovium initially regenerates normally but degenerates to rheumatoid synovial tissue over time
  - Preoperative evaluation of the cervical spine with radiographs is important.

Table 1-26 Sarcomere

Band	Description
A band	Contains actin and myosin
I band	Contains actin only
H band	Contains myosin only
M line	Interconnecting site of the thick filaments
Z line	Anchors the thin filaments

From Brinker MR, Miller MD: Fundamentals of Orthopaedics, Philadelphia, 1999, WB Saunders, p 11.

4. **Systemic lupus erythematosus** (SLE) (Tables 1-26 and 1-27; see also Table 1-25)
   - SLE is a chronic inflammatory disease of unknown origin.
     - Usually affects women (especially African Americans)
     - Probably related to the immune complex
     - Patients with SLE typically have positive antinuclear antibody (ANA) and HLA-DR3 titers and may have positive RF titers.
   - Manifestations include the following:
     - Fever
     - **Butterfly malar rash**
     - Pancytopenia
     - Pericarditis
     - Nephritis
     - Polyarthritis
   - Joint involvement is the most common feature.
     - Affecting more than 75% of patients with SLE
   - The arthritis in SLE typically manifests as acute, red, tender swelling of the PIP joints, MCP joints, carpus, knees, and other joints.
   - SLE is typically not as destructive as RA.
   - Treatment for SLE arthritis is usually the same medications as for RA.
   - Mortality in SLE is usually related to renal disease.
   - The differential diagnosis includes polymyositis and dermatomyositis.

Table 1-27 Agents That Affect Neuromuscular Impulse Transmission

Agent	Site of Action	Mechanism	Effect
Nondepolarizing drugs (curare, pancuronium, vecuronium)	Neuromuscular junction	Competitively binds to acetylcholine receptor to block impulse transmission	Paralytic agent (long-term)
Depolarizing drugs (succinylcholine)	Neuromuscular junction	Binds to acetylcholine receptor to cause temporary depolarization of muscle membrane	Paralytic agent (short-term)
Anticholinesterases (neostigmine, edrophonium)	Autonomic ganglia	Prevents breakdown of acetylcholine to enhance its effect	Reverses effect of nondepolarizing drugs; muscarinic effects (bronchospasm, bronchorrhea, bradycardia)

- These two conditions also manifest with symmetric weakness with or without a characteristic "heliotropic" rash of the upper eyelids.

5. Polymyalgia rheumatica
   - Common among elderly persons
   - Aching and stiffness of the shoulder and pelvic girdle, associated with malaise, headaches, and anorexia
   - Physical examination findings: usually unremarkable
   - Findings of laboratory studies:
     - Markedly elevated ESR
     - Anemia
     - Increased alkaline phosphatase level
     - Increased immune complexes
   - Usually treated symptomatically
     - Steroids for refractory cases
   - May be associated with temporal arteritis
     - Biopsy necessary for definitive diagnosis
     - Also requires timely treatment with high-dose steroids; if left untreated, may rapidly result in total blindness
6. **Juvenile rheumatoid arthritis** (see Tables 1-21 and 1-25)
   - **Seronegativity** denotes negative RF titers.
   - **Seropositivity** denotes positive RF titers.
     - The incidence of seropositivity is estimated to be less than 15% of JRA cases.
     - The incidence of chronic, active, and progressive disease is higher.
   - In early-onset JRA, onset of disease occurs before the teens; in late-onset JRA, onset of disease occurs during the teens or later.
   - Types include the following:
     - Systemic (20%)
     - Polyarticular (50%)
       - Five or more joints are involved.
       - Seronegative polyarticular JRA is more frequent in girls.
       - Seropositive polyarticular JRA is also more frequent in girls.
         - Exhibits destructive degenerative joint disease
         - Frequently develops into adult RA
     - Pauciarticular (30%)
       - Four or fewer joints are involved.
       - **Onset peaks at ages 2 to 4 years.**
       - Average duration of disease is 2 years, 9 months.
         - In 50% of cases, disease lasts less than 2 years.
       - Early-onset pauciarticular JRA has two distinctive characteristics:
         - More frequent in girls
         - Associated with iridocyclitis in 50% of cases (particularly in patients with a positive ANA titer)
       - Late-onset pauciarticular JRA has one distinctive characteristic:
         - Observed in boys more commonly than in girls
   - JRA may also be associated with an HLA locus.
     - HLA-DR2, HLA-DR4, HLA-DR5, HLA-DR8, and HLA-B27 in boys
   - Treatment:
     - High-dose aspirin
     - Occasionally gold or remittent agents (refractory polyarticular)
     - Frequent ophthalmologic examinations (with a slit lamp) for asymptomatic ocular involvement
     - Most common joint affected: the knee, followed by the finger/wrist, ankle, hip, and cervical spine
       - C-spine fusion or instability can occur
7. Relapsing polychondritis (see Table 1-21)
   - Rare disorder
     - Episodic inflammation
     - Diffuse, self-limiting arthritis
     - Progressive cartilage destruction with or without systemic vasculitis
   - Typically involves the ears (thickening of the auricle)
     - Also observed are inflammatory eye disorders, tracheal involvement, hearing disorders, and sometimes cardiac involvement.
   - May be an autoimmune disorder (affected by type II collagen)
   - Treatment is supportive
8. **Spondyloarthropathies/enthesopathies** (occur at ligament insertions into bone)
   - Characterized by a **positive HLA-B27** (sixth chromosome, D locus) titer and a **negative RF** titer
   - Ankylosing spondylitis (see Tables 1-21, 1-24, and 1-25)
     - Diagnostic criteria:
       - Bilateral sacroiliitis
       - With or without acute anterior uveitis
       - HLA-B27–positive male patient
     - Insidious onset of back pain
       - Associated morning stiffness
       - Hip pain
       - Third to fourth decades of life
     - Radiographic changes (Figure 1-55; see Table 1-23)
       - **Squaring of the vertebrae**
       - Vertical syndesmophytes

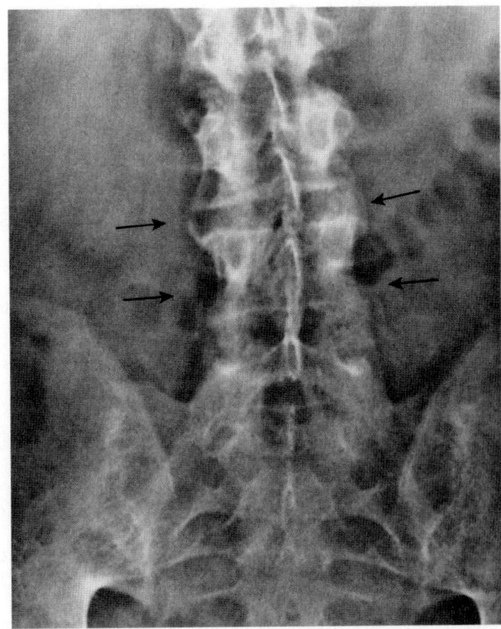

Figure 1-55 Anteroposterior radiograph of the lumbar spine and sacroiliac joints of a patient with ankylosing spondylitis, demonstrating typical marginal syndesmophytes *(arrows)*. Note bilateral involvement of the sacroiliac joints. (From Bullough PG, Vigorita VJ: *Atlas of orthopaedic pathology,* Philadelphia, 1984, Gower Medical, p 811.)

        - Obliteration of sacroiliac joints
        - "Whiskering" of the enthesis
    - Progressive spinal flexion deformities, advancing for approximately 20 years
        - Ascending ankylosis of the spine usually begins in the thoracolumbar spine, often causing the entire spine to become rigid.
    - Spinal manifestationsL
        - "Chin on chest" deformity (may require corrective osteotomy of the cervicothoracic junction)
        - Difficult cervical spine fractures, associated with epidural hemorrhage (high mortality rate)
            - Best diagnosed on a CT scan
            - Rate of neurologic involvement: 75%
        - Severe kyphotic deformities (corrected by means of a posterior closing wedge osteotomy)
        - Spondylodiscitis may develop in the late stage.
    - Other extraskeletal manifestations:
        - Iritis
        - Aortitis
        - Colitis
        - Arachnoiditis
        - Amyloidosis
        - Sarcoidosis
    - Pulmonary involvement (restriction of chest excursion [less than 2 cm]), hip involvement, and young age at onset: prognostic of poor outcome
    - Treatment
        - Initial
            - Physical therapy
            - NSAIDs (phenylbutazone is best but can cause bone marrow depression)
        - Bilateral THA
            - Often helps with lower spinal and hip flexion deformities, and pain or morning stiffness
        - Ankylosing spondylitis is often associated with heart disease and pulmonary fibrosis
- **Reiter's syndrome** (see Tables 1-21 and 1-23 through 1-25) (Figure 1-56)
    - Classical presentation is of a young man with the triad of conjunctivitis, urethritis, and oligoarticular arthritis.
        - Mnemonic: **"Can't see, pee, or bend the knee"**
    - Other common findings include the following:
        - Painless oral ulcers
        - Penile lesions
        - Pustular lesions on the extremities, palms, and soles (keratoderma blennorrhagicum)
        - Plantar heel pain
    - The arthritis usually causes sudden asymmetric swelling and pain in weight-bearing joints.
    - Recurrence is common and can lead to metatarsal head erosion and calcaneal periostitis.
    - Approximately 80% to 90% of patients with Reiter's syndrome are HLA-B27 positive.
        - Of patients with Reiter's syndrome, 60% with chronic disease have sacroiliitis.
    - Treatment includes NSAIDs, physical therapy, and possibly sulfa drugs.
- Psoriatic arthropathy (see Tables 1-21 and 1-23 through 1-25)
    - Affects approximately 5% to 10% of patients with psoriasis

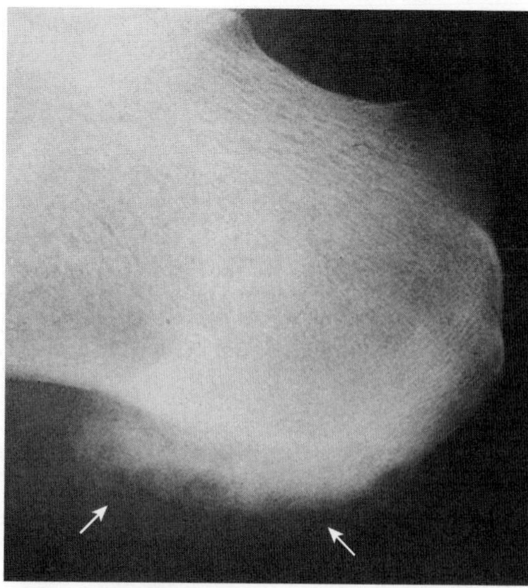

Figure 1-56 Lateral radiograph of the calcaneus of a patient with Reiter's syndrome, showing fluffy periosteal calcifications *(arrows).*

    - HLA-B27 is found in 50% of patients.
        - Many HLA loci may be involved.
    - Many forms exist; most patients have the oligoarticular form.
        - Asymmetrically affects small joints of the hands and feet
        - Nail pitting (also fragmentation and discoloration)
        - "Sausage" digits
        - "Pencil-in-cup" deformity (DIP involvement; Figure 1-57)
    - Treatment is similar to that for RA.
- Enteropathic arthritis (see Tables 1-21, 1-24, and 1-25)
    - Of patients with Crohn's disease and ulcerative colitis, 10% to 20% experience peripheral joint arthritis.
        - Five percent or more experience axial disease.
    - Nondeforming arthritis
        - Occurs more commonly in large, weight-bearing joints
    - Usually manifests as an acute monarticular synovitis that may precede any bowel symptoms
    - Approximately half of all affected persons are HLA-B27 positive.
    - Ten percent to 15% of cases are associated with ankylosing spondylitis.

9. Crystal deposition disease
    - **Gout** (Figure 1-58; see Table 1-21)
        - Disorder of nucleic acid metabolism causing hyperuricemia
            - **Deposition of monosodium urate crystals in joints**
        - Cause
            - The crystals activate inflammatory mediators.
                - These mediators include proteases, chemotactic factors, prostaglandins, leukotriene B_4, and free oxygen radicals.
                - The inflammatory mediators are inhibited by **colchicine.**

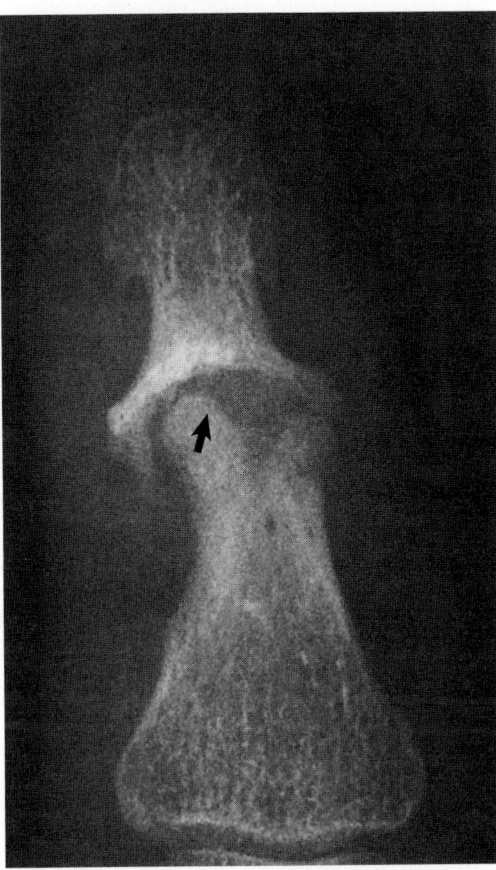

Figure 1-57 Anteroposterior radiograph of the distal interphalangeal joint of the foot in a patient with psoriatic arthritis, showing the classic pencil-in-cup deformity *(arrow)*.

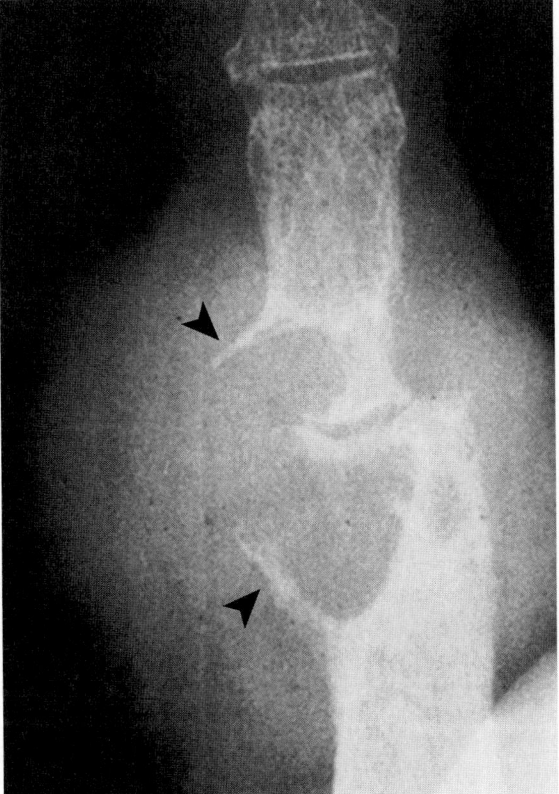

Figure 1-58 Anteroposterior radiograph of the proximal interphalangeal joint of a finger in a patient with gout. Note the soft tissue swelling, "punched out" periarticular erosions, and sclerotic overhangings bordering the joint *(arrowheads)*. (From Resnick D, Niwayama G: *Diagnosis of bone and joint disorders,* Philadelphia, 1981, WB Saunders, p 1478.)

  - The crystals also activate platelets, IL-1 production, and the complement system.
  - Phagocytosis is inhibited by phenylbutazone and indomethacin (Indocin).
  - Local polypeptides may inhibit the crystal inflammatory response by means of a glycoprotein "coating."
  - Gout may be precipitated by chemotherapy for myeloproliferative disorders.
- Diagnosis
  - Recurrent arthritis attacks, especially in men 40 to 60 years of age
    - Usually in the lower extremity, great toe (podagra)
  - Crystal deposition as tophi
    - Ear helix, eyelid, olecranon, Achilles tendon
    - Usually observed in the chronic form
  - Renal disease or stones
    - Kidneys are the second most commonly affected organ.
  - Radiographic findings:
    - Soft tissue changes
    - "Punched-out" periarticular erosions with sclerotic overhanging borders (see Figure 1-58)
  - Monosodium urate crystals—thin, tapered intracellular crystals that are strongly negatively birefringent (Figure 1-59) in joint aspirate—must be present for the diagnosis.
    - Elevated serum uric acid level is not diagnostic.
- Treatment:
  - **Initial treatment of acute attacks with indomethacin** (50 mg three times daily)
    - A rheumatology consultation is necessary afterwards.
    - Patients with gastrointestinal symptoms or a history of peptic ulcer disease should receive intravenous colchicine for acute attacks.

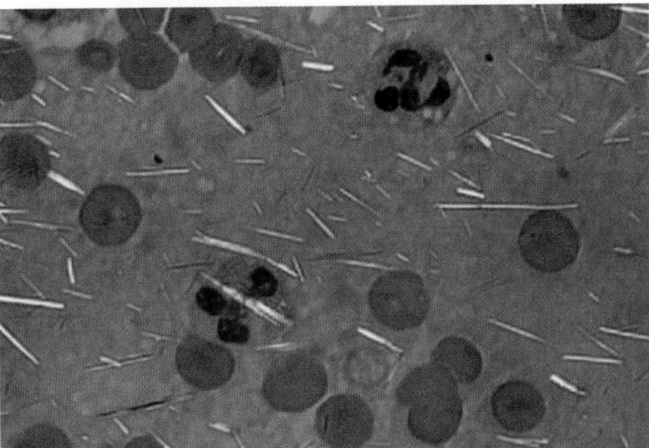

Figure 1-59 Monosodium gout crystals in synovial fluid under polarized light. (From McPherson RA, Pincus MR, editors: *Henry's clinical diagnosis and management by laboratory methods,* ed 21, Philadelphia, 2007, WB Saunders–Elsevier.)

- **Allopurinol** is used to lower the serum uric acid levels in hyperuricemic patients with chronic gout.
  - **It is a xanthine oxidase inhibitor;** xanthine oxidase is needed for the conversion of hypoxanthine to xanthine and xanthine to uric acid.
  - Also given before chemotherapy for myeloproliferative disorders
- Colchicine is used for prophylaxis after recurrent attacks.

- Chondrocalcinosis (see Table 1-21)
  - Caused by several disorders, including the following:
    - **Calcium pyrophosphate (dihydrate crystal) deposition disease (CPPD), or "pseudogout"**
      - A disorder of pyrophosphate metabolism
      - Occurs in older patients
      - Occasionally causes acute attacks, usually in the lower extremities, especially the **knee**, which can be mistaken for septic arthritis
      - Short, blunt, rhomboid-shaped crystals that are weakly positively birefringent (Figure 1-60) are observed in neutrophilic leukocytes in knee aspirate
    - Ochronosis
    - Hyperparathyroidism
    - Hypothyroidism
    - Hemochromatosis
  - Chondrocalcinosis of knee menisci: often related to a previous knee injury
  - Radiographs: fine linear calcification in hyaline cartilage and more diffuse calcification of menisci (Figure 1-61) and other fibrocartilage (triangular fibrocartilage complex, acetabular labrum)
  - NSAIDs often helpful
  - Intraarticular yttrium-90: injections have successfully reduced symptoms in chronic cases
- Calcium hydroxyapatite crystal deposition disease
  - Also associated with chondrocalcinosis and degenerative joint disease

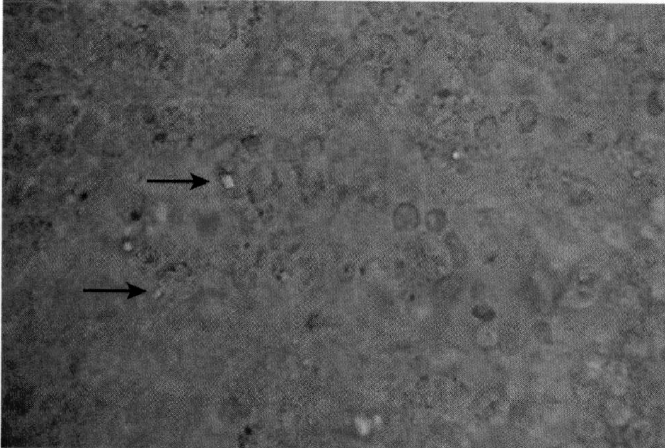

Figure 1-60 Calcium pyrophosphate crystals *(arrows)* in synovial fluid. (From Firestein GS et al, editors: *Kelley's textbook of rheumatology,* ed 8, Philadephia, 2008, WB Saunders.)

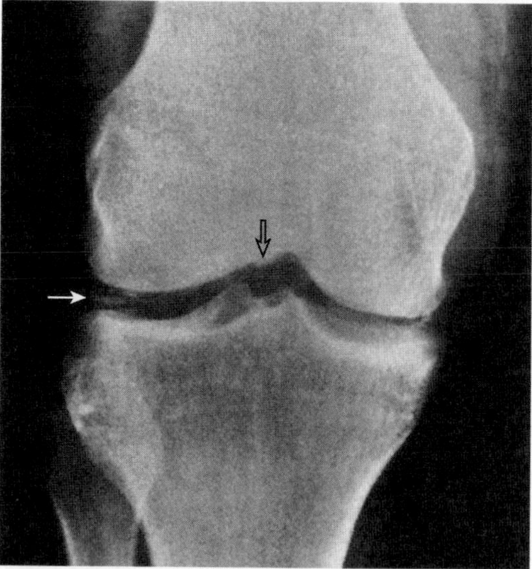

Figure 1-61 Anteroposterior radiograph demonstrating calcium pyrophosphate deposition disease (pseudogout) in the meniscus of the knee. Note calcification within the (fibrocartilage) meniscus *(solid arrow)* and articular involvement, with fine linear calcification of hyaline cartilage *(open arrow).* (From Weissman BNW, Sledge CB: *Orthopaedic radiology,* Philadelphia, 1986, WB Saunders, p 549.)

  - Destructive arthropathy commonly observed in the knee and shoulder
  - "Milwaukee shoulder": calcium phosphate deposition in the shoulder along with cuff tear arthropathy
  - Calcium hydroxyapatite crystals are too small to see with light microscopy
  - Treatment is generally supportive
- Birefringence
  - Positive: When long axis of crystal is parallel to the compensator (of the microscope), the crystal is blue.
  - Negative: When long axis of crystal is parallel to the compensator, the crystal is yellow.
    - When the crystal's long axis is perpendicular to the compensator, the color rules are reversed.
  - If the birefringence of the crystal is weak, the crystal appears dull.
  - If the birefringence of the crystal is strong, the crystal appears bright and shiny.

E. **Infectious arthritides**

1. Pyogenic arthritis (see Table 1-21)
   - Cause
     - Hematogenous spread
     - Extension of osteomyelitis
     - Posttraumatic (fight bites, open injuries)
     - Postoperative (iatrogenic)
   - Commonly occurs in children
   - Adults at high risk include the following:
     - Intravenous drug abusers
       - Especially when the sternoclavicular and sacroiliac joints are affected
     - Sexually active young adults
       - *Neisseria gonorrhoeae* infection (intracellular diplococci), especially if observed with skin papules
     - Patients with diabetes (the feet and lower extremities are mainly affected)
     - Patients with RA

- Histologic findings:
  - Synovial hyperplasia may be demonstrated.
  - Numerous PMNs are present.
  - Cartilage destruction is evident.
    - Can be direct (from proteolytic enzymes) or indirect (from pressure and lack of nutrition)
- Treatment:
  - Incision and drainage
  - Antibiotics for up to several weeks

2. Tuberculous arthritis (see Table 1-21)
   - Chronic granulomatous infection
     - *Mycobacterium tuberculosis*
     - Usually invades joints by hematogenous spread
   - **Spine and lower extremities most often involved**
   - Common in Mexico and Asia
   - Eighty percent of cases are monarticular
   - Characteristic radiographic findings:
     - Osteolytic changes on both sides of the joint
     - Subchondral osteoporosis
     - Cystic changes
     - Notchlike, bony destruction at the joint edge
     - Joint space narrowing
   - Diagnosis
     - Positive results of purified protein derivative test
     - Acid-fast bacilli and "rice bodies" (fibrin) in synovial fluid
     - Cultures may take several weeks to yield positive results
   - Histologic study: may demonstrate characteristic granulomas with Langerhans giant cells (peripheral nuclei)
   - Treatment:
     - Incision and drainage
     - Long-term (6 months) antibiotics (isoniazid, rifampin or rifabutin, pyrazinamide, and pyridoxine)
3. Fungal arthritis (see Table 1-21)
   - This condition is most common in neonates, **patients with acquired immunodeficiency syndrome (AIDS),** and drug abusers.
   - Pathogens include *Candida albicans.*
   - Potassium hydroxide (KOH) preparations of synovial fluid should be studied.
     - Helpful because cultures require prolonged incubation
   - Arthritis can be treated with fluconazole.
   - Amphotericin is often required.
     - Sometimes administered intraarticularly, with fewer side effects
4. **Lyme disease** (see Table 1-21)
   - Acute, self-limiting joint effusions
     - Especially in the shoulder and knee
     - Recur frequently
   - **Spirochete *Borrelia burgdorferi*** (*Borrelia garinii* in Europe).
     - Transmitted by **tick bites** (Ixodidae)
     - Endemic in half the United States
     - Transmission occurs in approximately 10% of bites by infected ticks
   - Sometimes called the "great mimicker"
   - Possible systemic signs:
     - Characteristic "bull's-eye" rash **(erythema migrans)**
     - Neurologic (Bell's palsy is common)
     - Cardiac symptoms
   - Three stages:
     - I: rash
     - II: neurologic symptoms
     - III: arthritis
   - Accumulation of immune complexes and cryoglobulins in the synovial fluid
   - Diagnosis:
     - Confirmed by enzyme-linked immunosorbent assay (ELISA) testing
     - Should be sought in endemic areas after a Gram stain and joint cultures of an infectious aspirate show no organisms
   - **Treatment:**
     - Doxycycline (most effective)
     - Amoxicillin
     - Cefuroxime
     - Erythromycin
     - Ceftriaxone for carditis

F. **Hemorrhagic effusions**

1. **Hemophilic arthropathy** (see Table 1-21)
   - **X-linked recessive disorder**
     - **Factor VIII deficiency**: hemophilia A (classic)
     - Factor IX deficiency: hemophilia B (Christmas disease)
   - Associated with repeated hemarthrosis caused by minor trauma
     - The condition leads to synovitis, cartilage destruction (enzymatic processes), and joint deformity.
     - Repeated episodes lead to replacement of the normal joint capsule with dense scar tissue.
   - Disease severity related to the degree of factor VIII deficiency:
     - Mild disease: levels of factor VIII are 5% to 25%
     - Moderate disease: 1% to 5%
     - Severe disease: 0% to 1%
   - Home factor treatment has reduced incidence substantially.
   - Diagnosis:
     - Most commonly involved: knee
       - Followed by elbow, ankle, shoulder, and spine
     - Joint swelling, decreased ROM, and pain
     - Concomitant infection: ruled out by examination of joint aspirate
     - Radiographic findings: may demonstrate variable changes
       - "Squared off" patella (Jordan's sign)
       - Widening of the intercondylar notch
       - Enlarged femoral condyles, appearing to "fall off" the tibia (Figure 1-62)
     - Ultrasonography: to diagnose and monitor intramuscular bleeding
       - Iliacus hematomas can cause femoral nerve palsies.
   - **Treatment:**
     - Correction of factor levels
       - Factor VIII: to 40% to 50% of normal levels
     - Splints and bracing
     - Compressive dressings
     - Analgesics
     - Steroids (occasionally helpful)
     - Surgical management
       - Synovectomy for recurrent hemarthroses refractory to medical treatment

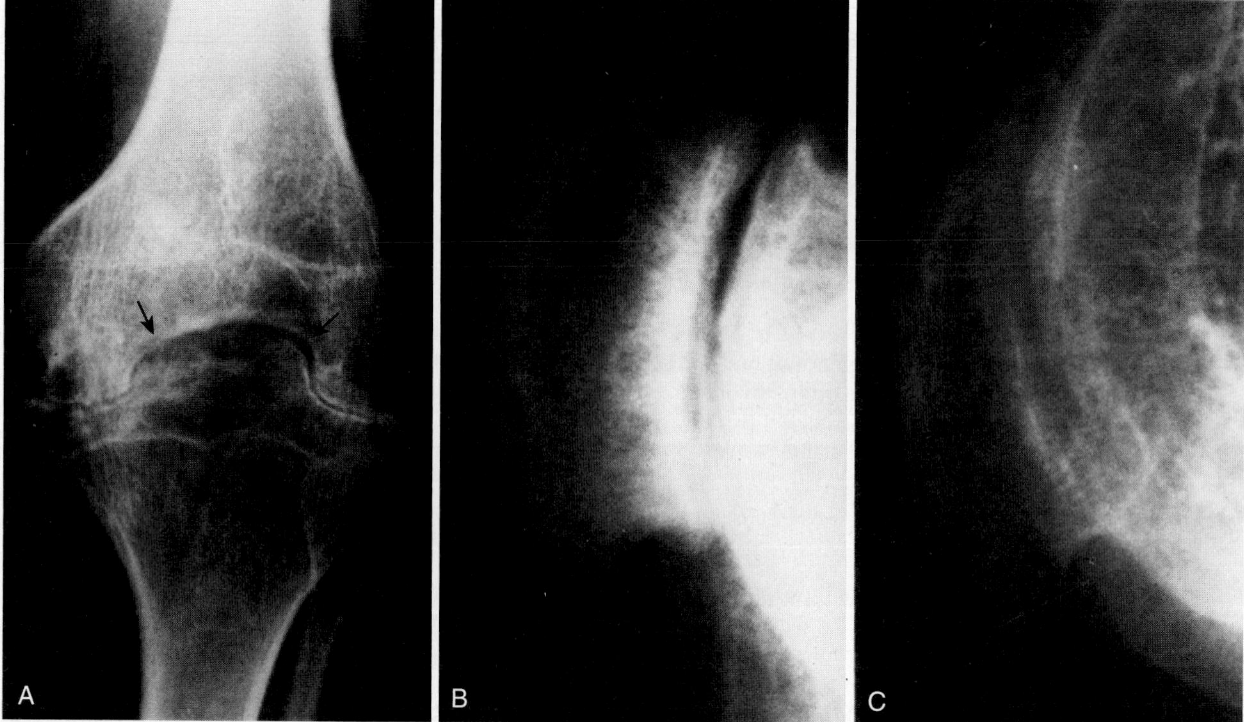

Figure 1-62 Radiographic changes of hemophilia. **A,** Anteroposterior radiograph of the knee, showing enlargement and ballooning of the distal femur, flattening of the distal femoral condyles, marked joint space narrowing, and severe widening of the intercondylar notch *(arrows).* **B** and **C,** Images showing the variation in radiographic changes that can occur in the patella; in **B,** the bone appears "squared off" (Jordan's sign), and in **C,** it appears elongated and thinned. (From Resnick D, Niwayama G: *Diagnosis of bone and joint disorders,* Philadelphia, 1981, WB Saunders, p 2025.)

- Reduces incidence of recurrent hemarthroses; causes less pain and swelling
- TJA for end-stage arthropathy
- Arthrodesis, especially for the ankle
- Preoperative screen for factor VIII inhibitors, specific IgG antibodies
  - Monoclonal recombinant factor VIII products are prone to induce action of inhibitors.
  - Inhibitors are present in 5% to 25% of affected patients and can develop any time.
  - Their presence is a relative contraindication to elective surgery.
  - Affected patient have no response to factor replacement therapy.
  - Other strategies to provide hemostasis are required.
- Maintenance of factor levels
  - Should be near 100% during the first postoperative week
  - At 50% to 75% the second week
- Synoviorthesis
  - Destruction of synovial tissue by intraarticular injection of a radioactive agent: colloidal phosphorus-32 chromic phosphate
  - For chronic hemophilic synovitis that is resistant to conventional treatment
- High incidence of human immunodeficiency virus (HIV) seropositivity (up to 90%)

2. Sickle cell disease
   - Hemoglobin SS is found in 1% of black North Americans.
   - This hemoglobin type leads to local infarction as a result of capillary stasis.
   - Bony infarcts and ischemic necrosis may occur in multiple bones.
     - Thalassemia does not produce infarcts or ischemic necrosis.
     - Osteonecrosis, particularly of the femoral head, is common among patients with sickle cell disease.
   - Dactylitis with metacarpal/metatarsal periosteal new bone formation may also be observed.
   - Osteomyelitis is not uncommon.
     - *Salmonella* species are the most characteristic infecting organisms.
     - *Staphylococcus* species are the most common infecting organisms.
     - *Salmonella* infection can spread from a gallbladder infection.
   - ESR is usually falsely low.
   - TJA results are poor because of ongoing negative bone remodeling.
3. Pigmented villonodular synovitis (PVNS) (Figure 1-63; see Table 1-21)
   - Synovial disease often affects young adults with PVNS.
   - PVNS is characterized by exuberant proliferation of villi and nodules.
   - Synovium is frequently rust colored or brown.
     - Extensive hemosiderin deposits are present.
   - Pain, swelling, synovitis, and a rust-colored or bloody effusion are common.
   - The knee is the most frequent site.
     - Occasional involvement of hip and ankle

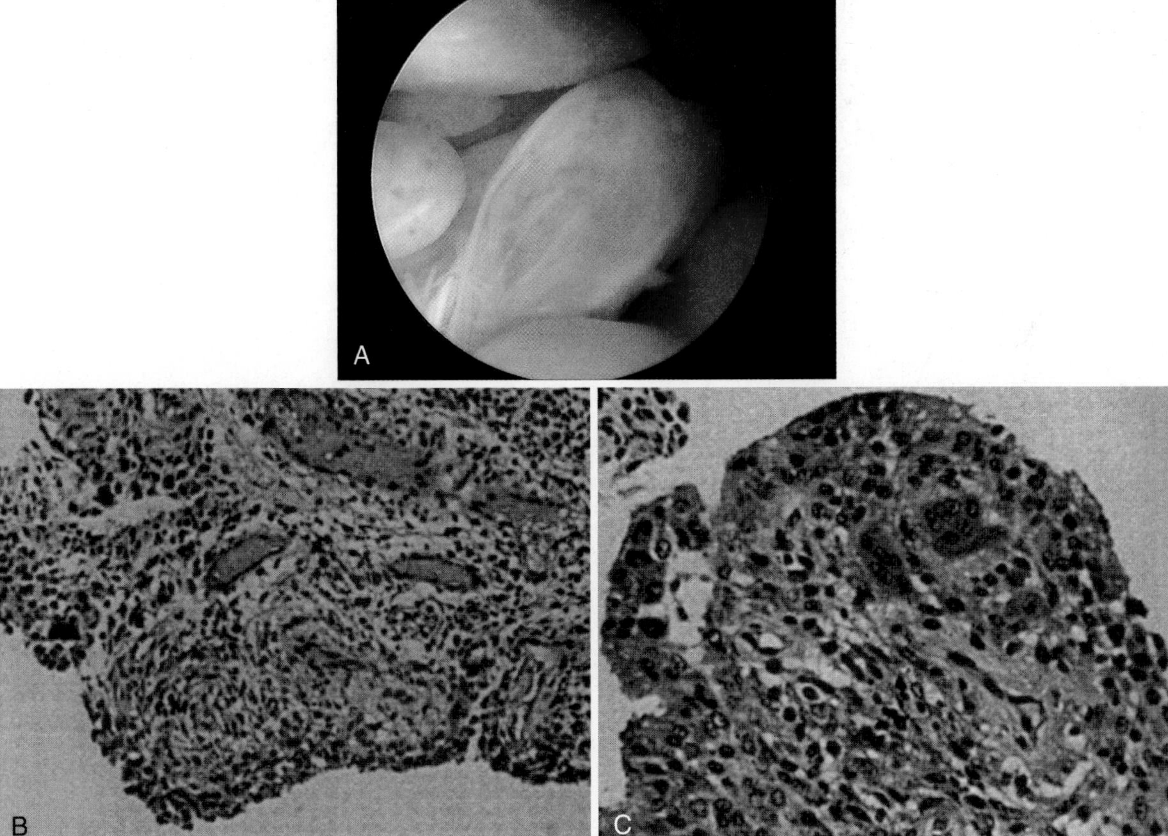

Figure 1-63 Localized pigmented villonodular synovitis. **A,** Arthroscopic view localized to the medial knee joint. **B,** Histologic view of vascular channels, giant cells, and blood pigments (hematoxylin and eosin stain, ×100). **C,** Histologic view of giant cells in synovial villus (hematoxylin and eosin stain, ×400).

- Radiographic findings:
  - Well-defined juxtacortical erosions with sclerotic margins
- Histologic findings:
  - Pigmented synovial histiocytes
  - Foam cells (lipid-laden histiocytes)
  - Multinucleated giant cells
- Treatment:
  - Surgical excision (total synovectomy) of the affected synovium may be performed.
  - Microscopic residual disease may be treated with intraarticular dysprosium (a radioisotope).
  - Localized PVNS necessitates only nodule resection.

SECTION 3 NEUROMUSCULAR AND CONNECTIVE TISSUES

I. SKELETAL MUSCLE

A. Noncontractile elements (Figure 1-64)

1. Muscle body
   - Epimysium surrounds individual muscle bundles.
   - Perimysium surrounds muscle fascicles.
   - Endomysium surrounds individual fibers.
2. **Myotendinous junction**
   - This is the weak link in the muscle, often the site of tears.
     - Especially with eccentric contractions
   - Sarcolemma filaments interdigitate with the basement membrane (type IV collagen) and tendon tissue (type I collagen).
   - Involution of muscle cells in this region provides maximum surface area for attachment.
   - Linking proteins and specialized membrane proteins are also present.
3. Sarcoplasmic reticulum
   - Stores calcium in intracellular membrane–bound channels
     - Includes T-tubules, which go to each myofibril
     - Also includes terminal cisternae, small storage areas (Figure 1-65)

B. Contractile elements (see Figure 1-64)

1. Derived from myoblasts
2. Each muscle composed of several muscle **fascicles**

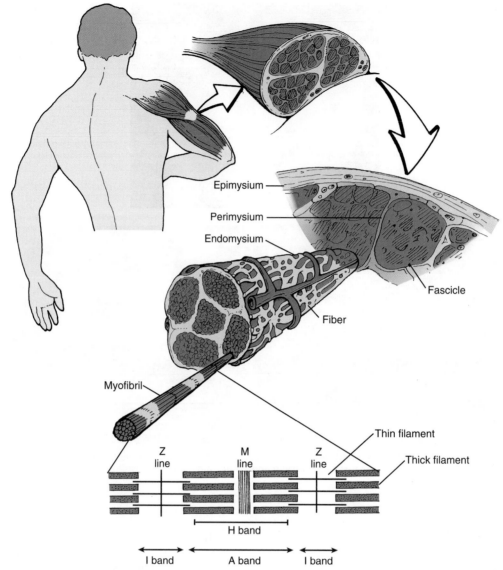

Figure 1-64 Skeletal muscle architecture. (From Brinker MR, Miller MD: *Fundamentals of orthopaedics,* Philadelphia, 1999, WB Saunders, p 10.)

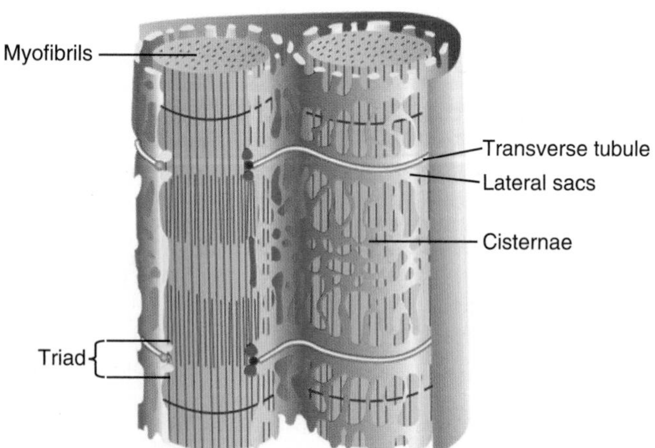

Figure 1-65 Sarcoplasmic reticulum. Action potentials travel down the transverse tubules, causing calcium release from the outer vesicles. (From DeLee JC, et al, editors: *DeLee and Drez's orthopaedic sports medicine: principles and practice,* ed 3, Philadephia, 2009, WB Saunders.)

3. Fascicles contain muscle **fibers**, the basic unit of contraction.
   - A muscle fiber is an elongated cell.
   - Fibers are usually parallel but can run oblique to one another (e.g., bipennate muscle).
   - Fiber architecture is specific for the required function.
4. Fibers are composed of **myofibrils** (1 to 3 μm in diameter and 1 to 2 cm long).
5. A myofibril is a collection of **sarcomeres.**
6. Sarcomeres are characterized as follows:
   - Thick **(myosin)** and thin **(actin)** filaments arranged to allow fibers to slide past each other
   - Arranged into bands and lines (see Figure 1-64, Table 1-26)
   - The H band: contains only thick (myosin) filaments
   - The I band: composed solely of thin (actin) filaments
   - The A band lies between I bands and contains the H band.
   - Thin filaments are attached to the Z line.

- ▫ Thin filaments extend across I bands and partially into the A band.
- ▫ Each sarcomere is bounded by two adjacent Z lines.

C. Action

1. Contraction is the following process:
   - Muscle tissue response to electrochemical or mechanical stimuli.
   - Tension develops.
2. Stimulus for contraction originates in the cell body of a nerve.
   - Carried toward the neuromuscular junction via an electrical impulse
   - Propagated down the length of the axon from spinal cord to muscle
3. The impulse reaches the **motor end plate,** a specialized synapse formed between muscle and nerves (Figure 1-66).
   - Acetylcholine (stored in presynaptic vesicles) is released.
4. Acetylcholine diffuses across the **synaptic cleft** (50 nm).
   - Acetylcholine binds to a specific receptor on the muscle membrane
     - ▫ Myasthenia gravis is a shortage of acetylcholine receptors.
     - ▫ Botulinum A injections reduce spasticity by blocking presynaptic acetylcholine release.
   - Acetylcholine binding depolarizes the sarcoplasmic reticulum.
     - ▫ This causes the release of calcium into the muscle cytoplasm.

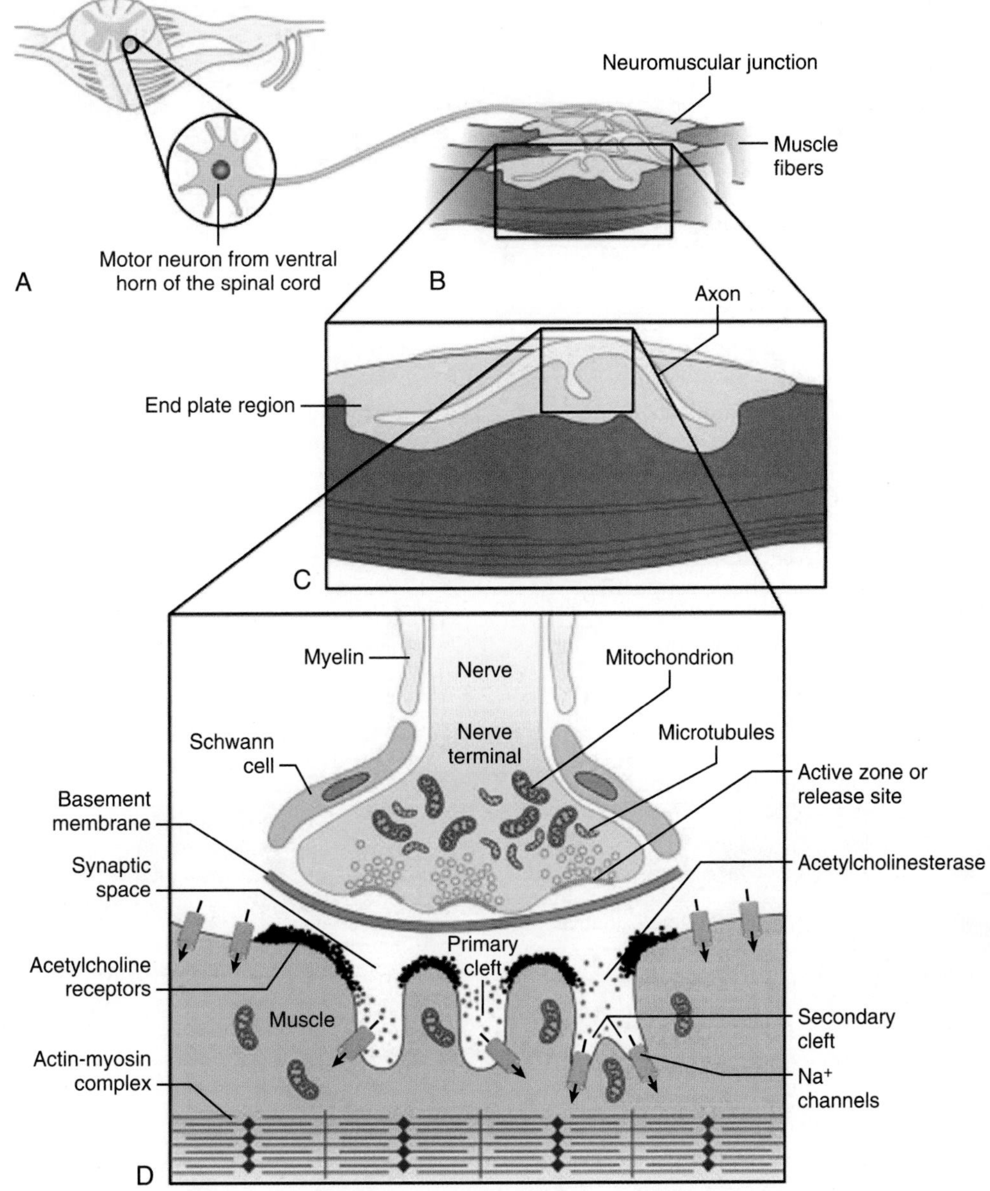

Figure 1-66 Structure of the adult motor end plate (neuromuscular junction). **A,** The motor nerve. **B,** The nerve branches that innervate many individual muscle fibers. **C,** The presynaptic boutons, which terminate on the muscle fiber. **D,** The nerve terminal. (From Miller RD, et al: *Miller's anesthesia,* ed 7, Philadelphia, 2010, Churchill Livingstone.)

Table 1-28 Types of Muscle Contractions

Type of Muscle Contraction	Definition	Example	Phases
Isotonic	**Muscle tension is constant** throughout the ROM. Muscle length changes throughout the ROM. This is a measure of dynamic strength.	Biceps curls with free weights	Concentric contraction: The muscle shortens during the contraction. Tension within the muscle is proportional to the externally applied load. An example of an isotonic concentric contraction is the "curl" (elbow moving toward increasing flexion) portion of a biceps curl. Eccentric contraction: The muscle lengthens during the contraction (internal force is less than external force). Eccentric contractions are the most efficient way to strengthen muscle but have the greatest potential for high muscle tension and muscle injury. An example of an isotonic eccentric contraction is "the negative" (elbow moving toward increasing extension) portion of a biceps curl.
Isometric	Muscle tension is generated, but the **muscle length remains unchanged.** This is a measure of static strength.	Pushing against an immovable object (such as a wall)	
Isokinetic	Muscle tension is generated as the muscle maximally contracts at a **constant velocity** over a full ROM. Isokinetic exercises are best for maximizing strength and are a measure of dynamic strength.	Isokinetic exercises require special equipment, such as a Cybex machine.	Concentric contraction Eccentric contraction

ROM, range of motion.

5. Calcium binds to troponin (on the thin filaments).
   - Causing change in position of tropomycin (also on the thin filaments)
   - Exposes the actin filament
6. Actin-myosin cross-bridges form.
   - With the breakdown of ATP, the thick and thin filaments slide past one another, contracting the muscle.
7. Certain agents affect impulse transmission (see Table 1-27).

D. Types of muscle contractions (Table 1-28)

E. Types of muscle fibers (Table 1-29)

1. **Slow-twitch (type I; oxidative; "red") fibers**
   - Aerobic
   - Have more mitochondria, enzymes, and triglycerides (energy source) than do type II fibers
   - Low concentrations of glycogen and glycolytic enzymes (adenosine triphosphatase [ATPase])
   - Mnemonic: "slow red ox"; type I fibers are characterized thus:

Table 1-29 Characteristics of Types of Human Skeletal Muscle Fibers

	TYPES		
Characteristic	Type I	Type IIA	Type IIB
Other names	Red, slow-twitch Slow oxidative	White, fast-twitch Fast oxidative glycolytic	Fast glycolytic
Speed of contraction	Slow	Fast	Fast
Strength of contraction	Low	High	High
Fatigability	Fatigue-resistant	Fatigable	Most fatigable
Aerobic capacity	High	Medium	Low
Anaerobic capacity	Low	Medium	High
Motor unit size	Small	Larger	Largest
Capillary density	High	High	Low

From Simon SR, editor: *Orthopaedic basic science,* Rosemont, Ill, 1994, American Academy of Orthopaedic Surgeons, p 100.

- Slower
- More vascular (red)
- Undergoing aerobic oxidation
- Enable performing endurance activities, posture, balance
- Are the first lost without rehabilitation

2. **Fast-twitch (type II; glycolytic; "white") fibers**
   - Anaerobic
   - Contract more quickly and have larger, stronger motor units (increased ATPase) than do type I fibers
     - However, are less efficient for these reasons
   - Develop a large amount of force per cross-sectional area
     - With high contraction speeds and quick relaxation times
   - Well suited for high-intensity, short-duration activities (e.g., sprinting)
     - Fatigue rapidly
   - Low intramuscular triglyceride stores
   - Types IIA and IIB fibers are associated with sprinting.
     - ATP–creatine phosphate system.
     - Subtypes are based on myosin heavy chains.

F. **Energetics (Figure 1-67)**

1. **ATP–creatine phosphate system (phosphagen system)**
   - For intense muscle activities lasting up to 20 seconds
     - For example, sprinting in a 100- or 200-m dash
   - Converts carbohydrates stored within the muscle fiber to energy
   - Does not use oxygen and does not produce lactate
   - Energy derived from high-energy phosphate bonds during hydrolysis:

$$\text{ATP} \rightarrow \text{Adenosine diphosphate (ADP)} + \text{Phosphate} + \text{Energy}$$

$$\text{ADP} \rightarrow \text{Adenosine monophosphate (AMP)} + \text{Phosphate} + \text{Energy}$$

2. **Lactic anaerobic system (lactic acid metabolism)** (Figure 1-68)
   - For intense muscle activities lasting 20 to 120 seconds
     - For example, a 400-m sprint
   - Involves hydrolysis of one glucose molecule to ultimately produce lactic acid plus energy
     - Converts two molecules of ADP to two molecules of ATP
3. **Aerobic system** (Figure 1-69; see also Figure 1-68)
   - The body depends on this system for muscle activities of longer duration and lower intensity.

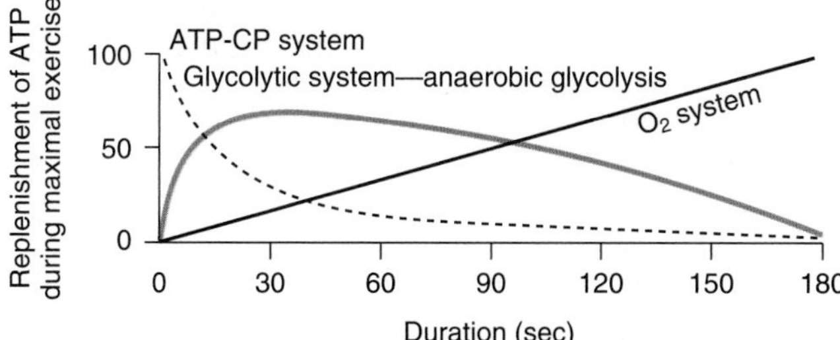

Figure 1-67 Energy sources for muscle activity. ATP, adenosine triphosphate; CP, creatine phosphate. (From Simon SR, editor: *Orthopaedic basic science,* Rosemont, Ill, 1994, American Academy of Orthopaedic Surgeons, p 102.)

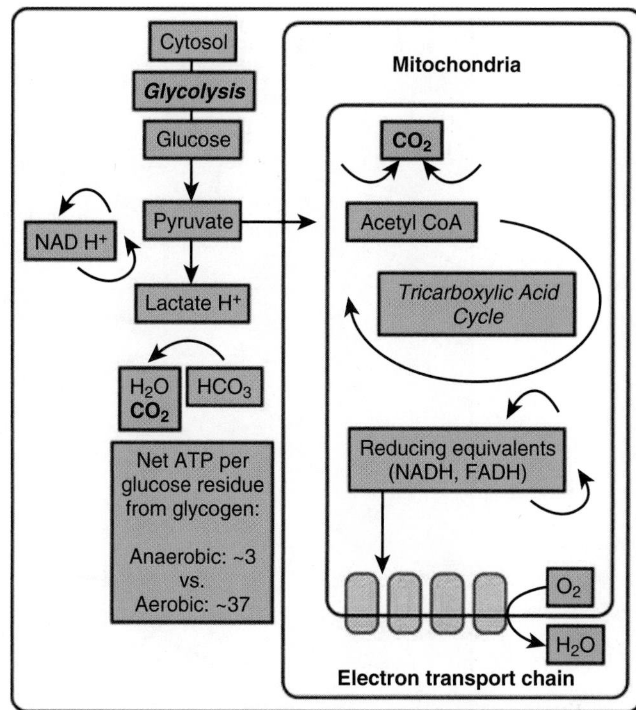

Figure 1-68 Adenosine triphosphate (ATP) production through anaerobic and aerobic breakdown of carbohydrates. Glycolysis and anaerobic metabolism occur in the cytoplasm; oxidative phosphorylation occurs in the mitochondria. CoA, coenzyme A; FADH, flavin adenine dinucleotide (reduced form); NAD, nicotinamide adenine dinucleotide; NADH, reduced form of NAD. (From Mason RJ, et al: *Murray and Nadel's textbook of respiratory medicine,* ed 5, Philadelphia, 2010, WB Saunders.)

   - When oxygen is available, the aerobic system replenishes ATP through oxidative phosphorylation and the Krebs (or citric acid or tricarboxylic acid) cycle.
     - Glucose or fatty acids are used to produce ATP.

G. **Athletes and training**

1. Distribution of fast-twitch versus slow-twitch fibers: genetically determined
   - However, specific training can selectively improve these fibers.
2. Endurance athletes typically have a higher percentage of slow-twitch fibers.
   - Sprinters and athletes in "strength"-type sports have more fast-twitch fibers.
3. **Endurance training**
   - Consists of decreased tension and increased repetitions
     - Induces hypertrophy of the slow-twitch fibers
     - Increases capillary density, mitochondria, and oxidative capacity
     - Increases resistance to fatigue
   - Also improves blood lipid profiles
4. **Strength training**
   - Consists of increased tension and decreased repetitions
     - This type of training increases myofibrils/fibers.
     - It induces hypertrophy (increased cross-sectional area) of fast-twitch (type II) fibers.
       - Skeletal muscle cross-sectional area is a reliably predictor of the potential for contractile force.

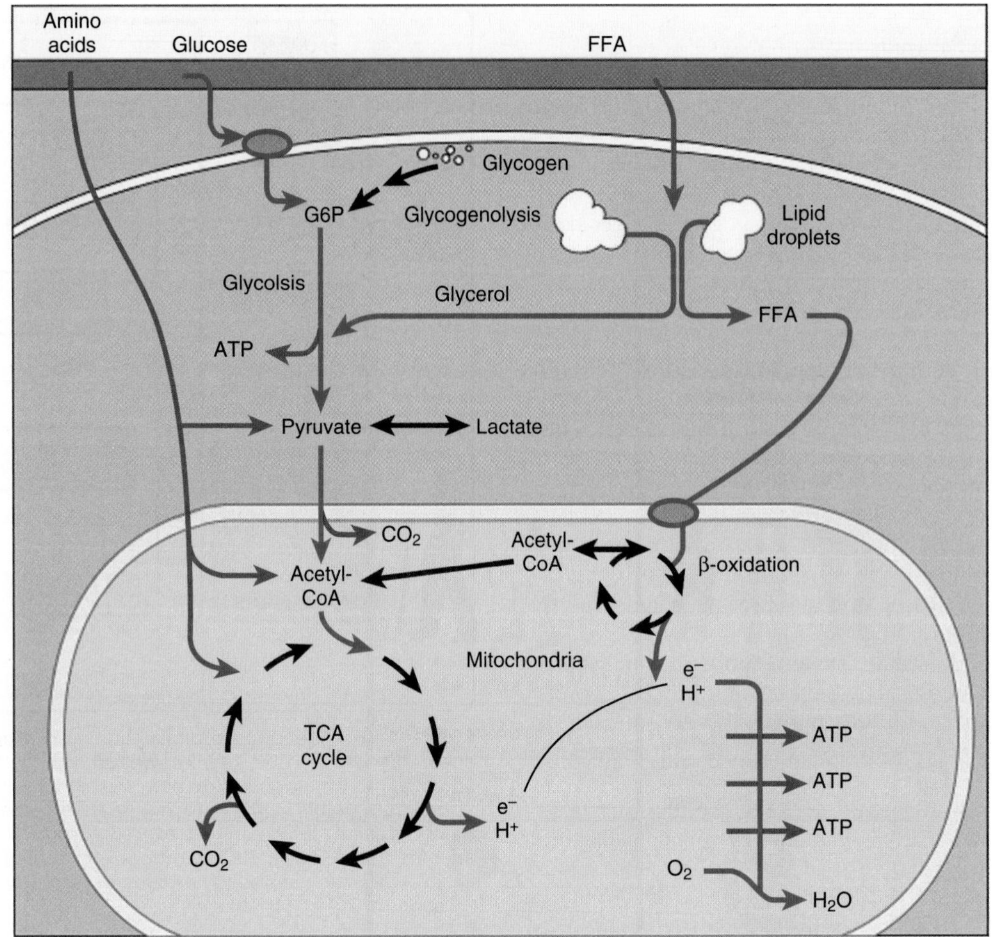

Figure 1-69 Energy metabolism: carbohydrates, fats, and proteins can enter the pathway to produce adenosine triphosphate (ATP). CoA, coenzyme A; FFA, free fatty acid; G6P, glucose-6-phosphate; TCA, tricarboxylic acid. (From DeLee JC, et al, editors: *DeLee and Drez's orthopaedic sports medicine: principles and practice*, ed 3, Philadephia, 2009, WB Saunders.)

- A well-conditioned muscle may be able to fire over 90% of its fibers simultaneously.
- Isokinetic exercises produce more strength gains than do isometric exercises.
- Isotonic exercises produce a uniform strength increase throughout joint ROM.
- Plyometric ("bounding") exercises consist of a muscle stretch followed immediately by a rapid contraction.
  - The stretch stores elastic energy, which increases the force of the concentric muscle contraction.
  - This is the most efficient method of improving power.
- Closed-chain exercise involves loading an extremity with the most distal segment stabilized or not moving.
  - Allows muscular cocontraction around a joint and minimizes joint shear (e.g., less stress on the anterior cruciate ligament [ACL])

5. Both endurance and strength training delay the lactate response to exercise.
6. Oxygen consumption (V_{O_2}) is an important consideration for athletes in training.
7. **Aerobic conditioning promotes cardiorespiratory fitness**
   - In contrast to resistance exercise, aerobic exercise increases stroke volume, which increases cardiac output.
   - To maintain health and reduce risk of disease for healthy adults:
     - 5 days per week, 30 minutes per session, moderate intensity (e.g., brisk walking)
     - Alternately, vigorous intensity exercise (e.g., jogging) 3 days a week for 20 minutes per session
     - More exercise needed to improve maximum aerobic capacity and performance
     - A significant decline in aerobic fitness ("detraining") occurs after only 2 weeks of no training
   - Aerobic conditioning lowers the incidence of back injury in workers and helps elderly persons remain ambulatory.
8. Anabolic (androgenic) steroids and growth hormone are widely used.
   - Anabolic (androgenic) steroids
     - Increase muscle strength
       - Increase messenger RNA and protein synthesis
       - Increase aggressive behavior that promotes increased weight training
     - Increase body weight
     - Side effects

- Testicular atrophy
- Irreversible deepening of the female voice
- Reduction in testosterone and gonadotropic hormones
- Growth retardation
- Oligospermia, azoospermia
- Gynecomastia
- Hypertension
- Striae
- Cystic acne
- Alopecia (irreversible)
- Liver tumors
- Raised low-density lipoprotein (LDL) levels and lower high-density lipoprotein (HDL) levels
- Abnormal amounts of the liver isoenzyme lactate dehydrogenase
- Do not increase aerobic power or capacity for muscular exercise
  - More effective than corticosteroids for long-term muscle strength recovery after contusion
- Pure testosterone extract has both anabolic and androgenic effects.
  - Anabolic effects include increased muscle development and mass, erythropoiesis.
- Testing for anabolic steroids is conducted by the International Olympic Committee through urine sampling.
- Abuse of the **growth hormone somatotropin** has adverse effects:
  - Selective hypertrophy of type I muscle fibers
  - Atrophy of type II fibers
  - Muscle hypertrophy with weakness and fatigue

9. Nutrition
   - **Weight reduction** with fluid and food restriction (wrestlers, boxers, and jockeys trying to "make weight") may result in several pathologic developments:
     - Reduced cardiac output
     - Increased heart rate
     - Smaller stroke volume
     - Lower oxygen consumption
     - Decreased renal blood flow
     - Electrolyte loss
   - **Carbohydrate loading** is often practiced by athletes.
     - Increasing carbohydrates and decreasing physical activity 3 days before an event (e.g., marathon)
   - **Fluid replacement** regimen is recommended for competitive athletes.
     - Consuming enough water to maintain prepractice weight, and maintaining a normal diet
   - Replacement of fluids, carbohydrates, and electrolytes is most effective when the fluid's osmolality is less than 10%.
     - Low-osmolality solutions enhance fluid absorption by the gut.
     - Glucose polymers minimize osmolality.
   - **Creatine supplements** are used by some athletes to enhance performance.
     - Creatine is converted to phosphocreatine, which acts as an energy reservoir for ATP in muscle.
     - Creatine supplementation can increase work produced in the first few maximum-effort anaerobic trials but does not increase peak force production.

- Treatment for heat cramps includes the following:
  - Passive stretching
  - Cooling
  - Fluid/electrolyte replacement

H. The "female athlete triad" (anorexia athletica)

1. **Amenorrhea**
   - Results from low body fat, energy imbalance, and changes in the hypothalamic-pituitary axis
2. **Osteoporosis**
   - Amenorrhea leads to bone demineralization.
3. **Anorexia**
4. Athletes with stress fracture and a history of amenorrhea should undergo bone mineral density testing.
5. Initial management
   - Energy balance: increase weight/food intake, decrease exercise
   - Possibly cyclic estrogens or progesterones
   - Possibly counseling for eating behaviors

I. Muscle injury

1. **Muscle strains**
   - These are the most common sports injury.
   - Most occur at the myotendinous junction.
   - They occur primarily in muscles crossing two joints (hamstring, gastrocnemius) that have increased type II fibers.
   - Initially there is inflammation and later fibrosis.
2. **Muscle tears**
   - Most occur at the myotendinous junction.
   - They often occur during a rapid (high-velocity) eccentric contraction.
     - Eccentric contractions develop the highest forces.
   - They typically heal with dense scarring.
   - Surgical repair of clean lacerations in the muscle midbelly usually results in minimal regeneration of muscle fibers distally, scar formation at the laceration, and recovery of about half the muscle strength.
   - Muscle activation (through stretching) allows twice the energy absorption before failure.
3. **Delayed-onset muscle soreness (DOMS)**
   - This phenomenon occurs 24 to 72 hours after intense exercise.
   - It may result from eccentric muscle contractions.
   - It may be associated with changes in the I band of the sarcomere.
   - NSAIDs relieve DOMS in a dose-dependent manner.
   - Massage has varying effects.
   - Other modalities (ice, stretching, ultrasonography, electrical stimulation) have not been shown to affect DOMS.
4. Denervation
   - This causes muscle atrophy and increased sensitivity to acetylcholine.
   - It leads to spontaneous fibrillations at 2 to 4 weeks after injury.
5. Spasticity: increased muscle reactivity to stretch

J. Immobilization

1. Immobilization changes the number of sarcomeres at the musculotendinous junction.
2. It accelerates granulation tissue response.
3. Immobilization in lengthened positions decreases contractures and maintains strength.
4. Atrophy results from disuse or altered recruitment.
   - Electrical stimulation can help offset these effects.

II. NERVOUS SYSTEM

A. Organization

1. Central nervous system
   - Improvement in function: may continue up to 6 months after a stroke and up to 18 months after traumatic brain injury
   - Spinal cord injury
     - Motor vehicle accident: the most common mechanism in adults
     - Spinal (neurogenic) shock
       - A state of vasodilation: paradoxic hypotension and bradycardia; absence of bulbocavernosus reflex
       - Occurs after cervical or upper thoracic spinal cord injury
       - Occurs because the descending sympathetic pathways are disrupted
       - Treated by positioning, pressor agents, and atropine
     - Patients with spinal cord injury may be given **methylprednisolone:**
       - If injury occurred less than 3 hours earlier: an initial bolus of 30 mg/kg over 15 minutes, followed by an infusion of 5.4 mg/kg/hr for 23 hours
       - If injury occurred between 3 and 8 hours earlier: an initial bolus of 30 mg/kg over 15 minutes, followed by an infusion of 5.4 mg/kg/hr for 47 hours
       - Decreases extent of cord hemorrhage
         - Does not affect cord edema
       - Considerable controversy regarding this protocol
       - May improve root function at the level of the injury
         - Spinal cord function may or may not improve.
       - Not indicated for nerve root deficits, brachial plexus deficits, or gunshot wounds
2. Peripheral nervous system (Figure 1-70)
   - Nerves
     - Axon bundles enclosed in a connective tissue sheath
   - Nerve fiber
     - Axon plus surrounding Schwann cell (myelin) sheath
     - Myelinated fibers
       - An axon 1 to 2 μm in diameter is considered myelinated.
       - Each myelinated axon is associated with one Schwann cell.
       - Conduction velocity is faster than in unmyelinated fibers.
     - Unmyelinated fibers

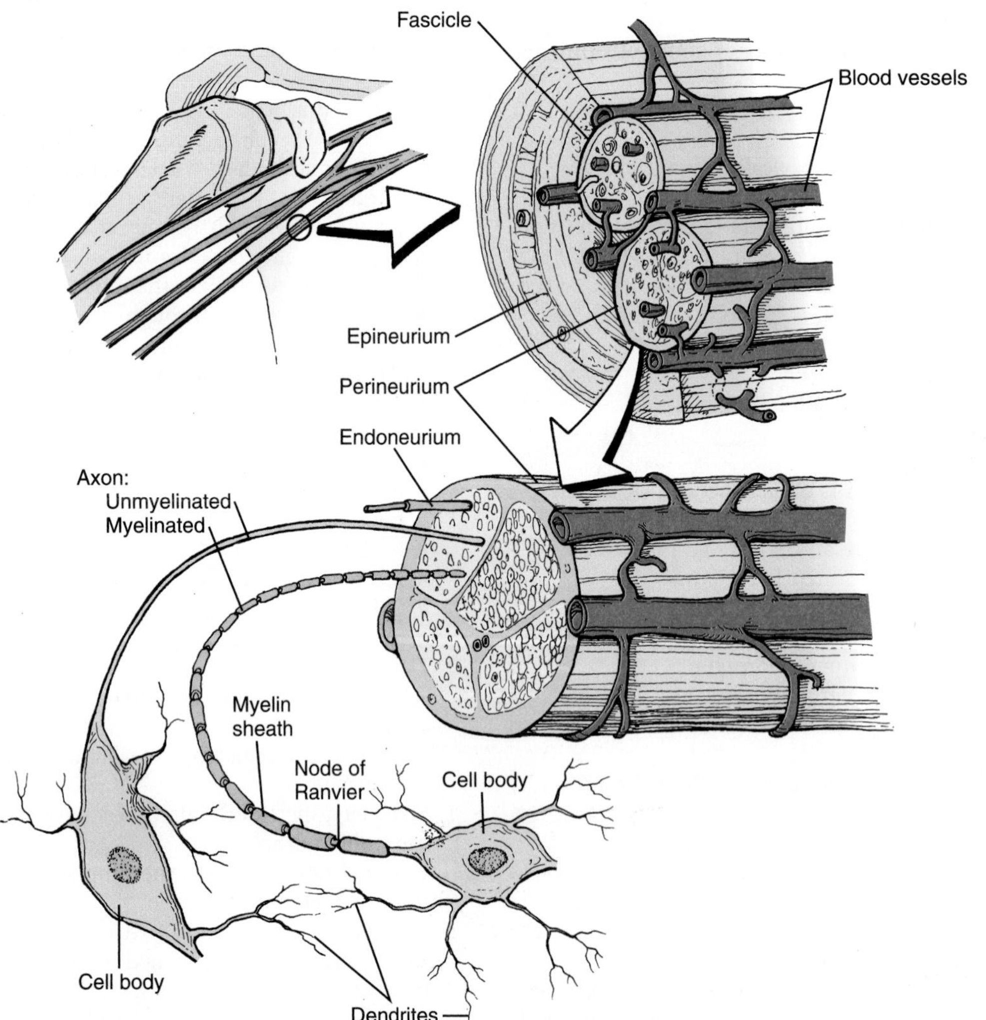

Figure 1-70 Nerve architecture. (From Brinker MR, Miller MD: *Fundamentals of orthopaedics,* Philadelphia, 1999, WB Saunders, p 13.)

- One Schwann cell surrounds several axons.
- Conduction velocity is relatively slow.

□ Afferent fibers

- Afferent fibers transmit from sensory receptors to the CNS.
- *Somatic afferent fibers* originate in receptors in muscle, skin, and sense organs of the head (vision, hearing, taste, smell).
- *Visceral afferent fibers* originate in viscera.

□ Efferent fibers

- Transmit from the CNS to the periphery.
- *Motor efferent fibers* innervate skeletal muscle fibers.
- *Somatic efferent fibers* innervate skin, skeletal muscle, and joints.
- *Autonomic efferent fibers* (splanchnic fibers) innervate viscera.

B. Histologic study and signal generation

1. Neuron (see Figure 1-70)
   - Cell body
     - □ Metabolic center
     - □ Accounts for less than 10% of neuron size
     - □ Gives rise to a single axon
   - Axon
     - □ Primary conducting vehicle of the neuron
     - □ Conveys electrical signals (over long distances) via action potentials
   - Dendrites
     - □ Thin processes branching from the cell body
     - □ Receive input (synaptic) from surrounding nerve cells
   - Presynaptic terminals
     - □ Transmit information from one neuron to another
       - To the cell body or dendrites of the "receiving" neuron
2. Glial cells (Figure 1-71)
   - **Schwann cells**
     - □ These cells are responsible for myelinating peripheral nerve axons.
       - Form an elongated double-membrane structure
     - □ Loss of the myelin sheath (demyelination) disrupts conduction of action potentials along the axon.
     - □ Myelin is 70% lipid and 30% protein.
   - Oligodendrocytes
     - □ Only in the CNS
     - □ Form myelin
   - Astrocytes
     - □ Only in the CNS
     - □ Most common of the glial cells
     - □ Have many functions but are primarily a supporting structure of the brain
3. Resting and action potentials
   - Resting potential
     - □ A resting potential results from unequal distribution of ions on either side of the neuronal cell membrane (lipid bilayer).

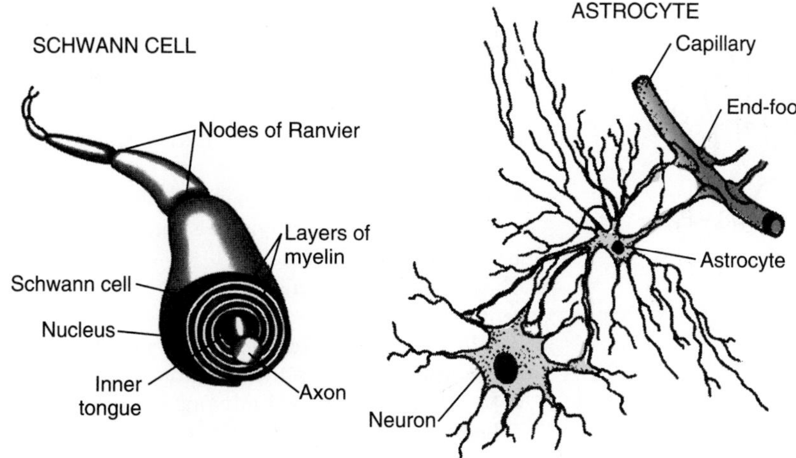

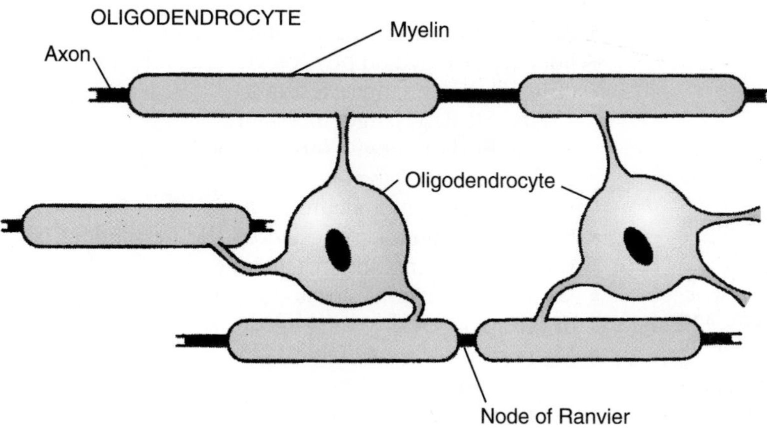

Figure 1-71 Glial cells include the Schwann cell, astrocytes, and oligodendrocytes. (From Simon SR, editor: *Orthopaedic basic science,* Rosemont, Ill, 1994, American Academy of Orthopaedic Surgeons, p 320.)

- The most plentiful ions are Na^+, K^+, Cl^-, and a group of organic ions (A^-).
- The resting potential is −50 to −80 mV.
  - The inside of a cell has negative charge in relation to the outside (Figure 1-72).

- Action potential
  - Action potentials transmit signals rapidly through electrical impulses to other neurons or effector organs (e.g., muscle).
  - Depolarization and the action potential result from increased cell membrane permeability to Na^+ in response to a stimulus.
  - Action potentials are related to three types of gated ion channels (Figure 1-73):
    - Voltage-gated channels
    - Mechanically gated channels
    - Chemical transmitter–gated channels
  - They are propagated through both passive current flow and active membrane changes (Figure 1-74).

C. **Sensory system**

1. **Sensory receptors** (located peripherally) receive messages from the environment and other parts of the body and transmit them to the CNS.

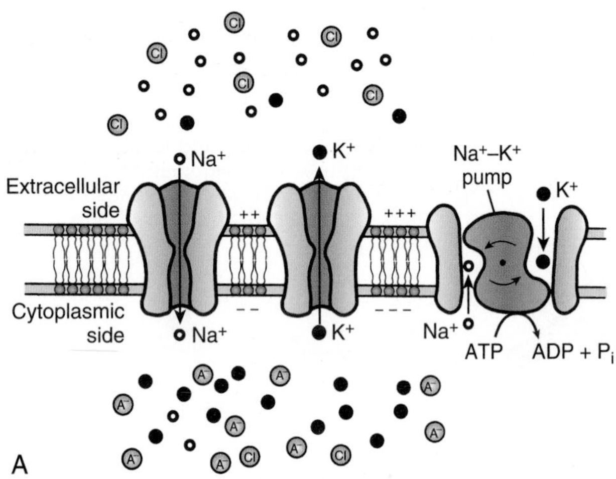

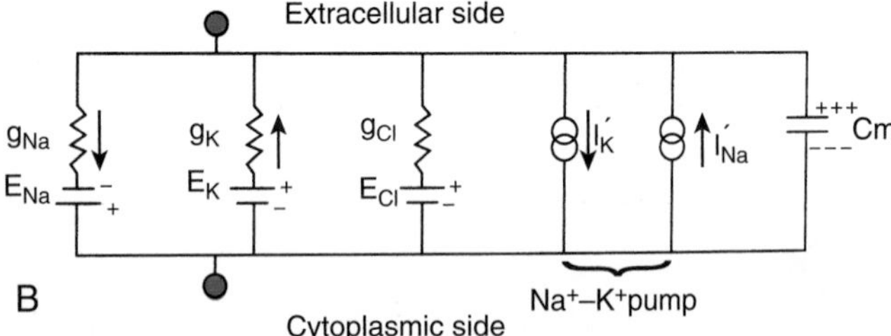

Figure 1-72 Electrolyte transport across cell walls. **A,** Passive fluxes of Na^+ and K^+ into and out of the cell are balanced by the energy-dependent sodium-potassium pump. **B,** Electrical circuit model of a neuron at rest. ADP, adenosine diphosphate; ATP, adenosine triphosphate; Cm, mutual capacitance; E_{Cl}, E_K, and E_{Na}, equilibrium potentials of chloride, potassium, and sodium, respectively; g_{Cl}, g_K, and g_{Na}, conductances of chloride, potassium, and sodium, respectively; I_K and I_{Na}, currents of potassium and sodium, respectively; P_i, inorganic phosphate. (From Simon SR, editor: *Orthopaedic basic science*, Rosemont, Ill, 1994, American Academy of Orthopaedic Surgeons, p 332.)

2. The four attributes of a stimulus are quality, intensity, duration, and location.
3. There are five sensory receptor types:
   - Photoreceptors (vision)
   - Mechanoreceptors (hearing, balance, mechanical stimuli)
   - Thermoreceptors (temperature)
   - Chemoreceptors (taste, smell)
   - Nociceptors (pain)
4. Neurogenic pain (and inflammatory) mediators are identifiable within the dorsal root ganglion of the lumbar spine.
5. The pain with osteoid osteoma is from prostaglandins secreted by the tumor itself.
6. Somatosensory system has the following characteristics:
   - Conveys three types of modalities: mechanical, pain, and thermal
   - Each mediated by a specific type of sensory receptor (Table 1-30)
   - Input transmitted to the spinal cord (or brainstem) via the **dorsal root ganglion** (Figure 1-75)

D. **Motor system**

1. Organized into four areas:
   - Spinal cord
   - Brainstem
   - Motor cortex
   - Premotor cortical areas (basal ganglia and cerebellum)
2. Spinal cord (see Figure 1-75)
   - White matter (peripheral)
     - Ascending and descending fiber tracts
     - Myelinated and unmyelinated axons
   - Gray matter (central)
     - Contains neuronal cell bodies, glial cells, dendrites, and axons (myelinated and unmyelinated)
     - Contains three types of neurons
       - Motoneurons (α and γ): Axons exit via ventral roots.
       - Interneurons: Axons remain in the spinal cord.
       - Tract cells: Axons ascend to supraspinal centers.
   - Spinal cord reflexes (Table 1-31)
     - These reflexes are "stereotyped responses" to a specific sensory stimulus.
     - **A reflex pathway** involves a sensory organ (receptor), an interneuron, and a motoneuron.
       - Monosynaptic reflex: Only one synapse is involved between receptor and effector.
       - Polysynaptic reflex: One or more interneurons are involved. Most human reflexes are polysynaptic.
3. Motor unit
   - An α-motoneuron and the muscle fibers it innervates
   - Four types, based on physiologic demands (Table 1-32):
     - Type S (slow, fatigue resistant)
     - Type FR (fast, fatigue resistant)
     - Type FI (fast, fatigue intermediate)
     - Type FF (fast, fatigable)
4. Upper and lower motoneurons
   - Upper motoneurons: located in the descending pathways of the cortex, brainstem, and spinal cord
   - Lower motoneurons: located in the ventral gray matter of the spinal cord
   - Motoneuron lesions (Table 1-33)
     - Spasticity is common in patients with an upper motoneuron lesion.

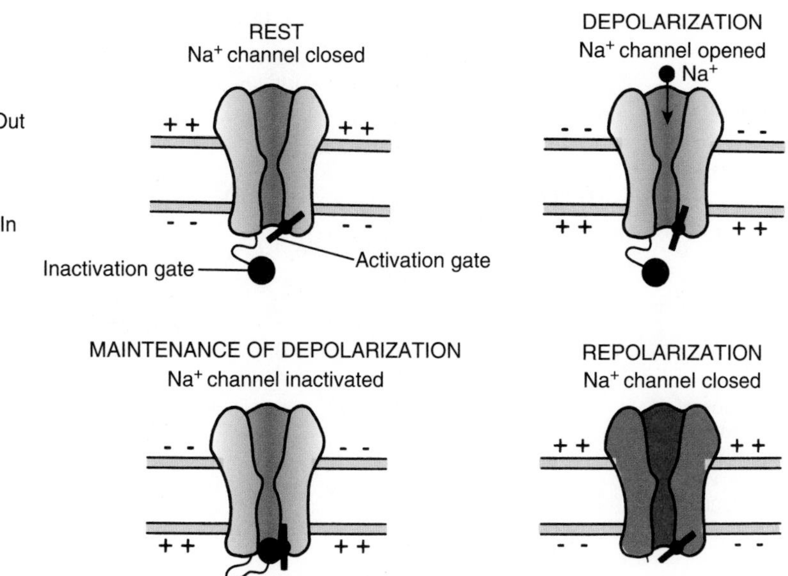

Figure 1-73 **Gated sodium channel response during an action potential.** (From Kandel ER, et al: *Principles of neural science,* ed 3, Norwalk, Conn, 1991, Appleton & Lange, p 14.)

E. Peripheral nerve

1. Morphologic features (see Figure 1-70):
   - A highly organized structure
     - Nerve fibers, blood vessels, and connective tissues
   - Axons coated with a fibrous tissue called **endoneurium**
     - Axons are grouped into nerve bundles called **fascicles.**
     - Fascicles are covered with connective tissue called **perineurium.**
   - Peripheral nerves: composed of one fascicle (monofascicular), a few fascicles (oligofascicular), or several fascicles (polyfascicular)
     - Surrounding areolar connective tissue **(epineurium)** is enclosed within an epineural sheath.
2. Nerve fibers (axons) (2 to 25 μm in diameter) (Table 1-34)
3. Conduction
   - As previously discussed, myelinated axons conduct action potentials rapidly.

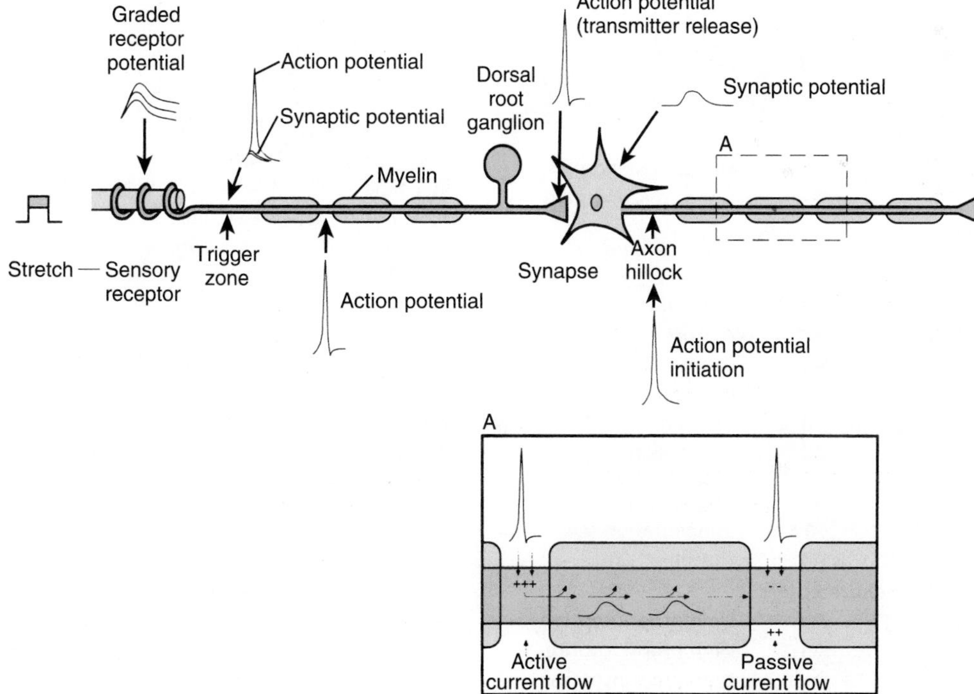

Figure 1-74 Propagation of action potentials. An action potential is propagated to the terminal region, where it triggers the release of a transmitter, which initiates a synaptic potential in the motoneuron. Action potential propagation results from the spread of local passive depolarizing currents between the nodes of Ranvier (A). At the nodes, voltage-gated channels open, producing an action potential. (From Simon SR, editor: *Orthopaedic basic science,* Rosemont, Ill, 1994, American Academy of Orthopaedic Surgeons, p 337.)

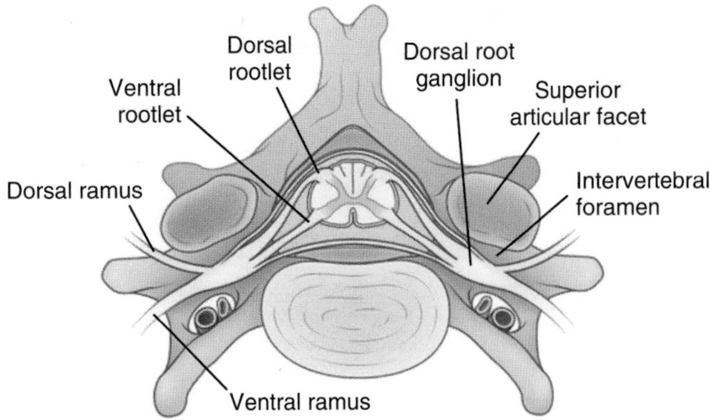

Figure 1-75 Spinal cord anatomy. Each spinal nerve has a dorsal (sensory) and a ventral (motor) root. Dorsal roots are branches from dorsal root ganglia cells; ventral roots are motor axons from cells in the ventral horn. (From Bradley WG, et al [editors]: *Neurology in clinical practice,* ed 5. Philadelphia, 2008, Butterworth-Heinemann.)

- □ Facilitated by **nodes of Ranvier** (gaps between Schwann cells)

4. Blood supply
   - Extrinsic: vessels in loose connective tissue surrounding the nerve trunk
   - Intrinsic: vascular plexuses in the epineurium, perineurium, and endoneurium

F. **Injury to the nervous system (Table 1-35)**

1. Types of injuries
   - Peripheral nerve injury leads to death of the distal axons and **Wallerian degeneration** (of myelin).
     - □ Extends to the somatosensory receptor

Table 1-30 Receptor Types

Receptor Type	Fiber Type	Quality
Nociceptors		
Mechanical	Aδ	Sharp, pricking pain
Thermal and mechanothermal	Aγ	Sharp, pricking pain
Thermal and mechanothermal	C	Slow, burning pain
Polymodal	C	Slow, burning pain
Cutaneous and Subcutaneous Mechanoreceptors		
Meissner's corpuscle	Aβ	Touch
Pacini's corpuscle	Aβ	Flutter
Ruffini's corpuscle	Aβ	Vibration
Merkel's receptor	Aβ	Steady skin indentation
Hair-guard, tylotrich hair	Aβ	Steady skin indentation
Hair down	Aβ	Flutter
Muscle and Skeletal Mechanoreceptors		
Muscle spindle, primary	Aα	Limb proprioception
Muscle spindle, secondary	Aβ	Limb proprioception
Golgi tendon organ	Aα	Limb proprioception
Joint capsule mechanoreceptor	Aβ	Limb proprioception

Adapted from Kandel ER, et al, editors: *Principles of neural science,* ed 3, Norwalk, Conn, 1991, Appleton & Lange, p 342.

Table 1-31 Summary of Spinal Reflexes

Segmental Reflex	Receptor Organ	Afferent Fiber
Phasic stretch reflex	Muscle spindle (primary endings)	Type Ia (large myelinated)
Tonic stretch reflex	Muscle spindle (secondary endings)	Type II (intermediate myelinated)
Clasp-knife response	Muscle spindle (secondary endings)	Type II (intermediate myelinated)
Flexion withdrawal reflex	Nociceptors (free nerve endings), touch and pressure receptors	Flexor-reflex afferents: small unmyelinated cutaneous afferents (Aδ, C and muscle afferent fibers, group III)
Autogenic inhibition	Golgi tendon organ	Type Ib (large myelinated)

From Simon SR, editor: *Orthopaedic basic science,* Rosemont, Ill, 1994, American Academy of Orthopaedic Surgeons, p 350.

Table 1-32 General Characteristics of Motor Unit Types

	MOTOR UNIT TYPES		
Parameter	*FF*	*FR*	*S*
Muscle Unit Physiology*			
Contraction time	Fastest	Slightly slower	Slowest
Sag	Present	Present	Absent
Maximum tension	Largest	Smaller	Smallest
Fatigue index	<0.25	<0.75-1.00	0.7-1.0
Muscle Unit Anatomy†			
Innervation ratio	2.9	2.1	1.0
Fiber cross-sectional area	1.3	0.98	1.0
Specific tension	1.4	1.2	1.0
Muscle Unit Metabolism			
Fiber type	FG	FOG	SO
Myosin heavy chain	IIB	IIA	I
Glycogen	High	High	Low
Hexokinase	Low	Intermediate	High
Glycolytic enzymes	High	High	Low
Oxidative enzymes	Low	High	High
Cytochrome c	Low	High	High
Capillary supply	Sparse	Rich	Very rich
Motoneuron			
Cell body size	Largest	Slightly smaller	Smallest
Conduction velocity	Fastest	Slightly slower	Slowest
After-hyperpolarization duration	Shortest	Slightly shorter	Longest
Input resistance	Lowest	Slightly higher	Highest

From Simon SR, editor: *Orthopaedic basic science,* Rosemont, Ill, 1994, American Academy of Orthopaedic Surgeons, p 344.

*Data relative to the FF unit.

†Data relative to the slow unit.

FF, fast, fatigable; FG, fast, glycolytic; FOG, fast, oxidative glycolytic; FR, fast, fatigue-resistant; S, slow, fatigue-resistant; SO, slow, oxidative.

Table 1-33 Findings in Upper and Lower Motoneuron Lesions

Findings	Upper Motoneuron Lesions	Lower Motoneuron Lesions
Strength	Decreased	Decreased
Tone	Increased	Decreased
Deep tendon reflexes	Increased	Decreased
Superficial tendon reflexes	Decreased	Decreased
Babinski's sign	Present	Absent
Clonus	Present	Absent
Fasciculations	Absent	Present
Atrophy	Absent	Present

From Simon SR, editor: *Orthopaedic basic science,* Rosemont, Ill, 1994, American Academy of Orthopaedic Surgeons, p 354.

Table 1-34 Types and Characteristics of Nerve Fibers

Type	Diameter (μm)	Myelination	Speed	Examples
A	10-20	Heavy	Fast	Touch
B	<3	Intermediate	Medium	Autonomic nervous system
C	<1.3	None	Slow	Pain

- Mechanical deformation of a compressed peripheral nerve is greatest in superficial regions and in zones between compressed and uncompressed segments.
- Nerve stretching can affect function.
  - Eight percent elongation diminishes microcirculation.
  - Fifteen percent elongation disrupts axons.
- The nucleus pulposus induces an inflammatory response when in contact with the nerve roots.
  - Leukotaxis
  - Increased vascular permeability
  - Decreased nerve conduction velocities

Table 1-35 Types and Characteristics of Nerve Injuries

Injury	Pathophysiologic Features	Prognosis
Neurapraxia	Reversible conduction block characterized by local ischemia and selective demyelination of the axon sheath	Good
Axonotmesis	More severe injury, with disruption of the axon and myelin sheath but leaving the epineurium intact	Fair
Neurotmesis	Complete nerve division, with disruption of the endoneurium	Poor

2. Nerve regeneration
   - Proximal axonal budding occurs after a 1-month delay.
     - Leads to regeneration at the rate of approximately 1 mm/day
     - Possibly 3 to 5 mm/day in children
   - Nerve regeneration is influenced by three processes:
     - Contact guidance (attraction of Schwann cell to the basal lamina)
     - Neurotrophism (factors enhancing growth)
     - Neurotropism (preferential attraction toward nerves rather than other tissues)
   - Pain is the first sensation to return.
3. Testing
   - Neurologic studies
     - Electromyography/nerve conduction study
     - May be useful for documenting the extent of injury
   - Cortical evoked potential testing
     - The most sensitive method of predicting neural compression
   - Histamine testing
     - In an brachial plexus injury, a positive histamine response implies that the reflex arc is intact.
     - A positive response also indicates that the lesion is proximal to the ganglion (preganglionic).

G. Nerve repair

1. Younger patients: better chance of recovery after operative repair of nerve transection
2. Proper alignment of nerve ends during surgical repair: crucial for maximizing potential for functional recovery
3. Direct muscular neurotization
   - Insertion of the proximal nerve stump into the affected muscle belly
   - Results in less than normal function but is indicated in selected cases
4. Epineural repair
   - Primary repair of the outer connective tissue layer at the site of injury
     - After resection of the proximal neuroma and distal glioma
   - Ensures proper rotation and lack of tension on the repair
5. Grouped fascicular repair
   - Identical to epineural repair, but reapproximates individual fascicles under microscopic guidance
   - Used for large nerves
   - Improved results over epineural repair have not been demonstrated

III. CONNECTIVE TISSUES

A. Tendons (Figure 1-76)

1. Dense, regularly arranged tissues that attach muscle to bone
2. Composition
   - Fascicles
     - Groups of collagen bundles
     - Separated by **endotenon** and surrounded by **epitenon**
   - Fibroblasts: the predominant cell type
     - Arranged in parallel rows (Figure 1-77)
     - Produce mostly **type I collagen** (85% of dry weight)
     - Also produce small amounts of type III collagen (5% dry weight)

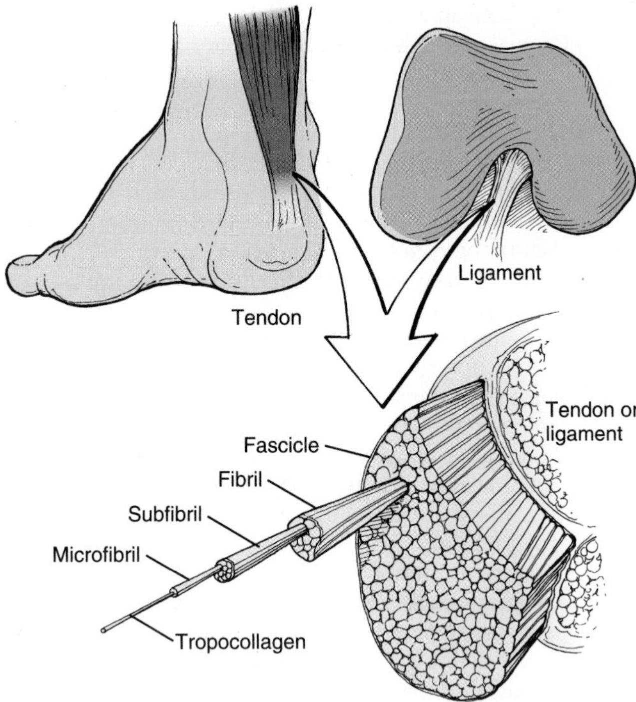

Figure 1-76 **Tendon and ligament architecture.** (From Brinker MR, Miller MD: *Fundamentals of orthopaedics,* Philadelphia, 1999, WB Saunders, p 15.)

3. Tendon inserts into bone by means of four transitional tissues (force dissipation)
   - Tendon
   - Fibrocartilage
   - Mineralized fibrocartilage (Sharpey's fibers)
   - Bone
4. Types
   - Paratenon-covered
     - Vascular tendons
     - Many vessels, rich capillary system (Figure 1-78)
     - High vascularity results in better healing
   - Sheathed

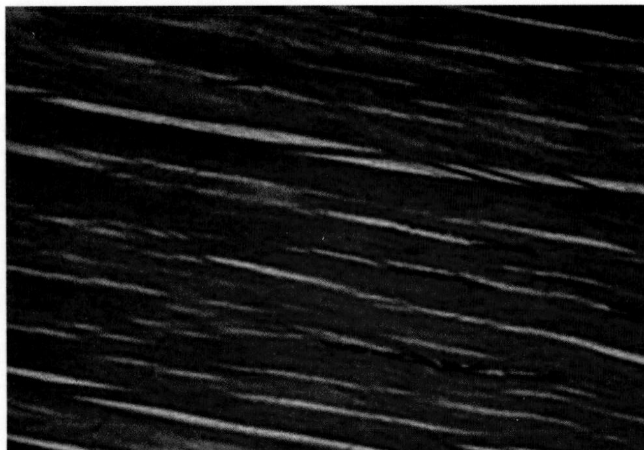

Figure 1-77 **Photomicrograph of a tendon, showing parallel rows of collagen bundles.** (From DeLee JC, et al, editors: *DeLee and Drez's orthopaedic sports medicine: principles and practice,* ed 3, Philadelphia, 2009, WB Saunders.)

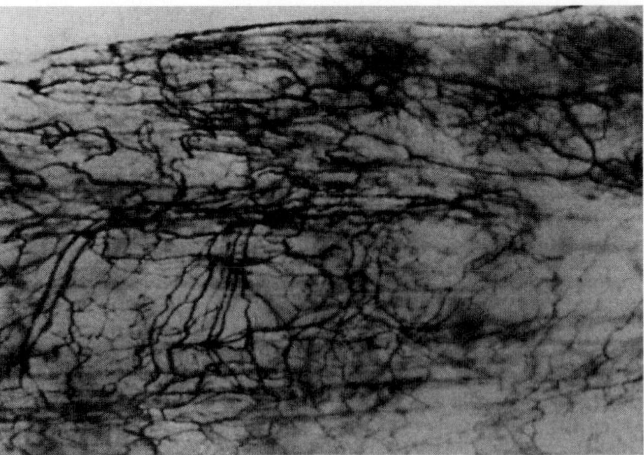

Figure 1-78 **India ink injection of rabbit calcaneal tendon (Spalteholtz's technique) demonstrates the vasculature of the paratenon.** (From Simon SR, editor: *Orthopaedic basic science,* Rosemont, Ill, 1994, American Academy of Orthopaedic Surgeons, p 50.)

     - A mesotenon (vinculum) carries a vessel that supplies only one tendon segment.
     - Avascular areas receive nutrition via diffusion (Figure 1-79).
5. Tendinous structures oriented along stress lines
6. Healing
   - Initiated by fibroblasts from the epitenon and macrophages
   - **Early healing with type III collagen**
     - Later converted to type I
   - The repair process affected by treatment
   - Surgical repairs: **weakest at 7 to 10 days**
     - Most of original strength regained at 21 to 28 days
     - **Maximum strength achieved at 6 months**
     - No evidence in favor of a trough (exposing the tendon to cancellous bone) over direct repair to cortical bone
   - Early mobilization
     - Increased ROM
     - However, decreased repair strength
   - Immobilization
     - Increased tendon substance strength
     - At the expense of ROM
     - Tends to decrease strength at tendon-bone interface
   - Bony avulsion: heals more rapidly than midsubstance tears

B. Ligaments (see Figure 1-76)

1. Attach bone to bone to stabilize joints
2. Composition
   - Primarily type I collagen **(90% of dry weight)**
   - Small amounts of type III collagen and elastin
   - Ultrastructure similar to that of tendons
     - Fibers more variable
     - **Higher elastin content**
     - "Uniform microvascularity," receives supply at insertion site
   - Contain mechanoreceptors and free nerve endings
     - May play a role in stabilizing joints
3. **Insertion**
   - Collagen sliding plays an important role in changes in ligament length (during growth and contracture).

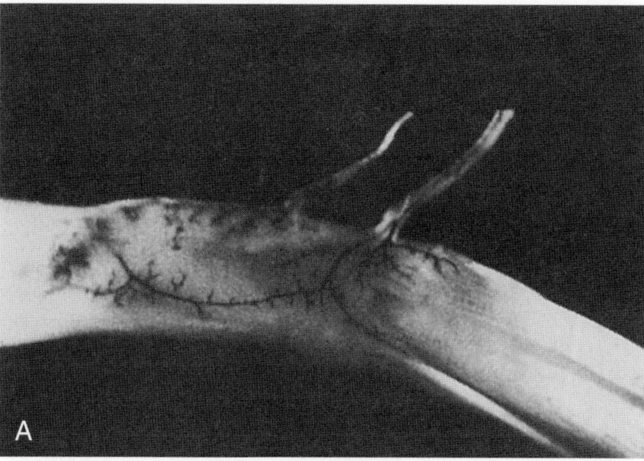

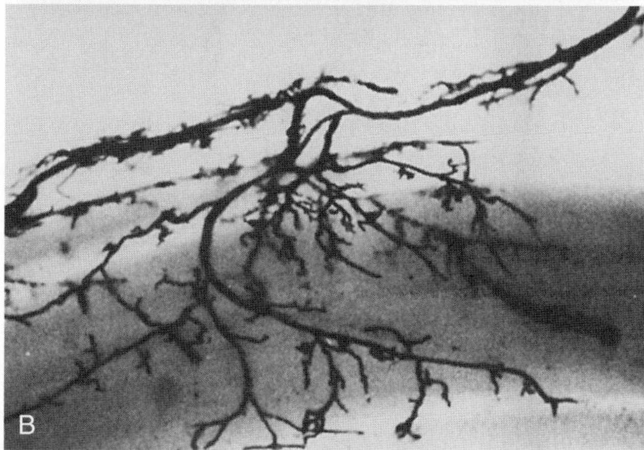

Figure 1-79 India ink specimens **(A, B)** demonstrating the vascular supply of the flexor tendons via vincula. **B,** Close-up of the specimen. (From Simon SR, editor: *Orthopaedic basic science,* ed 2, Rosemont, Ill, 1994, American Academy of Orthopaedic Surgeons, p 51.)

- **Ligament insertion into bone can be classified into two types:**
  - **Indirect insertion** (more common): superficial fibers
    - Insert at acute angles into the periosteum
  - **Direct insertion**: superficial and deep fibers
    - Deep fibers attach at 90-degree angles
    - **Ligament-to-bone transition in four phases: ligament, fibrocartilage, mineralized fibrocartilage, bone**

4. **Injury**
   - Most common ligament injury is rupture of sequential series of collagen fiber bundles.
     - Throughout the body of the ligament
     - Not localized to one specific area
   - Ligaments do not plastically deform.
     - They "break, not bend."
   - Midsubstance ligament tears are common in adults.
   - Avulsion injuries are more common in children.
     - Typically occurs between unmineralized and mineralized fibrocartilage layers
5. Healing
   - Three phases, as in bone
   - Benefits from normal stress and strain across the joint
     - Exercise increases mechanical and structural properties.
   - Local injection of corticosteroids: detrimental
   - **Early healing with type III collagen**
     - Later converted to type I
   - Immobilization
     - Adversely affects ligament strength: elastic modulus decreases
     - In rabbits, breaking strength reduced dramatically (66%) after 9 weeks of immobilization
     - Effects reverse slowly upon remobilization.

C. Intervertebral discs

1. Allow spinal motion and stability
2. Two components:
   - Central nucleus pulposus
     - A hydrated gel with compressibility
     - High glycosaminoglycan/low collagen content
   - Surrounding annulus fibrosis
     - Extensibility and increased tensile strength
     - High collagen/low glycosaminoglycan content
     - Superficial layer contains nerve fibers
3. Composition:
   - Water (85%)
   - Proteoglycans
   - Collagen type II in the nucleus pulposus
   - Collagen type I in the annulus fibrosis
4. **Avascular**
   - Nutrients and fluid diffuse through pores in hyaline cartilage end plates
5. **Aging disc**
   - Decreased water content
     - **A result of a lack of large proteoglycans and aggrecans**
     - **Also, decrease in proteoglycan concentration**
     - **Increase in keratin sulfate concentration**
   - Increase in collagen
6. Neuropeptides
   - Involved in sensory transmission, nociceptive transmission, neurogenic inflammation, and skeletal metabolism
   - Several types:
     - Substance P
     - Calcitonin gene–related peptide
     - Vasoactive intestinal peptide
     - C-flanking peptide of neuropeptide Y
7. Cigarette smoking: risk factor for degenerative disc disease

D. Soft tissue healing

1. Four phases:
   - Hemostasis
     - A primary platelet plug is formed within 5 minutes of injury.
     - Secondary clotting occurs through the coagulation cascade and fibrin within 10 to 15 minutes.
     - Fibronectin, a large glycoprotein, binds fibrin to cells and acts as a chemotactic factor.
     - Platelets release factors that activate the next phase of healing.
   - Inflammation
     - Macrophages cause débridement of injured/necrotic tissue within 1 week.
     - There are three stages:
       - Activation (immediate)
       - Amplification (in 48 to 72 hours)
       - Débridement (bacteria, phagocytosis, and matrix [biochemical])
     - Prostaglandins mediate the response.

- Organogenesis
  - Tissue modeling (in 7 to 21 days)
  - Differentiation of mesenchymal precursors into myofibroblasts
  - Angiogenesis
  - Further differentiation, which leads to the final stage of healing
- Remodeling (of individual tissue lines)
  - Continues for up to 18 months
  - Collagen realignment and cross-linking: increase tensile strength

2. Growth factors
   - Require activation, are redundant, have feedback loop mechanisms
   - Chemotactic factors (attracted cells)
     - Prostaglandins: PMNs
     - Prostanoids: PMNs
     - Complement: PMNs and macrophages
     - PDGF: macrophages and fibroblasts
     - Angiokines: endothelial cells
   - Competence factors: activate dormant (G_0) cells
     - PDGF
     - Prostaglandins
   - Progression factors: allow cell growth
     - Induce epidermal growth factor, IL-1, somatomedins
   - Inductive factors: stimulate differentiation
     - Angiokines
     - BMP
     - Specific tissue growth factors
   - Transforming factors: cause differentiation and proliferation
   - Permissive factors: enhancing factors
     - Fibronectin
     - Osteonectin

E. Soft tissue implants

1. Allografts
   - No donor-site morbidity
   - Incite an immune response
     - May transmit infection
     - **Risk of HIV exposure from a ligament allograft is 1:1,600,000**
   - Histologic recovery: slower and less predictable than that for autografts
   - Freeze-drying
     - Reduces the immunogenic response
     - Decreases strength
       - Deep freezing without drying does not affect strength.
   - Cryopreservation
     - Controlled rate freezing in a protective medium
     - Prevents ice crystal formation
     - Preserves some cell viability and protein structure
     - Strength at 6 months comparable to that for autograft
     - If not harvested under sterile conditions, cold ethylene oxide gas may have adverse affects **(graft failure).**
       - Particularly in conjunction with irradiation with more than 4 megarad
       - Irradiation with 2 megarad with ethylene oxide: apparently no significantly effect on mechanical properties
   - Fresh osteochondral allograft
     - **Osteoarticular allografts preserved with cryopreservation have no viable chondrocytes after clinical transplantation.**
     - Fresh allografts are stored in culture medium at 4° C for 14 days to allow for microbiologic and serologic testing.
     - Chondrocyte viability is maintained for up to 45 days, but there is a significant decrease after 28 days.
2. Synthetic ligaments
   - No initial period of weakness, in contrast to autografts or allografts
   - Subject to wear (debris)
   - Associated with **sterile joint effusions**
     - Increase in neutral proteinases (**collagenase** and gelatinase)
     - Chondrocyte activation factor (IL-1)

SECTION 4 CELLULAR AND MOLECULAR BIOLOGY, IMMUNOLOGY, AND GENETICS OF ORTHOPAEDICS

I. CELLULAR AND MOLECULAR BIOLOGY

A. Chromosomes

1. In the nucleus of every cell
   - In humans, 46 chromosomes in 23 pairs
   - Of these: 22 pairs of autosomes, 1 pair of sex chromosomes
2. Contain both deoxyribonucleic acid (DNA) and ribonucleic acid (RNA)
3. Each chromosome contains more than 150,000 **genes.**
4. Regulation of **gene expression:**
   - Relatively few genes are expressed for any given cell.
   - Genes determine each cell's unique biologic qualities.

B. DNA

1. All nuclear DNA resides in the 23 chromosome pairs.
2. DNA regulates cellular functions through **protein synthesis.**
   - DNA replication
   - Production of messenger RNA (mRNA)
   - Transcription of mRNA
   - Regulation of cell division
3. DNA has a double helix (double-stranded) structure.
   - **Two sugar molecules**
     - One on each strand
   - One nitrogenous base per sugar molecule (Figure 1-80)
     - Nitrogenous bases: adenine, guanine, cytosine, and thymine

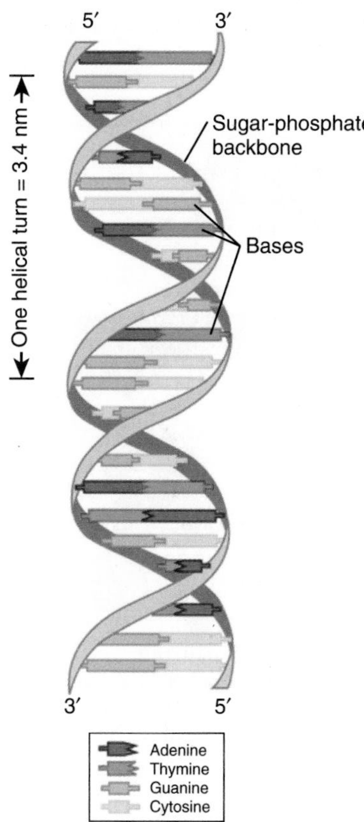

Figure 1-80 DNA structure. The two deoxyribose strands are connected by a pair of nucleotides (which form the rung of the ladder) that are in turn connected by hydrogen bonds. (From Jorde LB, et al, editors: *Medical genetics,* ed 2, St. Louis, 1999, Mosby.)

4. The sugar molecules within a strand are linked by phosphate groups.
5. The nitrogenous bases are linked across strands by hydrogen bonds.
   - Adenine is linked to thymine.
   - Guanine is linked to cytosine.

C. RNA

1. Important differences from DNA:
   - Ribose sugar
     - A hydroxyl group is attached to the pentose ring in the 2′ position, making RNA less stable.
   - Found in both nucleus and cytoplasm
   - Single-stranded
   - **Nitrogenous bases: adenine, guanine, cytosine, and uracil**
     - **No thymine**
   - Adenine is linked to uracil.

D. Nucleotide

1. A nucleotide consists of a DNA sugar molecule and phosphate group plus one nitrogenous base.
2. The nucleotide sequence in one strand of DNA determines the complementary nucleotide sequence in the other strand.
3. **Codons** are sequences of three nucleotides.
   - The genetic code is described in codons, or three-letter "words" (e.g., ACT = adenine-cytosine-thymine).
   - Each codon specifies one of the 20 amino acids that are the basic units of all proteins (Figure 1-81).

E. Gene

1. Portion of DNA that codes for a specific enzyme
   - "One gene equals one enzyme."

F. Transcription (Figure 1-82)

1. Transfer (via RNA polymerase) of the genetic code (amino acid sequence) for a specific protein from the respective gene in DNA to an mRNA molecule

G. Translation (Figure 1-83)

1. Building of a protein from mRNA through amino acids

H. Protein coding and regulation (Figure 1-84; see also Figure 1-83)

1. **Regulating DNA**
   - Large noncoding nucleotide sequences between functional sequences
   - Includes the **gene promoter** that is required for transcription
2. **Consensus sequences**
   - Binding sites for specific proteins involved in gene regulation
   - Named for a specific nucleotide sequence
3. **Gene enhancers**
   - Binding sites for proteins (transcription factors)
   - Involved in the regulation of transcription

I. Techniques used to study genetic (inherited) disorders

1. Restriction enzymes
   - Used to cut DNA at a precise, reproducible cleavage locations
   - Produce **restriction fragments**
     - Identify polymorphisms (alternative gene expressions)
   - **Linkage analysis**
     - Estimates the probability that a genetic trait or disease is associated with polymorphisms
2. Agarose gel electrophoresis
   - DNA (negatively charged) is suspended in agarose gel.
   - The gel is exposed to an electrical field.
   - DNA moves through the gel toward the positive pole of the field.
   - The gel acts as a "sieve":
     - Small DNA fragments move farther in a given time than do large fragments.
   - This technique is commonly used after and in conjunction with restriction enzymes.
3. DNA ligation
   - Method of attaching genes from human DNA to pieces of nonhuman DNA known as **plasmids**
   - Facilitates the study of specific genes
   - DNA fragments linked by ligation form **recombinant DNA**
4. Plasmid vectors
   - These are used to produce large quantities of a gene.
   - The gene is ligated to a plasmid (forming a recombinant plasmid).
   - The recombinant plasmid is inserted into a bacterium (the vector) by a process called **transformation.**
   - The recombinant plasmid replicates in the bacterium.
     - Increases the recombinant DNA and its gene
5. Cytogenetic analysis
   - Gross examination of chromosomes under microscope, with the use of techniques of banding and fluorescent in situ hybridization

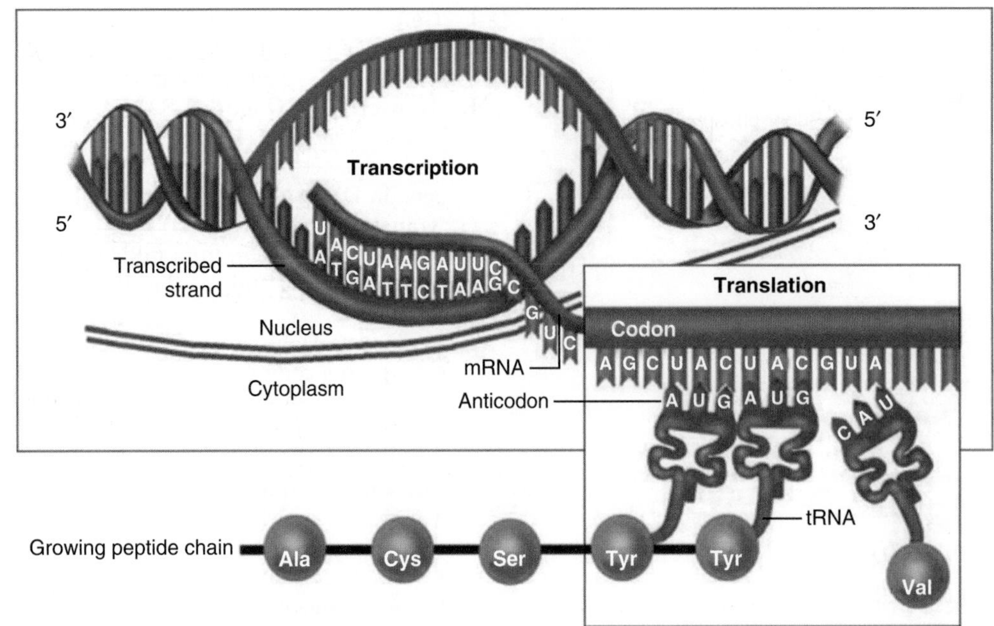

Figure 1-81 A genetic message begins as a double-stranded DNA molecule, which serves as the template for messenger RNA (mRNA). The mRNA, in groups of three nucleotides to a codon, directs the order of amino acids in protein. Ala, alanine; Cys, cysteine; Ser, serine; tRNA, transfer RNA; Tyr, tyrosine; Val, valine. (From Libby P, et al: *Braunwald's heart disease: a textbook of cardiovascular medicine,* Philadelphia, 2008, WB Saunders.)

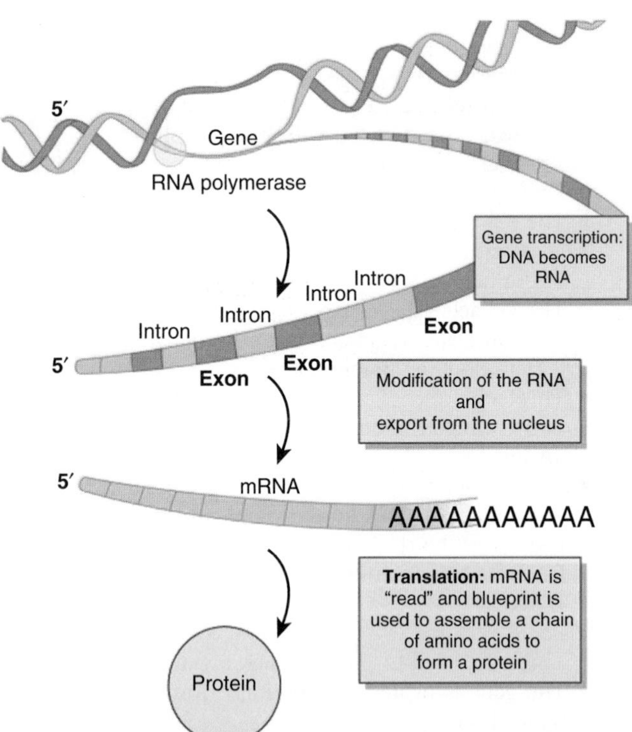

Figure 1-82 DNA information is transcribed into RNA in the nucleus. Messenger RNA (mRNA) is then transported to the cytoplasm, where ribosomes complete translation into proteins. (From Jorde LB, et al, editors: *Medical genetics,* ed 2, St. Louis, 1999, Mosby.)

First base	Second base U	Second base C	Second base A	Second base G
U	UUU UUC Phe UUA UUG Leu	UCU UCC UCA UCG Ser	UAU UAC Tyr UAA UAG TERM	UGU UGC Cys UGA TERM UGG Trp
C	CUU CUC CUA CUG Leu	CCU CCC CCA CCG Pro	CAU CAC His CAA CAG Gln	CGU CGC CGA CGG Arg
A	AUU AUC AUA Ile AUG Met	ACU ACC ACA ACG Thr	AAU AAC Asn AAA AAG Lys	AGU AGC Ser AGA AGG Arg
G	GUU GUC GUA GUG Val	GCU GCC GCA GCG Ala	GAU GAC Asp GAA GAG Glu	GGU GGC GGA GGG Gly

Figure 1-83 The genetic code for translation of the triplet nucleotide codons of messenger RNA into amino acids in proteins. Ala, alanine; Arg, arginine; Asn, asparagine; Asp, aspartate; Cys, cysteine; Gln, glutamine; Glu, glutamine; Gly, glycine; His, histidine; Ile, isoleucine; Leu, leucine; Lys, lysine; Met, methionine; Phe, phenylalanine; Pro, proline; Ser, serine; TERM, stop codon; Thr, threonine; Trp, tryptophan; Tyr, tyrosine; Val, valine. (From Libby P, et al: *Braunwald's heart disease: a textbook of cardiovascular medicine,* Philadelphia, PA, 2008, WB Saunders.)

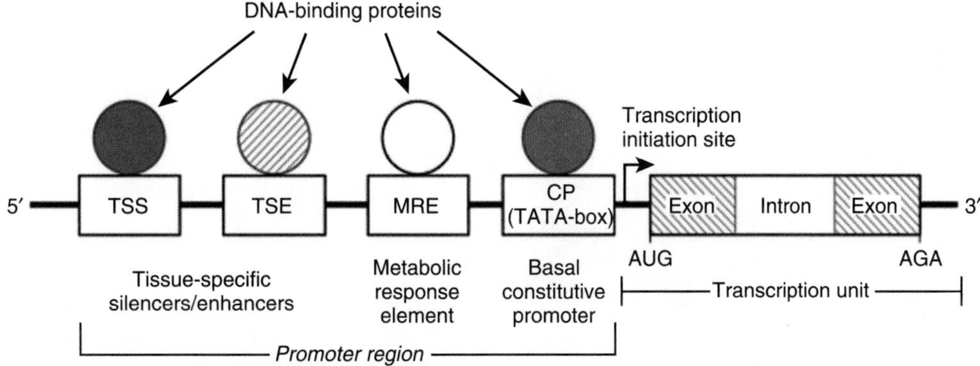

Figure 1-84 Protein coding and regulation. The transcription unit is the region of DNA composed of exons and introns that is transcribed into a messenger RNA (mRNA) precursor. The promoter region contains numerous short regulatory DNA sequences that are targets for interactions with specific DNA-binding proteins. These sequences consist of the basal constitutive promoter (CP) (TATA box), metabolic response elements (MRE) that modulate transcription, and tissue-specific enhancers (TSE) and silencers (TSS) that direct expression of specific subsets of genes to cells of a given phenotype. (From Kronenberg HM, et al: *Williams textbook of endocrinology,* ed 11, Philadelphia, 2008, WB Saunders.)

- **Used to detect chromosomal translocations, such as those observed in synovial sarcoma (translocation between chromosomes X and 18)**

6. Genomic screening (Figure 1-85)
7. Transgenic animals (Figure 1-86)
   - Such animals are bred to investigate the function of cloned genes.
   - A foreign gene (**transgene**) is inserted into a single-cell embryo.
   - The cell replicates.
     - The transgene is carried by every cell in the body.
8. Southern blotting (hybridization)
   - Restriction enzymes and agarose gel electrophoresis
   - Identifies a particular **DNA sequence** in an extract of mixed DNA
9. Northern blotting (hybridization)
   - Restriction enzymes and agarose gel electrophoresis

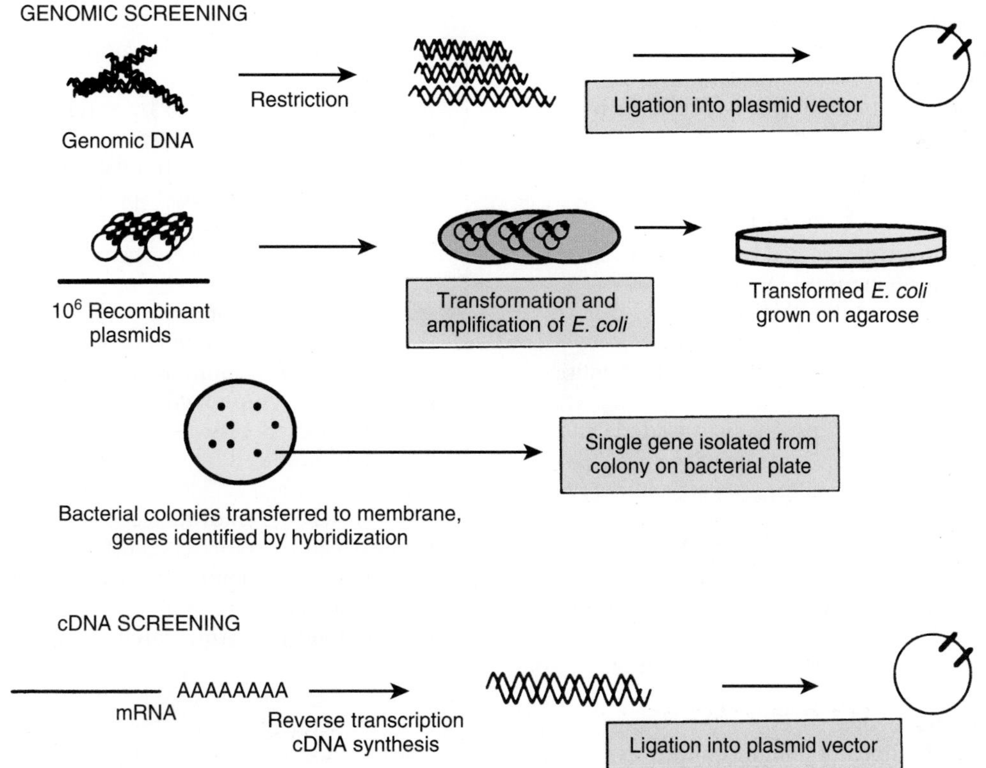

Figure 1-85 Genomic library of recombinant plasmids with fragments of all the DNA in the chromosome. The entire genome, restricted into small fragments, is ligated into plasmid vectors restricted by the same enzymes. These recombinant plasmids transform bacteria, which can be screened to isolate specific genes of interest. cDNA, complementary DNA; *E. coli, Escherichia coli;* mRNA, messenger RNA. (From Simon SR, editor: *Orthopaedic basic science,* Rosemont, Ill, 1994, American Academy of Orthopaedic Surgeons, p 227.)

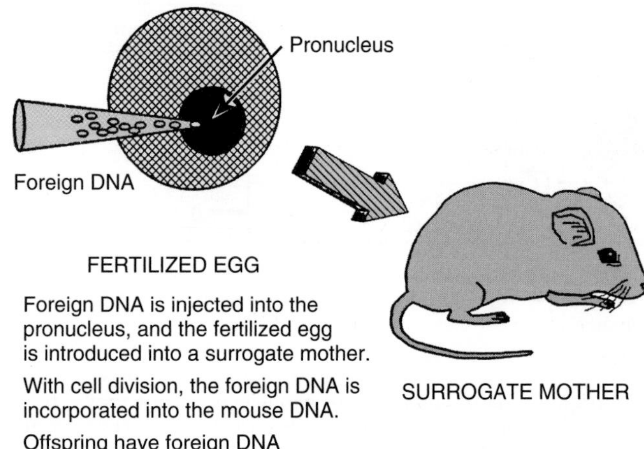

Pronucleus
Foreign DNA
FERTILIZED EGG
Foreign DNA is injected into the pronucleus, and the fertilized egg is introduced into a surrogate mother.
With cell division, the foreign DNA is incorporated into the mouse DNA.
Offspring have foreign DNA in every cell.
SURROGATE MOTHER

Figure 1-86 Transgenic mice. Recombinant DNA is injected into a fertilized mouse egg. The foreign DNA is incorporated into the chromosome, with cell division. As the egg develops into an embryo, every cell in the animal contains the foreign DNA. (From Simon SR, editor: *Orthopaedic basic science,* Rosemont, Ill, 1994, American Academy of Orthopaedic Surgeons, p 228.)

- Identifies a particular **RNA sequence** in an extract of mixed RNA

10. Western blotting
    - Sodium dodecyl sulfate–polyacrylamide gel electrophoresis (SDS-PAGE)
    - Identifies a particular **protein** in an extract of mixed proteins
11. **Polymerase chain reaction (PCR) amplification**
    - Repetitive synthesis (amplification) of a specific DNA sequence in vitro
      - The number of copies of DNA doubles each cycle.
    - Has gained widespread use
      - Prenatal diagnosis of sickle cell disease
      - Screening DNA for gene mutations
    - Reverse-transcription PCR (RT-PCR)
      - **Reverse transcriptase used to "reverse transcribe" RNA to complementary DNA**
      - Typically used to study RNA viruses

J. **Cloning**

1. The production of genetically identical biologic entities
2. Therapeutic cloning
   - DNA removed from a patient is inserted into an embryo.
   - Stem cells are removed from the growing embryo (which dies).
   - These cells are stimulated to differentiate into a specific tissue.
   - The specific tissue (or organ) is transplanted back into the patient.
     - Avoids the need for transplantation of an organ from another person
     - Avoids organ rejection
     - Avoids complications of immunosuppressive agents
3. Reproductive cloning
   - DNA is removed from a host and inserted into an embryo.
   - The embryo is then implanted into a healthy womb and allowed to develop.
   - The goal is to produce an animal that is genetically identical to the host.
4. Embryo cloning
   - One or more cells are removed from a fertilized embryo and stimulated to develop in utero.
   - The goal is to produce several genetically identical animals (e.g., twins or triplets).

II. IMMUNOLOGY

A. **Study of the body's defense mechanisms**

B. **Nonspecific (innate) immune response (Figure 1-87)**

1. **Inflammatory reaction**
   - Recognition of a foreign antigen
   - A result of a fracture, soft tissue injury, or foreign body
   - Release of histamine
     - Results in local vasodilation (exudate)
     - Phagocytic cells enzymatically digest "offending material"
2. Enhanced by activation of the complement system
3. Suppressed by anti-inflammatory medication

C. **Specific (adaptive) immune response (Figure 1-88)**

1. Includes **cell-mediated** and **humoral antibody–mediated** immune responses
2. Cells involved in specific immune responses (B and T cells)
   - Arise from primitive mesenchymal cells in the bone marrow
   - B lymphocytes mature in the lymph nodes
   - T lymphocytes
     - Originate in the bone marrow
     - Pass through the thymus during fetal development
     - Finally, move into the lymph nodes and blood
     - Include helper T cells, suppressor T cells, and killer T cells
3. Immune response evoked by **antigens**
   - **Macrophages and monocytes** process the antigen so that it will be able to stimulate lymphocytes.
   - Lymphocytes can mount specific reactions to millions of potential antigens.
     - They rearrange their genes (which no other cell can do).
     - They achieve antigenic diversity.
     - They produce millions of antibodies.
4. **Cell-mediated immune response** (Figure 1-89)
   - **Involves T lymphocytes and presentation of antigens by memory B cells and dendritic cells**
   - Protein produced by the gene rearrangement is fixed to the cell surface.
     - Acts as a receptor molecule
   - The T cell receptor acts indirectly on a foreign antigen.
     - Does not bond directly, as observed with B lymphocytes
5. **Humoral antibody–mediated immune response** (Figure 1-90)
   - These responses involve B lymphocytes.
     - Differentiate into plasma cells
     - Produce immunoglobulins against specific antigens
   - B lymphocytes are associated with immunoglobulins and the HLA system.
     - T lymphocytes are not.
   - Immunoglobulins are produced by plasma cells in a Y-shaped configuration (Figure 1-91).

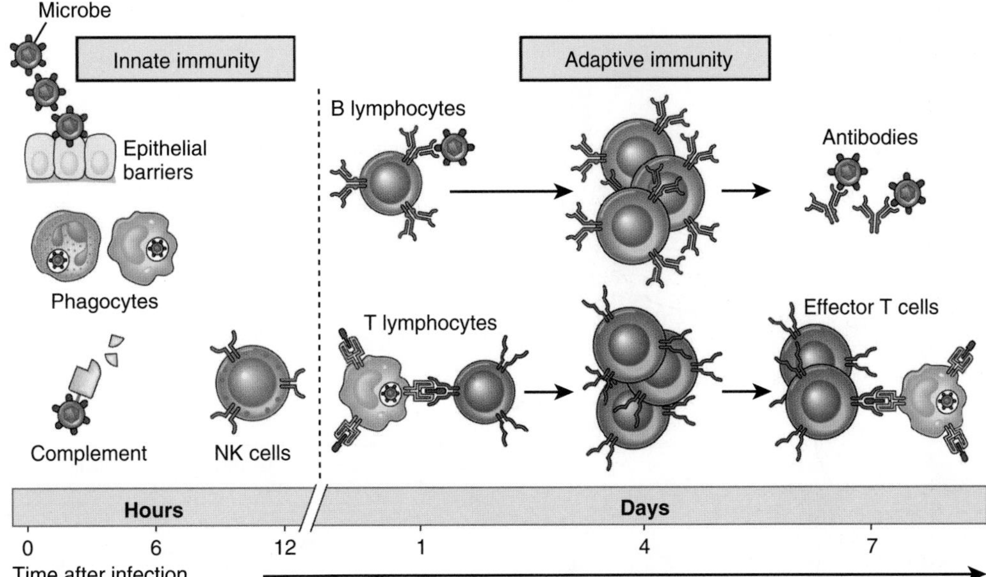

Figure 1-87 Innate and adaptive immunity. The mechanisms of innate immunity provide the initial defense against infections. Adaptive immune responses develop later and consist of activation of lymphocytes. NK, natural killer. (From Abbas AK, et al: *Cellular and molecular immunology,* ed 6, Philadelphia, 2009, WB Saunders.)

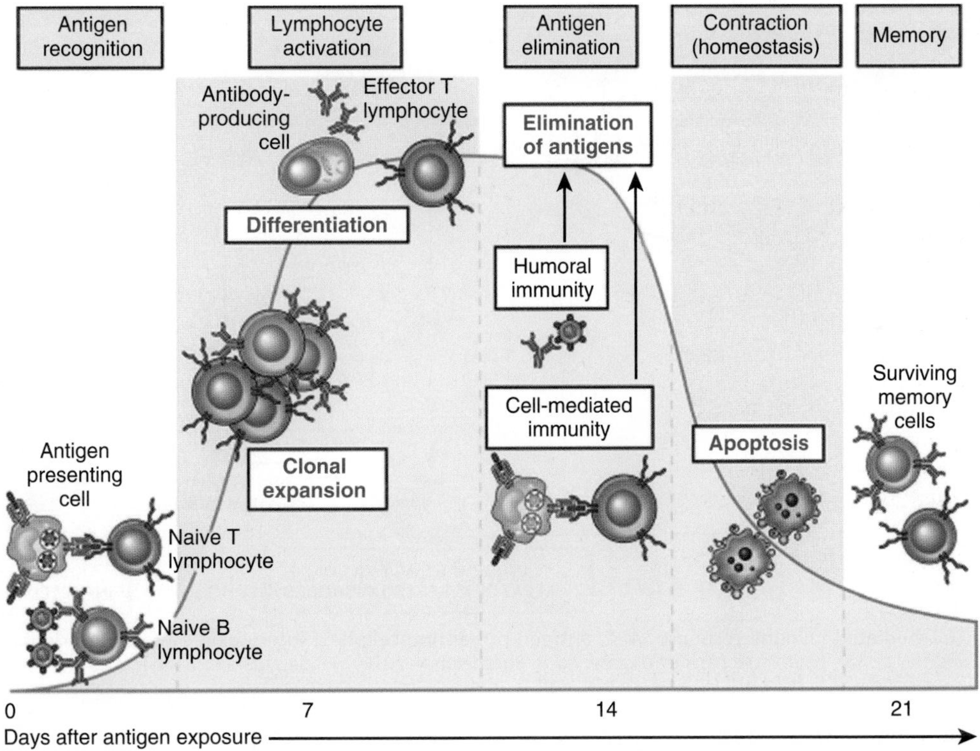

Figure 1-88 Phases of adaptive immune responses. Adaptive immune responses consist of distinct phases; the first three are the recognition of antigen, the activation of lymphocytes, and the elimination of antigen (the effector phase). The response contracts (declines) as antigen-stimulated lymphocytes die by apoptosis, which restores homeostasis, and the antigen-specific cells that survive are responsible for memory. (From Abbas AK, et al: *Cellular and molecular immunology,* ed 6, Philadelphia, 2009, WB Saunders.)

- Five classes of immunoglobulins have been described:
  - **Immunoglobulin A (IgA):** mucosal surfaces
  - **IgM:** produced earliest by fetus; largest; RF is an IgM
  - **IgG: most common; arises in response to infection**
  - **Immunoglobulin D (IgD):** acts as a receptor
  - **Immunoglobulin E (IgE):** allergic responses (e.g., to latex)

D. **Cytokines**

1. Proteins (or glycoproteins)
2. Cell products secreted in response to a foreign antigen
3. Produced by T cells
4. Regulate inflammatory and immune responses
5. Four broad categories:
   - Interferons

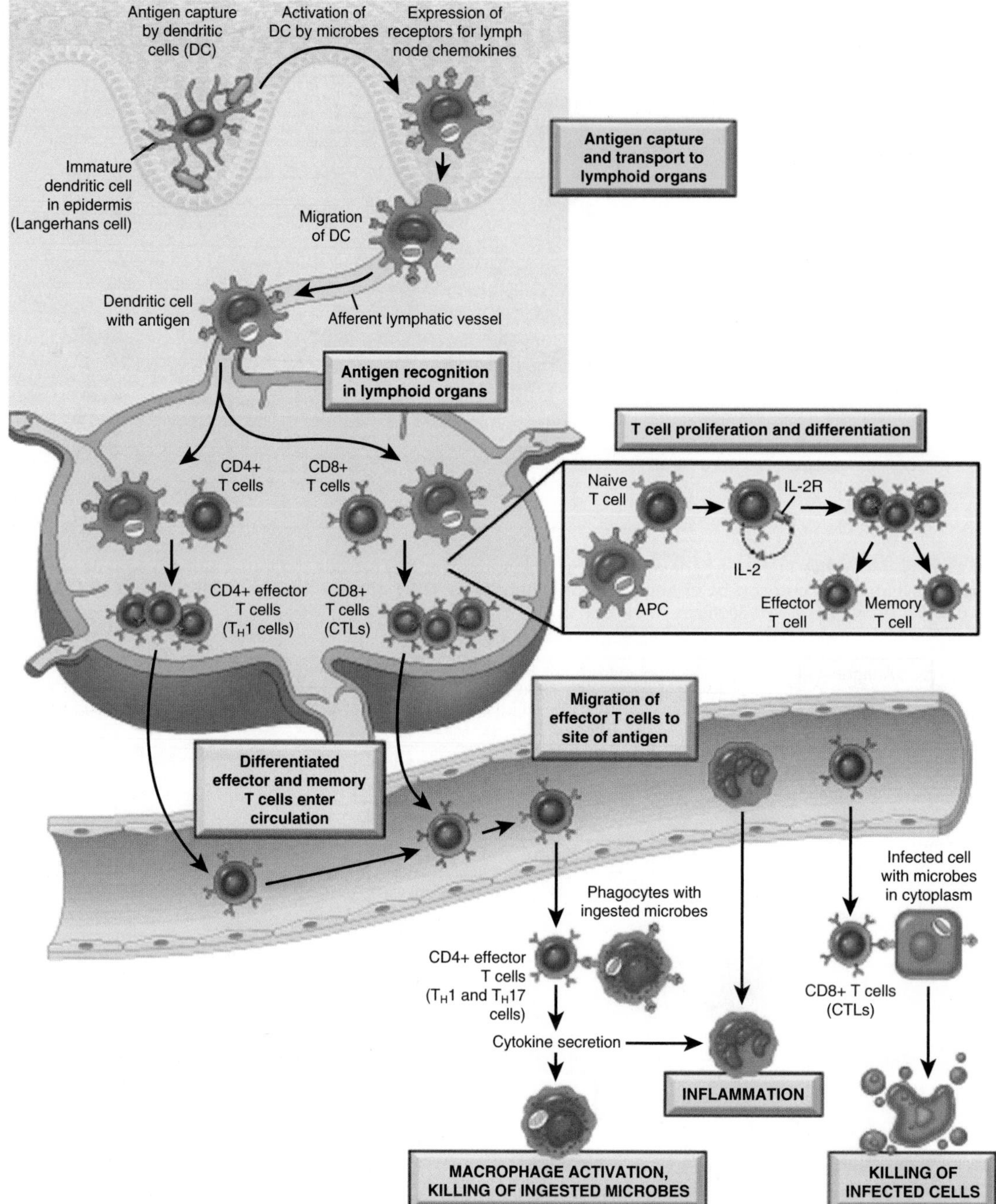

Figure 1-89 The cell-mediated immune response. APC, antigen-presenting cell; IL-2, interleukin-2; IL-2R, interleukin-2 receptor. (From Kumar V, et al: *Robbins and Cotran pathologic basis of disease,* ed 8, Philadelphia, 2010, WB Saunders.)

- Growth factors
- Colony-stimulating factors
- Interleukins

E. Complement system (Figure 1-92)

1. A group of 25 proteins
2. Acts in a cascading sequence
3. Amplifies an immune response

F. Immunogenetics

1. HLAs contribute to the specificity of immune recognition.
   - Associated with a variety of rheumatologic diseases
2. The HLA gene is located on chromosome 6 (short arm)
   - There are 6 class I loci and 14 class II loci.

G. Transplantation

1. Allogenic grafting
   - Transplantation between nonidentical members of the same species
2. Xenografting
   - Transplantation of tissues across species
3. Graft preparation
   - Freezing
     - Cellular response diminished
   - Freeze-drying (lyophilization)
     - Cellular response nearly undetectable

H. Oncologic features (Figure 1-93):

1. Cancer: characterized by abnormal, uncontrolled cell growth

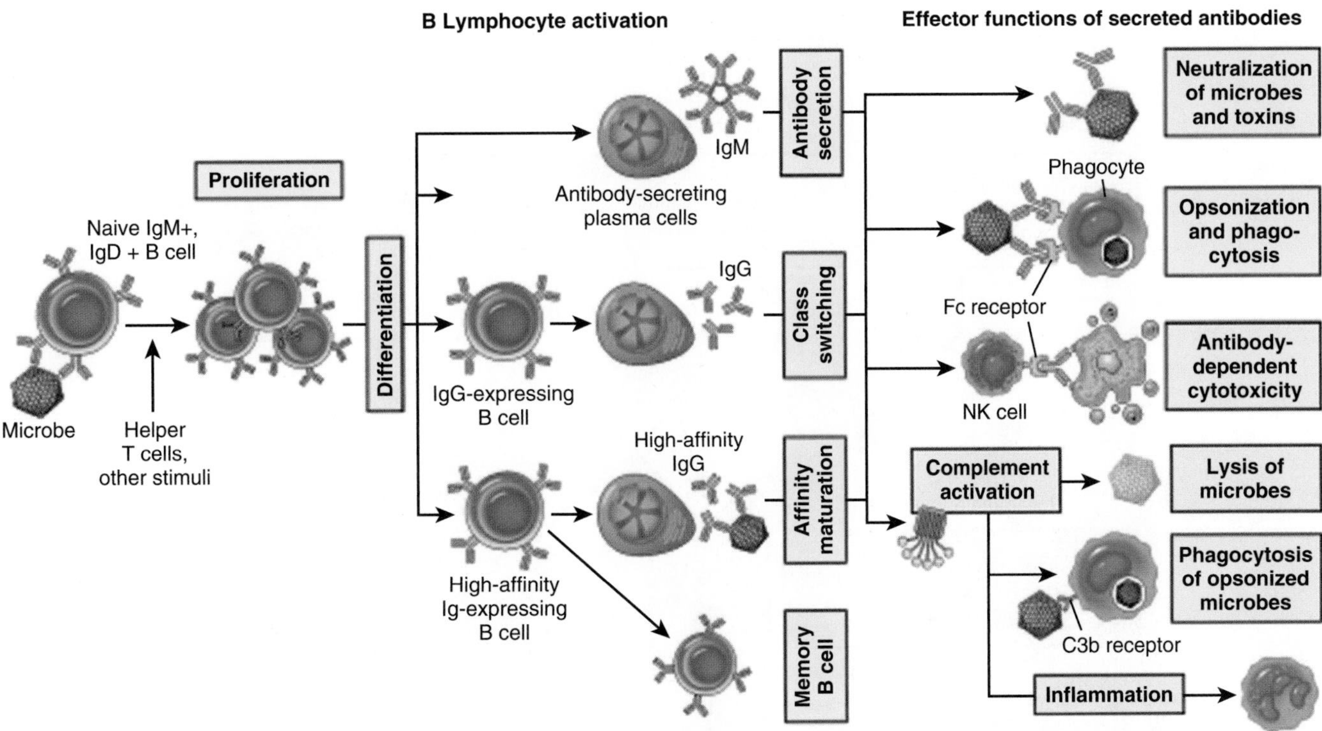

Figure 1-90 The humoral antibody response; activation of B cells and immunoglobulin production. Fc, crystallizable fragment; IgD, IgG, and IgM, immunoglobulins D, G, and M, respectively; NK, natural killer. (From Kumar V, et al: *Robbins and Cotran pathologic basis of disease,* ed 8, Philadelphia, 2010, WB Saunders.)

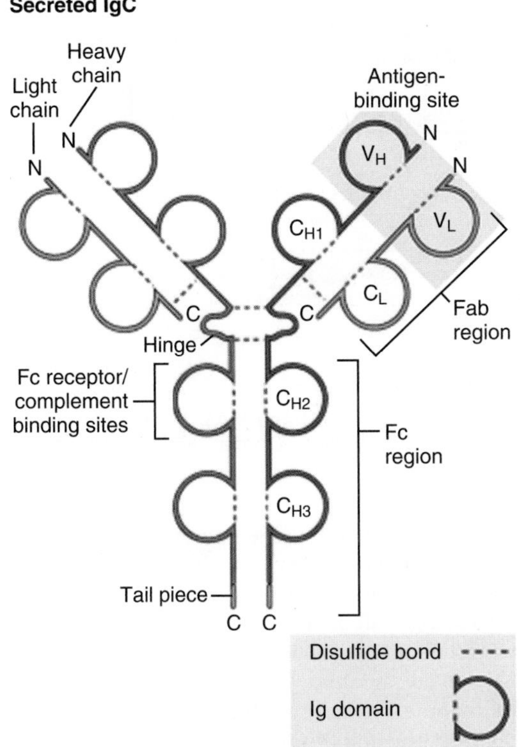

Figure 1-91 Basic subunit structure of the immunoglobulin molecule. C_H and C_L, constant regions; Fab, antigen-binding fragment; Fc, crystallizable fragment; IgC, immunoglobulin C; V_H and V_L, variable regions. (From Katz VL, et al: *Comprehensive gynecology,* ed 5, Philadelphia, 2007, Mosby.)

- This growth occurs a result of damage to the cell's DNA.
- The molecular approach is a way to discover mechanisms by which normal cells become cancer cells.

2. Malignancy: caused by various mechanisms
   - A point mutation in DNA
   - A gene deletion
   - A chromosomal translocation (resulting in gene rearrangement)
3. **Oncogenes**
   - These are growth control genes.
   - Improper oncogene expression results in unregulated cell growth, as observed in cancer cells.
4. **Antioncogenes (tumor suppressor genes)**
   - These genes suppress growth in damaged cells and thereby inhibit development of tumors.
   - **Loss of antioncogene function results in unregulated cell division and malignancy.**
5. **Metastases**
   - Sequence of events for primary tumor cells to metastasize to a distant organ
     - Progressive growth of the primary tumor
     - Neovascularization of the tumor
     - **Basement membrane erosion and invasion**
       - Matrix metalloproteinases degrade type IV collagen, which is present in the basement membrane
       - **They are thus believed to be important for tumor cell metastasis.**
     - Entry of tumor cells into adjacent blood vessels
     - Detachment of cells from the primary tumor

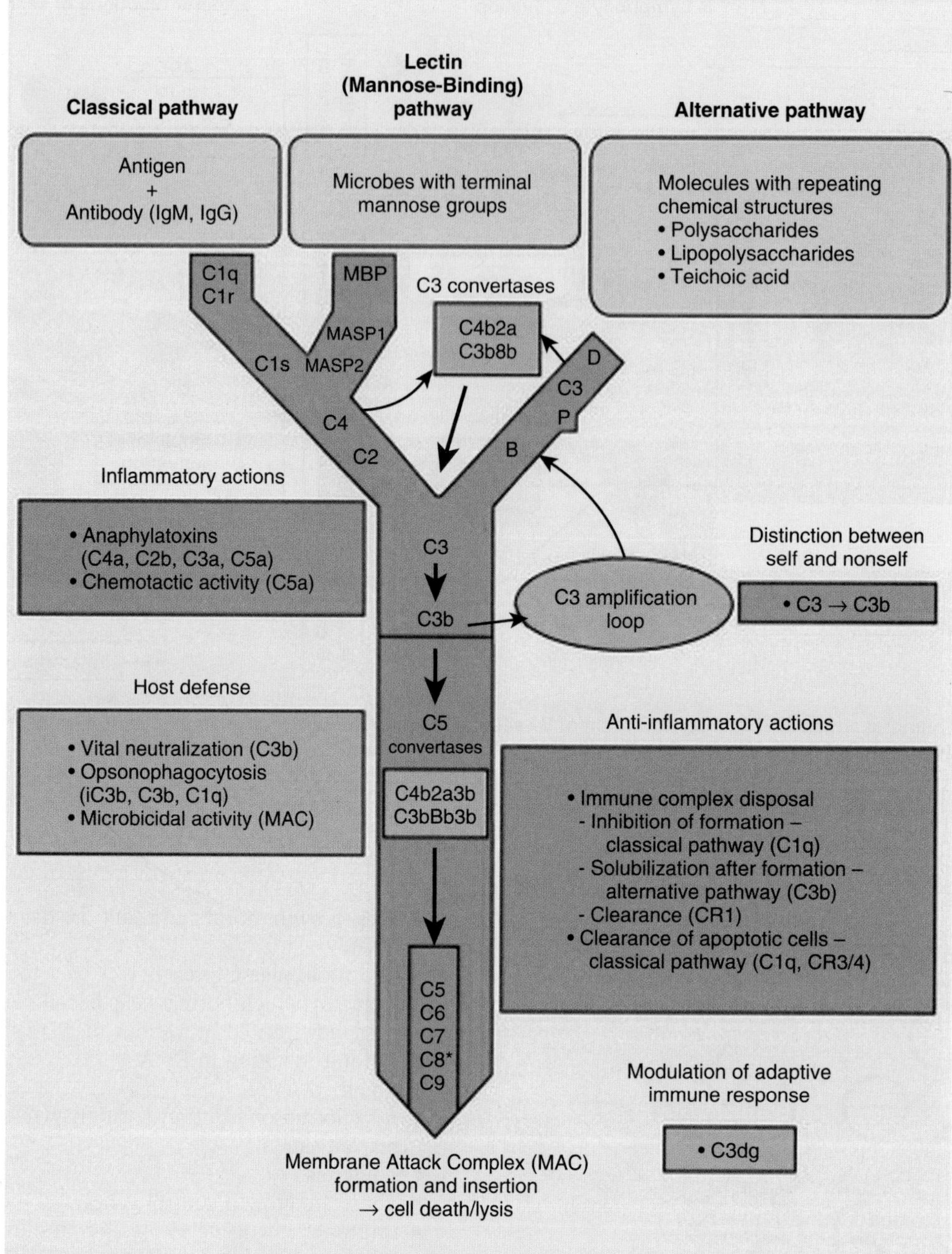

Figure 1-92 Complement cascade. IgG and IgM, immunoglobulins G and M, respectively; MASP1 and MASP2 , mannan-binding lectin serine proteases 1 and 2; MBP, mannose-binding protein. (Modified from Mandell GL, et al: *Mandell, Douglas, and Bennett's principles and practice of infectious diseases,* ed 7, Philadelphia, 2010, Churchill-Livingstone.)

- Embolization of tumor cells into the general circulation
- Attachment of tumor cells at a distant site
  - In bone, tumor cells attach through integrins to the endothelial layer.
- Invasion into vessel walls, with migration into surrounding parenchyma
- Progressive tumor growth at the new site

- **Most common sites of primary tumors that metastasize to bone**, in decreasing incidence:
  - Breast
  - Prostate
  - Lung
  - Kidney
  - Thyroid
- Most common soft tissue tumors that metastasize via lymphatic node system:
  - Rhabdomyosarcoma
  - Clear cell sarcoma
  - Epithelioid sarcoma
  - Synovial sarcoma

6. **Flow cytometry and cytofluorometry**
   - Quantify the amount of DNA in cells
   - Useful for quantifying abnormal (aneuploid) DNA in a malignant tumor
7. P-Glycoprotein: an energy-dependent cell-wall pump
   - Functions to eliminate toxins from the cytoplasm
   - Allows cells to develop resistance to chemotherapeutic agents

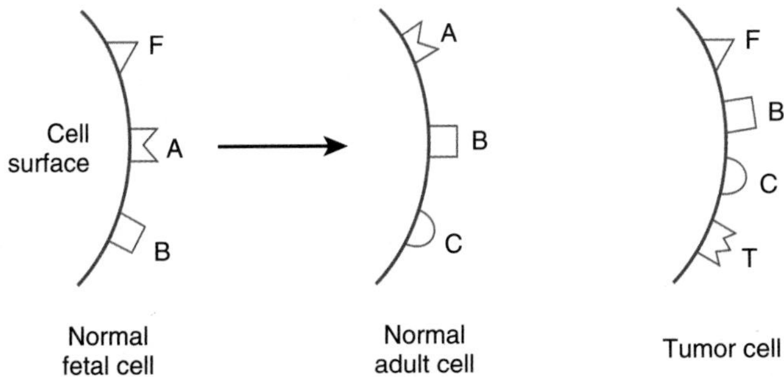

Figure 1-93 Tumor cells have cell surface antigens common to other normal cells that reflect the tissue of origin (antigens B and C). They may also demonstrate antigens normally present only on fetal cells (antigen F) and loose antigens common to the cell type of origin (antigen A). In addition, they acquire new tumor-associated antigens (antigen T). (From Friedlander GE: Immunology. In Albright JA, Brand RA, editors: *The scientific basis of orthopaedics,* ed 2, Norwalk, Conn, 1987, Appleton & Lange, p 502.)

III. GENETICS

A. Mendelian inheritance

1. Mendelian traits follow specific patterns of inheritance.
   - Controlled by a single gene pair ("monogenic")
2. An **allele** is one of several possible alternative forms of a gene.
   - Because chromosomes are paired, every gene has two copies (loci).
   - An individual is **homozygous** if the alleles on each of the paired chromosomes are identical.
   - An individual is **heterozygous** if the alleles differ.
3. **Phenotype** refers to the features (traits) exhibited because of genetic makeup.
4. **Genotype** refers to the presence or absence of particular genes, not the traits expressed.
5. Mendelian traits may be inherited by one of four modes (Table 1-36):
   - Autosomal dominant
   - Autosomal recessive
   - X-linked dominant
     - **Rare. All daughters of an affected father have the trait, but none of his sons do.**
   - **X-linked recessive**
6. Incidence of human mendelian disorders is approximately 1%.
7. Nonmendelian traits may be inherited through "polygenic" transmission.
   - Caused by the action of several genes
8. ***Anticipation* is said to occur when a genetic disease becomes progressively more severe in each subsequent generation.**

Table 1-36 Mendelian Inheritance

Inheritance Pattern	Description	Punnett Square(s)
Autosomal dominant*	Autosomal dominant disorders typically represent **structural defects.** The disorder is manifested in the heterozygous state (Aa). Of offspring, 50% are affected (assuming that only one parent is affected). Normal offspring do not transmit the condition. There is no gender preference.	A a a: Aa aa a: Aa aa
Autosomal recessive†	Autosomal recessive disorders typically represent **biochemical or enzymatic defects.** The disorder is manifested in the homozygous state (aa). Parents are unaffected (they are most commonly heterozygotes). Of offspring, 25% are affected (assuming that each parent is a heterozygote). There is no gender preference.	A a A: AA Aa a: Aa aa
X-linked dominant‡	X-linked dominant disorders are manifested in the heterozygous state (X′X or X′Y). Affected female (mating with unaffected male) transmits the X-linked gene to 50% of daughters and 50% of sons. Affected male (mating with unaffected female) transmits the X-linked gene to all daughters and no sons.	X Y X′: X′X X′Y X: XX XY X′ Y X: X′X XY X: X′X XY
X-linked recessive§	Heterozygote (X′Y) male manifests the condition. Heterozygote (X′X) female is unaffected. Affected male (mating with unaffected female) transmits the X-linked gene to all daughters (who are carriers) and no sons. Carrier female (mating with unaffected male) transmits the X-linked gene to 50% of daughters (who are carriers) and 50% of sons (who are affected).	X′ Y X: X′X XY X: X′X XY X Y X′: X′X X′Y X: XX XY

*"A" is the mutant dominant allele.
†"a" is the mutant recessive allele.
‡"X′" is the mutant dominant X allele.
§"X" is the mutant recessive X allele.

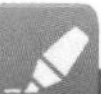

Table 1-37 Inheritance Patterns of Some Musculoskeletal Disorders

Autosomal Dominant	Autosomal Recessive	X-Linked Dominant	X-Linked Recessive
Achondroplasia Spondyloepiphyseal dysplasia (congenita form) Multiple epiphyseal dysplasia Metaphyseal chondrodysplasia (Schmid and Jansen types) **Hereditary multiple exostoses (HME)** Kniest dysplasia Malignant hyperthermia **Marfan's syndrome** Ehlers-Danlos syndrome Osteogenesis imperfecta (types I and IV) Osteochondromatosis Polydactyly **Osteopetrosis (tarda, mild form)**	Metaphyseal chondrodysplasia (McKusick type) Diastrophic dysplasia Laron's dysplasia Sickle cell anemia Hurler's syndrome Osteogenesis imperfecta (types II and III) Hypophosphatasia Hereditary vitamin D–dependent rickets Homocystinuria **Osteopetrosis (infantile, malignant form)**	**Hypophosphatemic rickets** **Leri-Weill dyschondrosteosis (bilateral Madelung's deformity)**	Spondyloepiphyseal dysplasia (tarda form) Hemophilia Hunter's syndrome **Duchenne's muscular dystrophy**

B. Mutations

1. Genetic disorders arise from alterations (mutations) in the genetic material.
2. Inherited mutations are passed from generation to generation.
3. A **sporadic mutation** may occur in the sperm or egg of the parents or in the embryo.

C. Chromosomal abnormalities

1. Disruptions in the normal arrangement or number of chromosomes
   - Aneuploidy: an abnormal number of chromosomes
     - Triploidy: three copies of chromosomes (69 chromosomes)
     - Tetraploidy: four copies of chromosomes (92 chromosomes)
     - Monosomy: one chromosome of one pair is absent (total: 45 chromosomes)
     - Trisomy: one chromosome pair has an extra chromosome (total: 47 chromosomes)
   - Deletion: a section of one chromosome (in a chromosome pair) is absent
   - Duplication: an extra section of one chromosome (in a chromosome pair) is present
   - Translocation: a portion of one chromosome is exchanged with a portion of another chromosome
   - Inversion: a broken portion of a chromosome reattaches to the same chromosome in the same location but in a reverse direction

D. The genetics of musculoskeletal conditions and abnormalities (Tables 1-37 and 1-38)

Text continued on p. 94

Table 1-38 Comprehensive Compilation of Inheritance Pattern, Defect, and Associated Gene in Musculoskeletal Disorders

Disorder	Inheritance Pattern	Defect	Associated Gene
Dysplasias			
Achondroplasia	Autosomal dominant	Defect in the fibroblast growth factor (FGF) receptor 3	***FGF3R***
Diastrophic dysplasia	Autosomal recessive	Mutation of a gene coding for a sulfate transport protein	DTDST
Kniest dysplasia	Autosomal dominant	Defect in type II collagen	COL 2A1
Laron's dysplasia (pituitary dwarfism)	Autosomal recessive	Defect in the growth hormone receptor	
McCune-Albright syndrome (polyostotic fibrous dysplasia, café-au-lait spots, precocious puberty)	Sporadic mutation	Germline defect in the Gsα protein	***Mutation of Gsα subunit of the receptor/adenylyl cyclase–coupling G proteins***
Metaphyseal chondrodysplasia (Jansen form)	Autosomal dominant		PTH; PTH-related protein
Metaphyseal chondrodysplasia (McKusick form)	Autosomal recessive		RMRP
Metaphyseal chondrodysplasia (Schmid-tarda form)	Autosomal dominant	Defect in type X collagen	COL 10A1

Table 1-38 Comprehensive Compilation of Inheritance Pattern, Defect, and Associated Gene in Musculoskeletal Disorders—cont'd

Disorder	Inheritance Pattern	Defect	Associated Gene
Multiple epiphyseal dysplasia	Autosomal dominant (most commonly)	Cartilage oligomeric matrix protein	COMP
Spondyloepiphyseal dysplasia	Autosomal dominant (congenita form) X-linked recessive (tarda form)	Defect in type II collagen	Linked to Xp22.12-p22.31, SEDL (tarda), and COL 2A1 (congenita)
Achondrogenesis	Autosomal recessive	Fetal cartilage fails to mature	
Apert syndrome	Sporadic mutation/ autosomal dominant		FGF2R
Chondrodysplasia punctata (Conradi-Hünerman)	Autosomal dominant		
Chondrodysplasia punctata (rhizomelic form)	Autosomal recessive	Defect in subcellular organelles (peroxisomes)	
Cleidocranial dysplasia (dysostosis)	Autosomal dominant	Mutation of a gene coding for a protein related to osteoblast function	**CBFA1**
Dysplasia epiphysealis hemimelica (Trevor's disease)	Unknown		
Ellis–van Creveld syndrome (chondroectodermal dysplasia)	Autosomal recessive		EVC
Fibrodysplasia ossificans progressiva	Sporadic mutation/ autosomal dominant		
Geroderma osteodysplastica (Walt Disney dwarfism)	Autosomal recessive		
Grebe chondrodysplasia	Autosomal recessive		
Hypochondroplasia	Sporadic mutation/ autosomal dominant		FGF3R
Kabuki makeup syndrome	Sporadic mutation		
Mesomelic dysplasia (Langer type)	Autosomal recessive		
Mesomelic dysplasia (Nievergelt type)	Autosomal dominant		
Mesomelic dysplasia (Reinhardt-Pfeiffer type)	Autosomal dominant		
Mesomelic dysplasia (Werner type)	Autosomal dominant		
Metatrophic dysplasia	Autosomal recessive		
Progressive diaphyseal dysplasia (Camurati-Engelmann disease)	Autosomal dominant		
Pseudoachondroplastic dysplasia	Autosomal dominant		COMP
Pyknodysostosis	Autosomal recessive		
Spondylometaphyseal chondrodysplasia	Autosomal dominant		
Spondylothoracic dysplasia (Jarcho-Levin syndrome)	Autosomal recessive		
Thanatophoric dwarfism	Autosomal dominant		FGF3R
Tooth-and-nail syndrome	Autosomal dominant		
Treacher Collins syndrome (mandibulofacial dysostosis)	Autosomal dominant		
Metabolic Bone Diseases			
Hereditary vitamin D–dependent rickets	Autosomal recessive	See Table 1-15	
Hypophosphatasia	Autosomal recessive	See Table 1-15	PHEX
Hypophosphatemic rickets (vitamin D–resistant rickets)	X-linked dominant	See Table 1-15	PHEX

Continued

Table 1-38 Comprehensive Compilation of Inheritance Pattern, Defect, and Associated Gene in Musculoskeletal Disorders—cont'd

Disorder	Inheritance Pattern	Defect	Associated Gene
Osteogenesis imperfecta	Autosomal dominant (types I and IV)	Defect in type I collagen (abnormal cross-linking)	COL IA1, COL IA2
	Autosomal recessive (types II and III)		COL IA1, COL IA2
Albright's hereditary osteodystrophy (pseudohypoparathyroidism)	Uncertain	PTH has no effect at the target cells (in the kidney, bone, and intestine)	
Infantile cortical hyperostosis (Caffey's disease)	Unknown		
Ochronosis (alkaptonuria)	Autosomal recessive	Defect in the homogentisic acid oxidase system	
Osteopetrosis	Autosomal dominant (mild, tarda form) Autosomal recessive (infantile, malignant form)		CLCN7, TC1RG1
Connective Tissue Disorders			
Marfan's syndrome	Autosomal dominant	Fibrillin abnormalities (some patients also have type I collagen abnormalities)	FBN1 or TGF-βR2
Ehlers-Danlos syndrome (there are at least 13 varieties)	Autosomal dominant (most common)	Defects in types I and III collagen have been described for some varieties; lysyl oxidase abnormalities	**COL 3A1 (for type III; most common)** **COL 1A2 (for type VII)**
Homocystinuria	Autosomal recessive	Deficiency of the enzyme cystathionine β-synthase	
Mucopolysaccharidosis			
Hunter's syndrome ("gargoylism")	X-linked recessive		
Hurler's syndrome	Autosomal recessive	Deficiency of the enzyme α-L-iduronidase	
Maroteaux-Lamy syndrome	Autosomal recessive		
Morquio's syndrome	Autosomal recessive		
Sanfilippo's syndrome	Autosomal recessive		
Scheie's syndrome	Autosomal recessive	Deficiency of the enzyme α-L-iduronidase	
Muscular Dystrophies			
Duchenne's muscular dystrophy	X-linked recessive	Defect on the short arm of the X chromosome	Dystrophin gene
Becker's dystrophy	X-linked recessive		
Fascioscapulohumeral dystrophy	Autosomal dominant		
Limb-girdle dystrophy	Autosomal recessive		
Steinert's disease (myotonic dystrophy)	Autosomal dominant		
Hematologic Disorders			
Hemophilia (A and B)	X-linked recessive	Hemophilia A: factor VIII deficiency Hemophilia B: factor IX deficiency	
Sickle cell anemia	Autosomal recessive	Hemoglobin abnormality (presence of hemoglobin S)	
Gaucher's disease	Autosomal recessive	***Deficient activity of the enzyme β-glucosidase (glucocerebrosidase)***	
Hemochromatosis	Autosomal recessive		
Niemann-Pick disease	Autosomal recessive	Accumulation of sphingomyelin in cellular lysosomes	
Smith-Lemli-Opitz syndrome	Uncertain		

Table 1-38 Comprehensive Compilation of Inheritance Pattern, Defect, and Associated Gene in Musculoskeletal Disorders—cont'd

Disorder	Inheritance Pattern	Defect	Associated Gene
Thalassemia	Autosomal recessive	Abnormal production of hemoglobin A	
von Willebrand's disease	Autosomal dominant		
Chromosomal Disorders with Musculoskeletal Abnormalities			
Down's syndrome		Trisomy of chromosome 21	
Angelman's syndrome		Chromosome 15 abnormality	
Clinodactyly		Associated with many genetic anomalies, including trisomy of chromosomes 8 and 21	
Edward's syndrome		Trisomy of chromosome 18	
Fragile X syndrome	X-linked trait (does not follow the typical pattern of an X-linked trait)		Xq27-28
Klinefelter's syndrome (XXY)		An extra X chromosome in affected boys and men	
Langer-Giedion syndrome	Sporadic mutation	Chromosome 8 abnormality	
Nail-patella syndrome	Autosomal dominant		LMX1B
Patau's syndrome		Trisomy of chromosome 13	
Turner's syndrome (XO)		One of the two X chromosomes missing in affected girls and women	SHOX
Neurologic Disorders			
Charcot-Marie-Tooth disease	Autosomal dominant (most common)	***Chromosome 17 defect for encoding peripheral myelin protein-22***	***PMP22***
Congenital insensitivity to pain	Autosomal recessive		
Dejerine-Sottas disease	Autosomal recessive		
Friedreich's ataxia	Autosomal recessive		
Huntington's disease	Autosomal dominant		
Menkes syndrome	X-linked recessive	Inability to absorb and use copper	
Pelizaeus-Merzbacher disease	X-linked recessive	Defect in the gene for proteolipid (a component of myelin)	
Riley-Day syndrome	Autosomal recessive		
Spinal muscular atrophy (Werdnig-Hoffman disease and Kugelberg-Welander disease)	Autosomal recessive		
Sturge-Weber syndrome	Sporadic mutation		
Tay-Sachs disease	Autosomal recessive	Deficiency in the enzyme hexosaminidase A	
Diseases Associated with Neoplasias			
Ewing's sarcoma			11;22 chromosomal translocation (EWS/FL11 fusion gene)
Multiple endocrine neoplasia (MEN) type I	Autosomal dominant		RET
MEN type II	Autosomal dominant		
MEN type III	Autosomal dominant	Chromosome 10 abnormality	
Neurofibromatosis (von Recklinghausen's disease) type 1 (NF1) and type 2 (NF2)	Autosomal dominant	***NF1: chromosome 17 defect; codes for neurofibromin*** NF2: chromosome 22 defect	NF1, NF2

Continued

Table 1-38 Comprehensive Compilation of Inheritance Pattern, Defect, and Associated Gene in Musculoskeletal Disorders—cont'd

Disorder	Inheritance Pattern	Defect	Associated Gene
Synovial sarcoma			(X;18) (p11;q11) chromosomal translocations (STT/ SSX fusion gene)
Miscellaneous Disorders			
Malignant hyperthermia	Autosomal dominant		
Osteochondromatosis	Autosomal dominant		
Postaxial polydactyly	Autosomal dominant		GLI3 (types A, A/B) GJA1 (type IV)
Camptodactyly	Autosomal dominant		
Cerebro-oculofacioskeletal syndrome	Autosomal recessive		
Congenital contractural arachnodactyly			Fibrillin gene (chromosome 5)
Distal arthrogryposis syndrome	Autosomal dominant		
Dupuytren's contracture	Autosomal dominant (with partial sex limitation)		
Fabry's disease	X-linked recessive	Deficiency of α-galactosidase A	
Fanconi's pancytopenia	Autosomal recessive		
Freeman-Sheldon syndrome (craniocarpotarsal dysplasia; whistling face syndrome)	Autosomal dominant Autosomal recessive		
GM1 gangliosidosis	Autosomal recessive		
Hereditary anonychia	Autosomal dominant		
Holt-Oram syndrome	Autosomal dominant		
Humeroradial synostosis	Autosomal dominant Autosomal recessive		
Klippel-Feil syndrome		Faulty development of spinal segments along the embryonic neural tube	
Klippel-Trénaunay-Weber syndrome	Sporadic mutation		
Krabbe's disease	Autosomal recessive	Deficiency of galactocerebroside β-galactosidase	
Larsen's syndrome	Autosomal dominant Autosomal recessive		
Lesch-Nyhan disease	X-linked trait	Absence of the enzyme hypoxanthine guanine phosphoribosyl transferase	
Madelung's deformity	Autosomal dominant		
Mannosidosis	Autosomal recessive	Deficiency of the enzyme α-mannosidase	
Maple syrup urine disease	Autosomal recessive	Defective metabolism of the amino acids leucine, isoleucine, and valine	
Meckel syndrome (Gruber's syndrome)	Autosomal recessive		
Möbius syndrome	Autosomal dominant		
Mucolipidosis (oligosaccharidosis)	Autosomal recessive	A family of enzyme deficiency diseases	
Multiple exostoses	Autosomal dominant		***EXT1: greater burden of disease and risk of malignancy*** ***EXT2/EXT3***
Multiple pterygium syndrome	Autosomal recessive		

Table 1-38 Comprehensive Compilation of Inheritance Pattern, Defect, and Associated Gene in Musculoskeletal Disorders—cont'd

Disorder	Inheritance Pattern	Defect	Associated Gene
Noonan's syndrome	Sporadic mutation		
Oral-facial-digital (OFD) syndrome			OFD I: X-linked dominant OFD II (Mohr's syndrome): autosomal recessive
Osler-Weber-Rendu syndrome (hereditary hemorrhagic telangiectasia)	Autosomal dominant		
Pfeiffer's syndrome (acrocephalosyndactyly)	Sporadic mutation/ autosomal dominant		FGF2R
Phenylketonuria	Autosomal recessive	Enzyme deficiency characterized by the inability to convert phenylalanine to tyrosine because of a chromosome 12 abnormality	
Phytanic acid storage disease	Autosomal recessive		
Progeria (Hutchinson-Gilford progeria syndrome)	Autosomal dominant		
Proteus syndrome	Autosomal dominant		
Prune-belly syndrome	Uncertain	Localized mesodermal defect	
Radioulnar synostosis	Autosomal dominant		
Rett's syndrome	Sporadic mutation/X-linked dominant		
Roberts syndrome (pseudothalidomide syndrome)	Sporadic mutation/ autosomal recessive		
Russell-Silver syndrome	Sporadic mutation (possibly X-linked)		
Saethre-Chotzen syndrome	Autosomal dominant		
Sandhoff disease	Autosomal recessive	Enzyme deficiency of hexosaminidases A and B	
Schwartz-Jampel syndrome	Autosomal recessive		
Seckel syndrome (so-called bird-headed dwarfism)	Autosomal recessive		
Stickler's syndrome (hereditary progressive arthro-ophthalmopathy)	Autosomal dominant	Collagen abnormality	
Thrombocytopenia-aplasia of radius (TAR) syndrome	Autosomal recessive		
Tarsal coalition	Autosomal dominant		
Trichorhinophalangeal syndrome	Autosomal dominant		
Urea cycle defects		A group of enzyme disorders characterized by high levels of ammonia in the blood and tissues	
Argininemia	Autosomal recessive		
Argininosuccinic aciduria	Autosomal recessive		
Carbamyl phosphate synthetase deficiency	Autosomal recessive		
Citrullinemia	Autosomal recessive		
Ornithine transcarbamylase deficiency	X-linked		
VATER association	Sporadic mutation		
Werner's syndrome	Autosomal recessive		
Zygodactyly	Autosomal dominant		

PTH, parathyroid hormone; TGF-βR2, transforming growth factor-β receptor 2; VATER, vertebral defects, imperforate anus, tracheoesophageal fistula, and radial and renal dysplasia.

SECTION 5 ORTHOPAEDIC INFECTIONS AND MICROBIOLOGY

I. MUSCULOSKELETAL INFECTIONS

The following is an overview. In general, the following recommendations for the initial treatment regimen are based on the presumed type of infection, as determined from clinical findings and symptoms. Definitive treatment should be based on final culture results when those results are available.

A. Soft tissue infections (Table 1-39) and bite injuries (Table 1-40)

1. **Necrotizing fasciitis**
   - Potentially lethal disease involving necrosis of subcutaneous fat and deep fascia
   - Diabetes mellitus: the most common risk factor, but half of cases occur in previously healthy patients
   - Clinical features:
     - Initial: swelling, edema, and disproportionate pain
     - Late: crepitus, bullae, "dishwater pus," systemic signs of sepsis
   - **Microbiologic findings:**
     - **Type 1: polymicrobial infection**
       - **Most common**
       - **Four to five species typically cultured, including non–group A streptococci, Enterobacteriaceae, and anaerobes**
     - Type 2: group A β-hemolytic streptococci
       - "Flesh eating" type
       - Commonly occurs in previously healthy individuals
     - Type 3: marine vibrios
       - Infection from puncture wound that is exposed to seawater or marine animals
       - *Vibrio vulnificus* is most virulent
     - Type 4: MRSA associated
   - Treatment:
     - Broad-spectrum antibiotics, prompt surgical débridement, aggressive systemic resuscitation, nutritional support
     - Amputation may be required
2. **Community-acquired MRSA**
   - **Increasingly prevalent as a pathogen for skin and soft tissue infection**
   - At risk groups:
     - Athletes
     - Intravenous drug abusers and homeless persons
     - Military recruits
     - Prisoners
   - Risk factors:
     - Previous antibiotic use within 1 year
     - Frequent skin-to-skin contact with others
     - Frequent sharing of personal items
     - Compromised skin integrity

B. Bone infections

1. **Osteomyelitis:** Infection of bone and bone marrow
   - May be caused by direct inoculation (open wound)
   - May also be caused by bloodborne organisms (hematogenous)
2. Microscopic organism causing chronic osteomyelitis: cannot be determined on the basis of the clinical picture and patient's age
   - Deep cultures are essential for specific microbiologic diagnosis.
   - Organisms isolated from sinus tract drainage typically do not accurately reflect the organisms present deep within the wound and within bone.
3. Acute hematogenous osteomyelitis
   - Causes and clinical features:
     - Caused by bloodborne organisms
     - Commonly in children (incidence higher in boys than in girls), typically in the metaphysis or epiphysis of the long bones
       - More common in lower extremity than in upper extremity
     - Vertebrae are most common sites in adults.
     - Radiographic changes include the following:
       - Soft tissue swelling (early)
       - Bone demineralization (10 to 14 days after infection)
       - **Sequestra (dead bone with surrounding granulation tissue) and involucrum (periosteal new bone) later**
     - Pain, loss of limb function, and soft tissue abscess may be present.
   - Diagnosis:
     - **Measurement of C-reactive protein is the most sensitive monitor of the course of infection in children**
       - **Has a short half-life, dissipates about 1 week after effective treatment**
     - ESR is elevated in 90% of cases.
       - Peaks after 3 to 5 days
     - WBC count may be elevated or blood or bone cultures may be positive.
       - This is true in fewer than 50% of cases.
     - Nuclear medicine studies may be helpful in equivocal cases.
     - **MRI** shows changes in bone and bone marrow before plain films do:
       - Decreased T1-weighted bone marrow signal intensity
       - Increased signal intensity on postgadolinium fat-suppressed T1-weighted images
       - Increased T2-weighted signal in relation to normal fat
   - Treatment:
     - Treatment may be summarized as follows:
       - Identify the organisms.
       - Select appropriate antibiotics.
       - Deliver antibiotics to the infected site.
       - Halt tissue destruction.
     - Empirical treatment should be administered before definitive culture findings become available.
       - **Newborn (up to 4 months of age)**
         - The most common infecting organisms are *S. aureus*, gram-negative bacilli, and group B streptococci.
         - Primary empirical therapy consists of nafcillin or oxacillin plus a third-generation cephalosporin.

Table 1-39 Soft Tissue Infections

Type	Affected Tissues	Clinical Findings	Organisms	Treatment
Cellulitis, erysipelas	Superficial, subcutaneous	Erythema; tenderness; warmth; lymphangitis; lymphadenopathy	Group A streptococci (most common) *Staphylococcus aureus* (less common)	Initial antibiotic treatment: penicillin G or penicillinase-resistant synthetic penicillins (nafcillin or oxacillin) Alternative therapies: erythromycin, first-generation cephalosporins, amoxicillin/clavulanate, azithromycin, clarithromycin, tigecycline, or daptomycin
Necrotizing fasciitis	Muscle fascia	Aggressive, life-threatening; may be associated with an underlying vascular disease (particularly diabetes) Commonly occurs after surgery, trauma, or streptococcal skin infection	Four types: 1) Groups A, C, and G streptococci 2) Clostridia 3) Polymicrobial (aerobic plus anaerobic) 4) Methicillin-resistant *S. aureus* (MRSA)	Necessitates extensive emergency surgical débridement (involving the entire length of the overlying cellulitis) and intravenous antibiotics Initial antibiotic treatments: penicillin G for streptococcal or clostridial infection; imipenem, doripenem, or meropenem for polymicrobial infections Add vancomycin or daptomycin if MRSA suspected
Gas gangrene	Muscle; commonly in grossly contaminated, traumatic wounds, particularly those that are closed primarily	Progressive, severe pain; edema (distant from the wound); foul-smelling, serosanguineous discharge; high fever; chills; tachycardia; confusion Clinical findings consistent with toxemia Radiographs typically show widespread gas in the soft tissues (facilitates rapid spread of the infection)	Classically caused by *Clostridium perfringens, Clostridium septicum*, or other histotoxic *Clostridium* species These gram-positive, anaerobic, spore-forming rods produce exotoxins that cause necrosis of fat and muscle and thrombosis of local vessels	Primary treatment: surgical (radical) débridement with fasciotomies Hyperbaric oxygen may be a useful adjuvant therapy, although its effectiveness remains inconclusive Initial antibiotic treatment: clindamycin plus penicillin G Alternative therapies include ceftriaxone or erythromycin
Toxic shock syndrome (TSS): staphylococcal	Toxemia, not septicemia In orthopaedics, TSS is secondary to colonization of surgical or traumatic wounds (even after minor trauma) TSS can be associated with tampon use through colonization of the vagina with toxin-producing *S. aureus*	Fever, hypotension, an erythematous macular rash with a serous exudate (gram-positive cocci are present) The infected wound may look benign, which may belie the seriousness of the underlying condition	Caused by toxins produced by *S. aureus*	Irrigation and débridement and intravenous antibiotics with intravenous immune globulin plus antibiotics Initial antibiotic treatment: penicillinase-resistant penicillins (nafcillin or oxacillin), vancomycin if MRSA Alternative therapies include first-generation cephalosporins Patients may also require emergency fluid resuscitation
Toxic shock syndrome (TSS): streptococcal	Toxemia, not a septicemia Commonly associated with erysipelas or necrotizing fasciitis	Similar to staphylococcal TSS	Toxins from Group A, B, C, or G *Streptococcus pyogenes*	Initial antibiotic treatment: clindamycin plus penicillin G Alternative therapies include ceftriaxone or clindamycin Intravenous immune globulin may be used; associated with decrease in organ failure, but no effect on all-cause mortality in children

Continued

Table 1-39 Soft Tissue Infections—cont'd

Type	Affected Tissues	Clinical Findings	Organisms	Treatment
Surgical wound infection	Varies		*S. aureus;* groups A, B, C, and G streptococci Other organism may be involved	Initial antibiotic treatment: trimethoprim-sulfamethoxazole or clindamycin MRSA species are best treated with vancomycin (alternatives for MRSA include daptomycin or ceftobiprole).
Marine injuries	Varies	History of fishing (or other marine activity) injury, with signs of infection Culture specimens at 30° C (60° F); organisms may take several weeks to grow on culture media	Marine injuries involve organisms that can cause indolent infections *Vibrio vulnificus* is the most likely organism in infected wounds that were exposed to brackish water or shellfish; can cause a devastating infection Consider atypical mycobacteria (e.g., *Mycobacterium marinum*) for injuries with indolent, low-grade infection	*V. vulnificus* is best treated with ceftazidime plus doxycycline; cefotaxime and ciprofloxacin are alternatives *M. marinum* is best treated with clarithromycin, minocycline, doxycycline, trimethoprim/sulfamethoxazole, or rifampin plus ethambutol

Table 1-40 Bite Injuries

Source of Bite	Organism	Primary Antimicrobial (or Drug) Regimen
Human	*Streptococcus viridans* (100%) *Bacteroides* species (82%) *Staphylococcus epidermidis* (53%) *Corynebacterium* species (41%) *S. aureus* (29%) *Peptostreptococcus* species *Eikenella* species	Early treatment (not yet infected): amoxicillin/clavulanate (Augmentin) With signs of infection: ampicillin/sulbactam (Unasyn), cefoxitin, ticarcillin/clavulanate (Timentin), or piperacillin-tazobactam Patients with penicillin allergy: clindamycin plus either ciprofloxacin or trimethoprim/sulfamethoxazole *Eikenella* organisms are resistant to clindamycin, nafcillin/oxacillin, metronidazole, and possibly to first-generation cephalosporins and erythromycin; susceptible to fluoroquinolones and trimethoprim/sulfamethoxazole; treat with cefoxitin or ampicillin
Dog	*Pasteurella canis* *S. aureus* *Bacteroides* species *Fusobacterium* species *Capnocytophaga* species	Amoxicillin/clavulanate (Augmentin) or clindamycin (adults); clindamycin plus trimethoprim/sulfamethoxazole (children) *P. canis* is resistant to doxycycline, cephalexin, clindamycin, and erythromycin Consider antirabies treatment Only 5% of dog bite wounds become infected
Cat	*Pasteurella multocida* *S. aureus* Possibly tularemia	Amoxicillin/clavulanate, cefuroxime axetil, or doxycycline Do not use cephalexin *P. multocida* is resistant to doxycycline, cephalexin, and clindamycin; many strains are resistant to erythromycin Of cat bite wounds, 80% become infected; culture
Rat	*Streptobacillus moniliformis* *Spirillum minus*	Amoxicillin/clavulanate or doxycycline Antirabies treatment is not indicated
Pig	Polymicrobial (aerobes and anaerobes)	Amoxicillin/clavulanate, third-generation cephalosporin, ticarcillin/clavulanate (Timentin), ampicillin/sulbactam, or imipenem-cilastatin
Skunk, raccoon, bat	Varies	Amoxicillin/clavulanate or doxycycline Antirabies treatment is indicated
Pit viper (snake)	*Pseudomonas* species Enterobacteriaceae *S. epidermidis* *Clostridium* species	Antivenom therapy Ceftriaxone Tetanus prophylaxis
Brown recluse spider	Toxin	Dapsone
Catfish sting	Toxins (may become secondarily infected)	Amoxicillin/clavulanate prophylaxis

Adapted from Gilbert DN, et al: *The Sanford guide to antimicrobial therapy,* Hyde Park, Vt, 2010, Antimicrobial Therapy, p 48.

- Alternative therapy: vancomycin plus a third-generation cephalosporin (primary if MRSA possible)
  - Patients may be afebrile; the best predictors are local signs in the extremity, including warmth.
  - Almost 70% of newborns with hematogenous osteomyelitis have positive blood cultures.
- **Children 4 months of age or older**
  - The most common infecting organisms are *S. aureus* and group A streptococci.
  - Primary empirical therapy consists of nafcillin or oxacillin.
    - Alternative therapy: vancomycin (primary if MRSA possible)
  - If Gram stain shows gram-negative bacilli, add a third-generation cephalosporin.
  - Immunization programs have almost eliminated *Haemophilus influenzae* bone infections that cause hematogenous osteomyelitis.
- **Adults 21 years of age or older**
  - **The most common infecting organism is *S. aureus*,** but a wide variety of other organisms have been isolated; **cultures are essential.**
  - Primary empirical therapy consists of nafcillin or oxacillin.
    - Alternative therapy: vancomycin (primary if MRSA possible)
- Sickle cell anemia
  - *Salmonella* infection is characteristic.
  - Primary empirical therapy consists of ciprofloxacin (only in adults).
    - Alternative therapy: levofloxacin (only in adults)
- Operative treatment may be necessary.
  - Start after cultures have been obtained by aspiration or surgical drainage.
  - Indications for operative intervention include the following:
    - Drainage of an abscess
    - Débridement of infected tissues to prevent further destruction
    - Refractory cases showing no improvement after nonoperative treatment

4. Acute osteomyelitis (after open fracture or open reduction with internal fixation)
   - Clinical findings may be similar to those of acute hematogenous osteomyelitis.
   - Treatment includes radical irrigation, débridement, and removal of orthopaedic hardware as necessary.
     - For open wounds, rotational or free flaps may be required.
   - The most common infecting organisms are *S. aureus, Pseudomonas aeruginosa,* and gram-negative bacilli.
   - Empirical therapy should be started before definitive cultures: vancomycin with a third-generation cephalosporin.
     - Alternative therapy is linezolid with a third-generation cephalosporin.
     - Antibiotic regimen should be adjusted after culture results become available.

Table 1-41 Chronic Osteomyelitis: Infected Host Types

Type	Description	Risk
A	Normal immune response; nonsmoker	Minimal
B	Local or mild systemic deficiency; smoker	Moderate
C	Major nutritional or systemic disorder	High

- In patients with acute osteomyelitis and vascular insufficiency or immunocompromise, the clinical picture is generally polymicrobial.

5. Chronic osteomyelitis
   - May result from inappropriately treated acute osteomyelitis, trauma, or soft tissue spread
   - Populations at high risk:
     - Elderly Cierny type C hosts (Table 1-41)
     - Immunosuppressed patients
     - Diabetic patients
     - Intravenous drug abusers
   - May be classified anatomically (Figure 1-94)
     - Skin and soft tissues are often involved.
     - Squamous cell carcinoma may develop in the sinus tract.
   - Periods of quiescence (of the infection) often followed by acute exacerbations
   - Diagnosis:
     - Nuclear medicine studies may help determine disease activity.
     - Accurate identification of organisms may require deep specimens from multiple foci.
     - *S. aureus,* Enterobacteriaceae, and *P. aeruginosa* are the most common infecting organisms.
   - Treatment:
     - Based on results of deep cultures and sensitivity testing
       - **Empirical therapy is not indicated.**

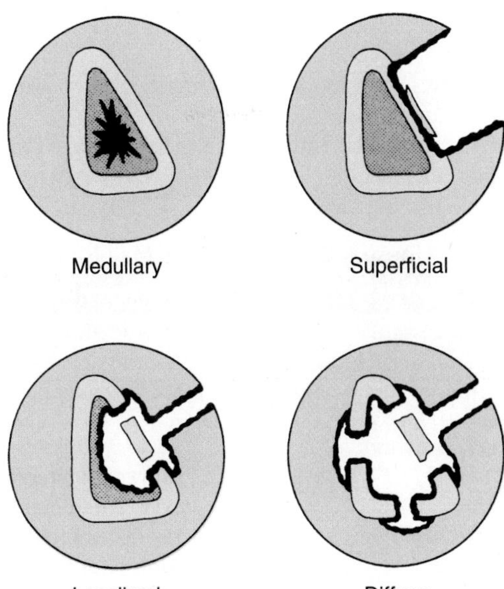

Figure 1-94 Cierny's anatomic classification of adult chronic osteomyelitis.

- Combined treatment:
  - Intravenous antibiotics (based on results of deep cultures)
  - Surgical débridement (complete removal of compromised bone and soft tissue)
  - Removal of retained hardware
    - Removing this hardware is the most important factor in eliminating infection.
    - Eliminating implant-associated infection is nearly impossible without removal of the implant.
    - Organisms grow in a **glycocalyx** (exopolysaccharide biofilm) that shields them from antibodies and antibiotics.
- After sterilization of the affected area, bone grafting and soft tissue coverage are often required.
- Unfortunately, amputation is required in certain cases.

6. Subacute osteomyelitis
   - Diagnosis
     - Usually discovered radiologically
       - Painful limp and no systemic (and often no local) signs or symptoms
       - **Brodie's abscess** (localized radiolucency usually observed in the metaphyses of long bones)
       - Sometimes difficult to differentiate from Ewing's sarcoma
     - May arise secondary to a partially treated acute osteomyelitis
       - Occasionally develops in a fracture hematoma
     - In contrast to acute osteomyelitis, WBC count and blood cultures are frequently normal
       - ESR, bone cultures, and radiographs are often useful.
     - Most commonly affects the femur and tibia
       - Unlike acute osteomyelitis, subacute osteomyelitis can cross the physis, even in older children.
   - Treatment:
     - Surgical curettage of Brodie's abscess in the metaphysis
       - When infection is localized to only the epiphysis, other lesions (e.g., chondroblastoma) must be ruled out.
     - Epiphyseal osteomyelitis: caused almost exclusively by *S. aureus*
     - Epiphyseal osteomyelitis: surgical drainage required if pus is present
       - Otherwise, intravenous antibiotics for 48 hours, followed by oral antibiotics for 6 weeks
7. Chronic sclerosing osteomyelitis
   - Unusual; primarily involves the diaphyseal bones of adolescents
   - Typified by intense proliferation of the periosteum, which leads to bony deposition
     - May be caused by anaerobic organisms
   - An insidious onset
     - Dense, progressive sclerosis on radiographs
     - Localized pain and tenderness are common
   - Malignancy must be ruled out
8. Chronic multifocal osteomyelitis
   - This condition is caused by an infectious agent; it appears in children without systemic symptoms.
     - Except for elevated ESR, laboratory values are often normal.
   - Radiographs demonstrate multiple metaphyseal lytic lesions.
     - Especially in the medial clavicle, distal tibia, and distal femur
   - It usually resolves spontaneously, necessitating only symptomatic treatment.
9. Osteomyelitis with unusual organisms (Table 1-42)
   - Radiographic findings:
     - Characteristic features in syphilis (*Treponema pallidum*): radiolucency in the metaphysis from granulation tissue
     - Characteristic features in tuberculosis: joint destruction on both sides of a joint
   - Histologic study can be helpful (e.g., in tuberculosis with granulomas).

C. Joint infections

1. **Septic arthritis**
   - Diagnosis
     - Septic arthritis commonly follows hematogenous spread or extension of metaphyseal osteomyelitis in children.
       - It can also be a complication of a diagnostic or therapeutic procedure
       - *Propionibacter acnes* infection can follow mini-open repair of the rotator cuff.
     - Most cases involve infants (hip) and children.
       - The most common infecting organism is *S. aureus*.
       - Group A streptococci are most common infecting organisms after varicella infection.

Table 1-42 Unusual Organisms That May Be Found in Osteomyelitis

Organism	Risk Factor	Symptoms/Signs/Findings	Treatment
Serratia marcescens	IV drug abuse	Axial skeleton	Cotrimoxazole
Pseudomonas aeruginosa	IV drug abuse	Nonspecific	Aminoglycoside
Brucella species (gram-negative)	Meat handling	Flat bones	Tetracycline/trimethoprim-sulfamethoxazole (Septra)
Salmonella organisms	Sickle cell disease	Asymptomatic	Ampicillin
Anaerobes	Skin contamination	Tissue culture	Clindamycin/cephalosporin
Fungi	Skin contamination	Special study	Amphotericin B
Treponema pallidum	Sexual contact	Nontender swelling	Penicillin
Mycobacteria	Tuberculosis Leprosy Fishermen	PPD/granuloma/culture at 30° C	PAS, isoniazid

IV, intravenous; PAS, *p*-aminosalicylic acid; PPD, purified protein derivative.

- The metaphyses of the proximal femur, proximal humerus, radial neck, and distal fibula are within their respective joint capsules.
  - Metaphyseal osteomyelitis can rupture into the joint in these areas.
- The most common sites at which septic arthritis follows acute osteomyelitis are the proximal femur and hip.
- Risk factors for adults:
  - RA (tuberculosis most characteristic, *S. aureus* most common)
  - Intravenous drug abuse (*Pseudomonas* most characteristic)

- Treatment:
  - Empirical antibiotic therapy (before results of definitive cultures are available).
    - **Newborn (up to 3 months of age)**
      - Most common infecting organisms: *S. aureus*, Enterobacteriaceae, group B streptococcus, *N. gonorrhoeae*
      - Adjacent bony involvement in approximately 70% of patients
      - Blood culture results commonly positive
      - Initial treatment: nafcillin or oxacillin plus a third-generation cephalosporin
        - Alternative treatment, or if MRSA is a concern: vancomycin with a third-generation cephalosporin
    - **Children (3 months to 14 years of age)**
      - Most common infecting organisms: *S. aureus, Streptococcus pyogenes, Streptococcus pneumoniae, H. influenzae,* and gram-negative bacilli
      - Initial treatment: vancomycin with a third-generation cephalosporin until culture results are available
    - **Sexually active adults who have acute monarticular septic arthritis**
      - Most common infecting organisms: *N. gonorrhoeae, S. aureus*, streptococci, and aerobic gram-negative bacilli
      - Empirical therapy when Gram stain result is negative: ceftriaxone, cefotaxime, or ceftizoxime
      - Vancomycin when Gram stain shows gram-positive cocci in clusters
    - **Adults who are not sexually active who have acute monarticular septic arthritis**
      - Most common infecting organisms: *S. aureus*, streptococci, and gram-negative bacilli
      - Empirical treatment driven by Gram stain results:
        - Gram negative: vancomycin plus a third-generation cephalosporin
        - Gram positive: vancomycin plus ciprofloxacin or levofloxacin
    - **Chronic monarticular septic arthritis**
      - Most common infecting organisms: *Brucella, Nocardia,* and *Mycobacteria* species and fungi
      - Treatment: organism-specific
    - **Polyarticular septic arthritis**
      - Most common infecting organisms: gonococci, *B. burgdorferi*, group A β-hemolytic streptococci (acute rheumatic fever), and viruses
  - Surgical drainage or daily aspiration
    - This protocol is the mainstay of treatment.
    - Open (or arthroscopic) drainage is required for septic hip joints.
    - Sacroiliac joint sepsis is unusual.
      - Best diagnosed from physical examination findings (flexion, abduction, and external rotation [FABER] most specific), ESR, bone scan, CT scan, and aspiration
    - A pannus similar to that of inflammatory arthritis can be observed in tuberculosis infections.
    - Late sequelae of septic arthritis include soft tissue contractures.
      - Can sometimes be treated with soft tissue procedures (such as a quadricepsplasty)

2. Septic bursitis
   - Most commonly caused by an *S. aureus* infection
   - Treatment: penicillinase-resistant synthetic penicillins
     - Vancomycin or linezolid if MRSA
3. Infected TJA
   - Prevention:
     - Perioperative intravenous antibiotics are most effective.
     - Also important:
       - Good operative technique
       - Laminar flow (avoiding obstruction between the air source and the operative wound)
       - Exhaust suits (“space suits”)
     - Preoperative joint aspiration for revision TKA appears to be useful in ruling out infection.
     - However, routine joint aspiration for revision THA results in a high incidence of false-positive culture findings.
   - Diagnosis:
     - ***Staphylococcus epidermidis*** is the most common pathogen in infection associated with an implant.
       - Next most frequent: *S. aureus* and group B streptococci
     - Signs:
       - Increased pain
       - Swelling
       - Erythema
       - Drainage
     - Tissue culture: most accurate test
       - Culture of joint aspirate
     - ESR: most sensitive indicator of infection
       - However, not specific
       - Elevated after surgery, even without infection
     - Measurement of specific C-reactive protein
       - However, this level also elevated after surgery
     - Preoperative skin ulcerations increase risk of infected TKA.
   - Treatment
     - **Acute** infections (within 2 to 3 weeks of arthroplasty):
       - The usual treatment is prosthesis salvage.
       - **Exchange only polyethylene components.**
         - Provided that the metallic components are stable
       - Synovectomy for an acute TKA infection is also beneficial.
     - Delayed or chronic TJA infections:
       - **Implant (and cement) removal is required.**

    - A staged exchange arthroplasty may be performed later, depending on the virulence of the organism.
  - An overlying glycocalyx formed by organisms
    - This makes infection control difficult without removal of the prosthesis and vigorous débridement.
    - However, according to Cierny, the host is more important than the organism in terms of risk (see Table 1-41).
  - Antibiotic-impregnated cement in revision arthroplasties and antibiotic spacers/beads in infected total joints: maybe useful
  - Reimplantation: successful at variable intervals
    - After thorough débridement
    - With use of polymethylmethacrylate (PMMA) with antibiotics
    - Use of frozen sections (to ensure that local tissues have less than 5 to 10 PMNs per high-power field) advocated by some authorities

D. Other infections

1. **Tetanus**
   - Tetanus is a potentially lethal neuroparalytic disease.
     - Caused by an exotoxin of ***Clostridium tetani***
   - Prophylaxis requires identifying a tetanus-prone wound and the patient's immunization history.
   - The following wounds are tetanus-prone:
     - Those more than 6 hours old
     - Those that have an irregular configuration
     - Those that have a depth of more than 1 cm or are the result of a projectile injury, crush injury, burn, or frostbite
     - Those that have devitalized tissue
     - Those that are grossly contaminated
   - Patients with tetanus-prone wounds and unknown tetanus status or fewer than three immunizations require the following prophylaxis:
     - Tetanus and diphtheria toxoids
     - Tetanus immune globulin (human)
   - Fully immunized patients with tetanus-prone wounds should be managed as follows:
     - Immune globulin is not required.
     - Tetanus toxoid should be administered in these cases:
       - The wound is severe or more than 24 hours old.
       - The patient has not received a booster immunization within the past 5 years.
   - Patients with non–tetanus-prone wounds should be managed as follows:
     - Tetanus toxoid only the following situations:
       - Immunization history is unknown.
       - Patient has received fewer than three doses of tetanus immunization.
   - Established tetanus should be treated as follows:
     - Primarily to control muscle spasms
       - Diazepam
     - Initial antibiotic therapy includes penicillin G or doxycycline; alternative therapy includes metronidazole
2. **Rabies**
   - Rabies is an acute infection characterized by CNS irritation.
     - May be followed by paralysis and death
   - The organism is a neurotropic virus present in the saliva of rabid animals.
   - With bites from presumably healthy dogs or cats bites, the animals should be observed for 10 days.
     - No need to start antirabies treatment immediately
     - If the animal begins to experience symptoms, one of the following:
       - Human rabies immune globulin with human diploid cell vaccine
       - Rabies vaccine absorbed (inactivated)
     - If the dog or cat is **suspected or known to be rabid**, immediate antirabies treatment
   - With bites from skunks, raccoons, bats, foxes, and most carnivores, the animals should be considered rabid.
     - The patient should be immunized immediately.
   - Animals whose bites rarely require antirabies treatment:
     - Mice, rats, chipmunks, gerbils, guinea pigs, hamsters, squirrels, and other rodents; rabbits and other lagomorphs
3. Puncture wounds of the foot
   - The most characteristic organism to cause infection as a result of a nail through the sole of a shoe is ***P. aeruginosa*** (unless the host is immunocompromised).
   - There is no standard prophylactic antibiotic treatment for a recent (hours-old) puncture through the sole of an athletic shoe.
     - Treatment may include removal of foreign bodies and tetanus prophylaxis.
   - Osteomyelitis can result from a puncture wound.
     - Develops in **1% to 2% of puncture wounds** through the sole of a shoe.
     - Treatment: ciprofloxacin or levofloxacin (except in children)
     - Alternative: ceftazidime or cefepime
4. Diabetic foot infections
   - Ulcer less than 2 cm in diameter, with superficial inflammation
     - No osteomyelitis
     - Most infecting common organisms: *S. aureus* (MRSA), *Streptococcus agalactiae,* and *S. pyogenes*
     - Suggested antibiotic treatment: oral trimethoprim-sulfamethoxazole; minocycline plus penicillin V potassium; second- or third-generation cephalosporin; or fluoroquinolone
   - Chronic, recurrent, limb-threatening "diabetic foot"
     - These infections can be life-threatening; **cultures** generally **reveal a polymicrobial picture** (including aerobic cocci, aerobic bacilli, and anaerobes).
     - Results of cultures from diabetic foot ulcers are unreliable.
       - Cultures from bone biopsy are required.
     - **Early or comparatively milder cases** can be treated as follows:
       - Oral treatment (one of the following regimens):
         - Ampicillin-clavulanate plus trimethoprim-sulfamethoxazole
         - Ciprofloxacin, levofloxacin, or moxifloxacin plus linezolid
         - Ertapenem
       - Parenteral treatment:

        - Vancomycin plus ampicillin-sulbactam, piperacillin-tazobactam, ticarcillin/clavulanate, or ertapenem
    - In **severe** cases or when the patient is septic, treatment is as follows:
        - Parenteral vancomycin plus one of the following:
            - β-lactam/β-lactamase inhibitor
            - Doripenem
            - Imipenem/cilastatin
            - Meropenem
    - Rapid surgical intervention with irrigation and débridement is essential.
        - Débridement helps differentiate a diabetic foot from necrotizing fasciitis or gas gangrene.

5. Paronychia
    - Infection/inflammation of the paronychial fold on the side of the nail
    - Caused by nail biting and manicuring
        - Most common infecting organism: *S. aureus*
            - Anaerobes are also common.
        - Initial antibiotic treatment: none; incision and drainage with culture
            - Alternative treatment: trimethoprim-sulfamethoxazole until culture results are available
    - Common among dentists, anesthesiologists, and wrestlers
        - In contact with the oral mucosa of other people
        - Most common infecting organism: herpes simplex (whitlow)
        - Commonly manifests with vesicles containing clear fluid
        - Gram stain and routine cultures yield negative results.
        - Treatment of choice: acyclovir
            - There is no need to débride the vesicles.
    - Common in dishwashers
        - Engaged in activities that involve prolonged immersion in water
        - Most common infecting organism: ***Candida*** organisms
        - Treatment: topical clotrimazole
            - Also avoiding immersion if possible
6. Fungal infections
    - Fungi are multicellular organisms with mycelia (branches) that induce a tissue hypersensitivity reaction.
    - They cause chronic granuloma, abscess, and necrosis.
    - Surgical treatment and **amphotericin B** administration are often required.
        - Oral ketoconazole is effective for some limited infections.
7. HIV infection
    - Incidence
        - Increased among homosexual men, patients with hemophilia, and intravenous drug abusers
            - HIV infection, however, may occur in any population.
        - Primarily affects lymphocyte and macrophage cell lines
            - **Decreases T helper cells (CD4 cells)**
    - AIDS
        - Diagnosis requires an HIV-positive test plus one of the following:
            - One of the opportunistic infections (such as pneumocystis)
            - CD4 count of less than 200 (normal = 700 to 1200)
    - Transmission
        - **Risk of seroconversion from a contaminated needlestick is 0.3%.**
            - Increases if the exposure involves a large amount of blood
            - Risk of seroconversion from mucous membrane exposure: 0.09%
        - Risk of HIV transmission from a large, frozen bone allograft is less than 1 per 1 million.
            - **Donor screening** is the most important factor in preventing viral transmission.
            - No cases of HIV conversion from fresh-frozen bone allograft have been reported **since 2001.**
        - The risk of transmission of HIV through a blood transfusion is estimated to be 1 per 500,000 per unit transfused.
            - Blood that is seronegative for HIV may nonetheless transmit HIV to a transfusion recipient; there is a delay (in the donor) between HIV infection and development of a detectable antibody.
    - Associated risks
        - HIV positivity is not a contraindication to performing required surgical procedures.
        - HIV-positive patients may be at increased risk for wound infections and nonwound complications (e.g., urinary tract infection, pneumonia).
        - Patients with HIV infection can develop secondary rheumatologic conditions such as Reiter's syndrome.
        - Fetal AIDS is transmitted across the placenta.
            - Affected children typically have a boxlike forehead, wide eyes, a small head, and growth failure.
8. Hepatitis
    - Hepatitis A
        - Common in areas with poor sanitation and public health concerns
        - Not a major problem regarding surgical transmission
    - Hepatitis B
        - Approximately 200,000 people are infected each year.
        - Currently, more than 12 million people in the United States are carriers.
            - 350 million carriers worldwide
        - Screening and vaccination have reduced the risk of transmission for health care workers.
        - Immune globulin is administered after exposure in nonvaccinated persons.
        - **The risk of transmission after allogenic blood transfusion is higher for hepatitis A than for HIV and hepatitis C.**
    - Hepatitis C (non-A, non-B)
        - The offending virus has been identified.
        - Recent advances in screening have decreased the risk of transfusion-associated infection.
            - **One per 103,000 transfusions**
        - Hepatitis C is also related to intravenous drug abuse.
        - **PCR** is the most sensitive method for early detection of infection.

9. **Cat-scratch fever (cat-scratch disease)**
   - Caused by ***Bartonella henselae,*** which infects the lymphatic system
     - Transmitted via a wound inflicted by a cat
   - Erythematous, painful lymphadenitis
   - Treatment: azithromycin
   - Alternative treatment:
     - Supportive only; needle aspiration of suppurative lymph nodes to relieve pain
     - **Do not perform incision and drainage** on the lesions
   - Resolves in 2 to 6 months
10. Allograft infection
    - May involve up to 20% of allografts
    - Aggressive measures are needed to control
11. Meningococcemia
    - Can develop in patients with multiple infarcts, such as **electrical burns**
12. Marjolin's ulcer
    - Squamous cell carcinoma
    - Develops in patients with chronic drainage from sinus tracts
    - Observed in untreated chronic osteomyelitis
13. Nutritional status and infection
    - Good nutrition decreases the incidence of postoperative infection.
    - Malnutrition is common after multiple trauma.
14. Postsplenectomy status
    - Patients are susceptible to streptococcal infections.

II. ANTIBIOTICS

A. Prophylactic treatment

1. Prevention of postoperative sepsis
   - For clean surgical cases, administer 1 hour preoperatively and continue for 24 hours postoperatively.
2. Perioperative use
   - First-generation cephalosporins in cases necessitating hardware
3. Shorter course of prophylactic antibiotics
   - Decreases the likelihood that bacteria will develop resistance

B. Initial care after an open traumatic wound

1. Types I and II open fractures
   - First-generation cephalosporins are the treatment of choice.
   - Some authorities suggest adding an aminoglycoside or a second-generation cephalosporin.
2. Type IIIA open fractures
   - First-generation cephalosporin plus an aminoglycoside
   - Penicillin added for grossly contaminated (type IIIB) open fractures

C. Antibiotic-resistant bacteria

1. Intrinsic resistance
   - Features of a cell that prevent antibiotics from acting on it
     - For example, absence of a metabolic pathway or enzyme
   - MRSA
     - Gene (mecA) produces the enzyme penicillin-binding protein 2a (PBP2a).
     - This enzyme prevents the normal enzymatic acylation of antibiotics.
2. Acquired resistance to antibiotics
   - A resistant strain emerges from a population that was previously sensitive.
   - Resistance is mediated by plasmids (extrachromosomal genetic elements) and transposons.

D. Spectrum of antimicrobial agents (Box 1-4)

E. Antibiotic indications and side effects (Table 1-43)

F. Mechanism of action of antibiotics (Table 1-44)

G. Other forms of antibiotic delivery

1. Antibiotic beads or spacers
   - PMMA is impregnated with antibiotics.
     - Usually an aminoglycoside
     - Useful for infected TJA or osteomyelitis with bony defects
     - Choice of antibiotic depends on the microorganism
     - Dosage depends on the antibiotic and type of PMMA
   - Antibiotics used with PMMA for infection include the following:
     - Tobramycin, gentamicin, cefazolin (Ancef) and other cephalosporins, oxacillin, cloxacillin, methicillin, lincomycin, clindamycin, colistin, fusidic acid (Fucidin), neomycin, kanamycin, and ampicillin
     - Chloramphenicol and tetracycline appear to become inactivated during polymerization.
   - Antibiotics elute from PMMA beads.
     - Exponential decline over a 2-week period
     - Cease to be present in significant levels by 6 to 8 weeks
   - Much higher local tissue concentrations can be achieved than by systemic administration, but with fewer problems.
     - Extremely high local concentrations can decrease cellular replication or cause cell death.
   - Increased surface area of PMMA (e.g., oval beads) enhances antibiotic elution.
   - Beads are inserted after thorough débridement.
   - Beads should always be removed.
     - PMMA may cause a foreign body reaction.
   - Adding 2 g of antibiotic powder per 40 g of powdered PMMA (simplex P) does not appreciably affect the compressive strength.
     - Maximum antibiotic without affecting strength is 5% total weight of PMMA.
     - Higher concentrations (4 to 5 g of antibiotic powder per 40 g of PMMA) significantly reduce compressive strength.
   - Antibiotic-impregnated cement spacers help prevent soft tissue contracture after removal of an infected TKA.
2. Osmotic pump
   - Delivers high concentrations of antibiotics locally
   - Used mainly for osteomyelitis
3. Home intravenous therapy
   - Cost-effective alternative for long-term intravenous antibiotics
   - Facilitated by a Hickman or Broviac indwelling catheter
4. Immersion solution
   - Contaminated bone (open fracture) may be sterilized by immersion in a chlorhexidine gluconate scrub and an antibiotic solution.

Box 1-4

Overview of Antimicrobial Agents

PENICILLINS

Natural

Penicillin G

Penicillin V potassium

Penicillinase-Resistant Penicillins

Methicillin (Staphcillin, Celbenin)

Nafcillin (Unipen, Nafcil)

Oxacillin (Prostaphlin, Bactocill)

Cloxacillin (Tegopen, Cloxapen)

Dicloxacillin (Dynapen, Pathocil)

Flucloxacillin (Floxapen, Ladropen, Staphcil)

Aminopenicillins

Ampicillin (Omnipen, Polycillin)

Amoxicillin (Amoxil)

Bacampicillin (Spectrobid)

Amoxicillin/clavulanate (Augmentin)

Ampicillin/sulbactam (Unasyn)

Antipseudomonal agents

Indanyl carbenicillin (Geocillin)

Ticarcillin (Ticar)

Ticarcillin/clavulanate (Timentin)

Mezlocillin (Mezlin)

Piperacillin (Pipracil)

Piperacillin/tazobactam (Zosyn)

CEPHALOSPORINS

First Generation

Cephalothin (Keflin, Seffin)

Cefazolin (Ancef, Kefzol)

Cephapirin (Cefadyl)

Cephradine (Velosef)

Cephalexin (Keflex, Keftab)

Cefadroxil (Duricef, Ultracef)

Second Generation

Cefaclor (Ceclor)

Cefamandole (Mandol)

Cefoxitin (Mefoxin)

Cefuroxime (Zinacef, Kefurox)

Cefuroxime axetil (Ceftin)

Cefmetazole (Zefazone)

Cefotetan (Cefotan)

Cefprozil (Cefzil)

Cefonicid (Monocid)

Loracarbef (Lorabid)

Ceftibuten (Cedax)

Third Generation

Cefdinir (Omnicef)

Cefditoren pivoxil (Spectracef)

Cefetamet pivoxil (Ro 15-8075)

Cefotaxime (Claforan)

Cefpodoxime proxetil (Vantin)

Cefoperazone (Cefobid, Claforan)

Ceftibuten (Cedax)

Ceftizoxime (Cefizox)

Ceftriaxone (Rocephin, Nitrocefin)

Ceftazidime (Fortaz, Tazicef, Tazidime)

Ceftriaxone (Rocephin)

Cefixime (Suprax)

Cefpodoxime proxetil (Vantin)

Fourth Generation

Cefpirome (HR 810)

Cefepime (Maxipime)

CARBAPENEMS

Ertapenem (Invanz)

Imipenem cilastatin (Primaxin)

Meropenem (Merrem)

MONOBACTAMS

Aztreonam (Azactam)

AMINOGLYCOSIDES

Amikacin (Amikin)

Gentamicin (Garamycin)

Kanamycin (Kantrex)

Neomycin

Netilmicin (Netromycin)

Tobramycin (Nebcin)

FLUOROQUINOLONES

Norfloxacin (Noroxin)

Ciprofloxacin (Cipro)

Ofloxacin (Floxin)

Enoxacin (Penetrex)

Gatifloxacin (Tequin)

Gemifloxacin (Factive)

Grepafloxacin (Raxar)

Lomefloxacin (Maxaquin)

Moxifloxacin (Avelox)

Pefloxacin

Levofloxacin (Levaquin)

Sparfloxacin (Zagam)

Trovafloxacin (Trovan)

MACROLIDES, AZALIDES, LINCOSAMIDES, KETOLIDES

Azithromycin (Zithromax)

Clarithromycin (Biaxin)

Dirithromycin (Dynabac)

Erythromycin

Telithromycin (Ketek)

Clindamycin (Cleocin)

OTHER ANTIBACTERIAL AGENTS

Chloramphenicol (Chloromycetin)

Colistin

Dalbavancin

Daptomycin (Cubicin)

Linezolid (Zyvox)

Quinupristin/dalfopristin (Synercid)

Rifampin (Rifadin, Rimactane)

Rifaximin (Xifaxan)

Tigecycline (Tygacil)

Vancomycin (Vancocin, Vancoled)

Teicoplanin (Targocid)

Doxycycline (Vibramycin)

Minocycline (Minocin)

Tetracycline (Terramycin)

Polymyxin B (Aerosporin)

Fusidic acid (Fucidin)

Fosfomycin (Monurol)

Sulfisoxazole (Gantrisin)

Trimethoprim/sulfamethoxazole (Bactrim, Septra)

Metronidazole (Flagyl)

ANTIFUNGAL AGENTS

Amphotericin B (Fungizone)

Fluconazole (Diflucan)

Flucytosine (Ancobon)

Ketoconazole (Nizoral)

Itraconazole (Sporanox)

Voriconazole

Caspofungin

Micafungin

ANTIMYCOBACTERIAL AGENTS

Amikacin (Amikin)

Capreomycin (Capastat)

Cycloserine (Seromycin)

Ethambutol (Myambutol)

Ethionamide

Isoniazid (INH [Nydrazid])

Pyrazinamide

Rifabutin (Mycobutin)

Rifampin (Rifadin)

Streptomycin

Thiacetazone

ANTIPARASITIC AGENTS

Albendazole (Zentel)

Atovaquone (Mepron)

Dapsone

Ivermectin (Stromectol)

Mefloquine (Lariam)

Nitazoxanide (Alinia)

Proguanil (Paludrine)

Pentamidine (Pentam 300)

Pyrimethamine (Daraprim)

Praziquantel (Biltricide)

Quinine

Tinidazole

ANTIVIRAL AGENTS

Abacavir (Ziagen)

Acyclovir (Zovirax)

Adefovir (Hepsera)

Amantadine (Symmetrel)

Amprenavir (Agenerase)

Atazanavir (Reyataz)

Cidofovir (Vistide)

Delavirdine (Rescriptor)

Didanosine (Videx)

Efavirenz (Sustiva)

Emtricitabine (Emtriva)

Enfuvirtide (Fuzeon)

Entecavir (Baraclude)

Famciclovir (Famvir)

Fosamprenavir (Lexiva)

Foscarnet (Foscavir)

Ganciclovir (Cytovene)

Indinavir (Crixivan)

Lamivudine (Epivir, Epivir-HBV)

Lopinavir/ritonavir (Kaletra)

Nelfinavir (Viracept)

Nevirapine (Viramune)

Oseltamivir (Tamiflu)

Ribavirin (Virazole)

Rimantadine (Flumadine)

Ritonavir (Norvir)

Saquinavir (Invirase, Fortovase)

Stavudine (Zerit)

Tenofovir (Viread)

Tipranavir (Aptivus)

Valacyclovir (Valtrex)

Zalcitabine (Hivid)

Zidovudine [AZT (Retrovir)]

Adapted from Gilbert DN, et al: *The Sanford guide to antimicrobial therapy 2006,* ed 36, Sperryville, Va, 2006, Antimicrobial Therapy, pp 59-81.

Table 1-43 Antibiotic Indications and Side Effects

Antibiotics	Sensitive Organisms	Complications/Other Information
Aminoglycosides	G–, PM	Auditory (most common) and vestibular damage is caused by destruction of the cochlear and vestibular sensory cells from drug accumulation in the perilymph and endolymph Renal toxicity Neuromuscular blockade
Amphotericin	Fungi	Nephrotoxic
Aztreonam	G–	Ineffective against anaerobes
Carbenicillin/ticarcillin/ piperacillin	Better against G– than for G+	Platelet dysfunction, increased bleeding times
Cephalosporins		Nausea, vomiting, diarrhea
First generation	Prophylaxis (surgical)	Cefazolin is the drug of choice
Second generation	Some G+, some G–	
Third generation	G–, fewer G+	Hemolytic anemia (bleeding diathesis [moxalactam])
Chloramphenicol	*Haemophilus influenzae,* anaerobes	Bone marrow aplasia
Ciprofloxacin	G–, methicillin-resistant *Staphylococcus aureus*	Tendon ruptures; cartilage erosion in children; antacids reduce absorption of ciprofloxacin; theophylline increases serum concentrations of ciprofloxacin
Clindamycin	G+, anaerobes	Pseudomembranous enterocolitis
Daptomycin	G+, methicillin-resistant *S. aureus*	Muscle toxicity
Erythromycin	G+	In cases of PCN allergy Ototoxic
Imipenem	G+, some G–	Resistance, seizure
Methicillin/oxacillin/ nafcillin	Penicillinase resistant	Same as penicillin; nephritis (methicillin); subcutaneous skin slough (nafcillin)
Penicillin	Streptococcal, G+	Hypersensitivity/resistance; hemolytic
Polymyxin/nystatin	GU	Nephrotoxic
Sulfonamides	GU	Hemolytic anemia
Tetracycline	G+	In cases of PCN allergy Stains teeth/bone (contraindicated up to age 8)
Vancomycin	Methicillin-resistant *S. aureus, Clostridium difficile*	Ototoxic; erythema with rapid IV delivery

G+, gram positive; G–, gram negative; GU, genitourinary; IV, intravenous; PM, polymicrobial; PCN, penicillin.

Table 1-44 Mechanism of Action of Antibiotics

Class of Antibiotic	Examples	Mechanism of Action
β-lactam antibiotics	Penicillin Cephalosporins	Inhibit cross-linking of polysaccharides in the cell wall by blocking transpeptidase enzyme
Aminoglycosides	Gentamicin Tobramycin	Inhibit protein synthesis (the mechanism is through binding to cytoplasmic 30S-ribosomal subunit)
Clindamycin and macrolides	Clindamycin Erythromycin Clarithromycin Azithromycin	Inhibit the dissociation of peptidyl-transfer RNA from ribosomes during translocation (the mechanism is through binding to 50S-ribosomal subunit)
Tetracyclines		Inhibit protein synthesis (binds to 50S-ribosomal subunit)
Glycopeptides	Vancomycin Teicoplanin	Interfere with the insertion of glycan subunits into the cell wall
Rifampin		Inhibits RNA polymerase F
Quinolones	Ciprofloxacin Levofloxacin Ofloxacin	Inhibit DNA gyrase
Oxazolidinones	Linezolid	Inhibits protein synthesis (binds to 50S-ribosomal subunits)

SECTION 6 PERIOPERATIVE PROBLEMS

I. PULMONARY PROBLEMS

A. Blood gas evaluation

1. Working formula for evaluating blood gases:

$$P_{O_2} = 7(F_{IO_2}) - P_{CO_2}$$

Where P_{O_2} is the expected partial pressure of oxygen in a healthy person, F_{IO_2} is the percentage of inspired oxygen, and P_{CO_2} is the partial pressure of carbon dioxide, the value of which is obtained by the blood gas assay.

Example: A 63-year-old man has an acute onset of shortness of breath 12 hours after a THA. A blood gas assay obtained 15 minutes after the patient is administered 60% oxygen (F_{IO_2} = 60) reveals the following **observed values:**

- P_{O_2} = 120
- P_{CO_2} = 60

However, the expected P_{O_2} = 7(60) − P_{CO_2} = 420 − P_{CO_2}. With a P_{CO_2} of 60, the expected (normal) P_{O_2} would therefore be

$$P_{O_2} = 420 - 60 = 360$$

The observed P_{O_2} (120) indicates an obvious problem with pulmonary status. To quantify the extent of the problem, calculate the **Aa gradient:**

$$\text{Aa gradient} = [\text{anticipated or normal } P_{O_2} \text{ (for a given } F_{IO_2})] - (\text{observed } P_{O_2})$$

Continuing with the example,

$$\text{Aa gradient} = (360) - (120) = 240$$

Finally, the **percent physiologic shunt** is calculated:

$$\text{Percent physiologic shunt} = \text{Aa gradient}/20$$

Therefore,

$$\text{Percent physiologic shunt} = 240/20 = 12\%$$

B. Thromboembolism

1. Common in patients who have undergone orthopaedic procedures
   - Especially those with procedures around the hip
2. Risk increases with many conditions (Box 1-5)
3. Deep venous thrombosis (DVT)
   - Pathophysiologic findings:
     - **Virchow's triad: endothelial damage, venous stasis, hypercoagulability**
     - **Tissue factor (thromboplastin) released in large amounts during orthopaedic procedures, triggering the coagulation cascade**
   - Diagnosis:
     - Clinical suspicion often more helpful than findings of physical examination (pain, swelling, Homan's sign)
       - Familial (factor V Leiden) thrombophilia
         - This condition is caused by an abnormality in factor V.
         - More than 50% of patients with familial thrombophilia will develop DVT with long bone fracture, TJA, or other risk.
     - Useful studies
       - Venography (the "gold standard")
         - Accuracy: 97% (70% for iliac veins)
       - Iodine-125 (^{125}I)–labeled fibrinogen
         - Artifact at the operative site causes false-positive findings.
       - Impedance plethysmography
         - Poor sensitivity
       - Duplex ultrasonography (B-mode)
         - Accuracy: 90% for DVT proximal to the trifurcation vessels
       - Doppler imaging
         - Immediate bedside tool, often the best first study
   - Prophylaxis:
     - The most important factor in decreasing morbidity and mortality
     - Common methods (Table 1-45):
       - Mechanical prophylaxis
         - Prevents venous stasis
         - Increases systemic release of endogenous fibrinolytic activity
       - Recommended options for 10-day treatment after knee or hip arthroplasty:
         - Low–molecular-weight heparin
         - Warfarin (targeted international normalized ratio of 2 to 3)
         - Fondaparinux
     - Warfarin (Coumadin)
       - Anticoagulation effects from inhibition of hepatic enzymes and vitamin K 2,3-epoxide reductase
       - Results in decarboxylation of the vitamin K–dependent protein factors
         - Factors II (prothrombin), VII (first affected), IX, and X

Box 1-5

Risk Factors for the Development of Thromboembolism

- History of thromboembolism
- Obesity
- Malignancy
- Aging
- Congestive heart failure (CHF)
- Use of a birth control pill
- Varicose veins
- Smoking
- General anesthetics (in contrast with continuous epidural)
- Increased blood viscosity
- Protein S deficiency
- Immobilization
- Paralysis
- Pregnancy

Table 1-45 Thromboembolism Prophylaxis

Method	Effect	Advantages	Disadvantages
Heparin			
Intravenous	Coagulation cascade: antithrombin III inhibitor	Reversible, effective	Control, embolization
Subcutaneous	Antithrombin III inhibitor	Reversible	No effect in extremity surgery
Warfarin (Coumadin)*	Coagulation cascade: vitamin K–dependent clotting factors	Most effective, oral	3-5 days to full effect, control
Aspirin	Inhibits platelet aggregation; inhibits thromboxane A_2 synthesis	Easy, no monitoring	Limited efficacy; not recommended as stand-alone option
Dextran	Dilutional	Effective	Fluid overload, bleeding
Pneumatic compression (and foot pumps)	Mechanical	Inexpensive, no bleeding	Bulky
Enoxaparin (Lovenox), a low–molecular-weight heparin	Inhibits clotting: targets factor Xa; forms complexes between antithrombin III and factors IIa and Xa	Fixed dose, no monitoring necessary, improved bioavailability	Bleeding

*See text for details.

        - Does not directly bind vitamin K or the clotting factors
            - **But inhibits posttranslational modification of vitamin K–dependent clotting factors**
        - Effects can be reversed with vitamin K or, more rapidly, with fresh-frozen plasma.
        - Rifampin and phenobarbital are antagonists to warfarin.
- Treatment:
    - Postoperative DVT necessitates initiation of heparin therapy.
        - Followed by later conversion to long-term (3-month) warfarin therapy
    - Treatment is recommended for all thigh DVTs.
        - Treatment of DVTs occurring below the popliteal fossa is controversial.
    - Preoperative DVT in a patient with lower extremity or pelvic trauma is an indication for placement of a vena cava filter.
    - **Virchow's triad** consists of events involved in venous thrombosis:
        - Venous stasis
        - Hypercoagulability
        - Intimal injury
    - Thromboembolism formation (Figure 1-95)

4. Pulmonary embolism
    - Approximately 700,000 people in the United States have an asymptomatic pulmonary embolism each year.
        - Of these cases, 200,000 are fatal.
        - The most important factor for survival is early diagnosis with prompt initiation of therapy.
        - DVT and fatal pulmonary embolism occur in varying frequencies in unprotected patients Table 1-46.
    - Pulmonary embolism should be suspected in postoperative patients with any of the following conditions:
        - An acute onset of pleuritic pain
        - Tachypnea (90%)
        - Tachycardia (60%)
    - Initial workup includes the following:
        - Electrocardiography
            - May show right bundle branch block
            - Shows right axis deviation in 25%
            - May also show slow-twitch depression or T-wave inversion in lead III
        - Chest radiography
            - Hyperlucency rare
        - Arterial blood gas measurements
            - Normal PO_2 does not rule out pulmonary embolism.
    - Nuclear medicine ventilation-perfusion scan (may be helpful)
        - Pulmonary angiography is the "gold standard" for diagnosis if there is any uncertainty.
    - Treatment:
        - Heparin therapy (continuous intravenous infusion) is initiated.
            - Followed by oral warfarin for 3 months
            - Monitored by measurements of partial thromboplastin time (PTT).

Table 1-46 Frequency of Deep Venous Thrombosis and Fatal Pulmonary Embolism (Diagnosed with Venography) in Unprotected Patients

	FREQUENCY (%)	
Procedure	Deep Venous Thrombosis	Fatal Pulmonary Embolism
Elective hip arthroplasty	70	2
Elective knee arthroplasty	80	1
Open meniscectomy	20	Unknown
Hip fracture	60	3.5
Spinal fracture with paralysis	100	≈1
Polytrauma patients	35	Unknown
Pelvic/acetabular fracture	20	Unknown

Adapted from Simon SR, editor: *Orthopaedic basic science,* Rosemont, Ill, 1994, American Academy of Orthopaedic Surgeons, p 489.

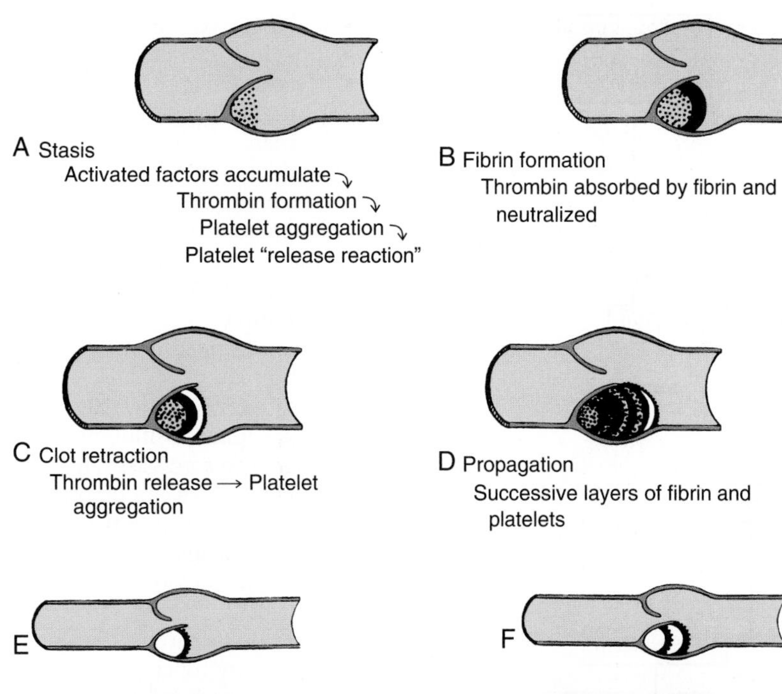

Figure 1-95 Venous thromboembolus formation. **A,** Stasis. **B,** Fibrin formation. **C,** Clot retraction. **D,** Propagation. **E through H,** Continuation of this process until the vessel is effectively occluded. (From Simon SR [editor]: *Orthopaedic basic science,* Rosemont, Ill, 1994, American Academy of Orthopaedic Surgeons, p 492.)

- Select cases necessitate more aggressive therapy.
  - Thrombolytic agents, vena cava filter, other surgical measures
- Heparin therapy is administered for 7 to 10 days, followed by oral warfarin for 3 months.
  - Monitored by measurements of prothrombin time

5. Coagulation (Figure 1-96)
   - A cascade of enzymatic reactions
     - Beginning with prothrombin-converting activity
     - Concluding with **fibrin** clot formation
       - As fibrinogen is cleaved by thrombin and converted to fibrin
   - Intrinsic pathway
     - Monitored by PTT
     - Activated when factor XII contacts the collagen of damaged vessels
   - Extrinsic pathway
     - Monitored by measurements of prothrombin time
     - Activated by thromboplastin release into the circulation after cellular injury
   - The bleeding-time test: a measure of platelet function
   - Fibrinolytic system dissolves clots.
     - Plasminogen is converted to plasmin.
       - With the help of tissue activators, factor XIIa, and thrombin)
     - Plasmin dissolves a fibrin clot.
   - Ginkgo biloba
     - Displaces platelet-activating factor from its receptor binding site
     - May lead to prolonged bleeding after THA

C. Acute respiratory distress syndrome (ARDS)

1. Acute respiratory failure is secondary to pulmonary edema.
   - Occurs after such events as trauma, shock, or infection
2. Causes include the following:
   - Pulmonary infection
   - Sepsis
   - Fat embolism
   - Microembolism
   - Aspiration
   - Fluid overload
   - Atelectasis
   - Oxygen toxicity
   - Pulmonary contusion
   - Head injury
   - Fluid overload, aspiration, and microscopic emboli may also contribute
3. Activation of the complement system leads to further progression.
4. Signs include the following:
   - Tachypnea
   - Dyspnea
   - Hypoxemia
   - Decreased lung compliance
5. Clinical diagnosis of ARDS after fracture of a long bone is best made with arterial blood gas measurements.
6. Normal supportive care is often unsuccessful.
   - A mortality rate of 50% is not uncommon.
7. Ventilation with positive end-expiratory pressure (PEEP) is important.
   - Steroids have not proven efficacious.

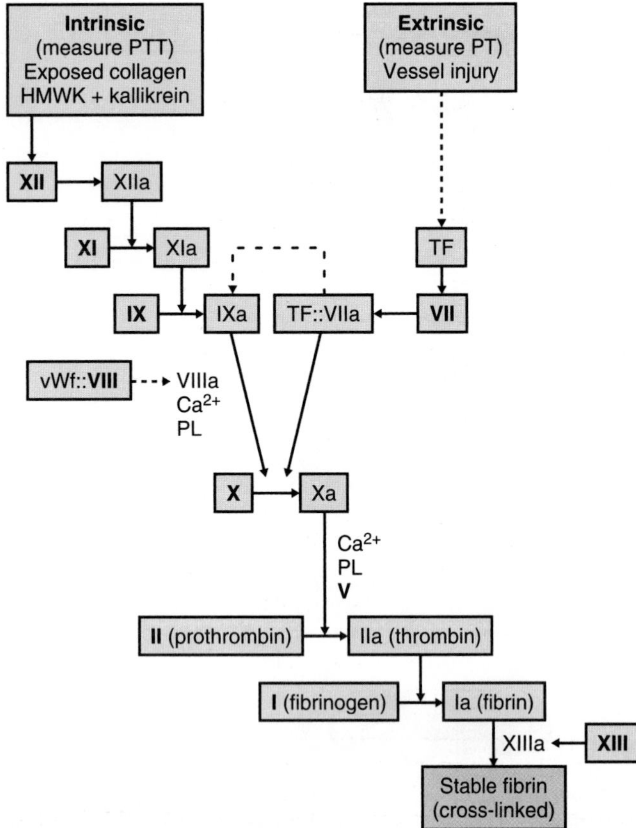

Figure 1-96 Coagulation cascade of factors I through XIII. HMWK, high-molecular-weight kininogens (bradykinin precursors); PL, platelet phospholipids; PT, prothrombin time; PTT, partial thromboplastin time; TF, tissue factor (thromboplastin); vWF, von Willebrand factor. (From Shannon MW, et al: *Haddad and Winchester's clinical management of poisoning and overdose,* ed 4, Philadelphia, 2007, WB Saunders.)

8. Early stabilization of fracture of a long bone (particularly femur) decreases risk of pulmonary complications.

D. Fat embolism (Figure 1-97)

1. Fat embolism usually occurs 24 to 72 hours after trauma.
   - Occurs in 3% to 4% of patients with long bone fractures
   - Fatal in 10% to 15% of cases
2. Early skeletal stabilization decreases incidence.
3. Onset may be heralded by any of the following:
   - **Hypoxemia (PaO_2 < 60 mm Hg)**
   - **CNS depression**
   - Petechiae: axillae, conjunctivae, palate
   - Tachypnea
   - Pulmonary edema
   - Tachycardia
   - Mental status changes
   - Confusion
4. Fat embolism may be caused by the following:
   - Bone marrow fat **(mechanical theory)**
   - Chylomicron changes, result of stress **(metabolic theory)**
   - Both these entities
5. A **ventilation-perfusion deficit** (hypoxemia) is consistent with ARDS.
   - Metabolism to free fatty acids
   - Initiation of the clotting cascade
   - Pulmonary capillary leakage
   - Bronchoconstriction
   - Alveolar collapse
6. Treatment is necessary:
   - Mechanical ventilation, **high levels of PEEP**
7. Steroids do not appear to have a prophylactic role.
8. Overreaming the femoral canal can decrease the incidence of fat embolism during TKA.
9. **Reamers** with a wider driver shaft increase risk of fat emboli during femoral reaming.

E. Pneumonia

1. Aspiration pneumonia can occur in the following scenarios:
   - In patients with decreased mentation
   - With supine positioning
   - With decreased gastrointestinal motility
2. Simple measures can be preventive.
   - Raising the head of the bed
   - Using antacids
   - Taking metoclopramide (Reglan)
3. Treatment
   - Appropriate intravenous antibiotics
   - Pulmonary toilet

F. Pulmonary complications of orthopaedic disorders

1. Severe scoliosis can cause pulmonary dysfunction.
2. Spontaneous pneumothorax is common in Marfan's syndrome.

II. OTHER MEDICAL (NONPULMONARY) PROBLEMS

A. Nutrition

1. Adequate nutrition should be ensured before elective surgery.
   - Malnutrition may be present in 50% of patients on a surgical ward.
2. Several indicators exist:
   - Anergy panels
   - Albumin levels
   - Transferrin level
   - Measurement of **arm muscle circumference** is the best indicator of nutritional status.
3. Complications of poor nutrition include the following:
   - Wound dehiscence and infection
   - Pneumonia
   - Sepsis
4. Lack of enteral feeding can lead to atrophy of the intestinal mucosae.
   - Leading in turn to bacterial translocation
5. Stress elevates nutritional requirements.
6. Provide full enteral or parenteral nutrition (nitrogen, 200 mg/kg/day) for patients who cannot tolerate normal intake.
   - Early elemental feeding through a jejunostomy tube can decrease complications in patients with multiple trauma.
   - Enteral protein supplements have proved effective in patients at risk of developing multiple organ system failure.
7. Starvation and stress produce metabolic changes (Table 1-47).

B. Myocardial infarction

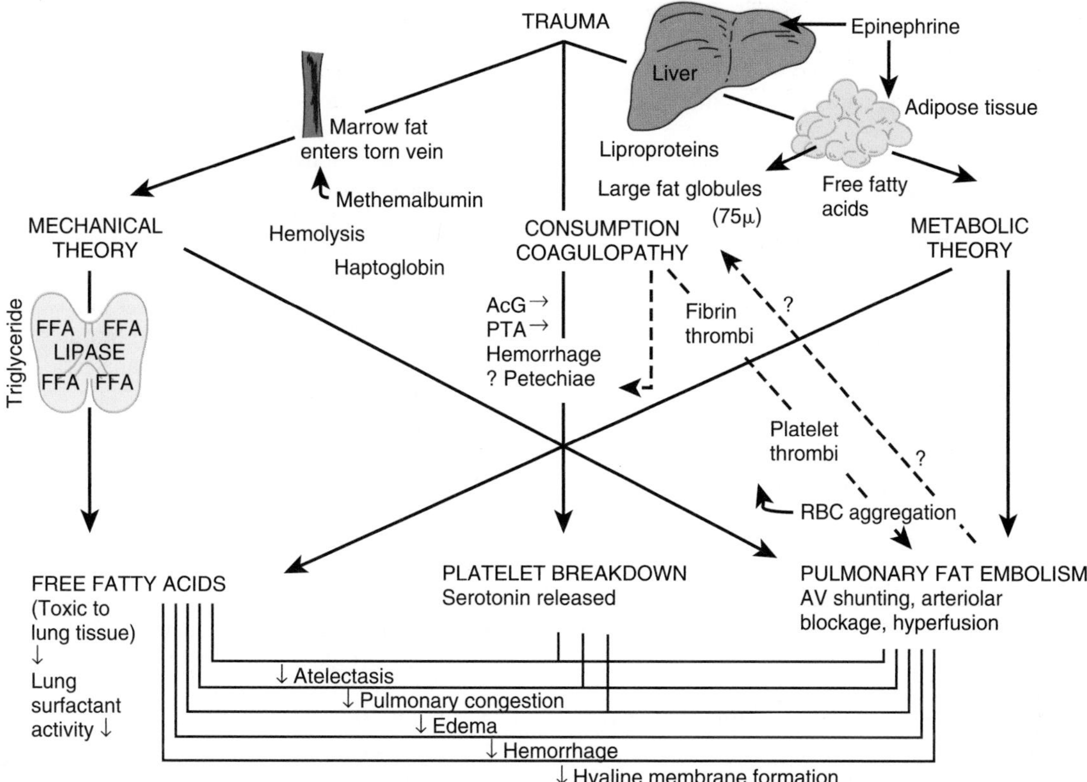

Figure 1-97 Pathologic events of fat embolism syndrome. AcG, accelerator globulin; AV, arteriovenous; FFA, free fatty acid; PTA, plasma thromboplastin antecedent. (From Simon SR, editor: *Orthopaedic basic science,* Rosemont, Ill, 1994, American Academy of Orthopaedic Surgeons, p 502.)

1. Classical presentation: radiating, acute chest pain and ECG changes
   - Monitoring warranted in an appropriate critical care environment
   - Cardiac enzymes and ECG monitoring needed on a continuing basis
2. Risk factors:
   - Increased age
   - Smoking
   - Elevated cholesterol
   - Hypertension
   - Aortic stenosis
   - History of coronary artery disease

C. **Gastrointestinal complications**
1. Range from ileus to upper gastrointestinal bleeding
   - Postoperative ileus common in diabetic patients with neuropathy
   - Risk approximately 1% after TJA

Table 1-47 Metabolic Changes of Starvation and Stress

	STARVATION		STRESS	
Metabolic Activity	Early	Late	Hypermetabolism	Multisystem
Energy expenditure	↓	↓↓	↑↑	Organ failure
Mediator activation	None	None	++	++
Metabolic responsiveness	Intact	Intact	Abnormal	Abnormal
Primary fuel	CHO	KB	"Mixed" (no KB)	"Mixed" (no KB)
Hepatic gluconeogenesis	↓	↓	↑	↑ or ↓
Hepatic protein synthesis	↓	↓	↑	↑ or ↓
Whole-body protein catabolism	Slight ↑	Slight ↑	↑↑	↑↑↑
Urinary nitrogen excretion	Slight ↑	Slight ↑	↑↑	↑↑↑
Malnutrition	Slow	Slow	Rapid	Rapid

Adapted from Simon SR, editor: *Orthopaedic basic science,* Rosemont, Ill, 1994, American Academy of Orthopaedic Surgeons, p 510.
↓, decreased; ↑, increased; ++, positive; CHO, carbohydrate; KB, ketone bodies.

2. Upper gastrointestinal bleeding more likely in patients with a history of ulcers, NSAID use, and smoking
   - Treatment: lavage, antacids, and H_2-blockers
   - Vasopressin (left gastric artery) for more serious cases
3. **Ogilvie's syndrome**, which includes cecal distension: can follow total joint replacement surgery
   - If cecum appears larger than 10 cm on an abdominal flat-plate radiograph, it must be decompressed (usually colonoscopically).

D. Decubitus ulcers

1. Associated with the following:
   - Advanced age
   - Critical illness
   - Neurologic impairment
2. Common sites: sacrum, heels, and buttocks
3. May be a source of infection and increased morbidity
4. Prevention is essential.
   - Frequent changing of position
   - Special mattresses
   - Treatment of systemic illness and malnutrition
5. Once ulcers established, débridement and sometimes soft tissue flaps necessary

E. Urinary tract infection (UTI)

1. UTIs are the most common nosocomial infection (6% to 8%).
2. They increase risk for joint sepsis after TJA.
3. Established UTIs should be treated preoperatively.
4. Perioperative catheterization (removed 24 hours postoperatively) may reduce the rate of postoperative UTI.

F. Prostatic hypertrophy

1. Causes postoperative urinary retention
2. Urologic referral preoperatively for the following reasons:
   - Suggestive findings of history and physical examination (prostate)
   - Urine flow studies: less than 17 mL/second peak flow rate

G. Acute tubular necrosis

1. Can cause renal failure in patients who have sustained trauma
2. Alkalization of urine important during early treatment of this disorder

H. Genitourinary injury

1. NSAIDs can affect the kidney.
   - Appropriate screening laboratory studies required at regular intervals
2. Retrograde urethrography best evaluates lower genitourinary injuries with displaced anterior pelvic fractures.

I. Shock

1. Capillary blood flow insufficient to perfuse vital tissues and organs
2. Hypovolemic shock ("volume loss")
   - Decreased cardiac output
   - Increased peripheral vascular resistance
   - Venous constriction
   - Tachycardia: most reliable early clinical finding
     - Drop in systolic blood pressure is a late finding.
3. Cardiogenic shock ("ineffective pumping")
   - Decreased cardiac output
   - Increased peripheral vascular resistance
   - Venous dilation
4. Vasogenic shock (pulmonary embolism or pericardial tamponade)
   - Arteriolar constriction
   - Venous dilation
5. Neurogenic shock/septic shock ("blood pooling")
   - Arteriolar, capillary, and venous dilation

J. Frostbite

1. Superficial
   - Treatment consists of the following:
     - General rewarming of the entire body
     - Immersion of the hands or feet in a warm-water bath (104° F [40° C]) for 15 to 30 minutes
   - Splinting, tetanus prophylaxis, analgesics, and antibiotics may be indicated.
   - Severe swelling may occur upon rewarming.
     - Monitor for compartment syndromes.
2. Deep
   - Débridement is often necessary.

K. Wound healing

1. Adequate healing after surgery is promoted by the following:
   - Transcutaneous oxygen tension higher than 30 mm Hg
   - Ischemic index (such as the ankle-brachial systolic index) of 0.45 or higher
   - Albumin level higher than 30 g/dL
   - Total lymphocyte count of 1500/mm^3

L. Anemia

1. Physiologic effects
   - Increased heart rate
   - Increased cardiac output
   - Increased coronary blood flow demand
   - Decreased peripheral resistance
   - Decreased blood viscosity

III. INTRAOPERATIVE CONSIDERATIONS

A. Anesthesia

1. Benefits
   - Regional anesthesia (disagreement in the literature):
     - May allow quicker recovery
     - May decrease blood loss
     - May produce fewer postoperative complications
       - Including a lower incidence of DVT/pulmonary embolism in THA
   - Controlled hypotension during surgery:
     - Helps with blood loss
     - Widely accepted, especially with THA and spinal arthrodesis
     - Nitroprusside, nitroglycerine, and isoflurane all effective
   - Fiber-optic bronchoscope: beneficial during surgery for patients with RA and others with cervical spine abnormalities
   - Local anesthetics for arthroscopy: also popular
2. **Malignant hyperthermia**
   - An autosomal dominant, hypermetabolic disorder of skeletal muscle
   - Can be triggered by various anesthetics in susceptible patients
     - Especially halothane and succinylcholine
     - Risk increased in Duchenne's muscular dystrophy, arthrogryposis, and osteogenesis imperfecta

- Involves impaired function of the sarcoplasmic reticulum and calcium homeostasis
  - Calcium transport affected by cell membrane defects
  - Leads to muscle rigidity and hypermetabolism
- Signs
  - First signs: increased end-tidal CO_2 and tachycardia
  - Masseter muscle spasm: often the first sign in children
  - Increased temperature
  - Rigidity
  - Acidosis
- Treatment:
  - Early diagnosis
  - **Dantrolene sodium**
    - Blocks calcium release by stabilizing the sarcoplasmic reticulum
    - Allows uptake of calcium
    - Decreases the intracellular concentration of calcium
  - Balancing of electrolytes
  - Increasing urinary output
  - Respiratory support
  - Cooling
- Muscle biopsy: the most accurate method for diagnosis
  - In vitro muscle fiber testing

B. Spinal cord monitoring

1. Usually involves testing the posterior column
   - The usefulness of monitoring other areas is under investigation.
2. Electrical monitoring
   - Somatosensory cortical evoked potentials (SCEPs)
   - Record summed input from stimulation of peripheral areas
   - Somatosensory spinal evoked potentials (SSEPs): more invasive but also more sensitive
   - Comparison of preoperative recordings (especially latency and amplitude) with readings at critical times during the procedure
3. The (Stagnara) wake-up test: the standard for monitoring
   - Lighten anesthesia.
   - Ask the patient to move selected extremities.

C. Tourniquet

1. Can injure the underlying nerves and muscles
   - Electromyographic abnormalities in up to 70% of patients after routine surgery
2. Prevention
   - Careful application
   - Wide cuffs
   - Lower pressures
     - 200 mm Hg in the upper extremity
     - 250 mm Hg in the lower extremity
     - Otherwise, 100 to 150 mm Hg above systolic blood pressure in the lower extremity
   - Double cuffs
3. Equilibrium reestablished within 5 minutes after 90 minutes of tourniquet use
   - Requires 15 minutes after 3 hours of tourniquet use

IV. OTHER PERIOPERATIVE PROBLEMS

A. Pain control

1. Acute pain: implies potential tissue damage; chronic pain (3 to 6 months) does not
2. Noxious stimuli transduced by nociceptors
   - Transmission along peripheral nerves
     - Types A and C fibers
   - To dorsal column, spinothalamic tract, thalamus
   - Transmission modulated by brainstem centers and endogenous opiates
3. Postoperative pain control: can be targeted at any step
   - Local prostaglandin inhibitors and long-acting local anesthetics target transduction of pain.
   - Perispinal opiates affect modulation.
   - Systemic opiates affect perception and modulation.
4. Local anesthetics
   - These agents cause transient, reversible loss of sensation in a confined area.
   - Local anesthetics interfere with nerve conduction (with the rate of rise of the depolarization phase of the action potential).
     - Cells fail to depolarize enough to fire after excitation.
   - Examples of such anesthetics are as follows:
     - Amides
       - Lidocaine (Xylocaine)
       - Bupivacaine (Marcaine)
     - Esters of *p*-aminobenzoic acid
       - Procaine (Novocain)
       - Butethamine (Monocaine)
     - Esters of meta-aminobenzoic acid
       - Cyclomethycaine (Surfacaine)
       - Metabutoxycaine (Primacaine)
     - Esters of benzoic acid
       - Cocaine
       - Ethyl aminobenzoate (Benzocaine)
5. NSAIDs
   - Anti-inflammatory, antipyretic, analgesic, and antiplatelet effects
     - Inhibit synthesis and release of prostaglandins
     - **Inhibit cyclooxygenase**
       - Cyclooxygenase catalyzes synthesis of cyclic endoperoxides.
       - **It is involved in forming prostaglandins from arachidonic acid.**
   - Acetaminophen
     - Does not affect cyclooxygenase activity
     - An antipyretic analgesic
     - Inhibits an IL-1β–dependent translocation, which inhibits prostaglandin synthesis
   - Cyclooxygenase inhibitors:
     - Two isoforms of cyclooxygenase:
       - COX-1
       - COX-2
     - In general, NSAIDs are drugs that inhibit both COX-1 and COX-2
       - Salicylates (e.g., aspirin)
       - Salicylate-like anti-inflammatory agents (e.g., ibuprofen)
       - Analgesic combinations and mixtures (e.g., codeine plus aspirin)
     - Example mechanisms by which NSAIDs inhibit cyclooxygenase:
       - Aspirin
         - Binds with a serine residue of cyclooxygenase
         - **Irreversible steric hindrance of the active site**

Table 1-48 Alternatives to Homologous (Blood Bank) Blood Transfusion

Type	Procedure	Notes
Autologous deposition	Requires a hemoglobin level of ≈11 (and a hematocrit level of 33%) and some lead time Iron supplementation during donation is routine	Allows storage of several units of blood before elective procedures in which significant blood loss is anticipated Significant cardiac disease, such as unstable angina, is a contraindication About 20% of patients who have undergone THA and donate 2 units of autologous blood require a homologous (from another donor) blood transfusion Significantly reduces hepatitis C risk Autologous blood that is seropositive for hepatitis can be reinfused, but warning labels and special handling and storage are required **Autologous donation is not recommended unless the risk with transfusion is greater than 10%**
"Cell saver"	Intraoperative autotransfusion	Usually requires 400 mL of blood loss to recover 1 unit (250 mL) Can be used for only 4 hours at one time
Autotransfusion	Allows postoperative drain recuperation and use	Reinfusion should begin within 6 hours of the beginning of collection to reduce febrile reaction risk
Acute preoperative normovolemic hemodilution	Immediate preoperative storage of autologous blood for intraoperative or postoperative use	Replace withdrawn autologous blood with crystalloid
Pharmacologic intervention	Desmopressin (antidiuretic hormone analog that increases levels of plasma factor VIII) Recombinant erythropoietin (stimulates erythrogenesis) Synthetic erythrocyte substitutes	
Judicious use of blood products	Platelet transfusion is used for massive bleeding or coagulopathies Fresh-frozen plasma is reserved for patients with massive bleeding and significantly abnormal results of coagulation tests Cryoprecipitate is used for hemophilia (less exposure than factor concentrates) and as a source of fibrinogen for consumptive coagulopathies	Platelet transfusion is based on clinical parameters rather than set platelet thresholds

THA, total hip arthroplasty.

- Ibuprofen
  - A reversible competitive cyclooxygenase inhibitor
- Indomethacin
  - Acts at the lipoxygenase side of the arachidonic metabolism pathway
  - Inhibits leukotriene inflammatory mediators
- **Side effects:**
  - Renal dysfunction
  - Gastrointestinal complications
    - Pain, dyspepsia
    - Peptic ulcer, perforation, bleeding, obstruction
      - Each year, these serious side effects occur in 2% to 4% of chronic users.
      - **Concurrent anticoagulant use is the most important risk factor, followed by age of more than 60 and a history of previous gastrointestinal disease.**
- **COX-2–specific inhibitors:**
  - Benefits
    - Do not inhibit functions of COX-1
      - **Maintain gastric mucosa**
      - Regulate renal blood flow
      - Influence platelet aggregation
    - Can be used perioperatively
      - No effect on platelet function
  - Label warning:
    - As of 2010, celecoxib (Celebrex) was the only COX-2 inhibitor available in the United States.
    - The package carries a label warning about increased risk of cardiovascular events.
  - Cyclooxygenase inhibitors: may delay or inhibit fracture healing
    - COX-2–specific inhibitors to a lesser extent

6. Substance P
   - Neuropeptide
   - Functions as a sensory neurotransmitter in CNS
     - Pain perception
7. Capsaicin
   - Pepper cream, obtained from red pepper
   - Believed to deplete neuropeptides in unmyelinated C fibers
     - Also depletes substance P from the spinal cord
   - Elevates threshold for painful stimuli

B. Transfusion

1. Transfusion reactions
   - Allergic reaction
     - Most common transfusion reaction
       - One per 150,000 transfusions
     - Occurs toward end of transfusion
       - Usually subsides spontaneously

- Symptoms:
  - Chills
  - Pruritus
  - Erythema
  - Urticaria
- Pretreatment:
  - Diphenhydramine (Benadryl) and hydrocortisone
  - May be appropriate in patients with a history of allergic reactions

- Febrile reaction
  - Also common
  - Occurs after initial transfusion of 100 to 300 mL of packed RBCs
  - Chills and fever
    - Caused by antibodies to foreign WBCs
  - Treatment:
    - Stop transfusion.
    - Administer antipyretics, as for allergic reaction.
- Hemolytic reaction
  - Less common but most serious
  - Occurs early in transfusion
  - Symptoms:
    - Chills
    - Fever
    - Tachycardia
    - Sensation of tightness in chest
    - Flank pain
  - Treatment:
    - Stop transfusion.
    - Administer intravenous fluids.
    - Conduct appropriate laboratory studies.
    - Monitor in intensive care unit.

2. Transfusion risks
   - Clerical error leading to transfusion reaction (hemolysis)
     - Occurs in 1 per 12,000 to 50,000 transfusions
     - **Most common transfusion adverse event**
   - Hepatitis C virus
     - Transmitted to 1 per 103,000 per unit transfused
   - Hepatitis B virus
     - Transmitted to 1 per 205,000 per unit transfused
   - Cytomegalovirus
     - Highest incidence; more than 70% of donors are seropositive
     - Not clinically important
   - Human T cell lymphotropic virus
     - Transmitted to 1 per 2,993,000 per unit transfused
   - HIV
     - Transmitted to 1 per 500,000 per unit transfused
   - Donor deferral for persons at high risk and more effective screening methods are helping manage these risks
3. Alternatives to homologous (blood bank) blood transfusion (Table 1-48)

C. Herbal medicines in the perioperative period

1. **Garlic, ginkgo biloba, and ginseng: increase risk of bleeding**
   - Mnemonic: all "Gs"
   - Ginseng also decreases anticoagulant activity of warfarin and may cause hypoglycemia
2. Ephedra: cardiovascular instability
3. Kava and valerian: potentiation of anesthetics

SECTION 7 IMAGING AND SPECIAL STUDIES

I. NUCLEAR MEDICINE

A. Bone scan

1. Technetium-99m phosphate complexes
   - Reflect increased blood flow and metabolism
   - Absorbed onto hydroxyapatite crystals in bone
     - Areas of infection, trauma, and neoplasia
2. Whole-body views and more detailed (pinhole) views possible
3. Evaluative uses:
   - Subtle fractures
   - Avascular necrosis
     - Hypoperfused early
     - Increased uptake in reparative phase
   - Osteomyelitis
     - Especially triple-phase study
     - Also in conjunction with gallium or indium scan
   - THA and TKA loosening
     - Especially femoral components
     - In conjunction with gallium scan to rule out infection
   - Patellofemoral overload
   - Osteochondritis dissecans of the talus
4. Phase studies
   - Three-phase (or even four-phase) studies
     - Helpful for reflex sympathetic dystrophy and osteomyelitis
     - Most reliable test for nondisplaced scaphoid fracture
   - **First phase** (blood flow, immediate)
     - Blood flow through the arterial system
   - **Second phase** (blood pool, 30 minutes)
     - Equilibrium of tracer throughout the intravascular volume
   - **Third phase** (delayed, 4 hours)
     - Displays sites of tracer accumulation
   - May be negative in pediatric septic arthritis

B. Gallium (Gallium-67 citrate) scan

1. Localizes in sites of **inflammation and neoplasia**
   - Exudation of labeled serum proteins
2. Delayed imaging required (24 to 48 hours or more)
3. Less dependent on vascular flow than is technetium
   - May identify foci otherwise missed
4. Difficulty differentiating cellulitis from osteomyelitis

C. Indium-111 scan

1. Labeled WBCS (leukocytes)
   - Collect in areas of **inflammation**
   - Do not collect in areas of neoplasia
2. Uses:
   - Acute infections (e.g., osteomyelitis)
   - Possibly TJA infections

D. Technetium-labeled WBC scan: similar to indium scan

E. Radiolabeled monoclonal antibodies

1. May identify primary malignancies and metastatic disease

F. DVT/pulmonary embolism scan

1. Radioactive iodine
   - Labels fibrinogen in clot on scanning
   - Inaccurate near surgical wounds
2. Lung scans: may help evaluate pulmonary blood flow
   - Limited at present

G. Single-Photon Emission Computed Tomography (SPECT)

1. Scintigraphy with CT to evaluate overlapping structures
   - Femoral head osteonecrosis
   - Patellofemoral syndrome
   - Spondylolysis

II. ARTHROGRAPHY (TABLE 1-49)

III. MAGNETIC RESONANCE IMAGING

A. Introduction

1. Excellent for evaluating soft tissues and bone marrow
2. Ineffective in evaluating trabecular bone and cortical bone
   - These tissues have virtually no hydrogen nuclei.
3. Used to evaluate osteonecrosis, neoplasms, infection, and trauma
4. Allows both axial and sagittal representations
5. Contraindications:
   - Pacemakers
   - Cerebral aneurysm clips
   - Shrapnel or hardware, in certain locations

B. Basic principles of MRI (Tables 1-50 through 1-52)

1. Radiofrequency pulses on tissues in a magnetic field
2. Images in any desired plane
   - No ionizing radiation
3. Nuclei with odd numbers of protons/neutrons (with a normally random spin) aligned parallel to a magnetic field
   - Field strength: 0.5 to 15 T (1 T = 10,000 G)
4. Nuclear magnetic moments of these particles deflected by radiofrequency pulses; results in an image
5. The use of surface coils decreases the signal-to-noise ratio.
   - Body coils are used for large joints.
   - Smaller coils are available.
6. Sequences developed to demonstrate the differences in T1 and T2 relaxation between tissues
7. **T1 images weighted toward fat**
   - Typical TR (time to repetition) values lower than 1000 ms
8. **T2 images weighted toward water**
   - Typical TR values higher than 1000 ms
9. Dark on T1- and bright on T2-weighted images
   - Water, cerebrospinal fluid, acute hemorrhage, soft tissue tumors
10. Other tissues showing similar intensity on both T1- and T2-weighted images:
    - Dark: cortical bone, rapid flowing blood, fibrous tissue
    - Gray: muscle and hyaline cartilage
    - Bright: fatty tissue, nerves, slow flowing (venous) blood, bone marrow
11. **T1-weighted images best for demonstrating anatomic structure**
    - **High signal-to-noise ratio**
12. T2-weighted images best for contrasting normal and abnormal tissues
13. **"Magic angle phenomena"**:
    - Tendon or ligament tissue oriented near 55 degrees to the field produces bright T1-weighted images
    - False appearance of pathologic process
    - Most common in shoulder, ankle, knee
14. Techniques for identifying contrast between fluid and nonfluid elements (e.g., bone, fat)
    - Spin tau inversion recovery (STIR)
    - Fat-suppressed T2-weighted images

C. Specific applications

1. Osteonecrosis
   - Highest sensitivity and specificity for early detection
     - Detects early marrow necrosis
     - Detects ingrowth of vascularized mesenchymal tissue
   - Specificity of 98% and high reliability for estimating age and extent of disease
   - Diseased marrow dark on T1-weighted images
     - Allows direct assessment of overlying cartilage
2. Infection and trauma
   - Excellent sensitivity to increased free water
   - Shows areas of infection and fresh hemorrhage
     - Dark on T1-weighted images, bright on T2-weighted images
   - Excellent (accurate and sensitive) for occult fractures
     - Particularly in hip in elderly patients
3. Neoplasms
   - MRI has many applications in the study of primary and metastatic bone tumors.
   - Primary tumors are well demonstrated.
     - Particularly tumors in soft tissue (extraosseous and marrow)
   - MRI is used in evaluating skip lesions and spinal metastases.
     - Nuclear medicine studies remain the procedure of choice for seeking metastatic foci in bone.
   - MRI demonstrates benign bony tumors.
     - Typically bright on T1-weighted images and dark on T2-weighted images
   - MRI also demonstrates malignant bony lesions.
     - Often bright on T2-weighted images
   - Differential diagnosis is best made on the basis of plain radiographs.
4. Spine
   - Disc disease is well demonstrated on T2-weighted images.
     - Degenerated discs lose water.
     - Such discs appear dark on T2-weighted studies.
     - Extent of herniation of discs is also well shown.
   - Recurrent disc herniation is best diagnosed with gadolinium MRI scan.
     - Differentiation from scar:
       - On T1-weighted image:
         - Scar: decreased signal
         - Free fragment: increased signal
         - Extruded disc: decreased signal
       - On T2-weighted image:
         - Scar: increased signal
         - Free fragment: increased signal
         - Extruded disc: decreased signal

Table 1-49 Arthrographic Findings

Anatomic Location	Conditions	Description
Shoulder		Technique can entail single or double contrast agents (better detail)
	Rotator cuff tear	Extravasation of contrast through the tear into the subacromial bursa
	Adhesive capsulitis	Demonstrates diminished joint capsule size and loss of the normal axillary fold May be therapeutic (distends the capsule)
	Recurrent dislocations	May demonstrate a distended capsule or disruption of the glenoid labrum Use with tomography or computed tomography to better demonstrate capsular or labral disease
	Other	Bicipital tendon abnormalities Articular disease Impingement syndrome
Elbow	Articular cartilage defects/loose bodies Osteochondral fractures	Especially helpful when used with tomography
Wrist	Posttraumatic ligament disruption	Communication between compartments is used to determine pathologic process, but communication is common in asymptomatic patients older than 40 years Communication at the radiocarpal and midcarpal joints: suspect scapholunate or lunoquitetral ligament tear Communication at the radiocarpal and distal radioulnar joints: suspect a triangular fibrocartilage complex (TFCC) tear
Hip		
Infants and children	"Septic" hip	Obtain aspirate and assess joint damage
	Developmental dysplasia of the hip	Degree of joint incongruity: interposed limbus
	Legg-Calvé-Perthes disease	Severity of deformity
Adolescents and adults	Arthritis	Cartilage destruction and loose bodies
	Osteochondral fractures, chondrolysis, and THA loosening	Digital subtraction arthrography can be useful for suspected loose THAs
Knee	Meniscal tears (except posterior horn of the lateral meniscus) and discoid lateral menisci	Can be useful for screening patients with equivocal history or findings Evaluation of cruciate ligaments yields less accurate findings than does evaluation of the menisci
	Articular cartilage evaluation	
	Loose bodies	Only air contrast is recommended for evaluation of loose bodies
	Pathologic synovial tissue	PVNS, popliteal cysts, synovial chondromatosis, plicae
Ankle	Acutely torn ligaments Chronic osseous and osteocartilaginous abnormalities	
Spine	Facet joints	May be useful combined with therapeutic injections (anesthetics and steroids)

PVNS, pigmented villonodular synovitis.

- Gadolinium–diethylenetriamine pentaacetic acid (DTPA) can be added in MRI studies.
  - Enhances edematous structures in T1-weighted images
  - Also used to differentiate scar from disc
- MRI is most sensitive for diagnosing early discitis.
  - Decreased signal on T1-weighted images, increased signal on T2-weighted images
- MRI can help evaluate the spine in asymptomatic persons.
  - Of subjects older than 40 years, 28% show cervical spine abnormality.
  - Of subjects younger than 40 years, 20% to 30% show evidence of lumbar disc herniation.
  - Of subjects older than 60 years, 93% show evidence of degeneration or bulging of lumbar discs.
  - Biochemical studies show degenerative disc changes as early as the second decade of life.

5. Bone marrow changes
   - Best demonstrated by MRI (poor specificity) (see Table 1-52)
6. Knee MRI
   - Arthrography with MRI
     - Accomplished with instillation of saline, which creates iatrogenic effusion
     - Improves joint definition
   - Knee derangements well demonstrated on MRI
     - ACL rupture correctly diagnosed in 95% of cases
     - Meniscal changes also demonstrated (Table 1-53)
     - **Best radiologic test for posterior cruciate ligament (PCL) rupture**

Table 1-50 Magnetic Resonance Imaging (MRI): Terminology

Term	Explanation
T1	Time constant of exponential growth of magnetism; T1 signal measures how rapidly a tissue gains magnetism
T2	Time constant of exponential decay of signal after an excitation pulse; a tissue with a long T2 signal (such as that with a high water content) maintains its signal (is bright on T2-weighted image)
T2*	Similar to T2 but includes the effects of magnetic field homogeneity
TR	Time to repetition; the time between successive excitation pulses; short TR is less than 80 ms, long TR is greater than 80
TE	Time to echo; the time that an echo is formed by the refocusing pulse; short TE is less than 1000 ms, long TE is greater than 1000
NEX	Number of excitations; higher NEX results in decreased noise with better images
FOV	Field of view
Spin-echo	A commonly used pulse sequence
FSE	Fast spin-echo; a type of pulse sequence
GRE	Gradient-recalled echo; a type of pulse sequence

Table 1-51 Signal Intensities on Magnetic Resonance Imaging

Tissue	Appearance on T1-Weighted Image	Appearance on T2-Weighted Image
Cortical bone	Dark	Dark
Osteomyelitis	Dark	Bright
Ligaments	Dark	Dark
Fibrocartilage	Dark	Dark
Hyaline cartilage	Gray	Gray
Meniscus	Dark	Dark
Meniscal tear	Bright	Gray
Yellow bone marrow (fatty-appendicular)	Bright	Gray
Red bone marrow (hematopoietic-axial)	Gray	Gray
Marrow edema	Dark	Bright
Fat	Bright	Gray
Normal fluid	Dark	Bright
Abnormal fluid (pus)	Gray	Bright
Acute blood collection	Gray	Dark
Chronic blood collection	Bright	Bright
Muscle	Gray	Gray
Tendon	Dark	Dark
Intervertebral disc (central)	Gray	Bright
Intervertebral disc (peripheral)	Dark	Gray

Modified from Brinker MR, Miller MD: *Fundamentals of orthopaedics*, Philadelphia, 1999, WB Saunders, p 24.

7. Shoulder MRI
   - Rotator cuff tears
     - Sensitivity and specificity: about 90%
     - Grade 0 tears: normal signal intensity
     - Grades 1, 2, and 3 tears: increased signal intensity
     - Morphologic features:
       - Grades 0 and 1 tears: normal
       - Grade 2 tears: abnormal
       - Grade 3 tears: discontinuity
   - Capsular/labral tears
     - Efficacy of MRI equals that of CT arthrography in presence of effusion.
8. MRI spectroscopy
   - May help measure metabolic changes
     - Especially ischemic changes

IV. OTHER IMAGING STUDIES

A. Computed tomography

1. Demonstrates details of bony anatomy better than any other study
2. Hounsfield units used to identify tissue types
   - −100 = air
   - −100 to 0 = fat
   - 0 = water
   - 100 = soft tissue
   - 1000 = bone
3. **Multiple-detector row arrays**
   - Improved resolution in the longitudinal axis
   - Decreased data acquisition times
   - Improved spatial resolution
   - Improved quality of reconstructing algorithms
   - Reduced artifact caused by hardware
4. Shows herniated nucleus pulposus better than myelography alone
   - CT may be helpful differentiating disc herniation from scar.
   - Intravenous contrast material is taken up in scar tissue but not in disc tissue.
5. Frequently used with contrast material
   - Arthrographic CT, myelographic CT
6. CT digital radiography (CT scanography)
   - Accurate demonstration of leg-length discrepancy with minimal radiation exposure
     - Particularly when joint contractures exist (lateral scanography)
7. Best demonstrates joint incongruity after closed reduction of hip dislocation
8. Useful for measuring the cross-sectional dural area in the workup of cervical spinal stenosis
   - Spinal stenosis is diagnosed if this area is **less than 100 mm^2.**
9. Important for evaluating subtalar joint injuries and diagnosing tarsal coalitions
   - Talocalcaneal tarsal coalitions also well visualized on axial (Harris) radiographs.
10. Dynamic CT scanning: test of choice for atlantoaxial rotatory subluxation
    - Grisel's syndrome: spontaneous atlantoaxial subluxation in conjunction with soft tissue inflammation in the neck, such as pharyngitis
11. Images distorted by metal implants

Table 1-52 MRI of Bone Marrow Disorders

Disorder	Pathologic Features	Examples	MRI Changes
Reconversion	Yellow→red	Anemia, metastasis	↓ T1-weighted intensity
Marrow infiltration		Tumor, infection	↓ T1-weighted intensity
Myeloid depletion		Anemia, chemotherapy	↓ T1-weighted intensity
Marrow edema		Trauma, CRPS	↓ T1-weighted intensity ↑ T2-weighted intensity
Marrow ischemia		Osteonecrosis	↓ T1-weighted intensity

↑, Increased; ↓, decreased; CRPS, complex regional pain syndrome; MRI, magnetic resonance imaging.

B. **Ultrasonography**
1. Shoulder
   - Diagnosing rotator cuff tears
2. Hip
   - Diagnosis and follow-up of developmental hip dysplasia
   - Identification of iliopsoas bursitis in adults
3. Knee
   - Determination of articular cartilage thickness
   - Identification of intra-articular fluid
4. Soft-tissue masses
5. Hematoma
6. Tendon rupture
7. Abscesses
8. Foreign body location
9. Intraspinal disorders in infants
10. Aorta
    - In patients at increased risk for aortic dilation or rupture
    - In patients with Marfan's syndrome
11. Fractures
    - To evaluate progression of fracture healing

C. **Guided biopsy**
1. Workup of musculoskeletal lesions
2. Commonly in conjunction with CT

D. **Myelography**
1. Procedure of choice for **extramedullary intradural pathologic processes**
2. Cervical radiculopathy
3. Subarachnoid cysts
4. Failed back syndrome
5. Can be used with other studies, such as CT

E. **Discography**
1. Use is controversial.
2. Helpful for evaluating symptomatic disc degeneration
3. Pathologic discs: reproduction of pain with injection and characteristic changes on discograms
4. Commonly used with CT

F. **Measurement of bone density (noninvasive)**
1. Single-photon absorptiometry
   - Cortical bone density is inversely proportional to quantity of photons passing through it.
   - Radioisotope ^{125}I emits a single-energy beam of photons.
     - ^{125}I passes through bone.

Table 1-53 Magnetic Resonance Imaging Changes of Meniscal Disease

Disease Group	Characteristics
I	Globular areas of hyperintense signal
II	Linear hyperintense signal
III	Linear hyperintense signal that communicates with the meniscal surface (tears)
IV	Vertical longitudinal tear/truncation

Table 1-54 Nerve Conduction Study Results

Condition	Latency	Conduction Velocity	Evoked Response
Normal study	Normal	Upper extremities: >45 m/sec; lower extremities: >40 m/sec	Biphasic
Axonal neuropathy	Increased	Normal or slightly decreased	Prolonged, decreased amplitude
Demyelinating neuropathy	Normal	Decreased (10%-50%)	Normal or prolonged, with decreased amplitude
Anterior horn cell disease	Normal	Normal (rarely decreased)	Normal or polyphasic, with prolonged duration and decreased amplitude
Myopathy	Normal	Normal	Decreased amplitude; may be normal
Neurapraxia			
Proximal to lesion	Absent	Absent	Absent
Distal to lesion	Normal	Normal	Normal
Axonotmesis			
Proximal to lesion	Absent	Absent	Absent
Distal to lesion	Absent	Absent	Normal
Neurotmesis			
Proximal to lesion	Absent	Absent	Absent
Distal to lesion	Absent	Absent	Absent

Modified from Jahss MH: *Disorders of the foot,* Philadelphia, 1982, WB Saunders.

Table 1-55 Electromyographic Findings

Condition	Insertional Activity	Activity at Rest	Minimal Contraction	Interference
Normal study	Normal	Silent	Biphasic and triphasic potentials	Complete
Axonal neuropathy	Increased	Fibrillations and positive sharp waves	Biphasic and triphasic potentials	Incomplete
Demyelinating neuropathy	Normal	Silent (occasional activity)	Biphasic and triphasic potentials	Incomplete
Anterior horn cell disease	Increased	Fibrillations, positive sharp waves, fasciculations	Large polyphasic potentials	Incomplete
Myopathy	Increased	Silent or increased spontaneous activity	Small polyphasic potentials	Early
Neurapraxia	Normal	Silent	None	None
Axonotmesis	Increased	Fibrillations and positive sharp waves	None	None
Neurotmesis	Increased	Fibrillations and positive sharp waves	None	None

Modified from Jahss MH: *Disorders of the foot,* Philadelphia, 1982, WB Saunders.

      - A sodium iodide scintillation counter detects the transmitted photons.
    - Denser bone attenuates the photon beam.
      - Fewer photons reach the scintillation counter.
    - This technique is best used in the appendicular skeleton.
      - Radius: diaphysis or distal metaphysis
    - Findings are unreliable in the axial skeleton.
      - Soft tissue depth alters the beam.
2. Dual-photon absorptiometry
    - Also an isotope-based method
    - Allows for measurement of the axial skeleton and the femoral neck
      - Accounts for soft tissue attenuation
3. Quantitative computed tomography
    - Preferred for measurement of trabecular bone density
      - Trabecular bone is at greatest risk for early metabolic changes.
    - Simultaneous scanning of phantoms of known density
      - Creating a standard calibration curve
    - Accuracy within 5% to 10%
    - Radiation dose higher than that for dual-energy X-ray aborptiometry **(DEXA)**
4. DEXA
    - Most accurate and reliable for predicting fracture risk
    - Radiation dose lower than that for quantitative CT
    - Measures bone mineral content and soft tissue components

G. Thermography

1. Maps body surface temperatures
2. Low specificity
3. Not recommended for clinical evaluation of the spine

V. ELECTRODIAGNOSTIC STUDIES

A. Nerve conduction studies

1. Evaluation of peripheral nerves
    - Sensory and motor responses along their courses
2. Nerve impulses stimulated and recorded by surface electrodes
    - Allows calculation of conduction velocity
3. Measures latency (time from stimulus onset to response) and response amplitude
4. Late responses (F wave, H reflex) allow evaluation of proximal lesions.
    - Impulse travels to the spinal cord and returns.
5. Somatosensory evoked potentials
    - Used to evaluate brachial plexus injuries
    - Used for spinal cord monitoring

B. Electromyography

1. Intramuscular needle electrodes to evaluate muscle units
2. Used to evaluate denervation
    - Fibrillations; earliest sign usually at 4 weeks
    - Sharp waves
    - Abnormal recruitment pattern

C. Interpretation

1. Peripheral nerve entrapment syndromes
    - Distal motor and sensory latencies longer than 35 m/second
    - Nerve conduction velocities shorter than 50 m/second
    - Changes over a distinct interval (Tables 1-54 and 1-55)

SECTION 8 BIOMATERIALS AND BIOMECHANICS

I. BASIC CONCEPTS

A. Definitions

1. Biomechanics
    - Science of forces, internal or external, on the living body
2. Statics
    - Action of forces on rigid bodies in a system in equilibrium
      - Either at rest or moving at a constant velocity
3. Dynamics
    - Bodies that are accelerating and the related forces
      - Kinematics
        - Study of motion (displacement, velocity, and acceleration) without reference to forces
      - Kinetics
        - Relates the effects of forces to motion

4. Kinesiology
   - Study of human movements and motions
     - Kinematics
     - Kinetics
     - Anatomy
     - Physiology
     - Motor control

B. Principal quantities

1. Basic quantities
   - Described by International System of Units (SI); metric system
     - Length: meters (m)
     - Mass (quantity of matter): kilograms (kg)
     - Time: seconds (sec)
2. Derived quantities: derived from basic quantities
   - Velocity
     - Time rate of change of displacement (meters/second)
     - Rate of translational displacement: *linear velocity*
     - Rate of rotational displacement: *angular velocity*
   - Acceleration
     - Time rate of change of velocity (meters/second^2)
     - Can also be linear or angular
   - Force
     - Action causing acceleration of a mass (body) in a certain direction
     - Unit of measure: newton (N) = kg • m/sec^2

C. Newton's laws

1. First law: inertia
   - If the net external force (F) acting on a body is zero, the body will remain at rest or move with a constant velocity.
   - This law allows static analysis: $\Sigma F = 0$ (sum of external forces equals zero).
2. Second law: acceleration
   - Acceleration (a) of an object of mass (m) is directly proportional to the force (F) applied to the object:

$$F = ma$$

   - This law is used in dynamic analysis.
3. Third law: reactions
   - For every action (force), there is an equal and opposite reaction (force).
   - This law leads to free-body analysis.
   - This law also assists in the study of interacting bodies.

D. Scalar and vector quantities

1. Scalar quantities
   - Have magnitude but no direction
   - Examples: volume, time, mass, and speed (not velocity)
2. Vector quantities
   - Have magnitude and direction
   - Examples: force and velocity
   - Vectors have four characteristics:
     - Magnitude (length of the vector)
     - Direction (head of the vector)
     - Point of application (tail of the vector)
     - Line of action (orientation of the vector)
   - Vectors can be added, subtracted, and split into components (resolved).
     - Resultant of two vectors: principle of "parallelogram of forces"
3. Tensors
   - Tensors are arrays of numbers or functions that represent the physical properties of a system
     - Scalars (e.g., mass) are tensors of rank 0.
     - Vectors (e.g., force) are tensors of rank 1.
     - Stress (force per unit area) is an example of a tensor of rank 2.
       - Stress has magnitude and direction and is determined over a plane (surface) rather than a line.
   - Higher order tensors represent properties more complex than can be represented by vectors.

D. Free-body analysis

1. Forces, moments, and free-body diagrams to analyze the action of forces on bodies
2. **Know how to solve these problems!**
3. Force
   - A mechanical push or pull (load) that causes external (acceleration) and internal (strain) effects
   - Unit of measure: the newton (N)
   - Force vectors (F): can be split into independent components for analysis
     - Usually in the x and y directions (F_x, F_y).
     - With angle (θ) between F_x and F_y.
   - Some elementary knowledge of trigonometry is helpful.
     - $F_x = F \cos \theta$
     - $F_y = F \sin \theta$
   - Also remember the following approximations:

$$\sin 30 = \cos 60 \cong 0.5$$

$$\sin 45 = \cos 45 \cong 0.7$$

$$\sin 60 = \cos 30 \cong 0.9$$

   - A *normal* force is perpendicular to the surface on which it acts.
   - A *tangential* force is parallel to the surface.
   - A *compressive* force shrinks a body in the direction of the force.
   - A *tensile* force elongates a body.
4. Moment (M)
   - Moment is the rotational effect of a force.
   - Moment = force (F) multiplied by the perpendicular distance (the moment arm or lever arm = d) from point of rotation:

$$M = F \times d$$

   - *Torque* is a moment from a force perpendicular to the long axis of a body, causing rotation.
   - A *bending moment* is from a force parallel to the long axis.
   - The ***mass moment of inertia* is the resistance to rotation.**
     - Product of mass times the square of the moment arm:

$$I = m \times d^2$$

     - Affects angular acceleration
5. Free-body diagram
   - A free-body diagram is a sketch of a body (or segments) isolated from other bodies, showing all forces acting on it.
   - The weight of each object acts through its center of gravity.
   - **Center of gravity in the human body is just anterior to S2.**

6. Free-body analysis
   - The following steps are used in the analysis:
     - Identify the system (objective, known quantities, assumptions).
     - Select a coordinate system.
     - Isolate free bodies (free-body diagram).
     - Apply Newton's laws; establish equilibrium ($\Sigma F = 0$ and $\Sigma M = 0$).
     - Solve for unknown quantities.
   - Assumptions
     - No change in motion
     - No deformation
     - No friction
   - Example (Figure 1-98)
     - Calculate biceps force (*B*) needed to hold the 20-N weight of the forearm:
       - Elbow flexed 90 degrees
       - Biceps insertion: 5 cm distal to the elbow
       - Center of gravity of the forearm: 15 cm distal to the elbow
       - *Answer:* 60 N
     - Also solve for the joint (compressive) force (*J*):
       - *Answer:* −40 N

E. Finite element analysis

1. Complex geometric forms and material properties are modeled.
2. A structure is modeled as a finite number of simple geometric forms.
   - Typically triangular or trapezoidal elements
3. A computer matches forces and moments between neighboring elements.
4. Finite element analysis is often used to estimate internal stresses and strains.
   - Example: stress/strain at bone-implant interface

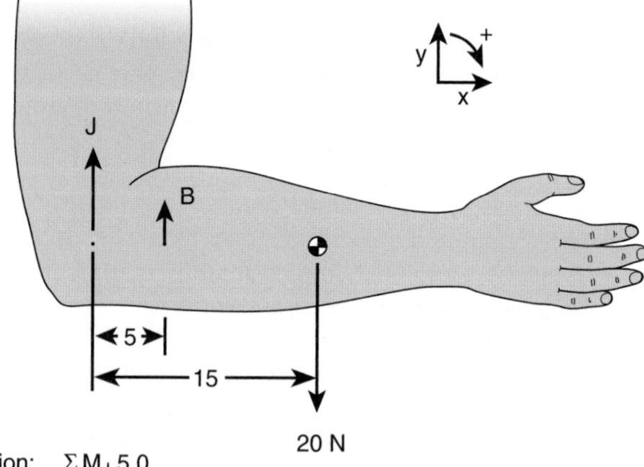

Solution: ΣM_J 5 0
2 B(.05) 20(.15) 5 0
.05 B 5 3
B 5 60N

ΣF_y 5 0
1 J 1 B 2 20 5 0
J 5 120 2 B
J 5 240N

Figure 1-98 Free-body diagram (see text for explanation). B, biceps force; J, joint compressive force; M, moment; N, newton (mass).

F. Other important basic concepts are as follows:

1. Work
   - The product of a force and the displacement it causes
   - Work (*W*) = force (*F*; vector components parallel to displacement) × distance (displacement produced by *F*)
   - Unit of measure: joule (J) = N • *m*
2. Energy
   - Ability to perform work (unit of measure is also joule)
   - Laws of conservation of energy:
     - Energy is neither created nor destroyed.
     - It is transferred from one state to another.
   - Potential energy
     - Stored energy
     - Potential of a body to do work as a result of its position or configuration (e.g., strain energy)
   - Kinetic energy
     - Energy caused by motion ($\frac{1}{2}mv^2$)
3. Friction (*f*)
   - Resistance to motion when one body slides over another
     - Produced at points of contact
   - Oriented opposite to the applied force
   - When applied force exceeds *f*, motion begins.
   - Proportional to coefficient of friction and applied normal (perpendicular) load
     - Independent of contact area and surface shape
4. Piezoelectricity
   - Electrical charge when a force deforms a crystalline structure (e.g., bone)
   - Concave (compression) side: charge is electronegative
   - Convex (tension) side: charge is electropositive

II. BIOMATERIALS

A. Strength of materials

1. Branch of mechanics
   - Study of relations between externally applied loads and resulting internal effects
2. Loads
   - Forces acting on a body
   - Compression, tension, shear, and torsion
3. Deformations
   - Temporary (elastic) or permanent (plastic) change in shape
   - Load changes produce deformational changes
4. **Elasticity**
   - Ability to return to resting length after undergoing lengthening or shortening
5. Extensibility
   - Ability to be lengthened
6. **Stress**
   - Intensity of internal force
     - **Stress = force/area**
     - *Internal* resistance of a body to a load
   - Unit of measure: pascal (Pa) = N/m^2
   - Helps in selection of materials
   - Normal stresses
     - Compressive or tensile
     - Perpendicular to the surfaces on which they act
   - Shear stresses
     - Parallel to the surfaces on which they act

- Cause a part of a body to be displaced in relation to another part
- Stress differs from *pressure:*
  - Pressure is the distribution of an *external* force to a solid body.
  - However, they share the same definition (force/area) and unit of measure (Pa).

7. **Strain**
   - Relative measure of deformation (six components) resulting from loading.
   - **Strain = change in length/original length**
   - Can also be normal or shear
   - Strain is a proportion; it has no units
   - *Strain rate*
     - Strain divided by time load is applied (units = sec^{-1}).
8. Hooke's law
   - Basically, stress is proportional to strain up to a limit.
     - The proportional limit
9. **Young's modulus of elasticity (*E*)**
   - Measure of material stiffness
     - Also a measure of the material's ability to resist deformation in tension
     - *E* = stress/strain
     - *E* is the slope in the elastic range of the stress-strain curve
   - The critical factor in load-sharing capacity
   - **Linearly perfect** elastic material
     - A straight stress-strain curve to the point of failure
     - Modulus = stress at failure (ultimate stress) divided by strain at failure (ultimate strain)
   - *E* is unique for every type of material
     - A material with a higher *E* can withstand greater forces than can material with a lower *E*.
10. Shear modulus
    - Ratio of shear stress to shear strain
    - A measure of stiffness
    - Unit of measure: pascal (Pa)
11. Stress-strain curve (Figure 1-99)
    - Derived by loading a body and plotting stress versus strain
      - The curve's shape varies by material.

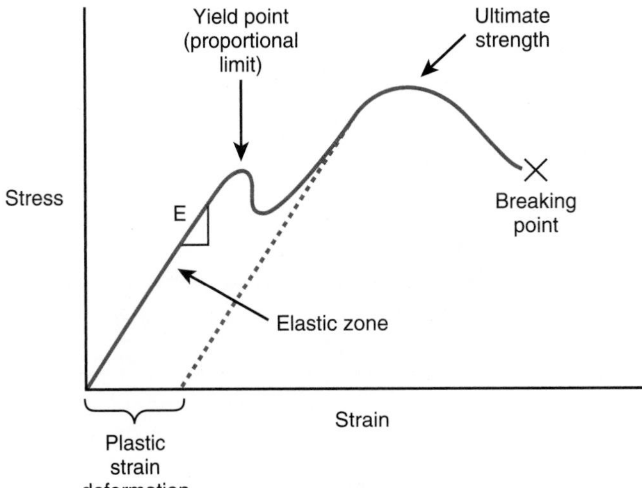

Figure 1-99 Stress-strain curve. *E,* Young's modulus of elasticity.

- Proportional limit
  - Transition point at which stress and strain are no longer proportional
    - The material returns to its original length when stress removed: elastic behavior.
- Elastic limit (yield point)
  - This is the transition point from elastic to plastic behavior.
  - Beyond this point, the material's structure is irreversibly changed.
  - The elastic limit equals 0.2% strain in most metals.
- **Plastic deformation**
  - Irreversible change after load is removed.
    - Occurs in the plastic range of the curve
    - After the elastic limit, before the breaking point
- Ultimate strength
  - Maximum strength obtained by the material
- Breaking point
  - Point at which the material fractures
  - If deformation between the elastic limit and breaking point is large, the material is *ductile.*
  - If this deformation is small, the material is *brittle.*
- **Strain energy** (toughness)
  - Capacity of material (such as bone) to absorb energy
  - **Area under the stress-strain curve**
  - Total strain energy = recoverable strain energy (resilience) + dissipated strain energy
  - A measure of the toughness of material
    - **Ability to absorb energy before failure**

B. Materials and structures

1. Material
   - Related to a substance or element
     - Mechanical properties:
       - Force
       - Stress
       - Strain
     - Rheologic properties:
       - Elasticity
       - Plasticity
       - Viscosity: resistance to flow or shear stress
       - Strength
   - **Brittle materials** (e.g., PMMA)
     - Stress-strain curve is linear up to failure.
     - These materials undergo only recoverable (elastic) deformation before failure.
     - They have little or no capacity for plastic deformation.
   - **Ductile materials** (e.g., metal)
     - These materials undergo large plastic deformation before failure.
     - Ductility is a measure of postyield deformation.
   - **Viscoelastic materials** (e.g., bone and ligaments)
     - Stress-strain behavior is **time-rate** dependent.
       - Properties depend on load magnitude and rate at which the load is applied.
     - A function of internal friction
     - These materials exhibit both fluid (viscosity) and solid (elasticity) properties.
     - Modulus increases as strain rate increases.
     - These materials exhibit **hysteresis.**
       - Loading and unloading curves differ.
       - Energy is dissipated during loading.
     - Most biologic tissues exhibit viscoelasticity.

- **Isotropic materials**
  - Mechanical properties are the same for all directions of applied load (e.g., as with a golf ball).
- **Anisotropic materials**
  - Mechanical properties vary with the direction of the applied load.
  - For example, bone is stronger with axial load than with radial load.
- Homogeneous materials
  - Have a uniform structure or composition throughout

2. Structure
   - Material, shape, and loading characteristics
   - Load deformation curve:
     - Constructed similarly to stress-strain curve
     - Slope in the elastic range is the rigidity of the structure
   - Bending rigidity of a rectangular structure:
     - Proportional to the base multiplied by the height cubed:

$$bh^3/12$$

   - Bending rigidity of a cylinder
     - Related to the fourth power of the radius
     - Intramedullary nails, half-pins
     - Closely related to area moment of inertia (*I*)
       - Resistance to bending
       - Function of width, thickness, and the polar moment of inertia (*J*)
       - *J*: resistance to torsion (twisting)
       - *I* and *J*: functions of the distribution of material in cross section
         - Distance squared of mass distribution from the center of mass
   - Deflection associated with bending
     - Proportional to applied force (*F*) divided by elastic modulus (*E*) and then multiplied by area moment of inertia (*I*):

$$\text{Deflection} = (F/E) \times (I)$$

3. Metals
   - Fatigue failure
     - Occurs with cyclic loading at stress below ultimate tensile strength
     - Depends on magnitude of stress and number of cycles
     - **Endurance limit**
       - Maximum stress under which the material will not fail regardless of number of loading cycles
       - If the stress is below this limit, the material may be loaded cyclically an infinite number of times (more than 10^6 cycles) without breaking.
       - Above this limit, fatigue life is expressed by the *S-n* curve:
         - Stress (*S*) versus the number of cycles (*n*)
   - Creep (cold flow)
     - Progressive deformation response to constant force over an extended period of time
     - Sudden stress followed by constant loading causes continued deformation
     - Can produce permanent deformity
     - May affect mechanical function (e.g., in TJA)
   - Corrosion (Table 1-56)
     - Chemical dissolving of metals
       - May occur in the body's high-saline environment
     - **Stainless steel (316 L)**
       - The metal most susceptible to both crevice corrosion and galvanic corrosion
       - Risk of galvanic corrosion highest between 316 L stainless steel and cobalt-chromium (Co-Cr) alloy
     - Modular components of THA
       - Direct contact between similar or dissimilar metals at the modular junctions
       - Results in corrosion products
         - Examples: metal oxides, metal chlorides
     - Corrosion can be decreased in the following ways:
       - Using similar metals
       - Proper implant design
       - Passivation by an adherent oxide layer
         - Effectively separates metal from solution
         - For example, stainless steel coated with chromium oxide
   - Types of metals
     - Orthopaedic implants
       - Three types of alloys: steel (iron-based), cobalt-based, titanium-based
       - 316 L stainless steel
         - Iron-carbon, chromium, nickel, molybdenum, manganese
         - Nickel: increases corrosion resistance and stabilizes molecular structure
         - Chromium: forms a passive surface oxide, improving corrosion resistance
         - Molybdenum: prevents pitting and crevice corrosion
         - Manganese: improves crystalline stability
         - "L" = low carbon: greater corrosion resistance
       - Cobalt alloys
         - Cobalt-chromium-molybdenum (Co-Cr-Mo)
           - 65% cobalt, 35% chromium, 5% molybdenum
           - Special forging process
           - Nickel may be added to improve ease of forging
       - **Titanium alloy** (Ti-6Al-4 V)
       - **Stiffness (*E*)** differences (Figure 1-100)
     - Problems with certain metals:
       - Wear
       - Stress shielding
         - Increased in metals with a higher *E*
       - Ion release

Table 1-56 Types of Corrosion

Corrosion	Description
Galvanic	***Dissimilar metals**; electrochemical destruction***
Crevice	Occurs in fatigue cracks with low O_2 tension
Stress	Occurs in areas with high stress gradients
Fretting	From small movements abrading outside layer
Other	For example, inclusion, intergranular

*Metals such as 316 L stainless steel and cobalt-chromium-molybdenum (Co-Cr-Mo) alloy produce galvanic corrosion.

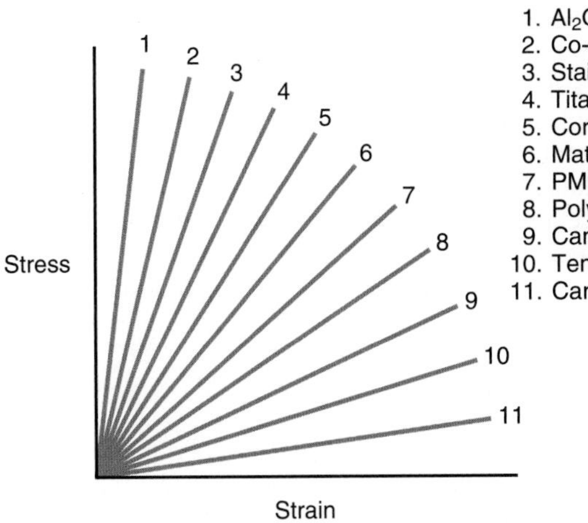

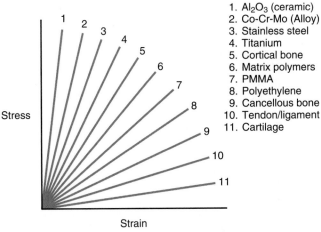

Figure 1-100 Comparison of Young's modulus (relative values, not to scale) for various orthopaedic materials. Al_2O_3, alumina; Co-Cr-Mo, cobalt-chromium-molybdenum; PMMA, polymethylmethacrylate.

- Co-Cr: macrophage proliferation and synovial degeneration
- Ions excreted through the kidneys

- **Titanium:** poor resistance to wear (notch sensitivity)
  - Particulate may incite a histiocytic response.
  - The relationship between titanium and neoplasms is uncertain.
  - Polishing, passivation, and ion implantation improve its fatigue properties.
  - Titanium is **extremely biocompatible:**
    - Rapidly forms an adherent oxide coating (self-passivation); decreases corrosion
    - A nonreactive ceramic coating
  - Other advantages of titanium are as follows:
    - Relatively low *E*
    - **Most closely emulates axial and torsional stiffness of bone**
    - High yield strength
- **Co-Cr alloy**
  - Generates less metal debris (in THA) than does titanium alloy
  - Problems with orthosis fabrication
  - Stainless steel: heavy
  - Aluminum: low endurance limit

4. Nonmetal materials
   - Polyethylene
     - Ultra–high-molecular-weight polyethylene (UHMWPE)
       - Polymer of long carbon chains
     - Used in weight-bearing components of TJAs
       - Acetabular cups, tibial trays
     - Wear characteristics superior to those of high-density polyethylene
       - Tough, ductile, resilient, resistant to wear, low friction
     - Polyethylene: viscoelastic and highly susceptible to abrasion
       - **Wear damage** to a UHMWPE articulating surface is most often caused by third-body inclusions.
     - UHMWPE: also thermoplastic
       - May be altered by temperature or high-dose radiation
     - Oxidative polyethylene degradation after γ-irradiation in air
       - This degradation is related to free radical formation.
         - Increases susceptibility to oxidation
       - **γ-Irradiation** increases polymer chain cross-links.
         - Greatly improves wear characteristics
         - However, reduces resistance to fatigue and fracture
         - Decreases elastic modulus, tensile strength, ductility, and yield stress
     - **Annealing**
       - Heating to below melting point
       - Decreases free radicals
       - Good mechanical properties; does not disrupt crystalline areas
     - Polyethylene is weaker than bone in tension and has a low *E*
     - Wear debris associated with a histiocytic osteolytic response.
       - **Particles with a size range of 0.1 to 1.0 μm are most reactive.**
       - This response is increased with thinner (less than 6 mm), flatter, carbon fiber–reinforced polyethylene.
     - Metal backing may help minimize plastic deformation of high-density polyethylene and loosening.
       - However, it decreases effective thickness.
     - Catastrophic wear of polyethylene tibial inserts associated with the following:
       - Varus knee alignment
       - Thin inserts (less than 6 mm)
       - Flat, nonconforming inserts
       - Heat treatments of the insert
     - Polyethylene wear debris: the main factor affecting THA longevity
       - Fatigue wear more prevalent in TKA than in THA.
     - Volumetric wear most affected by relative motion between the two surfaces in contact
   - **PMMA (bone cement)**
     - Used for fixation and load distribution for implants
       - Act as a grout, not an adhesive
       - Mechanically interlocks with bone
     - Reaches ultimate strength within 24 hours
     - Can be used as an internal splint for patients with poor bone stock
       - PMMA can be used as a temporary internal splint until the bone heals.
       - If the bone fails to heal, the PMMA will ultimately fail.
     - Poor tensile and shear strength
     - Is strongest in compression and has a low *E*
       - Not as strong as bone in compression
     - Reducing voids (porosity) increases cement strength and decreases cracking.
       - Vacuum mixing, centrifugation, good technique
       - Cement failure often caused by microfracture and fragmentation
     - Insertion can lead to a precipitous drop in blood pressure.

- Wear particles can incite a macrophage response.
  - Leads to prosthesis loosening
- Silicones
  - Polymers for replacement in non–weight-bearing joints
  - Poor strength and wear capabilities
    - Frequent synovitis with extended use
- Ceramics
  - Metallic and nonmetallic elements bonded ionically in a highly oxidized state
    - Good insulators (poor conductors)
    - Biostable (inert) crystalline materials such as Al_2O_3 (alumina) and ZrO_2 (zirconium dioxide)
    - Bioactive (degradable), noncrystalline substances such as bioglass
  - Typically **brittle** (no elastic deformation)
  - High modulus (*E*)
  - High compressive strength
  - Low tensile strength
  - **Low yield strain**
  - Poor crack resistance characteristics
    - Low resistance to fracture
  - Best wear characteristics, with polyethylene and a low oxidation rate
  - High surface wettability and high surface tension
    - Highly conducive to tissue bonding
    - Less friction and **diminished wear** ("smooth surface")
  - Small grain size allows an ultrasmooth finish
    - Less friction
  - Calcium phosphates (e.g., hydroxyapatite) may be useful as a coating (plasma sprayed) to increase attachment strength and promote bone healing.

5. Other materials
   - Investigational
     - Polylactic acid–coated carbon and new polymer composites with carbon fiber reinforcement
       - "Piles" of carbon fibers impregnated with matrix polymer (polysulfone or polyetherketone)
   - Bioabsorbable polymers induce foreign body reactions in many patients
6. Biomaterials
   - Possess certain unique characteristics
     - **Viscoelasticity**
     - Creep
     - Stress relaxation
       - Internal stress decreases with time.
       - Deformation remains constant.
   - Capable of self-adaptation and repair
     - Characteristics change with aging and sampling.
7. Comparison of common orthopaedic materials (see Figure 1-100)

C. Orthopaedic structures

1. Bone
   - Mechanical properties
     - Composite of collagen and hydroxyapatite
       - Collagen: low *E*, good tensile strength, poor compressive strength
       - Calcium apatite: stiff, brittle, good compressive strength
     - Anisotropic
       - Strongest in compression
       - Weakest in shear
       - Intermediate in tension
       - Resists rapidly applied loads better than slowly applied loads
     - **Mineral content** is the main determinant of the elastic modulus of cortical bone.
     - Cancellous bone is 25% as dense, 10% as stiff, and 500% as ductile as cortical bone.
       - Cortical bone excellent at resisting torque
       - Cancellous bone good at resisting compression and shear
     - Bone is dynamic
       - Able to self-repair
       - Changes with aging: stiffer and less ductile
       - Changes with immobilization: weaker
     - **Bone aging**
       - To offset loss in material properties, bone remodels to increase inner and outer cortical diameters.
       - Area moment of inertia increases.
         - Bending stresses decrease.
     - Stress concentration effects
       - Occur at defect points within bone or implant-bone interface (stress risers)
       - Reduce overall loading strength
     - **Stress shielding by load-sharing implants**
       - **Induces osteoporosis in adjacent bone**
         - **Decreases normal physiologic bone stresses**
       - Common under plates and at the femoral calcar in high-riding THAs
     - A hole 20% to 30% of bone diameter reduces strength up to 50%.
       - Regardless of whether it is filled with a screw
       - Area returns to normal 9 to 12 months after screw removal
     - Cortical defects can reduce strength 70% or more.
       - Oval defects less than rectangular defects
         - Smaller stress riser (concentration)
   - Fracture
     - Type is based on mechanism of injury.
     - **Tension**
       - Muscle pull, typically transverse
       - Perpendicular to load and bone axis
     - **Compression**
       - Axial loading of cancellous bone
       - Crush fracture
     - **Shear**
       - Commonly around joints
       - Load parallel to the bone surface
       - Fracture parallel to the load
     - **Bending**
       - Eccentric loading or direct blows
       - Begins on the tension side of the bone
       - Continues transversely/obliquely
       - Eventually bifurcates to produce a butterfly fragment
       - High-velocity bending: produces comminuted butterfly fracture
       - Four-point bending: produces segmental fracture
     - **Torsion**
       - Shear and tensile stresses around the longitudinal axis

- Most likely to result in a spiral fracture
- Torsional stresses proportional to the distance from the neutral axis to the periphery of a cylinder
  - Greatest stresses in a long bone under torsion are on the outer (periosteal) surface.
- Comminution
  - A function of the amount of energy transmitted to bone

2. Ligaments and tendons
   - These structures can sustain 5% to 10% tensile strain before failure.
     - In contrast, bone can sustain only 1% to 4% tensile strain.
     - Failure commonly results from tension rupture of fibers and shear failure among fibers.
   - Most ligaments can undergo plastic strain to the point that function is lost but structure remains in continuity.
   - Soft tissue implants have the following characteristics:
     - **Tendons**
       - Strong in tension only
       - *E* is 10% that of bone; increases with slower loading
       - Parallel fiber orientation
       - Demonstrate stress relaxation and creep
     - **Ligament fibers**
       - Oriented parallel if they resist major joint stress
         - More randomly if they resist forces from different directions
       - Stiffness = force/strain
         - As depicted on a force deformation graph
         - Similar to *E* but does not account for cross-sectional area
         - The bone-ligament complex is softer: less stiff implies decreased *E*.
       - Prolonged immobilization lowers yield point and tensile strength.
     - Stents
       - Internal splint devices:
         - Proplast Tendon Transfer Stabilizer
         - Gore-Tex prosthetic ligaments
         - Xenotech (bovine tendon)
         - Polyester implants
       - Stents do not allow adequate collagen ingrowth.
         - All eventually fail.
       - Synthetic ligaments produce wear particles.
         - Increase proteinases, collagenase, gelatinase, and chondrocyte activation factor
     - Ligament augmentation devices (LADs)
       - Kennedy LAD (polypropylene yarn) and Dacron LADs.
         - LADs do allow some fibrous ingrowth.
         - However, their use is limited.
     - Biodegradable tissue scaffolding
       - Immediate stability
       - Long-term replacement with host tissue
       - Carbon fiber and polylactic acid-coated carbon fiber devices
         - Limited success
         - Slow ingrowth is improved with polylactic acid coating.

3. Articular cartilage
   - Ultimate tensile strength is only 5% that of bone.
     - *E* is only 0.1% that of bone.
     - However, because of its viscoelastic properties, it is well-suited for compressive loading.
   - Articular cartilage is biphasic.
     - Solid phase depends on the structural matrix.
     - Fluid phase depends on deformation and shift of water within the solid matrix.
   - Relatively soft and impermeable solid matrix requires high hydrodynamic pressure to maintain fluid flow.
     - Significant support provided by the fluid component
     - Stress-shielding effect on the matrix

4. Metal implants
   - **Screws**
     - Have the following characteristics:
       - Pitch: distance between threads
       - **Lead:** distance advanced in one revolution
       - **Root diameter:** minimal/inner diameter is proportional to tensile strength
       - **Outer diameter:** determines holding power (pullout strength)
     - To maximize pullout strength
       - Large outer diameter
       - Small root diameter
       - Fine pitch
     - Pedicle screw pullout strength most affected by the degree of osteoporosis
   - **Plates**
     - Strength varies with material and moment of inertia.
     - Bending stiffness is proportional to the third power of the thickness (t^3).
       - Doubling thickness increases bending stiffness eightfold.
     - Plates are load-bearing devices.
       - Most effective on a fracture's tension side
     - Types include the following:
       - Static compression
         - Best in the upper extremity
         - Can be stressed for compression
       - Dynamic compression
         - For example, tension band plate
       - Neutralization
         - Resists torsion
       - Buttress
         - Protects bone graft
     - Stress concentration at open screw holes can lead to implant failure.
       - Screw holes that remain after removal of plate and screw represent a stress riser.
         - At risk for refracture
     - Blade plates
       - Increased resistance to torsional deformation
     - **Locking plates**
       - Absorb axial forces transmitted from screws
       - Do not require compression to bone; preserve periosteal blood supply
       - Biomechanical advantages for osteoporotic fractures without cortical contact
     - **Hybrid locking plates**
       - Both nonlocked and locked screws are used.

- Nonlocked screws assist in reduction.
- Locked screws create a fixed-angle device or can be used in patients with osteoporosis.

- **Intramedullary nails**
  - Load-sharing devices
    - Require high polar moment of inertia to maximize torsional rigidity and strength
  - Mechanical characteristics
    - **Torsional rigidity**
      - Amount of torque needed to produce a unit angle of torsional deformation
      - Depends on both material properties (shear modulus) and structural properties (polar moment of inertia)
    - **Bending rigidity**
      - Amount of force required to produce a unit amount of deflection
      - Depends on both material properties (elastic modulus) and structural properties (area moment of inertia, length)
      - Related to the fourth power of the nail's radius
        - Increasing nail diameter by 10% increases bending rigidity by 50%
    - Better at resisting bending forces than rotational forces
  - Reaming
    - Allows increased torsional resistance
      - Increased contact area
      - A larger nail; increased rigidity and strength
  - Unslotted nails
    - Smaller diameter
    - Stronger fixation
    - At the expense of flexibility
    - **Increased torsional stiffness:** greatest advantage of closed-section nails over slotted nails
  - Intramedullary nail insertion for femoral shaft fracture
    - Hoop stresses are lowest for a slotted titanium alloy nail with a thin wall.
    - Posterior starting points decrease hoop stresses and iatrogenic comminution of fractures.
    - Implant failure is more frequent with smaller-diameter, unreamed nails.
- External fixators
  - Conventional external fixators
    - Allowing fracture ends to come into contact is the most important factor for stability of fixation with external fixation.
    - Other factors to enhance stability (rigidity) include the following:
      - Larger-diameter pins (second most important factor)
      - Additional pins
        - Decreased bone-rod distance
      - Pins in different planes
        - Pins separated by more than 45 degrees
      - Increased mass of the rods or stacked rods
        - A second rod in the same plane increases resistance to bending.
      - Rods in different planes
      - Increased spacing between pins
        - Place central pins closer to the fracture site.
        - Place peripheral pins farther from the fracture site (near-near, far-far).
    - Tibial shaft fractures
      - Additional lag screws with external fixation are associated with a higher refracture rate than is external fixation alone.
  - **Circular (Ilizarov) external fixators**
    - Thin wires (usually 18 mm in diameter)
      - Fixed under tension (usually between 90 and 130 kg)
      - Circular rings
    - Half-pins may also be used
      - Offer better purchase in diaphyseal (not metaphyseal) bone
    - Optimum orientation of implants on the ring
      - At a 90-degree angle to each other
      - Maximizes stability
      - A 90-degree angle not always possible
        - Anatomic constraints, such as neurovascular structures
    - Bending stiffness of frame
      - Independent of the loading direction
      - Because the frame is circular
    - Each ring should have at least two implants
      - Wires or half-pins may be used.
      - The construct is most stable when an olive wire and a half-pin are at a 90-degree angle to each other on a ring.
      - Two wires are used on a ring.
        - One wire should be superior to the ring and one inferior.
        - Tensioned wires on the same side can cause the ring to deform.
  - Factors that enhance stability of circular external fixators:
    - Larger diameter wires (and half-pins)
    - Decreased ring diameter
    - Use of olive wires
    - Additional wires or half-pins, or both
    - Wires (or half-pins, or both) crossing at a 90-degree angle
    - Increased wire tension (up to 130 kg)
    - Placement of the two central rings close to the fracture site
    - Decreased spacing between adjacent rings
    - Increased number of rings
- **Total hip arthroplasty**
  - Evolving design has led to reduction in biomechanical constraints
  - Cemented versus cementless
    - Femoral components designed for use with or without cement
    - Cementless
      - Proximal porous coating: should be circumferential
      - Seals the diaphysis from wear debris
    - Cemented
      - Mantle less than 2 mm thick increases incidence of crack formation.
  - Stem length
    - Directly related to rigidity

- Metal heads: more neck-length options than ceramic heads
- Compressive and tensile stresses in adjacent structures can be minimized:
  - Broad medial surface
  - Broader lateral surface
  - Large moment of inertia
- Moment arms
  - Femoral component design must account for rotational forces.
    - Rotational torque in retroversion
      - Most responsible for initiating loosening in cemented femoral stems
      - Increased in femoral stems with a higher offset
- Femoral component
  - This can be used in cases of neutral or slight valgus angulation.
  - It decreases moment arm, cement stress, and abductor length.
  - Increasing offset moves the abductor attachment away from the joint center.
    - Increases the abductor moment arm
    - Reduces abductor force required in normal gait
    - Reduces resulting hip joint reaction force
    - Increases the bending moment (strain) on the implant
    - Increases strain on the medial cement mantle
- **Femoral head size**
  - Small (22-mm) components
    - Decrease ROM and stability
    - Decrease friction and torque and polyethylene volumetric wear
  - Large (36-mm) components
    - Increase ROM and stability
    - Increase friction and torque and polyethylene volumetric wear
    - Wear: less of an issue with modern bearings
- Durability
  - Survival of surface replacement hip arthroplasty is poor as a result of volumetric wear of polyethylene.
    - This wear is 4 to 10 times that of a THA when a 28-mm head is used.
  - Metal-backing acetabular components are used.
    - Decrease stress in cement and cancellous bone
  - Polyethylene on titanium makes a poor bearing surface.
    - Excessive volumetric wear
  - Titanium on weight-bearing surfaces is not recommended.
    - May lead to fretting, wear debris, and blackening of soft tissues
  - Wear synovitis can occur in TJA.
    - Associated with histiocyte injection of submicron polyethylene debris
  - UHMWPE serves as a "shock absorber."
    - Should be at least 6 mm thick to prevent creep
  - Ceramic femoral head on a ceramic acetabulum has the lowest coefficient of friction.
  - **Wear rates:**
    - UHMWPE in the acetabulum: 0.1 mm (100 μm) per year
    - Metal-on-metal bearings for THA: 0.002 to 0.005 mm (2 to 5 μm) per year
      - Smaller particles than UHMWPE, but more numerous
    - Ceramic bearing surfaces: 0.0005 to 0.0025 mm (0.5 to 25 μm) per year
  - Newer concepts
    - Computer design of THA stems
    - Modularity
      - Increased corrosion at modular metallic junction sites
      - Such as junction of the head and stem
    - Custom designs
    - More flexible stems
  - Forging of components appears to be superior to casting.
- **Total knee arthroplasty**
  - Design has evolved significantly.
    - Original designs did not account for human knee kinematics.
    - Appropriate compromise is sought between the following designs:
      - Total-contact designs
        - Excess stability (less motion)
        - Less wear
      - Low-contact designs
        - Less stability (better motion)
        - Increased wear
  - Metal alloys are typically used.
  - Cemented, cruciate ligament–substituting TKA designs are available.
    - Associated with low polyethylene wear rates
    - Minimal osteolysis
      - High tibiofemoral conformity
- Compression hip screws
  - Loading characteristics superior to those of blade plates
    - Higher angled plates subjected to lower bending loads
      - However, may be more difficult to insert
  - Sliding of the screw proportional to two aspects:
    - Angle of screw to side plate
    - Length of the screw in the barrel
- Implant fixation
  - Interference fit
    - Mechanical or press-fit components
      - Rely on formation of fibrous tissue interface
    - Loosening
      - Can occur if stability is not maintained and high-*E* substances are used
        - Increases bone resorption and remodeling
  - Interlocking fit
    - PMMA allows gradual transfer of stress to bone.
      - Microinterlocking of cement within cancellous bone
        - May not be achievable with cemented revision of previously cemented TKA
    - Aseptic loosening can occur over time.
    - Careful technique yields the best results.
      - Limiting porosities and gaps
      - Use of a 3- to 5-mm cement thickness
    - Other improvements are as follows:

      - Low-viscosity cement
      - Better bone bed preparation
      - Plugging and pressurization
      - Better (vacuum) cement mixing
  - Biologic fit
    - Tissue ingrowth
      - Fiber-metal composites
      - Void metal composites
      - Microbeads
      - Key: to create pore sizes of 100 to 400 μm (ideally 100 to 250 μm)
    - Mechanical stability required
    - Ingrowth typically limited to 10% to 30% of the surface area
    - Problems:
      - Fiber or bead loosening
      - Increased cost
      - Proximal bone resorption
        - Monocyte/macrophage-mediated
      - Corrosion
      - Decreased implant fatigue strength
    - Uncemented TJA
      - Bone ingrowth in the tibial component of TKA occurs adjacent to fixation pegs and screws.
      - Bone ingrowth depends on the avoidance of micromotion at the bone-implant interface.
        - Observed on radiographs as radiodense reactive lines about the prosthesis
    - Canal filling (maximal endosteal contact) of more fully coated femoral stems: important for bone ingrowth

5. Bone-implant unit
   - The composite structure of this unit has shared properties.
   - More accurate bone cross-section reconstruction with metallic support improves loading characteristics.
   - Plates should act as tension bands.
   - Materials with increased *E* may result in bone resorption.
   - Materials with decreased *E* may result in implant failure.
   - Placement of the implant initiates a race between bone healing and implant failure.

III. BIOMECHANICS

A. Joint biomechanics: general

1. Degrees of freedom
   - Rotations and translations each occur in the *x, y,* and *z* planes.
     - Thus, six parameters, or degrees of freedom, describe motion.
   - Translations may be relatively insignificant for many joints.
     - Are often ignored in biomechanical analyses
2. Joint reaction force (*R*)
   - *R* is the force within a joint in response to forces acting on the joint
     - Both intrinsic and extrinsic
     - Muscle contraction about a joint: the major contributing factor
   - *R* is correlated with predisposition to degenerative changes.
   - Joint contact pressure (stress) can be minimized:
     - Decrease *R*.
     - Increase contact area.
3. Coupled forces
   - In some joints, rotation about one axis causes obligatory rotation about another axis.
     - Such movements (and associated forces) are *coupled.*
     - Example: lateral bending of the spine accompanied by axial rotation
4. Joint congruence
   - Joint congruence is related to the fit of two articular surfaces.
     - A necessary condition for joint motion
   - It can be evaluated radiographically.
   - High congruence increases joint contact area.
   - Low congruence decreases joint contact area.
   - Movement out of a position of congruence increases stress in cartilage.
     - Allows less contact area for distribution of joint reaction force
     - Predisposes the joint to degeneration
5. **Instant center of rotation**
   - This is the point about which a joint rotates.
   - In some joints (knee), the instant center changes during the arc of motion, following a curved path.
     - Effect of joint translation and morphologic features
   - It normally lies on a line perpendicular to the tangent of the joint surface at all points of contact.
6. Rolling and sliding (Figure 1-101)
   - During motion, almost all joints roll and slide to remain in congruence.
   - Pure rolling:
     - Instant center of rotation is at the rolling surfaces.
     - Contacting points have zero relative velocity.
       - No "slipping" of one surface on the other
   - Pure sliding:
     - Occurs with pure translation or rotation about a stationary axis
     - No angular change in position
     - No instant center of rotation
       - "Slipping" of one surface on the other
7. Friction and lubrication
   - Friction: resistance between two objects as one slides over the other
     - Not a function of contact area
     - Coefficient of friction: 0 = no friction
   - Lubrication: decreases resistance between surfaces
     - Articular surfaces, lubricated with synovial fluid, have a coefficient of friction 10 times better than the best synthetic systems.
   - Coefficient of friction for **human joints: 0.002 to 0.04**
   - Coefficient of friction for metal-on-UHMWPE joint arthroplasty: 0.05 to 0.15
     - Not as good as human joints
   - Elastohydrodynamic lubrication
     - Primary lubrication mechanism for articular cartilage during dynamic function

B. Hip biomechanics

1. Kinematics
   - ROM (Table 1-57)

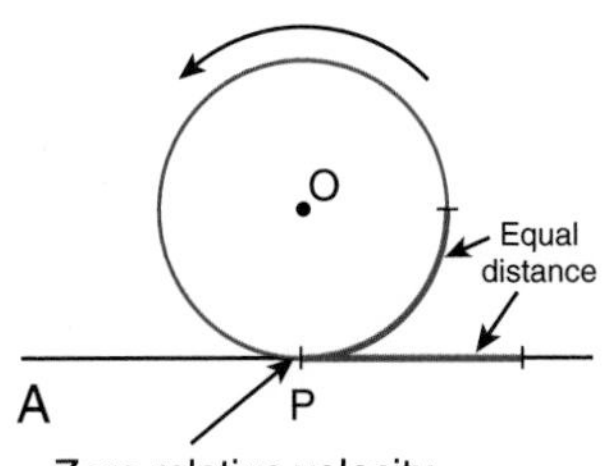

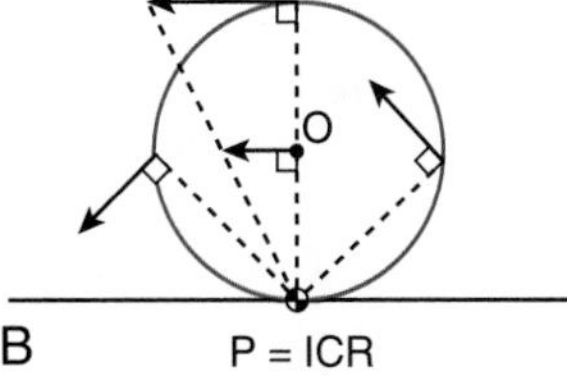

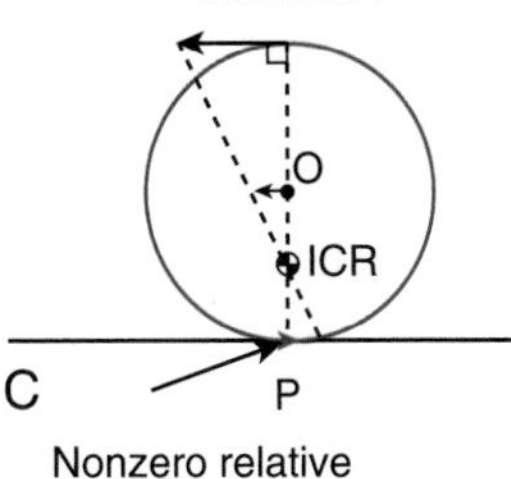

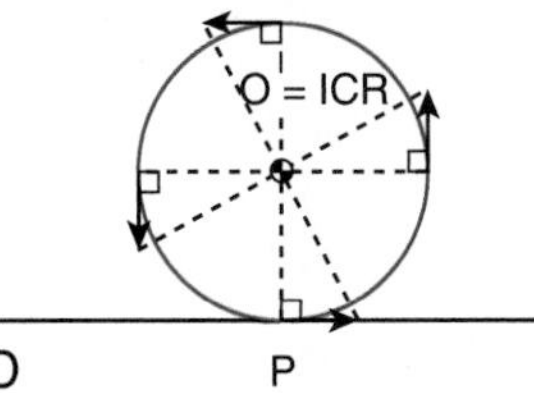

Figure 1-101 **A,** Rolling contact occurs when the circumferential distance of the rolling object equals the distance traced along the plane. This can occur only when there is no sliding: that is, when the relative velocity at the point of contact (P) is zero. **B,** For rolling contact, the point P of the wheel has zero velocity because it is in contact with the ground. Therefore, P is the instant center of rotation (ICR) of the wheel. This diagram shows the actual velocity of points along the wheel as it rolls along the ground. **C,** Rolling and sliding contact occurs when the relative velocity at the contact point is not zero. **D,** Pure sliding occurs when the wheel rotates about a stationary axis (O). In this case, the wheel would have no forward motion. (From Buckwalter JA, et al: *Orthopaedic basic science: biology and biomechanics of the musculoskeletal system,* ed 2, Rosemont, Ill, 2000, American Academy of Orthopaedic Surgeons, p 145.)

- Instant center
  - Simultaneous triplanar motion for this ball-and-socket joint makes analysis impossible.

2. Kinetics
   - **Joint reaction force** ***(R)*** in the hip can reach three to six times body weight *(W)*.
     - Primarily as a result of contraction of the muscles crossing the hip
   - Hip kinetics is demonstrated in Figure 1-102.
     - If *A* = 5 and *B* = 12.5, then according to standard free-body diagram analysis:

$$\Sigma M = 0 \text{ (sum of moments} = 0)$$
$$-5\,M_y + 12.5W = 0$$
$$M_y = 2.5W$$
$$\Sigma F_y = 0 \text{ (sum of forces} = 0)$$
$$-M_y - W + R_y = 0$$
$$R_y = 3.5W$$
$$R = R_y/(\cos 30 \text{ degrees})$$
$$R \cong 4W$$

   - An increase in the ratio of *A/B* decreases *R.*
     - For example, medialization of the acetabulum, long-neck prosthesis, or lateralization of the greater trochanter
     - If *A* = 7.5 and *B* = 10, *R* ≅ 2.3 *W.*
   - Both *R* and abductor moment are reduced by shifting body weight over the hip.
     - **Trendelenburg gait**
   - A cane in the contralateral hand produces an additional moment.
     - This can reduce *R* up to 60%.
     - Carrying a load in the ipsilateral hand also decreases *R* at the hip.
   - Energy expenditure is 264% of normal with a resection arthroplasty of the hip.
   - The hip and trunk generate 50% of the force during a tennis serve.
3. Other considerations
   - Stability
     - Deep-seated "ball-and-socket" joint is intrinsically stable.
   - Sourcil
     - Condensation of subchondral bone under superomedial acetabulum
     - *R* is maximal at this point.
   - Gothic arch
     - Remodeled bone supporting the acetabular roof
     - Sourcil at its base

Table 1-57 Hip Biomechanics: Range of Motion

Motion	Average Range (Degrees)	Functional Range (Degrees)
Flexion	115	90 (120 to squat)
Extension	30	
Abduction	50	20
Adduction	30	
Internal rotation	45	0
External rotation	45	20

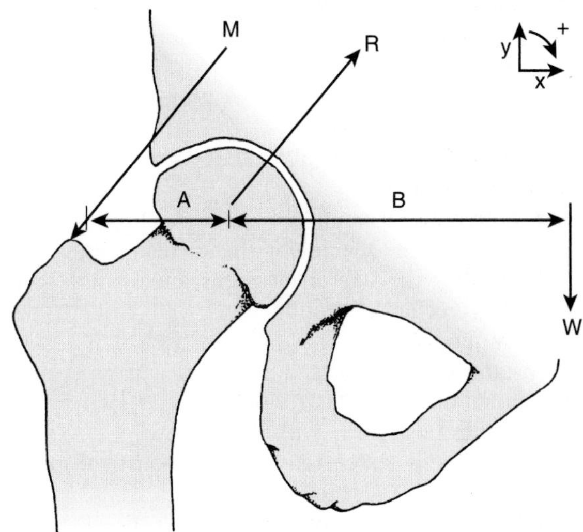

Figure 1-102 Free-body diagram of the hip (see text for explanation). M, moment; R, joint reaction force; W, work.

- Neck-shaft angle
  - Varus angulation
    - Decreases *R*
    - Increases shear across the neck
    - Leads to shortening of the lower extremity
    - Alters muscle tension resting length of the abductors
      - May cause a persistent limp
  - Valgus angulation
    - Increases *R*
    - Decreases shear
  - Neutral or valgus angulation better for THA
    - PMMA resists shear poorly
- Arthrodesis
  - **Position:** 25 to 30 degrees of flexion, 0 degrees of abduction and rotation
    - External rotation is better than internal rotation.
  - If the implant is fused in abduction, the patient will lurch over the affected lower extremity with an excessive trunk shift.
    - This will later result in lower back pain.
  - Effects:
    - Increases oxygen consumption
    - Decreases gait efficiency to approximately 50% of normal
    - Increases transpelvic rotation of the contralateral hip

C. **Knee biomechanics**

1. Kinematics
   - ROM
     - Ten degrees of extension (recurvatum) to 130 degrees of flexion.
       - Functional ROM is nearly full extension to about 90 degrees of flexion.
       - 117 degrees: required for squatting and lifting
       - 110 degrees: required for rising from a chair after TKA
     - Rotation varies with flexion.
       - At full extension, rotation is minimal.
       - At 90 degrees of flexion, ROM is 45 degrees of external rotation and 30 degrees of internal rotation.
     - Amount of abduction or adduction is essentially 0 degrees.
       - A few degrees of passive motion is possible at 30 degrees of flexion.
     - Knee motion is complex, about a changing instant center of rotation.
       - Polycentric rotation
     - Excursions of 0.5 cm for the medial meniscus and 11 cm for the lateral meniscus are possible during 120-degree arc of motion.
   - Joint motion
     - Instant center traces a J-shaped curve about the femoral condyle.
       - Moves posteriorly with flexion
     - Flexion and extension involve both **rolling and sliding.**
     - Femur internally rotates (external tibial rotation) during the last 15 degrees of extension.
       - **"Screw home" mechanism**
       - Related to different in radii of curvature for the medial and lateral femoral condyles and the musculature
     - **Posterior rollback** increases maximum knee flexion.
       - Tibiofemoral contact point moves posteriorly.
       - Normal rollback is compromised by PCL sacrifice, as in some TKAs.
     - Axis of rotation of the intact knee is in the medial femoral condyle.
     - Patellofemoral joint has sliding articulation.
       - Patella slides 7 cm caudally with full flexion.
       - Instant center is near the posterior cortex above the condyles.
2. Kinetics
   - Knee stabilizers
     - Ligaments and muscles play the major stabilizing role (Table 1-58).
       - ACL:
         - Typically subjected to peak loads of 170 N during walking
         - Up to 500 N with running
         - Ultimate strength in young patients: about 1750 N
         - Failures by serial tearing at 10% to 15% elongation
       - PCL: Sectioning increases contact pressures in the medial compartment and the patellofemoral joint.
   - Joint forces
     - Tibiofemoral joint
       - Knee joint surface loads
         - Three times body weight during level walking
         - Up to four times body weight with stair walking
       - Menisci
         - Help with load transmission
         - Bear one third to half body weight
         - Removal increases contact stresses
           - Up to four times the load transfer to bone
       - Quadriceps produces maximum anterior force on the tibia at 0 to 60 degrees of knee flexion.
     - Patellofemoral joint
       - Patella aids in knee extension.
         - Increases the lever arm
         - Stress distribution
       - It has the thickest cartilage in the entire body.
         - Bears the greatest load
         - Bears half the body weight with normal walking

Table 1-58 Knee Stabilizers

Direction	Structures
Medial	Superficial MCL (primary), joint capsule, medial meniscus, ACL/PCL
Lateral	Joint capsule, IT band, LCL (middle), lateral meniscus, ACL/PCL (90 degrees)
Anterior	ACL (primary), joint capsule
Posterior	PCL (primary), joint capsule; PCL tightens with internal rotation
Rotatory	Combinations: MCL checks external rotation; ACL checks internal rotation

ACL, anterior cruciate ligament; IT, iliotibial; LCL, lateral collateral ligament complex; MCL, medial collateral ligament complex; PCL, posterior cruciate ligament.

- Bears seven times the body weight with squatting and jogging
  - Loads proportional to ratio of quadriceps force to knee flexion
- In descending stairs, compressive force reaches two to three times body weight.
- **Patellectomy**
  - Length of the moment arm is decreased by the width of the patella: 30% reduction.
  - Power of extension is decreased by 30%.
- During TKA, the following enhance patella tracking:
  - External rotation of the femoral component
  - Lateral placement of the femoral and tibial components
  - Medial placement of the patellar component
  - Avoidance of malrotation of the tibial component
    - These actions avoid internal rotation.
- Axes of the lower extremity (Figure 1-103)
  - Mechanical axis of the lower extremity

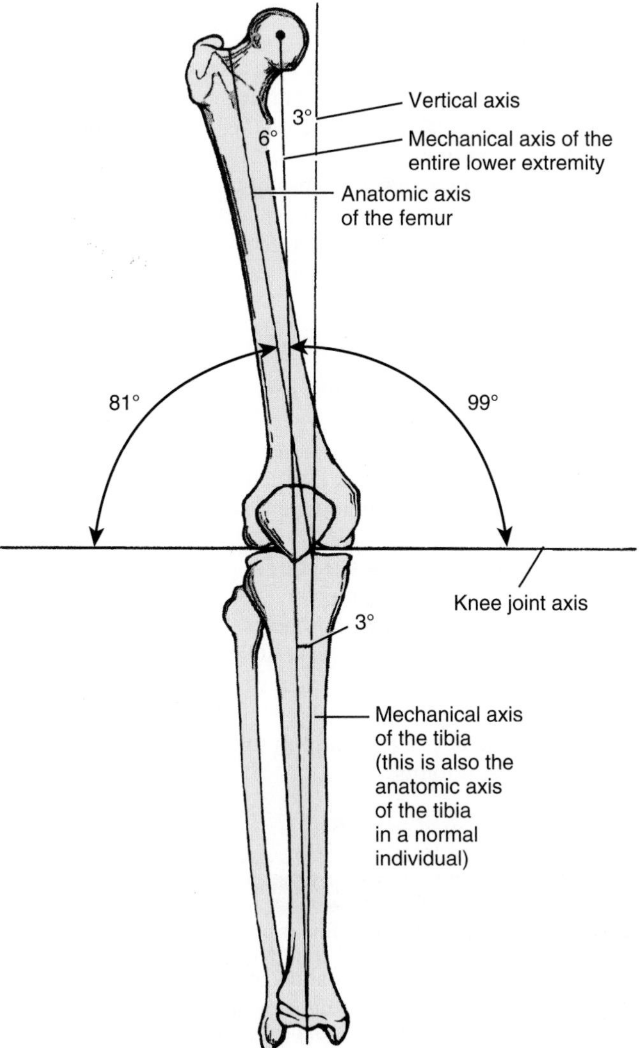

Figure 1-103 Axes of the lower extremity. (Modified from Helfet DL: Fractures of the distal femur. In Browner BD, et al, editors: *Skeletal trauma,* Philadelphia, 1992, WB Saunders, p 1645.)

    - Center of femoral head to center of ankle
    - Normally passes just medial to the medial tibial spine
  - Vertical axis
    - From the center of gravity to the ground
  - Anatomic axes
    - Along the shafts of the femur and tibia
    - Where these axes intersect at the knee, valgus angle is normal.
  - Mechanical axis of the femur
    - From center of the femoral head to center of the knee
  - Mechanical axis of the tibia
    - From center of the tibial plateau to center of the ankle
  - Relationships
    - Mechanical axis of the lower extremity is in 3 degrees of valgus angulation from the vertical axis.
    - Anatomic axis of the femur is in 6 degrees of valgus angulation from the mechanical axis.
      - Nine degrees versus the vertical axis
    - Anatomic axis of the tibia is in 2 to 3 degrees of varus angulation from the mechanical axis.
- Arthrodesis
  - Position: 0 to 7 degrees of valgus angulation, 10 to 15 degrees of flexion.

D. Ankle and foot biomechanics

1. Ankle

- Kinematics
  - Instant center of rotation within the talus
    - Lateral and posterior points at the tips of the malleoli
    - Change slightly with movement
  - Talus described as a cone
    - Body and trochlea wider anteriorly and laterally
    - Therefore, talus and fibula externally rotate slightly with dorsiflexion
  - Dorsiflexion and abduction are coupled.
  - ROM:
    - Dorsiflexion: 25 degrees
    - Plantar flexion: 35 degrees
    - Rotation: 5 degrees
- Kinetics
  - Tibiotalar articulation
    - Major weight-bearing surface of the ankle
    - Supports compressive forces up to five times body weight (*W*)
    - Shear (backward to forward) forces up to *Wt*
  - Large weight-bearing surface area decreases joint stress.
  - Fibular/talar joint transmits about one sixth of the force.
  - Highest net muscle moment occurs during terminal-stance phase of gait.
- Other considerations
  - Stability based on articulation shape (mortise maintained by talar shape) and ligament support
    - Stability is greatest in dorsiflexion.
    - During weight bearing, tibial and talar articular surfaces contribute most to stability.
  - Windlass action

- Full dorsiflexion is limited by the plantar aponeurosis.
- Further tension on the aponeurosis (toe dorsiflexion) raises the arch.
- A **syndesmosis screw** limits external rotation.
- Arthrodesis: neutral dorsiflexion, 5 to 10 degrees of external rotation, 5 degrees of hindfoot valgus angulation
  - Anticipate 70% loss of sagittal plane motion of the foot.

2. Subtalar joint (talus-calcaneus-navicular)
   - Axis of rotation:
     - In the sagittal plane: 42 degrees
     - In the transverse plane: 16 degrees
   - Functions like an oblique hinge
     - Pronation coupled with dorsiflexion, abduction, and eversion
     - Supination coupled with plantar flexion, adduction, and inversion
   - ROM
     - Pronation: 5 degrees
     - Supination: 20 degrees
     - Functional ROM: approximately 6 degrees
3. Transverse tarsal joint (talus-navicular, calcaneal-cuboid)
   - Motion based on foot position
     - Two axes of rotation: talonavicular and calcaneocuboid
   - Eversion (early stance)
     - The joint axes are parallel.
     - ROM is allowed.
   - Inversion (late stance)
     - External rotation of the lower extremity causes the joint axes to intersect.
     - Motion is limited.
4. Foot
   - Transmits 1.2 times body weight with walking
     - Three times body weight with running
   - Has three arches (Table 1-59)
   - Second metatarsal (Lisfranc) joint is "keylike."
     - Stabilizes the second metatarsal
     - Allows it to carry the most load with gait
     - First metatarsal bears the most load during standing.
   - Expected life of Plastazote shoe insert in active adults is less than 1 month.
     - Fatigues rapidly in compression and shear
     - Should be replaced frequently or supported with other materials, such as Spenco or PPT foam.

E. Spine biomechanics

1. Kinematics
   - ROM by anatomic segment (Table 1-60)

Table 1-60 Range of Motion of Spinal Segments

Level	Flexion/ Extension (Degrees)	Lateral Bending (Degrees)	Rotation (Degrees)	Instant Center
Occiput-C1	13	8	0	Skull, 2-3 cm above dens
C1-C2	10	0	45	Waist of odontoid
C2-C7	10-15	8-10	10	Vertebral body below
T-spine	5	6	8	Vertebra below/disc centrum
L-spine	15-20	2-5	3-6	Disc annulus

C, cervical; L, lumbar; T, thoracic.

   - Analysis based on the functional unit
     - **Motion segment:** two vertebrae and the intervening soft tissues
   - Six degrees of freedom exist about all three axes.
   - **Coupled motion**
     - Simultaneous rotation, lateral bending, and flexion or extension
     - Especially axial rotation with lateral bending
   - Instant center of rotation within the disc
   - Normal sagittal alignment of the lumbar spine: 55 to 60 degrees of lordosis
     - The lordosis exists because of the disc spaces (not the vertebrae).
     - Most lordosis occurs between L4 and S1.
     - Loss of disc space height can cause loss of normal lumbar lordosis.
   - Iatrogenic flat back syndrome of the lumbar spine
     - Result of a distraction force
2. Supporting structures
   - Anterior supporting structures
     - Anterior longitudinal ligament
     - Posterior longitudinal ligament
     - Vertebral disc
   - Posterior supporting structures
     - Intertransverse ligaments
     - Capsular ligaments and facets
     - Ligamentum flavum (yellow ligament)
   - Halo vest is the most effective device for controlling cervical motion.
     - Because of pin purchase in the skull
   - Apophyseal joints

Table 1-59 Arches of the Foot

Arch	Skeletal Components	Keystone	Ligament Support	Muscle Support
Medial longitudinal	Calcaneus, talus, navicular, three cuneiform bones, first to third metatarsals	Talus head	Spring (calcaneonavicular)	Tibialis posterior, flexor digitorum longus, flexor hallucis longus, adductor hallucis
Lateral longitudinal	Calcaneus, cuboid, fourth and fifth metatarsals		Plantar aponeurosis	Abductor digiti minimi, flexor digitorum brevis
Transverse	Three cuneiform bones, cuboid, metatarsal bases			Peroneus longus, tibialis posterior, adductor hallucis (oblique)

- Resist torsion during axial loading
  - Attached capsular ligaments resist flexion.
- Guide the motion segment
- Direction of motion determined by orientation of the facets of the apophyseal joint
  - Varies with each level
- Cervical spine facet
  - Orientation: 45 degrees to the transverse plane
  - Parallel to the frontal plane
- Thoracic spine facet
  - Orientation: 60 degrees to the transverse plane
  - Also 20 degrees to the frontal plane
- Lumbar spine facet
  - Orientation: 90 degrees to the transverse plane
  - Also 45 degrees to the frontal plane
  - They progressively tilt up (transverse) and inward (frontal)
- Cervical facetectomy of more than 50% causes loss of stability in flexion and torsion.
- Torsional load resistance in the lumbar spine:
  - Facets contribute 40%.
  - Disc contributes 40%.
  - Ligamentous structures contribute 20%.

3. Kinetics
   - Disc
     - Behaves viscoelastically
     - Demonstrates creep
       - Deforms with time
     - Demonstrates hysteresis
       - Absorbs energy with repeated axial loads
       - Later decreases in function
     - Compressive stresses highest in the nucleus pulposus
     - Tensile stresses highest in the annulus fibrosus
     - Stiffness increases with compressive load
     - Higher loads increase deformation and creep rate
     - Repeated torsional loading (shear forces)
       - Such repeated loading may separate the nucleus pulposus from the annulus and end plate.
       - This in turn may force nuclear material through an annular tear.
     - Loads increase with bending and torsional stresses.
     - After subtotal discectomy, extension is the most stable loading mode.
     - Disc pressures are lowest with lying supine, higher with standing, and highest with sitting.
     - **Carrying loads**
       - Disc pressures are lowest when the load is close to the body.
   - Vertebrae
     - Strength is related to bone mineral content and vertebrae size.
       - Increased in lumbar spine
     - Fatigue loading may lead to pars fractures.
     - Compression fractures occur at the end plate.
     - Vertebral body stiffness is decreased in osteoporosis.
       - Caused by loss of horizontal trabeculae
     - Spinal arthrodesis is helpful:
       - Increasing implant stiffness
         - Increases probability of successful fusion
         - Increases likelihood of decreased bone mineral content of the bridged vertebrae

F. Shoulder biomechanics (Table 1-61)

1. Kinematics
   - Scapular plane
     - Positioned 30 degrees anterior to the coronal plane
     - The preferred reference plane for ROM
   - Abduction requires external rotation of the humerus.
     - To prevent greater tuberosity impingement
     - With internal rotation contractures, abduction limited to 120 degrees
   - Abduction
     - Glenohumeral motion: 120 degrees
     - Scapulothoracic motion: 60 degrees
     - In ratio of 2 : 1
       - Varies over the first 30 degrees of motion
   - Scapulothoracic motion
     - Acromioclavicular joint movement during the early part
     - Sternoclavicular movement during the later portion
       - With clavicular rotation along the long axis
   - Surface joint motion in the glenohumeral joint is a combination of rotation, rolling, and translation.
2. Kinetics
   - Zero position
     - Abduction of 165 degrees in the scapular plane
     - Minimal deforming forces about the shoulder
     - Ideal position for reducing shoulder dislocations
       - Also for reducing "fractures with traction"
   - Free-body analysis of deltoid force (*D*) (Figure 1-104):

$$\Sigma M_0 = 0$$

$$3D - 0.05W(30) = 0$$

$$D = 0.5W$$

Table 1-61 Shoulder Biomechanics: Muscle Forces

Motion	Muscle Forces	Comments
Glenohumeral		
Abduction	Deltoid, supraspinatus	Cuff depresses head
Adduction	Latissimus dorsi, pectoralis major, teres major	
Forward flexion	Pectoralis major, deltoid (anterior), biceps	
Extension	Latissimus dorsi	
Internal rotation	Subscapularis, teres major	
External rotation	Infraspinatus, teres minor, deltoid (posterior)	
Scapular		
Rotation	Upper trapezius, levator scapulae (anterior), serratus anterior, lower trapezius	Works through a force couple
Adduction	Trapezius, rhomboid, latissimus dorsi	
Abduction	Serratus anterior, pectoralis minor	

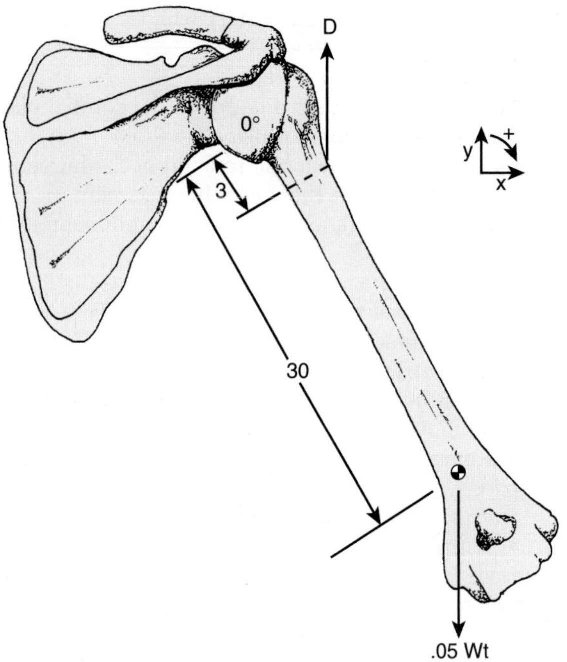

Figure 1-104 Free-body diagram of the deltoid force (D) (see text for explanation). Wt, weight of arm (N).

3. Stability
   - Limited about the glenohumeral joint
   - Humeral head surface area larger than glenoid area:
     - □ 48 × 45 mm versus 35 × 25 mm
   - Bony stability is limited.
     - □ Relies on humeral head inclination (125 degrees) and retroversion (25 degrees)
     - □ Also relies on slight glenoid retrotilt
   - **Inferior glenohumeral ligament** (superior band)
     - □ The most important static stabilizer
     - □ Superior and middle glenohumeral ligaments: secondary stabilizers to anterior humeral translation
   - Inferior subluxation prevented by negative intraarticular pressure.
   - Rotator cuff muscles
     - □ Dynamic contribution to stability
   - Arthrodesis: 15 to 20 degrees of abduction, 20 to 25 degrees of forward flexion, 40 to 50 degrees of internal rotation
     - □ Avoid excessive external rotation.
4. Other joints
   - Acromioclavicular joint
     - □ Scapular rotation through the conoid and trapezoid ligaments
     - □ Scapular motion through the joint itself
   - Sternoclavicular joint
     - □ Clavicular protraction/retraction in a transverse plane through the coracoclavicular ligament
     - □ Clavicular elevation and depression in the frontal plane
       - Also through the coracoclavicular ligament
     - □ Clavicular rotation around the longitudinal axis

G. Elbow biomechanics

1. Functions
   - A component joint of the lever arm when the hand is positioned
   - Fulcrum for the forearm lever
   - Weight-bearing joint in patients using crutches
   - Activities of daily living
2. Kinematics
   - Flexion and extension
     - □ 0 to 150 degrees
     - □ **Functional ROM: 30 to 130 degrees**
     - □ Axis of rotation: the center of the trochlea
   - Pronation and supination
     - □ Pronation: 80 degrees
     - □ Supination: 85 degrees
     - □ Functional pronation and supination: 50 degrees each
     - □ Axis: capitellum through radial head to ulnar head (forms a cone)
   - Carrying angle
     - □ Valgus angle at the elbow
     - □ For boys and men: 7 degrees; for girls and women, 13 degrees
     - □ Decreases with flexion
3. Kinetics
   - Forces at the elbow have short lever arms and are relatively inefficient (Figure 1-105):

$$\Sigma M_y = 0$$

$$-5B + 15Wt = 0$$

$$B = 3Wt$$

     - □ Results in large joint reaction forces
     - □ Subject the joint to degenerative changes
   - Flexion is accomplished primarily by the brachialis and biceps.
   - Extension is accomplished by the triceps.
   - Pronation is accomplished by pronators (teres and quadratus).
   - Supination is accomplished by the biceps and supinator.

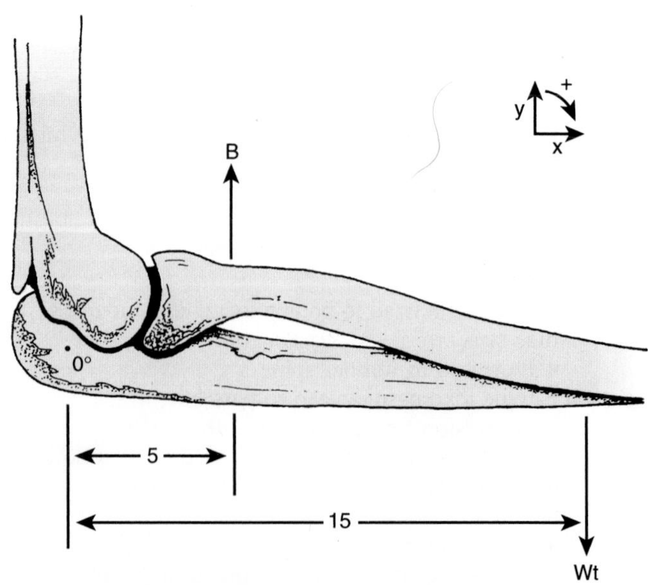

Figure 1-105 Free-body diagram of elbow flexion (see text for explanation). B, biceps force; Wt, weight of forearm.

- Static loads approach, and dynamic loads exceed, body weight.

4. Stability
   - Provided partially by articular congruity
   - Three necessary and sufficient constraints for stability:
     - Coronoid
     - Lateral (ulnar) collateral ligament (LCL)
     - Anterior band of the medial collateral ligament
     - **Most important:** anterior oblique fibers
     - Stabilizes against both valgus angulation and distractional force at 90 degrees
   - Most important secondary stabilizer against valgus stress: radial head
     - About 30% of valgus stability
     - Important at 0 to 30 degrees of flexion and pronation
   - In extension, capsule is the primary restraint to distractional forces.
   - Lateral stability is provided by lateral collateral ligament, anconeus, and joint capsule.
   - Unilateral arthrodesis: 90 degrees of flexion
   - Bilateral arthrodesis:
     - One elbow at 110 degrees of flexion for the hand to reach the mouth
     - Other at 65 degrees of flexion for perineal hygiene
   - Arthrodesis is difficult to perform and (fortunately) rarely required.
5. Forearm
   - Of the axial load, 17% is transmitted by the ulna.
   - Line of the center of rotation runs from radial head to distal ulna.

H. Wrist and hand biomechanics

1. Wrist
   - Part of an intercalated link system
   - Kinematics
     - Normal ROM
       - Flexion: 65 degrees
         - Functional: 10 degrees
       - Extension: 55 degrees
         - Functional: 35 degrees
       - Radial deviation: 15 degrees
         - Functional: 10 degrees
       - Ulnar deviation: 35 degrees
         - Functional: 15 degrees
     - Flexion and extension
       - Two-thirds radiocarpal
       - One-third intercarpal
     - Radial deviation
       - Primarily intercarpal movement
     - Ulnar deviation
       - Relies on radiocarpal and intercarpal motion
     - Instant center is usually the head of the capitate, but it varies.
   - **Columns** (Table 1-62)

Table 1-62 Columns of the Wrist

Column	Function	Comments
Central	Flexion-extension	Distal carpal row and lunate (link)
Medial	Rotation	Triquetrum
Lateral	Mobile	Scaphoid

   - Link system
     - A system of three links in a "chain":
       - Radius, lunate, and capitate
     - Less motion is required at each link.
       - However, it adds to instability of the chain.
     - Stability is enhanced by strong volar ligaments.
       - Also by the scaphoid, which bridges both carpal rows
   - Relationships
     - Carpal collapse
       - Ratio of carpal height to third metacarpal height: normally 0.54
     - Ulnar translation
       - Ratio of ulna-to-capitate length to third metacarpal height
       - Normal is 0.30
     - **Distal radius normally bears about 80% of distal radioulnar joint load.**
       - **Distal ulna bears 20%.**
       - **Ulnar load bearing increases with ulnar lengthening and decreases with ulnar shortening.**
     - Wrist arthrodesis is relatively common.
       - Dorsiflexion of 10 to 20 degrees is good for unilateral fusion.
       - Bilateral fusion:
         - Avoid if possible.
         - If necessary, fuse other wrist at 0 to 10 degrees of palmar flexion.
2. Hand
   - Kinematics
     - ROM
       - MCP joint
         - Universal joint, 2 degrees of freedom
         - Flexion: 100 degrees
         - Abduction-adduction: 60 degrees
       - PIP joints
         - Flexion: 110 degrees
       - DIP joints
         - Flexion: 80 degrees
   - Arches
     - Two transverse arches
       - Proximal through carpus
       - Distal through metacarpal heads
     - Five longitudinal arches
       - Through each of the rays
   - Stability
     - MCP joint
       - Volar plate and the collateral ligaments
       - **Collateral ligaments:** taut in flexion, lax in extension
     - PIP joints and DIP joints
       - Rely more on joint congruity
       - Large ratio of ligament to articular surface
   - Other concepts
     - Hand pulleys prevent bowstringing and decrease tendon excursion.
       - Bowstringing increases moment arms.
     - Sagittal bands allow MCP extension.
     - With hyperextension of the MCP, the intrinsic muscles must function to produce PIP extension, because the extension tendon is lax.
     - Normal grasp

- For boys and men: 50 kg
- For girls and women: 25 kg
- Only 4 kg needed for daily function
- Normal pinch
  - For boys and men: 8 kg
  - For girls and women: 4 kg
  - Only 1 kg needed for daily activities
- Kinetics
  - Joint loading with pinch mostly in MCP
    - Because they have large surface area, however, contact pressures (joint load/contact area) are lesser.
  - DIP joints have the most contact pressure.
    - Subsequently develop the most degenerative changes with time (Heberden's nodes).
  - Grasping contact pressures are lesser, focused on MCP.
    - Patients with MCP arthritis often had occupations in which grasping was required.
  - Compressive loads occur at the thumb with pinching.

Table 1-63 Recommended Positions of Flexion for Arthrodesis of the Joints of the Hand

Joint	Degrees of Flexion	Other Factors
MCP	20-30	
PIP	40-50	Less radial than ulnar
DIP	15-20	
Thumb CMC		
Thumb MCP	25	MC in opposition
Thumb IP	20	

CMC, carpometacarpal; DIP, distal interphalangeal; MC, metacarpal; MCP, metacarpophalangeal; PIP, proximal interphalangeal.

    - At interphalangeal joint: 3 kg
    - At MCP joint: 5 kg
    - At carpometacarpal joint: 12 kg
      - An unstable joint
      - Frequently leads to degeneration
  - Arthrodesis (Table 1-63)

TESTABLE CONCEPTS

SECTION 1 BONE

I. Histologic Features of Bone

- Osteoblasts are derived from undifferentiated mesenchymal stem cells, and RUNX2 is the multifunctional transcription factor that directs this process.
- Osteoblasts produce type I collagen (i.e., bone), alkaline phosphatase, osteocalcin, bone sialoprotein, and RANKL.
- Osteocytes are former osteoblasts surrounded by newly formed matrix. They constitute 90% of the cells in the mature skeleton, are important for control of extracellular calcium and phosphorous concentration, and are less active in matrix production than are osteoblasts.
- Osteoclasts are derived from hematopoietic cells in the macrophage lineage. RANKL is produced by osteoblasts, binds to immature osteoclasts, and stimulates differentiation into active, mature osteoclasts that result in an increase in bone resorption. Osteoprotegerin inhibits bone resorption by binding and inactivating RANKL.
- Osteoclasts bind to bone surfaces by means of integrins (vitronectin receptor), effectively sealing the space below, and then create a ruffled border and remove bone matrix by proteolytic digestion through the lysosomal enzyme cathepsin K.
- Bisphosphonates directly inhibit osteoclastic bone resorption. Nitrogen-containing bisphosphonates are up to 1000-fold more potent than non–nitrogen-containing bisphosphonates. Bisphosphonates function by inhibiting farnesyl pyrophosphate synthase in the mevalonate pathway. They are associated with osteonecrosis of the jaw, and in animal models, they have reduced the rate of spinal fusion.
- Bone matrix is 60% inorganic (mineral) components and 40% organic components. Calcium hydroxyapatite $Ca_{10}(PO_4)_6(OH)_2$ constitutes the majority of the inorganic matrix. Type I collagen is 90% of the organic component, and osteocalcin is the most abundant noncollagenous protein in bone.
- Wolff's law: Remodeling occurs in response to mechanical stress. Hueter-Volkmann law: Compressive forces inhibit growth, whereas tension stimulates it.
- There are three major types of bone formation. In enchondral formation, bone replaces a cartilage model. Intramembranous formation occurs without a cartilage model; aggregates of undifferentiated mesenchymal differentiate into osteoblasts, which form bone. In appositional formation, osteoblasts lay down new bone on existing bone; the groove of Ranvier supplies the chondrocytes.

II. Bone Injury and Repair

- There are three stages of fracture repair: inflammation, repair, and remodeling. Fracture healing type varies with treatment method. Closed treatment is through periosteal bridging callus and interfragmentary enchondral ossification. Compression plate treatment is through primary cortical healing.
- BMP-2 is used for acute open tibia fractures; BMP-7 is used for tibial nonunions. BMP-3 has no osteogenic activity.
  - NSAIDs adversely affect fracture healing and healing of lumbar spinal fusions. COX-2 activity is required for normal enchondral ossification during fracture healing.
- Bone grafts have three properties: Osteoconduction acts as a scaffold for bone growth; osteoinduction involves growth factors that stimulate bone formation; osteogenic grafts contain primitive mesenchymal cells, osteoblasts, and osteocytes.
- Calcium phosphate–based grafts are capable of osseoconduction and osseointegration. They have the highest compressive strength of any graft material. Calcium sulfate is osteoconductive but rapidly resorbed.

III. Conditions of Bone Mineralization, Bone Mineral Density, and Bone Viability

A. *Normal Bone Metabolism*

- The primary homeostatic regulators of serum calcium are PTH and 1,25$(OH)_2$-vitamin D_3. PTH results in increased serum Ca^{2+} level and decreased inorganic phosphate level.
- Bone mass peaks between 16 and 25 years of age. Physiologic bone loss affects trabecular bone more than cortical bone.
- Both urinary hydroxyproline and pyridinoline cross-links are elevated when there is bone resorption.

B. *Conditions of Bone Mineralization*

- The most common cause of hypercalcemia is malignancy. Initial treatment is with hydration, which causes a saline diuresis, along with loop diuretics.
- Renal osteodystrophy is a spectrum of disorders observed in chronic renal disease. The majority of cases are caused by phosphorous retention and secondary hyperparathyroidism.
- Rickets (in children) and osteomalacia (in adults) are caused by a failure of mineralization. In rickets, the width of the zone of provisional calcification is increased, which causes physeal widening and cupping.

C. *Conditions of Bone Mineral Density*

- Osteoporosis is a quantitative defect in bone. It is defined as a lumbar bone density of 2.5 or more standard deviations less than the peak bone mass of a healthy 25-year-old (T-score).
- Treatment of osteoporosis includes calcium supplements of 1000 to 1500 mg/day, as well as bisphosphonates.
- Scurvy results from ascorbic acid deficiency, which causes a decrease in chondroitin sulfate synthesis and ultimately defective collagen growth and repair. Widening in the zone of provisional calcification is observed.
- Osteogenesis imperfecta is caused primarily by a mutation in genes responsible for metabolism and synthesis of type I collagen.

D. *Conditions of Bone Viability*

- The causes of osteonecrosis are unclear, but there are numerous risk factors. Bone is weakest during the resorptive and remodeling phases. MRI provides the earliest positive findings and has the highest sensitivity and specificity.

Continued

SECTION 2 JOINTS

I. Articular Tissues

- Articular cartilage is composed of water (65% to 80% of wet weight), collagen (10% to 20% of dry weight but more than 50% of dry weight), proteoglycans (10% to 15% of wet weight), and chondrocytes (5% of wet weight). Collagen is 95% type II and contains hydroxyproline. Proteoglycans are composed of glycosaminoglycans and include chondroitin sulfate and keratin sulfate; these provide compressive and elastic strength.
- Chondrocytes are derived from mesenchymal precursors; the SOX-9 transcriptional factor is considered the "master switch."
- The effects of aging and osteoarthritis on cartilage are generally opposite except for proteoglycan content, which decreases in both conditions. In osteoarthritis, the water content is increased, proteoglycan content decreased, keratin sulfate concentration decreased, and proteoglycan degradation significantly increased.

II. Arthroses

- Charcot's arthropathy is an extreme form of osteoarthritis caused by disturbed sensory innervation. Diabetes is the most common overall cause and the most common cause of Charcot's disease in foot and ankle joints. The most common cause of Charcot's arthropathy in the upper extremity joints is syringomyelia, followed by Hansen's disease.
- Rheumatoid arthritis affects synovium and soft tissue first. Late synovial changes include hyperplastic cells, increased blood vessels and abundant lymphocytes. Pannus ingrowth denudes articular cartilage. There are no lymphocytes in pannus.
- DMARDs are increasingly being used in the treatment of RA and most, such as infliximab and etanercept, target TNF-α.
- Juvenile idiopathic arthritis includes both JRA and juvenile chronic arthritis. Juvenile idiopathic arthritis typically manifests before age 4 and commonly involves the knee, wrist, and hand. Slit-lamp examination is required twice yearly, because progressive iridocyclitis can lead to rapid loss of vision if left untreated.
- Gout results in deposition of monosodium urate crystals in joints. The classical radiographic finding is the appearance of punched-out periarticular erosions. Indomethacin is the initial treatment; allopurinol lowers serum acid levels chronically, and colchicine is used for prophylaxis.
- CPPD (pseudogout) is characterized by positively birefringent crystals and is a common cause of chondrocalcinosis.
- Hemophilic arthropathy is most commonly caused by factor VIII deficiency and most commonly involves the knee. Treatment is through correction of factor levels to 40% to 50% of normal.

SECTION 3 NEUROMUSCULAR AND CONNECTIVE TISSUES

I. Skeletal Muscle

- Slow-twitch (type I) muscle fibers are slower, more vascular (red), and undergo aerobic oxidation (mnemonic: "slow red ox").

II. Nervous System

- Schwann cells are responsible for myelinating peripheral nerve axons. Nodes of Ranvier are gaps between Schwann cells.
- Peripheral nerves have the following morphologic features: Axons are coated with endoneurium. Axons group into bundles called *fascicles* that are coated with perineurium. Peripheral nerves are composed of fascicles that are covered in epineurium.
- Upper motor neurons are located in the descending pathways of the cerebral cortex, brainstem, and spinal cord. Lower motor neurons are located in the ventral gray matter of the spinal cord and the periphery. Lesions in all motor neurons result in decreased strength and superficial tendon reflexes. Findings in upper versus lower motor neuron lesions are otherwise opposite; upper motor neuron lesions are characterized by increased tone, deep tendon reflexes, clonus, and the presence of Babinski's sign.

III. Connective Tissues

- Tendons insert into bone through four transitional tissues: tendon, fibrocartilage, mineralized fibrocartilage (Sharpey's fibers), and bone. Early tendon healing is with type III collagen. Repair is weakest at 7 to 10 days, and maximum strength is achieved at 6 months.
- Ligament insertion is classified into two types: indirect and direct insertion. In indirect insertion, which is more common, superficial fibers insert at acute angles into the periosteum. In direct insertion, both superficial and deep fibers insert through ligament, fibrocartilage, mineralized fibrocartilage (Sharpey's fibers), and bone.
- Both tendons and ligaments are primarily type I collagen with similar ultrastructure. Ligaments have fibers that are more variable and have a higher elastin content.
- Intervertebral discs are composed of water, proteoglycans, type II collagen in the nucleus pulposus, and type I collagen in the annulus fibrosis. The aging disc shows decreased water content as a result of decreases in proteoglycans and aggrecans.

SECTION 4 CELLULAR AND MOLECULAR BIOLOGY, IMMUNOLOGY, AND GENETICS OF ORTHOPAEDICS

I. Cellular and Molecular Biology

- Humans have 46 chromosomes that contain both DNA and RNA, which regulate cellular function through protein synthesis. RNA differs from DNA in that it is single stranded, contains a ribose sugar, and is found in the nucleus and cytoplasm, and uracil is substituted for thymine as a nitrogenous base.
- Transcription is through RNA polymerase and is the creation of an mRNA molecule from DNA. Translation is the building of a protein from mRNA with amino acids.
- A variety of techniques for studying genetic disorders exist. Cytogenetic analysis is gross examination of chromosomes under a microscope and is used to detect chromosomal translocations. In PCR amplification, a heat-stable DNA polymerase is used to amplify DNA sequences in vitro, which helps detect gene mutations and establish early diagnosis of certain diseases.

- Oncogenes are growth control genes. Improper expression results in unregulated cell growth. Antioncogenes are also termed *tumor suppressor genes,* and loss of function results in unregulated cell division.
- The key event in metastasis is erosion and invasion of the basement membrane, which enables entry of tumor cells into adjacent tissues and blood vessels.

II. Immunology

- The body's defenses can be broadly distinguished as innate and adaptive immunity. There are two types of adaptive immunity: humoral and cell-mediated.
- Humoral immunity is mediated by antibodies produced by B lymphocytes. IgG is the most common antibody type.
- Cell-mediated immunity is mediated by T lymphocytes and involves presentation of antigens by memory B cells and dendritic cells.

III. Genetics

- Traits may be passed along through mendelian or non-mendelian inheritance. Classic mendelian inheritance is through one of four modes: autosomal dominant, autosomal recessive, X-linked recessive, and (very rare) X-linked dominant. Only 1% of human disorders are inherited in a mendelian manner.
- Frequently tested mendelian inheritance patterns and associated genetic defect are as follows:
  - Autosomal dominant
    Achondroplasia: FGF receptor 3
    Cleidocranial dysplasia: CBFA1
    Charcot-Marie-Tooth (most common variety): PMP22
    Ehlers-Danlos (most common variety): COL
    Hereditary multiple exostoses: EXT1/EXT2/EXT3
    Neurofibromatosis: NF1, NF2
    Marfan's syndrome: FBN1
    Osteopetrosis (tarda form)
  - Autosomal recessive
    Diastrophic dysplasia: DTDST (sulfate transport protein)
    Gaucher's disease: lysosomal gluco-cerebrosidase
    Sickle cell disease: HbSS
    Osteopetrosis (malignant form)
    Thrombocytopenia-aplasia of radius (TAR) syndrome
  - X-linked recessive
    Duchenne's and Becker's muscular dystrophy: dystrophin
    Hemophilia: factor VIII or factor IX
  - X-linked dominant
    Hypophosphatemic rickets: PHEX
    Leri-Weill dyschondrosteosis: SHOX
  - Sporadic
    McCune-Albright syndrome: Gsα subunit of the receptor/adenylyl cyclase–coupling G proteins

SECTION 5 ORTHOPAEDIC INFECTIONS AND MICROBIOLOGY

I. Musculoskeletal Infections

- Necrotizing fasciitis involves subcutaneous fat and deep fascia. Diabetes is the most common risk factor. Polymicrobial infection is the most common cause; group A β-hemolytic streptococcal infections are most common in healthy individuals.
- Community-acquired MRSA is increasingly prevalent among athletes, military recruits, and prison populations.
- C-reactive protein is the most sensitive monitor of the course of infection; it has a short half-life and dissipates about 1 week after effective treatment.
- Most common causes of osteomyelitis by age or disease are as follows:
  - Ages 0 to 4 months: *S. aureus,* gram-negative bacilli, group B streptococcus
  - Ages 4 months to 21 years: *S. aureus,* group A streptococci
    Epiphyseal osteomyelitis: *S. aureus*
  - Ages after 21 years: *S. aureus,* coagulase-negative staphylococci
  - Patients with sickle cell disease: *S. aureus* and *Salmonella* organisms
  - Patients with open fracture: *S. aureus, P. aeruginosa,* and gram-negative bacilli
  - Diabetic patients: polymicrobial (both aerobic and anaerobic)
  - Intravenous drug abusers: *S. aureus, Serratia* species, *Pseudomonas* species
  - Meat handlers: *Brucella* species
  - Fishermen: *Mycobacterium* species
- Radiographic changes of osteomyelitis include sequestrum (dead bone with surrounding granulation tissue) and involucrum (periosteal new bone).
- Most common causes of septic arthritis are listed as follows by age or sexual activity status:
  - Ages 0 to 3 months: *S. aureus,* Enterobacteriaceae, group B streptococcus, *N. gonorrhoeae*
  - Ages 3 months to 14 years: *S. aureus, S. pyogenes, S. pneumoniae, H. influenzae,* and gram-negative bacilli
  - Sexually active adults: *N. gonorrhoeae, S. aureus*, streptococci, and aerobic gram-negative bacilli
  - Non–sexually active adults: *S. aureus*, streptococci, and gram-negative bacilli
- Tetanus is caused by *C. tetani.* Tetanus immune globulin is administered only when tetanus status is unknown or the patient has received fewer than three immunizations. Tetanus toxoid is given if wound is severe or occurred more than 24 hours previously *and* if the patient has received no booster vaccination within the previous 5 years.
- HIV is a single-stranded RNA retrovirus that results in decreased numbers of T helper (CD4 cells). The diagnosis of AIDS requires a positive result of an HIV test plus either a CD4 count higher than 200 or the presence of one of the opportunistic infections.
- The risk of acquiring disease from a needlestick from contaminated source is as follows:
  - Hepatitis B: 23% to 62% in unvaccinated persons
    Infection depends on hepatitis B e antigen status of source.
    Five percent to 10% of acute hepatitis B virus infections become chronic.
  - Hepatitis C: 1.8%
    Seventy percent to 85% of acute HCV infections become chronic.
  - HIV: 0.3%

Continued

II. Antibiotics

- Frequently tested antibiotic mechanisms of action are as follows:
  - β-Lactam antibiotics (penicillin and cephalosporins): inhibit cross-linking of polysaccharides in the cell wall by blocking transpeptidase enzyme
  - Vancomycin: interferes with the insertion of glycan subunits into the cell wall
  - Rifampin: inhibits RNA polymerase F
  - Clindamycin: binds to 50S ribosomal subunits and inhibits protein synthesis
  - Quinolones (ciprofloxacin): inhibit DNA gyrase
- Antibiotic resistance is mediated by plasmids and transposons. MRSA has the *mecA* gene that produces the enzyme penicillin-binding protein 2a, which prevents the normal enzymatic acylation of antibiotics.

SECTION 6 PERIOPERATIVE PROBLEMS

I. Pulmonary Problems

- Pathophysiologic effects of DVT are caused by Virchow's triad: endothelial damage, venous stasis, and hypercoagulability. Tissue factor (thromboplastin) is released in large amounts during orthopaedic procedures, triggering the coagulation cascade.
- Warfarin (Coumadin) inhibits posttranslational modification of vitamin K–dependent clotting factors (factors II, VII, IX, and X; proteins C and S).
- Fat embolism is the triad of hypoxemia, CNS depression, and petechiae. Early skeletal stabilization decreases the incidence.

II. Other Medical (Nonpulmonary) Problems

- There are four types of shock:
  - Hypovolemic: volume loss
  - Cardiogenic: infective pumping
  - Vasogenic: pulmonary embolism or pericardial tamponade
  - Neurogenic and septic: blood pooling

III. Intraoperative Considerations

- Malignant hyperthermia is an autosomal dominant condition. It is triggered by "-ane" inhalational agents, depolarizing muscle relaxants (succinylcholine), and amide-based local anesthetics. The first signs are increased end-tidal CO_2 and tachycardia. Treatment is with dantrolene sodium, which blocks calcium release by stabilizing the sarcoplasmic reticulum.

IV. Other Perioperative Problems

- NSAIDs inhibit cyclooxygenase, which is involved in forming prostaglandins from arachidonic acid. Gastrointestinal complications are common, and concurrent anticoagulant use is the most important risk factor, followed by age of more than 60 and a history of previous gastrointestinal disease. COX-2 inhibitors do not inhibit COX-1, which maintains gastric mucosa.
- The most common transfusion adverse event is a clerical error that leads to a transfusion reaction.
- Garlic, ginkgo biloba, and ginseng increase the risk of bleeding in the perioperative period.

SECTION 7 IMAGING AND SPECIAL STUDIES

- MRI basic principles are as follows:
  - T1 weighting: fat best demonstrates anatomic structure.
  - T2 weighting: water is best for contrasting normal and abnormal tissues.
  - The following appear dark on T1-weighted images and bright on T2-weighted images: water, cerebrospinal fluid, acute hemorrhage, and soft tissue tumors.

SECTION 8 BIOMATERIALS AND BIOMECHANICS

I. Basic Concepts

- Force is a mechanical push or pull (load) causing external (acceleration) and internal (strain) effects.
- Moment is the rotational effect of a force. The mass moment of inertia is the resistance to rotation.
- Human body center of gravity is just anterior to S2.

II. Biomaterials

- Stress is the intensity of internal force. Stress = force/area. Unit of measure: pascal (N/m^2).
- Strain is a measure of deformation resulting from loading. Strain is the change in length/original length. There is no standard unit of measure.
- Young's modulus of elasticity (E) is a measure of material stiffness (ability to resist deformation in tension): E = stress/strain. Materials with higher E withstand greater forces. The following materials are listed in order of high to low modulus: ceramic, cobalt-chrome, stainless steel, titanium, cortical bone, PMMA, polyethylene, cancellous bone, tendon/ligament, and cartilage.
- Strain energy (toughness) is the capacity of material to absorb energy before failure.
- Material types include the following:
  - Brittle: linear stress-strain curve with limited capacity for plastic deformation
    PMMA
  - Ductile: large plastic deformation before failure
    Metal
  - Viscoelastic: have time- and rate-dependent stress-strain behavior and exhibit hysteresis (loading and unloading curves differ)
    Bone, ligaments, and most biologic tissues
  - Isotropic: mechanical properties are the same for all directions of applied load
    Golf ball
  - Anisotropic: mechanical properties vary with direction of applied load
    Bone is stronger with axial load than with radial load.
- Galvanic corrosion occurs when dissimilar metals are in direct contact and result in corrosion products (metal oxides and chlorides). Risk of galvanic corrosion is highest between 316 L stainless steel and cobalt-chromium (Co-Cr) alloy.
- There are three major types of orthopaedically important alloys:
  - 316 L Stainless steel: iron-carbon, chromium, nickel, molybdenum, and manganese
  - Cobalt: cobalt, chromium, molybdenum, and nickel
  - Titanium: titanium, aluminum, and vanadium

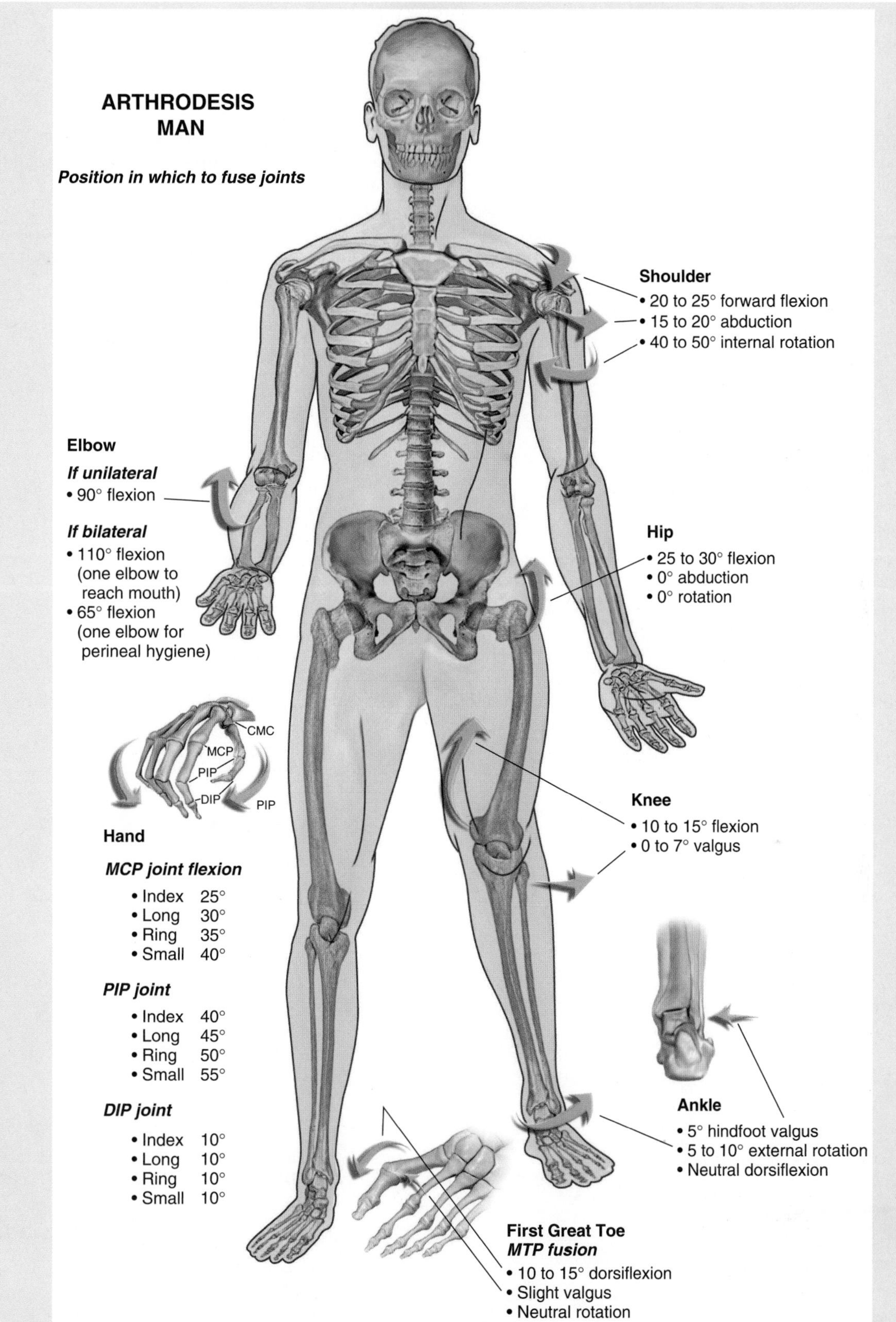

Figure 1-106 Recommended positions for arthrodesis of common joints. CMC, carpometacarpal; DIP, distal interphalangeal; MCP, metacarpophalangeal; MTP, metatarsophalangeal; PIP, proximal interphalangeal.

- PMMA bone cement acts as a grout, not an adhesive. It is strongest in compression and has poor tensile and shear strength.

III. **Biomechanics**

- Joint reaction force is the force generated within a joint in response to external force. Muscle contraction is the major contributing factor.
- Friction is the resistance between two objects as one slides over the other. Lubrication decreases resistance between surfaces. Elastohydrodynamic lubrication is the primary lubrication mechanism for articular cartilage during dynamic function.
- Principles of arthrodesis (Figure 1-106) are as follows:
  - Hip: 25 to 30 degrees of flexion, 0 degrees of abduction and rotation
  - Knee: 0 to 7 degrees of valgus angulation, 10 to 15 degrees of flexion
  - Ankle: neutral dorsiflexion, 5 to 10 degrees of external rotation, 5 degrees of hindfoot valgus angulation
  - Shoulder: 15 to 20 degrees of abduction, 20 to 25 degrees of forward flexion, 40 to 50 degrees of internal rotation
  - Elbow: 90 degrees of flexion if arthrodesis is unilateral. If it is bilateral: one elbow at 110 degrees of flexion for the hand to reach the mouth and the other at 65 degrees of flexion for perineal hygiene.
  - Wrist: 10 to 20 degrees of dorsiflexion for unilateral fusion. If arthrodesis is bilateral, fuse other side at 0 to 10 degrees of palmar flexion.

SELECTED BIBLIOGRAPHY

The selected bibliography for this chapter can be found on www.expertconsult.com.

Chapter 2

ANATOMY

Franklin D. Shuler and Matthew R. Schmitz

CONTENTS

SECTION 1 INTRODUCTION

I. OVERVIEW

A. Osteology: The human skeleton has 206 bones: axial skeleton (80) and appendicular skeleton (126)

1. Ossification:
   - Intramembranous (direct laying down of bone without a cartilage model [skull]) or enchondral (with a cartilage precursor [most bones]).
   - Enchondral growth begins in the diaphyses of long bones at primary ossification centers, most of which are present at birth (Table 2-1).
2. Secondary ossification centers usually develop in the periphery of bones and are important for growth and the treatment of childhood fractures.
3. Heterotopic ossification is the formation of bone tissue in an atypical, extraskeletal location.
4. Anatomic landmarks of the skeleton and their related structures are listed in Table 2-2.

B. Arthrology: Joints are commonly classified into three types on the basis of their freedom of movement

1. Synarthroses: joining of two bony elements with no motion during maturity; skull sutures
2. Amphiarthroses: have hyaline cartilage and intervening discs with limited motion; symphysis pubis
3. Diarthroses: characterized by hyaline cartilage, synovial membranes, capsules, and ligaments

C. Myology: classification based on the arrangement of muscle fibers

1. Parallel (e.g., rhomboids)
2. Fusiform (e.g., biceps brachii)
3. Oblique (with tendinous interdigitation): further classified as pennate, bipennate, multipennate
4. Triangular (e.g., pectoralis minor)
5. Spiral (e.g., latissimus dorsi)

D. Nerves

1. Peripheral nerves
   - Originate from the ventral rami of spinal nerves and are distributed via several plexuses (cervical, brachial, lumbosacral)
   - The mnemonic "SAME" can be used to help understand the function of nerves: **s**ensory = **a**fferent; **m**otor = **e**fferent.
   - Efferent (motor) fibers carry impulses from the central nervous system to muscles.
   - Afferent (sensory) fibers carry information toward the central nervous system.
2. Autonomic nerves
   - Control visceral structures
   - Consist of the parasympathetic (craniosacral) and sympathetic (thoracolumbar) divisions
     - Preganglionic neurons of parasympathetic nerves:
       - Arise in the nuclei of **cranial nerves** III, VII, IX, and X and in the S2, S3, and S4 segments of the spinal cord
       - Synapse in peripheral ganglia
     - Preganglionic neurons in the sympathetic system
       - Located in the spinal cord (T1 to L3)
       - Synapse in chain ganglia adjacent to the spine and collateral ganglia along major abdominal blood vessels

E. Vessels: arteries, veins, and lymphatic vessels

1. Of primary concern is avoiding major injury to these structures.
2. Courses and relationships are important and are highlighted in this chapter.

Table 2-1 Summary of Ossification Patterns

Bone	Ossification Center	Age at Appearance	Age at Fusion
Scapula	Body (primary)	8 wk (fetal)	
	Coracoid (tip)	1 yr	
	Coracoid	15 yr	
	Acromion	15 yr	
	Acromion	16 yr	
	Inferior angle	16 yr	
	Medial border	16 yr	
Clavicle	Medial (primary)	5 wk (fetal)	25 yr
	Lateral (primary)	5 wk (fetal)	
	Sternal	19 yr	
Humerus	Body (primary)	8 wk (fetal)	Blends at 6 yr and unites at 20 yr
	Head	1 yr	
	Greater tuberosity	3 yr	
	Lesser tuberosity	5 yr	
	Capitulum	2 yr	Blends and unites with body at 16-18 yr
	Medial epicondyles	5 yr	
	Trochlea	9 yr	
	Lateral epicondyles	13 yr	
Ulna	Body (primary)	8 wk (fetal)	
	Distal ulna	5 yr	20 yr
	Olecranon	10 yr	16 yr
Radius	Body (primary)	8 wk (fetal)	
	Distal radius	2 yr	17-20 yr
	Proximal radius	5 yr	15-18 yr
Pelvis	Ilium (primary)	2 mo	15 yr
	Ischium (primary)	4 mo	15 yr
	Pubis (primary)	6 mo	15 yr
	Acetabulum	12 yr	15 yr
Tibia	Body (primary)	7 wk (fetal)	
	Proximal (secondary)	Birth	20 yr
	Distal (secondary)	2 yr	18 yr
Fibula	Body (primary)	8 wk (fetal)	
	Proximal (secondary)	3 yr	25 yr
	Distal (secondary)	2 yr	20 yr

Table 2-2 Skeletal Grooves, Notches, and Points

Region	Groove or Notch	Important Related Structures
Hand	Hook of hamate	Ulnar nerve
	Trapezial groove	Tendon of flexor carpi radialis
Wrist	Distal ulna	Extensor carpi ulnaris
	Radial styloid	Extensor pollicis longus
Elbow	Medial supracondylar process	Median nerve, brachial artery
Shoulder	Scapular notch	Suprascapular nerve
	Supraglenoid tubercle	Long head of biceps brachii
	Infraglenoid tubercle	Long head of triceps brachii
Hip	Anterior-superior iliac spine	Sartorius
	Anterior-inferior iliac spine	Direct head of rectus femoris
	Ischial spine	Coccygeus, levator ani
	Lesser sciatic foramen	Pudendal nerve
	Piriformis fossa	Obturator externus
	Tip of greater trochanter	Piriformis
	Quadrate tubercle	Quadratus femoris
	Lesser trochanter	Psoas minor
Knee	Hunter's canal	Femoral artery becomes popliteal artery
	Adductor tubercle	Adductor magnus
	Gerdy tubercle	Iliotibial band
	Fibular neck	Common peroneal nerve
Foot	Henry's knot	Intersection of flexor digitorum longus and flexor hallucis longus
	Sustentaculum tali	Spring ligament: flexor hallucis longus (inferior)
	Base of fifth metatarsal	Peroneus brevis/plantar aponeurosis
	Tuberosity of navicular	Tibialis posterior
	Cuboid groove	Peroneus longus
	Sinus tarsi	Ligamentum cervicis tali and extensor digitorum brevis

SECTION 2 UPPER EXTREMITY

Table 2-3 summarizes upper extremity innervation. Table 2-4 summarizes standard surgical approaches to the upper extremity.

I. SHOULDER

A. Osteology

1. Scapula
   - Spans the second through seventh ribs and serves as an attachment for 17 muscles and four ligaments
   - Glenoid is retroverted approximately 5 degrees.
   - Scapular spine: separates supraspinatus from infraspinatus.
   - Coracoid: Attachments to the coracoid include the coracoacromial ligament, coracoclavicular ligaments (conoid and trapezoid [lateral]), conjoined tendon (coracobrachialis and short head of biceps), and pectoralis minor.
   - Acromion
   - Suprascapular notch has the superior transverse scapular ligament separating the suprascapular artery (superior) from the suprascapular nerve (inferior).
   - Spinoglenoid notch has both the artery and nerve inferior to the inferior transverse scapular ligament; **long-term nerve compression at the spinoglenoid notch (i.e., ganglion; assume labral disease) results in infraspinatus atrophy.**
2. Clavicle
   - It is the fulcrum for lateral movement of the arm.
   - It has a double curvature (sternal-ventral, acromial-dorsal) and serves as an attachment for the upper extremity.

Table 2-3 Summary of Upper Extremity Innervation

Nerves	Muscles Innervated
Musculocutaneous (lateral cord)	Coracobrachialis, biceps, brachialis
Axillary (posterior cord)	Deltoid, teres minor
Radial (posterior cord)	Triceps, brachioradialis, extensor carpi radialis longus and brevis
Posterior interosseous	Supinator, extensor carpi ulnaris, extensor digitorum, extensor digiti minimi, abductor pollicis longus, extensor pollicis longus and brevis, extensor indicis proprius
Median (medial and lateral cord)	Pronator teres, flexor carpi radialis, palmaris longus, flexor digitorum superficialis, abductor pollicis brevis, supinator head of flexor pollicis brevis, opponens pollicis, first and second lumbrical muscles
Anterior interosseous	Flexor digitorum profundus (first and second), flexor pollicis longus, pronator quadratus
Ulnar (medial cord)	Flexor carpi ulnaris, flexor digitorum profundus (third and fourth), palmaris brevis, abductor digiti minimi, opponens digiti minimi, flexor digiti minimi, third and fourth lumbrical muscles, interossei, adductor pollicis, deep head of flexor pollicis brevis

- **The clavicle is the first bone in the body to ossify (at 5 weeks of gestation) and the last to fuse (medial epiphysis at 25 years of age; see Table 2-1). Fracture of the clavicle is the most common musculoskeletal birth injury.**

B. Arthrology: one major articulation (glenohumeral joint) and several minor articulations (sternoclavicular, acromioclavicular, scapulothoracic joints)

1. Glenohumeral joint (Figure 2-1): Spheroidal, ball and socket, with the greatest joint range of motion; motion is at the expense of stability with static and dynamic restraints.
   - Static restraints include the articular anatomy, glenoid labrum, negative pressure, capsule, and ligaments.
   - Dynamic restraints include the rotator cuff and biceps tendon, and scapulothoracic motion is restrained.
   - Important glenohumeral stabilizers summarized in Table 2-5
2. Sternoclavicular joint:
   - This joint is double-gliding, with an articular disc.
   - Ligaments include the anterior and posterior sternoclavicular ligaments, an interclavicular ligament, and a costoclavicular ligament.
   - The sternoclavicular joint rotates 30 degrees with shoulder motion.
3. Acromioclavicular joint:
   - Plane/gliding joint with a fibrocartilaginous disc
   - Ligaments (Figure 2-2):

Table 2-4 Standard Orthopaedic Surgical Approaches to the Upper Extremity

Region	Approach	Eponym	Muscular Interval 1 (Nerve)	Muscular Interval 2 (Nerve)	Structures at Risk
Shoulder	Anterior	Henry's	Deltoid (axillary)	Pectoralis major (medial and lateral pectoral)	Musculocutaneous nerve; cephalic vein
	Lateral		Deltoid: splitting (axillary)	Deltoid: splitting (axillary)	Axillary nerve
	Posterior		Infraspinatus (suprascapular)	Teres minor (axillary)	Axillary nerve; posterior circumflex humeral artery
Proximal humerus	Anterolateral		Deltoid (axillary)	Pectoralis major (medial and lateral pectoral)	Anterior circumflex humeral artery (radial and axillary from retraction)
Distal humerus	Anterolateral		Triceps and brachialis (radial and musculocutaneous)	Brachioradialis (radial)	Radial nerve
	Lateral		Triceps (radial)	Brachioradialis (radial)	Radial nerve
Humerus	Posterior		Long head of triceps (radial)	Lateral head of triceps (radial) with split of medial deep head of triceps	Radial nerve and deep brachial artery
Elbow	Anterolateral	Henry's	Brachialis and pronator teres (musculocutaneous and median)	Brachioradialis (radial)	Lateral antebrachial cutaneous nerve; radial nerve
	Posterolateral	Kocher's	Anconeus (radial)	Extensor carpi ulnaris (PIN)	PIN
	Medial		Brachialis (musculocutaneous)	Triceps and pronator teres (radial and median)	Ulnar nerve
Forearm	Anterior	Henry's	Brachioradialis (radial)	Pronator teres and flexor carpi radialis (median)	PIN
	Dorsal	Thompson's	Extensor carpi radialis brevis (radial)	Extensor digitorum and extensor pollicis longus (PIN)	PIN
	Ulnar		Extensor carpi ulnaris (PIN)	Flexor carpi ulnaris (ulnar)	Ulnar nerve and artery
Wrist	Dorsal		Third compartment (PIN)	Fourth compartment (PIN)	
Scaphoid	Volar	Russé's	Flexor carpi radialis or through sheath (median)	Radial artery	Radial artery
	Dorsolateral	Matti's	First compartment (PIN)	Third compartment (PIN)	Superficial radial nerve; radial artery

PIN, posterior interosseous nerve.

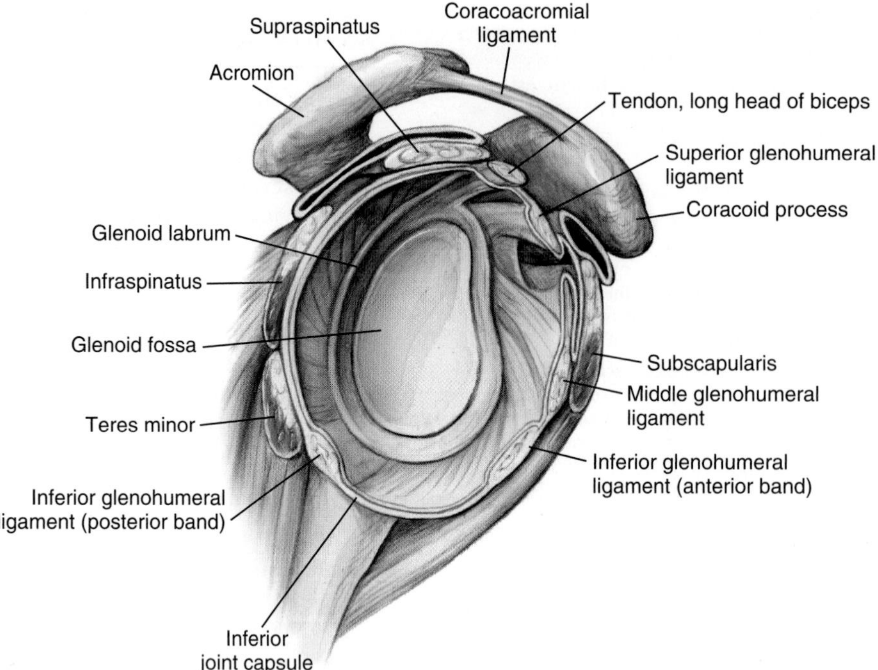

Figure 2-1 **Glenohumeral ligaments and rotator cuff muscles. The rotator interval is between the anterior border of the supraspinatus and the superior border of the subscapularis. This interval helps limit flexion and external rotation of the shoulder. Within the rotator interval is the superior glenohumeral ligament, the primary restraint both in inferior translation of the adducted shoulder and in external rotation of the adducted or slightly abducted arm. The middle glenohumeral ligament, absent in up to 30% of shoulders, is the primary stabilizer in anterior translation, with the arm slightly abducted (45 degrees). The inferior glenohumeral ligament complex is the primary stabilizer for anterior and inferior instability in abduction. The inferior glenohumeral ligament complex is composed of the anterior and posterior bands of the inferior glenohumeral ligament.** (From Miller MD, et al: *Orthopaedic surgical approaches,* Philadelphia, 2008, Saunders, Figure SA-4.)

- ▫ Acromioclavicular ligament: prevents anteroposterior displacement
- ▫ Coracoclavicular ligaments: prevent superior displacement of the distal clavicle (trapezoid [anterolateral] and conoid [posteromedial and stronger])

- When the arm is maximally elevated, about 5 to 8 degrees of rotation is possible at the acromioclavicular joint, although the clavicle rotates approximately 40 to 50 degrees.

4. Scapulothoracic joint:
   - Though not a true joint, this attachment allows scapular movement against the posterior rib cage.
   - Fixed primarily by the scapular muscular attachments.
   - Glenohumeral motion in comparison with scapulothoracic motion is in a 2:1 ratio.
5. Intrinsic ligaments of the scapula:
   - Superior transverse scapular ligament (which separates the suprascapular nerve [inferior] and vessels [superior] at the suprascapular notch; mnemonic: "Army over Navy" for artery over nerve)
   - Inferior transverse scapular ligament (spinoglenoid notch)
   - Coracoacromial ligament
     - ▫ Frequent cause of impingement.
     - ▫ **The coracoacromial ligament is important for superoanterior restraint in rotator cuff deficiencies and should be preserved during débridement of painful massive rotator cuff tears that cannot be surgically repaired.**
     - ▫ The acromial branch of the thoracoacromial artery runs on the medial aspect of the coracoacromial ligament.

Table 2-5 Glenohumeral Stabilizers

Structure	Function
Coracohumeral ligament	Primary restraint in inferior translation of the adducted arm and to external rotation
Glenoid labrum	Increases surface area, static stabilizer
Superior glenohumeral ligament	Primary restraint in external rotation of the adducted or slightly abducted arm Primary restraint in inferior translation of the adducted arm
Middle glenohumeral ligament (absent up to 30% of shoulders)	Primary stabilizer in anterior translation, with the arm abducted to 45 degrees
Inferior glenohumeral ligament complex	Primary stabilizer for anterior and inferior translation in abduction

C. Muscles (Figure 2-3)

1. Muscles connecting the upper limb to the vertebral column: trapezius, latissimus, both rhomboid muscles, and levator scapulae
2. Muscles connecting the upper limb to the thoracic wall: both pectoralis muscles, subclavius, and serratus anterior
3. Muscles acting on the shoulder joint itself: deltoid, teres major, and the four rotator cuff muscles (supraspinatus, infraspinatus, teres minor, subscapularis)

Table 2-6 Muscles of the Shoulder

Muscle	Origin	Insertion	Action	Innervation
Trapezius	SP C7-T12	Clavicle, scapula (acromion, SP)	Rotating scapula	Cranial nerve XI
Latissimus dorsi	SP T6-S5, ilium	Humerus (ITG)	Extending, adducting, internally rotating humerus	Thoracodorsal nerve
Rhomboid major	SP T2-T5	Scapula (medial border)	Adducting scapula	Dorsal scapular nerve
Rhomboid minor	SP C7-T1	Scapula (medial spine)	Adducting scapula	Dorsal scapular nerve
Levator scapulae	Transverse process C1-C4	Scapula (superior medial)	Elevating, rotating scapula	C3, C4 nerves
Pectoralis major	Sternum, ribs, clavicle	Humerus (lateral ITG)	Adducting, internally rotating arm	Medial and lateral pectoral nerves
Pectoralis minor	Ribs 3-5	Scapula (coracoid)	Protracting scapula	Medial pectoral nerve
Subclavius	Rib 1	Inferior clavicle	Depressing clavicle	Upper trunk nerves
Serratus anterior	Ribs 1-9	Scapula (ventral medial)	Preventing winging	Long thoracic nerve
Deltoid	Lateral clavicle, scapula	Humerus (deltoid tuberosity)	Abducting arm	Axillary nerve
Teres major	Inferior scapula	Humerus (medial ITG)	Adducting, internally rotating, extending arm	Lower subscapular nerve
Subscapularis	Ventral scapula	Humerus (lesser tuberosity)	Internally rotating arm, providing anterior stability	Upper and lower subscapular nerves
Supraspinatus	Superior scapula	Humerus (GT)	Abducting and externally rotating arm, providing stability	Suprascapular nerve
Infraspinatus	Dorsal scapula	Humerus (GT)	Providing stability, externally rotating arm	Suprascapular nerve
Teres minor	Scapula (dorsolateral)	Humerus (GT)	Providing stability, externally rotatjng arm	Axillary nerve

GT, greater tuberosity; ITG, intertubercular groove; SP, spinous process.

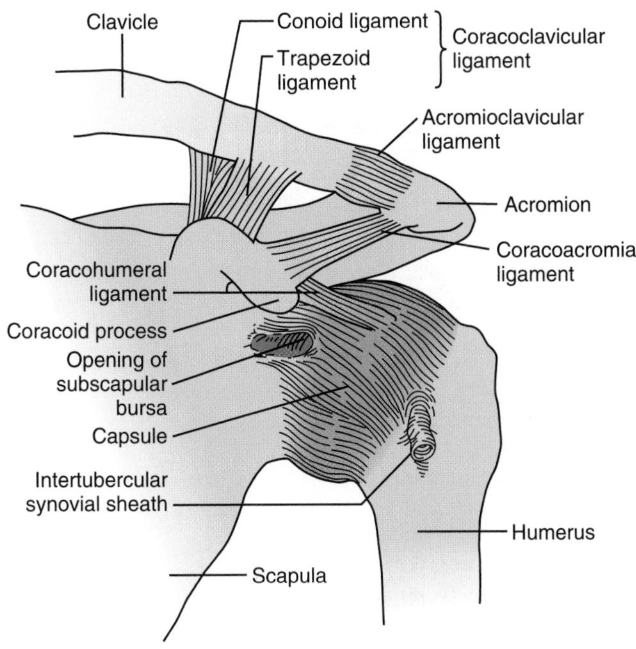

Figure 2-2 Ligaments about the shoulder. The acromioclavicular ligaments (superior, inferior, anterior, and posterior) prevent anteroposterior translation of the distal clavicle. The superior ligament is the most important and is reinforced by fibers from the trapezius and deltoid muscles. The coracoclavicular ligaments—conoid (posteromedial) and trapezoid (anterolateral)—prevent superior translation of the distal clavicle. The coracoacromial ligament should be preserved in massive rotator cuff defects because it provides superior restraint to the humeral head. Bleeding encountered during release of the coracoacromial ligament comes from the acromial branch of the thoracoacromial artery (second part of axillary artery; see Figure 2-6). (Adapted from Jenkins DB: *Hollinshead's functional anatomy of the limbs and back*, ed 6, Philadelphia, 1991, Saunders, p 71.)

- The rotator cuff muscles depress and stabilize the humeral head against the glenoid; all attach to the greater tuberosity except the subscapularis, which has a lesser tuberosity insertion (shoulder internal rotator).
- **The shoulder internal rotators (pectoralis major, latissimus dorsi, teres major, and subscapularis) are stronger than the external rotators (teres minor and infraspinatus), which is why posterior shoulder dislocations are more common than anterior dislocations after electrical shock and seizures.**
- Table 2-6 presents the specific characteristics of these muscles, and Figure 2-4 and Table 2-7 describe the four layers of shoulder musculature.

D. Nerves

1. Anatomy of brachial plexus (Figure 2-5)
   - The brachial plexus is formed from the ventral primary rami of C5 to T1 and lies under the clavicle between the scalenus anterior and scalenus medius.
   - Dorsal rami of C5 to T1 innervate the dorsal neck musculature and skin.
   - Brachial plexus consists of roots, trunks, divisions, cords, and branches (mnemonic: "**R**on **T**aylor **d**rinks **c**old **b**eer").

Table 2-7 Shoulder-Supporting Anatomic Layers

Layer	Structures
I	Deltoid; pectoralis major; trapezius
II	Clavipectoral fascia; conjoined tendon, short head of biceps, and coracobrachialis
III	Deep layer of subdeltoid bursa; rotator cuff muscles (supraspinatus, infraspinatus, teres minor, subscapularis [SITS])
IV	Glenohumeral joint capsule; coracohumeral ligament

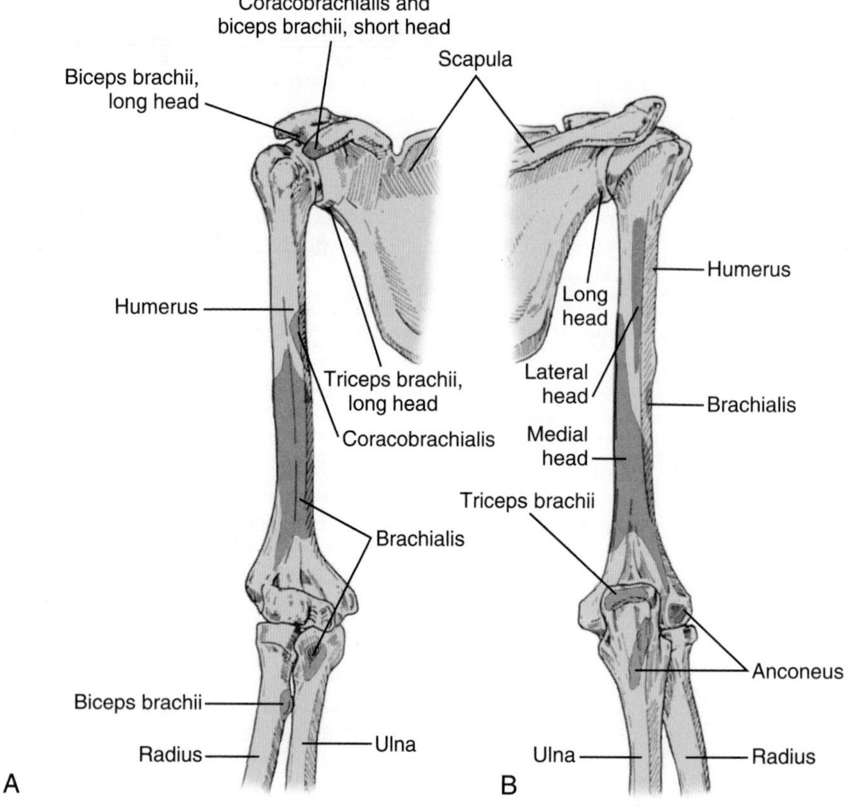

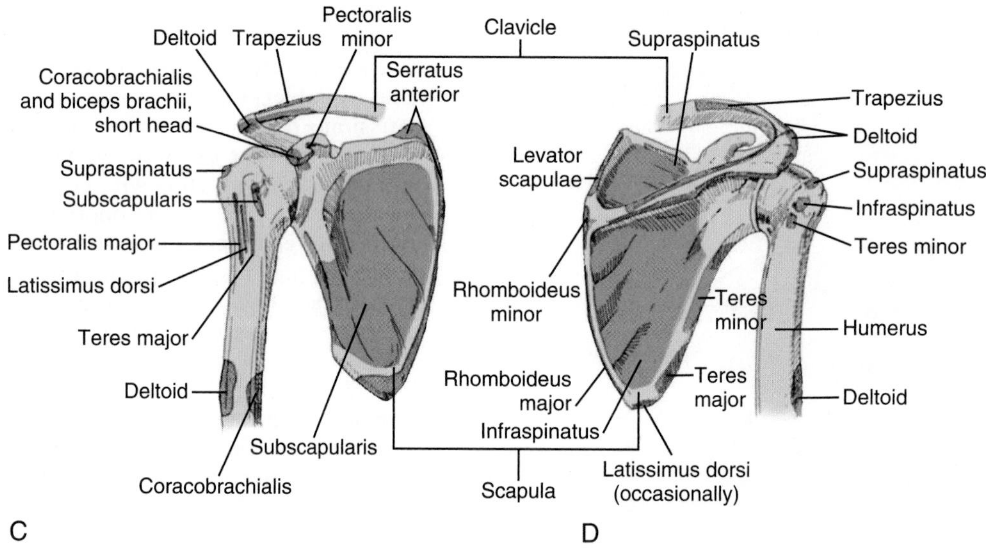

Figure 2-3 Origins and insertions of the muscles about the shoulder and upper arms **(A, B)** and shoulder girdle **(C, D)**. **A,** Anterior view. **B,** Posterior view. **C,** Anterior view. **D,** Posterior view. (From Jenkins DB: *Hollinshead's functional anatomy of the limbs and back,* ed 6, Philadelphia, 1991, Saunders, Figure 5-3.)

- Five roots (C5 to T1, although contributions from C4 and T2 can be small)
- Three trunks (upper, middle, lower)
- Six divisions (two from each trunk)
- Three cords **(named because of their anatomic relationship to the axillary artery: posterior, lateral, and medial); the termination of each cord is shown in Table 2-8**
- Multiple branches: four preclavicular branches (from roots and upper trunk):
  - Dorsal scapular nerve
  - Long thoracic nerve
  - Suprascapular nerve
  - Nerve to the subclavius

2. Muscle innervation: innervation of all rotator cuff muscles derived from C5 and C6 of the brachial plexus (Table 2-9; see also Table 2-3)
3. Brachial plexus injury
   - Preganglionic brachial plexus lesions
     - Proximal to the dorsal root ganglion

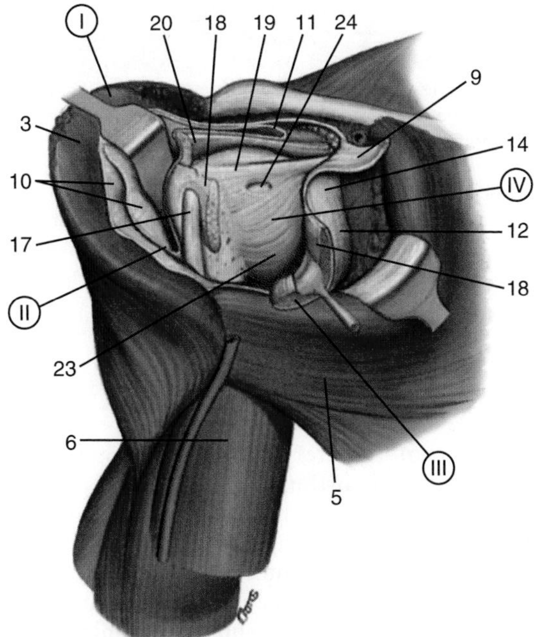

Figure 2-4 Anterior aspect of the right shoulder, depicting the four layers (circled Roman numerals). In this illustration, the lateral retractor is placed deep to layer II, demonstrating the ease of dissection in the plane of the bursa around the lateral aspect of the proximal humerus. The subscapularis and supraspinatus (layer III) have been reflected, disclosing layer IV (capsule and coracohumeral ligament). The usual shape and position of the defect in the rotator interval (if present) are depicted and show variability. 3, Deltoid; 5, pectoralis major; 6, biceps; 9, coracoacromial ligament; 10, fasciae (layer II); 11, deep layer of subdeltoid bursa; 12, conjoined tendon; 14, tip of coracoid process; 17, biceps brachii long head; 18, deep layer of subdeltoid bursa and subscapularis; 19, coracohumeral ligament; 20, supraspinatus under deep bursa layer; 23, joint capsule; 24, hiatus in capsule. (From Cooper DE, et al: Supporting layers of glenohumeral joint, *Clin Orthop* 289:151, 1993.)

Table 2-8 Brachial Plexus Cord Terminations

Cord	Termination
Lateral	Musculocutaneous nerve* Lateral pectoral nerve
Posterior	Radial and axillary nerve* Upper and lower subscapular nerve Thoracodorsal nerve
Medial	Ulnar nerve* Medial pectoral nerve Medial brachial cutaneous nerve Medial antebrachial cutaneous nerve
Medial and lateral	Median nerve*

*Major branches.

Table 2-9 Rotator Cuff Muscle Innervation: All C5 and C6 Muscle Innervation

Muscles Innervated	Nerves
External Rotators	
Supraspinatus	Suprascapular nerve (C5, C6)
Infraspinatus	Suprascapular nerve (C5, C6)
Teres minor	Axillary nerve (C5, C6)
Internal Rotator	
Subscapularis	Upper (C5) and lower (C5, C6) subscapular nerve

  - Produce **medial** scapular winging (because of paralysis of the preclavicular long thoracic nerve with resultant serratus anterior dysfunction) and Horner's syndrome (injury to brachial plexus at C8 to T1 involving the inferior/stellate ganglion)
- Postganglionic brachial plexus injuries
  - Do not produce Horner's syndrome, a winged scapula, diaphragmatic paralysis, or rhomboid paralysis
- Obstetric brachial plexus palsy (Table 2-10)
- Injury to the spinal accessory nerve (cranial nerve XI)
  - Causes trapezius dysfunction and scapular-trapezius winging **(lateral winging)**
  - Results in shoulder depression with scapular translation laterally and the inferior angle rotated laterally because of the unopposed pull of the serratus anterior

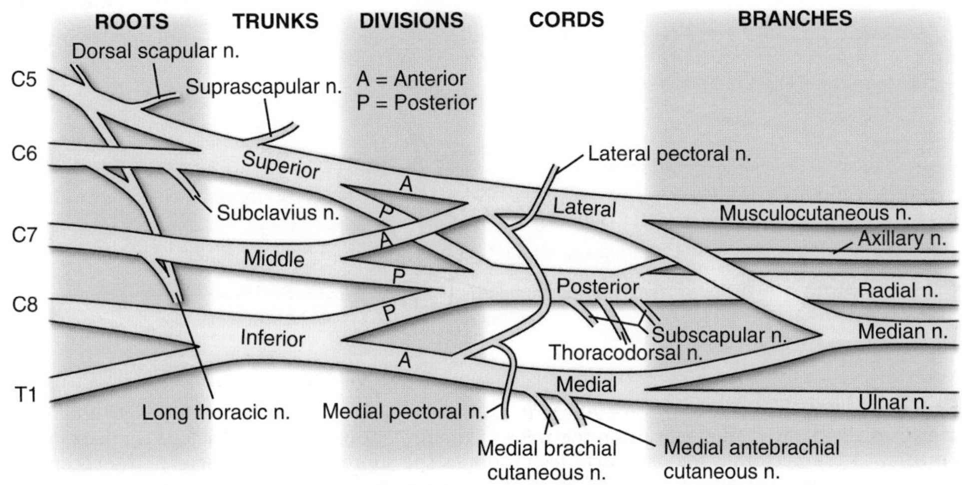

Figure 2-5 Brachial plexus. There are four preclavicular/supraclavicular branches: the long thoracic nerve (serratus anterior muscle), dorsal scapular nerve (rhomboid muscle), suprascapular nerve (supraspinatus and infraspinatus muscles), and nerve to the subclavius. (From Miller MD, et al: *Orthopaedic surgical approaches,* Philadelphia, 2008, Saunders, Figure SA-7.)

Table 2-10 Obstetric Brachial Plexus Palsies

Palsy Type	Roots	Deficit	Prognosis
Erb-Duchenne	C5, C6	Weakness of deltoid, rotator cuff, elbow flexors, and wrist and hand extensors "Waiter's tip"	Best
Klumpke's	C8, T1	Weakness of wrist flexors and intrinsic apparatus, Horner's syndrome	Poor
Total plexus	C5-T1	Flaccid arm	Worst

- Injury to the long thoracic nerve **(C5 to C7)**
  - Causes serratus anterior dysfunction and **medial scapular winging**
  - Results in superior elevation with scapular translation medially and the inferior angle rotated medially

E. **Vessels**

1. Subclavian artery
   - The left subclavian artery arises directly from the aorta, and the right subclavian artery arises from the brachiocephalic trunk.
   - It then emerges between the scalenus anterior and medius muscles and becomes the axillary artery at the outer border of the first rib.
2. Axillary artery (Table 2-11, Figure 2-6)
   - This artery is conceptualized as divided into three parts on the basis of its physical relationship to the pectoralis minor muscle (the first part is medial to it, the second is under it, and the third is lateral to it).

Table 2-11 Axillary Artery Branches

Part	Branch	Course
I	Supreme thoracic	Medial to serratus anterior and pectoral muscles
II	Thoracoacromial	Four branches: deltoid, acromial, pectoralis, clavicular
	Lateral thoracic	Descends to serratus anterior
III	Subscapular	Two branches: thoracodorsal and circumflex scapular (triangular space)
	Anterior humeral circumflex	Blood supply to humeral head: arcuate artery lateral to bicipital groove
	Posterior humeral circumflex	Branch in the quadrangular space accompanying the axillary nerve

- **Each part of the artery has as many branches as the number of that portion (e.g., the second part has two branches: thoracoacromial and lateral thoracic).**
- The third part of the axillary artery, at the origin of the anterior and posterior humeral circumflex arteries, is the most vulnerable to traumatic vascular injury.

F. **Surgical approaches to the shoulder (Table 2-12; see Table 2-4):**

1. Anterior (Henry's) approach (Figure 2-7)
   - Interval: deltoid (axillary nerve) and the pectoralis major (medial and lateral pectoral nerves)
   - Dissection:
     - Dissect the cephalic vein, and retract it laterally with the deltoid, thereby exposing the underlying subscapularis.
     - Then divide the subscapularis (preserving the most inferior fibers in order to protect the axillary nerve); then the shoulder capsule is visualized.

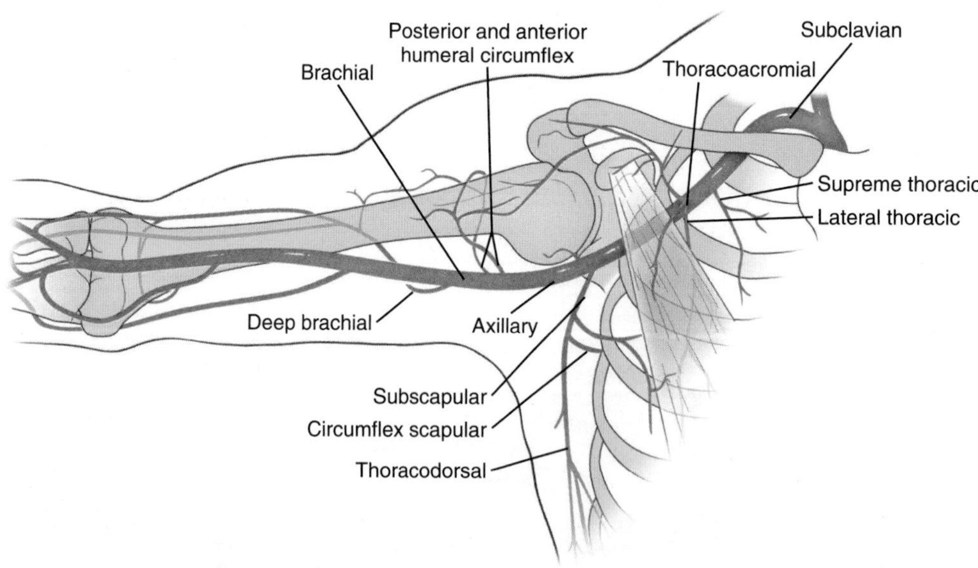

Figure 2-6 Branches of the axillary artery. At the point where the subclavian artery passes beneath the clavicle, it becomes the axillary artery. The axillary artery is divided into three sections on the basis of their relationship to the pectoralis minor muscle. The first part of the axillary artery is medial to the pectoralis minor muscle and supplies the supreme thoracic artery. The second part is beneath the muscle and supplies the thoracoacromial artery and the lateral thoracic artery. The third part is lateral to the muscle and supplies the subscapular artery and the posterior and anterior humeral circumflex arteries. The third part of the axillary artery, at the origin of the anterior and posterior humeral circumflex arteries, is the part most vulnerable to traumatic vascular injury. (From Miller MD, et al: *Orthopaedic surgical approaches,* Philadelphia, 2008, Saunders, Figure SA-9.)

Table 2-12 Surgical Approaches to the Shoulder

Approach	Interval	Structures at Risk
Anterior (Henry's)	Deltoid (axillary nerve) and pectoralis major (medial and lateral pectoral nerve)	Axillary nerve limits inferior exposure; place arm in adduction and external rotation Musculocutaneous nerve: avoid vigorous retraction and medial dissection to the conjoined tendon/ coracobrachialis
Lateral	Deltoid splitting (axillary nerve)	Avoid deltoid split >5 cm below acromion, to avoid damaging axillary nerve
Posterior	Infraspinatus (suprascapular nerve) and teres minor (axillary nerve)	Dissection inferior to the teres minor puts quadrangular space structures at risk: axillary nerve and posterior humeral circumflex artery Avoid excessive medial retraction on infraspinatus, which can injure suprascapular nerve

- □ A leash of three vessels (one artery and the superior and inferior venae comitantes) marks the lower border of the subscapularis.
- ▪ Risks:
  - □ Musculocutaneous nerve (lateral cord brachial plexus)
    - ▪ Protect by avoiding vigorous retraction of the conjoined tendon and avoiding dissection medial to the coracobrachialis.
    - ▪ This nerve usually penetrates the biceps/ coracobrachialis 5 to 8 cm below the coracoid, but it enters these muscles proximal to this 5-cm "safe zone" in almost 30% of shoulders.
    - ▪ Palsy of the musculocutaneous nerve would affect the coracobrachialis, biceps brachii, and brachialis muscles, and it would affect sensation in the lateral antebrachial cutaneous nerve (termination of the musculocutaneous nerve).
  - □ Axillary nerve
    - ▪ Just inferior to the shoulder capsule
    - ▪ Protected during procedures in this area with adduction and external rotation of the arm

2. Lateral approach
   - ▪ Interval: none; this is a deltoid-splitting approach
   - ▪ Dissection:
     - □ Either split the deltoid muscle or subperiosteally dissect it from the acromion.
     - □ The supraspinatus tendon is exposed, which allows for repairs of the rotator cuff.
   - ▪ Risks:
     - □ Deltoid should not be split more than 5 cm below the acromion, in order to avoid injury to the axillary nerve (posterior cord brachial plexus exiting from quadrangular space).

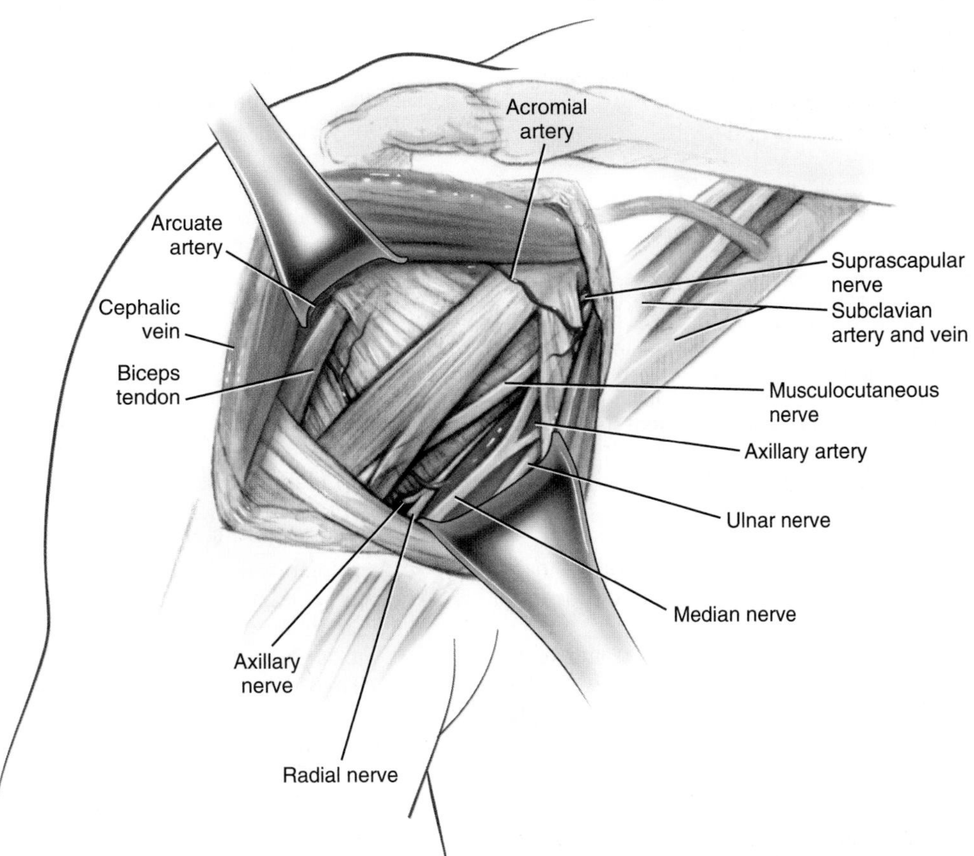

Figure 2-7 Anterior (Henry's) surgical approach to the shoulder. In this approach, the interval between the deltoid (axillary nerve) and the pectoralis major (medial and lateral pectoral nerves) is explored. To prevent injury to the musculocutaneous nerve, avoid excessive medial retraction (see medial retractor) on the coracobrachialis or avoid dissection medial to this muscle. Also avoid the axillary nerve, which is inferior to the shoulder capsule. Positioning the arm in adduction and external rotation helps displace the axillary nerve from the surgical field. (From Miller MD, et al: *Orthopaedic surgical approaches,* Philadelphia, 2008, Saunders, Figure SA-12.)

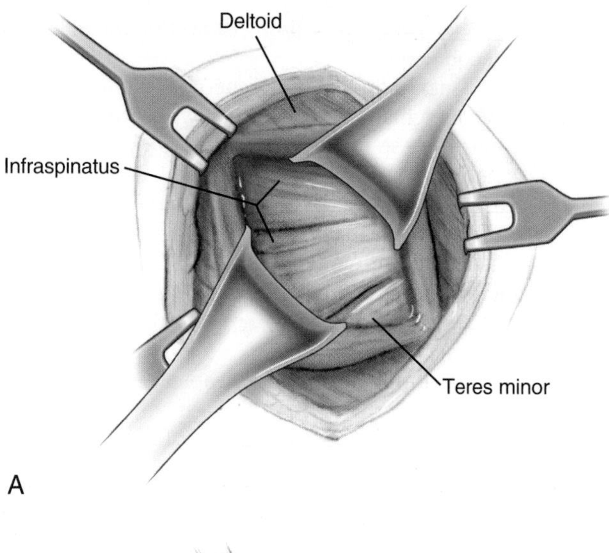

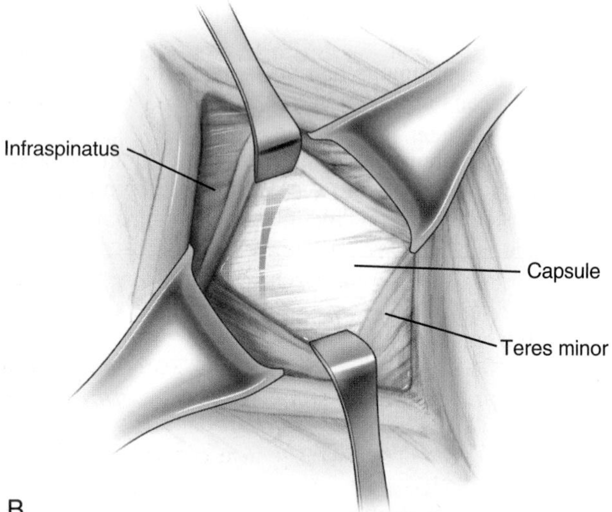

Figure 2-8 Posterior approach to the shoulder. **A,** Superficial exposure. **B,** Deep exposure. In this approach, the interval between the infraspinatus (suprascapular nerve) and the teres minor (axillary nerve) is explored. Do not dissect below the teres minor. Dissections below the teres minor place the structures in the quadrangular space at risk for injury: the posterior humeral circumflex artery and the axillary nerve. Also, to prevent suprascapular nerve palsy, avoid excessive retraction of the infraspinatus. (From Miller MD, et al: *Orthopaedic surgical approaches,* Philadelphia, 2008, Saunders, Figures SA-24 and SA-25.)

- ▫ If dissection extends more than 5 cm inferiorly, denervation of the deltoid can occur in its anterior portion.

3. Posterior approach (Figure 2-8)
   - Interval: infraspinatus (suprascapular nerve) and teres minor (axillary nerve)
   - Dissection: Split the posterior deltoid, thereby exposing the interval between the infraspinatus and teres minor; the posterior capsule lies immediately beneath it.
   - Risks: Both the axillary nerve and the posterior circumflex humeral artery run in the quadrangular space below the teres minor, so it is important to stay above this muscle. Excessive medial retraction of the infraspinatus can injure the suprascapular nerve.

G. Arthroscopy (discussed in Chapter 4, Sports Medicine)

1. Anterior-superior portal: musculocutaneous nerve at risk for injury
2. Anterior-inferior portal: must be above the subscapularis and lateral to the conjoined tendon
3. Posterior portal (inferior portals may put the axillary nerve at risk for injury)

II. ARM

A. Osteology: humerus

1. Humeral head:
   - Articulates with the smaller scapular glenoid cavity
   - Retroverted 30 degrees (in relation to the transepicondylar axis of the humerus)
   - Scapular glenoid: retroverted 5 degrees
2. Anatomic neck, directly below the humeral head, serves as an attachment for the shoulder capsule.
3. Surgical neck is lower and is more often involved in fractures.
4. Greater tuberosity is lateral to the humeral head.
   - Serves as the attachment for the supraspinatus, infraspinatus, and teres minor muscles (anterior to posterior, respectively)
5. Lesser tuberosity, located anteriorly, has only one muscular insertion: the last rotator cuff muscle, the subscapularis.
6. Bicipital groove (for the tendon of the long head of the biceps brachii) is a bony groove between the two tuberosities.
7. Humeral shaft has a posterior spiral groove (for the radial nerve) adjacent to the deltoid tuberosity and approximately 13 cm above the articular surface of the trochlea.
8. Distally, the humerus flares into medial and lateral epicondyles.
   - Forms half of the elbow joint
   - Medial spool-shaped trochlea (which articulates with the olecranon of the ulna)
   - Lateral globular capitellum (which opposes the radial head)
   - Normal articular alignment of the distal humerus has a 7-degree valgus tilt (carrying angle)

B. Arthrology

1. Joints
   - Elbow is composed of a hinge joint (the humeroulnar articulation) and a pivot joint (the humeroradial articulation) (Table 2-13).
   - Axis of rotation for the elbow is centered through the trochlea and capitellum and passes through a point anteroinferior on the medial epicondyle.
   - Elbow joint has capsuloligamentous tissues (Figure 2-9) that are a key source of testable material.
     - ▫ Capsule allows maximum distension at approximately 70 to 80 degrees of flexion, which is why patients with effusion hold their arms in this position, which is most comfortable.

Table 2-13 Elbow Joint Articulations

Articulation	Components
Humeroulnar	Trochlea and trochlear notch
Humeroradial	Capitulum and radial head
Proximal radioulnar	Radial notch and radial head

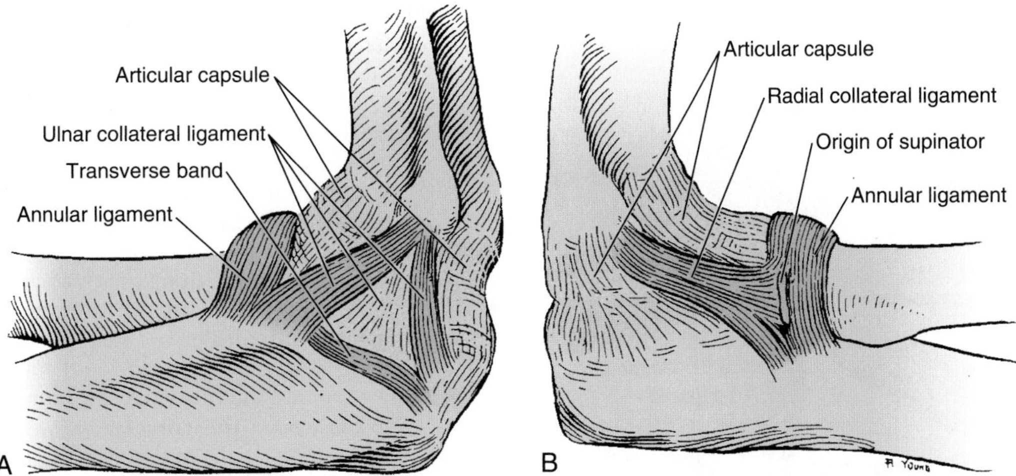

Figure 2-9 Elbow ligaments. **A,** Medial view. The most important portion of the medial collateral ligament is the anterior bundle or ulnar collateral ligament. **B,** Lateral view. The most important portion of the lateral collateral ligament complex is the lateral ulnar collateral ligament (LUCL) or radial collateral ligament. A deficiency of the LUCL results in posterolateral rotatory instability. (From Jenkins DB: *Hollinshead's functional anatomy of the limbs and back,* ed 6, Philadelphia, 1991, Saunders, p 108.)

- Anterior capsule attaches at a point approximately 6 mm distal to the tip of the coronoid.
  - Coronoid tip is an intraarticular structure that is visualized during elbow arthroscopy.

2. Ligaments (Table 2-14)
   - The medial collateral ligament (MCL) (anterior, posterior, and transverse bundles) arises from the anteroinferior portion of the medial humeral epicondyle and provides stability in valgus stress.
     - **The anterior bundle is the most important in helping resist valgus forces and attaches 18 mm distal to the coronoid tip.**
     - Valgus stability with the arm in pronation suggests that the anterior bundle of the MCL is intact.
   - The lateral or radial collateral ligament (annular, radial, and ulnar parts) originates on the lateral humeral epicondyle near the axis of elbow rotation.
     - **The lateral ulnar collateral ligament (LUCL) is an essential elbow stabilizer and runs from the lateral epicondyle to the ulna crista supinatoris (supinator crest).**
     - **A deficiency of the LUCL is manifested as posterolateral rotatory instability of the elbow (see Table 2-14).**

Table 2-14 Elbow Ligaments

Ligament	Components	Comments
Medial collateral	Anterior bundle of MCL (ulnar collateral); posterior bundle; transverse bundle (Cooper ligament)	Anterior bundle (strongest of all elbow ligaments): anterior band taut from 60 degrees of flexion to full extension, posterior band taut from 60-120 degrees of flexion
Lateral collateral	LUCL; annular ligament; quadrate (annular ligament to radial neck) and oblique cord	Deficiency of LUCL results in posterolateral rotator instability

LUCL, lateral ulnar collateral ligament; MCL, medial collateral ligament.

C. **Muscles: four muscles of the arm controlling elbow motion (Table 2-15)**

1. Flexors (biceps, brachialis, and brachioradialis); the brachialis attaches to the coronoid at 11 mm distal to the tip
2. Extensors (triceps); also helps form borders for three important spaces (Figure 2-10 and Table 2-16)
   - **Triangular space:** bordered by teres minor (superiorly), teres major (inferiorly), and long head of biceps brachii (laterally)
     - Contains the circumflex scapular vessels
   - **Quadrangular space:** bordered by the teres minor (superiorly) and teres major (inferiorly); medial border formed by the long head of the triceps, and lateral border formed by the humerus
     - **Transmits the posterior humeral circumflex vessels and the axillary nerve**
   - **Triangular interval:** immediately inferior to the quadrangular space and bordered by the teres major

Table 2-15 Muscles of the Arm

Muscle	Origin	Insertion	Action	Innervation
Coracobrachialis	Coracoid	Mid-humerus (medial)	Flexion, adduction	Musculocutaneous
Biceps brachii	Coracoid (short head) Supraglenoid (long head)	Radial tuberosity	Supination, flexion	Musculocutaneous
Brachialis	Anterior humerus	Ulnar tuberosity (anterior)	Flexing forearm	Musculocutaneous, radial
Triceps brachii	Infraglenoid (long head) Posterior humerus (lateral head) Posterior humerus (medial head)	Olecranon	Extending forearm	Radial

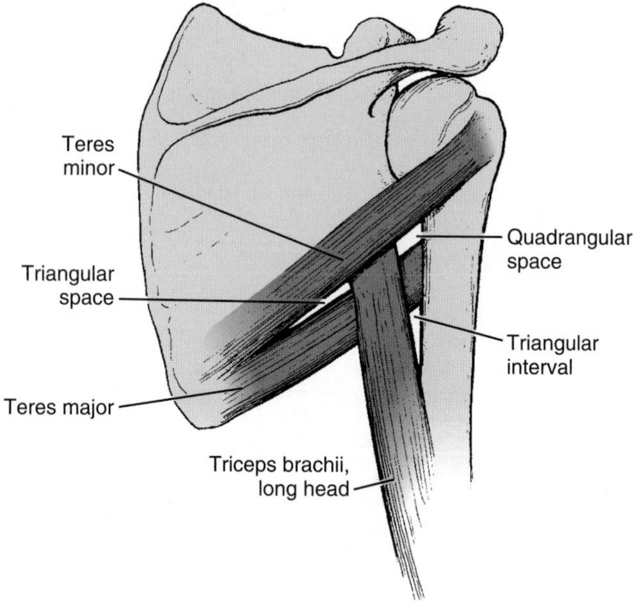

Figure 2-10 Borders of key spaces and intervals, posterior view: quadrangular space (containing the axillary nerve and posterior humeral circumflex artery), triangular space (circumflex scapular vessels), and triangular interval (radial nerve and profunda brachii artery). (From Kaplan EB: *Surgical approaches to the neck, cervical spine, and upper extremity,* Philadelphia, 1966, Saunders, p 53.)

(superiorly), long head of the triceps (medially), and lateral head of the triceps or the humerus (laterally)
- □ Through this interval, **the profunda brachii artery and radial nerve can be seen**

D. **Nerves**

1. Anatomy
   - Four major nerves traverse the arm; two give off branches to arm musculature, and two innervate the distal musculature (Figure 2-11). Most of the cutaneous innervation of the arm arises directly from the brachial plexus.

Table 2-16 Shoulder Spaces and Intervals

Space	Borders	Nerve	Vessel
Quadrangular (quadrilateral) space	Superior: lower border of teres minor Lateral: surgical neck of humerus Medial: long head of triceps Inferior: upper border of teres major	Axillary	Posterior humeral circumflex artery
Triangular space	Superior: lower border of teres minor Lateral: long head of triceps Medial: teres major		Circumflex scapular artery
Triangular interval	Superior: lower border of teres major Lateral: shaft of humerus Medial: long head of triceps	Radial	Profunda brachii artery

- Musculocutaneous nerve (lateral cord):
  - □ Pierces the coracobrachialis 5 to 8 cm distal to the coracoid
  - □ Branches to supply the coracobrachialis, the biceps, and the brachialis
  - □ Gives off a branch to the elbow joint before it becomes the lateral antebrachial cutaneous nerve of the forearm, which is located deep to the cephalic vein
- Radial nerve (posterior cord):
  - □ Spirals around the humerus (medial to lateral) in the spiral groove at a distance of approximately **13 cm from the trochlea**
  - □ Emerges on the lateral side of the arm after piercing the lateral intermuscular septum approximately **7.5 cm above the trochlea** between the brachialis and brachioradialis anterior to the lateral epicondyle (where it supplies the anconeus muscle)
- Median nerve (medial and lateral cords):
  - □ Accompanies the brachial artery along the arm, crossing it during its course (lateral to medial)
  - □ Supplies some branches to the elbow joint but has no branches in the arm itself
- Ulnar nerve (medial cord):
  - □ Passes medial to the brachial artery in the arm and then runs behind the medial epicondyle of the humerus, where it is superficial
  - □ Also has branches to the elbow but none to the arm
- Cutaneous nerves:
  - □ Supraclavicular nerve (C3 and C4) supplies the upper shoulder.
  - □ Axillary nerve supplies the shoulder joint and the overlying skin.
  - □ Medial, lateral, and dorsal brachial cutaneous nerves supply the balance of the cutaneous innervation of the arm.
  - □ Lateral antebrachial cutaneous nerve is the termination of the musculocutaneous nerve (Figure 2-12 summarizes the dermatome patterns).

2. Compressive neuropathies (Table 2-17)
3. Muscle innervation (see Table 2-3)

E. **Vessels**

1. Brachial artery
   - Originates at the lower border of the tendon of the teres major and continues to the elbow, where it bifurcates into the radial and ulnar arteries (see Figure 2-11)
   - Lies medial in the arm, curving laterally to enter the cubital fossa
   - Cubital fossa: formed by the distal humerus proximally, the brachioradialis laterally, and the pronator teres medially
2. Principal branches
   - Deep brachial (also known as the *profunda,* this artery accompanies the radial nerve posteriorly in the triangular interval)
   - Superior and inferior ulnar collateral arteries
   - The nutrient and muscular branches
   - The supratrochlear artery (the least flexible branch)
   - These collateral vessels can bind up the brachial artery with distal humerus fractures

F. **Surgical approaches to the humerus. (Table 2-18)**

1. Anterolateral approach to the humerus (Figure 2-13)

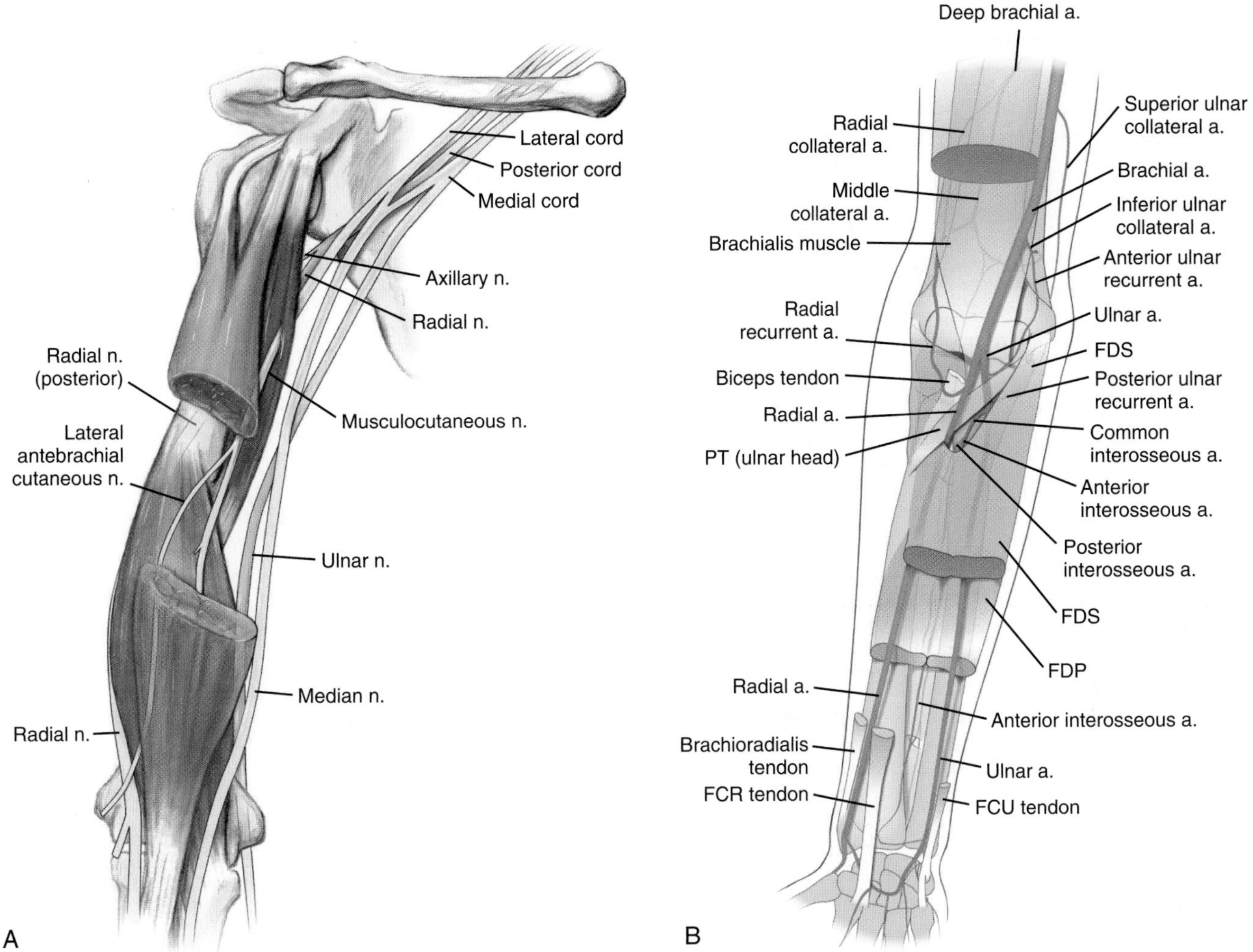

Figure 2-11 Principal nerves **(A)** and arteries **(B)** of the upper extremity. FCR, flexor carpi radialis; FCU, flexor carpi ulnaris; FDP, flexor digitorum profundus; FDS, flexor digitorum superficialis; PT, pronator teres. (From Miller MD, et al: *Orthopaedic surgical approaches,* Philadelphia, 2008, Saunders, Figures SA-8 and EF-12.)

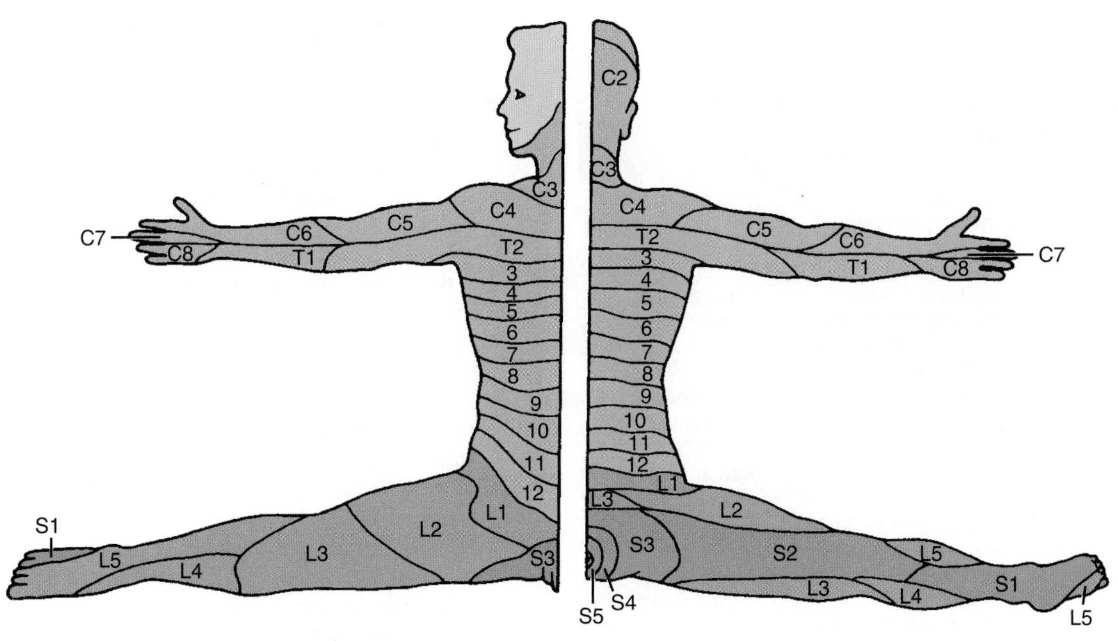

Figure 2-12 Dermatome patterns.

Table 2-17 Nerve Compression Syndromes of the Arm and Forearm

Syndrome	Nerve Involved	Sites of Compression
Pronator	Median	Supracondylar process of humerus and ligament of Struthers Lacertus fibrosis (bicipital aponeurosis) Pronator teres Arch of flexor digitorum superficialis
AIN	AIN of median	Deep head of pronator teres Flexor digitorum superficialis Aberrant vessels Accessory muscles (i.e., Gantzer's muscles)
Cubital tunnel	Ulnar	Arcade of Struthers Medial intermuscular septum Medial epicondyle Cubital tunnel Proximal edge of flexor carpi ulnaris (Osborne fascia) Deep flexor pronator aponeurosis
PIN Radial tunnel	PIN of radial	Fibrous bands Recurrent leash of Henry Extensor carpi radialis brevis Arcade of Frohse (proximal edge of superficial head of supinator) Supinator distal margin
Superficial radial nerve	Superficial radial	Between the brachioradialis and extensor carpi radialis longus

AIN, anterior interosseous nerve; PIN, posterior interosseous nerve.

- Interval: deltoid (axillary nerve) and pectoralis major (medial and lateral pectoral nerves) proximally and between the fibers of the brachialis (radial and musculocutaneous nerves) distally
- Dissection:
  - Proximal approach: the anterior circumflex humeral vessels may need to be ligated

Table 2-18 Surgical Approaches to the Humerus

Approach	Interval	Structures at Risk
Anterolateral—proximal	Proximal—deltoid (axillary nerve) and pectoralis major (medial and lateral pectoral nerve) Distal—brachialis (radial and musculocutaneous nerve)	Radial nerve; axillary nerve; anterior humeral circumflex artery
Posterior	Triceps (radial nerve); lateral and long heads	Radial nerve; deep brachial artery
Anterolateral—distal	Brachialis (musculocutaneous and radial nerve) and brachioradialis (radial nerve)	Radial nerve
Lateral	Triceps (radial nerve) and brachioradialis (radial nerve)	Radial nerve with proximal extension

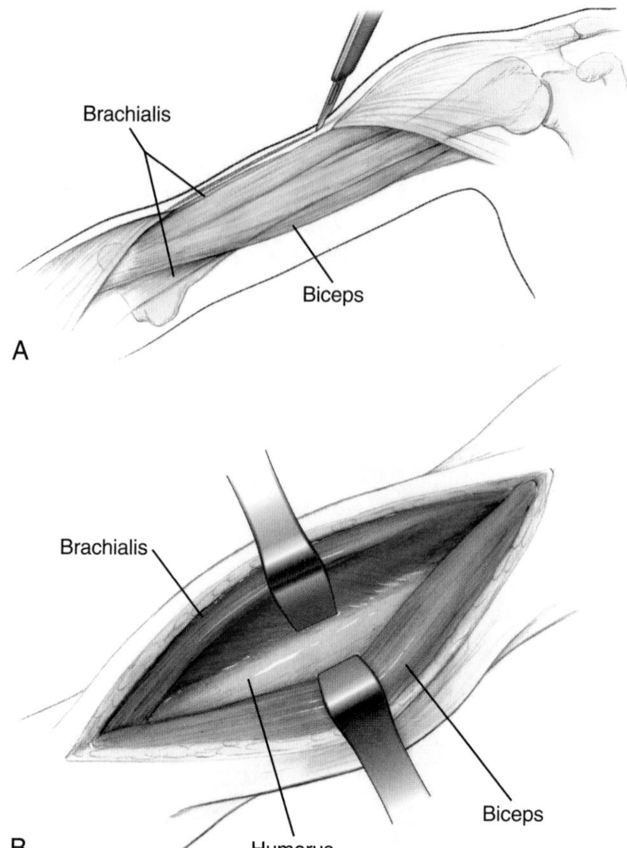

Figure 2-13 Anterolateral approach to the humerus. **A,** Superficial exposure. **B,** Deep exposure. This approach can be extended proximally into the deltopectoral approach. (From Miller MD, et al: *Orthopaedic surgical approaches*, Philadelphia, 2008, Saunders, Figures SA-43 and SA-44.)

  - Distal approach: between the biceps and brachialis laterally, or the brachialis can be split because of its dual innervation
- Risks: The radial and axillary nerves are at risk for injury mainly because of forceful retraction.

2. Posterior approach to the humerus (Figure 2-14)
   - Interval: none; this is a triceps-splitting approach
   - Dissection:
     - Superficial approach: Dissect between the lateral and long heads of the triceps.
     - Deep approach: Split the medial head of the triceps.
   - Risks:
     - Radial nerve: limits proximal extension of approach
       - Identify and protect the radial nerve as it passes from medial to lateral in the proximal part of the exposure.
     - Ulnar nerve: jeopardized unless subperiosteal dissection of the humerus is performed meticulously

G. Surgical approaches to the elbow (Table 2-19)

1. Posterior approach to the elbow (Figure 2-15)
   - Interval: none
   - Dissection:
     - Detach the extensor mechanism of the elbow to obtain excellent exposure for many elbow fractures.
     - Predrill the olecranon osteotomy (best done with a chevron cut 2 cm distal to the tip), and protect the ulnar nerve.

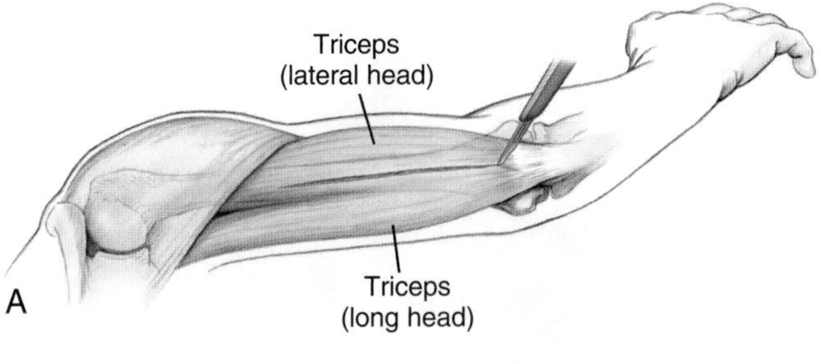

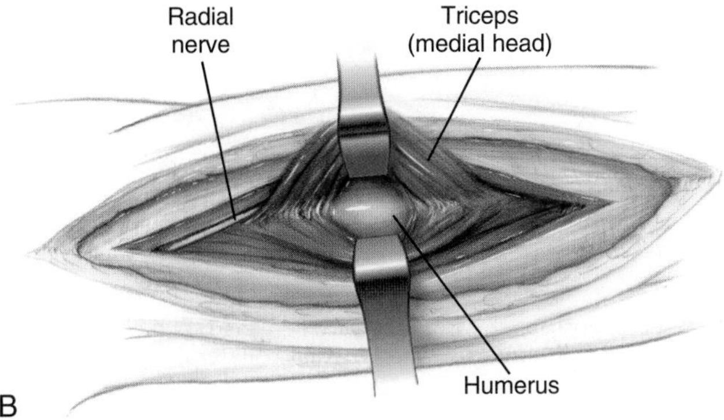

Figure 2-14 Posterior approach to the humerus. **A,** Superficial exposure. **B,** Deep exposure. The medial (deep) head of the triceps is split in this approach. (From Miller MD, et al: *Orthopaedic surgical approaches,* Philadelphia, 2008, Saunders, Figures SA-45 and SA-47.)

Table 2-19 Surgical Approaches to the Elbow

Approach	Interval	Structures at Risk
Posterior	Detach triceps or olecranon osteotomy	Ulnar nerve Olecranon nonunion
Medial	Proximally: brachialis (musculocutaneous nerve) and triceps (radial nerve) Distally: brachialis and pronator teres (median nerve)	Ulnar nerve; medial antebrachial cutaneous nerve
Anterolateral (Henry's)	Proximally: brachialis (musculocutaneous nerve) splitting Distally: pronator teres (median nerve) and brachioradialis (radial nerve)	Lateral antebrachial cutaneous nerve; radial nerve Ligation of radial recurrent artery; protect brachial artery To reduce risk: **supinate forearm**
Posterolateral (Kocher's)	Anconeus (radial nerve) and extensor carpi ulnaris (PIN of radial nerve)	PIN (pronation moves PIN anteriorly and radially) To reduce risk: **pronate forearm**

PIN, posterior interosseous nerve.

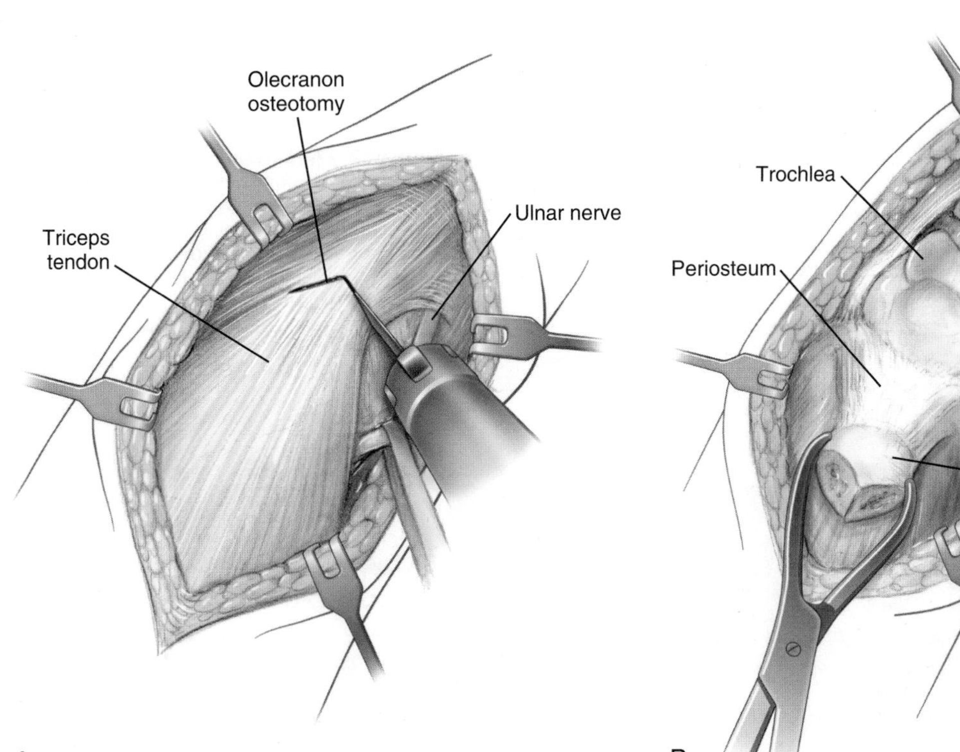

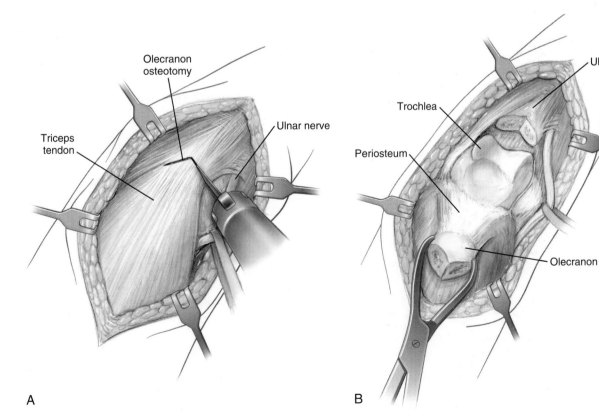

Figure 2-15 Posterior approach to the elbow. **A,** Superficial exposure. **B,** Deep exposure. An olecranon osteotomy is shown. (From Miller MD, et al: *Orthopaedic surgical approaches,* Philadelphia, 2008, Saunders, Figures EF-46 and EF-47.)

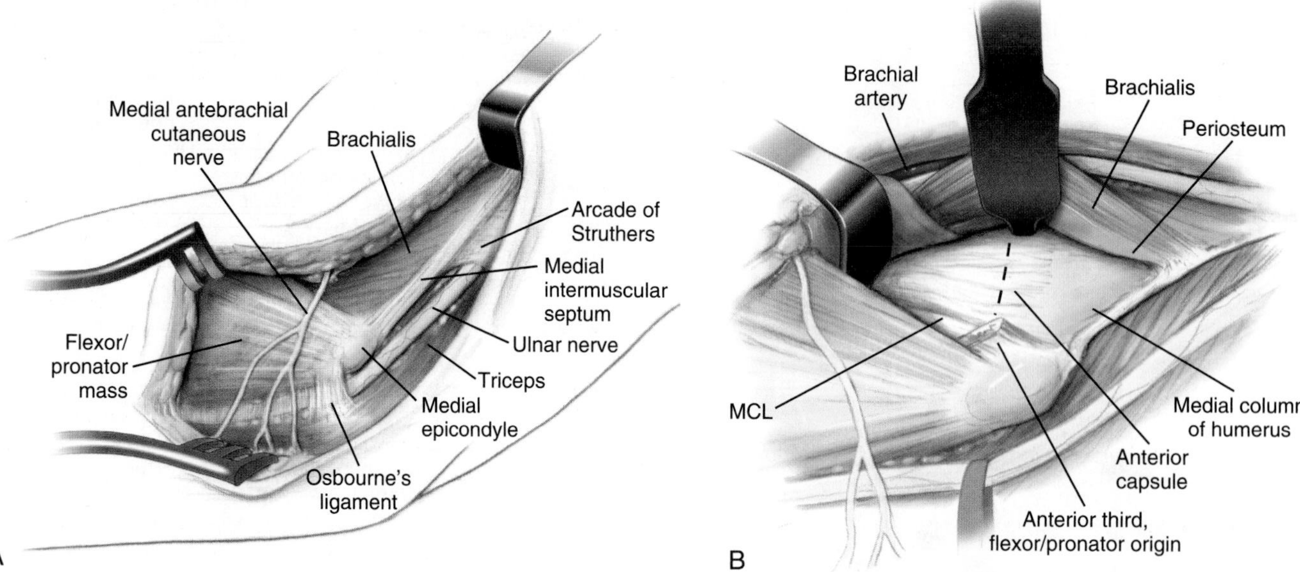

Figure 2-16 Medial approach to the elbow. **A,** Superficial exposure. **B,** Deep exposure. The interval between the brachialis (musculocutaneous nerve) and triceps (radial nerve) can be used to access the anterior distal humerus. MCL, medial collateral ligament. (From Miller MD, et al: *Orthopaedic surgical approaches,* Philadelphia, 2008, Saunders, Figures EF-23 and EF 26.)

    - In an alternative approach, split the triceps and leave the olecranon intact.
  - Risks:
    - Ulnar nerve can be injured with dissection or excessive retraction.
    - Radial nerve limits the proximal extension along the humerus.
2. Medial approach to the elbow (Figure 2-16)
  - Interval: between the brachialis (musculocutaneous nerve) and the triceps (radial nerve) proximally and between the brachialis and pronator teres (median nerve) distally.
  - Dissection: Incise the anterior third of the flexor pronator mass to reach the anterior elbow capsule.
  - Risks: The ulnar and medial antebrachial cutaneous nerves are in the field and must be protected.
3. Lateral or posterolateral (Kocher's) approach to the elbow (Figure 2-17)
  - Interval: between the anconeus (radial nerve) and the origin of the main extensor (extensor carpi ulnaris, posterior interosseous nerve [PIN])
  - Dissection: Pronate the arm to move the PIN anteriorly and radially, and approach the radial head through the proximal supinator fibers.

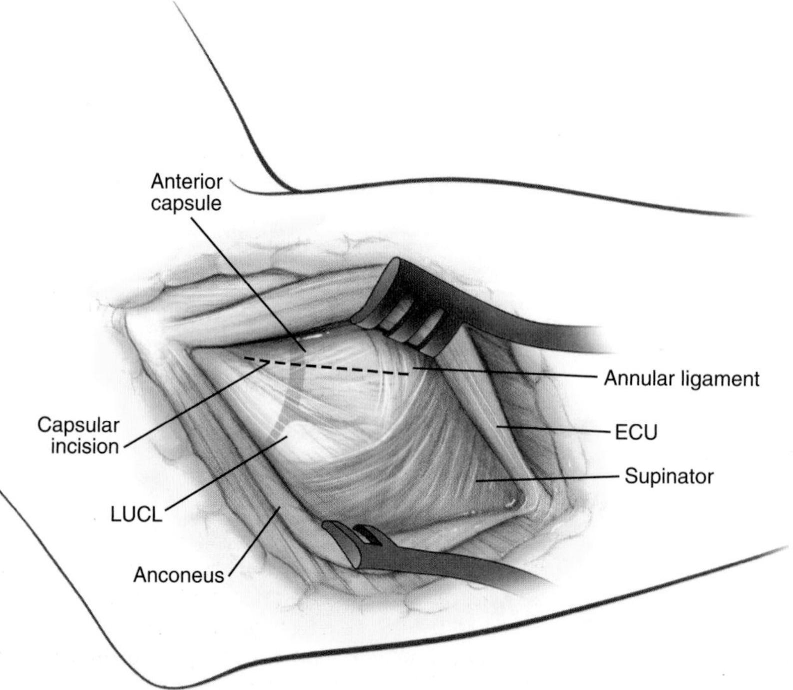

Figure 2-17 Lateral approach to the elbow. This approach explores the interval between the anconeus (radial nerve) and the extensor carpi ulnaris (ECU) (posterior interosseous nerve [PIN]). Arm pronation helps move the PIN away from the surgical field. LUCL, lateral ulnar collateral ligament. (From Miller MD, et al: *Orthopaedic surgical approaches,* Philadelphia, 2008, Saunders, Figure EF-32.)

- Risks: Extending this approach distal to the annular ligament increases the risk for injury to the PIN.

4. Proximal extension of lateral approach
   - Interval: along lateral intercondylar ridge, between triceps and extensor carpi radialis longus (ECRL) (brachioradialis nerve)
   - Dissection: Subperiosteally expose the anterior humerus and lateral column.
   - Risks: retractor placed under brachialis anteriorly to protect radial nerve, distally limited by PIN

H. Arthroscopy: portals for elbow arthroscopy

1. Anterolateral portal (risk for injury to the radial nerve)
2. Anteromedial portal (risk for injury to the medial antebrachial cutaneous and median nerves)
3. Posterolateral portals

I. Cross-sectional anatomy of shoulder and arm (Figure 2-18)

III. FOREARM

A. Osteology: includes the ulna and radius, which articulate with the humerus (principally the ulna) and carpi (principally the radius)

1. Ulna
   - Proximally, the ulna is composed of two curved processes, the olecranon and the coronoid processes, with an intervening trochlear notch.
   - Distally, the ulna tapers and ends in a lateral head and a medial styloid process.
2. Radius
   - Proximally, the radius is composed of a head with a central fovea, neck, and proximal medial radial tuberosity (for insertion of the biceps tendon).
   - It has a gradual bend (convex laterally) and gradually increases in size distally; **restoration of the radial bow (and length) is paramount in the fixation of radial shaft fractures.**
   - Distally, the radius is composed of the carpal articular surface, an ulnar notch, a dorsal tubercle (Lister's tubercle, which is at the level of the scapholunate joint), and a lateral styloid process.

B. Arthrology: proximally includes the elbow joint (discussed earlier) and distally includes the wrist

1. **Distal radioulnar articulation (most stable in supination)**
2. Radiocarpal joint
   - This joint is ellipsoid and involves the distal radius and the scaphoid, lunate, and triquetrum.
   - It is usually located at the level of the crease of the proximal wrist flexion.
   - Covered by a loose capsule, the wrist relies heavily on ligaments, **especially volar ligaments**, for stability.
   - Ligaments about this joint are the volar and dorsal radiocarpal ligaments and the ulnar and radial collateral ligaments.
3. Triangular fibrocartilage complex (Figure 2-19): originates from the most ulnar portion of the radius and extends into the caput ulnae and the wrist aspect of the ulna to the base of the fifth metacarpal; **includes the components listed in Table 2-20**

C. Muscles (Figure 2-20 and Table 2-21): arranged according to both location and function

Table 2-20 Components of the Triangular Fibrocartilage Complex

Component	Origin	Insertion
Dorsal and volar radioulnar ligament	Ulnar radius	Caput ulnae
Articular disc	Radius/ulna	Triquetrum
Prestyloid recess	Disc	Meniscus homolog
Meniscus homolog	Ulna/disc	Triquetrum/ulnar collateral ligament
Ulnar collateral ligament	Ulna	Fifth metacarpal

1. Volar flexors (superficial and deep)
2. Dorsal extensors (superficial and deep): **tennis elbow (lateral epicondylitis) involves primarily the extensor carpi radialis brevis (ECRB)**

D. Nerves

1. Anatomy: nerves of upper arm continue into the forearm (Figure 2-21, Table 2-22)
   - Radial nerve
     - This nerve is anterior to the lateral epicondyle.
     - It runs between the brachialis and brachioradialis and divides into the anterior and deep (PIN) branches.
     - **The PIN splits the supinator and supplies all of the extensor muscles, except the mobile wad (brachioradialis, ECRB, ECRL).**
     - Compression of the PIN can occur at six places (see in the section "Compressive Neuropathies of the Forearm").
     - The superficial branch of the radial nerve passes to the dorsal radial surface of the hand in the distal third of the forearm by passing between the brachioradialis and ECRL.
   - Median nerve
     - This nerve is medial to the brachial artery at the elbow and superficial to the brachialis muscle.
     - In the forearm, the median nerve **splits the two heads of the pronator teres** and then runs between the flexor digitorum superficialis (FDS) and flexor digitorum profundus (FDP).
     - It becomes more superficial at the flexor retinaculum, where it continues into the hand.
     - It has branches to all the superficial flexor muscles of the forearm except the flexor carpi ulnaris (FCU).
     - The anterior interosseous branch, which runs between the flexor pollicis longus (FPL) and FDP, supplies all the deep flexors except the ulnar half of the FDP.
   - Ulnar nerve
     - Enters the forearm **between the two heads of the FCU**, which it supplies
     - Runs between the FCU and FDP, innervating the ulnar half of this muscle
     - Lies more superficial at the wrist and enters the hand through the Guyon canal
   - Cutaneous nerves (see Figure 2-12)
     - Lateral antebrachial cutaneous nerve: the continuation of the musculocutaneous nerve that passes lateral to the cephalic vein after emerging laterally from between the biceps and brachialis at the elbow
     - Medial antebrachial cutaneous nerve: a branch from the medial cord of the brachial plexus

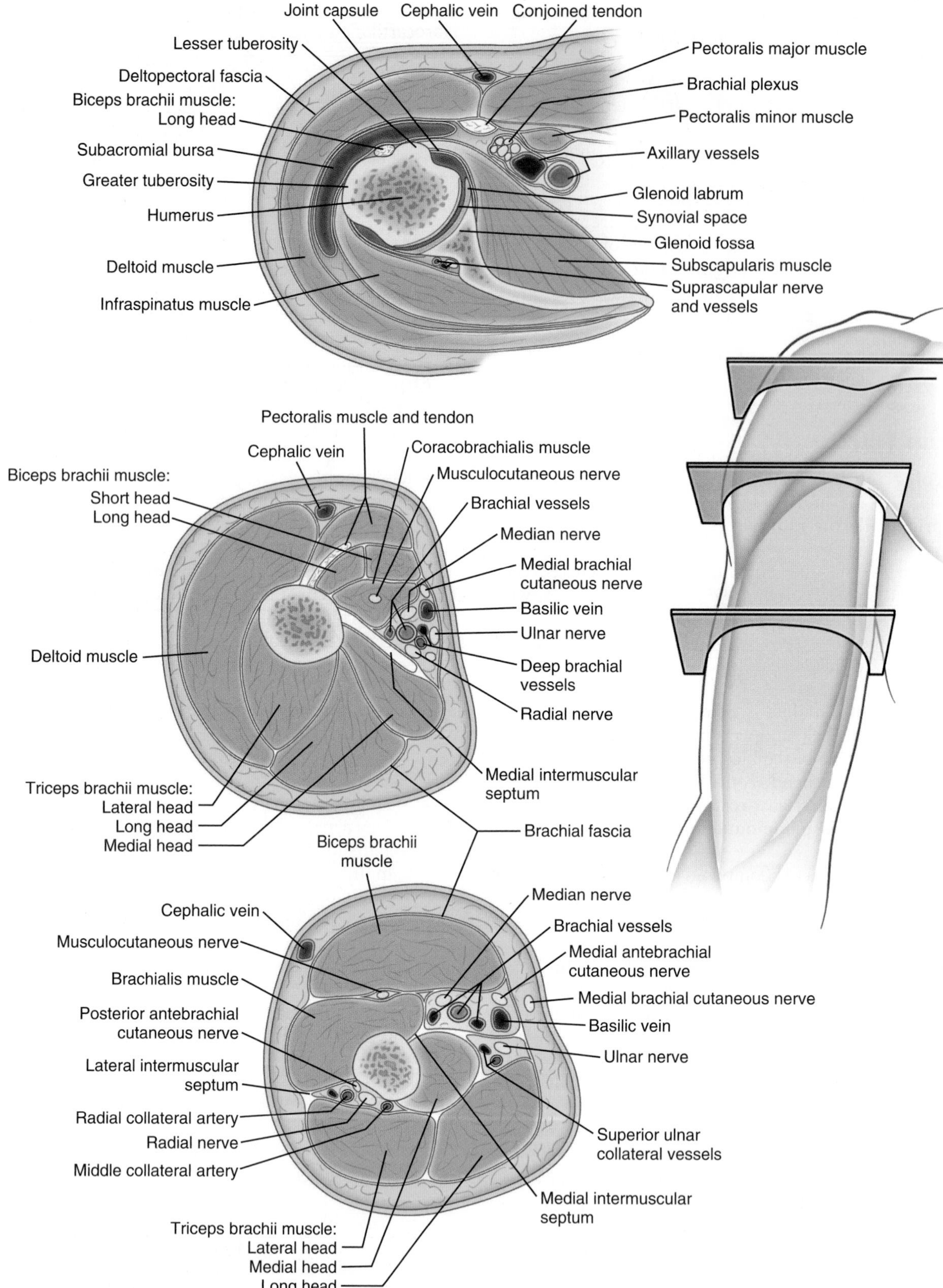

Figure 2-18 Cross-sectional view of the anatomy of the shoulder and arm. (From Miller MD, et al: *Orthopaedic surgical approaches,* Philadelphia, 2008, Saunders, Figure SA-10.)

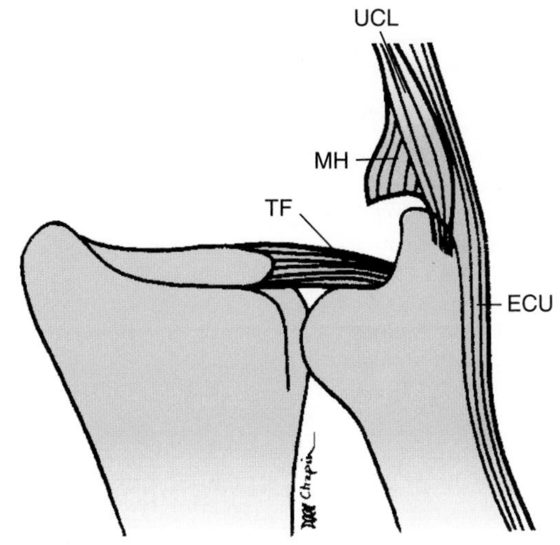

Figure 2-19 Triangular fibrocartilage complex. ECU, extensor carpi ulnaris; MH, meniscal homolog; TF, transverse fibers (radio-ulnar ligament); UCL, ulnar collateral ligament. (From Weissman BN, Sledge CB: *Orthopedic radiology,* Philadelphia, 1986, Saunders, p 115.)

- Posterior antebrachial cutaneous nerve:a branch of the radial nerve given off in the arm

2. Compressive neuropathies of the forearm (see Table 2-17)
   - An example of key testable material on compressive neuropathies would be to determine which muscle is last to return to function after the alleviation of PIN palsy.
   - PIN innervates the supinator, extensor carpi ulnaris, extensor digitorum, extensor digiti minimi, abductor pollicis longus (APL), extensor pollicis longus (EPL), extensor pollicis brevis (EPB), and extensor indicis proprius, in that order.
   - **Last muscle to return to function after PIN compression (extensor indicis proprius) is the most distally innervated muscle.**
3. Innervation of the forearm (Table 2-23)

E. Vessels (see Figure 2-11)

1. Brachial artery
   - Enters cubital fossa (bordered by the two epicondyles, the brachioradialis, and the pronator teres and overlying the brachialis and supinator)

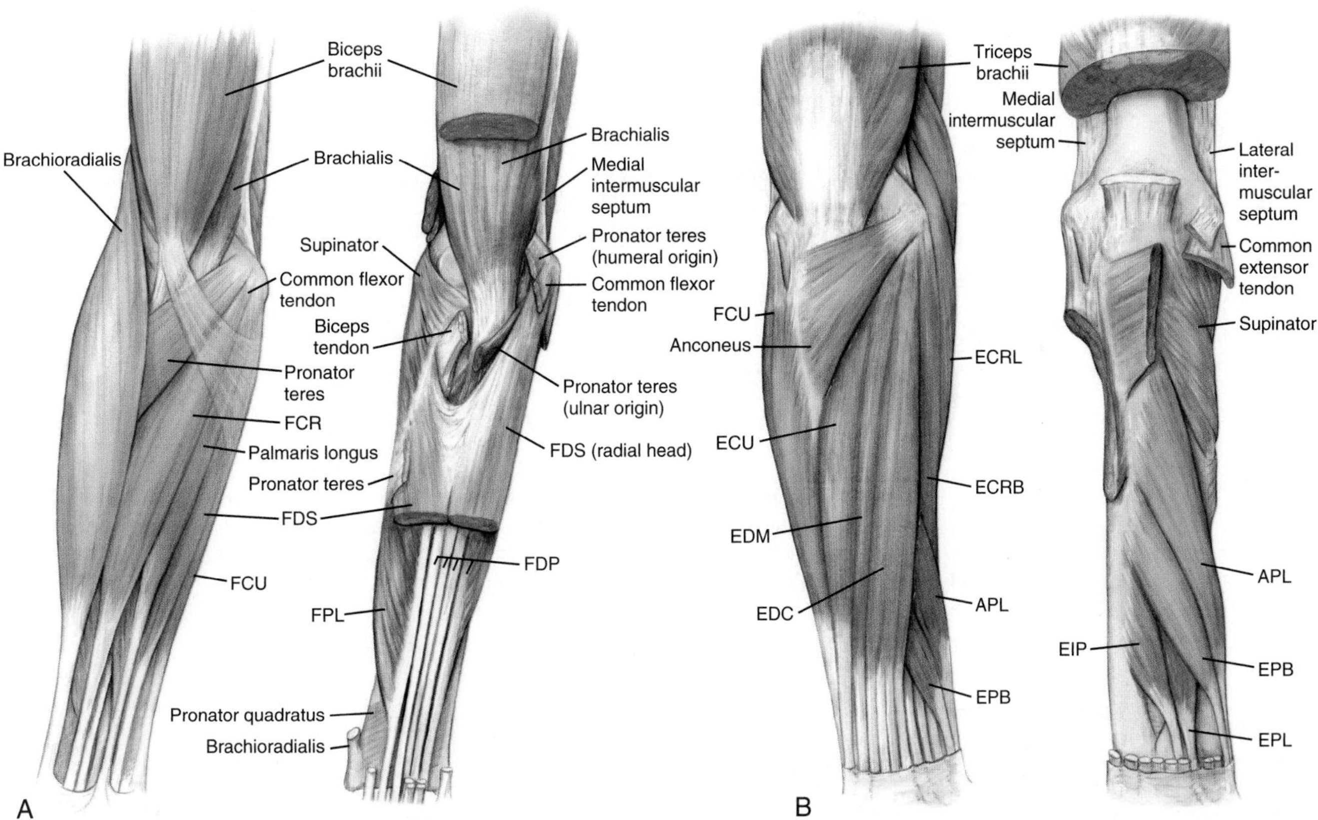

COMMON ABBREVIATIONS	
FCR	Flexor carpi radialis
FCU	Flexor carpi ulnaris
FDP	Flexor digitorum profundus
FDS	Flexor digitorum superficialis
FPL	Flexor pollicis longus

COMMON ABBREVIATIONS			
APL	Abductor pollicis longus	EDM	Extensor digiti minimi
ECRB	Extensor carpi radialis brevis	EIP	Extensor indicis profundus
ECRL	Extensor carpi radialis longus	EPB	Extensor pollicis brevis
ECU	Extensor carpi ulnaris	EPL	Extensor pollicis longus
EDC	Extensor digitorum communis		

Figure 2-20 Muscles of the forearm. **A,** Anterior view. **B,** Posterior view. (From Miller MD, et al: *Orthopaedic surgical approaches,* Philadelphia, 2008, Saunders, Figures EF-4 and EF-5.)

Table 2-21 Muscles of the Forearm

Muscle	Origin	Insertion	Action	Innervation
Superficial Flexors				
Pronator teres	Medial epicondyle and coronoid	Mid-lateral radius	Pronating, flexing forearm	Median nerve
Flexor carpi radialis	Medial epicondyle	Second and third metacarpal bases	Flexing wrist	Median nerve
Palmaris longus	Medial epicondyle	Palmar aponeurosis	Flexing wrist	Median nerve
Flexor carpi ulnaris	Medial epicondyle and posterior ulna	Pisiform	Flexing wrist	Ulnar nerve
Flexor digitorum superficialis	Medial epicondyle, proximal anterior ulna and anterior radius	Base of middle phalanges	Flexing PIP joint	Median nerve
Deep Flexors				
Flexor digitorum profundus	Anterior and medial ulna	Base of distal phalanges	Flexing DIP joint	Median–anterior interosseous/ulnar nerves
Flexor pollicis longus	Anterior and lateral radius	Base of distal phalanges	Flexing IP joint, thumb	Median–anterior interosseous nerve
Pronator quadratus	Distal ulna	Volar radius	Pronating hand	Median–anterior interosseous nerve
Superficial Extensors				
Brachioradialis	Lateral supracondylar humerus	Lateral distal radius	Flexing forearm	Radial nerve
Extensor carpi radialis longus	Lateral supracondylar humerus	Second metacarpal base	Extending wrist	Radial nerve
Extensor carpi radialis brevis	Lateral epicondyle of humerus	Third metacarpal base	Extending wrist	Radial nerve
Anconeus	Lateral epicondyle of humerus	Proximal dorsal ulna	Extending forearm	Radial nerve
Extensor digitorum	Lateral epicondyle of humerus	Extensor aponeurosis	Extending digits	Radial–posterior interosseous nerve
Extensor digiti minimi	Common extensor tendon	Small finger extensor carpi ulnaris	Extending small finger	Radial–posterior interosseous nerve
Extensor carpi ulnaris	Lateral epicondyle of humerus	Fifth metacarpal base	Extending/adducting hand	Radial–posterior interosseous nerve
Deep Extensors				
Supinator	Lateral epicondyle of humerus, ulna	Dorsolateral radius	Supinating forearm	Radial–posterior interosseous nerve
Abductor pollicis longus	Dorsal ulna/radius	First metacarpal base	Abducting/extending thumb	Radial–posterior interosseous nerve
Extensor pollicis brevis	Dorsal radius	Thumb proximal phalanx base	Extending thumb MCP joint	Radial–posterior interosseous nerve
Extensor pollicis longus	Dorsolateral ulna	Thumb dorsal phalanx base	Extending thumb IP joint	Radial–posterior interosseous nerve
Extensor indicis proprius	Dorsolateral ulna	Index finger extensor apparatus (ulnarly)	Extending index finger	Radial–posterior interosseous nerve

DIP, distal interphalangeal joint; IP, interphalangeal joint; PIP, proximal interphalangeal joint; MCP, metacarpophalangeal joint.

Table 2-22 Neuroanatomic Relationships in the Forearm

Nerve	Relationships
Radial	Between brachialis and brachioradialis
Posterior interosseous	Splits supinator
Superficial radial	Between brachioradialis and extensor carpi radialis longus
Median	Medial to brachial artery at elbow
Anterior interosseous	Splits pronator teres and runs between flexor digitorum superficialis and flexor digitorum profundus Between flexor pollicis longus and flexor digitorum profundus
Ulnar	Between flexor carpi ulnaris and flexor digitorum profundus

- Then divides at the level of the radial neck into the radial and ulnar arteries (Table 2-24)

2. Radial artery
   - This artery initially runs on the pronator teres, deep to the brachioradialis.
   - It continues to the wrist between this muscle and the flexor carpi radialis (FCR).
   - Forearm branches include the recurrent radial (see earlier discussion) and muscular branches.
3. Ulnar artery: larger of the two branches
   - This artery is covered by the superficial flexors proximally (between the FDS and FDP).
   - Distally, the artery lies on the FDP, between the tendons of the FCU and FDS.

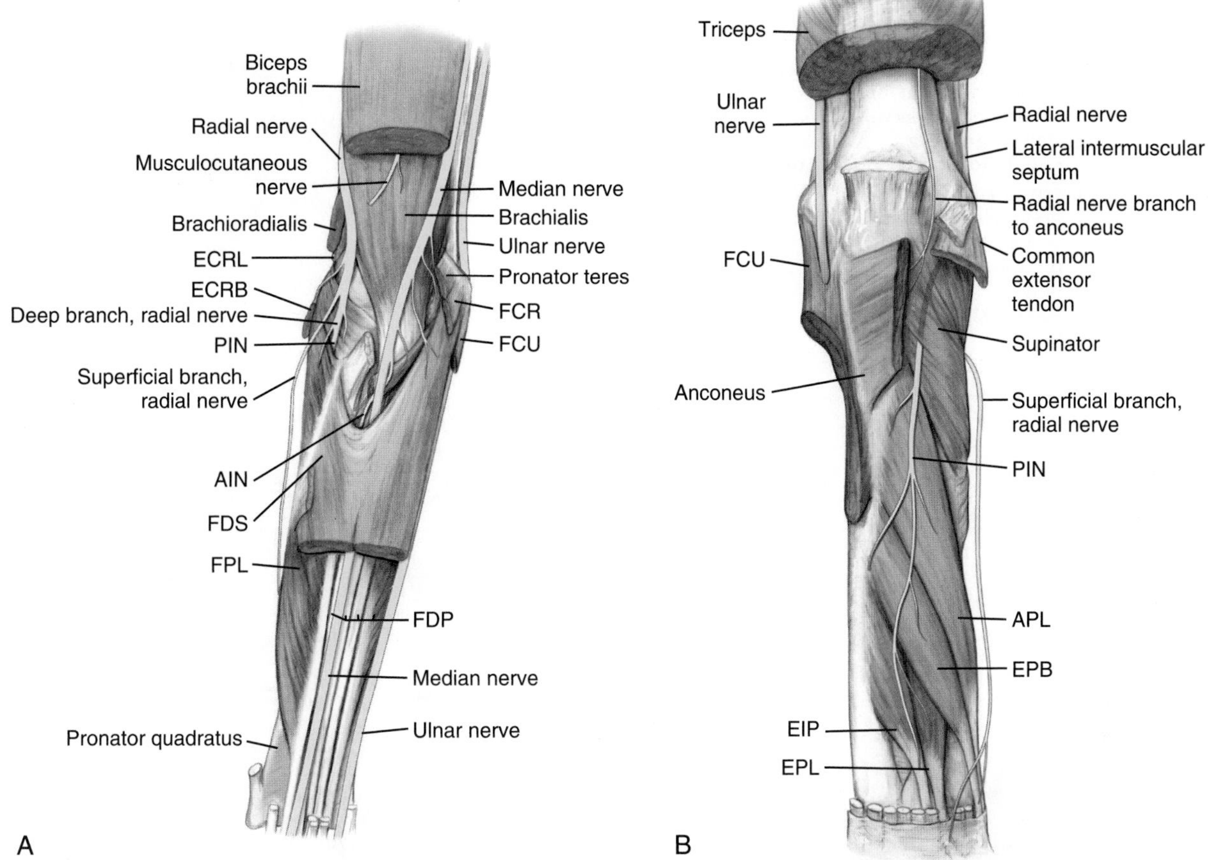

Figure 2-21 Nerves of the forearm. **A,** Anterior view. **B,** Posterior view. APL, abductor pollicis longus; ECRB, extensor carpi radialis brevis; ECRL, extensor carpi radialis longus; EIP, extensor indicis proprius; EPB, extensor pollicis brevis; EPL, extensor pollicis longus; FCR, flexor carpi radialis; FCU, flexor carpi ulnaris; FDP, flexor digitorum profundus; FDS, flexor digitorum superficialis; FPL, flexor pollicis longus. (From Miller MD, et al: *Orthopaedic surgical approaches,* Philadelphia, 2008, Saunders, Figures EF-6 and EF-7.)

Table 2-23 Innervation of the Forearm

Nerves	Muscles Innervated
Radial Nerve	
Radial (posterior cord)	Triceps, brachioradialis, extensor carpi radialis longus, extensor carpi radialis brevis
Posterior interosseous	Supinator, extensor carpi ulnaris, extensor digitorum, extensor digiti minimi, abductor pollicis longus, extensor pollicis longus, extensor pollicis brevis, extensor indicis proprius
Median Nerve	
Median (medial and lateral cord)	Pronator teres, flexor carpi radialis, palmaris longus, flexor digitorum superficialis, abductor pollicis brevis, superficial head of flexor pollicis brevis, opponens pollicis, first and second lumbrical muscles
Anterior interosseous	Flexor digitorum profundus (first and second), flexor pollicis longus, pronator quadratus
Ulnar Nerve	
Ulnar (medial cord)	Flexor carpi ulnaris, flexor digitorum profundus (third and fourth), pollicis brevis, abductor digiti minimi, opponens digiti minimi, flexor digiti minimi, third and fourth lumbrical muscles, interossei, adductor pollicis, deep head of flexor pollicis brevis

- **Forearm branches include the anterior and posterior recurrent ulnar (discussed earlier), the common interosseous (with anterior and posterior branches), and several muscular and nutrient arteries.**

F. **Surgical approaches to the forearm (Table 2-25)**

1. Anterior (Henry's) approach (Figure 2-22)
   - Interval: between the brachioradialis (radial nerve) and pronator teres or FCR distally (median nerve)
   - Dissection:
     - Proximally: Isolate and ligate the leash of Henry (radial artery branches) proximally, and strip the supinator from its insertion subperiosteally; **supination of the forearm displaces the PIN ulnarly.**

Table 2-24 Vascular Anatomic Relationships in the Forearm

Artery	Relationships
Radial	On pronator teres deep to brachioradialis Enters wrist between brachioradialis and flexor carpi radialis
Ulnar	Proximally between FDS and FDP Distally on FDP between flexor carpi ulnaris and FDS

FDP, flexor digitorum profundus; FDS, flexor digitorum superficialis.

Table 2-25 Surgical Approaches to the Forearm

Approach	Interval	Structures at Risk
Anterior (Henry's)	Brachioradialis (radial nerve) and pronator teres (median nerve) Distally: flexor carpi radialis (median nerve)	Ligate leash of Henry (radial artery branches) Superficial branch of radial nerve
Dorsal posterior (Thompson's)	Extensor carpi radialis brevis (radial nerve) and extensor digitorum communis (PIN) Distally: extensor pollicis longus	PIN: avoid excessive retraction of supinator
Ulnar	Extensor carpi ulnaris (PIN) and flexor carpi ulnaris (ulnar nerve)	

PIN, posterior interosseous nerve.

- Middle third: Pronate the forearm and incise the insertion of the pronator teres subperiosteally.
- Distally: Dissect off the FPL and pronator quadratus.

- Risks:
  - The superficial branch of the radial nerve must be protected (retract laterally) with the brachioradialis.

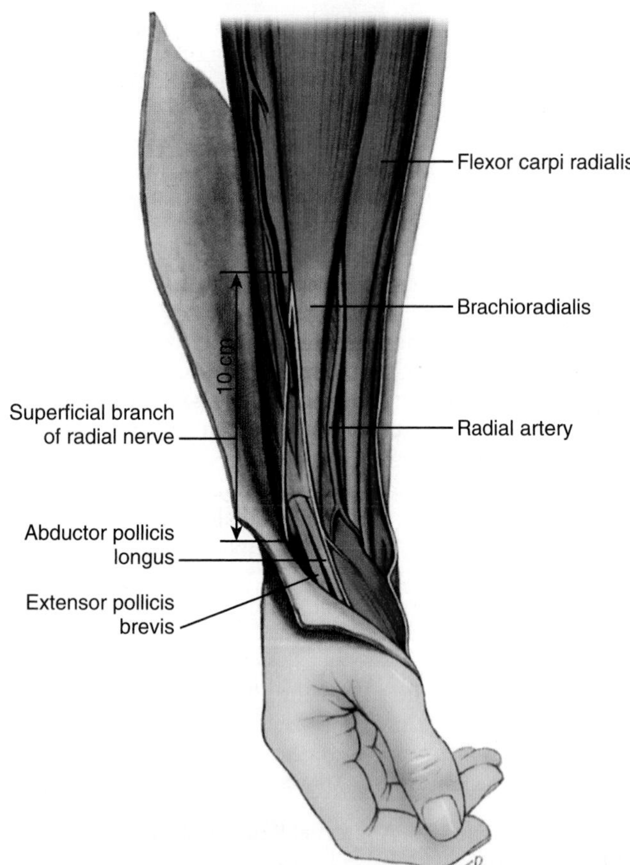

Figure 2-22 Anterior (Henry's) surgical approach to the forearm. In this approach, the interval between the brachioradialis (radial nerve) and the pronator teres or flexor carpi radialis (median nerve) is explored. Protect the superficial radial nerve, which lies underneath the brachioradialis. (Modified from Kaplan EB: *Surgical approaches to the neck, cervical spine, and upper extremity,* Philadelphia, 1966, Saunders, p 92.)

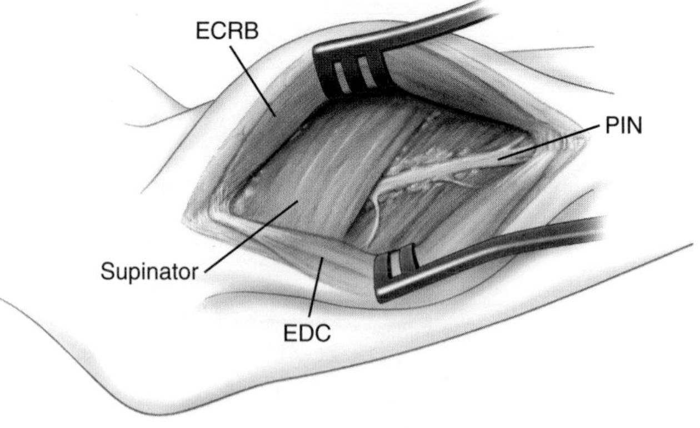

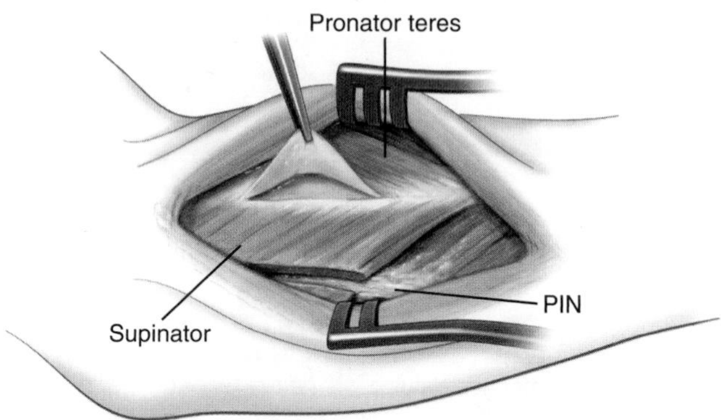

Figure 2-23 Dorsal (posterior; Thompson's) approach to the forearm. In this approach, the interval between the extensor carpi radialis brevis (radial nerve) and the extensor digitorum communis (posterior interosseous nerve [PIN]) is explored. ECRB, extensor carpi radialis brevis; EDC, extensor digitorum communis. (From Miller MD, et al: *Orthopaedic surgical approaches,* Philadelphia, 2008, Saunders, Figures EF-65 and EF-68.)

  - The radial artery is at risk for injury proximally because it courses medial to the biceps tendon and distally with retraction of the brachioradialis.
  - The PIN can be injured during deep dissection of proximal exposure.

2. Dorsal (posterior; Thompson's) approach (Figure 2-23)
   - Interval: between the ECRB (radial nerve) and extensor digitorum or EPL distally (PIN)
   - Dissection:
     - Identify the PIN as it exits the supinator before the forearm is supinated, and reflect the supinator off the anterior surface of the proximal radius.
     - Distally, retract the APL and EPB to gain access to the middle and distal portions of the radius.
   - Risks: The PIN must be identified and protected.
3. Exposure of the ulna
   - Interval: between the extensor carpi ulnaris (PIN) and the FCU (ulnar nerve)
   - Dissection: Strip muscles from the ulna subperiosteally.
   - Risks: FCU stripped subperiosteally to protect ulnar nerve and artery

G. Cross-sectional diagrams of proximal forearm (Figure 2-24), mid-forearm (Figure 2-25), and distal forearm (Figure 2-26)

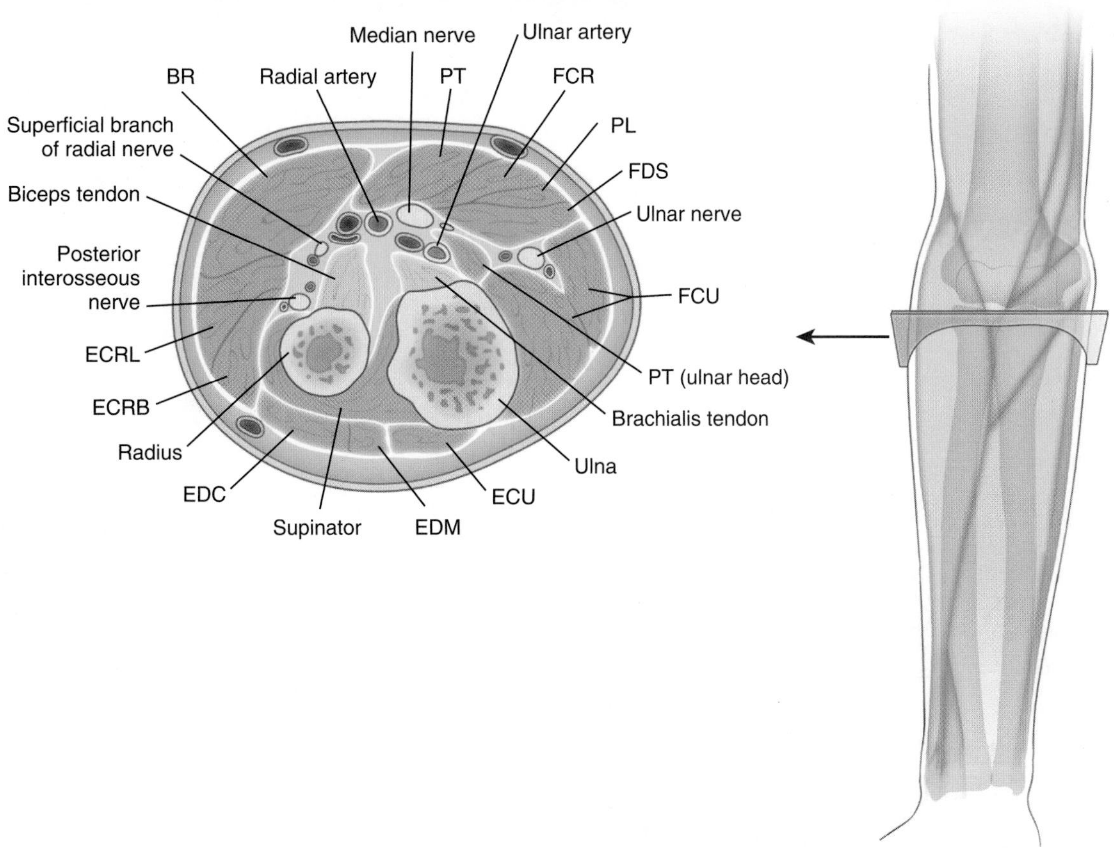

Figure 2-24 Cross-sectional view of the proximal forearm. BR, brachioradialis; ECRB, extensor carpi radialis brevis; ECRL, extensor carpi radialis longus; ECU, extensor carpi ulnaris; EDC, extensor digitorum communis; EDM, extensor digiti minimi; FCR, flexor carpi radialis; FCU, flexor carpi ulnaris; FDS, flexor digitorum superficialis; PL, palmaris longus; PT, pronator teres. (From Miller MD, et al: *Orthopaedic surgical approaches,* Philadelphia, 2008, Saunders, Figure EF-13.)

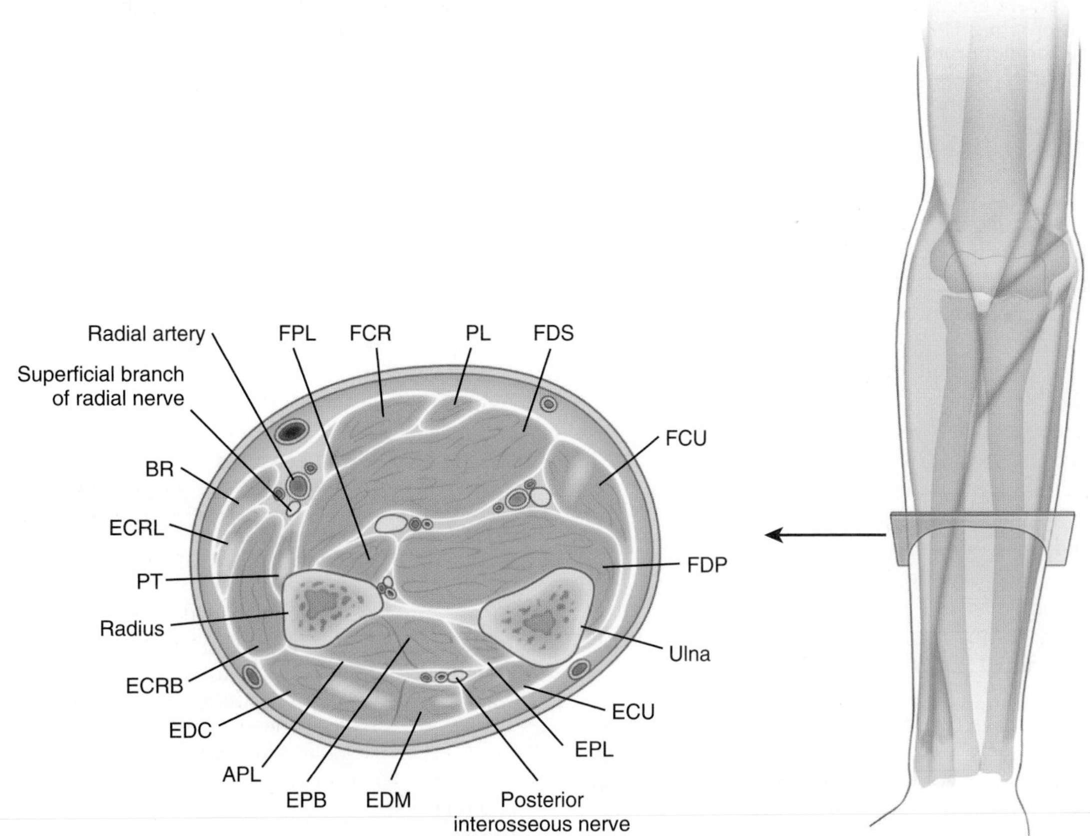

Figure 2-25 Cross-sectional view of the mid-forearm. APL, abductor pollicis longus; BR, brachioradialis; ECRB, extensor carpi radialis brevis; ECRL, extensor carpi radialis longus; ECU, extensor carpi ulnaris; EDC, extensor digitorum communis; EDM, extensor digiti minimi; EPB, extensor pollicis brevis; EPL, extensor pollicis longus; FCR, flexor carpi radialis; FCU, flexor carpi ulnaris; FDP, flexor digitorum profundus; FDS, flexor digitorum superficialis; FPL, flexor pollicis longus; PL, palmaris longus; PT, pronator teres. (From Miller MD, et al: *Orthopaedic surgical approaches,* Philadelphia, 2008, Saunders, Figure EF-13.)

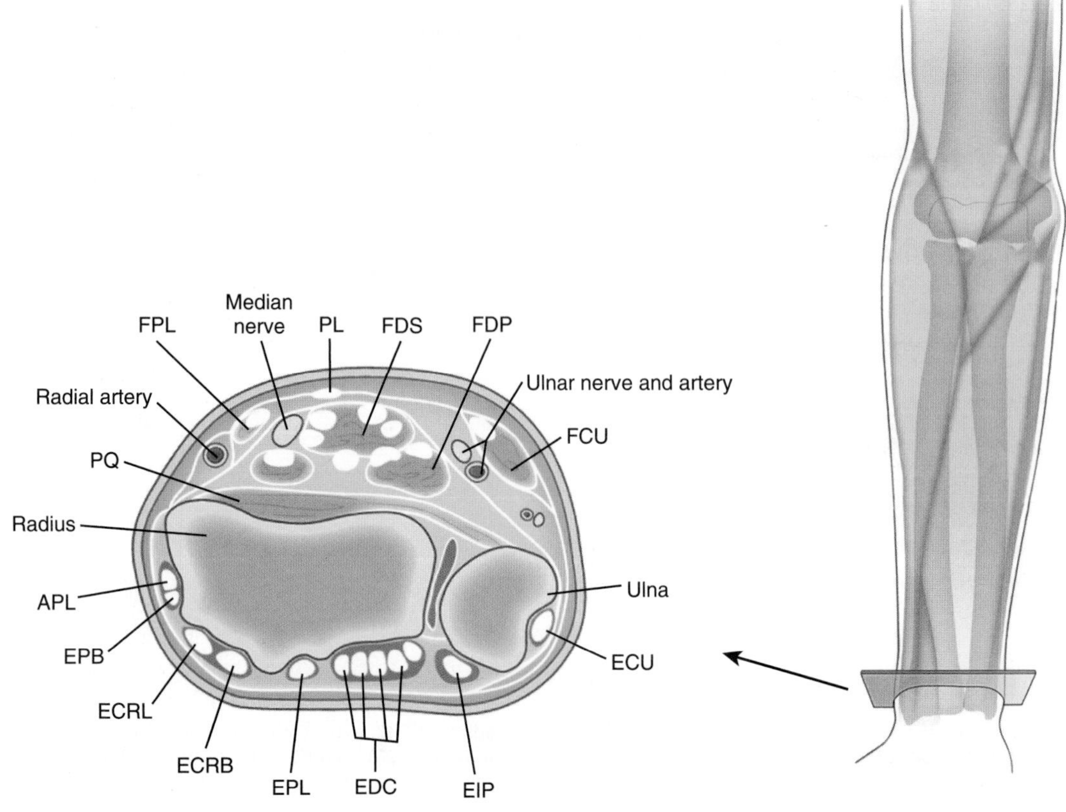

Figure 2-26 Cross-sectional view of the distal forearm proximal to the distal radioulnar joint. APL, abductor pollicis longus; ECRB, extensor carpi radialis brevis; ECRL, extensor carpi radialis longus; ECU, extensor carpi ulnaris; EDC, extensor digitorum communis; EIP, extensor indicis proprius; EPB, extensor pollicis brevis; EPL, extensor pollicis longus; FCU, flexor carpi ulnaris; FDP, flexor digitorum profundus; FDS, flexor digitorum superficialis; FPL, flexor pollicis longus; PL, palmaris longus; PQ, pronator quadratus. (From Miller MD, et al: *Orthopaedic surgical approaches,* Philadelphia, 2008, Saunders, Figure EF-13.)

IV. WRIST AND HAND*

A. Osteology

1. Carpal bones
   - Ossification begins at the capitate (usually present at 1 year of age) and proceeds in a counterclockwise direction, according to posteroanterior radiographs of the right hand.
   - Hamate is the second carpus to ossify (by ages 1 to 2 years).
   - Triquetrum (by age 3 years)
   - Lunate (by ages 4 to 5 years)
   - Scaphoid (by age 5 years)
   - Trapezium (by age 6 years)
   - Trapezoid (by age 7 years)
   - Pisiform, which is a large sesamoid bone, is the last to ossify (by age 9 years).
   - Several key features are important to recognize in the individual carpal bones (Table 2-26).
2. Metacarpals
   - These bones have two ossification centers:
     - One for the body (primary center of ossification), which ossifies at 8 weeks of gestation (like most long bones)
     - One at the neck, which usually appears before 3 years of age
   - First metacarpal is a primordial phalanx, and its secondary ossification center is located at the base (like those of the phalanges).
   - Several characteristics allow the identification of the individual metacarpals (Table 2-27).

Table 2-26 Carpal Features

Carpal Bone	Distinctive Features	Number of Articulations
Scaphoid	Tubercle (TCL, APB), distal vascular supply	5
Lunate	Half-moon–shaped	5
Triquetrum	Pyramid-shaped	3
Pisiform	Spheroidal (TCL, FCU)	1
Trapezium	FCR groove, tubercle (opponens, APB, flexor pollicis brevis, TCL)	4
Trapezoid	Wedge-shaped	4
Capitate	Largest bone, central location	7
Hamate	Hook (TCL)	5

APB, abductor pollicis brevis; FCR, flexor carpi radialis; FCU, flexor carpi ulnaris; TCL, transverse carpal ligament.

*See Chapter 7, Hand and Upper Extremity.

Table 2-27 Metacarpal Features

Metacarpal	Distinctive Features
I (Thumb)	Short, stout; base is saddle-shaped
II (Index)	Longest, largest base; medial at base
III (Middle)	Styloid process
IV (Ring)	Small quadrilateral base, narrow shaft
V (Small)	Tubercle at base (extensor carpi ulnaris)

3. Phalanges
   - Each hand has 14 phalanges (three for each finger and two for the thumb), which are similar.
   - All have secondary ossification centers at their bases that appear at ages 3 years (proximal), 4 years (middle), and 5 years (distal).
   - Bases of the proximal phalanges are oval and concave, with the smaller heads ending in two condyles.
   - Middle phalanges have two concave facets at their bases and pulley-shaped heads.
   - Distal phalanges are smaller and have palmar ungual tuberosities distally.

B. **Arthrology**

1. Radiocarpal (wrist) joint
   - The wrist is an ellipsoid joint and made up of the distal radius, scaphoid, lunate, triquetrum, and ligamentous structures (Table 2-28).
   - **The palmar/volar radiocarpal ligament is the strongest supporting structure, although it has a weak area on the radial side (the space of Poirier) that lends less support to the scaphoid, lunate, and trapezoid** (Figure 2-27).
2. Intercarpal joints
   - Proximal row
     - Scaphoid, lunate, and triquetrum form gliding joints.
     - Two dorsal intercarpal ligaments connect the scaphoid and lunate and the lunate and triquetral bones.
     - Two palmar intercarpal ligaments connect the scaphoid and lunate and the lunate and triquetral bones.
     - **Dorsal intercarpal ligaments are stronger.**
     - Interosseous ligaments are narrow bundles connecting the scaphoid and lunate and the lunate and triquetral bones.
   - Pisiform articulation
     - The pisotriquetral joint has a thin articular capsule.
     - The ulnar collateral and palmar radiocarpal ligaments also connect the pisiform proximally.
     - The pisohamate ligament and pisometacarpal ligaments help extend the pull of the FCU.
   - Distal row
     - This row includes trapezium, trapezoid, capitate, and hamate gliding joints.
     - Dorsal intercarpal ligaments connect the trapezium with the trapezoid, the trapezoid with the capitate, and the capitate with the hamate.
     - Palmar ligaments do the same.
     - Interosseous ligaments are much thicker in the distal row, connecting the capitate and hamate (strongest), the capitate and trapezoid, and the trapezium and trapezoid (weakest).
   - Midcarpal joint
     - Transverse articulations between the proximal and distal rows are reinforced by palmar and dorsal intercarpal ligaments and carpal collateral ligaments.
     - The radial ligament is stronger.

Table 2-28 Radiocarpal Wrist Ligaments

Structure	Attachments	Distinctive Features
Articular capsule	Surrounds joint	Reinforced by volar and dorsal radiocarpal ligament
Volar (radiocarpal ligament)	Radius, ulna, scaphoid, lunate, triquetrum, capitate	Oblique ulnar, strong
Dorsal radiocarpal ligament	Radius, scaphoid, lunate, triquetrum	Oblique radial, weak
Ulnar collateral ligament	Ulna, triquetrum, pisiform, transverse carpal ligament	Fan-shaped, two fascicles
Radial collateral ligament	Radius, scaphoid, trapezium, transverse carpal ligament	Radial artery adjacent

3. Carpometacarpal (CMC) joints
   - Thumb CMC joint
     - Highly mobile saddle-shaped joint
     - Supported by a capsule and radial, palmar, and dorsal CMC ligaments
   - Finger CMC joints
     - Gliding joints with capsules, dorsal CMC ligaments (strongest), palmar CMC ligaments, and interosseous CMC ligaments
4. Metacarpophalangeal joints
   - Ellipsoid and covered by palmar (volar plate), collateral, and deep transverse metacarpal ligaments
5. Interphalangeal joints
   - Hinge joints, with capsules and obliquely oriented collateral ligaments
6. Other important structures
   - Extensor retinaculum
     - This structure covers the dorsum of the wrist and contains six synovial sheaths (Figure 2-28).
     - Orientation of the extensor tendons at the wrist is a key testable item (Table 2-29).
     - The first dorsal compartment contains the APL and the EPB.
     - The EPB tendon is ulnar to the APL tendon **(the APL frequently has multiple tendon slips, which should be addressed during release for de Quervain's tenosynovitis).**
     - In the second dorsal compartment, the ECRL tendon is radial to the ECRB tendon. **Thus, the EPL tendon is ulnar to the ECRB tendon at the wrist level.**
     - The anatomic snuffbox is bordered by tendons of the first and third dorsal wrist compartments; the EPB tendon serves as the radial snuffbox border, and the EPL tendon serves as the ulnar border.
     - **The posterior interosseous nerve is contained within the floor of the fourth dorsal wrist compartment.**

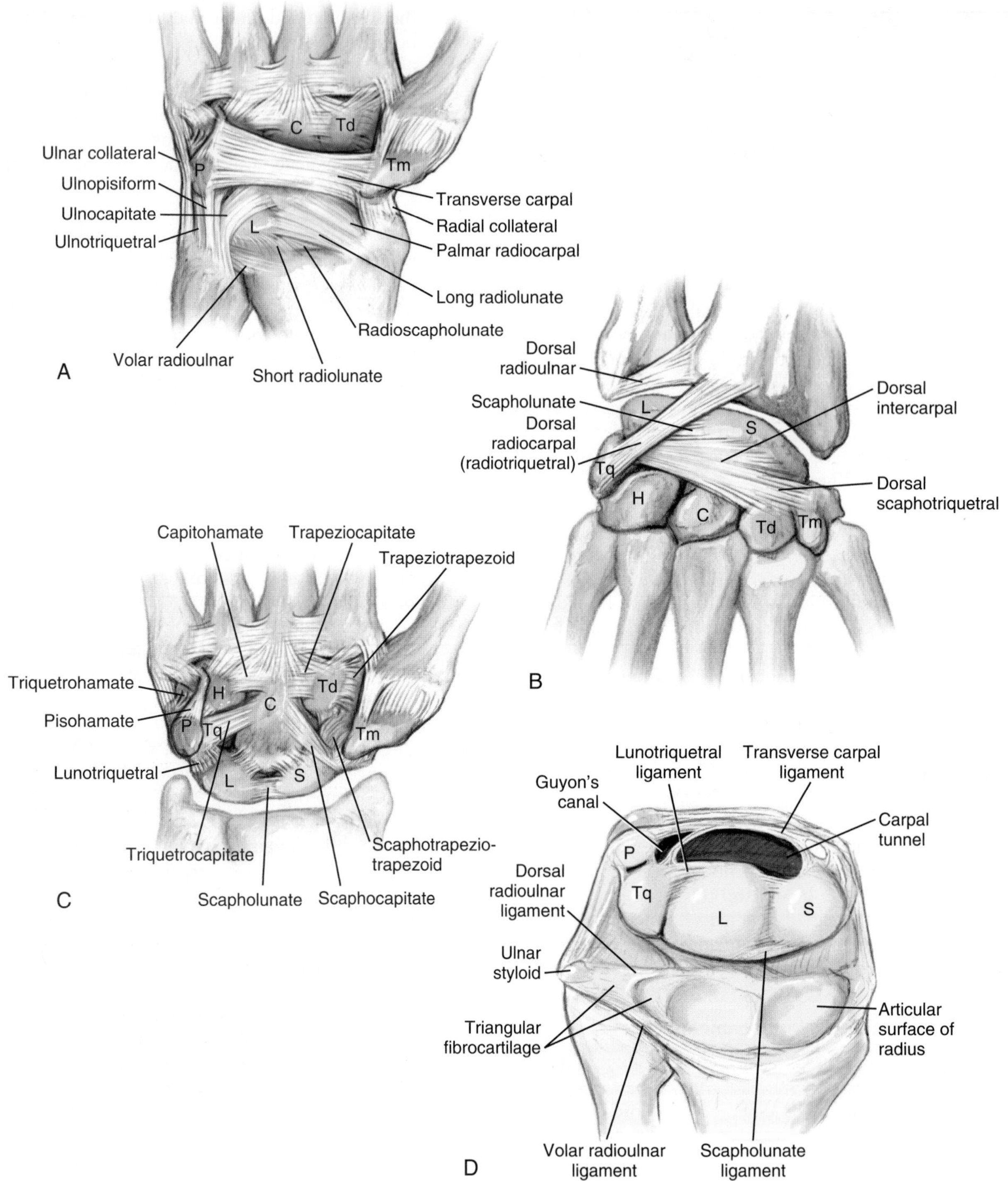

Figure 2-27 Hand and wrist ligaments. **A,** Volar ligaments (radioulnar, radiocarpal, ulnocarpal, and transverse carpal). **B,** Dorsal ligaments. **C,** Volar ligaments (short intercarpal). **D,** Joint opened volarly and hyperextended. C, capitate; H, hamate; L, lunate; P, pisiform; S, scaphoid; Td, trapezoid; Tm, trapezium; Tq, triquetrum. (From Miller MD, et al: *Orthopaedic surgical approaches,* Philadelphia, 2008, Saunders, Figure HW-2.)

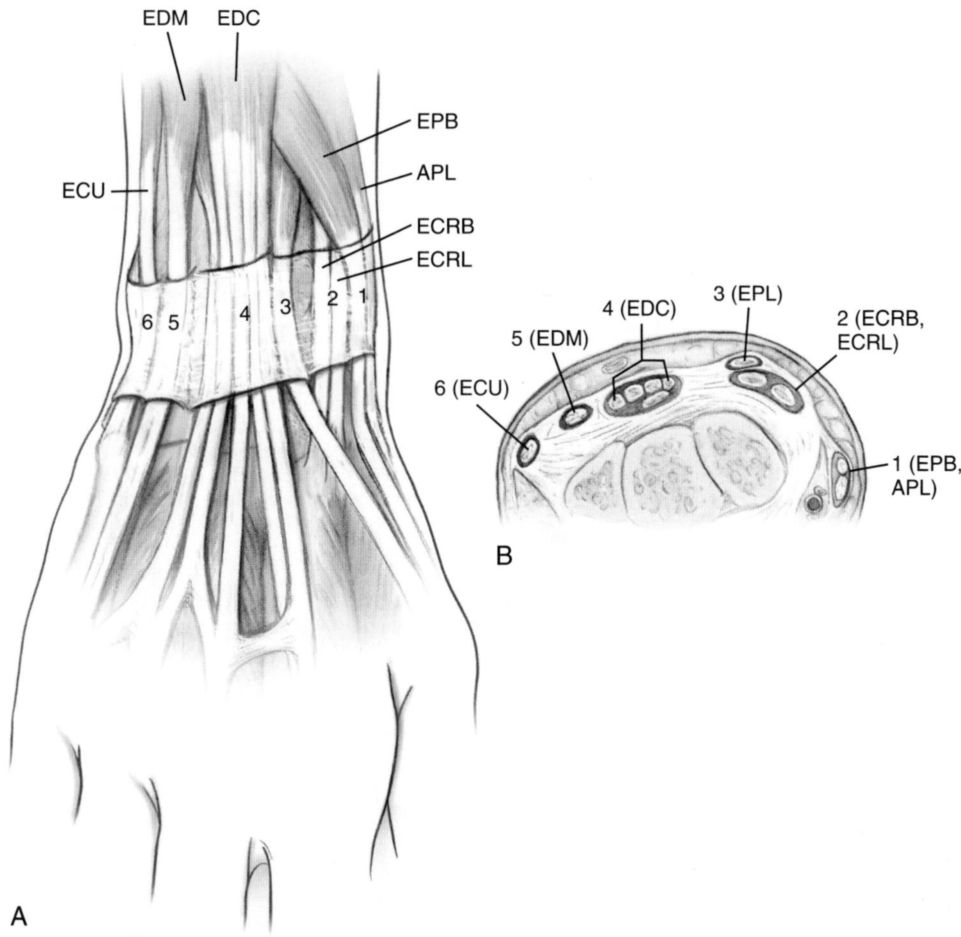

Figure 2-28 Extensor compartments of the wrist (1 to 6). See Table 2-29. APL, abductor pollicis longus; ECRB, extensor carpi radialis brevis; ECRL, extensor carpi radialis longus; ECU, extensor carpi ulnaris; EDC, extensor digitorum communis; EDM, extensor digiti minimi; EPB, extensor pollicis brevis; EPL, extensor pollicis longus. (Modified from Miller MD, et al: *Orthopaedic surgical approaches,* Philadelphia, 2008, Saunders, Figure HW-6.)

Table 2-29 Dorsal Wrist Compartments

Compartment	Contents	Pathologic Condition
I	Abductor pollicis longus, extensor pollicis brevis	De Quervain's tenosynovitis
II	Extensor carpi radialis longus, brevis	Extensor tendinitis (intersection syndrome)
III	Extensor pollicis longus	Rupture at Lister's tubercle (after wrist fractures) Drummer's tendinitis of the wrist
IV	Extensor digitorum communis, extensor indicis proprius	Extensor tenosynovitis
V	Extensor digiti minimi	Rupture (rheumatoid arthritis: Vaughn-Jackson syndrome)
VI	Extensor carpi ulnaris	Snapping at ulnar styloid

- Transverse carpal ligament (TCL)
  - This is one component of the flexor retinaculum, which serves as the roof of the carpal tunnel (Figure 2-29).
  - It is attached medially to the pisiform and the hook of the hamate and laterally to the tuberosity of the scaphoid and the ridge of the trapezium.
  - Carpal tunnel decreases in volume with wrist flexion.
  - **This tunnel contains the median nerve and nine tendons (one FPL, four FDS, and four FDP).**
  - In the tunnel, the FDS tendons of the middle and ring fingers are volar to the tendons of the index and small fingers.
  - The flexor retinaculum also forms the floor of Guyon's canal, which is bordered as well by the hook of the hamate and the pisiform and is covered by the volar carpal ligament; the ulnar nerve can become entrapped in this canal (Figure 2-30).
- Triangular fibrocartilage complex
  - This complex is formed by the triangular fibrocartilage, ulnocarpal ligaments (volar ulnolunate and ulnotriquetral ligaments), and a meniscal homolog.
  - Injury to this structure is a common cause of ulnar wrist pain (see Figure 2-19).
- Intrinsic apparatus (Table 2-30)

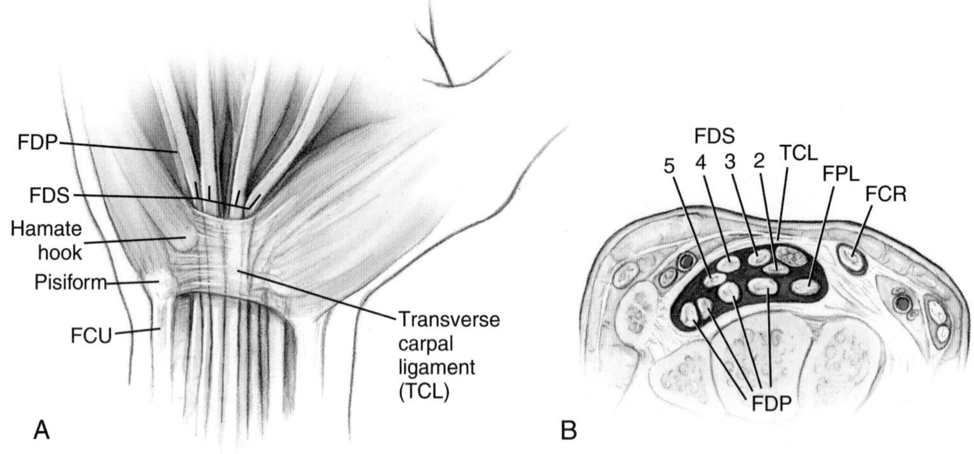

Figure 2-29 Components of the carpal tunnel. **A,** Palmar view. **B,** Cross-sectional view. The roof of the carpal tunnel is the flexor retinaculum, which is composed of the deep forearm fascia, the transverse carpal ligament (TCL), and the distal aponeurosis between the thenar and hypothenar muscles. The carpal tunnel contains the median nerve and nine tendons: one flexor pollicis longus (FPL) and four each of flexor digitorum superficialis (FDS) and flexor digitorum profundus (FDP) tendons. The FPL is dorsal to the flexor carpi radialis and is the most radial tendon within the carpal tunnel. The FPL is volar to the flexor carpi radialis, which is the most dorsal radial tendon passing under the flexor retinaculum. FCU, flexor carpi ulnaris. (From Miller MD, et al: *Orthopaedic surgical approaches,* Philadelphia, 2008, Saunders, Figure HW-6.)

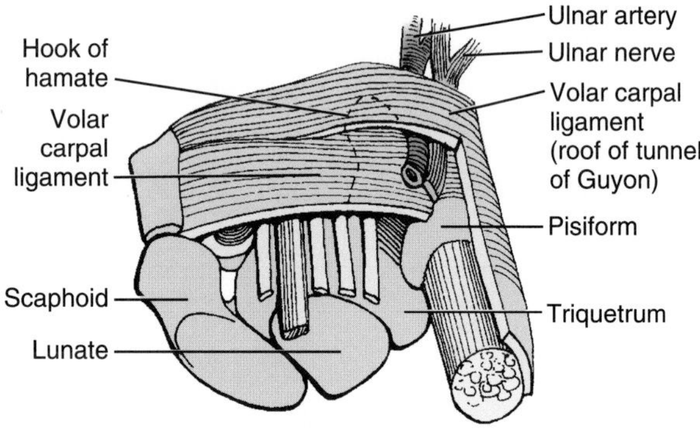

Figure 2-30 The carpal tunnel is formed by the transverse carpal ligament on the volar side and the carpal bones on the floor and sides. Guyon's canal is formed by the volar carpal ligament (roof), the hamate (lateral wall), and the pisiform (medial wall). (From DeLee JC, Drez D Jr: *Orthopaedic sports medicine: principles and practice,* vol 1, Philadelphia, 1994, Saunders, p 932.)

Table 2-30 Intrinsic Apparatus

Structure	Attachments	Significance
Sagittal bands	Covers MCP joint	Allows MCP extension
Transverse (sagittal)	Volar plate fibers	Allows MCP flexion (interossei)
Lateral bands	Covers PIP joint	Allows PIP extension (lumbrical muscles)
Oblique retinacular ligament (Landsmeer)	A4 pulley, terminal tendon	Allows DIP extension (passive)

A4, annular 4; DIP, distal interphalangeal; MCP, metacarpophalangeal; PIP, proximal interphalangeal.

Table 2-31 Muscles of the Hand and Wrist

Muscle	Origin	Insertion	Action	Innervation
Thenar Muscles				
Abductor pollicis brevis	Scaphoid, trapezoid	Base of proximal phalanx, radial side	Abducting thumb	Median nerve
Opponens pollicis	Trapezium	Thumb metacarpal	Abducting, flexing, rotating (medially)	Median nerve
Flexor pollicis brevis	Trapezium, capitate	Base of proximal phalanx, radial side	Flexing MCP joint	Median, ulnar nerves
Adductor pollicis	Capitate, second and third metacarpals	Base of proximal phalanx, ulnar side	Adducting thumb	Ulnar nerve
Hypothenar Muscles				
Palmaris brevis	TCL, palmar aponeurosis	Ulnar palm	Retracting skin	Ulnar nerve
Abductor digiti minimi	Pisiform	Base of proximal phalanx, ulnar side	Abducting small finger	Ulnar nerve
Flexor digiti minimi brevis	Hamate, TCL	Base of proximal phalanx, ulnar side	Flexing MCP joint	Ulnar nerve
Opponens digiti minimi	Hamate, TCL	Small-finger metacarpal	Abducting, flexing, rotating (laterally)	Ulnar nerve
Intrinsic Muscles				
Lumbrical	Flexor digitorum profundus	Lateral bands (radial)	Extending proximal interphalangeal joint	Median, ulnar nerves
Dorsal interosseous	Adjacent metacarpals	Proximal phalanx base/ extensor apparatus	Abducting, flexing MCP joint	Ulnar nerve
Volar interosseous	Adjacent metacarpals	Proximal phalanx base/ extensor apparatus	Adducting, flexing MCP joint	Ulnar nerve

MCP, metacarpophalangeal; TCL, transverse carpal ligament.

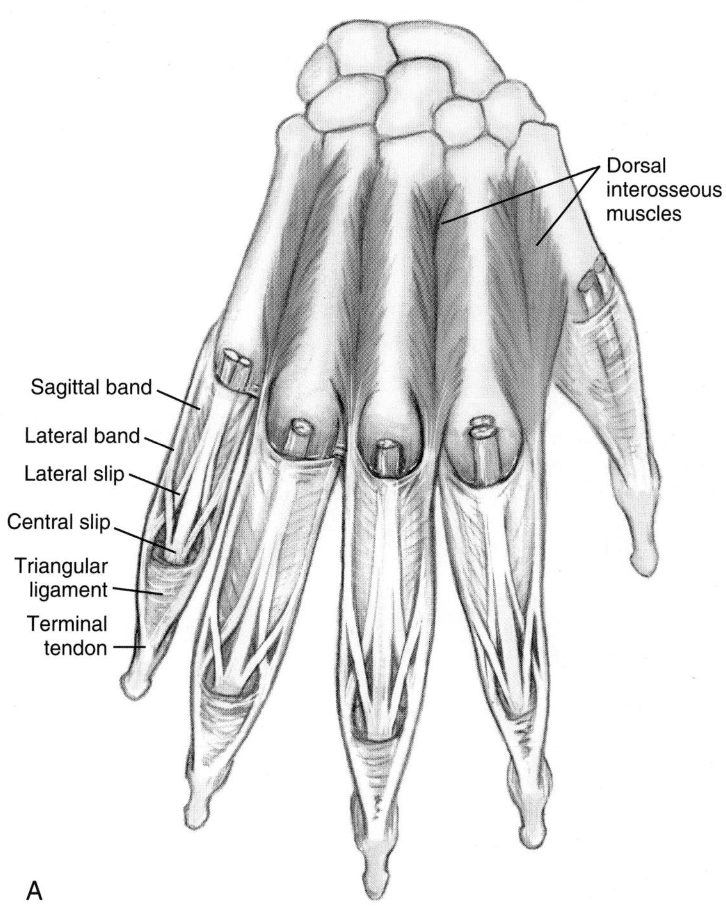

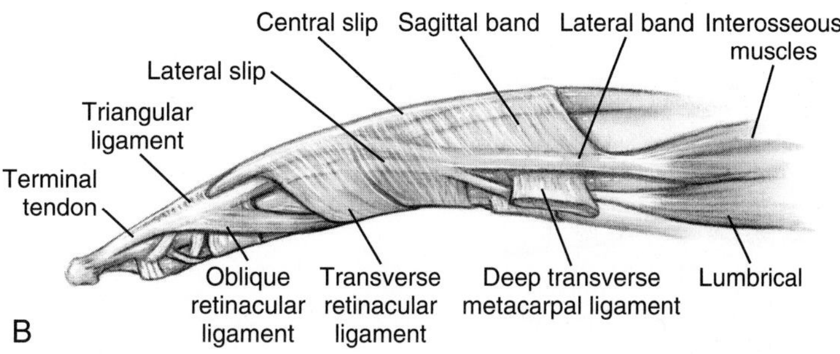

Figure 2-31 Dorsal extensor apparatus. **A,** Dorsal view. **B,** Lateral view. (From Miller MD, et al: *Orthopaedic surgical approaches,* Philadelphia, 2008, Saunders, Figure HW-4.)

- Complex arrangement of structures that surround the digits (Figure 2-31)
- Flexor sheath (Figure 2-32)
  - This covers the flexor tendons in the finger, protecting and nourishing the tendons (vincula).
  - It forms five annular pulleys (A1 to A5) with three intervening cruciate attachments (C1 to C3).
  - **A2 and A4 pulleys originate from bone, whereas A1, A3, and A5 pulleys originate from the palmar plates of the metacarpal, proximal interphalangeal, and distal interphalangeal joints.**
  - **The A2 pulley, overlying the proximal phalanx, is the most critical to function, followed by A4, which covers the middle phalanx.**
  - The A1 pulley is involved in trigger digits.

C. Muscles (Table 2-31); origins and insertions (Figure 2-33)

D. Nerves (Figure 2-34)

1. Anatomy
   - Median nerve
     - This nerve enters the wrist just under the TCL, between the FDS and FCR.
     - The palmar cutaneous branch, which arises proximal to the TCL between the palmaris longus and FCR, innervates the thenar skin.
     - The deep (muscular) branch runs radially and innervates the thenar muscles.
     - The digital nerves innervate the lumbrical muscles and the volar aspect of the radial three and a half digits.

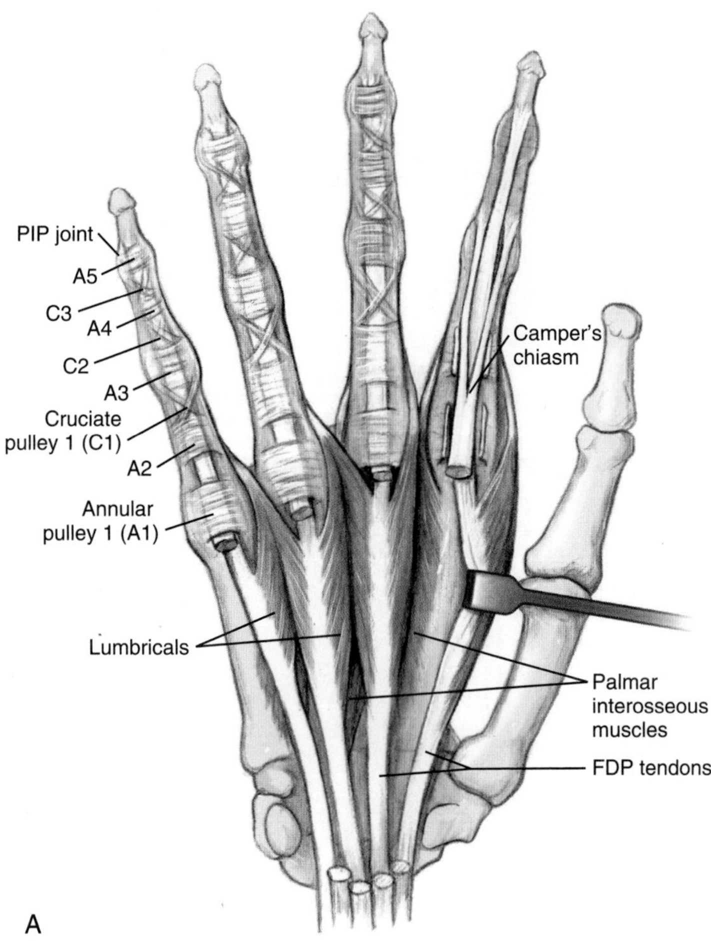

Figure 2-32 Flexor pulleys. The annular 1 (A1) pulley is the source of trigger digits. DIP, distal interphalangeal; FDP, flexor digitorum profundus; MP, metacarpal; PIP, proximal interphalangeal. (From Miller MD, et al: *Orthopaedic surgical approaches,* Philadelphia, 2008, Saunders, Figure HW-4.)

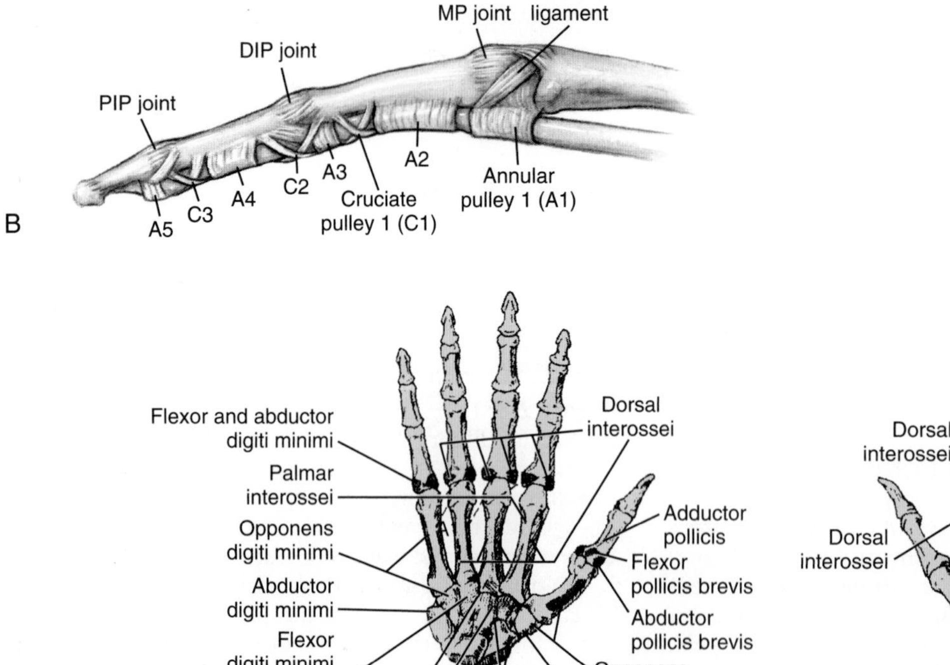

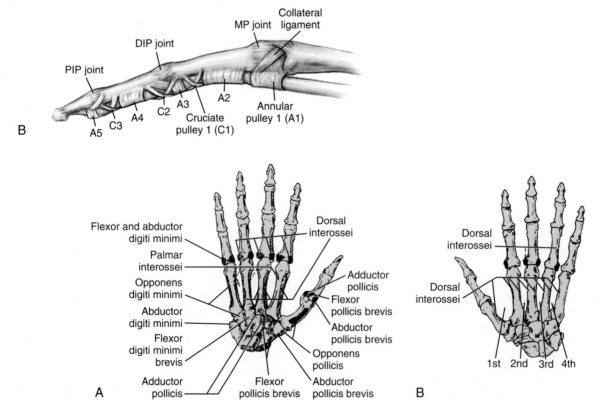

Figure 2-33 Origins and insertions of muscles of the wrist and hand. **A,** Dorsal view. **B,** Volar view. (From Jenkins DB: *Hollinshead's functional anatomy of the limbs and back,* ed 6, Philadelphia, 1991, Saunders, Figure 11-9.)

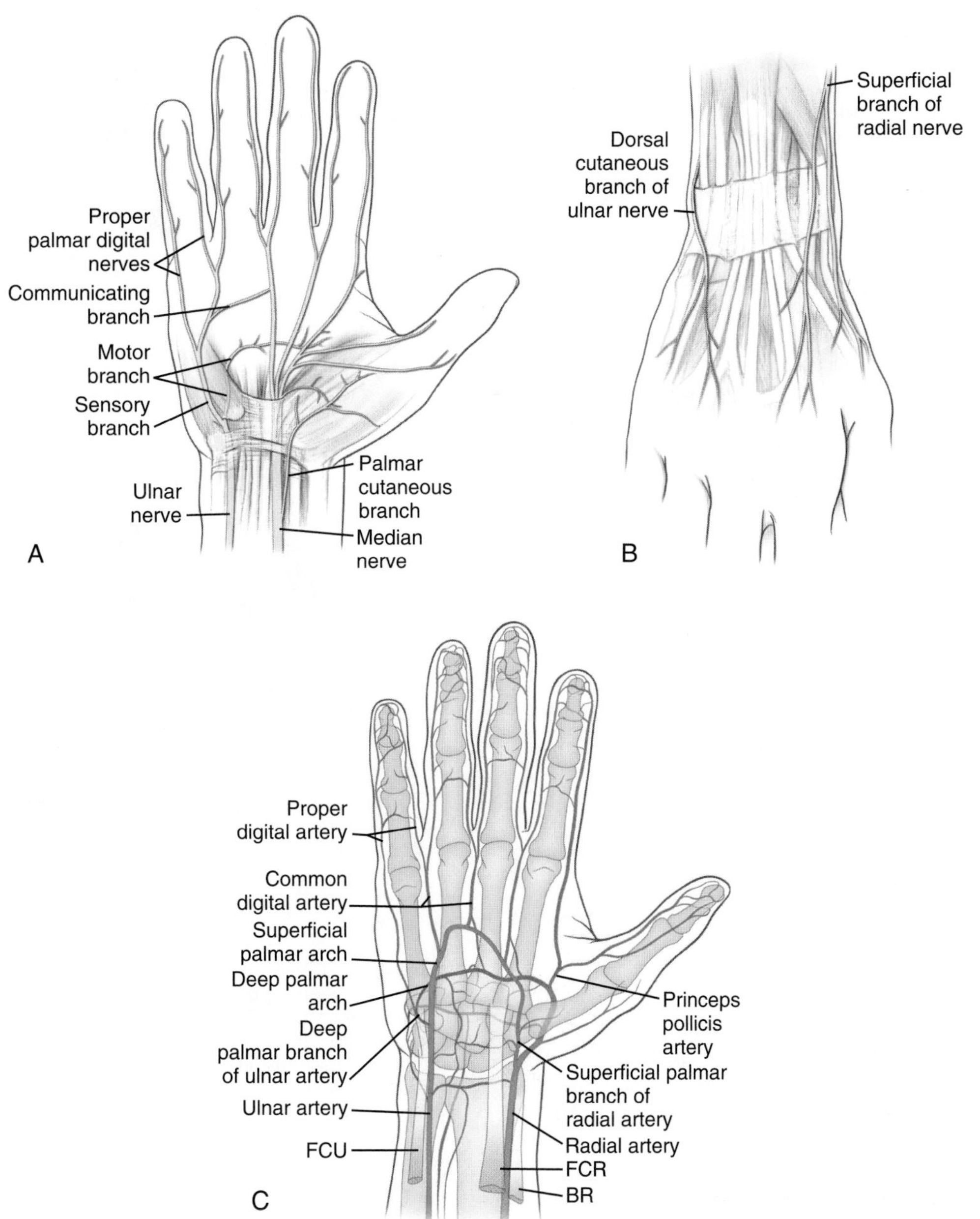

Figure 2-34 Nerves and vessels of the hand. **A,** Palmar view of nerves. **B,** Dorsal view of nerves in wrist. **C,** Palmar view of the arteries. BR, brachioradialis; FCR, flexor carpi radialis; FCU, flexor carpi ulnaris. (From Miller MD, et al: *Orthopaedic surgical approaches,* Philadelphia, 2008, Saunders, Figures HW-7 and HW-8.)

- Ulnar nerve
  - This nerve enters the wrist through Guyon's canal and divides into a superficial branch (palmaris brevis and skin) and a deep branch.
  - The deep branch travels with the deep palmar arch and passes between the abductor digiti minimi and flexor digiti minimi brevis, giving off motor branches to the deep musculature (three hypothenar muscles, two ulnar lumbrical muscles, all interossei, and the adductor pollicis) and terminating in digital nerves for the ulnar one and a half digits.
  - The dorsal cutaneous branch swings dorsally at the wrist and can be injured by either arthroscopic portal placement or surgical incision.
- Sensation to the thumb
  - Provided by five branches: lateral antebrachial cutaneous nerve, superficial and dorsal digital branches of the radial nerve, and digital and palmar branches of the median nerve

2. Innervation of the wrist and hand (Table 2-32)

E. Vessels (see Figure 2-34)

1. Radial artery
   - At the wrist, the radial artery reaches the dorsum of the carpus by passing between (1) the FCR and (2) the APL and EPB tendons (snuffbox).
   - Before that, it gives off a superficial palmar branch that communicates with the superficial arch (ulnar artery).
   - **It forms the deep palmar arch in the hand.**

Table 2-32 Innervation of the Wrist and Hand

Nerve	Muscles Innervated
Median (medial and lateral cord)	Abductor pollicis brevis, superficial head of flexor pollicis brevis, opponens pollicis, first and second lumbrical muscles
Ulnar (medial cord)	Abductor digiti minimi, opponens digiti minimi, flexor digiti minimi, third and fourth lumbrical muscles, interossei, adductor pollicis, deep head of flexor pollicis brevis

- The dorsal carpal branch of the radial artery enters the scaphoid dorsally and distally.

2. Ulnar artery
   - At the wrist, the ulnar artery lies on the TCL.
   - It gives off a deep palmar branch (which anastomoses with the deep arch) and **then forms the superficial palmar arch (which is distal to the deep arch).**
3. Digital arteries
   - These arteries arise from the superficial palmar arch and run dorsal to the nerves.

F. **Surgical approaches to the wrist and hand (Table 2-33)**

1. Dorsal approach to the wrist (Figure 2-35)
   - Interval: between the third and fourth extensor compartments (EPL and extensor digitorum)
   - Dissection:
     - Incise the extensory retinaculum between the third and fourth compartments.
     - Protect and retract these tendons to allow access to the distal radius and the dorsal radiocarpal joint.
     - Transpose the EPL, and incise the dorsal capsule.
   - Risks: Do not violate the interosseous scapholunate ligament.
2. Carpal tunnel release (Figure 2-36)
   - Incision is usually made in line with the fourth ray to avoid the palmar cutaneous branch of the median nerve.
   - Dissection through the TCL must be performed carefully in order to avoid injury to the median nerve or its motor branch.
3. Volar (Russé's) approach to the scaphoid
   - Interval: between the FCR and radial artery
   - An approach through the radial aspect of the FCR sheath: often easier and protects the radial artery
4. Dorsolateral approach to the scaphoid

Table 2-33 Surgical Approaches to the Wrist

Approach	Interval	Structures at Risk
Dorsal wrist	Third (extensor pollicis longus) and fourth (extensor digitorum communis) compartments	Transection of the innervation of the posterior interosseous nerve to the wrist capsule can be performed
Volar wrist	Flexor carpi radialis	Palmar cutaneous branch of median nerve
Volar scaphoid	Flexor carpi radialis and radial artery	Radial artery
Dorsolateral scaphoid	First and third compartments	Superficial radial nerve and radial artery

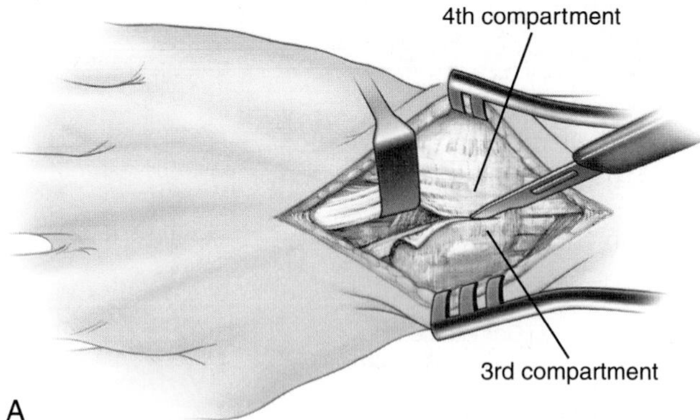

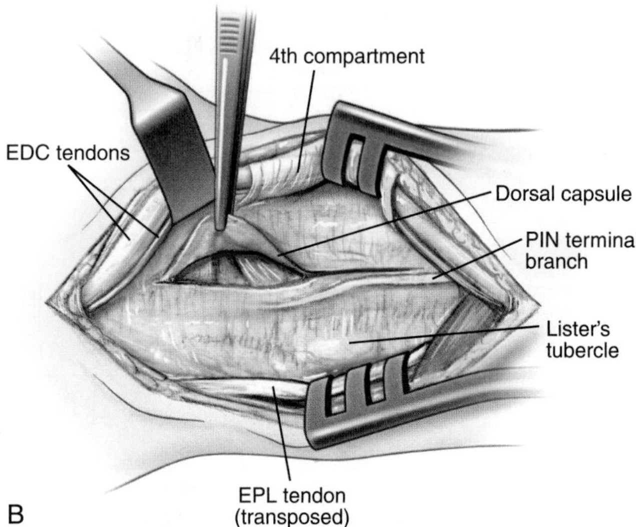

Figure 2-35 Dorsal surgical approach to the wrist. **A,** Superficial exposure. **B,** Deep exposure. In this approach, the interval between the third (extensor pollicis longus) and fourth (extensor digitorum communis) dorsal wrist compartments is explored. EDC, extensor digitorum communis; EPL, extensor pollicis longus; PIN, posterior interosseous nerve. (From Miller MD, et al: *Orthopaedic surgical approaches,* Philadelphia, 2008, Saunders, Figures HW-13 and HW-14.)

   - Using an incision within the anatomic snuffbox (first and third dorsal wrist compartment) helps protect the superficial radial nerve and radial artery (deep).
5. Volar approach to the flexor tendons (Bunnell's)
   - Zigzag incisions across the flexor creases help to expose the flexor sheaths.
   - Digital sheaths should be avoided.
6. Midlateral approach to the digits
   - Good for stabilization of fractures and neurovascular exposure
   - Requires a laterally placed incision at the dorsal extent of the interphalangeal creases
   - Exposure of the digital neurovascular bundle: volar to the incision

G. **Arthroscopy**

1. The placement of portals used for wrist arthroscopy is based on the dorsal compartments.
2. The 1-2 portal (risk for injury to radial artery), 6-R portal, and 6-U portal (radial and ulnar to the sixth compartment; risk for injury to the ulnar nerve and artery) carry the highest risk for damage.
3. The commonly used 3-4 and 4-5 portals are safer.

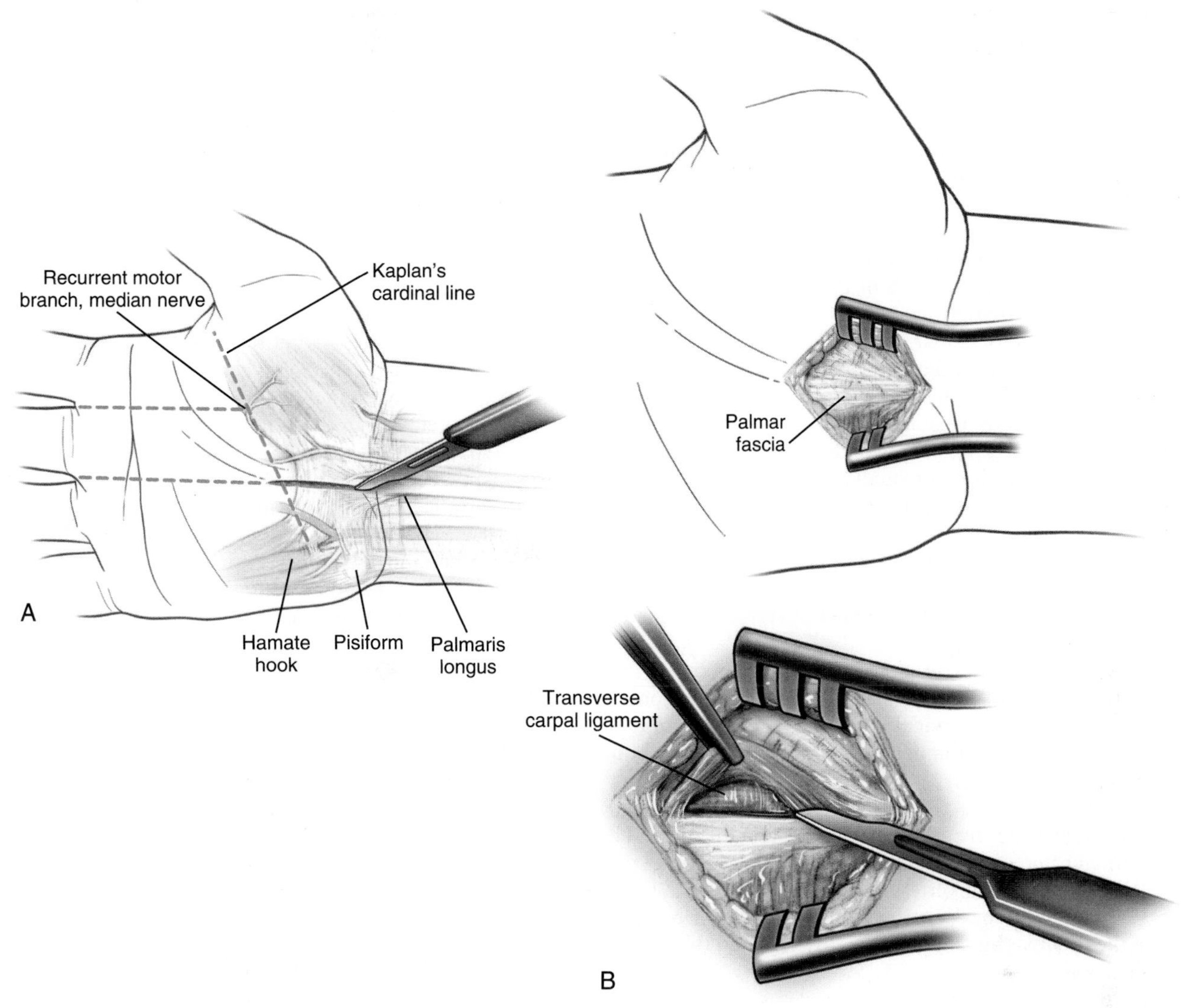

Figure 2-36 Carpal tunnel surgical approach. **A,** Incision. **B,** Superficial exposure. **C,** Deep exposure. (From Miller MD, et al: *Orthopaedic surgical approaches,* Philadelphia, 2008, Saunders, Figures HW-27 and HW-28.)

SECTION 3 SPINE

I. SPINE

A. Osteology

1. **Thirty-three vertebrae:** 7 cervical, 12 thoracic, 5 lumbar, 5 fused sacral, and 4 fused coccygeal
   - Normal curves are cervical lordosis, thoracic kyphosis, lumbar lordosis, and sacral kyphosis.
   - **Vertebral bodies generally increase in width in a craniocaudad direction, with the exception of T1 to T3.**
   - Important spine topographic landmarks are listed in Table 2-34.
2. Cervical spine
   - The atlas (C1) has no vertebral body and no spinous process.
     - C1 has two concave superior facets that articulate with the occipital condyles.

Table 2-34 Spine Vertebral Bodies

Topographic Landmark	Spinal Level
Mandible	C2-C3
Hyoid cartilage	C3
Thyroid cartilage	C4-C5
Cricoid cartilage	C6
Vertebra prominens	C7
Scapular spine	T3
Distal tip of scapula	T7
Iliac crest	L4-L5

- **Highest percentage of neck flexion and extension occurs at the occiput-C1 articulation (50% of the total).**
- **Axis (C2) develops from five ossification centers, with an initial cartilaginous junction between the dens and vertebral body (subdental synchondrosis) that fuses at 7 years of age.**
  - The base of the dens narrows because of the transverse ligament.
- **Atlantoaxial articulation is responsible for the majority of neck rotation; 50% of total rotation occurs at the C1-C2 articulation.**
- Atlantoaxial joint is diarthrodial.
  - *Pannus* in rheumatoid arthritis can affect this articulation and result in instability (see Chapter 8, Spine).
  - Cervical spine clearance including radiographs is recommended for elective orthopaedic procedures in patients with rheumatoid arthritis.
- C2 to C7 vertebrae have foramina in each transverse process and bifid spinous processes (except for the C7 nonbifid posterior spinous process [vertebral prominens]).
- The vertebral artery travels in the transverse foramina of C6 to C1.
- Carotid (Chassaignac's) tubercle is found at C6.
- **The diameter of the cervical spine canal is normally 17 mm, and the cervical cord may become compromised when the diameter is reduced to less than 13 mm.**

3. Thoracic spine
   - Unique features include costal facets (present on all 12 vertebral bodies and the transverse processes of T1 to T9) and a rounded vertebral foramen.
   - **Thoracic vertebral articulation with the rib cage makes this the most rigid region of the axial skeleton.**
4. Lumbar spine
   - Lumbar vertebrae are the largest vertebrae and are higher anteriorly than posteriorly, significantly contributing to the lumbar lordosis.
     - Lumbar lordosis ranges from 55 to 60 degrees, with the apex at L3; 66% of lordosis occurs in the region from L4 to the sacrum.
     - Lumbar vertebrae contain short laminae and pedicles.
     - Mammillary processes (separate ossification centers) project posteriorly from the superior articular facet.
     - **Spondylolysis is a defect in the pars interarticularis and the most common cause of back pain in children and adolescents.**
5. Sacrum
   - The sacrum is formed from the fusion of five spinal elements.
   - The sacral promontory is an anterosuperior portion that projects into the pelvis.
   - Four pairs of pelvic sacral foramina located both anteriorly and posteriorly transmit respective ventral and dorsal branches of the upper four sacral nerves.
   - The sacral canal opens caudally into the sacral hiatus.
6. Coccyx
   - The coccyx is formed from the fusion of the lowest four spinal elements.
   - It attaches dorsally to the gluteus maximus, the external anal sphincter, and the coccygeal muscles.

B. Arthrology

1. Spinal ligaments
   - Anterior longitudinal ligament (ALL)
     - Strong
     - Thickest at center of vertebral body and thinnest at periphery
     - Characterized by separate fibers extending from one to five levels
     - Resists hyperextension
   - Posterior longitudinal ligament
     - Weaker than the anterior longitudinal ligament
     - Extends from occiput (tectorial membrane) to the posterior sacrum
     - Separated from the center of the vertebral body by a space that allows passage of the dorsal branches of the spinal artery and veins
     - Hourglass-shaped, with the wider (yet thinner) sections located over the discs; **ruptured discs tend to be lateral to these expansions**
   - Ligamentum flavum
     - Strong, yellow, elastic ligament connecting the laminae
     - Runs from the anterior surface of the superior lamina to the posterior surface of the inferior lamina and is constantly in tension
     - Hypertrophy of the ligamentum flavum is said to contribute to nerve root compression.
   - Supraspinous, interspinous, and intertransverse ligaments
     - Ligamentous capsules overlying the zygapophyseal joints; the intertransverse ligaments contribute little to interspinous stability.
     - Supraspinous ligament lies dorsal to the spinous processes, and interspinous ligament lies between the spinous processes.
       - Supraspinous ligament begins at C7 and is in continuity with the ligamentum nuchae (which runs from C7 to the occiput).

1. Spine stability (Denis model): the three-column system (Table 2-35)
2. Specialized ligaments
   - Atlanto-occipital joint
     - Composed of two articular capsules (anterior and posterior) and the tectorial membrane (a cephalad extension of the posterior longitudinal ligament)
     - Further stabilization by the ligamentous attachments to the dens
   - Atlantoaxial joint

Table 2-35 Denis Model of Spine Columns

Column	Composition
Anterior	Anterior longitudinal ligament, anterior two thirds of annulus and vertebral body
Middle	Posterior third of body and annulus, posterior longitudinal ligament
Posterior	Pedicles, facets and facet capsules, spinous processes, posterior ligaments that include interspinous and supraspinous ligaments, ligamentum flavum

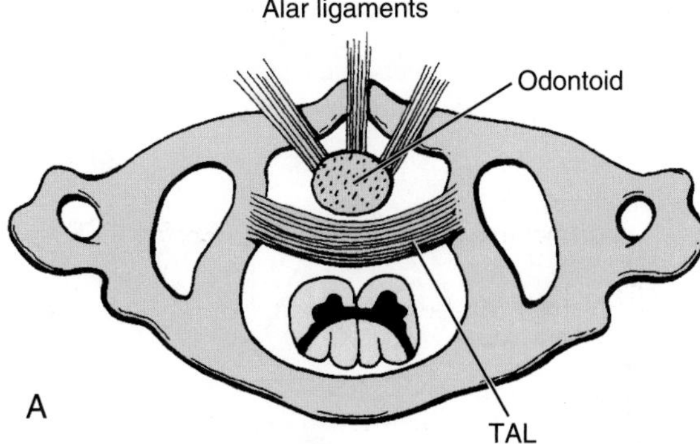

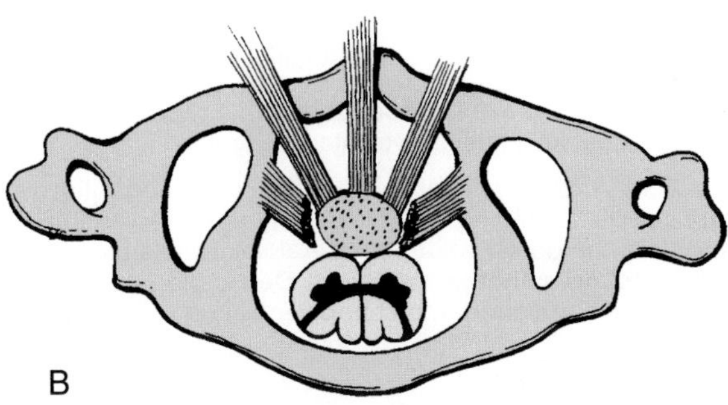

Figure 2-37 The atlantoaxial complex as seen from above **(A).** **The disruption of the transverse axial ligament (TAL) with intact alar ligaments results in C1-C2 instability without cord compression (B).** (From DeLee JC, Drez D Jr: *Orthopaedic sports medicine: principles and practices,* vol 1, Philadelphia, 1994, Saunders, p 432. **B,** Redrawn from Hensinger RN: Congenital anomalies of the atlantoaxial joint. In Sherk HH, editor: *The cervical spine,* ed 2, Philadelphia, 1989, JB Lippincott, the Cervical Spine Research Society Editorial Committee, p 242.)

- **The transverse ligament is the major stabilizer of the atlantoaxial joint.**
- This articulation is further stabilized by the apical ligament (longitudinal), which, together with the transverse axial ligament, composes the cruciate ligament.
- In addition, a pair of alar ("check") ligaments runs obliquely from the tip of the dens to the occiput (Figure 2-37).
- **An atlanto-dens interval of more than 7 to 10 mm or a posterior space of less than 13 mm is a relative contraindication to elective orthopaedic surgery, and the spine should be stabilized first.**
- Common measurements in C1-C2 disorders are covered in Figure 8-2.

- Iliolumbar ligament
  - This stout ligament connects the transverse process of L5 with the ilium.
  - Tension on this ligament in patients with unstable vertical shear pelvic fractures can lead to avulsion fractures of the transverse process.

4. Facet (apophyseal) joints
   - The orientation of the facets of the spine dictates the plane of motion at each relative level.
   - Facet orientation varies with the spinal level (Table 2-36).

Table 2-36 Orientation of Spine Facets

Spinal Level	Orientation of Sagittal Facet	Orientation of Coronal Facet
Cervical	35 Degrees at C2, increasing to 55 degrees at C7	Neutral, 0 degrees
Thoracic	60 Degrees at T1, increasing to 70 degrees at T12	20 Degrees posterior
Lumbar	137 Degrees at L1, decreasing to 118 degrees at L5	45 Degrees anterior

   - In the cervical spine, the superior articular facet is anterior and inferior to the inferior articular process of the vertebra above; the nerve roots exit near the superior articulating process.
   - In the lumbar spine, the superior articular facet is anterior and lateral to the inferior articular facet.

5. Intervertebral discs
   - Fibrocartilaginous
   - Annulus fibrosus: obliquely oriented composed of type I collagen
   - Central nucleus pulposus: made of type II collagen and softer than the annulus
   - Nucleus pulposus: high polysaccharide content and approximately 88% water
   - Aging: results in the loss of water and conversion to fibrocartilage
   - **Intervertebral discs: account for 25% of the total height of the spinal column**
   - Attach to the vertebral bodies by hyaline cartilage, which is responsible for the vertical growth of the column
   - **Intradisc pressure: position dependent: pressure is lowest in supine position and highest in the sitting position and flexed forward with weights on the hands**

C. Muscles (Table 2-37)

1. Neck: functional classification (anterior and posterior regions)
   - Anterior neck region
     - This region contains the superficial platysma muscle (cranial nerve VII innervated), stylohyoid and digastric muscles (cranial nerve VII innervated) above the hyoid, and "strap" muscles below the hyoid.
     - Strap muscles include the sternohyoid and omohyoid in the superficial layer and the thyrohyoid and sternohyoid in the deep layer; all are innervated by the ansa cervicalis (C1 to C3).
     - The sternocleidomastoid muscle (cranial nerve XI and ansa) runs obliquely across the neck, rotating the head to the contralateral side.

Table 2-37 Spinal Muscle Relationships

Muscle	Relationships
Longus capitis	Anterior to longus colli Posterior to sympathetic chain
Longus colli	Anterior to vertebral artery Posterior to longus capitis

- The anterior triangle (borders: sternocleidomastoid, midline of the neck, and lower border of the mandible) is the largest area.
- Three smaller triangles are as follows:
  - Submandibular
  - Carotid (bordered by the posterior aspect of the digastric and omohyoid and used for the anterior approach to C5)
  - Posterior (bordered by the trapezius muscle, sternocleidomastoid muscle, and clavicle)
- Posterior neck region
  - Posterior neck muscles form the borders of the suboccipital triangle.
  - The superior and inferior heads of the obliquus capitis muscle and the rectus capitis posterior major muscle form this triangle.
  - The vertebral artery and the first cervical nerve are within this triangle, and the greater occipital nerve (C2) is superficial.

2. Back
   - Blanketed by the trapezius (superiorly) and latissimus dorsi (inferiorly)
   - Rhomboid muscles and levator scapulae are deep to this layer.
   - Deep muscles: the erector spinae and transversospinalis
     - Erector spinae run from the transverse and spinous processes of the inferior vertebrae to the spinous processes of the superior vertebrae.
     - They stabilize and extend the back.
     - All of the deep back musculature is innervated by dorsal primary rami of the spinal nerves.

D. Nerves

1. Spinal cord
   - General anatomy
     - The spinal cord extends from the brainstem to the inferior border of L1, where it terminates as the conus medullaris.
     - A small filum terminale continues distal with the surrounding nerve roots contained within a common dural sac (cauda equina) to its termination in the coccyx.
     - The spinal cord is enclosed within the bony spinal canal with variable amounts of space (greatest in the upper cervical spine).
     - The cord also varies in diameter (widest at the origin of the plexuses).
     - In cross-section, the cord is observed to have both geographic and functional boundaries (Figure 2-38). It is divided in the midline anteriorly by a fissure and posteriorly by the sulcus.
   - Functional anatomy: The functions of the ascending (sensory) and descending (motor) tracts are summarized in Table 2-38.
     - The posterior funiculi (*dorsal columns*) are located dorsally and receive ascending fibers, which deliver deep tactile, proprioceptive, and vibratory sensations.
     - The *lateral spinothalamic tract* transmits sensations of pain and temperature.
       - Site for chordotomy to alleviate intractable pain
     - Descending in the *lateral corticospinal tract* are fibers that transmit instructions for voluntary muscle contraction.

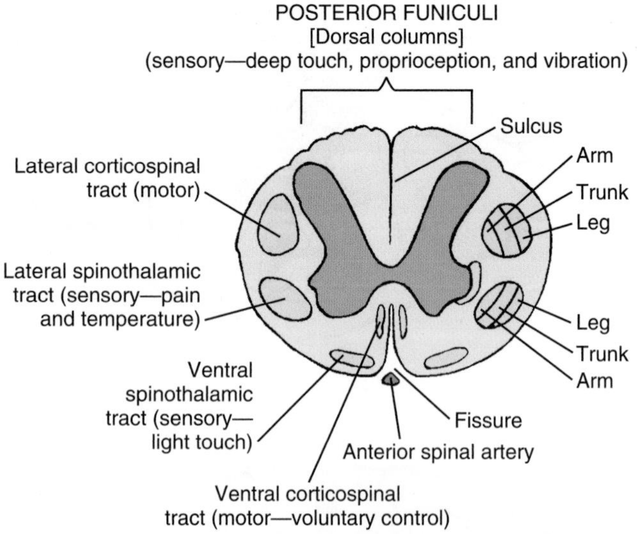

Figure 2-38 Cross-sectional view of the spinal cord, illustrating functions of the ascending and descending tracts. Ascending tracts (sensory) are the dorsal columns, lateral spinothalamic tract, and ventral (anterior) spinothalamic tract. Descending tracts (motor) are the lateral corticospinal tract and ventral (anterior) corticospinal tract.

       - Sacral structures are the most peripheral in the lateral corticospinal tracts; cervical structures are more medial.
       - **This is why central cord syndrome affects the upper extremities more than the lower extremities.**
     - The *ventral (anterior) spinothalamic tract* transmits light tactile sensation.
     - *Ventral (anterior) corticospinal tract* delivers cortical messages of voluntary contraction.
     - Deficits associated with patterns of incomplete spinal cord injury are predictable from the anatomy of the ascending and descending tracts.
     - The prognosis with incomplete spinal cord injury is unaffected by the presence or absence of the bulbocavernosus reflex.
     - Incomplete spinal cord injury patterns are summarized in Table 2-39.
     - Spinal cord injury distal to the conus medullaris may permanently interrupt the bulbocavernosus reflex.
2. Nerve roots (Figure 2-39)
   - There are 31 pairs of spinal nerves: 8 cervical, 12 thoracic, 5 lumbar, 5 sacral, and 1 coccygeal.

Table 2-38 Spinal Cord Tracts

Direction	Tracts	Function
Ascending (sensory)	Dorsal columns	Deep touch, proprioception, vibratory
	Lateral spinothalamic	Pain and temperature
	Anterior spinothalamic	Light touch
Descending (motor)	Lateral corticospinal	Voluntary motor
	Anterior corticospinal	Voluntary motor

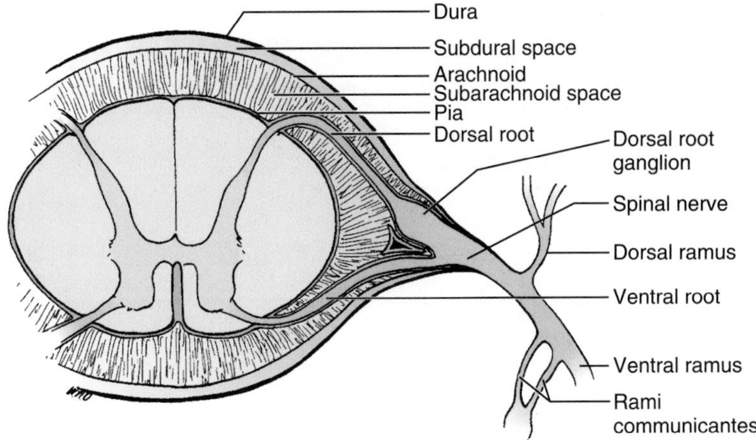

Figure 2-39 Spinal nerves. The facet joints are innervated by the medial branch of the dorsal primary ramus and by the sinovertebral nerve. (From Jenkins DB: *Hollinshead's functional anatomy of the limbs and back,* ed 6, Philadelphia, 1991, Saunders, p 205.)

- Within the subarachnoid space, the dorsal root (and ganglia) and ventral roots converge to form the spinal nerve.
  - The nerve becomes "extradural" as it approaches the intervertebral foramen (the dura becomes epineurium) at all levels above L1.
  - Below this level, the nerves are contained within the cauda equina.
- After exiting the foramen, the spinal nerve gives off dorsal primary rami, which supply the muscles and skin of the neck and back regions.
- Innervation of structures within the spinal canal—including the periosteum, meninges, vascular structures, and articular connective tissue—is from the *sinuvertebral nerve.*
- Ventral rami supply the anteromedial trunk and limbs.
- With the exception of the thoracic nerves, the ventral rami are grouped in plexuses before delivering sensorimotor functions to a general region.
- **In the cervical spine, the numbered nerve exits at a level above the pedicle of the corresponding vertebral level (e.g., the C2 nerve exits at the level of vertebrae C1 to C2).**
- **In the lumbar spine, the nerve root traverses the respective disc space above the named vertebral body and exits the respective foramen under the pedicle (Figure 2-40).**
- Herniated discs usually impinge on the traversing nerve root and facet joint.
  - For example, a disc herniation at the level of L4 to L5 would cause compression of the traversing L5 nerve root, resulting in a positive tension sign (straight-leg raise) and diminished strength in the hip abductors and extensor hallucis longus (EHL) and pain and numbness in the lateral leg to the dorsum of the foot (see Figure 2-12).
  - A far lateral disc herniation at the level of L4 to L5 would compress the exiting L4 nerve root, resulting in a positive tension sign (femoral nerve stretch test) and L4 nerve compromise.
- **The L5 nerve root is relatively fixed to the anterior sacral ala and can be damaged by sacral fractures and errant, anteriorly placed iliosacral screws.**
- Key testable neurologic levels are listed in Table 2-40.

Table 2-39 Patterns of Incomplete Spinal Cord Injury

Pattern of Injury	Functional Deficit	Recovery
Central (most common)	Upper extremity affected more than lower extremity, usually quadriparetic with sacral sparing; flaccid paralysis of upper extremity and spastic paralysis of lower extremity	75%
Anterior	Complete motor deficit	**10% (worst prognosis)**
Brown-Séquard	Unilateral cord injury with ipsilateral motor deficit, contralateral pain, and temperature deficit (two levels below injury)	>90% recovery

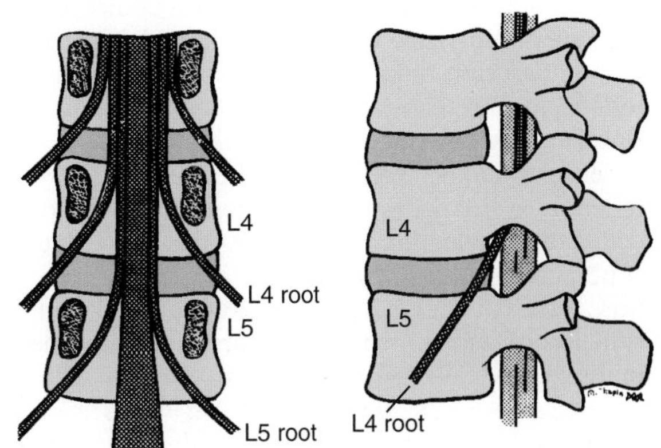

Figure 2-40 Locations of the lumbar spine nerve root in relation to vertebral landmarks. Central disc herniation between L4 and L5 would compress the traversing root and therefore affect L5. A far lateral disc herniation between L4 and L5 would affect the L4 exiting root. In the cervical spine, the numbered nerve exits at a level above the pedicle of the corresponding vertebral level. (From Weissman BN, Sledge CB: *Orthopedic radiology,* Philadelphia, 1986, Saunders, p 283.)

Table 2-40 Key Testable Neurologic Levels

Neurologic Level	Representative Muscle	Reflex
C5	Deltoid	Biceps
C6	Wrist extension	Brachioradialis
C7	Wrist flexion	Triceps
C8	Finger flexion	
T1	Interossei	
L4	Tibialis anterior	Patellar
L5	Toe extensors	
S1	Peroneal	Achilles

- Nerve root compression: A summary of the findings of nerve root compression is highlighted in Chapter 8, Spine (Tables 8-2 [cervical] and 8-7 [lumbar]). Dermatomes are key testable items (see Figure 2-12).

3. Sympathetic chain
   - Cervical sympathetic chain posterior and medial to the carotid sheath
     - Anterior to the longus capitis muscle
     - Cross-sectional relationships in the carotid sheath are key testable material; contents include the internal carotid artery, common carotid artery, internal jugular vein, and cranial nerve X (vagus nerve).
   - Three ganglia of cervical sympathetic chain: superior, middle, and inferior (Table 2-41)
     - **Disruption of the inferior ganglia can lead to Horner's syndrome (ptosis, miosis [pupillary constriction], and anhidrosis).**
     - Can be seen with preganglionic brachial plexus lesions
   - Sympathetic ganglia: 11 in the thoracic region, 4 in the lumbar region, and 4 in the sacral region

E. Vessels

1. Spinal blood supply from segmental arteries
   - Located at vertebral midbodies via the aorta (which lies on the left side of the vertebral column; the inferior vena cava and azygos vein are on the right).
   - Primary supply to the dura and posterior elements is from the dorsal branches.
   - Ventral branches supply the vertebral bodies via the ascending and descending branches, which are delivered underneath the posterior longitudinal ligament in four separate ostia.
2. Vertebral artery (a branch of the subclavian artery)
   - Ascends through the transverse foramina of C1 to C6 (anterior to and not through C7) posterior to the longus colli muscle and then posterior to the lateral masses; courses along the cephalic surface of the posterior arch of C1 (atlas); and passes ventromedially around the spinal cord and through the foramen magnum before uniting at the midline basilar artery

Table 2-41 Cervical Sympathetic Ganglia

Ganglion	Location	Comments
Superior	C2-C3	Largest
Middle	C6	Variable
Inferior	C7-T1	Stellate

   - **The distance from the spinous process of C1 laterally to the vertebral artery is 2 cm** (a safe distance for dissections would therefore be less than 2 cm).
3. **Artery of Adamkiewicz (great anterior medullary artery)**
   - Enters through the left intervertebral foramen in the lower thoracic spine from T8 to T12; it supplies the interior two thirds of the anterior cord
4. Spinal cord arterial supply
   - From the anterior and posterior spinal arteries and segmental branches of the vertebral artery and dorsal arteries, which travel via the dorsal and ventral rootlets to the respective dorsal and anterolateral portions of the cord.
   - Disruption of the anterior longitudinal artery can result in loss of function of the anterior two-thirds of the cord.
5. Venous drainage of the vertebral bodies
   - Primarily through the central sinusoid located on the dorsum of each vertebral body

F. Surgical approaches to the spine (Table 2-42, Figure 2-41)

1. Anterior approach to the cervical spine
   - Incision: transverse and based on the desired level (e.g., for C5, the carotid triangle should be entered)
   - Dissection
     - Retract the platysma with the skin.
     - Expose the pretracheal fascia to explore the interval between the carotid sheath—which contains the internal and common carotid arteries, the internal jugular vein, and the vagus nerve (cranial nerve X)—and the trachea.
     - Incise the prevertebral fascia sharply, and the retract the longus colli muscle gently (protecting the recurrent laryngeal nerve, a branch of the vagus nerve that lies outside the sheath) to expose the vertebral body. The anterior surface of the vertebral body is exposed.
   - Risks: **Injury to the recurrent laryngeal nerve with right-sided approaches (paralysis is identified by a hoarse, scratchy voice caused by unilateral vocal cord paralysis, visualized with direct laryngoscopy).**

Table 2-42 Surgical Approaches to the Spine

Approach	Interval	Structures at Risk
Anterior cervical	Carotid sheath and the trachea	Recurrent laryngeal nerve Sympathetic ganglion
Posterior cervical	Midline approach between paracervical muscle	Vertebral artery
Anterior thoracic	Transverse between ribs two levels above surgical site	Intercostal neurovascular bundle; to avoid, dissect over top of rib
Posterior thoracolumbar	Midline approach over spinous processes	Posterior primary rami and segmental vessels; protect nerve root
Anterior lumbar (transperitoneal)	Between segmentally innervated rectus abdominis	Presacral plexus of parasympathetic nerve

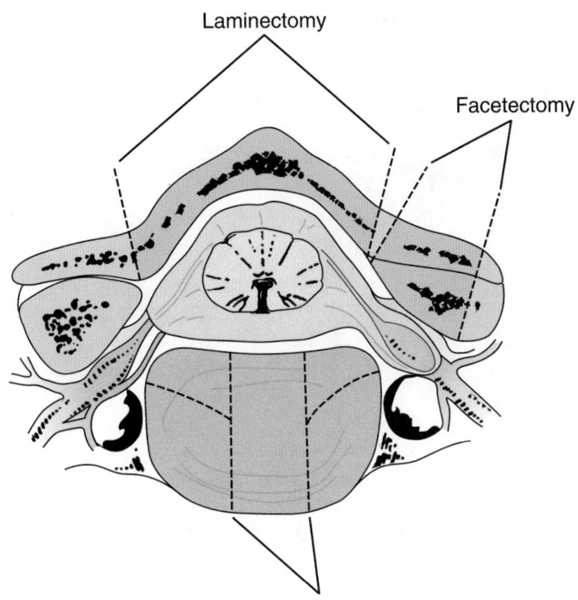

Figure 2-41 Surgical procedures on the cervical spine. (From Rothman RH, Simeon FA: *The spine,* ed 2, Philadelphia, 1982, Saunders, p 484.)

- □ Recurrent laryngeal nerve arises from the vagus at the level of the subclavian artery on the right; the left arises at the level of the aortic arch.
- □ Anterior cervical approaches from the lower left side increase the risk for injury to the thoracic duct, which is posterior to the carotid sheath.
- □ **When the longus muscles are dissected subperiosteally, the stellate ganglion is also protected (avoiding Horner's syndrome).**
- □ **Postoperatively, the upper airway is at risk for edema, vocal cord paralysis, and hematoma.**

2. Posterior approach to the cervical spine
   - ▪ Incision: midline
   - ▪ Dissection:
     - □ After a midline approach through the ligamentum nuchae, reflect the superficial (trapezius) and intermediate (splenius, semispinalis, longissimus capitis) layers laterally; the vertebrae are exposed.
     - □ Access to the spinal canal is through laminectomy or facetectomy.
   - ▪ Risks:
     - □ The vertebral artery is especially vulnerable as it leaves the foramen transversarium and travels superiorly and medially to pierce the atlanto-occipital membrane at its lateral angle.
     - □ The greater occipital nerve (C2) and the third occipital nerve (C3) should also be protected in the suboccipital region.
     - □ **Postoperative C5 palsy is the most common complication with a posterior approach.**
3. Anterior (transthoracic) approach to the thoracic spine
   - ▪ Incision: transverse, made approximately two ribs above the level of interest
   - ▪ Dissection:
     - □ Dissect over the top of the rib to avoid injuring the intercostal neurovascular bundle (which lies on the inferior internal surface of the rib).
     - □ Further dissect the rib, and remove it from the surgical field.
     - □ The right-sided approach is favored in order to avoid the aorta, segmental arteries, artery of Adamkiewicz, and thoracic duct (in the upper thoracic spine on the left side of the esophagus and behind the carotid sheath).
   - ▪ Risks:
     - □ The esophagus, aorta, venae cavae, and pleura of the lungs should be identified and protected.
     - □ Intercostal neuralgia is the most common complication.
4. Posterior approach to the thoracolumbar spine
   - ▪ Incision: straight, midline, over the spinous processes and carried down through the thoracolumbar fascia
   - ▪ Dissection:
     - □ Use the plane between the two segmentally innervated erector spinae muscles.
     - □ Subperiosteally dissect the paraspinal musculature from the attached spinous processes, thereby exposing the posterior elements.
     - □ Perform partial laminectomy to allow greater exposure of the cord and discs.
     - □ Place pedicle screws at the junction of the lateral border of the superior facet and the middle of the transverse process.
     - □ Angle these screws 15 degrees medially and in line with the slope of the vertebra, as seen on lateral radiographs.
   - ▪ Risks: injury to the posterior primary rami (near the facet joints) and segmental vessels (anterior to the plane connecting the transverse processes)
5. Anterior approach to the lumbar spine (transperitoneal)
   - ▪ Incision: longitudinal, from below the umbilicus to just above the pubic symphysis
   - ▪ Dissection:
     - □ Split the rectus abdominis muscles, and incise the peritoneum.
     - □ Protect and retract the bladder distally and the bowel cephalad, and incise the posterior peritoneum longitudinally over the sacral promontory.
     - □ The aortic bifurcation is revealed; ligate the middle sacral artery.
     - □ The L5-S1 disc space is exposed.
   - ▪ Risks: Injury to the lumbar plexus, particularly the superior hypogastric plexus of the sympathetic plexus that lies over the L5 vertebral body, can cause sexual dysfunction and retrograde ejaculation. (Ejaculation is predominantly a sympathetic nervous system function and erection predominantly a parasympathetic nervous system function.)
6. Anterolateral approach to the lumbar spine (retroperitoneal)
   - ▪ Incision: oblique, centered over the twelfth rib to the lateral border of the rectus abdominis muscle
   - ▪ Dissection:
     - □ Incise the external oblique, internal oblique, and transversus abdominis muscles in line with the skin incision.
     - □ Elevate the retroperitoneal fat, thereby revealing the psoas major muscle and genitofemoral nerve.

- Ligate the segmental lumbar vessels, and mobilize the aorta and venae cavae to expose the desired vertebral level.
- **The great vessels typically bifurcate at the L4-L5 disc level; therefore, use a larger area of dissection than would be used for operating on the L5-S1 disc level, which lies below the bifurcation of the aorta.**

- Risks: injury to the sympathetic chain (medial to the psoas and lateral to the vertebral body) and ureters (between the peritoneum and psoas fascia)

7. Anatomy important in placement of halo pins
   - The optimal position for the placement of anterolateral halo pins is approximately 1 cm superior to the orbital rim in the outer two thirds of the orbit below the equator of the skull (Figure 2-42).
   - With this pin position, the temporal fossa and temporalis muscle are situated laterally, and the supraorbital nerve, supratrochlear nerve, and frontal sinus are situated medially.
   - **The supraorbital nerve is lateral to the supratrochlear nerve, which lies anterior to the frontal sinus.**
   - The most commonly injured cranial nerve with halo traction is the abducens (cranial nerve VI); injury is recognized from the loss of lateral gaze.

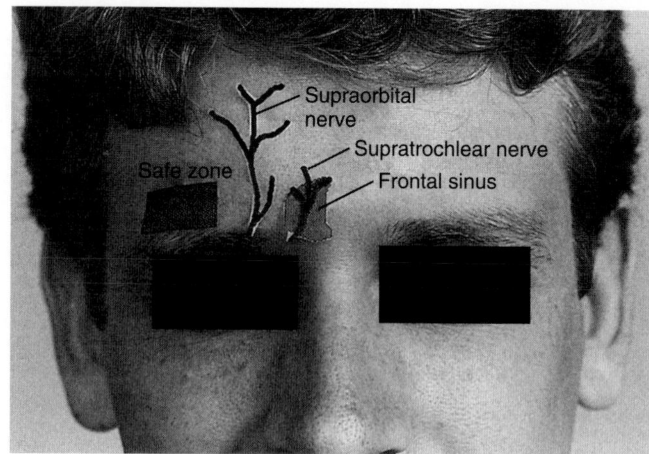

Figure 2-42 Safe placement of halo pins. The safe zone for halo pin placement is highlighted. From lateral to medial are the supraorbital nerve and the supratrochlear nerve, which overlies the frontal sinus.

SECTION 4 LOWER EXTREMITY AND PELVIS

Table 2-43 summarizes lower extremity neurology. Table 2-44 summarizes lower extremity innervation. Table 2-45 summarizes standard surgical approaches to the lower extremity.

I. PELVIS AND HIP

A. Osteology

1. The pelvic girdle is composed of two innominate (coxal) bones that articulate with the sacrum.
2. Each innominate bone is composed of three united bones: the ilium, ischium, and pubis.
3. The ilium has two important anterior prominences:
   - Anterior-superior iliac spine
     - Palpable at the lateral edge of the inguinal ligament
     - Origin of the sartorius muscle and the transverse and internal abdominal muscles
   - Anterior-inferior iliac spine
     - Less prominent
     - **Provides the origin of the direct head of the rectus femoris and the iliofemoral ligament (Y ligament of Bigelow)**
4. The ilium also has a posterior-superior iliac spine, which is usually located 4 to 5 cm lateral to the S2 spinous process.

Table 2-43 Important Neurologic Features of Lower Extremity

Joint	Function	Neurologic Level
Hip	Flexion	T12-L3
	Extension	S1
	Adduction	L2-L4
	Abduction	L5
Knee	Flexion	L5, S1
	Extension	L2-L4
Ankle	Dorsiflexion	L4, L5
	Plantar flexion	S1, S2
	Inversion	L4
	Eversion	S1

Table 2-44 Innervation of Lower Extremity

Nerves	Muscles Innervated
Femoral	Iliacus, psoas, quadriceps femoris (rectus femoris, vastus lateralis, vastus intermedius, and vastus medialis)
Obturator	Adductor brevis, adductor longus, adductor magnus (along with tibial nerve), gracilis
Superior gluteal	Gluteus medius, gluteus minimus, tensor fascia lata
Inferior gluteal	Gluteus maximus
Sciatic	Semitendinosus, semimembranosus, biceps femoris (long head [tibial division] and short head [peroneal division]), adductor magnus (with obturator nerve)
Tibial	Gastrocnemius, soleus, tibialis posterior, flexor digitorum longus, flexor hallucis longus, medial and lateral plantar nerves
Deep peroneal	Tibialis anterior, extensor digitorum longus, extensor hallucis longus, peroneus tertius, extensor digitorum brevis
Superficial peroneal	Peroneus longus, peroneus brevis

Table 2-45 Standard Orthopaedic Surgical Approaches to the Lower Extremity

Region	Approach	Eponym	Muscular Interval 1 (Nerve)	Muscular Interval 2 (Nerve)	Structures at Risk
Iliac crest	Posterior		Gluteus maximus (inferior gluteal)	Latissimus dorsi (thoracodorsal)	Clunial n., superior gluteal artery, sciatic n.
	Anterior		Tensor fascia lata, gluteus medius, and gluteus minimus (superior gluteal)	External abdominal oblique (segmental)	ASIS/LFCN
Hip	Anterior	Smith-Peterson	Sartorius and rectus femoris (femoral)	Tensor fascia lata and gluteus medius (superior gluteal)	LFCN, femoral n., ascending branch of LFCA
	Anterolateral	Watson-Jones	Tensor fasciae latae (superior gluteal)	Gluteus medius (superior gluteal)	Femoral n., a., and v./ profunda femoris a.
	Lateral	Hardinge's	Splits gluteus medius (superior gluteal)	Splits vastus lateralis (femoral)	Femoral n., a., and v./ LFCA (transverse branch)
	Posterior	Moore-Southern	Splits gluteus maximus (inferior gluteal)	N/A	Sciatic, inferior gluteal a.
	Medial	Ludloff's	Adductor longus and adductor brevis (anterior division of obturator)	Gracilis and adductor magnus (obturator and tibial)	Anterior division of obturator n./MFCA
Thigh	Lateral		Vastus lateralis (femoral)	Vastus lateralis (femoral)	Perforating branch of profunda femoris a.
	Posterolateral		Vastus lateralis (femoral)	Hamstrings (sciatic)	Perforating branch of profunda femoris a.
	Anteromedial		Rectus femoris (femoral)	Vastus medialis (femoral)	Medial superior geniculate a.
Distal femur	Posterior		Biceps femoris (sciatic)	Vastus lateralis (femoral)	Sciatic n./PFCN
Knee	Medial parapatellar		Vastus medialis (femoral)	Rectus femoris (femoral)	Infrapatellar branch of saphenous n.
	Medial		Vastus medialis (femoral)	Sartorius (femoral)	Infrapatellar branch of saphenous n.
	Lateral		Iliotibial band (superior gluteal)	Biceps femoris (sciatic)	Peroneal n./popliteus tendon
	Posterior		Semimembranosus and lateral gastrocnemius (tibial)	Biceps and lateral gastrocnemius (tibial)	Medial sural cutaneous n./tibial n./peroneal n.
	Lateral		Vastus lateralis (femoral)	Biceps femoris (sciatic)	Peroneal n./ lateral superior geniculate a.
Tibia	Posterolateral		Gastrocnemius, soleus, flexor hallucis longus (tibial)	Peroneus brevis and peroneus longus (superior peroneal)	Lesser saphenous v./ posterior tibial a.
	Anterior		Tibialis anterior (peroneal)	Periosteum	Long saphenous v.
Ankle	Anterior		Extensor hallucis longus (deep peroneal)	Extensor digitorum longus (deep peroneal)	Superficial and deep peroneal n./anterior tibial a.
Medial malleolus	Posterior		Tibialis posterior	Flexor digitorum longus	Saphenous n. and v.
Ankle	Posterolateral		Peroneus brevis (superior peroneal)	Flexor hallucis longus (tibial)	Sural n./small saphenous v.
Distal fibula	Lateral		Peroneus tertius (deep peroneal)	Peroneus brevis (superior peroneal)	Sural n.
Foot	Anterolateral		Peroneal muscles (superior peroneal)	Extensor digitorum and peroneus tertius (deep peroneal)	Deep peroneal n./ anterior tibial a.
	Posteromedial		Tibialis posterior or flexor digitorum longus	Flexor digitorum longus or flexor hallucis longus	Posterior tibial a./tibial n.

a., artery; ASIS, anterior-superior iliac spine; LFCA, lateral femoral circumflex artery; LFCN, lateral femoral cutaneous nerve; MFCA, medial femoral circumflex artery; n., nerve; N/A, not applicable; PFCN, posterior femoral cutaneous nerve; v., vein.

5. The greater sciatic notch is located posterior and superior to the acetabulum.
6. The iliopectineal eminence is an anteriorly raised region that represents the union of the ilium and pubis.
   - The iliopsoas muscle traverses a groove between this eminence and the anterior-inferior iliac spine.
7. **The acetabulum is anteverted (15 degrees) and obliquely oriented (45 degrees caudally).**
   - The posterosuperior articular surface is thickened to accommodate weight bearing.
   - The inferior surface is deficient and contains the acetabular, or cotyloid, notch, which is bound by the transverse acetabular ligament.
8. The proximal femur is composed of the femoral head, femoral neck, and greater and lesser trochanters.
   - **The femoral neck is anteverted approximately 14 degrees in relation to the femoral condyles.**
   - The angle of the femoral neck shaft averages 127 degrees.
9. The hip trabecular architecture is illustrated in Figure 2-43.

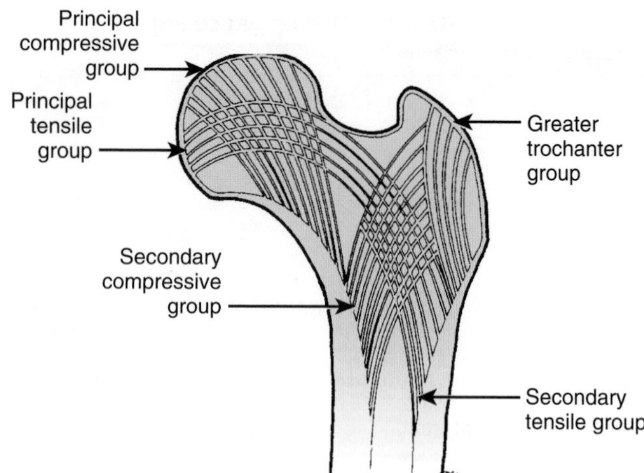

Figure 2-43 Hip trabeculae. **Trabecular patterns help determine the presence of osteopenia and displacement of femoral neck fractures.** (From DeLee JC: Fractures and dislocations of the hip. In Rockwood CA Jr, et al, editors: *Fractures in adults,* ed 3, Philadelphia, 1991, JB Lippincott, p 1488.)

B. Arthrology
1. Hip
   - The hip is a ball-and-socket type of diarthrodial joint.
   - Stability is based primarily on the bony architecture.
   - The acetabulum is deepened by the fibrocartilaginous labrum.
   - The joint capsule extends anteriorly across the femoral neck to the trochanteric crest.
     - However, it extends posteriorly only partially across the femoral neck.
     - The basocervical and intertrochanteric crest regions are left extracapsular (Figure 2-44).
   - Three ligaments compose the capsule anteriorly.
     - **The iliofemoral ligament (Y ligament of Bigelow) is the strongest ligament in the body and attaches the anterior-inferior iliac spine to the intertrochanteric line in an inverted Y manner.**
     - The remaining anterior ligaments, the ischiofemoral and pubofemoral ligaments, are weaker but provide additional stability.
   - Ligamentum teres:
     - Arises from the apex of the cotyloid notch and attaches to the fovea of the femoral head
     - Transmits an arterial branch of the posterior division of the obturator artery to the femoral head (less significant in adults)

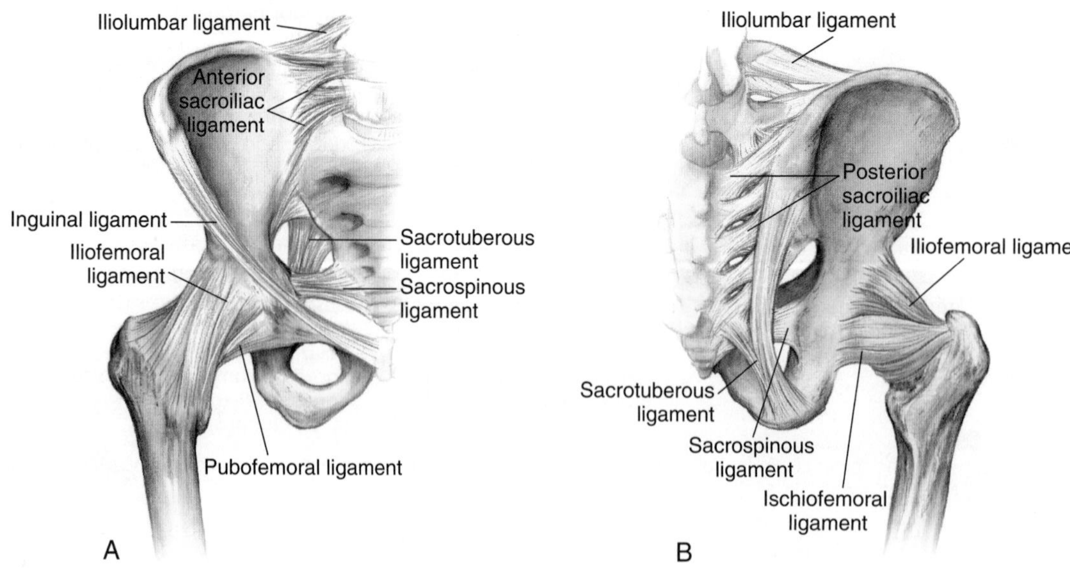

Figure 2-44 Hip capsuloligamentous structures. **A,** Anterior view. The anterior femoral neck is intracapsular. **B,** Posterior view. Because the posterior capsule extends only partially across the femoral neck, the posterior basocervical and intertrochanteric crest regions are extracapsular. (From Miller MD, et al. *Orthopaedic surgical approaches,* Philadelphia, 2008, Saunders, Figures HP-5 and HP-6.)

Table 2-46 Age-Dependent Changes to Blood Supply to Femoral Head

Age	Blood Supply
Birth to 4 yr	Primary medial and lateral circumflex arteries (from deep femoral artery) Ligamentum teres with posterior division of obturator artery
4 yr to adult	Negligible amount from lateral circumflex artery Minimal amount from ligamentum teres Posterosuperior and posteroinferior retinacular from medial femoral circumflex artery
Adult	Medial femoral circumflex to lateral epiphyseal artery

- The blood supply to the femoral head changes with age (Table 2-46), which helps explain why the standard starting point for antegrade femoral nailing is undesirable for pediatric femur fractures.
  - **Using the piriformis as a starting point would damage the posterosuperior retinacular vessels, causing avascular necrosis of the femoral head.**
  - In adults, completely transecting the quadratus femoris muscle in the posterior acetabular approach should be avoided in order to avert damage to the main blood supply to the femoral head–medial femoral circumflex artery.

2. Sacroiliac joint
   - Supported by three groups of ligaments: posterior and anterior sacroiliac ligaments and interosseous ligaments
3. Symphysis pubis
   - Connects the two hemipelvises anteriorly and is united with a fibrocartilaginous disc and supported by the superior and arcuate pubic ligaments
4. Other ligaments
   - These include the sacrospinous and sacrotuberous ligaments, which outline the boundaries for the greater and lesser sciatic foramina (see Figure 2-44).
   - **The sacrospinous ligament (anterior sacrum to the ischial spine) constitutes the inferior border of the greater sciatic foramen and the superior border of the lesser sciatic foramen, effectively separating the greater and lesser sciatic foramina.**
   - The sacrotuberous ligament (posterolateral sacrum to the ischial tuberosity) forms the inferior border of the lesser sciatic foramen.
   - The piriformis, sciatic nerve, and other important structures exit the greater sciatic foramen.
   - The short external rotators of the hip exit the lesser sciatic foramen.

C. **Muscles (Table 2-47; Figure 2-45)**

1. Hip flexor muscles are the iliopsoas, rectus femoris, and sartorius.

Table 2-47 Muscles of the Pelvis and Hip

Muscle	Origin	Insertion	Nerve	Segment
Flexors				
Iliacus	Iliac fossa	Lesser trochanter	Femoral	L2-L4 (P)
Psoas	Transverse processes of L1-L5	Lesser trochanter	Femoral	L2-L4 (P)
Pectineus	Pectineal line of pubis	Pectineal line of femur	Femoral	L2-L4 (P)
Rectus femoris	Anterior inferior iliac spine, acetabular rim	Patella and tibial tubercle	Femoral	L2-L4 (P)
Sartorius	Anterior superior iliac spine	Proximal medial tibia	Femoral	L2-L4 (P)
Adductors				
Posterior adductor magnus	Inferior pubic ramus/ischial tuberosity	Linea aspera/adductor tubercle	Obturator (P) and sciatic (tibial)	L2-L4 (A)
Adductor brevis	Inferior pubic ramus	Linea aspera/pectineal line	Obturator (P)	L2-L4 (A)
Adductor longus	Anterior pubic ramus	Linea aspera	Obturator (A)	L2-L4 (A)
Gracilis	Inferior symphysis/pubic arch	Proximal medial tibia	Obturator (A)	L2-L4 (A)
External Rotators				
Gluteus maximus	Ilium, posterior gluteal line	Iliotibial band/gluteal sling (femur)	Inferior gluteal	L5-S2 (P)
Piriformis	Anterior sacrum/sciatic notch	Proximal greater trochanter	Piriformis	S12 (P)
Obturator externus	Ischiopubic rami/obturator	Trochanteric fossa	Obturator	L2-L4 (A)
Obturator internus	Ischiopubic rami/obturator membrane	Medial greater trochanter	Obturator internus	L5-S2 (A)
Superior gemellus	Outer ischial spine	Medial greater trochanter	Obturator internus	L5-S2 (A)
Inferior gemellus	Ischial tuberosity	Medial greater trochanter	Obturator femoris	L4-S1 (A)
Quadratus femoris	Ischial tuberosity	Quadrate line of femur	Obturator femoris	L4-S1 (A)
Abductors				
Gluteus medius	Ilium between posterior and anterior gluteal lines	Greater trochanter	Superior gluteal	L4-S1 (P)
Gluteus minimus	Ilium between anterior and inferior gluteal lines	Anterior border of greater trochanter	Superior gluteal	L4-S1 (P)
Tensor fasciae latae (tensor fasciae femoris)	Anterior iliac crest	Iliotibial band	Superior gluteal	L4-S1 (P)

A, anterior; P, posterior.

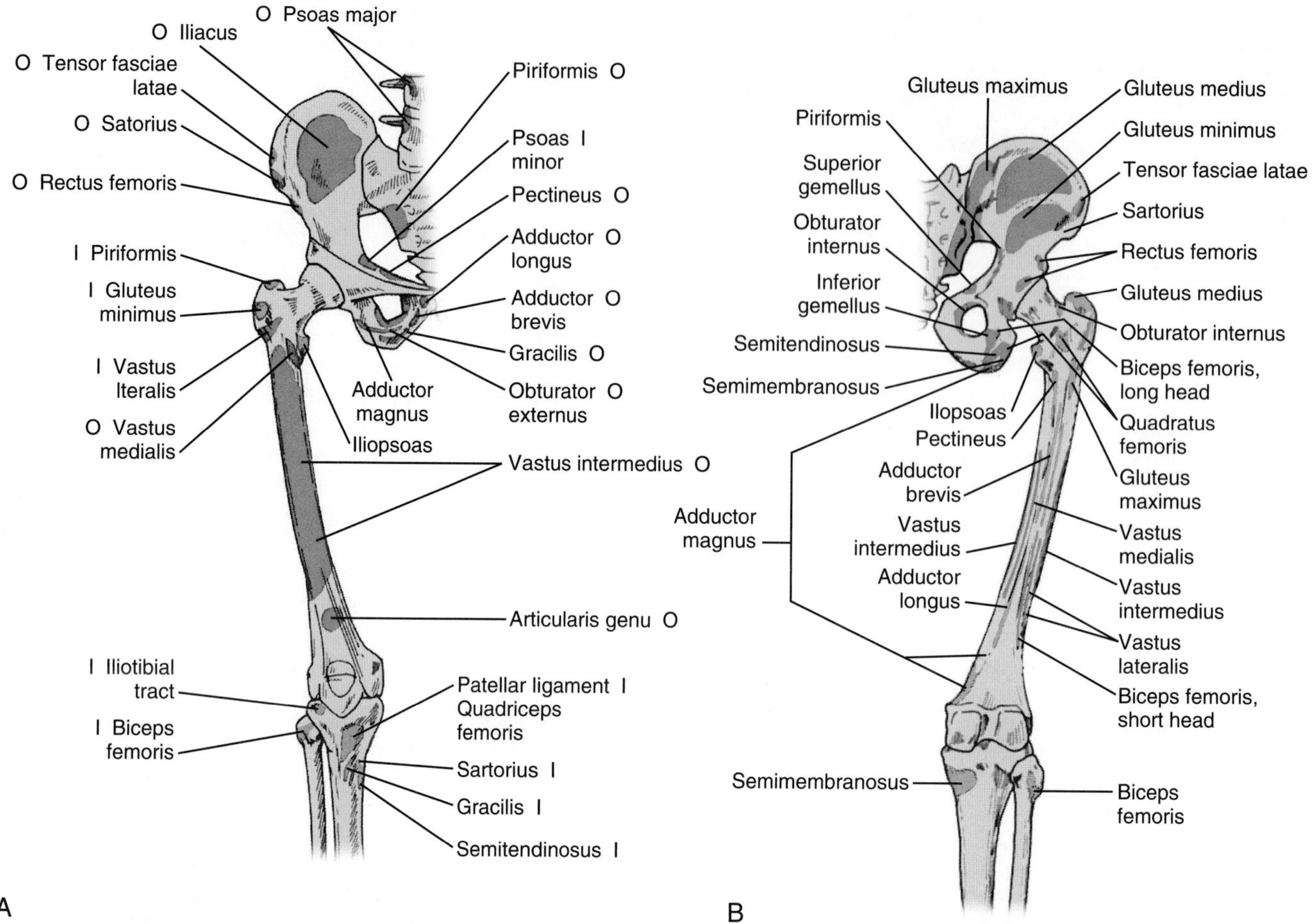

Figure 2-45 Origins (O; *red areas*) and insertions (I; *blue areas*) of muscles of the hip and leg. **A,** Anterior view. **B,** Posterior view. (Adapted from Jenkins DB: *Hollinshead's functional anatomy of the limbs and back,* ed 6, Philadelphia, 1991, Saunders, Figures 16-7 and 17-3.)

2. Hip extensor muscles are the gluteus maximus and hamstrings (semitendinosus, semimembranosus, and long head of biceps femoris).
3. Hip abduction results primarily from the actions of the gluteus medius and minimus. The tensor fasciae latae also helps with abduction in a flexed hip.
4. Hip adduction results primarily from the actions of the adductor brevis, adductor longus, adductor magnus, pectineus, and gracilis.
5. Hip external rotation results from the action of the obturator internus, obturator externus, superior and inferior gemellus, quadratus femoris, and piriformis.
6. Hip internal rotation is provided by secondary actions of the anterior fibers of the gluteus medius and gluteus minimus and by the tensor fasciae latae, semimembranosus, semitendinosus, pectineus, and posterior part of the adductor magnus.

D. **Nerves (see Table 2-44)**

1. Lumbosacral plexus (Figure 2-46; Table 2-48)
   - This plexus is composed of ventral rami from T12 to S3 and lies posterior to the psoas muscle.
   - The sciatic nerve (L4 to S3) has an anterior preaxial tibial nerve division and a postaxial peroneal nerve division.
     - The spatial orientation of the sciatic nerve also places the peroneal division more lateral than the tibial division.
     - This orientation makes it more vulnerable to injury at the time of surgery.
     - **The most common neural injury at the time of primary total hip arthroplasty is the peroneal division of the sciatic nerve.**
     - The only muscle innervated by the peroneal division of the sciatic nerve above the level of the fibular neck is the short head of the biceps femoris.
     - The peroneal division of the sciatic nerve runs on the deep surface of the long head of the biceps femoris.
2. Anatomic spatial relationships
   - The lumbar plexus is found on the anterior surface of the quadratus lumborum under (and within) the substance of the psoas major muscle.
   - The genitofemoral nerve pierces the psoas and then lies on the anteromedial surface of the psoas.
   - The femoral nerve lies between the iliacus and psoas muscles.
   - The lateral femoral cutaneous nerve lies on the surface of the iliacus muscle and exits the pelvis under the lateral attachment of the inguinal ligament.
   - Virtually all the important nerves about the hip leave the pelvis by way of the sciatic foramen.
   - The major reference point for the greater sciatic nerve and related structures in the hip is the piriformis muscle (the "key" to the sciatic foramen).

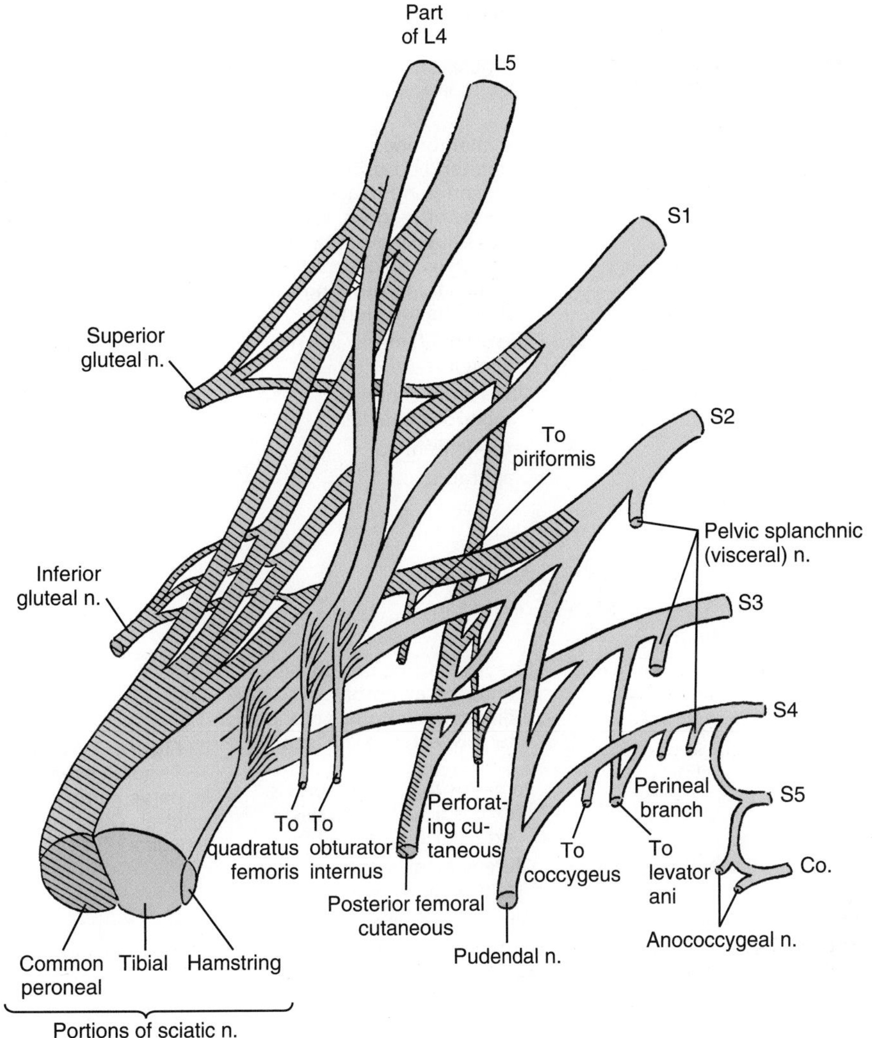

Figure 2-46 Lumbosacral plexus. The anterior division is *unshaded,* and the posterior division is *shaded.* Co., coccyx; Post., posterior; quadr, quadriceps. (From Jenkins DB: *Hollinshead's functional anatomy of the limbs and back,* ed 6, Philadelphia, 1991, Saunders, p 256.)

  - The superior gluteal nerve and artery lie superior to the piriformis, and virtually everything else leaves inferior to the muscle.
  - **Mnemonic for lateral to medial nerves: "POP'S IQ" (pudendal, obturator internus, postfemoral cutaneous, sciatic, inferior gluteal, quadratus femoris).**
- Two nerves leave the greater sciatic foramen and reenter the pelvis via the lesser foramen:
  - The pudendal nerve
  - The nerve to the obturator internus
- Anteriorly, the great nerves and vessels enter the thigh (and into the femoral triangle) under the inguinal ligament (Figure 2-47).
  - The borders of this triangle include the sartorius laterally, the pectineus medially, and the inguinal ligament superiorly.
  - Within the triangle, in a lateral-to-medial direction, are the femoral **n**erve, **a**rtery, and **v**ein **a**nd the **l**ymphatic vessels (mnemonic: "NAVAL").
  - The floor of the femoral triangle (again in a lateral-to-medial direction) is made up of the iliacus, psoas, pectineus, and adductor longus.
- The femoral nerve descends between the iliacus and psoas and delivers numerous branches to muscle, overlying skin, and the hip joint.
  - A spontaneous iliacus hematoma may irritate the femoral nerve because of its proximity.
  - **Hip pain can also manifest as a result of Pott's disease (tuberculous spondylitis) of the spine because of the attachment of the iliopsoas to the lumbar spine.**
- At the apex of the femoral triangle, the saphenous nerve branches off and travels under the sartorius muscle.
- The obturator nerve exits the pelvis via the obturator canal.
  - It splits into anterior and posterior divisions within the canal.
  - The anterior division proceeds anteriorly to the obturator externus and posteriorly to the pectineus, supplying the adductor longus, adductor brevis, and gracilis; it then delivers cutaneous branches to the medial thigh.
  - The posterior division supplies the obturator externus, adductor brevis, and upper part of the adductor

Table 2-48 Lumbosacral Plexus Divisions and Innervations

Nerve	Level	Muscles Innervated
Anterior Division		
Tibia	L4-S3	Semimembranosus, semitendinosusbiceps brachii (long head), adductor magnus, superior gemellus, soleus, plantaris, popliteus, tibialis posterior, flexor digitorum longus, flexor hallucis longus
Quadratus femoris	L4-S1	Quadratus femoris, inferior gemellus
Obturator internus	L5-S2	Obturatorius internus, superior gemellus
Pudendal	S2-S4	Sensory: perineal
Motor: bulbocavernosus, urethra, urogenital		Diaphragm
Coccygeus	S4	Coccygeus
Levator ani	S3-S4	Levator ani
Posterior Division		
Peroneal	L4-S2	Biceps (short head), tibialis anterior, extensor digitorum longus, peroneus tertius, extensor hallucis longus Peroneus longus and brevis, extensor hallucis brevis, extensor digitorum brevis
Superior gluteal	L4-S1	Gluteus medius and minimus, tensor fascia lata
Inferior gluteal	L5-S2	Gluteus maximus
Piriformis	S2	Piriformis
Posterior femoral cutaneous	S1-S3	Sensory: posterior thigh

magnus, and it delivers other branches to the knee joint.

- Pain from the hip can be referred to the knee as a result of the continuation of the obturator nerve anteriorly, which can provide sensation to the medial side of the knee.
- Retractors placed behind the transverse acetabular ligament can injure the obturator nerve and artery.

E. Vessels (Figure 2-48)

1. The aorta branches into the common iliac **arteries anterior to the L4 vertebral body.**
2. The common iliac vessels in turn divide into the internal (or hypogastric [medial] and external [lateral]) iliac vessels at the S1 level.
3. Important internal iliac artery branches are as follows:
   - Obturator (the posterior branch supplies the transverse acetabular ligament)
   - Superior gluteal (can be injured in the sciatic notch)
   - Inferior gluteal (supplies the gluteus maximus and the short external rotators)
   - Internal pudendal (reenters the pelvis through the lesser sciatic notch) (Figure 2-49)
   - **Obturator artery and vein jeopardized by anteroinferior screws and acetabular retractors**

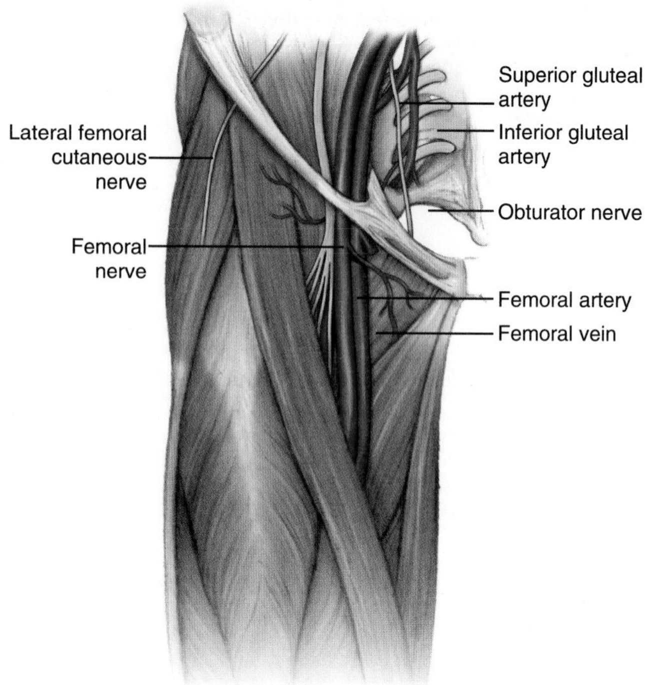

Figure 2-47 Femoral triangle. **The order of structures of the femoral canal from lateral to medial: iliopsoas/iliacus, femoral nerve, femoral artery, femoral vein, and pectineus.** (From Miller MD, et al: *Orthopaedic surgical approaches,* Philadelphia, 2008, Saunders, Figure HP-24.)

4. The corona mortis is an anastomotic connection between the inferior epigastric branch of the external iliac vessels and the obturator vessels in the obturator canal.
   - Can lead to life-threatening bleeding if injured
5. The external iliac artery continues under the inguinal ligament to become the femoral artery.
   - **Can be injured by the placement of acetabular screws in the anterosuperior quadrant during total hip arthroplasty**
   - A summary of the key issues for acetabular screw placement is shown in Table 2-49.
6. The femoral artery enters the femoral triangle.
   - Delivers the profunda femoris, which supplies the anteromedial portion of the thigh
   - Also gives off the femoral artery perforators; these perforators pierce the lateral intermuscular septum to supply the vastus lateralis muscle
   - The profunda femoris has two other important branches:
     - The lateral femoral circumflex, which travels obliquely and deep to the sartorius and rectus femoris

Table 2-49 Placement Zones for Acetabular Screws

Acetabular Zone	Structures at Risk
Posterior-superior	None (safe zone)
Posterior-inferior	None (safe zone)
Anterior-superior	External iliac artery and vein
Anterior-inferior	Anterior inferior obturator nerve; obturator artery and vein

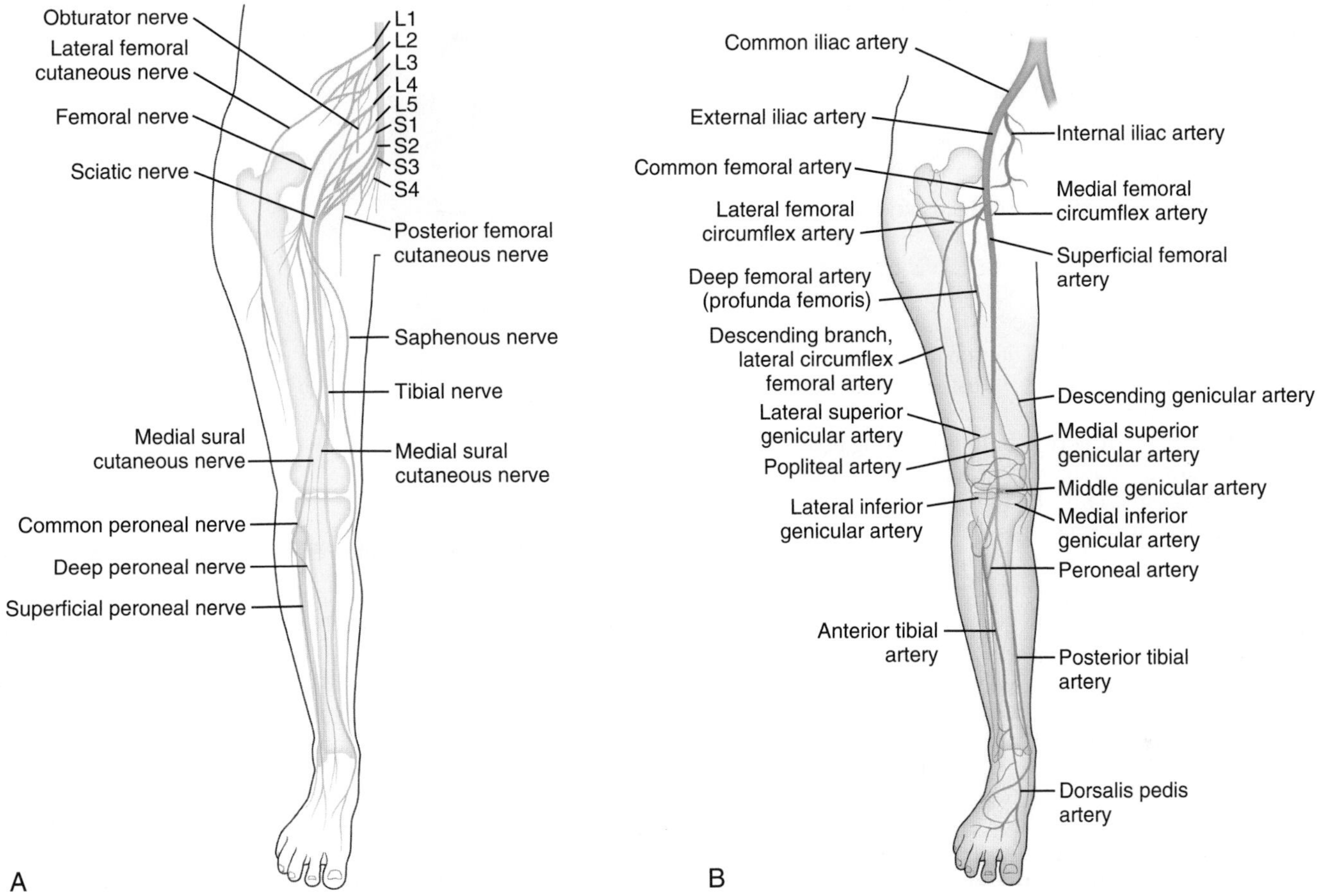

Obturator nerve
Lateral femoral cutaneous nerve
Femoral nerve
Sciatic nerve
L1
L2
L3
L4
L5
S1
S2
S3
S4
Posterior femoral cutaneous nerve
Saphenous nerve
Tibial nerve
Medial sural cutaneous nerve
Medial sural cutaneous nerve
Common peroneal nerve
Deep peroneal nerve
Superficial peroneal nerve
A
Common iliac artery
External iliac artery
Internal iliac artery
Common femoral artery
Medial femoral circumflex artery
Lateral femoral circumflex artery
Superficial femoral artery
Deep femoral artery (profunda femoris)
Descending branch, lateral circumflex femoral artery
Descending genicular artery
Lateral superior genicular artery
Medial superior genicular artery
Popliteal artery
Middle genicular artery
Lateral inferior genicular artery
Medial inferior genicular artery
Peroneal artery
Anterior tibial artery
Posterior tibial artery
Dorsalis pedis artery
B

Figure 2-48 Nerves **(A)** and vessels **(B)** of the lower extremity. (From Miller MD, et al: *Orthopaedic surgical approaches,* Philadelphia, 2008, Saunders, Figures KL-8 and KL-9.)

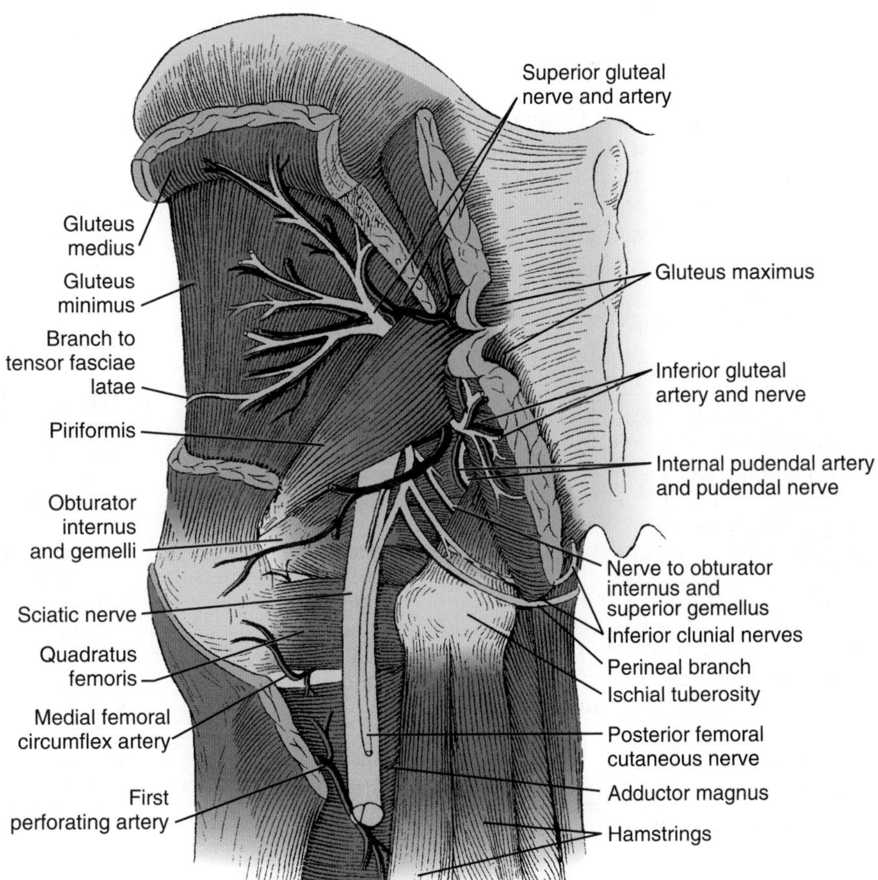

Figure 2-49 Posterior hip anatomy. Note relationship of structures to the piriformis muscle. (From Jenkins DB: *Hollinshead's functional anatomy of the limbs and back,* ed 6, Philadelphia, 1991, Saunders, p 260.)

Superior gluteal nerve and artery
Gluteus medius
Gluteus minimus
Gluteus maximus
Branch to tensor fasciae latae
Inferior gluteal artery and nerve
Piriformis
Internal pudendal artery and pudendal nerve
Obturator internus and gemelli
Nerve to obturator internus and superior gemellus
Sciatic nerve
Inferior clunial nerves
Quadratus femoris
Perineal branch
Ischial tuberosity
Medial femoral circumflex artery
Posterior femoral cutaneous nerve
First perforating artery
Adductor magnus
Hamstrings

- It delivers an ascending branch (at risk for injury during anterolateral approaches) that proceeds to the greater trochanteric region.
- Its descending branch travels laterally under the rectus femoris.

- The medial femoral circumflex, which supplies most of the blood to the femoral head
  - Runs between the pectineus and iliopsoas
  - Then, in the interval, runs between the obturator externus and adductor brevis muscles
  - Finally in the interval, runs between the adductor magnus and brevis
  - Proceeds distally anterior to the quadratus femoris on its cranial edge just distal to the obturator externus
  - Particularly at risk for injury during psoas tenotomy during an anteromedial approach for developmental dysplasia of the hip

7. The cruciate anastomosis is the confluence of the ascending branch of the first perforating artery, the descending branch of the inferior gluteal artery, and the transverse branches of the medial and lateral femoral circumflex arteries.
   - Lies at the inferior margin of the quadratus femoris muscle
8. The superficial femoral artery continues on the medial side of the thigh (between the vastus medialis and adductor longus) toward the adductor (Hunter's) canal.
   - Becomes the popliteal artery in the popliteal fossa in the posteromedial thigh

F. Surgical approaches to the pelvis and hip (Table 2-50)

1. Anterior (Smith-Peterson) approach to the hip (Figure 2-50)
   - Interval: between the sartorius (femoral nerve) and tensor fasciae latae (superior gluteal nerve)
   - Dissection:
     - **Retract the lateral femoral cutaneous nerve anteriorly, and ligate the ascending branch of the lateral femoral circumflex artery (which lies superficial to the rectus).**
     - For deeper dissection, approach the interval between the gluteus medius and rectus femoris.

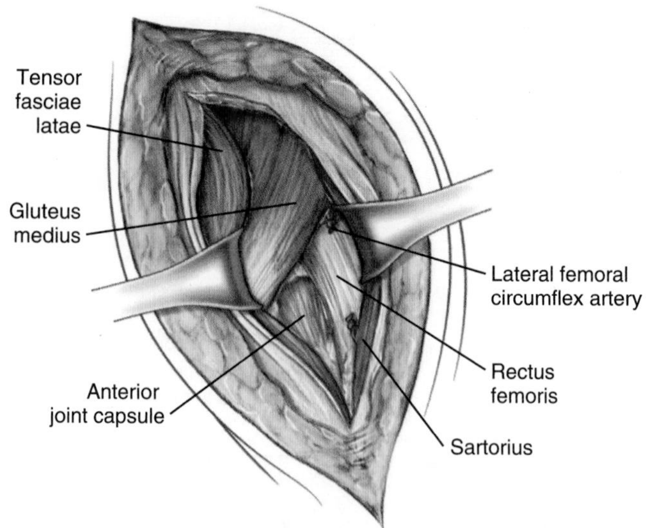

Figure 2-50 **Anterior (Smith-Peterson) surgical approach to the hip. In this approach, the interval between (1) the sartorius and rectus femoris (femoral nerve) and (2) the tensor fasciae latae and gluteus medius (superior gluteal nerve) is explored. The ascending branch of the lateral femoral circumflex artery is ligated.** (From Miller MD, et al: *Orthopaedic surgical approaches,* Philadelphia, 2008, Saunders, Figure HP-49.)

     - Detach the origin of both heads of the rectus femoris.
     - Retract the rectus medially and the gluteus medius laterally.
     - Dissect any attachments of the iliopsoas to the inferior capsule, and perform a capsulotomy.
   - Risks:
     - Lateral femoral cutaneous nerve, which is located anterior or medial to the sartorius muscle, about 6 to 8 cm below the anterior-superior iliac spine, can be injured.
     - Reflection of the conjoined rectus tendon too distally can increase the risk of injury to the descending branch of the lateral femoral circumflex artery.
     - The superficial circumflex artery, which penetrates the tensor fasciae latae just anterior to the lateral femoral cutaneous nerve, can be injured.

Table 2-50 Surgical Approaches to the Hip

Approach	Interval	Structures at Risk
Anterior (Smith-Peterson)	Sartorius and rectus femoris (femoral nerve) and tensor fasciae latae and gluteus medius (superior gluteal nerve)	Lateral femoral cutaneous nerve (6-8 cm below anterior-inferior iliac spine, anterior or medial to sartorius) Ascending branch of lateral femoral circumflex artery (lies superficial to rectus femoris muscle): ligation
Anterolateral (Watson-Jones)	Tensor fasciae latae (superior gluteal nerve) and gluteus medius (superior gluteal nerve)	Femoral nerve: because of excessive medial retraction Descending lateral femoral circumflex artery: injury
Lateral (Hardinge's)	Gluteus medius (superior gluteal nerve) and vastus lateralis (femoral nerve)	Femoral nerve, artery, and vein Lateral femoral circumflex artery
Posterior (Moore-Southern)	Gluteus maximus (inferior gluteal nerve) and gluteus medius/tensor fasciae latae (superior gluteal nerve)	Sciatic nerve and inferior gluteal artery, during the gluteus maximus muscle split Medial femoral circumflex artery: ligation if quadratus femoris transected
Medial (Ludloff's)	Adductor longus and adductor brevis (obturator nerve) and gracilis and adductor magnus (obturator/tibial nerve)	Anterior division of obturator nerve Medial femoral circumflex artery Deep external pudendal artery

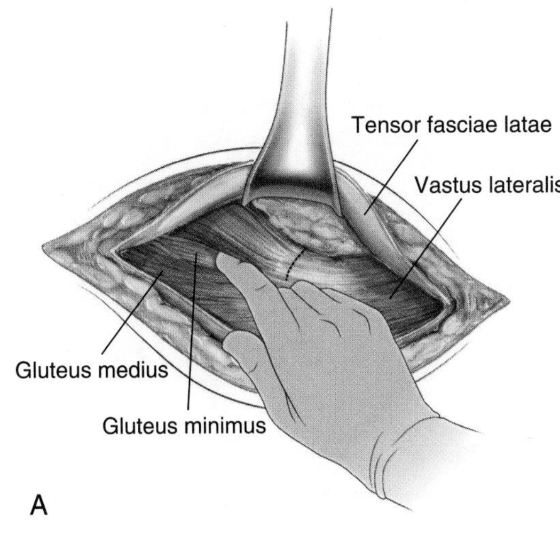

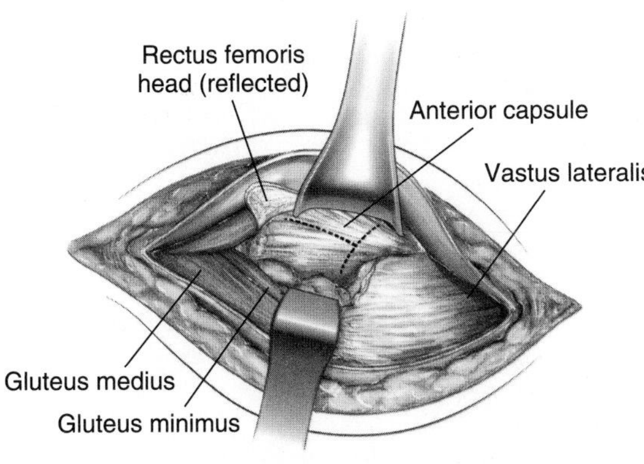

Figure 2-51 **Anterolateral (Watson-Jones) approach to the hip. A, Superficial exposure. B, Deep exposure. In this approach, the interval between the tensor fasciae latae (superior gluteal nerve) and the gluteus medius (superior gluteal nerve) is explored.** (From Miller MD, et al: *Orthopaedic surgical approaches,* Philadelphia, 2008, Saunders, Figures HP-80 and HP-81.)

- Femoral nerve and vessels can sometimes be injured by aggressive medial retraction of the sartorius.

2. Anterolateral (Watson-Jones) approach to the hip (Figure 2-51)
   - Interval: There is no true interneural plane, but the intermuscular plane between the tensor fasciae latae and gluteus medius is used.
   - Dissection:
     - Split the fasciae latae, to expose the vastus lateralis.
     - Detach the anterior third of the gluteus medius from the greater trochanter and the entire gluteus minimus.
     - Dissect the reflected head of the rectus femoris (and capsular attachment of the iliopsoas, if necessary), and retract medially to gain access to the capsule.
   - Risks:
     - Femoral nerve can be injured by excessive medial retraction.
     - Denervation of the tensor fascia latae can occur if the intermuscular interval is exploited too superiorly (the superior gluteal nerve lies about 5 cm above the acetabular rim).
     - Injury to the descending branch of the lateral femoral circumflex artery can occur with anterior and inferior dissection.
3. Lateral (Hardinge's) approach to the hip (Figure 2-52)
   - Interval: splitting of the gluteus medius and vastus lateralis in tandem
   - Dissection:
     - Incise the skin and the fascia lata to expose the gluteus medius and the vastus lateralis.
     - Incise the gluteus medius from the greater trochanter, leaving a cuff of tissue and the posterior half to two thirds attached.
     - Extend this incision to split the gluteus medius proximally.
     - Split the vastus lateralis distally along its anterior fourth down to the femoral shaft.
     - Detach the gluteus minimus from its insertion.
     - The hip capsule is now exposed for further dissection.
   - Risks: injury to the femoral nerve and possible denervation of the gluteus medius (superior gluteal nerve) if the split is too proximal (more than 5 cm proximal to the greater trochanter)
4. Posterior (Moore's or Southern's) approach to the hip (Figure 2-53)
   - Interval: splitting the fibers of the gluteus maximus
   - Dissection:
     - Incise the skin and the fascia lata along the posterior border of the femur, and then split the fibers of the gluteus maximus bluntly.
     - Expose the short external rotators close to their insertions into the greater trochanter, and reflect them laterally to protect the sciatic nerve and expose the posterior hip capsule.
     - A portion of the quadratus femoris may be taken down with the short external rotators, but be aware of the significant bleeding that can come from the inferior portion of this muscle (ascending branches of the medial femoral circumflex artery).
   - Risks:
     - Sciatic neurapraxia if the sciatic nerve is not properly protected by the short external rotators
     - Damage to the inferior gluteal artery during the splitting of the gluteus maximus
5. Medial (Ludloff's) approach to the hip (Figure 2-54)
   - Interval:
     - Between the adductor longus and gracilis superficially
     - Between the adductor brevis (anterior) and magnus (posterior) at the deep level
   - Risks:
     - **Anterior division of the obturator nerve and medial femoral circumflex artery (between the adductor brevis and the adductor magnus/pectineus)**
     - Deep external pudendal artery (anterior to the pectineus near the adductor longus origin) is also at risk proximally for injury.
6. Acetabular approaches: used primarily for open reduction with internal fixation (ORIF) of pelvic fractures
   - These approaches are basically extensions of incisions for exposure of the hip (discussed earlier).

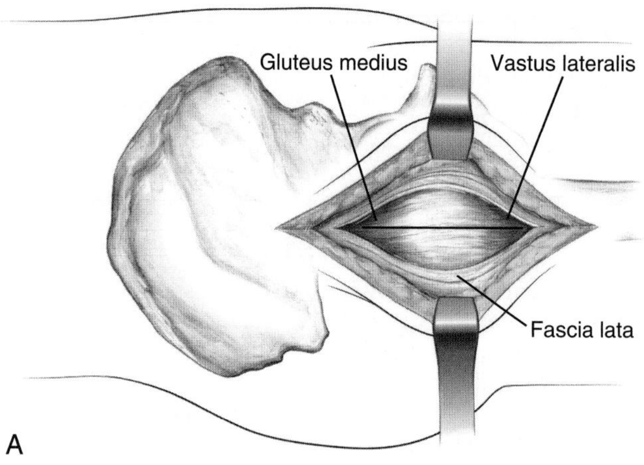

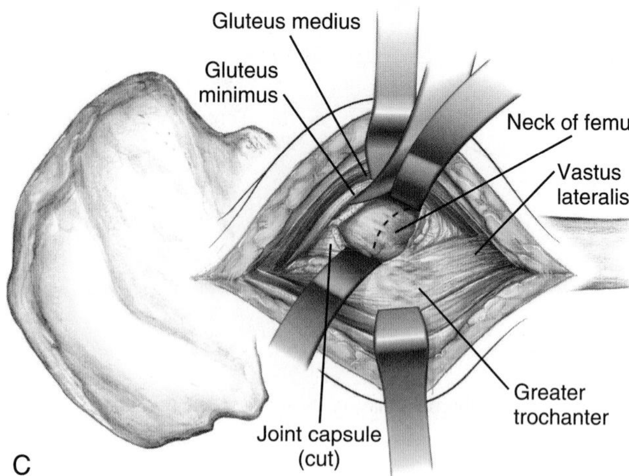

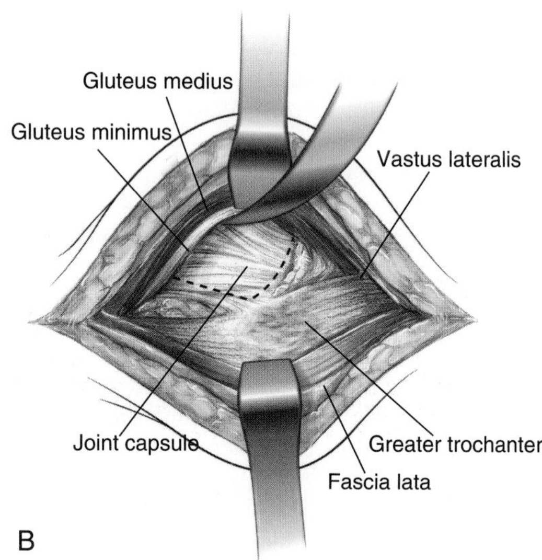

Figure 2-52 Lateral (Hardinge's) approach to the hip. **A,** Superficial exposure. **B,** Deep exposure. **C,** Close-up view of deep exposure. In this approach, the interval between the gluteus medius (superior gluteal nerve) and the vastus lateralis (femoral nerve) is explored. (From Miller MD, et al: *Orthopaedic surgical approaches,* Philadelphia, 2008, Saunders, Figures HP-72, HP-73, and HP-74.)

- The Kocher-Langenbeck incision is a posterolateral approach that provides access to the posterior column/acetabulum.
- The ilioinguinal incision relies on mobilization of the rectus abdominis and iliacus.
  - ▫ This incision exposes the anterior column (Figure 2-55).
  - ▫ Three windows are available with this approach:
    - The first window gives access to the internal iliac fossa, the anterior sacroiliac joint, and the upper portion of the anterior column.
    - The second window (between the iliopectineal fascia and the external iliac vessels) provides access to the pelvic brim from the anterior sacroiliac joint to the lateral portion of the superior pubic ramus.
    - The third window (below the vessels and the spermatic cord) gives access to the symphysis pubis.
- The extended iliofemoral incision allows access to both columns by reflecting the gluteal muscles and tensor posteriorly and dividing the obturator internus and piriformis.

G. **Arthroscopy**

1. The portals for hip arthroscopy include the anterolateral and posterolateral portals (adjacent to the superior border of the greater trochanter) and the anterior portal (risk for injury to the femoral and lateral femoral cutaneous nerves).

H. **Cross-sectional anatomy (Figures 2-56, 2-57, and 2-58)**

II. THIGH

A. **Osteology of the femur**

1. Introduction
   - The neck-shaft angle averages approximately 127 degrees, although it begins at 141 degrees in the fetus.
   - Femoral anteversion varies from 1 to 40 degrees but averages 14 degrees.
   - The femur has an anterior bow.
   - There are two femoral condyles:
     - ▫ The medial condyle is larger.
     - ▫ The more prominent medial epicondyle supports the adductor tubercle.

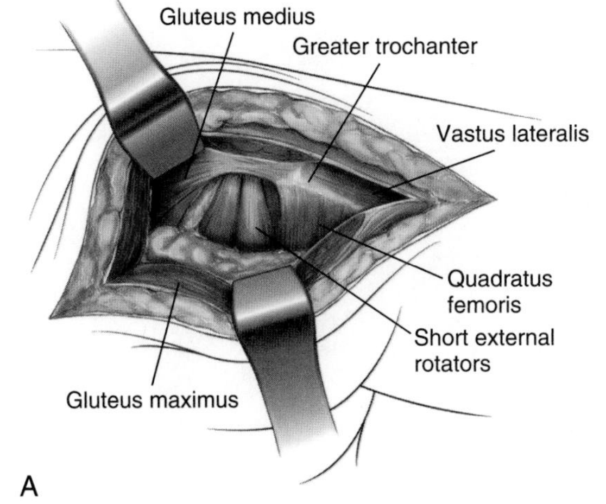

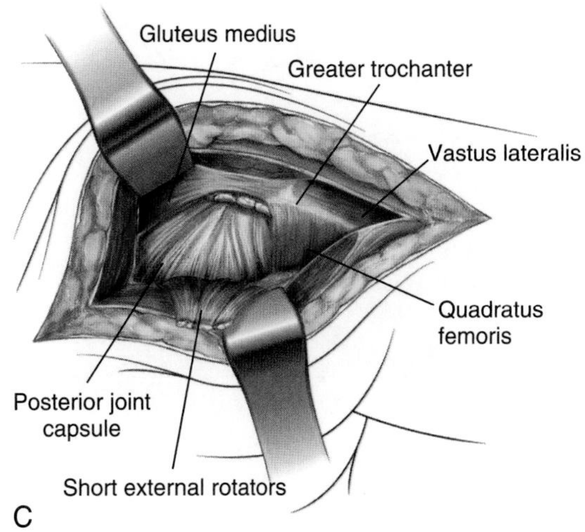

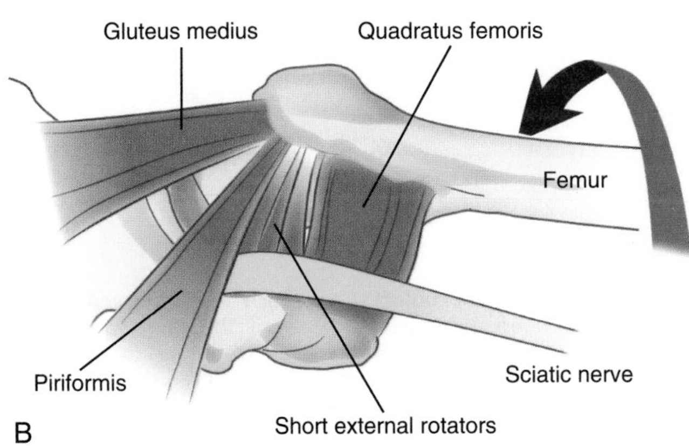

Figure 2-53 Posterior (Moore's or Southern's) approach to the hip. **A,** Superficial exposure. **B,** Relationship of muscles to bones. **C,** Deep exposure. In this approach, the interval between the gluteus maximus (inferior gluteal nerve) and the gluteus medius/tensor fascia lata (superior gluteal nerve) is explored. (From Miller MD, et al: *Orthopaedic surgical approaches,* Philadelphia, 2008, Saunders, Figures HP-58, HP-59, and HP-60.)

2. Ossification: the important areas of femoral ossification include the head and the distal femur.
   - The femoral head is usually not present at birth but appears as one large physis that includes both trochanters at about the age of 11 months and fuses at age 18 years.
   - **Slipped capital femoral epiphysis occurs through the femoral head physis (zone of hypertrophy).**
   - The distal femoral epiphysis is present at birth and fuses at age 19 years.

B. Muscles (Figures 2-59, 2-60, and 2-61; Table 2-51)

1. Anterior thigh

Table 2-51 Muscles of the Thigh

Muscle	Origin	Insertion	Innervation
Anterior Thigh			
Vastus lateralis	Iliotibial line/greater trochanter/lateral linea aspera	Lateral patella	Femoral
Vastus medialis	Iliotibial line/medial linea aspera/supracondylar line	Medial patella	Femoral
Vastus intermedius	Proximal anterior femoral shaft	Patella	Femoral
Posterior Thigh			
Biceps femoris (long head)	Medial ischial tuberosity	Fibular head/lateral tibia	Tibial
Biceps (short head)	Lateral linea aspera/lateral intermuscular septum	Lateral tibial condyle	Peroneal
Semitendinosus	Distal medial ischial tuberosity	Anterior tibial crest	Tibial
Semimembranosus	Proximal lateral ischial tuberosity	Oblique popliteal ligament Posterior capsule Posterior/medial tibia Popliteus Medial meniscus	Tibial

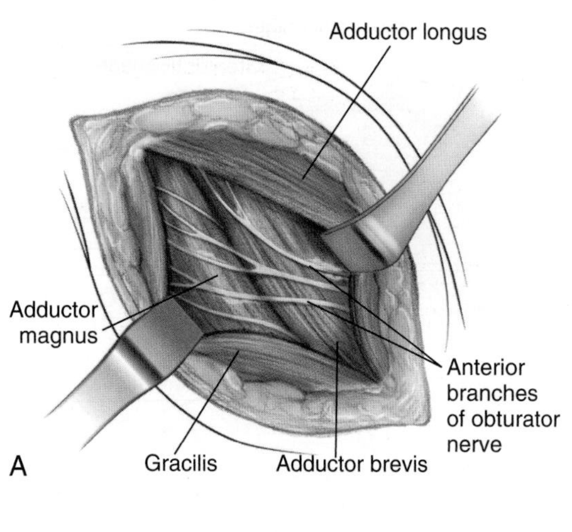

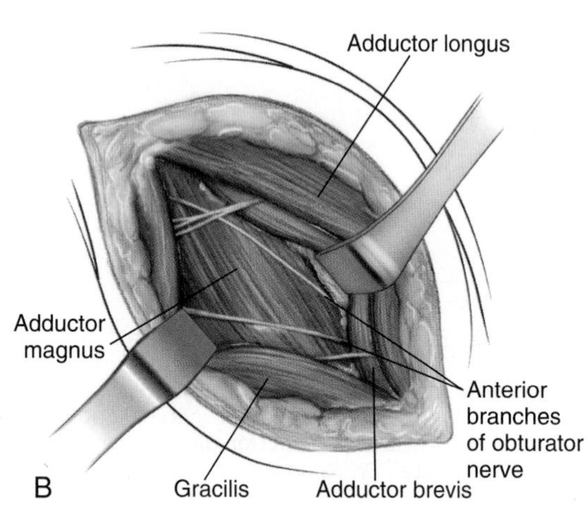

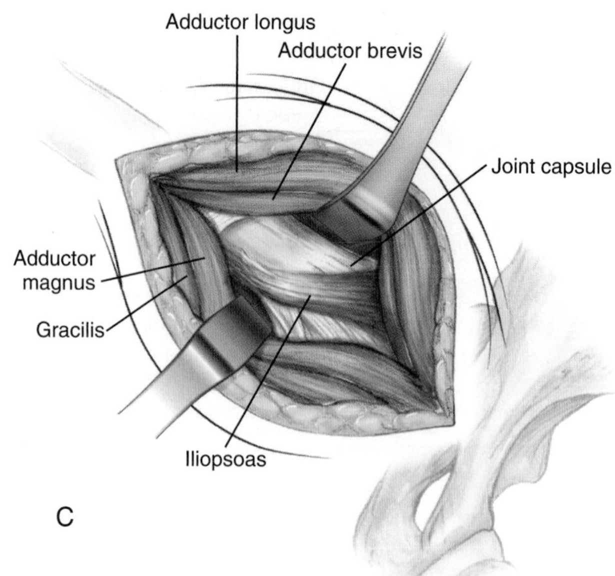

Figure 2-54 Medial (Ludloff's) approach to the hip. **A,** Superficial exposure. **B,** Deep exposure. **C,** View of the joint capsule. In this approach, the interval between the adductor longus (obturator nerve) and the gracilis (obturator nerve) is explored. (From Miller MD, et al: *Orthopaedic surgical approaches,* Philadelphia, 2008, Saunders, Figures HP-65, HP-66, and HP-67.)

2. Medial thigh (see Table 2-47 for adductors)
3. Posterior thigh

C. Nerves (also see the preceding discussion on the pelvis and hip and the following discussion on the knee and leg)

1. Anatomy
   - The sciatic nerve (L4 to S3)
     - Emerges from its foramen anterior to the piriformis muscle (through the piriformis in 2% of people) and lies posterior to the other short external rotators
     - Descends below the gluteus maximus and proceeds posteriorly to the adductor magnus and between the long head of the biceps femoris and semimembranosus
     - Before it emerges from the popliteal fossa, it divides into the common peroneal nerve and the tibial nerve.
     - **The peroneal division has one innervation in the thigh: the short head of the biceps femoris.**
     - The common peroneal nerve diverges laterally and traverses the lateral knee region under cover of the biceps femoris.
     - The tibial nerve emerges into the popliteal fossa laterally, proceeds posteriorly to the vessel, and then descends between the heads of the gastrocnemius.
   - The femoral nerve (L2 to L4)
     - This is the largest branch of the lumbar plexus and supplies the thigh muscles.
     - Largest branch of the femoral nerve is the saphenous nerve.
     - **The infrapatellar branch of the saphenous nerve supplies the skin of the medial side of the front of the knee and patellar ligament and can be damaged during total knee replacement surgery.**
   - The lateral femoral cutaneous nerve (L2 to L3)
     - Supplies the skin and fascia on the surface of the anterolateral thigh from the greater trochanter to the knee
     - Can be damaged by acetabular approaches that dissect around its course underneath the lateral end of the inguinal ligament
   - The obturator nerve (L2 to L4)
     - Can be damaged during various hip and acetabular approaches (by screw placement in the anteroinferior quadrant), resulting in a decrease in sensation in the medial thigh and loss of hip adductor function
     - Has two branches after it passes through the obturator foramen:
       - The anterior branch (adductor longus, adductor brevis, gracilis) and the posterior branch (obturator

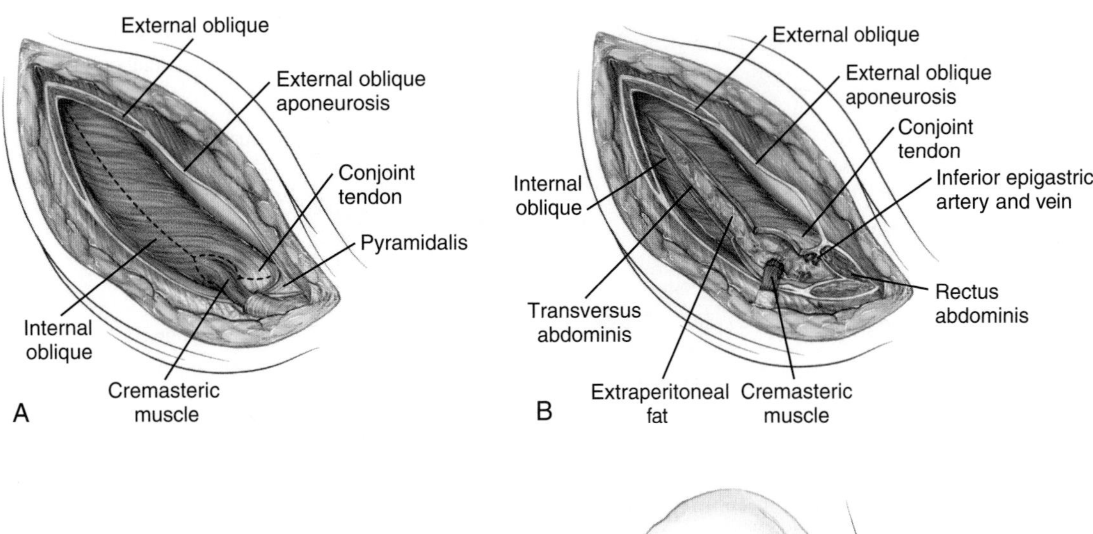

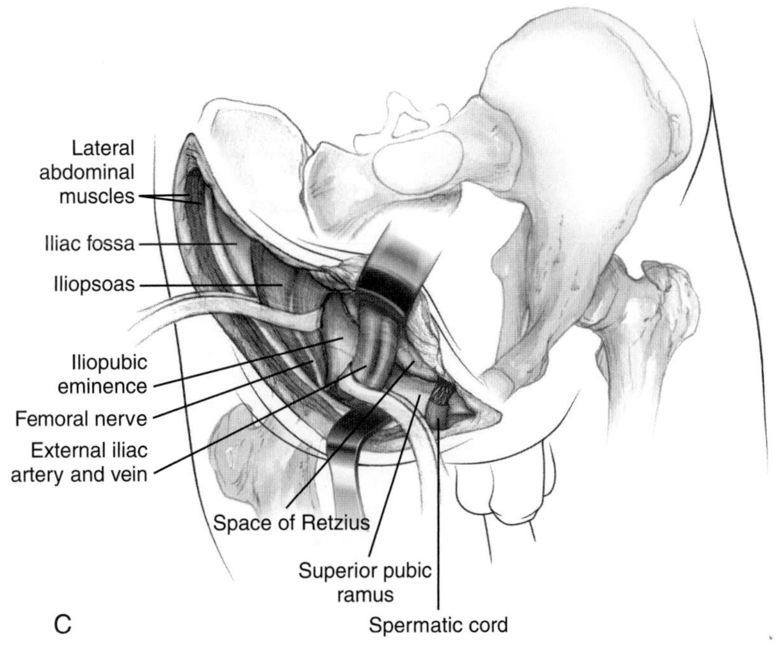

Figure 2-55 The ilioinguinal approach. **A,** Dissection through the external oblique fascia and around the inguinal ring. **B,** Dissection around the spermatic cord (men and boys) or round ligament (women and girls) and through the transversus abdominis. **C,** The three working windows of the approach. The first window of the ilioinguinal approach gives access to the internal iliac fossa, the anterior sacroiliac joint, and the upper portion of the anterior column. The second window of the ilioinguinal approach gives access to the pelvic brim from the anterior sacroiliac joint to the lateral extremity of the superior pubic ramus. The quadrilateral surface and posterior column are accessible beyond the pelvic brim. The third window gives access to the symphysis pubis and retropubic space of Retzius, medial to the spermatic cord and femoral vessels. (Modified from Miller MD, et al: *Orthopaedic surgical approaches,* Philadelphia, 2008, Saunders, Figures HP-39, HP-40, and HP-41.)

externus, adductor magnus, adductor brevis [variable])

- **The anterior branch of the obturator nerve can provide sensation to the medial side of the knee and can be a source of referred pain from hip pathology.**

2. Innervation (Table 2-52; see also Table 2-44)

D. Vessels (also see the preceding discussion on the pelvis and hip and the following discussion on the knee and leg)

1. Anatomy
   - The external iliac artery becomes the femoral artery after it traverses the inguinal ligament, arriving at the femoral triangle.

Table 2-52 Innervation of the Thigh

Nerve	Components	Muscles Innervated
Femoral	L2-L4	Iliacus, psoas major (lower part), sartorius, pectineus, quadriceps, articularis genus
Obturator	L2-L4	Obturator externus, hip adductors (brevis, longus, magnus), gracilis
Sciatic	L4-S3	Peroneal division: short head of biceps femoris Tibial division: hamstrings (semitendinosus, semimembranosus), part of adductor magnus, long head of biceps femoris

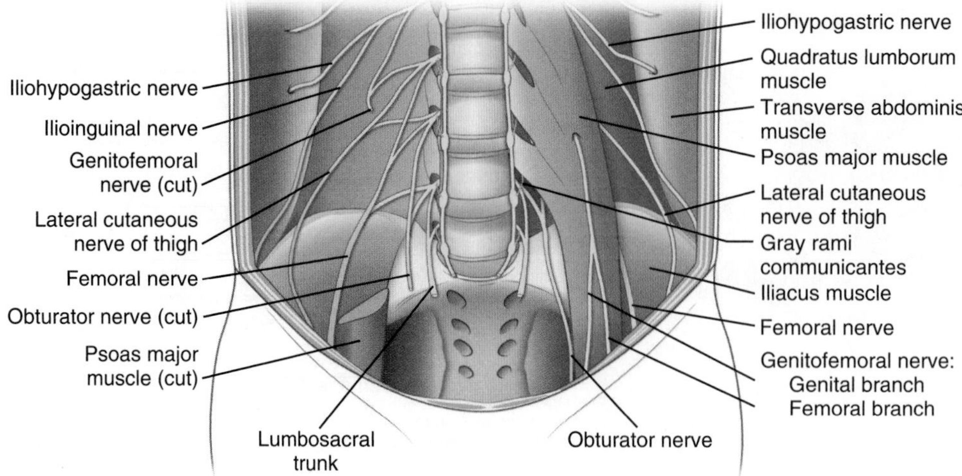

Figure 2-56 Cross-sectional coronal view of anatomy of the pelvis and lumbosacral region. (From Miller MD, et al: *Orthopaedic surgical approaches,* Philadelphia, 2008, Saunders, Figure HP-18.)

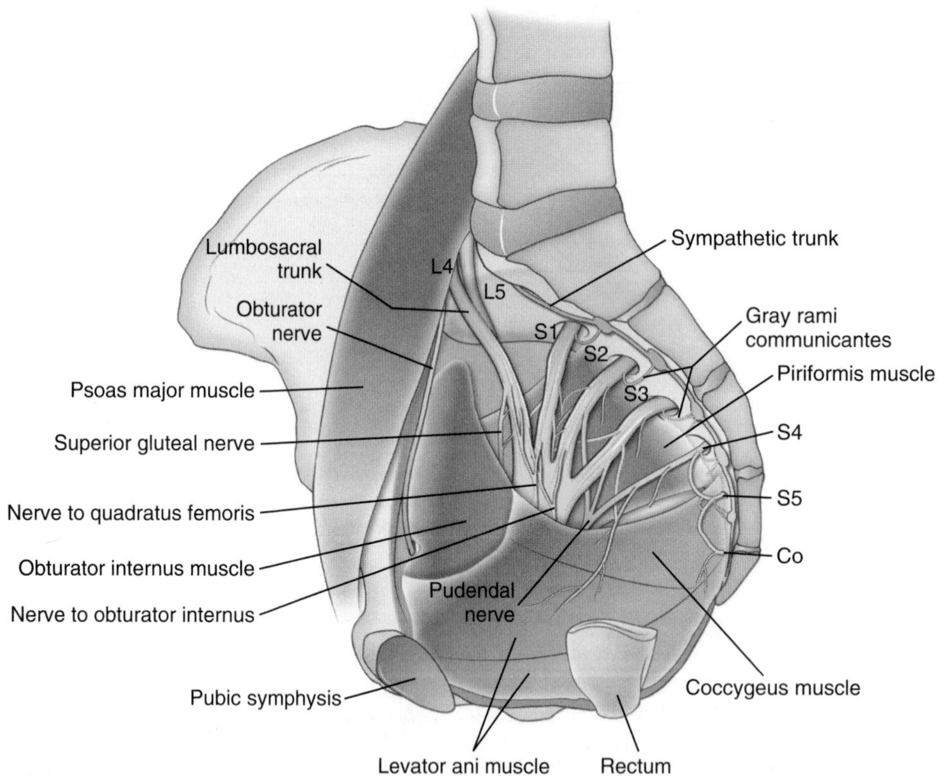

Figure 2-57 Cross-sectional sagittal view of anatomy of the pelvis and lumbosacral region. (From Miller MD, et al: *Orthopaedic surgical approaches,* Philadelphia, 2008, Saunders, Figure HP-19.)

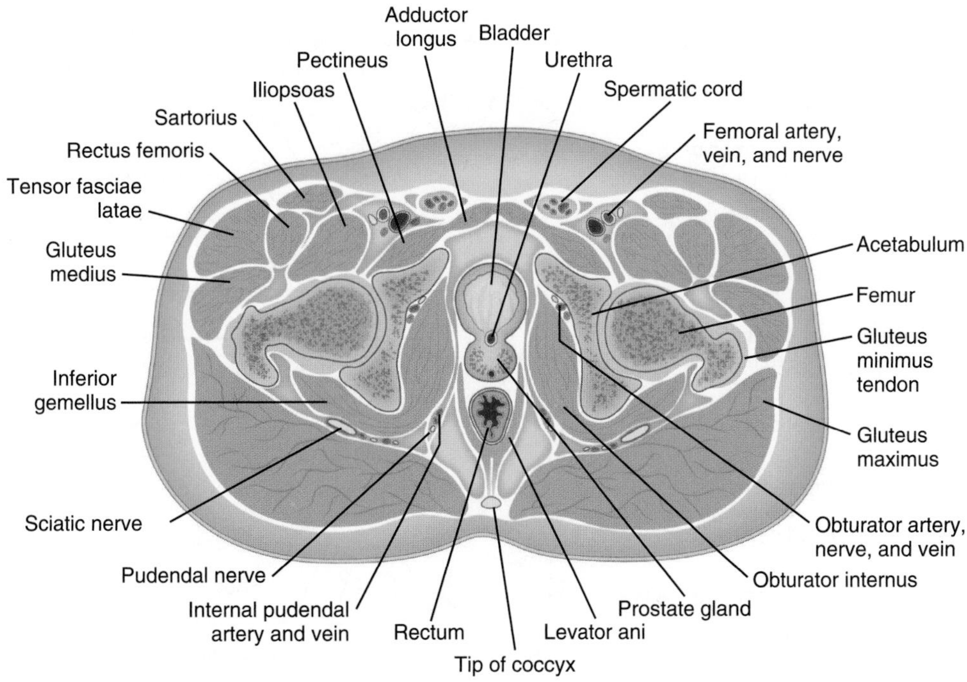

Figure 2-58 Cross-sectional transverse view of anatomy of the proximal femur and pelvis at the level of the hip joint. Note the course of the obturator internus. (From Miller MD, et al: *Orthopaedic surgical approaches,* Philadelphia, 2008, Saunders, Figure HP-23.)

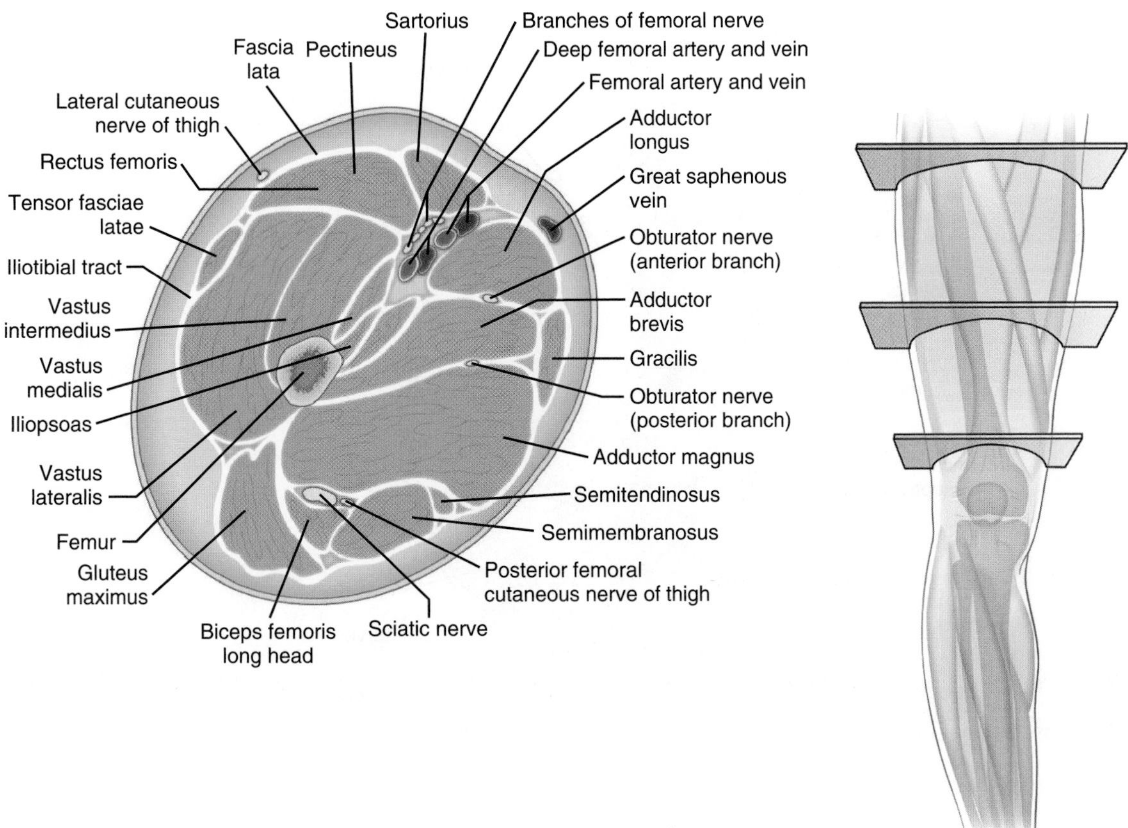

Figure 2-59 Cross-sectional view of the proximal thigh. (From Miller MD, et al: *Orthopaedic surgical approaches,* Philadelphia, 2008, Saunders, Figure HP-20.)

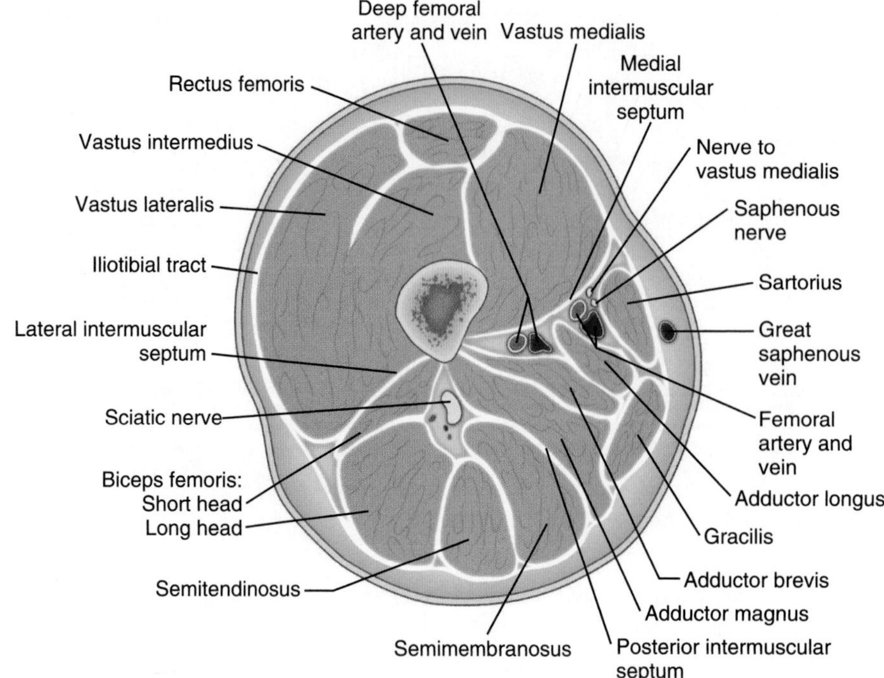

Figure 2-60 Cross-sectional view of the middle thigh. Note the relationship of the sciatic nerve to the two heads of the biceps femoris. (From Miller MD, et al: *Orthopaedic surgical approaches,* Philadelphia, 2008, Saunders, Figure HP-21.)

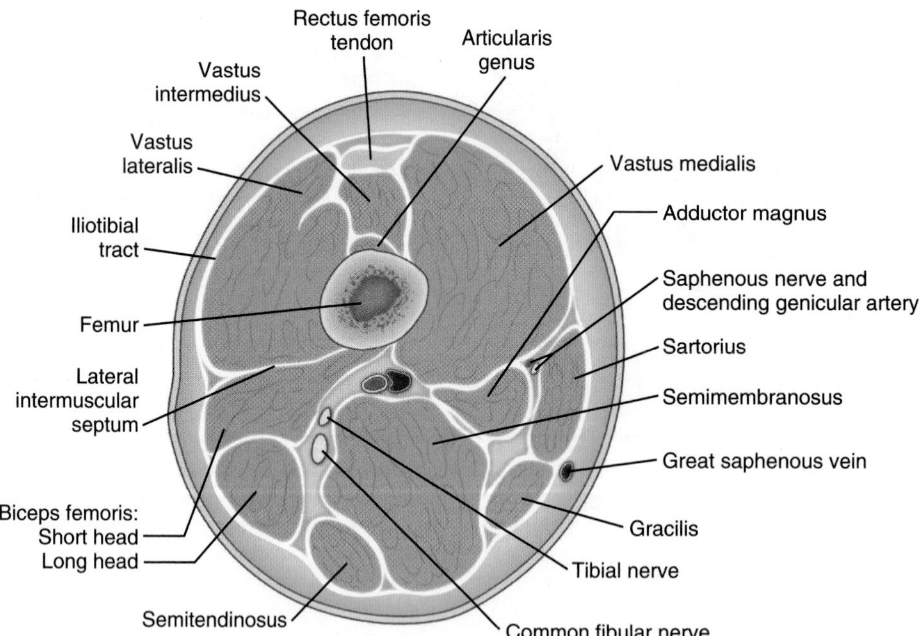

Figure 2-61 Cross-sectional view of the distal thigh. (From Miller MD, et al: *Orthopaedic surgical approaches,* Philadelphia, 2008, Saunders, Figure HP-22.)

- The femoral artery branches to become the deep femoral artery and the superficial femoral artery.
  - The deep femoral artery gives rise to the medial and lateral femoral circumflex arteries.
    - The medial femoral circumflex artery is the major blood supply to the femoral head in the adult and lies anterior to the quadratus femoris muscle.
  - After giving off the profunda femoris (described earlier), the superficial femoral artery descends under cover of the sartorius muscle and proceeds between the adductor group and the vastus medialis into the adductor canal.
    - At the level above the medial femoral condyle, the artery gives off a descending geniculate branch, then passes through a defect in the adductor magnus (adductor hiatus), and finally emerges in the popliteal fossa.
    - The vein is usually posterior to the artery.
- The obturator artery is a branch of the internal iliac artery.
  - Its **posterior branch supplies the ligamentum teres acetabular artery. This artery is an important source of blood to the femoral head from birth to the age of 4 years.**
- The internal iliac artery also supplies the superior and inferior gluteal arteries.

2. Vessels at risk for injury (Table 2-53)

E. Surgical approaches to the thigh (Table 2-54)

1. Lateral approach to the thigh
   - Used for ORIF of intertrochanteric and femoral neck fractures; can be extended for access to shaft and supracondylar fractures
   - Interval: none
   - Dissection:
     - Split the fascia lata in line with the femoral shaft.
     - If necessary, include part of the tensor fasciae latae.
     - Then bluntly dissect the vastus lateralis in line with its fibers, or dissect the fibers of the intermuscular septum.
     - Identify and cauterize the various perforators from the profunda femoris.
2. Posterolateral approach to the thigh
   - Interval: between the vastus lateralis (femoral nerve) and hamstrings (sciatic nerve)

Table 2-53 Thigh Vessels at Risk During Surgical Procedures

Approach	Vascular Structures at Risk
Anterior hip (Smith-Peterson)	Ascending branch of lateral femoral circumflex artery (superficial to rectus femoris muscle)
Anterolateral hip (Watson-Jones)	Descending branch of lateral femoral circumflex artery
Medial hip (Ludloff's)	Medial femoral circumflex artery and deep external pudendal artery (at risk for injury during percutaneous tenotomy of adductor longus)
Lateral and posterolateral thigh	Perforators from profunda femoris artery
Anteromedial distal femur	Medial superior geniculate artery

Table 2-54 Surgical Approaches to the Thigh

Approach	Interval	Structures at Risk
Lateral	Vastus lateralis (femoral nerve)	Perforators from the profunda femoris artery
Posterolateral	Vastus lateralis (femoral nerve) and hamstrings (sciatic nerve)	Perforators from the profunda femoris artery
Anteromedial (distal)	Rectus femoris (femoral nerve) and vastus medialis (femoral nerve)	Medial superior geniculate artery, infrapatellar branch of saphenous nerve
Posterior	Biceps femoris (sciatic nerve) and vastus lateralis (femoral nerve)	Posterior femoral cutaneous nerve (between biceps and semitendinosus) and sciatic nerve

   - Dissection: Incise the fascia under the iliotibial band and retract the vastus superiorly. Continue anteriorly to the lateral intermuscular septum with blunt dissection until the periosteum over the linea aspera is reached.
   - Risks: This dissection entails risk for injury in the series of perforating vessels from the profunda femoris that pierce the lateral intermuscular septum to reach the vastus. If they are approached without care, vessels can retract and bleed underneath the septum.
3. Anteromedial approach to the distal femur
   - Interval: between the rectus femoris and vastus medialis (femoral nerve) and extending to a point medial to the patella
   - Dissection:
     - Retract the rectus laterally.
     - Explore the interval to reveal the vastus intermedius.
     - It may be necessary to open the knee joint.
     - If so, incise the medial patellar retinaculum and split a portion of the quadriceps tendon just lateral to the medial border.
     - After identifying the vastus intermedius, split it along its fibers to expose the femur.
   - Risks:
     - The medial superior geniculate artery and the infrapatellar branch of the saphenous nerve can be injured because both cross the site of exposure.
     - In addition, an adequate cuff of tissue must be left for a strong patellar retinacular repair; otherwise, there is a risk of lateral subluxation of the patella.

F. Cross-sectional anatomy (see Figures 2-59, 2-60, and 2-61)

III. KNEE AND LEG

A. Osteology

1. Patella: the largest sesamoid bone
   - Serves three functions:
     - Serves as a fulcrum for the quadriceps
     - Protects the knee joint
     - Enhances lubrication and nutrition of the knee
   - An accessory or "bipartite" patella may represent failure of fusion of the superolateral corner of the patella and is commonly confused with patellar fractures.

2. Tibia
   - The tibia articulates with the distal femur by means of proximal medial facet (oval and concave) and lateral facet (circular and convex).
   - The Gerdy tubercle lies on the lateral side of the proximal tibia and is the insertion of the iliotibial tract.
   - Tibial shaft is triangular in cross-section and tapers to its thinnest point at the junction of the middle and distal thirds before widening again to form the tibial plafond.
   - Distally, the tibia forms an inferior quadrilateral surface for articulation with the talus and the pyramid-shaped medial malleolus.
   - Laterally, the fibular notch forms an articulation with the fibula.
3. Fibula
   - The styloid process of the head serves as the attachment for the fibular collateral ligament and the biceps tendon.
   - Lying just below the head, the neck of the fibula is grooved by the common peroneal nerve.
   - The expanded distal fibula is known as the *lateral malleolus* and extends beyond the distal margin of the medial malleolus.
     - Together with the inferior distal surface of the tibia, these structures make up the ankle mortise.

B. Arthrology

1. Knee
   - Enclosed in a capsule that has posteromedial and posterolateral recesses **extending 15 mm distal to the subchondral surface of the tibial plateau (be careful to avoid intraarticular pin placement).**
   - Medial and lateral femoral condyles articulate with the corresponding tibial facets.
   - Menisci
     - Serve to deepen the concavity of the facets, help protect the articular surface, and assist in rotation of the knee (Figure 2-62).
     - Peripheral thirds of the menisci are vascular and can be repaired; the inner two thirds are nourished by synovial fluid.
     - **The medial meniscus tears three times more often than the more mobile lateral meniscus.**
       - The saphenous nerve must be protected during repairs to the medial meniscus.
     - The lateral meniscus is associated with meniscal cysts and discoid menisci and is the most common site of tears in acute injuries to the anterior cruciate ligament (ACL).
       - The peroneal nerve must be protected during repairs to the lateral meniscus.
   - Ligaments
     - Stability of the knee is enhanced by a complex arrangement of ligaments (Table 2-55).
     - The cruciate ligaments are crucial for anteroposterior stability, and the collateral ligaments provide varus and valgus stability.
     - Each cruciate ligament is made up of two portions, or bundles.
     - **The anterior bundles of the ACL and posterior cruciate ligament (PCL) are tight in flexion.**
     - The PCL has an anterolateral bundle, and the ACL has an anteromedial bundle.
     - Mnemonic: "PAL" (**P**CL has **a**ntero**l**ateral bundles)
       - Thus, the ACL is composed of an anteromedial portion that is tight in flexion and a posterolateral portion that is tight in extension.
       - The PCL has an anterolateral portion that is tight in flexion and a posteromedial portion that is tight in extension.
     - The PCL lies between the ligament of Humphrey (anterior) and the Wrisberg ligament (posterior).
     - The posterolateral corner comprises the arcuate ligament, popliteus, posterolateral capsule, lateral

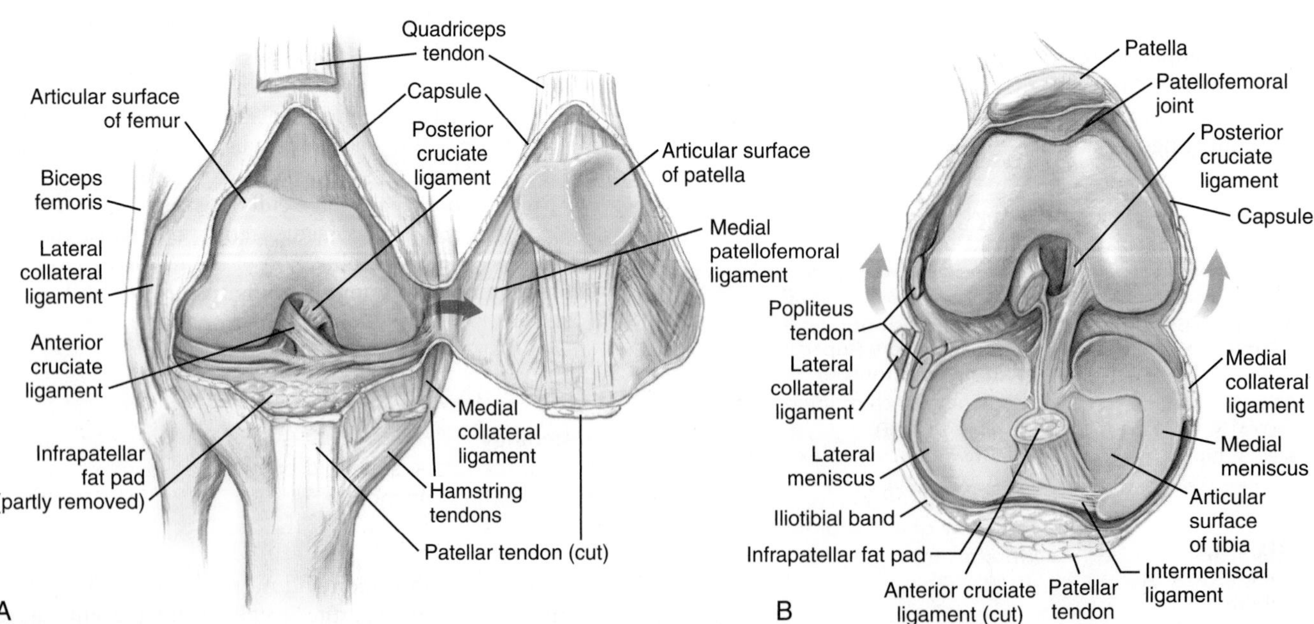

Figure 2-62 Menisci and ligaments of the knee. **A,** Anterior view. **B,** Superior view. (From Miller MD, et al: *Orthopaedic surgical approaches,* Philadelphia, 2008, Saunders, Figures KL-4 and KL-5.)

Table 2-55 Ligaments of the Knee

Ligament	Origin	Insertion	Function
Retinacular	Vastus medialis and vastus lateralis	Tibial condyles	Forms anterior capsule
Posterior fibers	Femoral condyles	Tibial condyles	Forms posterior capsule
Oblique popliteal	Semimembranosus tendon	Lateral femoral condyle/posterior capsule	Strengthens capsule
Deep MCL	Medial epicondyle	Medial meniscus	Holds medial meniscus to femur
Superficial MCL	Medial epicondyle	Medial condyle of tibia	Resists valgus force
Arcuate	Lateral femoral condyle, over popliteus	Posterior tibia/fibular head	Posterior support
Lateral collateral	Lateral epicondyle	Lateral fibular head	Resists varus force
Anterior cruciate	Anterior intercondylar tibia	Posteromedial lateral femoral condyle	Limits hyperextension/sliding
Posterior cruciate	Posterior sulcus of tibia	Anteromedial femoral condyle	Prevents hyperflexion/sliding
Coronary	Meniscus	Tibial periphery	Meniscal attachment
Wrisberg	Posterolateral meniscus	Medial femoral condyle (behind posterior cruciate ligament)	Stabilizes lateral meniscus
Humphrey	Posterolateral meniscus	Medial femoral condyle (in front)	Stabilizes lateral meniscus
Transverse meniscal	Anterolateral meniscus	Anteromedial meniscus	Stabilizes menisci

MCL, medial collateral ligament.

collateral ligament, popliteofibular ligament, and lateral head of the gastrocnemius.

- **Isolated injuries to the PCL cause the greatest instability at 90 degrees of knee flexion.**
- **Combined injuries of the PCL and posterolateral corner result in increasing instability as the knee is flexed from 30 to 90 degrees.**
- **Isolated injuries of the posterolateral corner result in increasing instability that is most notable at 30 degrees; instability decreases as the knee is flexed to 90 degrees.**

- Muscles and tendons
  - Several muscles and tendons traverse the knee, giving it dynamic stability.
  - The hamstring tendons used for autograft ACL reconstruction are the gracilis and semitendinosus.

2. Superior tibiofibular joint: strengthened by the anterior and posterior ligaments of the head of the fibula

C. **Muscles of the leg**

1. These muscles are commonly divided into groups on the basis of compartments (anterior, lateral, superficial posterior, and deep posterior) (Table 2-56).

Table 2-56 Muscles of the Leg

Muscle	Origin	Insertion	Action	Innervation
Anterior Compartment				
Tibialis anterior	Lateral tibia	Medial cuneiform, first metatarsal	Dorsiflexing, inverting foot	Deep peroneal (L4) nerve
Extensor hallucis longus	Mid-fibula	Great toe, distal phalanx	Dorsiflexing, extending toe	Deep peroneal (L5) nerve
Extensor digitorum longus	Tibial condyle/fibula	Toe, middle and distal phalanges	Dorsiflexing, extending toe	Deep peroneal (L5) nerve
Peroneus tertius	Fibula and extensor digitorum longus tendon	Fifth metatarsal	Everting, dorsiflexing, abducting foot	Deep peroneal (S1) nerve
Lateral Compartment				
Peroneus longus	Proximal fibula	Medial cuneiform, first metatarsal	Everting, plantar flexing, abducting foot	Superficial peroneal (S1) nerve
Peroneus brevis	Distal fibula	Tuberosity of fifth metatarsal	Everting foot	Superficial peroneal (S1) nerve
Superficial Posterior Compartment				
Gastrocnemius	Posterior medial and lateral femoral condyles	Calcaneus	Plantar flexing foot	Tibial (S1) nerve
Soleus	Fibula/tibia	Calcaneus	Plantar flexing foot	Tibial (S1) nerve
Plantaris	Lateral femoral condyle	Calcaneus	Plantar flexing foot	Tibial (S1) nerve
Deep Posterior Compartment				
Popliteus	Lateral femoral condyle, fibular head	Proximal tibia	Flexing, internally rotating knee	Tibial (L5, S1) nerve
Flexor hallucis longus	Fibula	Great toe, distal phalanx	Plantar flexing great toe	Tibial (S1) nerve
Flexor digitorum longus	Tibia	Second to fifth toes, distal phalanges	Plantar flexing toes, foot	Tibial (S1, S2) nerve
Tibialis posterior	Tibia, fibula, interosseous membrane	Navicular, medial cuneiform	Inverting/plantar flexing foot	Tibial (L4, L5) nerve

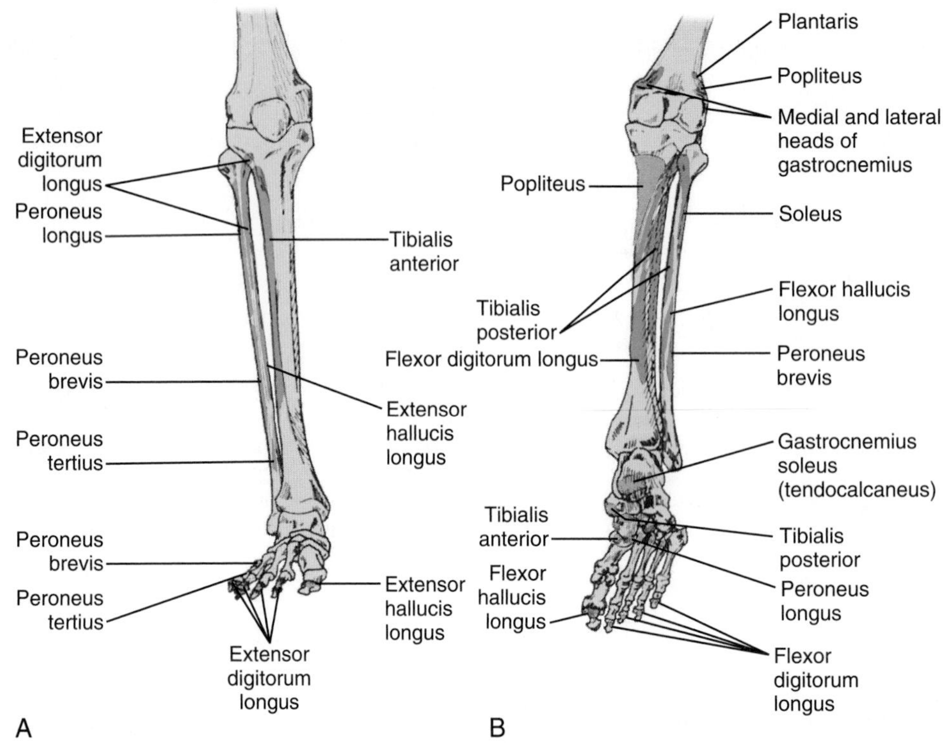

Figure 2-63 Skeletal origins and insertions of leg and foot muscles. **A,** Anterior view. **B,** Posterior view. (From Jenkins DB: *Hollinshead's functional anatomy of the limbs and back,* ed 6, Philadelphia, 1991, Saunders, Figure 19-3.)

- The posterior compartments are supplied by the tibial nerve and contain preaxial muscles.
- The anterior and lateral compartments are supplied by the common peroneal nerve (anterior supplied by the deep peroneal nerve, and lateral supplied by the superficial peroneal nerve) and contain postaxial muscles.

2. The origins and insertions are noted in Figure 2-63.
3. The popliteal fossa is bordered by the gastrocnemius muscles, the semimembranosus, and the biceps; the plantaris muscle makes up the floor of the fossa.
4. **Four compartment releases of the leg are key testable material and are summarized in Table 2-57. The saphenous nerve (termination of the femoral nerve) is subcutaneous.**

Table 2-57 Compartment Releases of Leg

Compartment	Muscles	Neurovascular Structures Released
Anterior	Tibialis anterior, extensor hallucis longus, extensor digitorum longus, peroneus tertius	Deep peroneal nerve and anterior tibial artery
Lateral	Peroneus longus and brevis	Superficial peroneal nerve
Superficial posterior	Gastrocnemius-soleus complex, plantaris	Sural nerve
Deep posterior	Popliteus, flexor hallucis longus, flexor digitorum longus, tibialis posterior	Posterior tibial artery and vein, tibial nerve, peroneal artery and vein

D. Nerves (Figure 2-64)

1. Anatomy
   - Tibial nerve (L4 to S3; see Table 2-44)
     - Continues in the thigh deep to the long head of the biceps femoris and enters the popliteal fossa
     - Crosses over the popliteus muscle and splits the two heads of the gastrocnemius, passing deep to the soleus on its course to the posterior aspect of the medial malleolus
     - Terminates as the medial and lateral plantar nerves
     - Muscular branches supply the posterior leg along its course (superficial and deep posterior compartments.
   - Common peroneal nerve (L4 to S2)
     - **The smaller terminal division of the sciatic nerve, this nerve runs laterally along the popliteal fossa in the interval between the medial border of the biceps and the lateral head of the gastrocnemius.**
     - It winds around the neck of the fibula and runs deep to the peroneus longus, where it divides into the superficial and deep branches.
     - It can be injured with traction and by lateral meniscal repair.
   - Superficial peroneal nerve
     - Runs along the border between the lateral and anterior compartments in the leg, supplying muscular branches to the peroneus longus and brevis (lateral compartment; see Table 2-56)
     - Terminates in two cutaneous branches (medial dorsal and intermediate dorsal cutaneous nerves) supplying the dorsal foot
     - Supplies dorsal medial sensation to the great toe

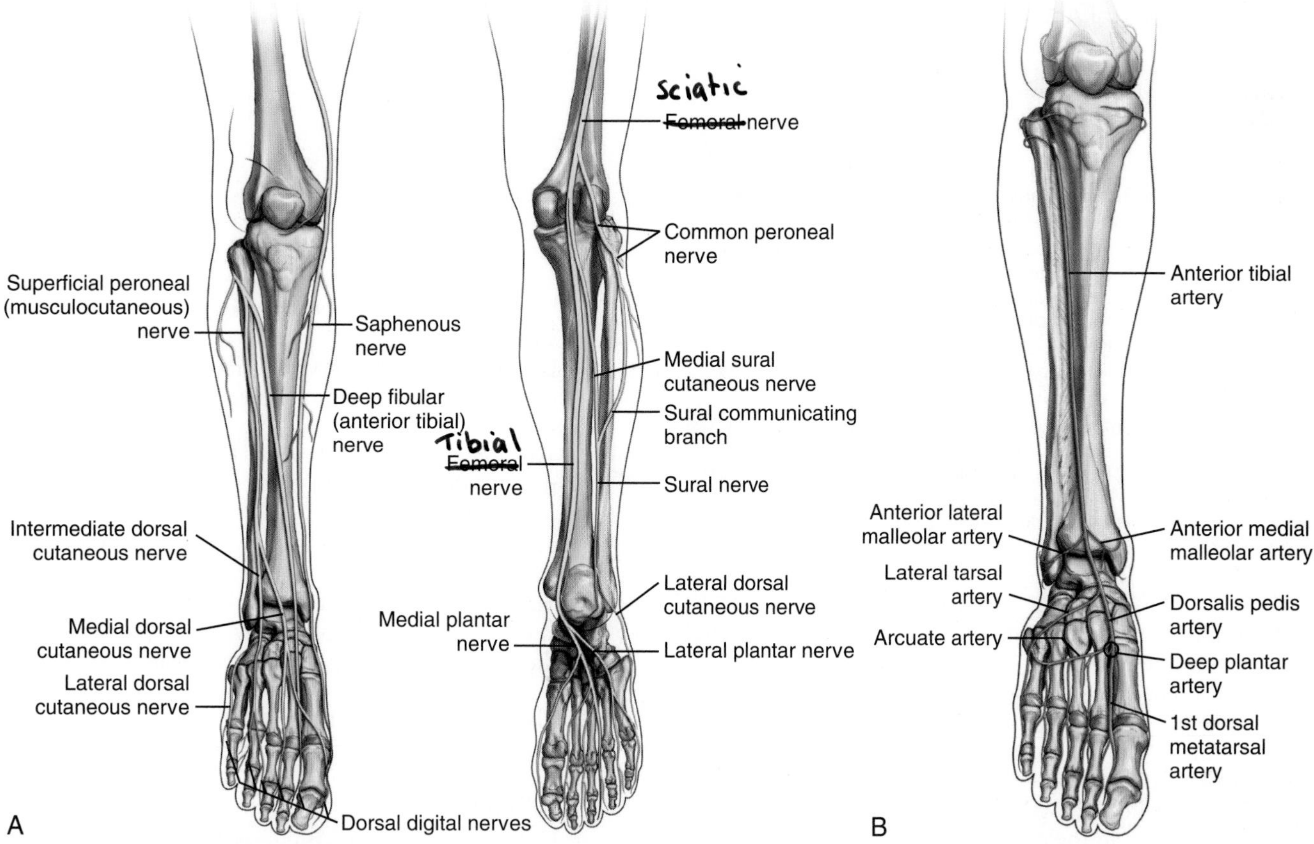

Figure 2-64 Nerves and vessels of the leg. A, Nerves. B, Vessels. (From Miller MD, et al: *Orthopaedic surgical approaches,* Philadelphia, 2008, Saunders, Figures FA-22 and FA-23.)

- Deep peroneal nerve
  - Sometimes known as the *anterior tibial nerve,* this nerve runs along the anterior surface of the interosseous membrane, supplying the musculature of the anterior compartment: tibialis anterior, EHL, extensor digitorum longus, and peroneus tertius (see Table 2-45).
  - Sensation to the first web space is provided by the deep peroneal nerve.
- Cutaneous nerves (see Figure 2-12)
  - The saphenous nerve (L3 to L4) is the continuation of the femoral nerve of the thigh, and it becomes subcutaneous on the medial aspect of the knee between the sartorius and gracilis.
    - It is sometimes injured during procedures about the knee, such as meniscal repair.
    - It supplies sensation to the medial aspect of the leg and foot.
  - The sural nerve (S1 to S2) is formed by cutaneous branches of both the tibial (medial sural cutaneous) and common peroneal (lateral sural cutaneous) nerves.
    - It is often used for nerve grafting.
    - Inadvertent cutting of this nerve can cause painful neuroma.
    - It lies on the lateral aspect of the leg and foot.

2. Innervation (see Table 2-44 and 2-56)

E. Vessels (see Figure 2-64)

1. The branches of the popliteal artery (the continuation of the femoral artery) supply the leg.
   - The popliteal artery enters the popliteal fossa between the biceps and semimembranosus and descends underneath the tibial nerve, terminating between the medial and lateral heads of the gastrocnemius and dividing into the anterior and posterior tibial arteries.
     - Several genicular branches are given off in the popliteal fossa, **including the medial and lateral geniculate arteries (which supply the menisci) and the middle geniculate artery (which supplies the cruciate ligaments).**
     - Superior lateral geniculate artery can be injured during lateral-release procedures.
     - Descending geniculate artery (a branch of the femoral artery proximal to Hunter's canal) supplies the vastus medialis at the anterior border of the intermuscular septum.
     - Inferior geniculate artery passes between the popliteal tendon and fibular collateral ligament in the posterolateral corner of the knee.
2. Anterior tibial artery:
   - First branch of the popliteal artery
   - Passes between the two heads of the tibialis posterior and the interosseous membrane to lie on the anterior surface of that membrane between the tibialis anterior and EHL
   - Terminates as the dorsalis pedis artery
3. Posterior tibial artery:
   - Continues in the deep posterior compartment of the leg, coursing obliquely to pass behind the medial malleolus

Table 2-58 Surgical Approaches to the Knee and Leg

Approach	Interval	Structures at Risk
Medial parapatellar knee	Through quadriceps tendon	Infrapatellar branch of saphenous nerve
Medial knee	Sartorius and medial patellar retinaculum	Saphenous nerve and vein
Lateral knee	Iliotibial band (superior gluteal nerve) and biceps femoris (sciatic nerve)	Common peroneal nerve Popliteus tendon Lateral inferior geniculate artery
Anterior tibia	Elevation of tibialis anterior	
Posterolateral tibia	Soleus and flexor hallucis longus (tibial nerve) and peroneal muscles (peroneal nerve)	Peroneal artery

- Terminates by dividing into the medial and lateral plantar arteries
- Main branch: the peroneal artery
  - Given off 2.5 cm distal to the popliteal fossa and continues in the deep posterior compartment lateral to its parent artery between the tibialis posterior and flexor hallucis longus (FHL)
  - Terminates in the calcaneal branches

F. Surgical approaches to the knee and leg (Table 2-58)

1. Medial parapatellar approach to the knee
   - Dissection: Use a midline incision and a medial parapatellar capsular incision.
   - Risks: The infrapatellar branch of the saphenous nerve is sometimes cut with incisions that stray too far medially, leading to painful neuroma.
2. Medial approach to the knee (Figure 2-65)
   - Interval: between the sartorius and medial patellar retinaculum
   - Dissection: Three layers are commonly recognized (from superficial to deep): (1) the pes anserinus tendons, (2) the superficial MCL, and (3) the deep MCL and capsule.
   - Risks: The saphenous nerve and vein must be identified and protected.
3. Lateral approach to the knee (Figure 2-66)
   - Interval: between the iliotibial band (superior gluteal nerve) and the biceps (sciatic nerve)
   - Dissection:
     - Develop interval between the iliotibial band and biceps for identification of lateral collateral ligament and popliteus.
     - Develop a second interval within the iliotibial band to identify the lateral femoral epicondyle.
   - Risks:
     - The common peroneal nerve, located near the posterior border of the biceps, must be isolated and retracted.
     - The popliteus tendon is also at risk for injury and should be identified.
     - The lateral inferior geniculate artery is posterior to the lateral collateral ligament between the lateral head of the gastrocnemius and the posterolateral capsule; it must also be identified and cauterized.
     - The superior lateral geniculate artery is located between the femur and vastus lateralis.
4. Posterior approach to the knee
   - Dissection:
     - Use an S-shaped incision, beginning laterally and ending medially (distally).
     - Expose the popliteal fossa by using the small saphenous vein and medial sural cutaneous nerves as landmarks.
     - If greater exposure is necessary, detach the two heads of the gastrocnemius.
     - In an alternative approach, mobilize the medial head of the gastrocnemius (lateral to the semimembranosus) and retract it laterally, using its muscle belly to protect the neurovascular structures.

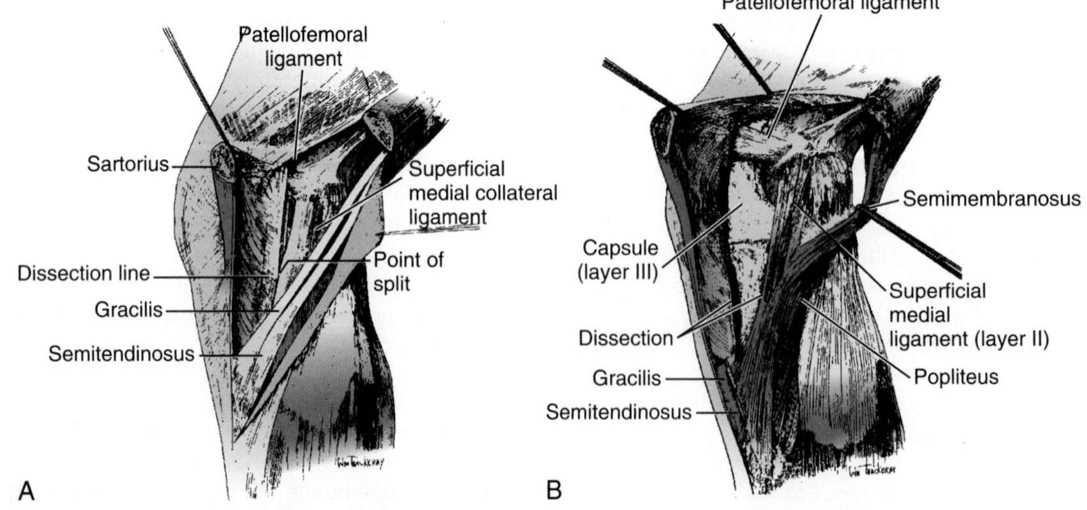

Figure 2-65 Medial structures of the knee. **A,** Superficial exposure. **B,** Deep exposure. (From Warren LF, Marshall JL: The supporting structures and layers of the medial side of the knee, *J Bone Joint Surg Am* 61:58, 1979.)

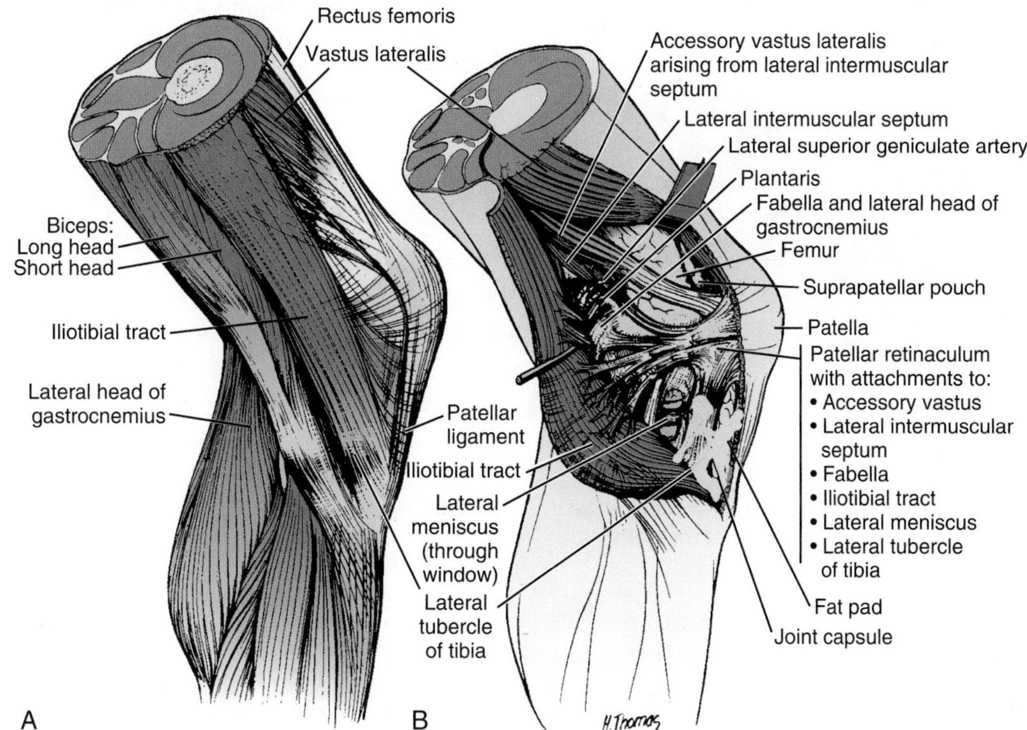

Figure 2-66 Lateral structures of the knee. **A,** Superficial exposure. **B,** Deep exposure. (From Seebacher JR, et al: The structure of the posterolateral aspect of the knee, *J Bone Joint Surg Am* 64:533, 1982.)

- Risks: The popliteal vessels and tibial nerve are at risk for injury.

5. Anterior approach to the tibia
   - This approach may be used for ORIF of fractures and bone grafting; it relies on subperiosteal elevation of the tibialis anterior.
6. Posterolateral approach to the tibia (for bone grafting)
   - Interval: between the soleus and the FHL (tibial nerve) and the peroneal muscles (superficial peroneal nerve)
   - Dissection: Detach the FHL from its origin on the fibula, and detach the tibialis posterior from its origin along the interosseous membrane to reach the tibia.
   - **Risks: The neurovascular structures in the posterior compartment (including the peroneal artery) are protected by the muscle bellies of the tibialis posterior and FHL medially to laterally and between soleus and tibialis posterior anteriorly to posteriorly.**
7. Approach to the fibula
   - This approach is through the same interval as the posterolateral approach to the tibia, but it stays more anterior and relies on isolation and protection of the common peroneal nerve in the proximal dissection.

G. Arthroscopy

1. The arthroscopic portals for knee arthroscopy commonly include the inferomedial and inferolateral portals and a proximal (medial or lateral) portal.
2. Posterior portals can place certain neurovascular structures (lateral, common peroneal nerve; medial, saphenous nerve and vein) at risk for injury.

IV. ANKLE AND FOOT

A. Osteology

1. Anatomy
   - The 26 bones of the foot include 7 tarsal bones, 5 metatarsals, and 14 phalanges.
   - The foot is divided into the hindfoot (talus and calcaneus), midfoot (navicular, cuboid, and three cuneiforms), and forefoot (metatarsals and phalanges).
2. Tarsals: This network of bones includes the talus, calcaneus, cuboid, navicular, and three cuneiforms.
   - Talus
     - The talus articulates with the tibia and fibula in the ankle mortise and with the calcaneus and navicular distally
     - It is made up of a body that is wider anteriorly, with three articular surfaces—the trochlea (including surfaces for the malleoli articulations), and the posterior and middle calcaneal facets—and a posterior process (for the posterior talofibular ligament).
     - The neck of the talus connects with the head, which in turn articulates with the navicular distally and the calcaneus inferiorly.
     - The talus has no muscular attachments but has a groove posteriorly for the tendon of the FHL.
     - Two thirds of the talus is covered with cartilage.
     - **The primary blood supply to the talar body is from the artery of the tarsal canal (posterior tibial artery).**

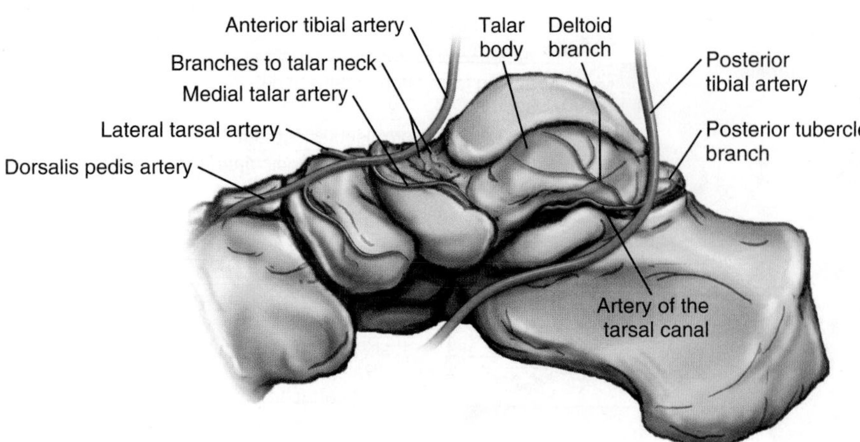

Figure 2-67 Arterial supply to the talus. (From Miller MD, et al: *Orthopaedic surgical approaches,* Philadelphia, 2008, Saunders, Figure FA-26.)

- Other blood supply is from the superior neck vessels (anterior tibial artery) and the artery of the tarsal sinus (dorsalis pedis) (Figure 2-67).
- Calcaneus
  - The calcaneus has three surfaces that articulate with the talus: a large posterior facet, an anterior facet, and a middle facet.
  - Distally, an articular surface receives the cuboid bone.
  - The sustentaculum tali is an overhanging horizontal eminence on the anteromedial surface of the calcaneus.
  - The sustentaculum tali supports the middle articular surface above it and has an inferior groove for the FHL tendon.
- Cuboid
  - Lying on the lateral aspect of the foot, the cuboid is grooved on the plantar surface by the peroneus longus and has four facets for articulation with the calcaneus, the lateral cuneiform, and the fourth and fifth metatarsals.
- Navicular
  - The most medial tarsal bone, the navicular lies between the talus and the cuneiforms.
  - Proximally, the surface is oval and concave for its articulation with the head of the talus.
  - Distally, the navicular has three articular surfaces, one for each of the cuneiforms.
  - The medial plantar projection serves as the insertion for the posterior tibial tendon.
- Cuneiforms
  - Three bones (medial, intermediate, and lateral)
  - Articulate with the navicular and posterior cuboid (lateral cuneiform) and the first three metatarsals
  - **The intermediate cuneiform does not extend as far distally as the medial cuneiform, which allows the second metatarsal to "key" into place.**

3. Metatarsals
   - Five bones, numbered from a medial to lateral direction, span the distance between the tarsal bones and phalanges.
   - In general, their shape and function are similar to those of the metacarpals of the hand.
   - The first metatarsal has a plantar crista that articulates with the fibular and tibial sesamoids contained within the flexor hallucis brevis tendon.
4. Phalanges
   - The phalanges of the foot are similar to those of the hand.
   - The great toe has two phalanges, and the remaining digits have three.
5. Ossification
   - Each tarsal has a single ossification center except for the calcaneus, which has a second center posteriorly.
   - The calcaneus, talus, and usually the cuboid are present at birth.
   - The lateral cuneiform appears during the first year, the medial cuneiform during the second year, and the intermediate cuneiform and navicular during the third year.
   - The posterior center for the calcaneus usually appears during the eighth year.
   - The second through fifth metatarsals have two ossification centers:
     - A primary center in the shaft
     - A secondary center for the head, which appears at ages 5 to 8 years
   - The phalanges and first metatarsal have secondary centers at their bases that appear proximally during the third or fourth year and distally during the sixth or seventh year.

B. Arthrology

1. Inferior tibiofibular joint
   - Formed by the medial distal fibula and the notched lateral distal tibia
   - Supported by four ligaments: the anterior and posterior inferior tibiofibular ligaments, a transverse tibiofibular ligament, and an interosseous ligament
   - **The anteroinferior tibiofibular ligament is an oblique band that connects the bones anteriorly. Avulsion of this ligament may result in a Tillaux fracture.**
2. Ankle joint (Figure 2-68; Table 2-59)
   - Formed by the malleoli and talus
   - The MCL (deltoid ligament) comprises two layers:
     - The superficial layer: tibionavicular and tibiocalcaneal
     - The deep layer: anterior and posterior tibiotalar
   - The lateral fibular ligaments are the anterior talofibular ligament, calcaneofibular ligament, and posterior talofibular ligament.
     - The anterior talofibular ligament is the weakest and is intracapsular (intracapsular thickening).

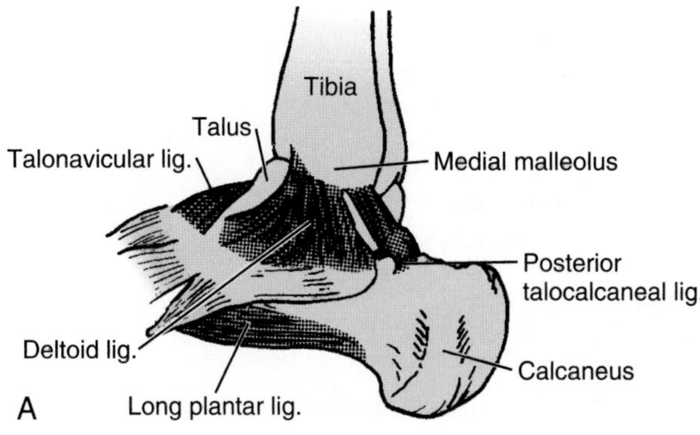

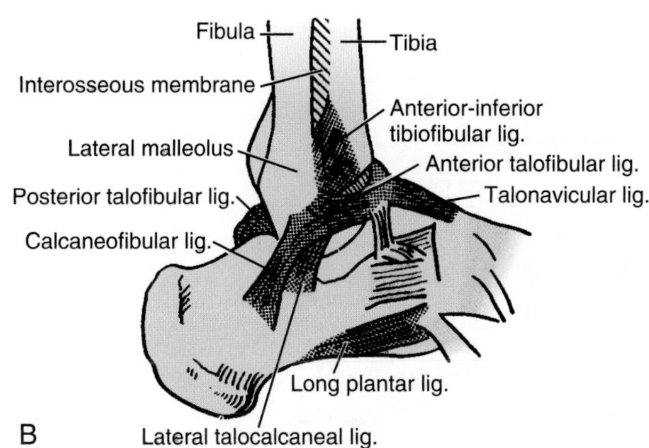

Figure 2-68 Ankle ligaments. **A,** Medial view. **B,** Lateral view. (From Weissman BN, Sledge CB: *Orthopedic radiology,* Philadelphia, 1986, Saunders, pp 593-594.)

- **The position of the ankle is critical when the lateral ligament complex is tested. Plantar flexion tightens the anterior talofibular ligament, and inversion with neutral flexion tightens the calcaneofibular ligament.**

3. Subtalar joint
   - Talar plantar facets articulate with the calcaneus.
   - Stability is derived from four ligaments: the medial ligament, the lateral ligament, the interosseous talocalcaneal ligament, and the cervical ligament.
4. Intertarsal joints (Figure 2-69): Several ligamentous structures are important (Table 2-60).
5. Other joints
   - Tarsometatarsal joints are gliding joints supported by dorsal, plantar, and interosseous ligaments.
   - The base of the first metatarsal is not ligamentously connected to the second metatarsal.

Table 2-59 Ankle Joint Ligaments

Ligament	Origin	Insertion
Capsule	Tibia	Talus
Deltoid	Medial malleolus	Medial malleolus
Tibionavicular	Medial malleolus	Navicular tuberosity
Tibiocalcaneal	Medial malleolus	Sustentaculum tali
Posterior tibiotalar	Medial malleolus	Inner side of talus
Anterior tibiotalar	Medial malleolus	Medial surface of talus
Anterior tibiofibular	Lateral malleolus	Transversely to talus anteriorly
Posterior tibiofibular	Lateral malleolus	Transversely to talus posteriorly
Calcaneofibular	Lateral malleolus	Obliquely to calcaneus posteriorly

- **The Lisfranc ligament connects the medial (shortest) cuneiform to the second (longest) metatarsal.**
  - In about 20% of patients, it exists as a plantar and dorsal structure.
- The deep transverse metatarsal ligaments interconnect the metatarsal heads.
  - The digital nerve courses in a plantar direction under the transverse metatarsal ligament and is the spot where interdigital neuritis (Morton's neuroma, usually the second or third interdigital space) occurs.
  - In addition, the transverse metatarsal ligament attaches the second metatarsal head to the fibular sesamoid.
  - This ligament holds the hallucal sesamoids in place and gives the appearance of sesamoid subluxation when the first metatarsal moves medially in hallux valgus.
- The plantar and collateral ligaments support the metatarsophalangeal joints.
- The primary stabilizing structure of the metatarsophalangeal joint is the plantar plate.
- Interphalangeal joints are supported mainly by their capsules.

C. **Muscles**

1. Anatomy
   - The origins and insertions of muscles are shown in Figure 2-70, and the muscles and tendons about the foot and ankle are shown in Figure 2-71. The tendons are arranged about the toe as shown in Figure 2-72. The major tendons crossing the ankle joint include the following:

Table 2-60 Ligaments of the Intertarsal Joints

Ligament	Common Name	Origin	Insertion
Interosseous talocalcaneal	Cervical	Talus	Calcaneus
Calcaneocuboid/calcaneonavicular	Bifurcate	Calcaneus	Cuboid and navicular
Calcaneocuboid-metatarsal	Long plantar	Calcaneus	Cuboid and first to fifth metatarsals
Plantar calcaneocuboid	Short plantar	Calcaneus	Cuboid
Plantar calcaneonavicular	Spring	Sustentaculum tali	Navicular
Tarsometatarsal	Lisfranc	Medial cuneiform	Second metatarsal base

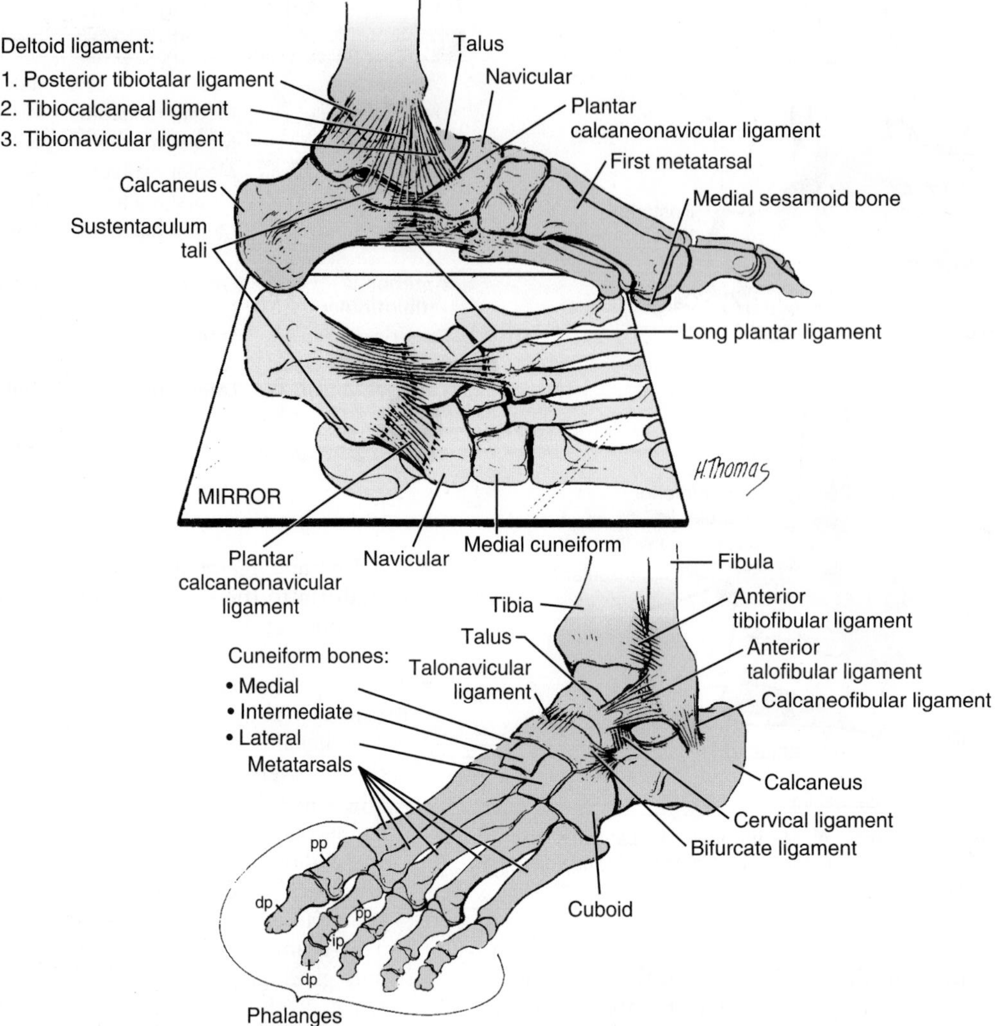

Figure 2-69 Ligaments of the foot. **A,** Medial view with inferior view highlighted with mirror. **B,** Lateral oblique view. (From Jahss MH: *Disorders of the foot,* Philadelphia, 1982, Saunders, p 14.)

- Posterior: Achilles
- Lateral: peroneal tendons with longus (superficial) and brevis (deep)
- Anterior (from a lateral to medial direction): peroneus tertius, extensor digitorum longus, EHL, tibialis anterior
- Medial (mnemonic: "**T**om, **D**ick, and **H**arry": **t**ibialis posterior, flexor **d**igitorum longus, and flexor **h**allucis longus)

2. Achilles tendon: Maximum anteroposterior dimension on magnetic resonance imaging is 8 mm.
3. The arrangement of muscles and tendons in the foot is best considered in layers (Table 2-61; Figure 2-73).
   - On the plantar surface, the intrinsic muscles dominate the first and third layers.
   - Extrinsic tendons are more important in the second and fourth layers.
4. There is one dorsal intrinsic muscle of the foot: the extensor digitorum brevis (EDB) (innervated by the lateral terminal branch of the deep peroneal nerve).
5. **Plantar heel spurs originate in the flexor digitorum brevis (medial plantar nerve innervation).**
6. The lumbrical muscles are located plantar to the transverse metatarsal ligament, and interosseous tendons are dorsal.
7. Key testable material depends on which muscles are active during the different periods of the gait cycle (see Chapter 10, Rehabilitation).
8. **The posterior tibial tendon is the initiator of hindfoot inversion during gait (Chapter 10). This explains why a person cannot perform a single-stance toe rise with posterior tibial tendon deficiency and a normal Achilles tendon.**
9. Neuromuscular interactions are listed in Table 2-62.

D. **Nerves (see Figure 2-48)**

1. Anatomy: The nerves of the ankle and foot are branches of the proximal nerves, discussed earlier.
   - Tibial nerve
     - The tibial nerve supplies all intrinsic foot muscles except the EDB (deep peroneal nerve).

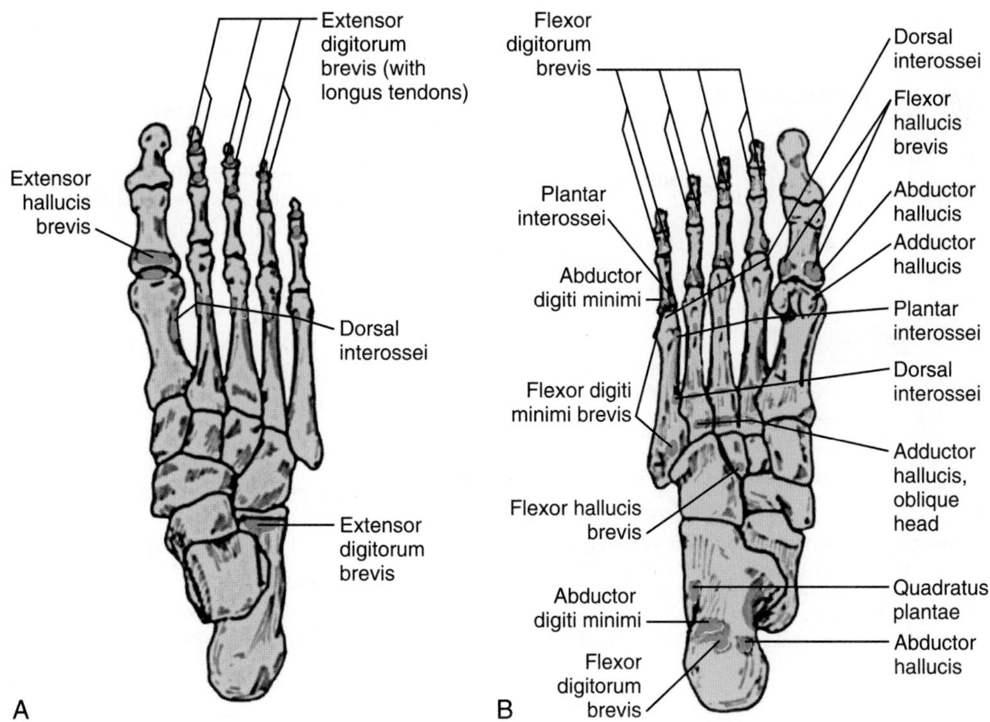

Figure 2-70 Origins and insertions of the muscles of the foot. **A,** Dorsal view. **B,** Plantar view. (From Jenkins DB: *Hollinshead's functional anatomy of the limbs and back,* ed 6, Philadelphia, 1991, Saunders, Figure 20-7.)

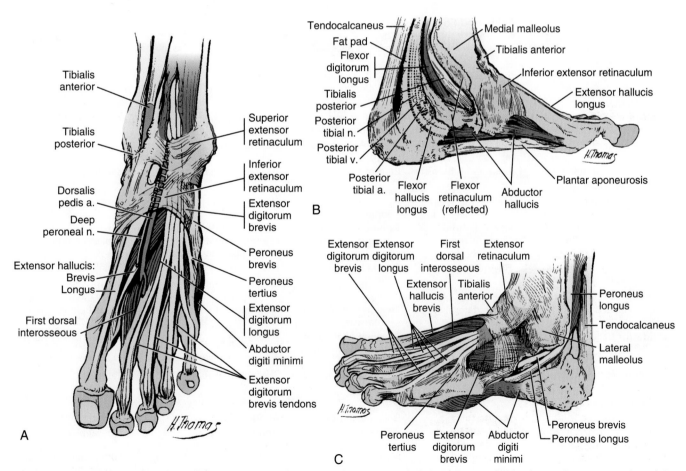

Figure 2-71 Muscles and tendons of the foot and ankle. **A,** Dorsal view. **B,** Medial view. **C,** Lateral view. (From Jahss MH: *Disorders of the foot,* Philadelphia, 1982, Saunders, pp 18-20.)

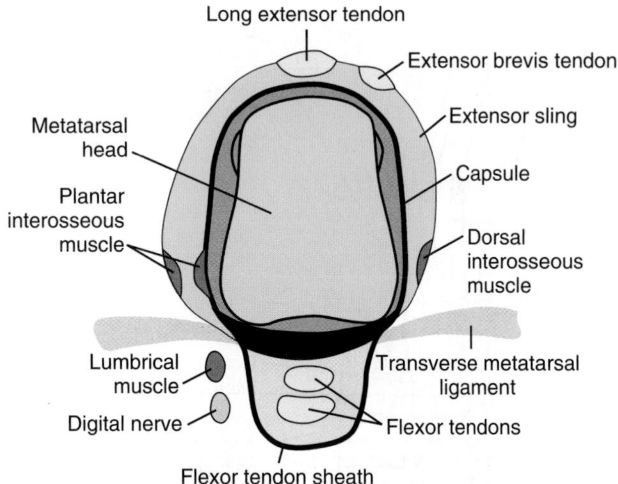

Figure 2-72 Cross-sectional view of the toe at the metatarsal head. The lumbrical muscles are plantar to the transverse ligament (with the digital nerve), and the interossei are dorsal to this ligament. The interossei and lumbrical muscles (except the first lumbrical muscle [medial plantar nerve]) are innervated by the lateral plantar nerve. (From Jahss MH: *Disorders of the foot,* Philadelphia, 1982, Saunders, pp 623.)

- **The tibial nerve splits into two branches (the medial and lateral plantar nerves) under the flexor retinaculum.**
  - **Both of these nerves run in the second layer of the foot.**
  - **The medial plantar nerve runs deep to the abductor hallucis, and the lateral plantar nerve runs obliquely under the cover of the quadratus plantae.**
  - **The most proximal branch of the lateral plantar nerve is the nerve to the abductor digit quinti (Baxter's nerve).**
- The distribution of the sensory and motor branches of the plantar nerves is similar to that in the hand.
  - The medial plantar nerve (like the median nerve of the hand) supplies plantar sensation to the medial three and a half digits and motor sensation to only a few plantar muscles (flexor hallucis brevis, abductor hallucis, flexor digitorum brevis, and the first lumbrical muscle).
  - The lateral plantar nerve (like the ulnar nerve in the hand) supplies plantar sensation to the lateral one

Table 2-61 Muscles of the Ankle and Foot

Muscle	Origin	Insertion	Action	Innervation
Dorsal Layer				
Extensor digitorum brevis	Superolateral calcaneus	Base of proximal phalanges	Extending	Deep peroneal nerve
First Plantar Layer				
Abductor hallucis	Calcaneal tuberosity	Base of great toe, proximal phalanx	Abducting great toe	Medial plantar nerve
Flexor digitorum brevis	Calcaneal tuberosity	Distal phalanges of second to fifth toes	Flexing toes	Medial plantar nerve
Abductor digiti minimi	Calcaneal tuberosity	Base of small toe	Abducting small toe	Lateral plantar nerve
Second Plantar Layer				
Quadratus plantae	Medial and lateral calcaneus	Flexor digitorum longus tendon	Helping flex distal phalanges	Lateral plantar nerve
Lumbrical muscles	Flexor digitorum longus tendon	Extensor digitorum longus tendon	Flexing metatarsophalangeal joint, extending interphalangeal joint	Medial and lateral plantar nerves
Flexor digitorum longus and flexor hallucis longus	Tibia/fibula	Distal phalanges of digits	Flexing toes, inverting foot	Tibial nerve
Third Plantar Layer				
Flexor hallucis brevis	Cuboid/lateral cuneiform	Proximal phalanx of great toe	Flexing great toe	Medial plantar nerve
Adductor hallucis	Oblique: second to fourth metatarsals	Proximal phalanx of great toe (lateral)	Adducting great toe	Lateral plantar nerve
Flexor digiti minimi brevis	Base of fifth metatarsal head	Proximal phalanx of small toe	Flexing small toe	Lateral plantar nerve
Fourth Plantar Layer				
Dorsal interosseous	Metatarsal	Dorsal extensors	Abducting	Lateral plantar nerve
Plantar interosseous	Third to fifth metatarsals	Proximal phalanges medially	Adducting toes	Lateral plantar nerve
(peroneus longus and tibialis posterior)	Fibula/tibia	Medial cuneiform/navicular	Everting/inverting foot	Superficial peroneal/tibial nerve

Note: For abduction and adduction in the foot, the second toe serves as the reference.

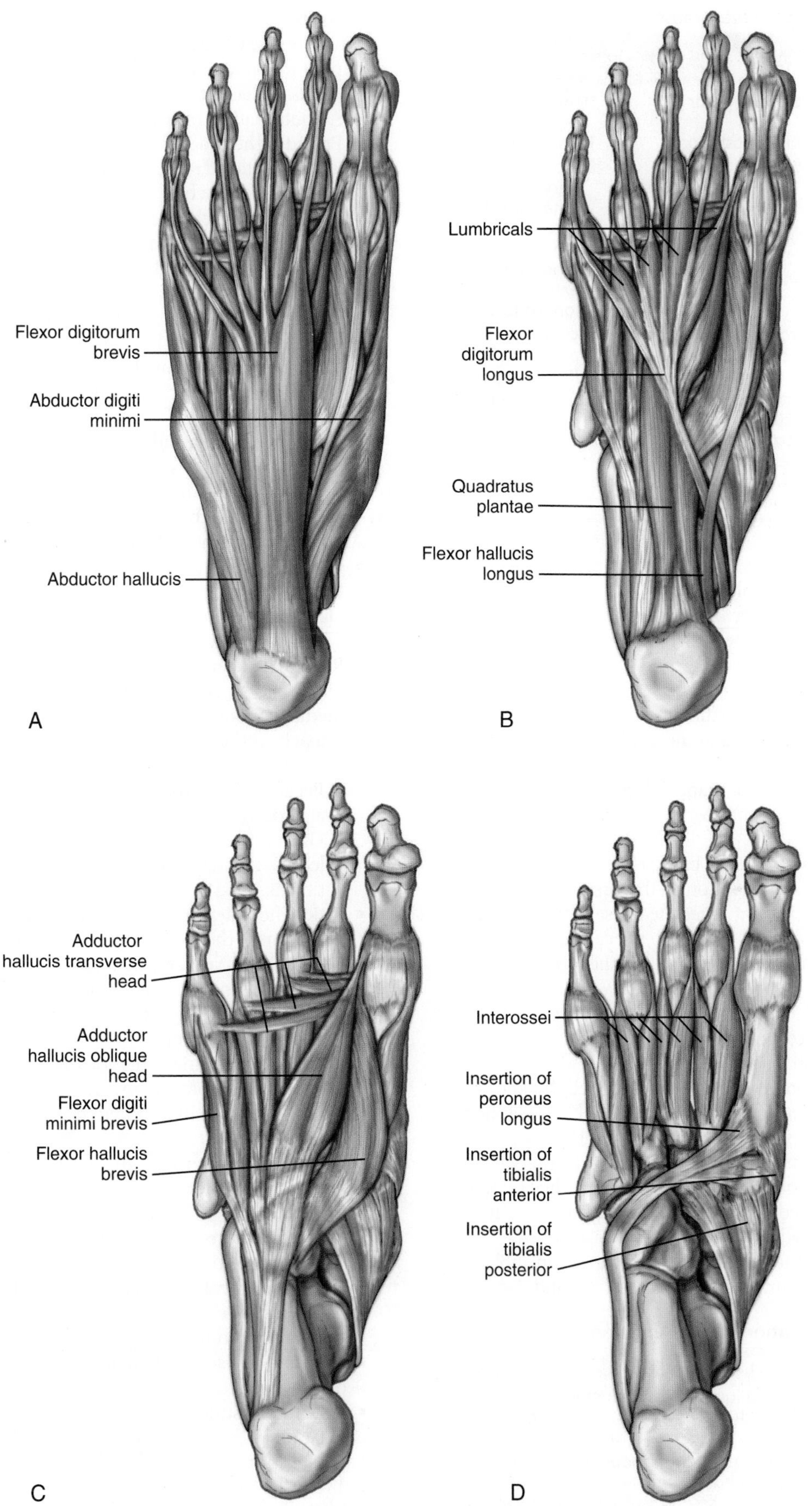

Figure 2-73 Four layers of the plantar surface of the foot. **A,** First layer. **B,** Second layer. **C,** Third layer. **D,** Fourth layer. (From Miller MD, et al: *Orthopaedic surgical approaches,* Philadelphia, 2008, Saunders, Figures FA-17 to FA-20.)

Table 2-62 Foot Neuromuscular Interactions

Foot Function	Muscle	Innervation
Inversion	Tibialis anterior	Deep peroneal nerve (L4)
	Tibialis posterior	Tibial nerve (S1)
Dorsiflexion	Tibialis anterior, extensor digitorum longus, extensor hallucis longus	Deep peroneal nerve: tibialis anterior (L4), extensor digitorum longus, and extensor hallucis longus (L5)
Eversion	Peroneus longus and peroneus brevis	Superficial peroneal nerve (S1)
Plantar flexion	Gastrocnemius-soleus complex, flexor digitorum longus, flexor hallucis longus, tibialis posterior (also hindfoot inverter)	Tibial nerve (S1)

and a half digits and the remaining intrinsic muscles of the foot (Table 2-63).
- The digital nerve of the third web space consists of branches from both the medial and lateral plantar nerves.

- Common peroneal nerve
  - This nerve splits into the superficial and deep branches in the leg and has terminal branches in the foot as well.
  - The lateral terminal branch of the deep peroneal nerve ends in the proximal dorsal foot by supplying the EDB muscle.
  - The medial terminal branch of the deep peroneal nerve supplies sensation to the first web space.
  - The medial and intermediate dorsal cutaneous nerves of the superficial peroneal nerve supply the bulk of the remaining sensation to the dorsal aspect of the foot.
  - The dorsal intermediate branch is at risk for injury during placement of the arthroscopic portal of the anterolateral ankle (discussed later).
  - All sensation in the foot is supplied by the sciatic nerve, except in the medial ankle and foot (saphenous nerve [termination of femoral nerve]).
  - The dorsal medial cutaneous nerve (a branch of the superficial peroneal nerve) crosses the EHL in a lateral-to-medial direction and supplies sensation to the dorsomedial aspect of the great toe.

2. Neuromuscular interactions are summarized in Table 2-62.
3. Innervation is summarized in Tables 2-44 and 2-63.

Table 2-63 Innervation of the Ankle and Foot

Nerves	Muscles Innervated
Medial plantar	Flexor hallucis brevis, abductor hallucis, flexor digitorum brevis, first lumbrical muscle
Lateral plantar	Pronator quadratus, abductor digiti minimi, flexor digiti minimi, adductor hallucis, interossei, second to fourth lumbrical muscles

E. **Vessels**

1. Like the nerves that run with them, two main arteries supply the ankle and foot.
2. Dorsalis pedis artery:
   - A continuation of the anterior tibial artery of the leg
   - Provides the blood supply to the dorsum of the foot via its lateral tarsal, medial tarsal, arcuate, and first dorsal metatarsal branches
   - Its largest branch, the deep plantar artery, runs between the first and second metatarsals and contributes to the plantar arch (see Figure 2-66, *A*).
3. Posterior tibial artery:
   - Divides into the medial and lateral plantar branches under the abductor hallucis muscle
   - The larger lateral branch receives the deep plantar artery and forms the plantar arch in the fourth layer of the plantar foot.

F. Important neurovascular relationships may be observed in a coronal section (Figure 2-74) and a transverse section (Figure 2-75) at the ankle joint.

G. **Surgical approaches (Table 2-64)**

1. Anterior approach to the ankle
   - Interval: between the EHL and extensor digitorum longus (both deep peroneal nerve)
   - Dissection: Before incising the extensor retinaculum, carefully protect the superficial peroneal nerve.
   - Risks: The deep peroneal nerve and anterior tibial artery, which lie directly in this interval, must be retracted medially along with the EHL.
2. Approach to the medial malleolus
   - Dissection:
     - Because it is superficial, use an anterior or posterior approach.
     - Use a posteromedial approach behind the medial malleolus through the tendon sheath of the posterior tibialis.
   - Risk: The anterior approach jeopardizes the saphenous nerve and the long saphenous vein; the posterior approach jeopardizes the structures running behind the medial malleolus in the following order: posterior **t**ibial tendon, F**D**L, posterior tibial **v**ein, posterior tibial **a**rtery, posterior tibial **n**erve, and F**H**L (mnemonic: "**T**om, **D**ick, and **v**ery **a**ngry **n**ervous **H**arry").
3. Posteromedial approach to the ankle and foot: used for release of clubfoot in children
   - Dissection:
     - Begin this approach medial to the Achilles tendon, and follow the curve distally along the medial border of the foot.
     - Use the posterior tibialis tendon as a landmark for the location of the subluxated navicular in the clubfoot.
   - Risk: Care must be taken to protect the posterior tibial nerve and artery and their branches.
4. Lateral approach to the ankle
   - Dissection: Use a subcutaneous approach for ORIF of distal fibula fractures.
   - Risks: The sural nerve (posterolateral) and the superficial peroneal nerve (anterior) must be avoided.
5. Lateral approach to the hindfoot: used for triple arthrodesis
   - Interval: between the peroneus tertius (deep peroneal nerve) and peroneal tendons (superficial peroneal nerve)

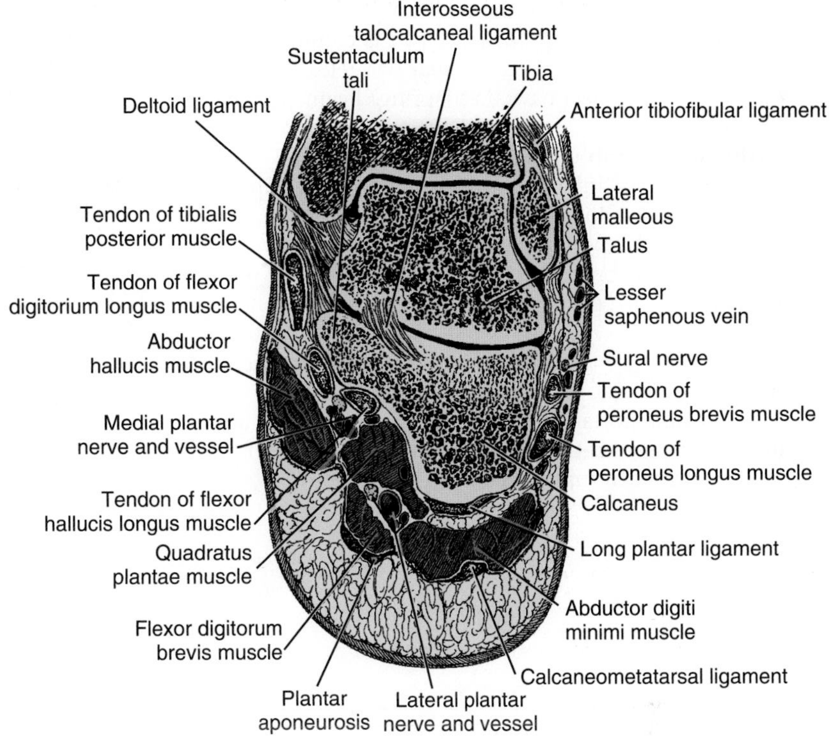

Figure 2-74 Vertical (coronal) section of the ankle. Note the groove of the flexor hallucis longus under the sustentaculum tali of the calcaneus. (From Woodburne RT, Burkel WE: *Essentials of human anatomy,* ed 9, Oxford, UK, 1994, Oxford University Press.)

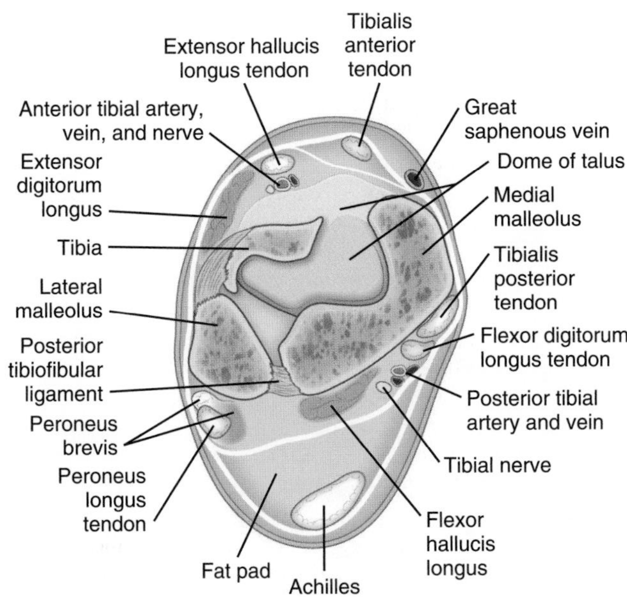

Figure 2-75 Transverse (axial) cross-sectional view of the ankle. Note the relationship of the peroneal nerves in relation to one another and the tibialis posterior tendon, flexor digitorum longus (FDL), and flexor hallucis longus (FHL) in relation to the neurovascular structures. (From Miller MD, et al: *Orthopaedic surgical approaches,* Philadelphia, 2008, Saunders, Figure FA-28.)

- Dissection: Remove the fat pad covering the sinus tarsi, and reflect the EDB from its origin to expose the joints.
- Risks:
  - The lateral branch of the deep peroneal nerve (which supplies the EDB) must be protected in this approach.
  - Deep penetration with an instrument used in this approach can injure the FHL.

Table 2-64 Surgical Approaches to the Foot and Ankle

Approach	Interval	Structures at Risk
Anterior ankle	Extensor hallucis longus (deep peroneal nerve)	Superficial and deep peroneal nerve
Extensor digitorum longus (deep peroneal nerve)	Anterior tibial artery	
Anterior medial ankle		Saphenous nerve and vein
Distal fibula		Sural nerve (posterolateral) and superficial peroneal nerve (anterior with variable position)
Lateral hindfoot	Peroneus tertius (deep peroneal nerve) and peroneal tendons (superficial peroneal nerve)	Lateral branch of deep peroneal nerve
Anterolateral midfoot	Release of extensor digitorum brevis	Calcaneal navicular ligament

6. Anterolateral approach to the midfoot
   - Dissection: In this approach, which is commonly used for excision of a calcaneonavicular bar, release the EDB.
   - Risk: The calcaneal navicular (spring) ligament may be injured.

H. Arthroscopy (Table 2-65)

1. The portals used in ankle arthroscopy can put important structures at risk for injury.
2. The anterolateral portal can jeopardize the dorsal intermediate cutaneous branch of the superficial peroneal nerve.
3. The anteromedial portal can damage the greater saphenous vein.
4. Anterior central portals are no longer recommended because of the risk to the dorsalis pedis artery.
5. Posteromedial portals can injure the posterior tibial artery and are consequently not recommended, and posterolateral portals can injure the sural nerve.

Table 2-65 Portals for Ankle Arthroscopy

Portal	Location	Structures at Risk
Anterolateral	Medial to lateral malleolus, lateral to peroneus tertius	Dorsal intermediate cutaneous branch of superficial peroneal nerve
Anteromedial	Medial to tibialis anterior tendon, lateral to medial malleolus	Saphenous nerve and vein
Posterolateral	Medial to peroneal tendons, lateral to Achilles tendon	Sural nerve and small saphenous vein
Anterior central	Medial to extensor digitorum communis, lateral to extensor hallucis longus	Deep peroneal nerve and anterior tibial artery

TESTABLE CONCEPTS

SECTION 2 UPPER EXTREMITY

- Long-term nerve compression at the spinoglenoid notch (i.e., ganglion; consider labral disease) results in infraspinatus atrophy.
- The clavicle is the first bone in the body to ossify (at 5 weeks of gestation) and the last to fuse (medial epiphysis at 25 years of age; see Table 2-1). Fracture of the clavicle is the most common musculoskeletal birth injury.
- The coracoacromial ligament is important to superoanterior restraint in rotator cuff deficiencies and should be preserved when painful massive rotator cuff tears that cannot be surgically repaired are débrided.
- The shoulder internal rotators (pectoralis major, latissimus dorsi, and subscapularis) are stronger than the external rotators (teres minor and infraspinatus), which is why posterior shoulder dislocations are more common than anterior dislocations after electrical shock and seizures.
- The axillary artery is divided into three parts on the basis of its physical relationship to the pectoralis minor. Each part of the artery has as many branches as the number of that portion (e.g., the second part has two branches: thoracoacromial and lateral thoracic).
- The anterior bundle of the elbow MCL is the most important in helping resist valgus forces and attaches 18 mm distal to the coronoid tip.
- The LUCL of the elbow is an essential elbow stabilizer and runs from the lateral epicondyle to the ulna crista supinatoris (supinator crest). A deficiency of the LUCL is manifested as posterolateral rotatory instability of the elbow (see Table 2-14).
- Restoration of the radial bow (and length) is paramount in the fixation of radial shaft fractures to regain full range of motion in the elbow and wrist.
- Tennis elbow (lateral epicondylitis) involves primarily the ECRB.
- The PIN splits the supinator and supplies all of the extensor muscles, except the mobile wad (brachioradialis, ECRB, ECRL).
- The ulnar nerve splits the two heads of the FCU as it enters the forearm, and the median nerve splits the two heads of the pronator teres.
- In the proximal portion of Henry's anterior approach to the forearm, supination of the forearm moves the PIN ulnarly.
- The palmar/volar radiocarpal ligament is the strongest supporting structure of the wrist ligaments, although it has a weak area on the radial side (the space of Poirier) that provides less support to the scaphoid, lunate, and trapezoid.
- In the dorsal extensor compartments of the wrist, the APL frequently has multiple tendon slips, which need to be addressed during the release for de Quervain's tenosynovitis.
- In the second dorsal compartment, the ECRL tendon is radial to the ECRB tendon; thus the EPL tendon is ulnar to the ECRB tendon at the wrist level.
- The A2 pulley, overlying the proximal phalanx, is the most important one, followed by A4, which covers the middle phalanx; the A1 pulley is involved in trigger digits.
- The radial artery forms the deep palmar arch in the hand, whereas the ulnar artery forms the superficial palmar arch.

SECTION 3 SPINE

- The highest percentage of neck flexion and extension (50% of total) occurs at the occiput-C1 articulation.
- The atlantoaxial articulation is responsible for the majority of neck rotation; 50% of total rotation occurs at the C1-C2 articulation.
- Pannus in rheumatoid arthritis can involve the diarthrodial atlantoaxial joint and produce instability. Obtain preoperative cervical spine radiographs before elective surgical procedures.
- The vertebral artery travels in the transverse foramina of C1 to C6.
- The most common cause of back pain in children and adolescents is spondylolysis, a defect in the pars interarticularis.
- The annulus fibrosis contains type I collagen while the softer nucleus pulposus contains type II collagen and is approximately 88% water.
- Intradiscal pressure is position dependent: It is lowest in the supine position and highest in sitting (flexed forward with weights in hands).
- The lateral corticospinal tracts are oriented with the sacral structures most peripheral; cervical structures, those more medial. This is why central cord syndrome affects the upper extremities more than the lower extremities (see Figure 2-38).
- The distance from the spinous process of C1 laterally to the vertebral artery is 2 cm.
- For cervical halo pin placement, the anterolateral pin should be 1 cm superior to the orbital rim in the outer two thirds of the orbit below the equator of the skull. As a result, the pin would be lateral to the supraorbital nerve and medial to the temporal fossa and temporalis muscle.

SECTION 4 LOWER EXTREMITY AND PELVIS

- The acetabulum is anteverted (15 degrees) and obliquely oriented (45 degrees caudally).
- The femoral neck is anteverted approximately 14 degrees in relation to the femoral condyles.
- The iliofemoral ligament (Y ligament of Bigelow) is the strongest ligament in the body and attaches the anterior-inferior iliac spine to the intertrochanteric line in an inverted Y manner.
- The most common neural injury at the time of primary total hip arthroplasty is the peroneal division of the sciatic nerve.
- The sacrospinous ligament attaches to the ischial spine and separates the greater and lesser sciatic notches into foramina.
- The major reference point for the greater sciatic nerve and related structures in the hip is the piriformis muscle (the "key" to the sciatic foramen); the superior gluteal nerve and artery lie above the piriformis, and virtually everything else leaves below the muscle.

- Remember the mnemonic "POP'S IQ" for structures leaving the pelvis below the piriformis (lateral to medial nerves): **P**udendal, **O**bturator internus, **P**ostfemoral cutaneous, **S**ciatic, **I**nferior gluteal, **Q**uadratus femoris.
- The aorta branches into the common iliac arteries anterior to the L4 vertebral body.
- The corona mortis is an anastomotic connection between the inferior epigastric branch and the obturator vessels in the obturator canal that can lead to life-threatening bleeding if injured.
- During hip arthroplasty, anteroinferior screws and acetabular retractors jeopardize the obturator artery and vein; the external iliac artery can be injured by the placement of acetabular screws in the anterosuperior quadrant.
- Slipped capital femoral epiphysis occurs through the femoral head epiphysis (zone of hypertrophy).
- The peroneal division of the sciatic nerve has one innervation in the thigh: the short head of the biceps femoris.
- The infrapatellar branch of the saphenous nerve supplies the skin of the medial side of the front of the knee and patellar ligament and can be damaged during total knee replacement surgery.
- The anterior branch of the obturator nerve can provide sensation to the medial side of the knee and can be a source of referred pain from hip disease.
- The knee is enclosed in a capsule that has posteromedial and posterolateral recesses extending 15 mm distal to the subchondral surface of the tibial plateau (be careful to avoid intraarticular pin placement).
- The medial meniscus tears three times more often than the more mobile lateral meniscus.
- The lateral meniscus is associated with meniscal cysts and discoid menisci and is the most common site of tears in acute injuries to the ACL.
- Isolated injuries to the PCL cause the greatest instability at 90 degrees of knee flexion.
- Combined PCL and posterolateral corner injuries result in increasing instability as the knee is flexed from 30 to 90 degrees.
- Isolated posterolateral corner injuries result in increasing instability that is most notable at 30 degrees; instability decreases as the knee is flexed to 90 degrees.
- The saphenous nerve (termination of the femoral nerve) is subcutaneous and can be injured during four-compartment fasciotomies.
- The primary blood supply to the talar body is from the artery of the tarsal canal (posterior tibial artery).
- The intermediate cuneiform does not extend as far distally as the medial cuneiform, which allows the second metatarsal to "key" into place.
- The anteroinferior tibiofibular ligament is an oblique band that connects the bones anteriorly. Avulsion of this ligament may result in a Tillaux fracture.
- The position of the ankle is critical when the lateral ligament complex is tested: plantar flexion tightens the anterior talofibular ligament, and inversion with neutral flexion tightens the calcaneofibular ligament.
- The Lisfranc ligament connects the medial (shortest) cuneiform to the second (longest) metatarsal.
- The digital nerve courses in a plantar direction under the transverse metatarsal ligament and is the spot where interdigital neuritis (Morton's neuroma, usually the second or third interdigital space) occurs.
- Plantar heel spurs originate in the flexor digitorum brevis (medial plantar nerve innervation).
- The posterior tibial tendon is the initiator of hindfoot inversion during gait (Chapter 10). This explains why a person cannot perform a single-stance toe rise with posterior tibial tendon deficiency and a normal Achilles tendon.

SELECTED BIBLIOGRAPHY

The selected bibliography for this chapter can be found on www.expertconsult.com.

Chapter 3

PEDIATRIC ORTHOPAEDICS

Todd A. Milbrandt and Daniel J. Sucato

CONTENTS

CONTENTS—cont'd

SECTION 1 BONE DYSPLASIAS (DWARFISM)

I. INTRODUCTION

A. Definition: *Dysplasia* means abnormal development.

1. Shortening of the involved bones affects specific portions of the growing bone (Figure 3-1); hence the term *dwarfism*. Most forms of dwarfism are related to gene defects (single or multiple genes; Table 3-1).

B. The term *proportionate dwarfism* implies a symmetric decrease in both trunk and limb length (e.g., as occurs with mucopolysaccharidoses).

C. Disproportionate dwarfism:

1. Short-trunk variety (e.g., Kniest syndrome–spondyloepiphyseal)
2. Short-limb variety (e.g., achondroplasia, diastrophic dysplasia)
   - Short-limb dwarfism can be subclassified by the region of the limb that is short (e.g., rhizomelic-proximal, mesomelic-middle, acromelic-distal).
   - All types of dwarfism are summarized in Table 3-2.

II. ACHONDROPLASIA

A. Introduction and etiology

1. Achondroplasia is the most common form of disproportionate dwarfism.
2. **Autosomal dominant condition; 80% of cases caused by a spontaneous mutation in the fibroblast growth factor receptor 3 (FGFR3)**
3. This disproportionate, short-limbed form of dwarfism is caused by abnormal endochondral bone formation that is more affected than appositional growth.
4. Anatomically, achondroplasia is categorized as a physeal dysplasia.
5. **Caused by failure in the cartilaginous proliferative zone of the physis.** Achondroplasia is a quantitative, not a qualitative, cartilage defect.
6. It may be associated with advanced paternal age.

B. Signs and symptoms

1. Normal trunk and short limbs (rhizomelic) with hypotonia
2. Frontal bossing, button noses, small nasal bridges, trident hands (inability to approximate extended middle and ring fingers) (Figure 3-2).
3. Thoracolumbar kyphosis (which usually resolves around the age at ambulation)
4. **Lumbar stenosis (most likely to cause disability) and excessive lordosis (short pedicles with decreased interpedicular distances)**
   - Neurologic symptoms are usually related to nerve root or spinal cord compression, which can occur at any level, including the foramen magnum (which may cause periods of apnea).
5. Radial head subluxation
6. Normal intelligence but delayed motor milestones
7. Although sitting height may be normal, standing height is below the third percentile.

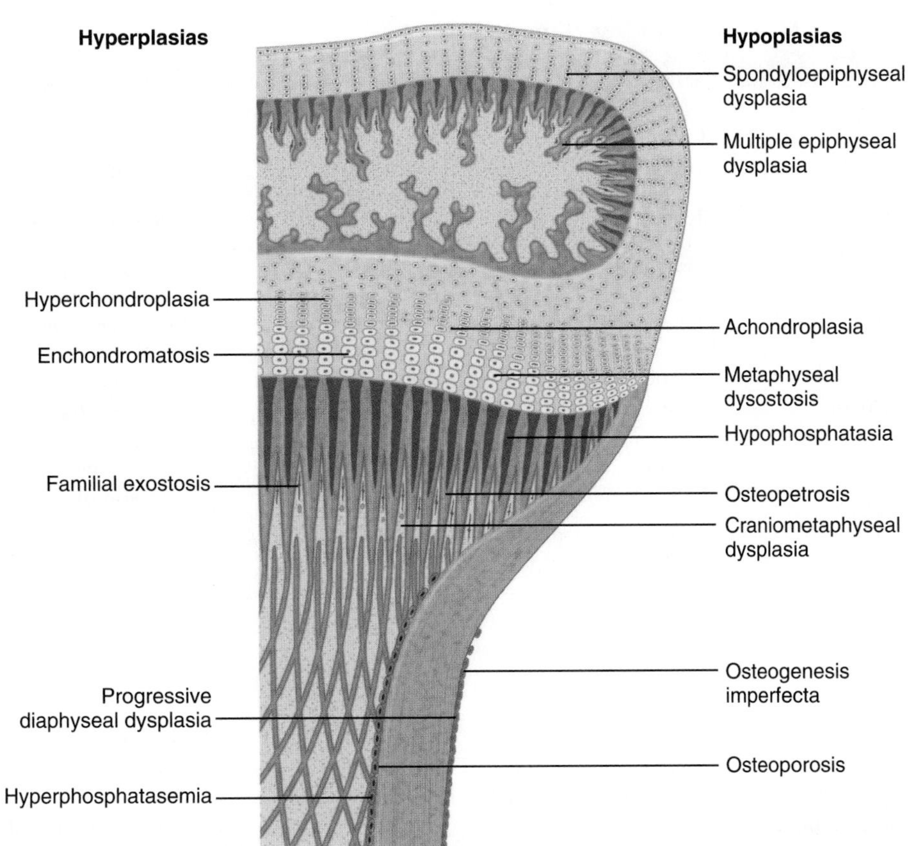

Figure 3-1 Locations of abnormalities that lead to dysplasias. (Adapted from Rubin P: *Dynamic classification of bone dysplasias,* Chicago, 1964, Year Book Medical Publishers.)

Table 3-1 Pediatric Congenital Disorders and Associated Genetic Defects

Disorder	Genetic Defect	Disorder	Genetic Defect
Achondroplasia	FGFR3	Hypophosphatemic rickets	PEX
Hypochondroplasia	FGFR3	Marfan syndrome	Fibrillin-1
Thanatophoric dysplasia	FGFR3	Osteogenesis imperfecta	Collagen type I
Pseudoachondroplasia	COMP	Ehlers-Danlos syndrome	
Multiple epiphyseal dysplasia type I	COMP	Types I and II	Collagen type V
Multiple epiphyseal dysplasia type II	Collagen type IX	Type IV	Collagen type IV
Spondyloepiphyseal dysplasia congenita	Collagen type II	Types VI and VII	Collagen type I
Kniest syndrome	Collagen type II	Duchenne/Becker muscular dystrophies	Dystrophin
Stickler syndrome (hereditary arthro-ophthalmopathy)	Collagen type II	Limb-girdle dystrophies	Sarcoglycan and dystroglycan complex
Diastrophic dysplasia	Sulfate transporter gene	Charcot-Marie-Tooth disease	PMP22
Schmid metaphyseal chondrodysplasia	Collagen type X	Spinal muscular atrophy	Survival motor neuron protein
Jansen metaphyseal chondrodysplasia	PTHRP	Myotonic dystrophy	Myotonin
Craniosynostosis	FGFR2	Friedreich ataxia	Frataxin
Cleidocranial dysplasia	CBFA1	Neurofibromatosis	Neurofibromin
		McCune-Albright syndrome	cAMP

cAMP, cyclic adenosine monophosphate; CBFA1, transcription factor for osteocalcin; COMP, cartilage oligomeric matrix protein; FGFR3 and FGFR2, fibroblast growth factor receptors 3 and 2; PEX, period-extender gene; PMP22, peripheral myelin protein-22; PTHRP, parathyroid hormone–related peptide.

Table 3-2 Summary of Major Types of Dwarfism

Dwarfism Type	Genetic Defect	Inheritance	Pathognomonic Feature
Achondroplasia	FGFR3	AD	Trident hands and lumbar kyphosis
Pseudoachondroplasia	COMP	AD	Normal facies and cervical instability
Spondyloepiphyseal dysplasia	Type II collagen	Congenita: AD Tarda: X-linked recessive	Epiphyseal fragmentation with spine involvement
Kniest syndrome	Type II collagen	AD	Retinal detachment and dumbbell-shaped bone
Jansen metaphyseal chondroplasia	PTHRP	AD	Hypercalcemia with metaphyseal expansion
Schmid metaphyseal chondroplasia	Type X collagen	AD	Coxa vara with proximal femur involvement
McKusick metaphyseal chondroplasia	Unknown COMP	AR	Odontoid hypoplasia
Multiple epiphyseal dysplasia	Type II collagen	AD	Bilateral hip involvement
Mucopolysaccharidosis (see Table 3-3)			
Diastrophic dysplasia	Sulfate transport protein	AR	Cauliflower ears and kyphoscoliosis
Cleidocranial dysplasia	CBFA1	AD	Aplasia of clavicles and coxa vara

AD, autosomal dominant; AR, autosomal recessive; CBFA1, transcription factor for osteocalcin; COMP, cartilage oligomeric matrix protein; FGFR3, fibroblast growth factor receptor 3; PTHRP, parathyroid hormone–related peptide.

8. Radiographic findings
   - **Spine: narrowed interpedicular distance in the distal spine (L1 to S1), with pedicular shortening, T12/L1 wedging, generalized posterior vertebral scalloping**
   - **Pelvis: wider than it is deep ("champagne glass" pelvic outlet)**

C. Treatment

1. Lumbar stenosis: decompression and fusion of the spine for a developing neurologic deficit (usually in children older than age 10)
2. Foramen magnum stenosis: decompression
3. Progressive kyphosis: if fail bracing, anterior and posterior fusion are indicated for residual kyphosis greater than 60 degrees by age 5 years.
4. Genu varum: Tibial osteotomies or hemiepiphysiodesis
5. Limb lengthening through callodiastasis (lengthening through a metaphyseal corticotomy) have been well described, with a high rate of complications.
   - Controversial

D. Pseudoachondroplasia: This disorder is clinically similar to achondroplasia.

1. **Genetics: The inheritance pattern is autosomal dominant with a defect on chromosome 19 within the cartilage oligometric matrix protein (COMP).**
2. Signs and symptoms:
   - Normal facies
   - Orthopaedic manifestations include cervical instability; scoliosis with increased lumbar lordosis; significant lower extremity bowing; and hip, knee, and elbow flexion contractures with precocious osteoarthritis.
3. Radiographic findings: metaphyseal flaring and delayed epiphyseal ossification

III. SPONDYLOEPIPHYSEAL DYSPLASIA

A. Clinical features

1. Must be differentiated from multiple epiphyseal dysplasia (MED)
2. MED and spondyloepiphyseal dysplasia involve abnormal epiphyseal development in the upper and lower extremities.
3. **The distinguishing feature of spondyloepiphyseal dysplasia is the added typical spine involvement.**
   - Scoliosis: typically with a sharply curved apex over a small number of vertebrae
4. Retinal detachment and respiratory problems are common.

B. Causes

1. Genetic defect is within the gene encoding **type II collagen.**

IV. CHONDRODYSPLASIA PUNCTATA

A. Clinical features

1. Characterized by multiple punctate calcifications seen on radiographs during infancy
2. The autosomal dominant form (Conradi-Hünermann) has a wide variation of clinical expression.
3. Autosomal recessive, rhizomelic form is usually fatal during the first year of life.
   - Cataracts, asymmetric limb shortening that may necessitate surgical correction, and spinal deformities are common.

V. KNIEST SYNDROME

A. Clinical features

1. Autosomal dominant; short-trunked, disproportionate dwarfism with joint stiffness/contractures, scoliosis, kyphosis, dumbbell-shaped femora, and hypoplastic pelvis and spine
2. Otitis media and hearing loss are frequent.

B. Causes

1. Defect within type II collagen

C. Radiographic findings

1. Osteopenia and dumbbell-shaped bones

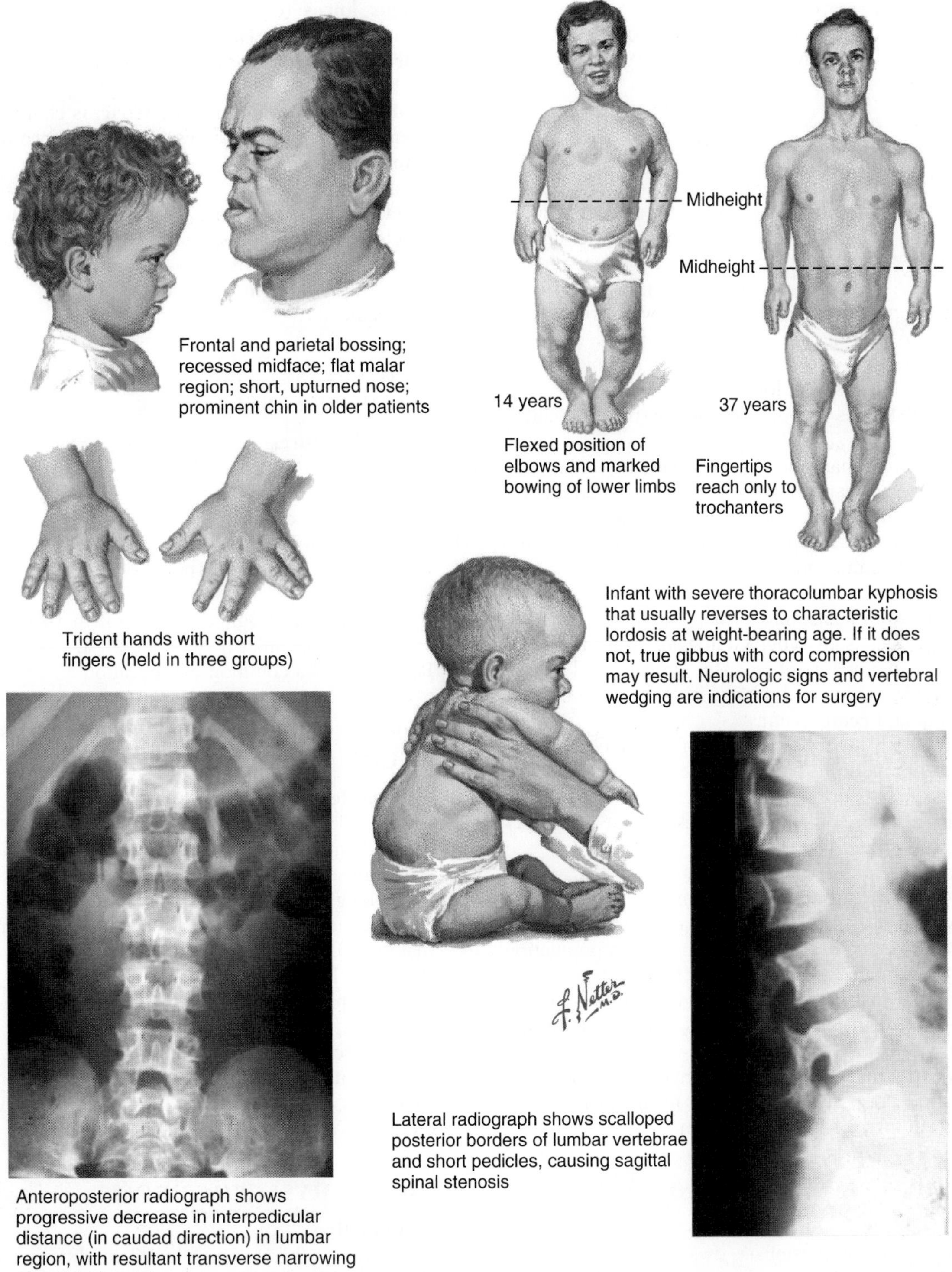

Frontal and parietal bossing; recessed midface; flat malar region; short, upturned nose; prominent chin in older patients
Midheight
Midheight
14 years
37 years
Flexed position of elbows and marked bowing of lower limbs
Fingertips reach only to trochanters
Trident hands with short fingers (held in three groups)
Infant with severe thoracolumbar kyphosis that usually reverses to characteristic lordosis at weight-bearing age. If it does not, true gibbus with cord compression may result. Neurologic signs and vertebral wedging are indications for surgery
F. Netter M.D.
Lateral radiograph shows scalloped posterior borders of lumbar vertebrae and short pedicles, causing sagittal spinal stenosis
Anteroposterior radiograph shows progressive decrease in interpedicular distance (in caudad direction) in lumbar region, with resultant transverse narrowing of vertebral canal

Figure 3-2 Clinical features of achondroplasia. Note the space between the middle and ring fingers. (From Greene WB: *Netter's orthopaedics,* Philadelphia, 2005, WB Saunders, Figure 3-6.)

D. **Treatment**
1. Early therapy for joint contractures is required. Reconstructive procedures may be required for early hip degenerative arthritis.

VI. METAPHYSEAL CHONDRODYSPLASIA

A. **Clinical features**
1. Heterogeneous group of disorders characterized by metaphyseal changes of tubular bones with normal epiphyses

B. **Causes**
1. The defect appears to be in the proliferative and hypertrophic zones of the physis.

C. **Types**
1. Jansen (rare): most severe form
   - Genetic defect is in **parathyroid hormone–related peptide.**
   - Autosomal dominant inheritance; retardation, markedly short-limbed dwarfism with wide eyes, monkey-like stance, and hypercalcemia.
   - Striking bulbous metaphyseal expansion of long bones is a distinctive radiographic finding.
2. Schmid type
   - More common, less severe form
   - Genetic defect is in **type X collagen,** transmitted by autosomal dominant inheritance; short-limbed dwarfism not diagnosed until patient is older, as a result of coxa vara and genu varum.
   - Predominantly involves the proximal femur. Gait is often Trendelenburg, and patients have increased lumbar lordosis.
   - Condition often confused with rickets, but laboratory test results are normal.
3. McKusick type
   - Autosomal recessive inheritance; cartilage-hair dysplasia (hypoplasia of cartilage and small diameter of hair) is observed most commonly among the Amish population and in Finland.
   - Atlantoaxial instability is common (odontoid hypoplasia). Ankle deformity develops as a result of fibular overgrowth distally.
   - Affected patients may have abnormal immunocompetence and have an increased risk for malignancies, intestinal malabsorption, and megacolon.

VII. MULTIPLE EPIPHYSEAL DYSPLASIA

A. **Clinical features**
1. Short-limbed, disproportionate dwarfism that often is not manifested until between the ages of 5 and 14. It must be differentiated from spondyloepiphyseal dysplasia. A mild form (Ribbing) and a more severe form (Fairbanks) exist.

B. **Causes**
1. **Most common gene mutation is in COMP.**

C. **Radiologic findings**
1. MED is characterized by irregular, delayed ossification at multiple epiphyses (Figure 3-3).
2. Short, stunted metacarpals and metatarsals, irregular proximal femora, abnormal ossification (tibial "slant sign" and flattened femoral condyles, patella with double layer), **valgus knees** (early osteotomy should be considered), waddling gait, and early hip arthritis are common.
3. **The proximal femoral involvement can be confused with Perthes disease.**
   - **MED is bilateral and symmetric, is characterized by early acetabular changes, and is not accompanied by metaphyseal cysts.**

D. **Treatment**
1. **Obtain bone survey to differentiate between MED and single epiphyseal dysplasia, as well as to identify all areas of involvement.**
2. Treat limb alignment and perform early joint replacement.

VIII. DYSPLASIA EPIPHYSEALIS HEMIMELICA (TREVOR DISEASE)

A. **Clinical features**
1. An epiphyseal osteochondroma
2. Most commonly seen at the knee and ankle
3. Usually affects only one joint

B. **Radiologic findings**
1. Calcifications are seen within the joint.

C. **Treatment**
1. Excision of the prominent overgrowth (if symptomatic) and later osteotomies may be required.
2. Recurrence is a common complication.

IX. PROGRESSIVE DIAPHYSEAL DYSPLASIA (CAMURATI-ENGELMANN DISEASE)

A. **Clinical features**
1. Autosomal dominant inheritance.
2. Affected children are often "late walkers" (because of associated muscle weakness), with symmetric cortical thickening of long bones.
3. The tibia, femur, and humerus are most often involved (in that order), affecting only the diaphyseal portion of bone.
4. Watch for leg-length inequality.

B. **Radiographic findings**
1. Widened, fusiform diaphyses with increased bone formation and sclerosis

C. **Treatment**
1. Salicylates, nonsteroidal anti-inflammatory drugs (NSAIDs), and steroids for refractory cases

X. MUCOPOLYSACCHARIDOSIS

A. **Introduction**
1. In contrast to the aforementioned conditions, these forms of dwarfism are easily differentiated on the basis of the presence of complex sugars in the urine.
2. The accumulation of mucopolysaccharides, as a result of a hydrolase enzyme deficiency, produces a proportionate dwarfism.

B. **Types (Table 3-3)**
1. **Morquio syndrome** (autosomal recessive)
   - **Most common form;** manifests by ages 18 months to 2 years with waddling gait, genu valgum ("knock-knees"), thoracic kyphosis, cloudy corneas, and normal intelligence
   - Urinary excretion of **keratan sulfate**

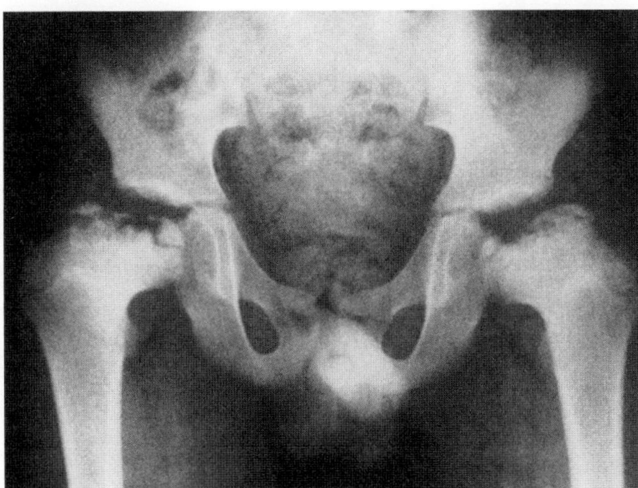

Figure 3-3 Multiple epiphyseal dysplasia. Radiograph of the pelvis in a 6-year-old patient shows abnormal bilateral femoral heads. (From Benson M, et al: *Children's orthopaedics and fractures,* New York, 1994, Churchill Livingstone, p 52.)

- Bony changes include a thickening skull; wide ribs; anterior beaking of vertebrae; a wide, flat pelvis; coxa vara with unossified femoral heads; and bullet-shaped metacarpals.
- **C1-C2 instability (caused by odontoid hypoplasia) can be seen with Morquio syndrome, manifesting with myelopathy and necessitating decompression and cervical fusion.**

2. Hurler syndrome (autosomal recessive inheritance)
   - Most severe form
   - Urinary excretion of **dermatan/heparan sulfate**
   - Mental retardation
   - Bone marrow transplantation has increased the life span for patients with this disorder.
3. Hunter syndrome (sex-linked recessive inheritance)
   - Urinary excretion of dermatan/heparan sulfate
   - Mental retardation
   - Bone marrow transplantation has increased the life span for patients with this disorder.
4. Sanfilippo syndrome (autosomal recessive inheritance)
   - Urinary excretion of heparan sulfate
   - Associated with mental retardation
   - Bone marrow transplantation has increased the life span for patients with this disorder

XI. DIASTROPHIC DYSPLASIA

A. Clinical features
1. **Autosomal recessive inheritance;** severe, short-limbed dwarfism
2. **Cleft palate (59% of cases)**
3. Severe joint contractures (especially hip and knee)
4. **Cauliflower ears (80% of cases),** hitchhiker's thumb
5. **Rigid clubfeet**

B. Causes
1. **Deficiency in sulfate transport protein**

C. Radiologic findings
1. Spine radiographs reveal **cervical kyphosis** (often severe, necessitating immediate treatment), thoracolumbar kyphoscoliosis (83% of cases), spina bifida occulta, and atlantoaxial instability.

D. Treatment
1. Quadriplegia is a major concern with deformities of the cervical spine.
   - Must fuse early
2. Surgical release of clubfoot deformities
3. Osteotomies for contractures
4. Spinal fusion often required

XII. CLEIDOCRANIAL DYSPLASIA (DYSOSTOSIS)

A. Clinical features
1. Autosomal dominant inheritance
2. Proportionate dwarfism that affects bones formed by intramembranous ossification (clavicles, cranium, pelvis)

B. Causes
1. **Defect in transcription factor for osteocalcin (CBFA1)**

C. Radiologic findings
1. **Hypoplasia or aplasia of the clavicle (no intervention necessary)** (Figure 3-4)
2. Delayed closure of skull sutures
3. Frontal bossing
4. **Coxa vara**
5. Delayed ossification of the pubis
6. Wormian-type bone

D. Treatment
1. Consider intertrochanteric valgus osteotomy if neck-shaft angle is less than 100 degrees.

XIII. DYSPLASIAS ASSOCIATED WITH BENIGN BONE GROWTH

A. These conditions include multiple hereditary exostosis (osteochondromatosis), fibrous dysplasia, Ollier disease (enchondromatosis), and Maffucci syndrome (enchondromatosis and hemangiomas). These entities are discussed in Chapter 9, Orthopaedic Pathology.

Table 3-3 Mucopolysaccharidoses

Syndrome	Inheritance	Intelligence	Cornea	Urinary Excretion	Other
Hurler	AR	Below normal	Cloudy	Dermatan/heparan sulfate	Worst prognosis
Hunter	XR	Below normal	Clear	Dermatan/heparan sulfate	
Sanfilippo	AR	Below normal	Clear	Heparin sulfate	Normal development until 2 yr of age
Morquio	AR	Normal	Cloudy	Keratan sulfate	Most common

AR, autosomal recessive; XR, X-linked recessive.

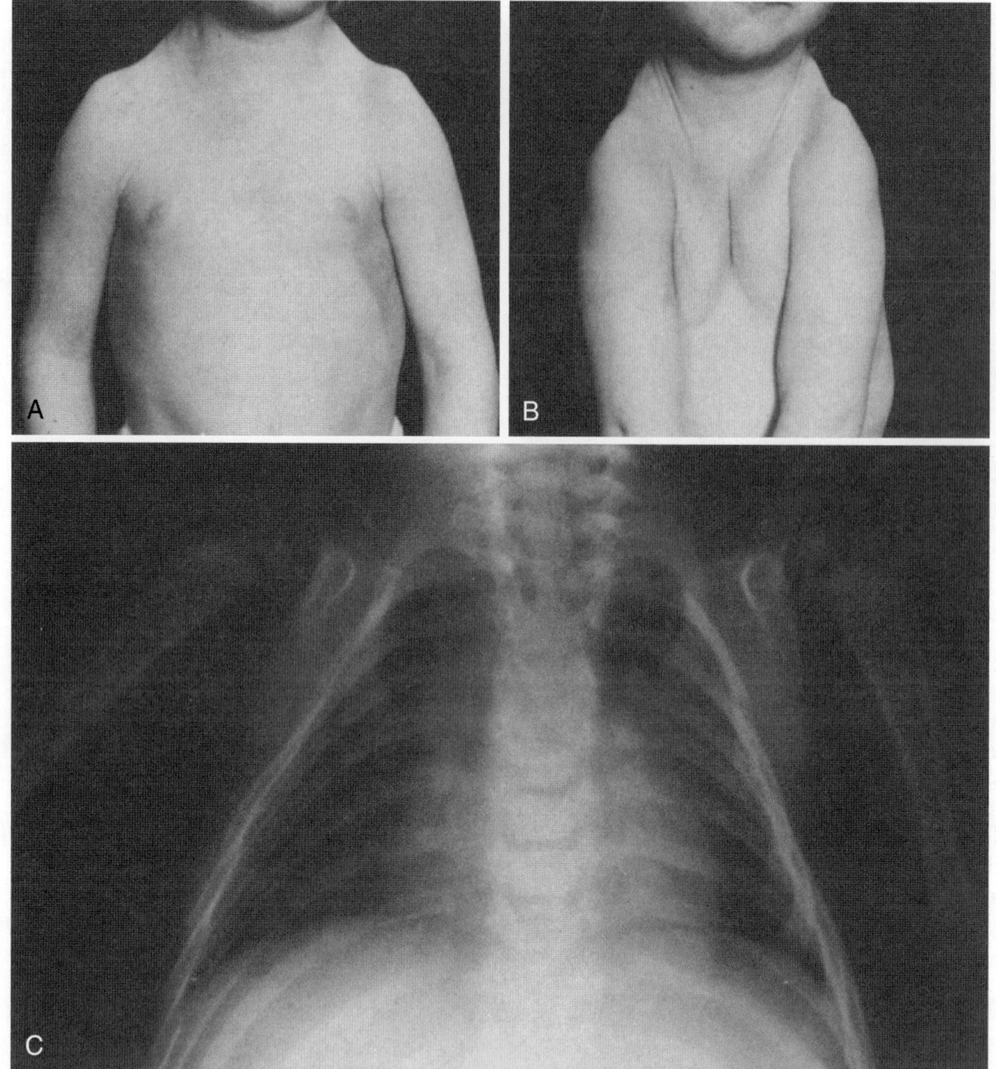

Figure 3-4 Cleidocranial dysostosis. **A,** Clinical photograph, showing the shoulders in normal position. **B,** Clinical photograph, showing the shoulders approximated. **C,** Radiograph of the chest and shoulders, showing bilateral aplasia of the clavicles. (From Benson M, et al: *Children's orthopaedics and fractures,* New York, 1994, Churchill Livingstone, p 364.)

SECTION 2 CHROMOSOMAL AND TERATOLOGIC DISORDERS

I. DOWN SYNDROME (TRISOMY 21)

A. Clinical features

1. Usually characterized by ligamentous laxity, hypotonia, mental retardation, heart disease with atrial septal defect (50% of cases), endocrine disorders (hypothyroidism and diabetes), and premature aging
2. Orthopaedic problems include metatarsus primus varus, pes planus, spinal abnormalities (**atlantoaxial instability** [Figure 3-5], scoliosis [50% of cases], spondylolisthesis [6% of cases]), **hip instability** (open reduction with or without osteotomy is usually required), slipped capital femoral epiphysis (SCFE) (hypothyroidism should be sought), **patellar dislocation,** and symptomatic planovalgus feet.
3. Atlantoaxial instability may be subtle but commonly manifests as a loss or change in motor milestones.

B. Causes

1. Trisomy 21 is the most common chromosomal abnormality; its incidence increases with maternal age.
2. Chromosome 21 is the location of genes that encode for type VI collagen (*COL6A1* and *COL6A2*).
   - Abnormal type VI collagen is thought to be cause for generalized joint laxity and other orthopaedic problems in Down syndrome.

C. Radiologic studies

1. Lower extremity radiographs are needed to evaluate for patella dislocations and genu valgum.
2. Anteroposterior and frog-leg pelvic views to evaluate for SCFE

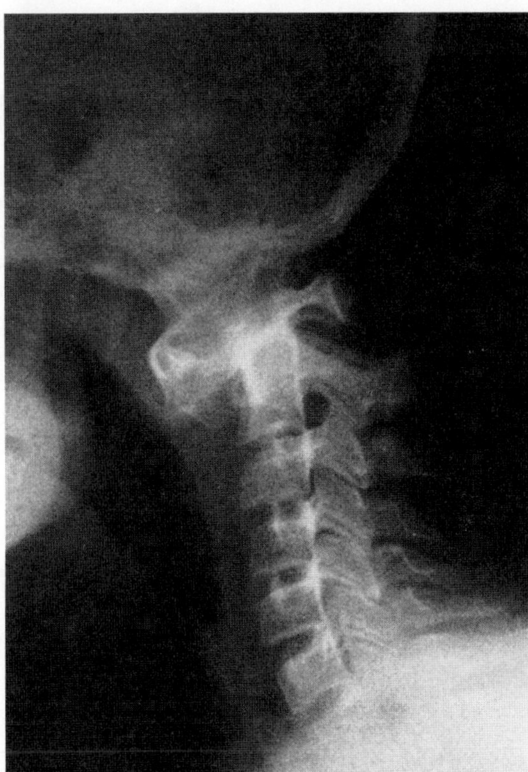

Figure 3-5 **Gross atlantoaxial instability in an 11-year-old with Down syndrome. His gait was clumsy, and he had poor coordination of his extremities. Therefore, he underwent posterior stabilization.** (From Benson M, et al: *Children's orthopaedics and fractures,* New York, 1994, Churchill Livingstone, p 590.)

3. Flexion-extension radiographs of the cervical spine to evaluate atlantoaxial instability

D. **Treatment**

1. **Screening for cervical spine instability:**
   - Usefulness is **controversial**.
     - Exception: possibly preoperative assessment before administration of anesthetic
   - Special Olympics requires cervical spine x-ray screening for participation in selected sports.
2. **Children with asymptomatic instability should avoid contact sports, diving, and gymnastics.**
3. Children with symptomatic instability often require surgery, but the rate of wound healing problems and infection is high.
   - Cervical instability with neurologic symptoms: fusion with autologous bone graft and instrumentation, with consideration of halo immobilization
   - Scoliosis: bracing for 25- to 30-degree curves, surgery for 50- to 60-degree curves
   - **Hip: initially may be treated with closed reduction, but capsulorraphy, pelvis osteotomy, and femoral osteotomy may be required.**
   - Patellar instability: if symptomatic, then lateral release, medial reefing, or bony realignment of the patellar tendon should be considered.

II. TURNER SYNDROME

A. **Clinical features**

1. Affected patients are female and have short stature, lack of sexual development, webbed neck, and cubitus valgus.
2. Idiopathic scoliosis is common. Growth hormone therapy can exacerbate scoliosis.
3. Malignant hyperthermia is common with anesthetic use.
4. Must be differentiated from Noonan syndrome (same appearance except for normal gonadal development, mental retardation, and more severe scoliosis)

B. **Causes**

1. 45,XO Genotype

C. **Radiologic findings**

1. Genu valgum and shortening of the fourth and fifth metacarpals, which usually necessitate no treatment

D. **Treatment**

1. Monitor for osteoporosis.

III. PRADER-WILLI SYNDROME

A. **Clinical features**

1. Floppy, hypotonic infant who grows up to be an intellectually impaired, obese adult with an insatiable appetite
2. Growth retardation
3. Hypoplastic genitalia

B. **Causes**

1. Partial chromosome 15 deletion (missing portion from father)

C. **Radiologic findings**

1. Hip dysplasia and juvenile-onset scoliosis

IV. MENKES SYNDROME

A. **Clinical features**

1. Characteristic "kinky" hair
2. May be differentiated from occipital horn syndrome (which also affects copper transport) in that the latter is characterized by bony projections from the occiput of the skull

B. **Causes**

1. Sex-linked recessive disorder of copper transport

C. **Radiologic findings**

1. Skull (wormian bones), long bones (metaphysial spurring), and ribs (anterior flaring and multiple fractures)

V. RETT SYNDROME

A. **Clinical features**

1. Progressive impairment and stereotaxic, abnormal hand movements (like those in autism)
2. Manifests in girls at 6 to 18 months of age
3. Loss of developmental milestones that is rapid and then stabilizes

B. **Causes**

1. Family of deletion mutations of the X-linked gene encoding a protein called methyl-CpG-binding protein 2 (MECP2)

C. **Radiologic findings**

1. Scoliosis with a C-shaped curve that is unresponsive to bracing

D. Treatment

1. Spinal instrumentation must include all of the kyphosis and the scoliosis.
2. Spasticity results in joint contractures, which are treated as they are in cerebral palsy.

VI. BECKWITH-WIEDEMANN SYNDROME

A. Clinical features

1. Organomegaly, omphalocele, and a large tongue
2. **Orthopaedic manifestations include hemihypertrophy with spastic cerebral palsy.**
3. **There is a predisposition to Wilms tumor (patient must be screened regularly with kidney ultrasonography).**

B. Causes

1. Spasticity is thought to be the result of infantile hypoglycemic episodes secondary to pancreatic islet cell hypertrophy.

C. Treatment

1. Growth arrest may be necessary in large limb.

VII. TERATOGEN-INDUCED DISORDERS

A. Fetal alcohol syndrome: Maternal alcoholism can cause growth disturbances, central nervous system dysfunction, dysmorphic facies, hip dislocation, cervical spine vertebral and upper extremity congenital fusions, congenital scoliosis, and myelodysplasia. Contractures respond to physical therapy.

B. Maternal diabetes: This may lead to heart defects, sacral agenesis, and anencephaly. Careful management of pregnant diabetic women is essential.

C. Other teratogens: These include drugs (e.g., aminopterin, phenytoin, thalidomide), trace metals, maternal conditions, infections, and intrauterine factors; they may also lead to orthopaedic manifestations in affected children.

SECTION 3 HEMATOPOIETIC DISORDERS

I. GAUCHER DISEASE

A. Clinical features

1. Osteopenia
2. Bone pain (Gaucher crisis), and bleeding abnormalities
3. Hepatosplenomegaly (characteristic finding)
4. Types
   - Type I, most commonly in persons of Ashkenazi Jewish descent
   - Type II, infantile
   - Type III, chronic neuropathic

B. Causes

1. Aberrant autosomal recessive, lysosomal storage disease characterized by accumulation of cerebroside in cells of the reticuloendothelial system. The cause is a deficiency of the enzyme **β-glucocerebrosidase.**

C. Radiologic findings

1. Metaphyseal enlargement (failure of remodeling), femoral head necrosis (may be confused with Perthes disease or MED), "moth-eaten" trabeculae, patchy sclerosis, and Erlenmeyer flask deformity of the distal femora (70% of cases)

D. Treatment

1. Treatment is supportive; new enzyme therapy is available but is extremely expensive.

II. NIEMANN-PICK DISEASE

A. Autosomal recessive disorder

B. Caused by an accumulation of sphingomyelin in reticuloendothelial system cells

C. Occurs commonly in Jews of eastern European descent

D. Marrow expansion and cortical thinning are common in long bones; coxa valga is also seen.

III. SICKLE CELL ANEMIA

A. Clinical features

1. Sickle cell disease (affects 1% of African Americans) is more severe but less common than sickle cell trait (8% prevalence).
2. Bone infarction is more common than acute osteomyelitis in children with sickle cell disease who present with acute musculoskeletal pain.
3. ***Salmonella* infection is more commonly seen in children with sickle cell disease. Despite this tendency, *Staphylococcus aureus* infection is still the most common cause of osteomyelitis in affected patients.**
4. Dactylitis (acute hand/foot swelling) is also common.

B. Causes

1. Mutation in the β-globin gene, resulting in sickle hemoglobin (HbS) production. When the cell becomes deoxygenated, HbS molecules assemble into fibers that produce a sickle-shaped red blood cell.
2. Crises usually begin at ages 2 to 3 years, are caused by substance P, and may lead to characteristic bone infarctions.

C. Radiologic findings

1. Growth retardation or skeletal immaturity, **osteonecrosis of femoral and humeral heads,** osteomyelitis (often in diaphysis), biconcave "fish" vertebrae, acetabular protrusio, and septic arthritis are common in this disorder.
2. **Differentiating bone infarction and osteomyelitis:**
   - **Sequential bone marrow tests and bone scans within 24 hours of hospital admission**
   - Gadolinium-enhanced T1-weighted magnetic resonance imaging (MRI) sequences

D. Treatment

1. Aspiration and culture may be necessary to differentiate infarction from osteomyelitis.

2. Preoperative oxygenation and exchange transfusion are helpful for affected patients requiring surgery. Hydroxyurea has produced dramatic relief of pain when used for bone crises.

IV. THALASSEMIA

A. Similar to sickle cell anemia in manifestation

B. Most commonly observed in people of Mediterranean descent

C. Common symptoms include bone pain and leg ulceration

D. Radiographic findings: long-bone thinning, metaphyseal expansion, osteopenia, and premature physeal closure

V. HEMOPHILIA

A. Clinical features

1. Hemarthrosis manifests with painful swelling and decreased range of motion (ROM) of affected joints.
2. The knee is the joint most commonly affected.
3. Deep intramuscular bleeding is also common and can lead to the formation of a pseudotumor (blood cyst), which can occur in soft tissue or bone.
   - **Intramuscular hematomas can lead to compression of adjacent nerves.**
     - The classic scenario is an iliacus hematoma that causes femoral nerve paralysis and mimics bleeding into the hip joint.

B. Causes

1. X-linked recessive disorder with decreased amounts of factor VIII (hemophilia A), abnormal factor VIII with platelet dysfunction (von Willebrand disease), or decreased amounts of factor IX (hemophilia B, Leyden, or Christmas disease)
2. Can be mild (5% to 25% of normal amounts of factor present), moderate (1% to 5% available), or severe (<1% present)

C. Radiologic findings

1. Squaring of the patellae and condyles, epiphyseal overgrowth with leg-length discrepancy
2. Generalized osteopenia with resulting fractures
3. Cartilage atrophy, resulting from enzymatic matrix degeneration and chondrocyte death, is frequent.

D. Treatment

1. Acute treatment of hemarthrosis is crucial and should begin immediately with administration of factor VIII or factor IX. Administration should continue for 3 to 7 days after cessation of bleeding and should be followed by physical therapy.
2. Home transfusion therapy has reduced the severity of the arthropathy with the advantage of immediate treatment when bleeding occurs.
3. Aspiration of a hemarthrosis is controversial.
4. **Treatment of the sequelae**
   - **Synovectomy**
     - **Indicated for hemarthroses that recur despite optimal medical management**
     - Arthroscopy has better results with motion and duration of hospitalization than does open synovectomy.
     - Radiation synovectomy: useful in patients with antibody inhibitors and poor medical management
   - Contracture release and osteotomies
   - Total joint arthroplasty for hemophilic arthropathy
5. **Factor VIII levels should be increased for prophylaxis in the following situations: vigorous physical therapy (20% of patients), treatment of hematoma (30%), acute hemarthrosis or soft tissue surgery (>50%), and skeletal surgery (approaching 100% preoperatively and maintained at >50% for 10 days postoperatively).**
6. **Immunoglobulin G** (IgG) antibody inhibitors are present in 4% to 20% of hemophiliac patients; their presence is a relative contraindication to surgery.
7. Because of the amount of blood component therapy needed to treat this disorder, a large percentage of older hemophiliac patients are seropositive for human immunodeficiency virus (HIV).

VI. LEUKEMIA

A. Clinical features

1. The most common malignancy of childhood. Acute lymphocytic leukemia represents 80% of cases of leukemia.
2. Incidence peaks at 4 years of age.
3. One fourth to one third of affected children have musculoskeletal complaints (back, pelvic, leg pains).

B. Radiologic findings

1. Bony changes include demineralization of bones, periostitis, and occasionally lytic lesions. Radiolucent "leukemia" lines may be seen in the metaphyses of affected bones in older affected children.

C. Treatment

1. Management of leukemia includes chemotherapy, which may predispose the patient to pathologic fractures.

SECTION 4 METABOLIC DISEASE/ARTHRITIDES*

I. RICKETS

A. Clinical features

1. Short stature
2. Limb angulation (usually varus)
3. Bone pain

B. Causes

1. Deficiency of calcium (and sometimes phosphorus), affecting mineralization at the epiphyses of long bones
2. Histologic findings: Widened osteoid seams and "Swiss cheese" trabeculae are characteristic in bone.
3. **Growth plate abnormalities include enlarged and distorted maturation zone (zone of hypertrophy)** and a poorly defined zone of provisional calcification.

*See Chapter 1, Basic Sciences.

C. Radiologic findings

1. **Classical findings in this disorder include brittle bones with physeal cupping/widening, bowing of long bones**, transverse radiolucent Looser lines, ligamentous laxity, flattening of the skull, enlargement of costal cartilages (rachitic rosary), and dorsal kyphosis (cat back) (Figure 3-6).

D. Treatment

1. Several varieties of rickets are based on the underlying abnormality (e.g., gastrointestinal, kidney, diet, and organ); they are discussed in detail in Chapter 1, Basic Sciences.

II. OSTEOGENESIS IMPERFECTA

A. Clinical features

1. Bone fragility (brittle "wormian" bone), short stature
2. Scoliosis
3. Tooth defects (dentinogenesis imperfecta)
4. Hearing defects

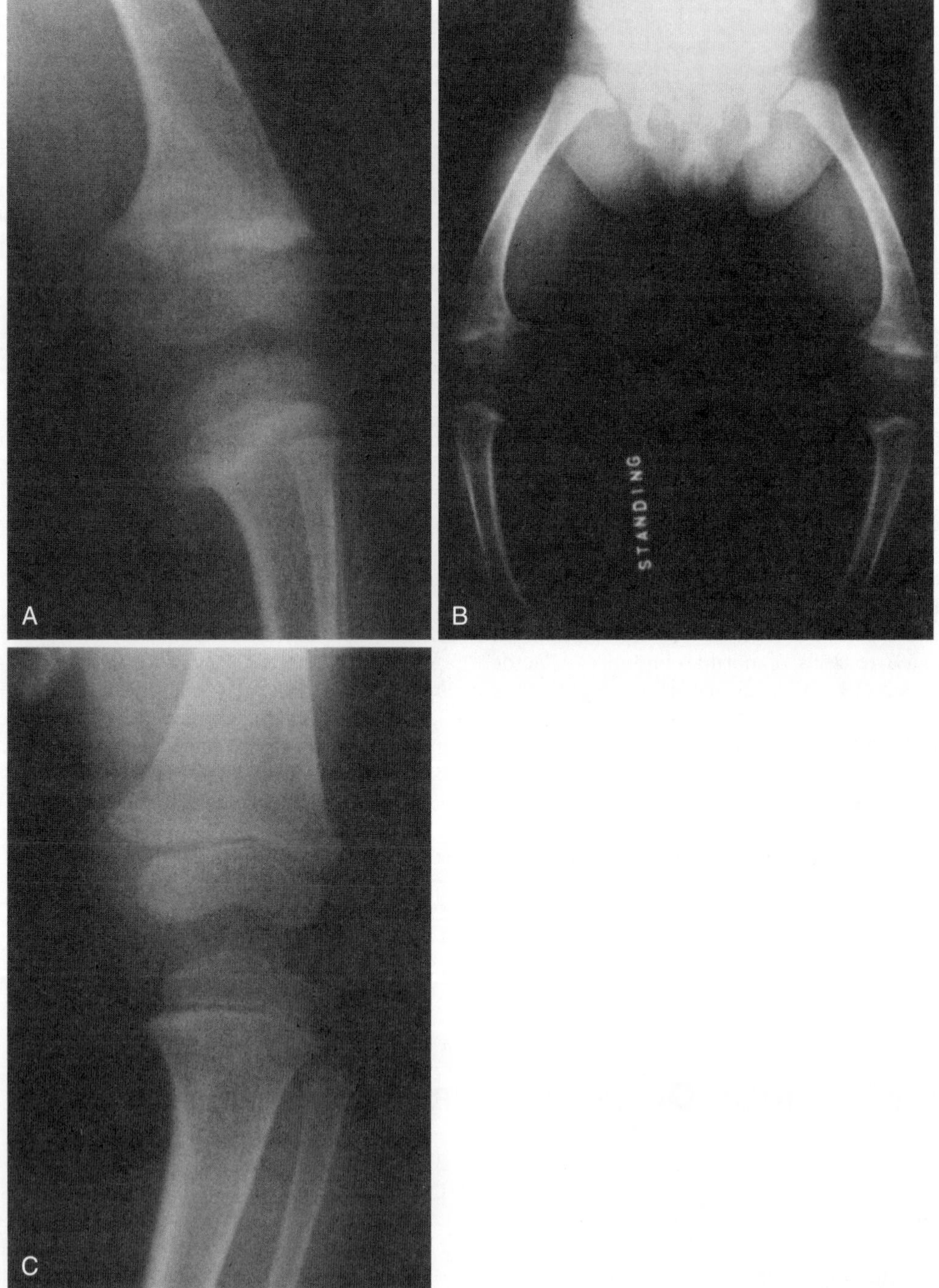

Figure 3-6 Rickets. **A,** Hazy metaphysis with cupping in an affected young boy. **B,** Accentuated genu varum is present. **C,** With vitamin D replacement therapy, the bone lesions healed in 6 months. (From Herring JA, editor: *Tachdjian's pediatric orthopaedics,* ed 4, Philadelphia, 2008, WB Saunders, p 1921.)

5. Blue sclerae in types I and II
6. Ligamentous laxity
7. **Basilar invagination is common in more severe clinical phenotypes.**
8. Fractures are common:
   - Healing is normal, but bone typically does not remodel.
   - Fractures occur less frequently with advancing age (usually cease at puberty).
   - Compression fractures (codfish vertebrae) are also common.

B. Causes

1. **Defect in type I collagen (*COL1A2* gene) that causes abnormal cross-linking and leads to decreased collagen secretion**
2. Histologic findings: increased diameters of haversian canals and osteocyte lacunae, increased numbers of cells, and replicated cement lines, which result in the thin cortices seen on radiographs
3. Classification
   - Four types have been identified (Sillence, 1981), although the disorder is probably best considered as a continuum with different inheritance patterns and severity (Table 3-4).

C. Radiologic findings

1. Thin cortices and generalized osteopenia

D. Treatment

1. Fracture management and long-term rehabilitation
2. Bracing of extremities early to prevent deformity and minimize fractures
3. Sofield osteotomies—"shish kebab" multiple long-bone osteotomies with either fixed-length Rush rods or telescoping (Bailey-Dubow or Fassier-Duval) intramedullary rods—are sometimes required for progressive bowing of long bones.
4. Fractures in children younger than 2 years are treated similarly to those in children without osteogenesis imperfecta. After age 2, telescoping intramedullary rods can be considered.
5. Bisphosphonates have been shown to decrease the number of fractures in these patients.
   - **Iatrogenic osteopetrosis can occur with high-dose, long-term use of bisphosphonates.**
6. Scoliosis is common, and bracing is ineffective treatment. Surgery is necessary for scoliosis deformities exceeding 50 degrees, and a large blood loss is to be expected.

Table 3-4 Osteogenesis Imperfecta

Type	Inheritance	Sclerae	Features
IA, IB	AD	Blue	Onset at preschool age (tarda); hearing loss; involvement of teeth (type IA only)
II	AR	Blue	Lethal; concertina femur, beaded ribs
III	AR	Normal	Fractures at birth, progressively short stature
IVA, IVB	AD	Normal	Milder form; normal hearing, involvement of teeth (type IVA only)

AD, autosomal dominant; AR, autosomal recessive.

III. IDIOPATHIC JUVENILE OSTEOPOROSIS

A. Clinical features

1. Rare, self-limiting disorder that appears between the ages of 8 and 14 years with osteopenia, growth arrest, and bone and joint pain.
2. This disorder must be differentiated from other causes of osteopenia (e.g., osteogenesis imperfecta, malignancy, Cushing disease).

B. Causes

1. Serum calcium and phosphorus levels are normal.

C. Radiologic findings

1. Possible multiple vertebral body microfractures

D. Treatment

1. Bracing for vertebral body fractures
2. Typically, this disorder resolves spontaneously 2 to 4 years after the onset of puberty.

IV. OSTEOPETROSIS

A. Clinical features

1. Bone pain
2. **Loss of the medullary canal can cause anemias and encroachment on the optic and oculomotor nerves, which in turn causes blindness.**

B. Causes

1. **Failure of osteoclastic resorption, probably secondary to a defect in the thymus, leading to dense bone (so-called "marble" bone)**
2. The mild form is autosomal dominant; the "malignant" form is autosomal recessive.

C. Radiologic findings

1. "Rugger jersey" spine (Figure 3-7)
2. Marble bone
3. Erlenmeyer flask deformity of the proximal humerus and distal femur

D. Treatment

1. Healing is normal, but amount of time for healing may be prolonged.
2. **Bone marrow transplantation** may be helpful for treating the malignant form (see Chapter 1, "Basic Sciences").

V. INFANTILE CORTICAL HYPEROSTOSIS (CAFFEY DISEASE)

A. Clinical features

1. Soft tissue swelling and bony cortical thickening (especially the jaw and ulna) that follow a febrile illness in infants 0 to 9 months old.
2. This disorder may be differentiated from trauma (and child abuse) on the basis of single-bone involvement.
3. Infection, scurvy, tumor, and progressive diaphyseal dysplasia may be included in the differential diagnosis.

B. Radiologic findings

1. Characteristic periosteal reaction

C. Treatment

1. The condition is benign and self-limiting.

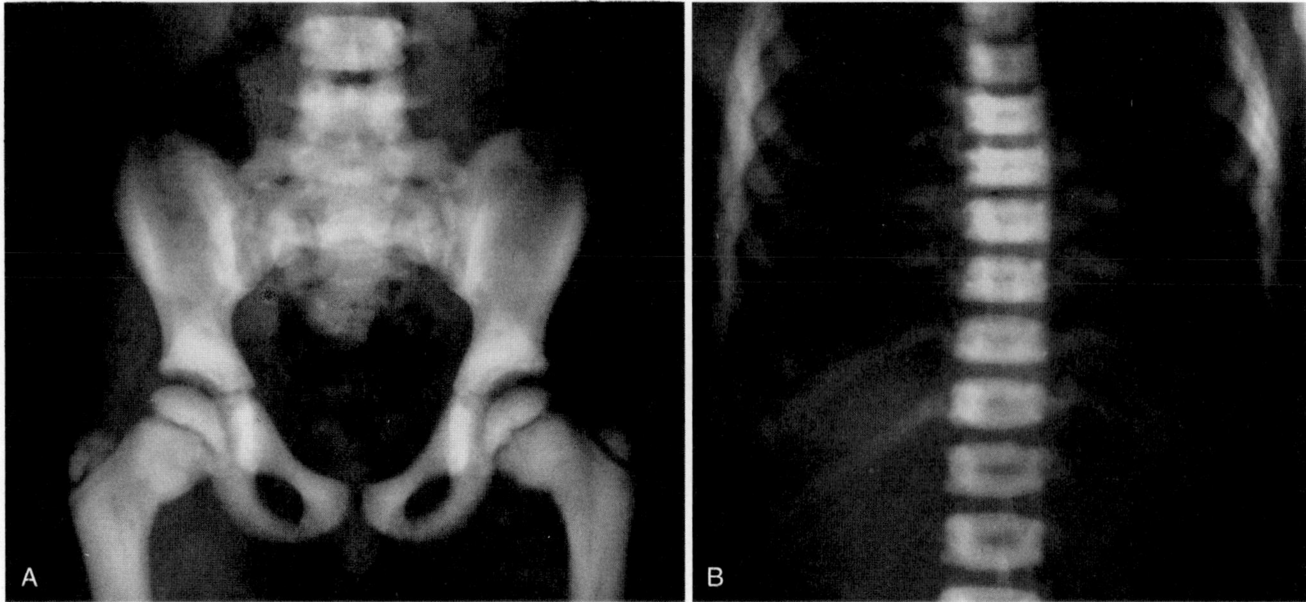

Figure 3-7 Osteopetrosis. **A,** The bones are diffusely dense in the pelvis. **B,** In the spine, the centers of the vertebral bodies are relatively lucent, resulting in a "rugger jersey" (horizontally striped shirt) appearance on radiographs. (From Dormans JP, editor: *Pediatric orthopaedics and sports medicine: requisites,* Philadelphia, 2004, Mosby.)

VI. MARFAN SYNDROME

A. Clinical features

1. Arachnodactyly (long, slender fingers; "peeking thumb sign"), pectus deformities, scoliosis (50% of cases), **acetabular protrusio (15% to 25%)**, cardiac abnormalities (aortic dilation), and ocular abnormalities (superior lens dislocation in 60%)
2. Dural ectasia and meningocele
3. Joint laxity

B. Causes

1. Defect in **fibrillin-1 (FBN1)**
2. **Autosomal dominant inheritance**

C. Radiologic findings

1. Scoliosis
2. Acetabular protrusio

D. Treatment

1. Joint laxity is treated conservatively.
2. **Bracing for scoliosis is ineffective.**
3. Curves may necessitate anterior and posterior fusion.
4. Echocardiographic and cardiologic evaluation are required before surgery.
5. Acetabular protrusio should be observed unless the patient has severe symptoms.

VII. EHLERS-DANLOS SYNDROME

A. Clinical features

1. Hyperextensibility of "cigarette paper" skin
2. Joint hypermobility and dislocation
3. Soft tissue and bone fragility, and soft tissue calcification
4. Classification
   - Of types I to XI, types II and III are the most common and least disabling.

B. Causes

1. Autosomal dominant disorder of collagen V (coexpressed with collagen I)

C. Radiologic findings

1. Dislocations may be shown.
2. Kyphoscoliosis may be found.

D. Treatment

1. Physical therapy, orthoses, and arthrodesis when soft tissue procedures fail

VIII. HOMOCYSTINURIA

A. Clinical features

1. Osteoporosis, a marfanoid-like habitus (but with stiffening joints)
2. Inferior lens dislocation
3. Differentiated from Marfan syndrome on the basis of the direction of lens dislocation and the presence of osteoporosis in homocystinuria
4. Central nervous system effects, including mental retardation, are common in this disorder.

B. Causes

1. Autosomal recessive inborn error of methionine metabolism (decreased enzyme cystathionine β-synthase). Accumulation of the intermediate metabolite homocysteine in the production of the amino acid cysteine.
2. The diagnosis is made by demonstrating increased homocysteine in urine (cyanide-nitroprusside test).

C. Treatment

1. Early treatment with vitamin B_6 and a diet with decreased amounts of methionine are often successful.

IX. JUVENILE IDIOPATHIC ARTHRITIS

A. Includes both juvenile rheumatoid arthritis and juvenile chronic arthritis

B. Clinical features

1. Persistent noninfectious arthritis lasting 6 weeks to 3 months and diagnosed after other possible causes have been ruled out

2. Affects girls more than boys and typically manifests before age 4 years
3. Commonly involves the knee, wrist (flexed and ulnar deviated) and hand (fingers extended, swollen, radially deviated)
4. To confirm the diagnosis, one of the following must be present: rash, presence of rheumatoid factor, **iridocyclitis,** cervical spine involvement, pericarditis, tenosynovitis, intermittent fever, or morning stiffness.
5. In 50% of affected patients, symptoms resolve without sequelae; 25% of patients are slightly disabled, and 20% to 25% have crippling arthritis, blindness, or both.

C. **Radiologic findings**

1. **Cervical spine involvement can lead to kyphosis, facet ankylosis, and atlantoaxial subluxation.**
2. Lower extremity problems include flexion contractures (hip and knee flexed, ankle dorsiflexed), subluxation, and other deformities (hip protrusio, valgus knees, equinovarus feet).

D. **Treatment**

1. Medical therapy involves less high-dose steroids and salicylates and more specific immunomodulating drugs (infliximab).
2. Surgical interventions include joint injections and (rarely) synovectomy (for chronic swelling refractory to medical management). Arthrodesis and arthroplasty may be required for severe juvenile idiopathic arthritis.
3. **Slit-lamp examination is required twice yearly, as progressive iridocyclitis can lead to rapid loss of vision if left untreated.**

X. ANKYLOSING SPONDYLITIS

A. **Clinical features**

1. Typically affects adolescent boys with asymmetric, lower extremity, large-joint arthritis; heel pain; and sometimes eye symptoms
2. Hip and back pain (cardinal symptoms) may develop later.
3. **Limitation of chest wall expansion is a more specific finding than is a positive HLA-B27 test result.**

B. **Causes**

1. The HLA-B27 test yields positive results in 90% to 95% of patients with ankylosing spondylitis or Reiter syndrome, but the result is also positive in 4% to 8% of all white Americans; thus, its usefulness as a screening tool is limited.

C. **Radiologic findings**

1. Bilateral, symmetric sacroiliac erosion, followed by joint space narrowing, subsequent ankylosis, and late vertebral scalloping (bamboo spine)

D. **Treatment**

1. NSAIDs and physical therapy

SECTION 5 BIRTH INJURIES

I. BRACHIAL PLEXUS PALSY

A. **Clinical features**

1. In 2 per 1000 births, an injury is still associated with stretching or contusion of the brachial plexus.
2. Typically present with internal rotation contracture of the shoulder and with elbow and wrist flexion contractures.
   - **Progressive glenoid dysplasia occurs in 70% of children with significant internal rotation contracture.**
3. Hand function is variable, according to level of brachial plexus deformity.
4. Three types are commonly recognized (Table 3-5).

B. **Causes**

1. Large size of neonate, shoulder dystocia, forceps delivery, breech position, and prolonged labor

C. **Radiologic studies**

1. Investigations have focused on the position of the humeral head within the glenoid.
   - Posterior subluxation with erosion of the glenoid should be prevented.
2. Axillary lateral view of the shoulder should be obtained to evaluate position of humeral head.
3. **Consider computed tomographic (CT) scanning instead of MRI of the shoulder if surgical reconstruction is planned.**

D. **Treatment**

1. The key to the success of therapy is maintaining passive ROM and awaiting return of motor function (up to 18 months).
2. More than 90% of cases eventually resolve without intervention.
   - **Lack of biceps function 6 months after injury and the presence of Horner syndrome carry a poor prognosis.**
3. Options include releasing contractures (Fairbanks), **latissimus and teres major transfer to the shoulder external rotators** (L'Episcopo), tendon transfers for elbow flexion (Clark pectoral transfer and Steindler flexorplasty), proximal humerus rotational osteotomy (Wickstrom), and microsurgical nerve grafting.
4. Release of the subscapularis tendon for internal rotation contracture, if performed by age 2 years, may result in improved active external rotation of the shoulder, with muscle transfer to assist in active external rotation.

Table 3-5 Brachial Plexus Palsy

Type	Roots	Deficit	Prognosis
Erb-Duchenne palsy	C5, C6	Deltoid, cuff, elbow flexors, wrist and hand dorsiflexors; "waiter's tip" deformity	Best
Total plexus	C5, T1	Sensory and motor; flaccid arm	Worst
Klumpke palsy	C8, T1	Wrist flexors, intrinsic muscles; Horner syndrome	Poor

II. CONGENITAL MUSCULAR TORTICOLLIS

A. Clinical features

1. It is associated with other "molding disorders," such as hip dysplasia and metatarsus adductus (up to 20% association with hip dysplasia).
2. Fibrosis of the muscle and a palpable mass are noted within the first 4 weeks of life.
3. This is a diagnosis of exclusion, inasmuch as other causes for the torticollis must be evaluated:
   - Infection, congenital spinal deformity, rotatory subluxation of cervical spine, hearing loss and optic dysfunction

B. Causes

1. A congenital deformity resulting from contracture of the sternocleidomastoid muscle, perhaps from an intrauterine compartment syndrome involving this muscle.

C. Imaging studies

1. Anteroposterior and lateral views of the cervical spine are needed.
2. Ultrasonography has been shown to differentiate between mild fibrosis of the sternocleidomastoid muscle and severe fibrosis.

D. Treatment

1. Most patients (90%) respond to passive stretching within the first year of life.
   - **Rotate the infant's chin to the ipsilateral shoulder while simultaneously tilting the head toward the contralateral shoulder.**
   - A physical therapist can assist in ensuring that the infant makes progress,
   - **Ultrasound demonstration of severe fibrosis is associated with failure of nonoperative management.**
2. Surgery (Z-plasty of the sternocleidomastoid muscle) may be required if torticollis persists beyond the first year.

III. CONGENITAL PSEUDARTHROSIS OF THE CLAVICLE

A. Clinical features

1. Failure of union of the medial and lateral ossification centers of the right clavicle
2. Manifests as an enlarging, painless, nontender mass

B. Causes

1. May be related to pulsations of the underlying subclavian artery

C. Radiologic findings

1. Anteroposterior view of the clavicle reveals rounded sclerotic bone at the pseudarthrosis site.

D. Treatment

1. Surgery (open reduction, internal fixation with bone grafting) is indicated for unacceptable cosmetic deformities or with significant functional symptoms (mobility of the fragments and winging of the scapula) at ages 3 to 6 years.
2. Successful union is predictable (in contrast to congenital pseudarthrosis of the tibia).

SECTION 6 CEREBRAL PALSY

I. INTRODUCTION

A. This nonprogressive neuromuscular disorder. with onset before age 2 years, results from injury to the immature brain.

B. The cause is usually not identifiable but can include prematurity (most common), prenatal intrauterine factors, perinatal infections (toxoplasmosis, other infections, rubella, cytomegalovirus infection, and herpes simplex), anoxic injuries, and meningitis.

C. This upper motor neuron disease results in a mixture of muscle weakness and spasticity.

D. Initially, the abnormal muscle forces cause dynamic deformity at joints.

1. Persistent spasticity can lead to contractures, bony deformity, and ultimately joint subluxation/dislocation.

E. MRI of the brain commonly reveals periventricular leukomalacia.

II. CLASSIFICATION

A. Cerebral palsy can be classified on the basis of physiology (according to the movement disorder), anatomy (according to geographic distribution), or function.

B. Physiologic classification (Figure 3-8):

1. Spastic
   - Increased muscle tone and hyperreflexia with slow, restricted movements because of simultaneous contraction of agonist and antagonist
   - Most common and is most amenable to improvement of musculoskeletal function by operative intervention
2. Athetosis
   - Constant succession of slow, writhing, involuntary movements
   - Less common and more difficult to treat
3. Ataxia
   - Inability to coordinate muscles for voluntary movement, resulting in an unbalanced, wide-based gait
   - Less amenable to orthopaedic treatment
4. Mixed
   - Typically involves a combination of spasticity and athetosis with total body involvement

C. Anatomic classification (see Figure 3-8):

1. **Hemiplegia**
   - **Involves the upper and lower extremities on the same side, usually with spasticity**
   - "Handedness" often develops early
   - All children with hemiplegia are eventually able to walk, regardless of treatment.

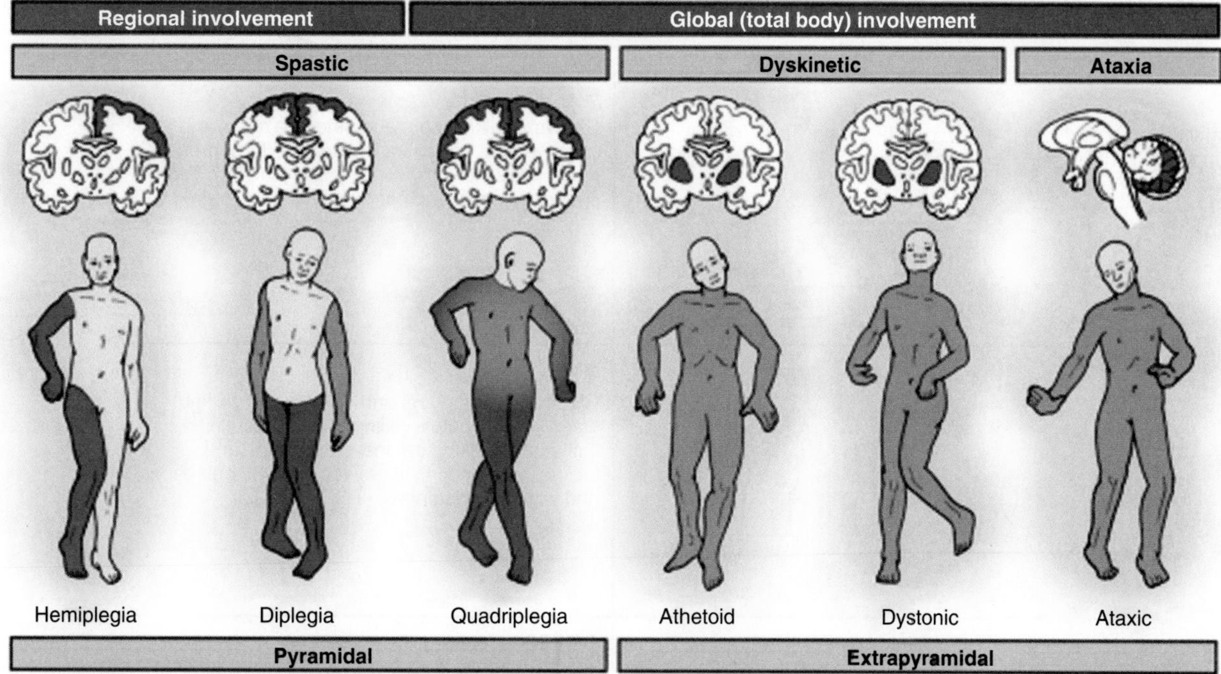

Figure 3-8 Classification of cerebral palsy. Although overlaps in terminology exist, cerebral palsy can be classified according to distribution (regional versus global involvement; hemiplegic, diplegic, quadriplegic), physiologic type (spastic, dyskinetic/dystonic, dyskinetic/athetoid, ataxic), or presumed neurologic substrate (pyramidal, extrapyramidal). (Redrawn from Pellegrino L: Cerebral palsy. In Batshaw ML, editor: *Children with disabilities,* ed 4, Baltimore, 1997, Paul H. Brookes.)

2. **Diplegia**
   - **The lower extremity is involved more extensively than the upper extremity.**
   - Most diplegic patients eventually walk.
   - IQ may be normal; strabismus is common.
3. Total involvement (quadriplegia)
   - Extensive involvement, low IQ, and a high mortality rate
   - Affected patients usually unable to walk

D. Functional classification

1. Gross motor and functional classification system (GMFCS) (Figure 3-9)
   - Classification is based on walking ability and need for assistive devices.
   - Functional loss over time or after surgery can be monitored with GMFCS.

III. ORTHOPAEDIC ASSESSMENT

A. Examination

1. Based on examination and thorough birth and developmental history
2. **A patient's locomotor profile is based on the persistence of primitive reflexes; the presence of two or more usually means the child will not be able to ambulate.**
   - **Commonly tested reflexes include the Moro startle reflex (normally disappears by age 6 months) and the parachute reflex (normally disappears by age 12 months).**
   - **The ability to sit independently by age 2 years is highly prognostic of ability to walk.**

IV. SPASTICITY TREATMENT

A. Botulinum toxin

1. Intramuscular botulinum A toxin can temporarily decrease dynamic spasticity.
2. The mechanism of action of botulinum toxin is a presynaptic blockade at the neuromuscular junction.
3. The effectiveness of botulinum toxin is limited to 6 months; therefore, it is not a permanent cure for spasticity.
4. It is used to maintain joint motion during rapid growth when a child is too young for surgery.

B. Dorsal rhizotomy

1. Selective dorsal root rhizotomy is a neurosurgical procedure designed to decrease lower extremity spasticity.
2. The procedure includes resection of dorsal rootlets that do not exhibit a myographic or clinical response to stimulation.
3. **It is performed primarily in ambulatory patients with spastic diplegia to help reduce spasticity and complement orthopaedic management.**
4. It requires multilevel laminoplasty, which may lead to late spinal instability and deformity.

C. Systemic medication

1. Oral baclofen is used as adjunct therapy to control overall tone.
   - Provides decreased tone in all extremities by inhibiting signals through the γ-aminobutyric acid (GABA) pathway.
   - Negative effects include increased somnolence and decreased alertness during the day.

GMFCS FOR CHILDREN AGED 6–12 YEARS: DESCRIPTORS AND ILLUSTRATIONS

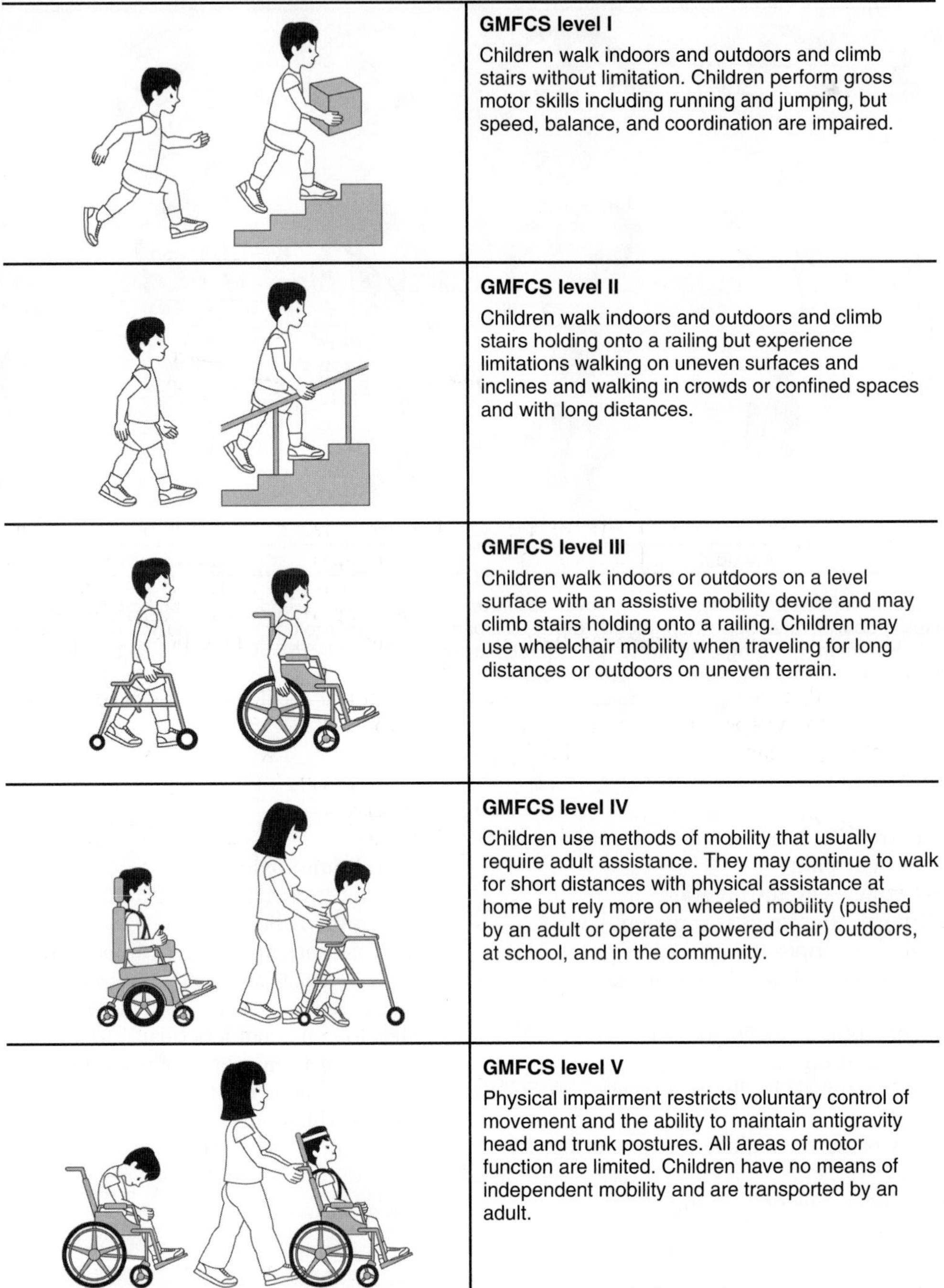

GMFCS level I
Children walk indoors and outdoors and climb stairs without limitation. Children perform gross motor skills including running and jumping, but speed, balance, and coordination are impaired.
GMFCS level II
Children walk indoors and outdoors and climb stairs holding onto a railing but experience limitations walking on uneven surfaces and inclines and walking in crowds or confined spaces and with long distances.
GMFCS level III
Children walk indoors or outdoors on a level surface with an assistive mobility device and may climb stairs holding onto a railing. Children may use wheelchair mobility when traveling for long distances or outdoors on uneven terrain.
GMFCS level IV
Children use methods of mobility that usually require adult assistance. They may continue to walk for short distances with physical assistance at home but rely more on wheeled mobility (pushed by an adult or operate a powered chair) outdoors, at school, and in the community.
GMFCS level V
Physical impairment restricts voluntary control of movement and the ability to maintain antigravity head and trunk postures. All areas of motor function are limited. Children have no means of independent mobility and are transported by an adult.

Figure 3-9 Gross motor and functional classification system (GMFCS) for children ages 6 to 12 years: descriptors and illustrations. (Illustrations copyrighted by Kerr Graham, Bill Reid, and Adrienne Harvey, The Royal Children's Hospital, Melbourne Eastern Resource Centre, Melbourne, Australia.)

D. Baclofen pump

1. Surgical implantation of a pump that provides only local delivery of baclofen to an area of the spinal cord
   - Pump then delivers a much lower dose of baclofen.
   - Pump is then refilled when empty.
2. No systemic delivery; thus, less somnolence
3. May exacerbate scoliosis progression
4. Wound problems common in thin children

V. GAIT DISORDERS

A. Evaluation

1. Findings are usually the impetus for the orthopaedic consultation.
2. In many hemiplegic patients, toe walking is the only manifestation.
3. Three-dimensional computerized gait analysis with dynamic electromyography and force-plate studies have

Table 3-6 Surgical Options for Gait Disorders

Problem	Diagnostic Findings	Surgical Option
Hip flexion	Positive result of Thomas test	Psoas tenotomy or recession
Spastic hip	Decreased abduction, uncovered femoral head	Adductor release, osteotomy (late)
Hip adduction	Scissoring gait	Adductor release
Femoral anteversion	Prone internal rotation increased	Osteotomy, VDRO, hamstring lengthening
Knee flexion	Increased popliteal angle	Hamstring lengthening
Knee hypertension	Recurvatum	Rectus femoris lengthening
Stiff-leg gait	Electromyographic study of hamstring and quadriceps; continuous passive knee flexion decreased with hip extension	Distal rectus transfer to hamstrings
Talipes equinus	Toe walking	Achilles tendon lengthening
Talipes varus	Appearance in standing position	Split–anterior or split–posterior tibialis transfer (on the basis of EMG findings)
Talipes valgus	Appearance in standing position	Peroneal lengthening, Grice subtalar fusion, calcaneal lengthening osteotomy
Hallux valgus	Appearance on examination and radiographs	Osteotomy, metatarsophalangeal fusion

EMG, electromyographic; VDRO, varus derotation osteotomy.

allowed a more scientific approach to preoperative decision making and postoperative analysis of the results of surgery for cerebral palsy.

B. **Treatment**

1. Lengthening of continuously active muscles and transfer of muscles out of phase are often helpful. Surgeries should usually be done at multiple levels to best correct the problem. In general, surgery is performed at ages 4 to 5 years. A few generalized guidelines are given in Table 3-6.

VI. SPINAL DISORDERS

A. **Evaluation**

1. These disorders most commonly involve scoliosis, which can be severe, making proper wheelchair sitting difficult.
2. The risk for scoliosis is highest in children with total body involvement (spastic quadriplegic).
3. Surgical indications include curves greater than 45 to 50 degrees, worsening pelvic obliquity, or wheelchair seating problems.
4. Curves are classified in two groups (Figure 3-10):
   - Group I curves are double curves with thoracic and lumbar components and little pelvic obliquity.
   - Group II curves are larger lumbar or thoracolumbar curves with marked pelvic obliquity.

B. **Treatment**

1. Treatment is tailored to the needs of the patient and must involve all caregivers.
2. Small curves with no loss of function or large curves in severely involved patients may necessitate only observation.
3. Group I curves in ambulatory patients are treated as idiopathic scoliosis with posterior fusion and instrumentation. Group I curves in sitting patients and group II curves may necessitate posterior fusion with segmental posterior instrumentation from the upper thoracic spine to the pelvis (Luque-Galveston technique), with or without anterior fusion.
4. Kyphosis is also common and may necessitate fusion and instrumentation.

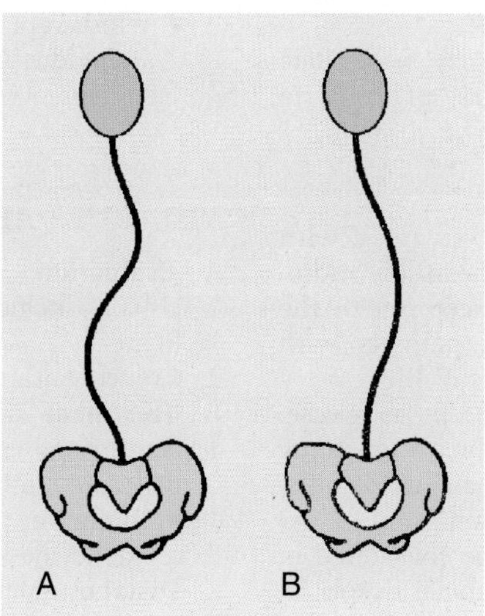

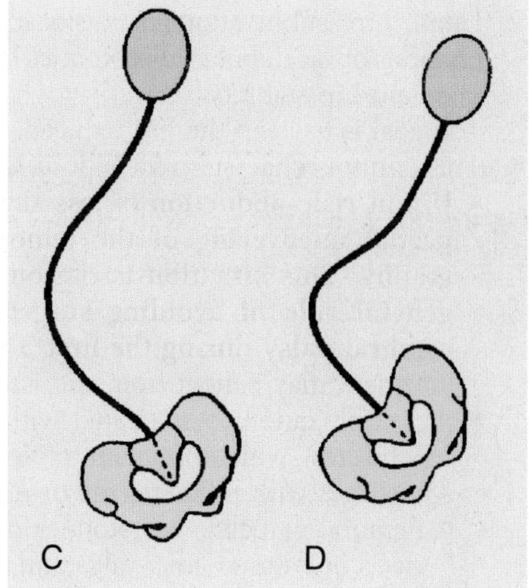

Figure 3-10 Curve patterns of scoliosis in cerebral palsy. Group I curves **(A, B)** are double curves with thoracic and lumbar components. If there is little pelvic obliquity **(A)**, the curve may be well balanced. If the thoracic curve is more significant **(B)**, there may be some imbalance. Group II curves **(C, D)** are large lumbar or thoracolumbar curves with marked pelvic obliquity. There may be a short fractional curve between the end of the curve and the sacrum **(C)**, or the curve may continue into the sacrum **(D)**, with the sacral vertebrae forming part of the curve. (Adapted from Weinstein SL: *The pediatric spine: principles and practice,* New York, 1994, Raven Press.)

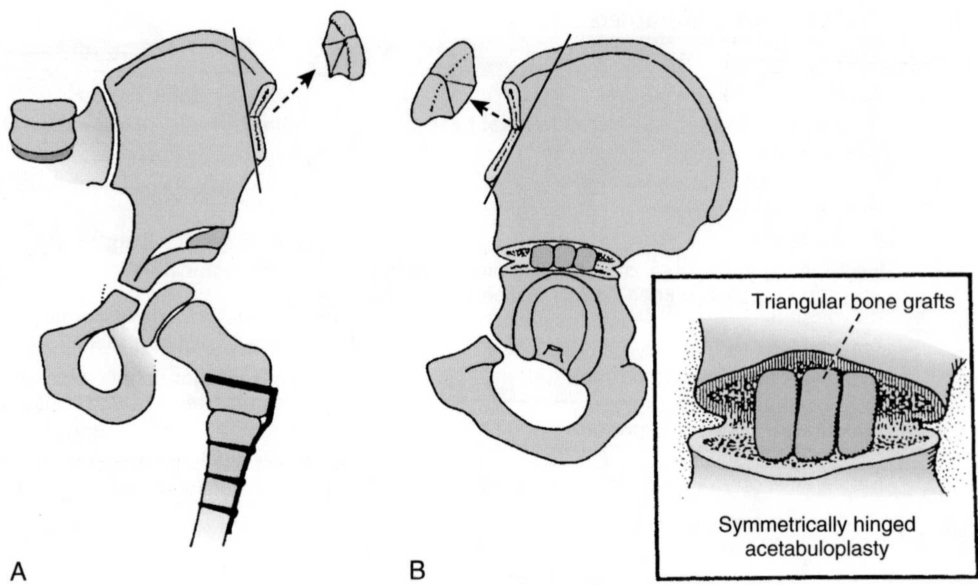

Figure 3-11 Placement of graft for Dega acetabuloplasty. **A,** Bone graft is obtained from the anterosuperior iliac crest and shaped into three small triangles, whose bases are 1 cm long. **B,** The grafts are placed in the osteotomy site; the largest is placed in the area where maximal improvement of coverage is desired. The triangular wedges are packed close to each other to prevent collapse, turning, or dislodgment; the result is a symmetric hinging on the *triradiate cartilage* **(inset).** With the medial wall of the pelvis maintained, the elasticity of the osteotomy keeps the wedges in place. No pins are necessary to maintain the osteotomy. (Adapted from Mubarak SJ, et al: One-stage reconstruction of the spastic hip, *J Bone Joint Surg Am* 74:1352, 1992.)

5. It is important to assess nutritional status (albumin < 3.5 g/dL and white blood cell [WBC] count < 1500/μL) preoperatively and to consider gastrostomy tube placement before spinal surgery if indicated.

VII. HIP SUBLUXATION AND DISLOCATION

A. Evaluation

1. In many children, pathologic processes of the hip are asymptomatic.
2. Caregivers may describe a pain response.
3. Difficulty with abduction for peroneal care is the most common problem.

B. Treatment

1. Initial treatment is with a soft tissue release (adductor/psoas) plus abduction bracing.
2. Later, hip subluxation or dislocation may necessitate femoral or acetabular osteotomies (Dega), or both, to maintain hip stability.
3. The goal is to keep the hip reduced.
4. This entity is characterized by four stages:
   - **Hip at risk: abduction of less than 45 degrees, with partial uncovering of the femoral head on radiographs. This situation is the only exception to the general rule of avoiding surgery in patients with cerebral palsy during the first 3 years of life.**
     - Patient may benefit from adductor and psoas release.
   - Hip subluxation: best treated with adductor tenotomy in children with abduction of less than 20 degrees, sometimes with psoas release or recession.
     - Femoral or pelvic osteotomies may be considered in cases of femoral coxa valga and acetabular dysplasia, which is usually lateral and posterior.
   - Spastic dislocation: **Patients may benefit from open reduction, femoral shortening, varus derotation osteotomy, Dega osteotomy** (Figure 3-11), **triple osteotomy, or Chiari osteotomy.**
     - The type of pelvic osteotomy indicated is best determined in a three-dimensional CT scan, which demonstrates the area of acetabular deficiency (anterior, lateral, or posterior) and the congruency of the joint surfaces.
     - **Addressing both hips can prevent dislocation of opposite hip.**
     - Late dislocations may best be left untreated or treated with a Schanz abduction osteotomy or a modified Girdlestone resection arthroplasty (resection below the lesser trochanter).
   - Windswept hips: characterized by abduction of one hip and adduction of the contralateral hip
     - Bilateral femoral osteotomies to achieve a more varus angle can assist in maintaining reduction.

VIII. KNEE ABNORMALITIES

A. Evaluation

1. Usually includes hamstring contractures and decreased ROM
2. Crouch gait in spastic diplegia patients

B. Treatment

1. Hamstring lengthening is often helpful (sometimes increases lumbar lordosis).
   - To prevent peroneal nerve injury, be careful not to overextend the knee in the operating room.
2. **Distal transfer of an out-of-phase rectus femoris muscle to the semitendinosus or gracilis muscle is indicated**

when there is loss of knee flexion during the swing phase of gait.

IX. FOOT AND ANKLE ABNORMALITIES

A. Equinovalgus foot

1. Most common in spastic diplegia
2. Causes
   - Caused by spastic peroneal muscles, contracted heel cords, and ligamentous laxity
3. Treatment
   - Peroneus brevis lengthening is often helpful in correcting moderate valgus angulation. Lateral column-lengthening calcaneal osteotomy is used to correct hindfoot valgus angulation.

B. Equinovarus foot

1. **Most common in spastic hemiplegia**
2. Causes
   - Overpull of the posterior or anterior tibialis tendons (or both)
3. Treatment
   - Lengthening of the posterior tibialis is rarely sufficient.
   - Transfers
     - Likewise, transfer of an entire muscle (posterior or anterior tibialis) is rarely recommended.
     - **Split-muscle transfers are helpful when the affected muscle is spastic during both the stance and swing phases of gait. The split–posterior tibialis transfer (rerouting half of the tendon dorsally to the peroneus brevis) is used in cases with spasticity of the muscle, flexible varus foot, and weak peroneal muscles.**
     - Complications include decreased foot dorsiflexion. Split–anterior tibialis transfer (rerouting half of its tendon laterally to the cuboid) is used in patients with spasticity of the muscle and a flexible varus deformity.
     - Most often it is coupled with Achilles tendon lengthening and posterior tibial tendon intramuscular lengthening (Rancho procedure) to treat the fixed equinus contracture.

X. HAND MANAGEMENT

A. Hand management is discussed in Chapter 7, Hand, Upper Extremity, and Microvascular Surgery.

SECTION 7 NEUROMUSCULAR DISORDERS

I. ARTHROGRYPOTIC SYNDROMES

A. Arthrogryposis multiplex congenita (amyoplasia): nonprogressive disorder with multiple joints that are congenitally rigid (Figure 3-12). This disorder can be myopathic, neuropathic, or both and is associated with a decrease in anterior horn cells and other neural elements of the spinal cord. Intelligence is normal.

1. Evaluation
   - Evaluation should include neurologic studies, enzyme tests, and muscle biopsy (at 3 to 4 months of age).
   - Affected patients typically have normal facies, normal intelligence, multiple joint contractures, and no visceral abnormalities.
   - Upper extremity involvement usually includes adduction and internal rotation of the shoulder, extension of the elbow, and flexion and ulnar deviation of the wrist. The elbow has no creases. These patients have an ability to use the feet as functional appendages.
   - Lower extremity involvement includes teratologic hip dislocations, knee contractures, resistant clubfeet, and vertical talus.
   - The spine may be involved, with characteristic C-shaped (neuromuscular) scoliosis (33% of cases).
2. Treatment
   - Upper extremity
     - Passive manipulation and serial casting
     - **Active elbow flexion achieved through anterior triceps transfer and posterior soft tissue release**
     - Osteotomies are also considered after 4 years of age to allow independent eating.

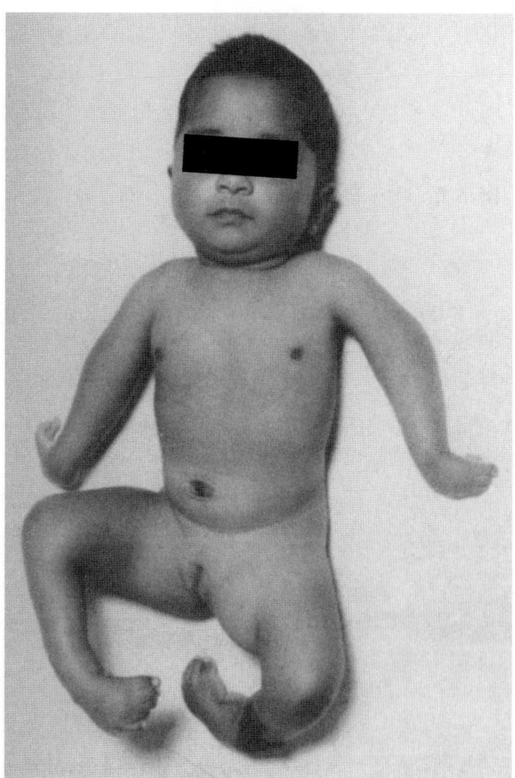

Figure 3-12 Arthrogryposis. Typical appearance of a child in whom all four limbs are affected. Note the lack of creases at the elbows, the flexion contractures at the knees, and the severe clubfoot deformities. (From Benson M, et al: *Children's orthopaedics and fractures,* New York, 1994, Churchill Livingstone, p 321.)

- One upper extremity should be left in extension at the elbow for positioning and perineal care and the other elbow in flexion for feeding.
- Lower extremity
  - **Hip dislocation:**
    - **Unilateral: medial open reduction with possible femoral shortening**
    - **Bilateral: typically left unreduced because ambulation is often preserved**
  - Knee contractures are treated with early (at ages 6 to 9 months) soft tissue releases (especially hamstrings).
  - **The foot deformities (clubfoot and vertical talus) are initially treated with a soft tissue release, but later recurrences may necessitate bone procedures (talectomy).** The goal is for the foot to be stiff and plantigrade in order to wear shoes and possibly ambulate.
  - Knee contractures should be corrected before hip reduction in order to maintain the reduction.
- Spine
  - Fusion if curve is large (>50 degrees) or progressive
  - May impede function and ambulatory ability

B. Distal arthrogryposis syndrome

1. Evaluation
   - Autosomal dominant disorder that affects predominantly the hands and feet
   - Ulnarly deviated fingers (at metacarpal joints), metacarpal and proximal interphalangeal flexion contractures, and adducted thumbs with web space thickening are common.
   - Clubfoot and vertical talus deformities are common in the feet.
2. Treatment
   - Comprehensive releases are more often required combined with boney surgery.

C. Larsen syndrome

1. Evaluation
   - Similar to arthrogryposis in clinical appearance, but joints are less rigid.
   - Characterized primarily by multiple joint dislocations (including bilateral congenital knee dislocations), flattened facies, scoliosis, and clubfeet.
   - Cervical kyphosis (watch for late myelopathy) is important to recognize early.
   - Affected patients have normal intelligence.
2. Treatment
   - Posterior cervical fusion for progressive cervical kyphosis
   - Knee reduction may necessitate femoral shortening and excision of collateral ligaments.
   - Open hip reduction is required.

D. Multiple pterygium syndrome

1. Evaluation
   - Autosomal recessive disorder whose name means "little wing" in Greek
   - Characterized by cutaneous flexor surface webs (knee and elbow), congenital vertical talus, and scoliosis
2. Treatment
   - Care must be taken when the webs are elongated because of the superficial nature of the neurovascular bundle.

II. MYELODYSPLASIA (SPINA BIFIDA)

A. Introduction

1. Causes
   - Disorder of incomplete spinal cord closure or rupture of the developing cord secondary to hydrocephalus
2. Classification:
   - Spina bifida occulta: defect in the vertebral arch, with confined cord and meninges
   - Meningocele: sac without neural elements protruding through the defect
   - Myelomeningocele: in spina bifida, the sac with neural elements protrudes through the skin
   - Rachischisis: neural elements exposed, with no covering
     - Function is related primarily to the level of the defect and the associated congenital abnormalities.
     - **The myelodysplasia level is based on the lowest functional level** (Table 3-7). L4 is a key level because the quadriceps can function and allow independent ambulation around the community (Figure 3-13).

B. Evaluation

1. Diagnosis
   - **Can be diagnosed in utero (increased levels of α-fetoprotein)**
   - Related to a folate deficiency in utero
   - A type II Arnold-Chiari malformation is the most common comorbid condition.
2. Central axis
   - Sudden changes in function (rapid increase of scoliotic curvature, spasticity, new neurologic deficit, or increase in urinary tract infections) can be associated with tethered cord, hydrocephalus (most common), or syringomyelia.

Table 3-7 Levels of Myelodysplasia

	CHARACTERISTICS				
Level	Hip	Knee	Feet	Orthosis	Extent of Ambulation
L1	External rotation/flexed	—	Equinovarus	HKAFO	Nonfunctional
L2	Adduction/flexed	Flexed	Equinovarus	HKAFO	Nonfunctional
L3	Adduction/flexed	Recurvatum	Equinovarus	KAFO	Household
L4	Adduction/flexed	Extended	Cavovarus	AFO	Household, some community
L5	Flexed	Limited flexion	Calcaneal valgus	AFO	Community
S1	—	—	Foot deformities	Shoes	Near normal

AFO, ankle-foot orthosis; HKAFO, hip-knee-ankle-foot orthosis; KAFO, knee-ankle-foot orthosis.

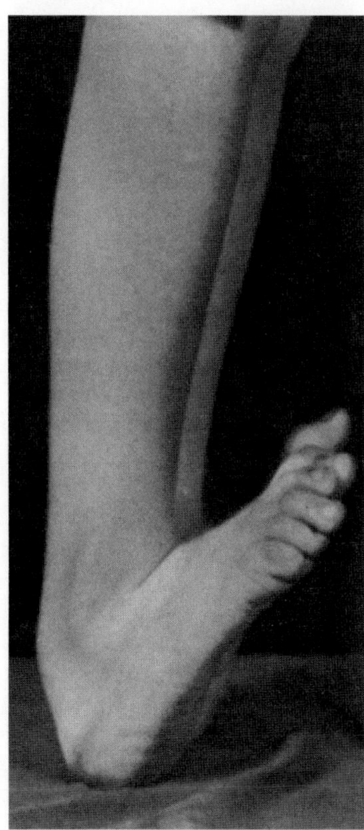

Figure 3-13 Myelodysplasia below L5. Typical posture of a leg and foot in an affected child. The feet assume a progressive calcaneus posture that necessitates surgical correction. (From Herring JA, editor: *Tachdjian's pediatric orthopaedics,* ed 4, Philadelphia, 2008, WB Saunders.)

- Head CT scans (70% of myelodysplastic patients have hydrocephalus) and myelography or spinal MRI are required.

3. Fractures
   - **Fractures are also common in myelodysplasia, most often about the knee and hip in children 3 to 7 years of age, and can frequently be diagnosed only by noting redness, warmth, and swelling.**
   - Fractures are commonly misdiagnosed as infection in these patients.
   - Fractures are treated conservatively, with a well-padded splint.
   - Fractures usually heal, with abundant callus.

C. **Treatment principles**

1. Careful observation of patients with myelodysplasia is important. Several myelodysplasia "milestones" have been developed to assess progress (Table 3-8).
2. Treatment involves a team approach (urologist, orthopaedist, neurosurgeon, and developmental pediatrician) to allow maximal function consistent with the patient's level and other abnormalities.
3. Proper use of orthoses is essential in patients with myelodysplasia. The determination of ambulation potential is based on the level of the deficit and motivation of the child.
4. Surgery for myelodysplasia focuses on balancing of muscles and correction of deformities.
5. **Increased attention has been focused on latex sensitivity in myelodysplastic patients. A latex-free environment is necessary to prevent life-threatening allergic reactions.**

Table 3-8 Milestones in Myelodysplasia

Age (Months)	Function	Treatment
4-6	Head control	Positioning
6-10	Sitting	Supports/orthoses
10-12	Prone mobility	Prone board
12-15	Upright stance	Standing orthosis
15-18	Upright mobility	Trunk/extremity orthosis

D. **Hip pathology**

1. A wide spectrum of hip disease occurs, including flexion contractures, hip subluxation and dislocation, developmental dysplasia of the hip (DDH), and abduction or external rotation contracture. In general, management of the hip in patients with myelomeningocele is controversial.
2. Flexion contractures:
   - Occur in patients with thoracic/high lumbar myelomeningocele as a result of unopposed hip flexors or in patients who sit most of the time
   - Treatment
     - Anterior hip release with tenotomy of the iliopsoas, sartorius, rectus femoris, and tensor fasciae latae
     - For patients with lesions at the low lumbar level, the psoas should be preserved for independent ambulation.
     - Hip abduction contracture can cause pelvic obliquity and scoliosis; it is treated with proximal division of the tensor fasciae latae and distal iliotibial band release (Ober-Yount procedure).
     - Adduction contractures are treated with adductor myotomy.
3. Hip dislocation
   - Caused by paralysis of the hip abductors and extensors with unopposed hip flexors and adductors
     - Hip dislocation is most common at the level of L3 to L4.
   - Treatment
     - **Containment is controversial, but in general, it is considered essential only in patients with a functioning quadriceps.**
     - **Redislocation may occur no matter what treatment is used to maintain the reduction.**
     - Principles of treatment should follow those for any paralytic hip dislocation:
       - Concentric reduction
       - Bony abnormality correction (femoral anteversion with valgus, posterior acetabular insufficiency)
       - Muscle balance correction by means of transfer or release (flexor-adductor, extensor-abductor balance)
     - Late dislocation at the low lumbar level may be caused by a tethered cord, which must be released before the hip is reduced.
     - **The functional outcome of thoracic-level myelomeningocele is independent of whether the hips are in proper postion or dislocated.**
       - **Management should focus on limiting soft tissue contractures.**

E. Knee problems

1. Usually include quadriceps weakness (usually treated with knee-ankle-foot orthoses)
2. Flexion deformities are not problematic in patients who use wheelchairs but can be treated with hamstring release and posterior capsular release.
3. Recurvatum is rarely a problem and can be treated early with serial casting and knee-ankle-foot orthoses. Tenotomies (quadriceps lengthening) are sometimes required.
4. Valgus deformities are usually not a problem. Sometimes iliotibial band release, guided growth, or osteotomies are needed.

F. Ankle and foot deformities

1. **Objectives: (1) for feet to be braceable and plantigrade and (2) muscle balance**
2. Calcaneal deformity (see Figure 3-13)
   - Often caused by unopposed action of the tibialis anterior in patients with paralysis at the lower lumbar level
   - Predisposes to heel ulcers that can result in osteomyelitis of the calcaneus
   - Passive stretching is initial treatment, but tibialis anterior transfer to the calcaneus is often required. At time of transfer, do not fix the foot in equinus position, as this predisposes to distal tibial metaphyseal fracture.
3. **Valgus foot and ankle**
   - **Valgus ankle deformity is common** in ambulatory patients with the deformity in the distal tibia or subtalar joint (or both). Surgical correction is warranted when pressure sores are present and orthotics fail to hold correction.
   - **For skeletally immature patients: distal tibial hemiepiphysiodesis or Achilles tendon–fibular tenodesis**
   - For skeletally mature patients: distal tibial osteotomy
   - In subtalar region valgus, ankle-foot orthoses are often helpful, but tendon release (anterior tibialis, Achilles), posterior tibialis lengthening, and other procedures may be required. Triple arthrodesis should be avoided in most myelodysplastic patients and is used only for severe deformities with sensate feet.
4. Rigid clubfoot
   - Secondary to retained activity or contracture of the tibialis posterior and tibialis anterior; common in patients with L4-level lesions
   - **Treatment consists of complete subtalar release through a transverse (Cincinnati) incision, lengthening of the tibialis posterior and Achilles tendons, and transfer of the tibialis anterior tendon to the dorsal midfoot.**
   - Talectomy may be appropriate for refractory clubfoot.

G. Spine problems

1. Lumbar kyphosis or other congenital malformation of the spine as a result of a lack of segmentation or formation (i.e., hemivertebrae, diastematomyelia, unsegmented bars).
   - Treatment of kyphosis is based on problems with skin breakdown or necessity of using upper extremities to hold up their torso.
   - Resection of the kyphosis (kyphectomy) with local fusion or fusion to the pelvis with instrumentation is required in severe cases (Figure 3-14).
2. Scoliosis can also occur with severe lordosis as a result of muscular imbalance that is caused by thoracic-level paraplegia.
   - Nearly all patients with thoracic-level paraplegia develop scoliosis.
   - Bracing is generally unsuccessful in treating these spinal deformities.
   - Rapid curve progression can be associated with hydrocephalus or a **tethered cord,** which may be manifested as lower extremity spasticity or an increase in urinary tract infections.
   - Severe, progressive curves necessitate surgical treatment.
     - Segmental Luque sublaminar wiring with fixation to the pelvis (Galveston technique) or fixation to the front of the sacrum (Dunn technique) may be used (see Figure 3-14).
     - Infection rates are high because of frequent septicemia and poor skin quality over the lumbar spine.

H. Pelvic obliquity

1. Result of prolonged unilateral hip contractures or scoliosis
2. Treatment
   - Custom seat cushions, thoracolumbosacral orthosis, spinal fusion, and ultimately pelvic osteotomies may be required.

III. MYOPATHIES (MUSCULAR DYSTROPHIES)

A. Introduction

1. These noninflammatory, inherited disorders are characterized by progressive muscle weakness.
2. Treatment focuses on physical therapy, orthoses, genetic counseling, and surgery.
3. Several types of muscular dystrophy are classified on the basis of their inheritance patterns.

B. Duchenne muscular dystrophy

1. Causes
   - Markedly elevated **creatine phosphokinase** level and absence of **dystrophin protein** on muscle biopsy and DNA testing.
   - A muscle biopsy sample shows foci of necrosis and connective tissue infiltration.
   - **Sex-linked recessive inheritance**
   - Occurs in young boys
2. **Physical findings manifested as muscle weakness (proximal groups weaker than distal),** clumsy walking, decreased motor skills, lumbar lordosis, calf pseudohypertrophy, a positive Gowers sign (rises by walking the hands up the legs to compensate for gluteus maximus and quadriceps weakness; Figure 3-15). Hip extensors are typically the first muscle group affected.
3. Treatment
   - Goals are to keep patients ambulatory as long as possible.
   - Patients lose independent ambulation by age 10; although it is controversial, the use of knee-ankle-foot orthoses and release of contractures can extend walking ability for 2 to 3 years.
   - Patients are usually wheelchair dependent by age 15 years.

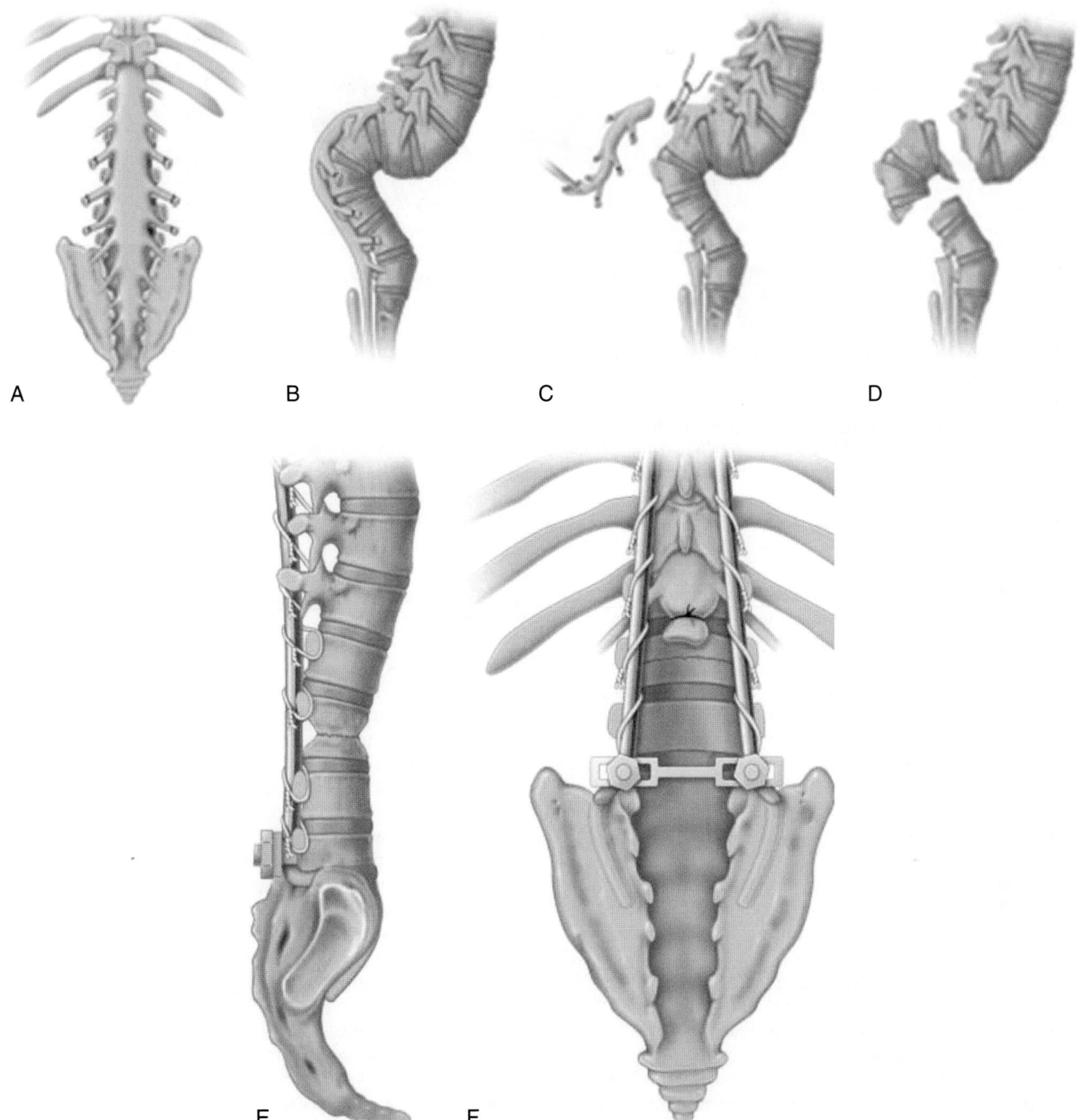

Figure 3-14 **Lumbar kyphectomy in patients with myelomeningocele. Fixation to the pelvis is accomplished with the Dunn-McCarthy technique.** (From Herring JA, editor: *Tachdjian's pediatric orthopaedics,* ed 4, Philadelphia, 2008, WB Saunders.)

- Patients usually die of cardiorespiratory complications before age 20.
- Newer medical treatment includes high-dose steroids, which have been shown to prevent scoliosis formation and prolong walking ability.
- Scoliosis:
  - With no muscle support, scoliosis rapidly progresses in virtually all patients by age 14 years.
  - Patients can become bedridden by age 16 as a result of spinal deformity and are unable to sit for more than 8 hours.
  - Forced vital capacity decreases by 4% each year and another 4% for every 10 degrees of thoracic scoliosis.
  - Scoliosis should be treated early (at 25 to 30 degrees of curvature) before pulmonary and cardiac function deteriorate.
  - The surgical approach includes posterior spinal fusion with segmental instrumentation to include the pelvis.

4. Differential diagnosis
   - **Becker muscular dystrophy** (also sex-linked recessive with a decrease in dystrophin)

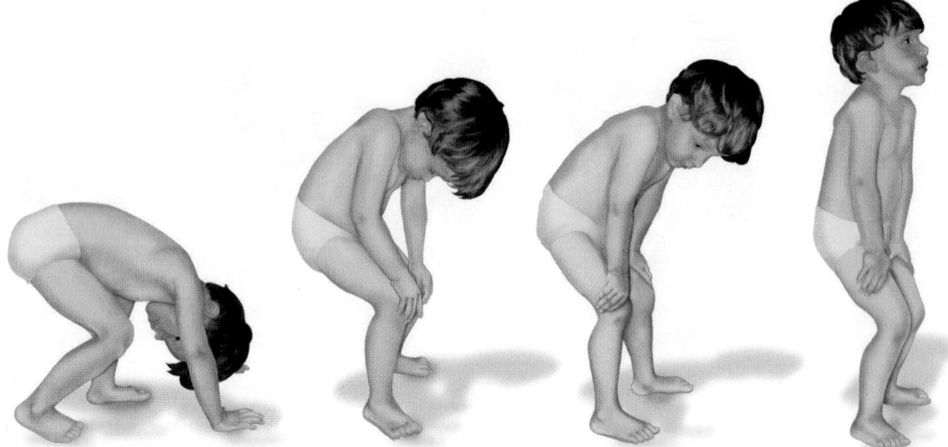

Figure 3-15 Gowers sign. The child rises from the floor by "walking up" the thighs with his hands—a functional test for quadriceps muscle weakness. Note the bulky calf. (Redrawn from Herring JA, editor: *Tachdjian's pediatric orthopaedics,* ed 3, Philadelphia, 2002, WB Saunders, p 85.)

- Found in boys with red/green color-blindness, with a similar but less severe picture
- The diagnosis of Becker muscular dystrophy applies to patients with the same examination findings but who live beyond 22 years without respiratory support.

C. Facioscapulohumeral muscular dystrophy

1. Causes and findings
   - Autosomal dominant disorder typically observed in patients 6 to 20 years of age with facial muscle abnormalities, normal creatine phosphokinase level, and winging of the scapula
2. Treated with stabilization by means of scapulothoracic fusion

D. Limb-girdle muscular dystrophy

1. Causes and findings
   - Autosomal recessive disorder seen in patients 10 to 30 years of age with pelvic or shoulder girdle involvement and increased creatine phosphokinase values

E. Other muscular dystrophies

1. Gowers (distal involvement; high incidence in Sweden); ocular, oculopharyngeal (high incidence among French Canadians)

IV. POLYMYOSITIS AND DERMATOMYOSITIS

A. Causes

1. Manifest with a febrile illness that may be acute or insidious
2. Females predominate and typically exhibit photosensitivity and increased creatine phosphokinase and erythrocyte sedimentation rate (ESR) values.
3. Muscles are tender, brawny, and indurated. Biopsy findings demonstrate the pathognomonic inflammatory response.

B. Treatment

1. Anti–tumor necrosis factor medication can decrease symptoms and control flares.

V. HEREDITARY NEUROPATHIES

A. Disorders associated with multiple central nervous system lesions

B. Friedreich ataxia

1. Causes and findings
   - Autosomal recessive disorder with problems with the frataxin gene
   - Spinocerebellar degenerative disease with mean onset between 7 and 15 years of age
   - Manifests with staggering, wide-based gait; nystagmus; cardiomyopathy; a cavus foot; and scoliosis
   - Involves motor and sensory defects, with an increase in polyphasic potentials on electromyograms
   - Use of a wheelchair is needed by age 15, and death occurs between ages 40 and 50, usually from cardiomyopathy.
2. Treatment
   - Foot deformities treated with plantar release with or without metatarsal and calcaneal osteotomies early, and triple arthrodesis later
   - Spine fusion when curves progress to 50 degrees, and number of levels should be interpreted as if a curve is a neuromuscular curve. Bracing is ineffective.

C. Hereditary sensory motor neuropathies: a group of inherited neuropathic disorders with similar characteristics (Table 3-9)

D. Charcot-Marie-Tooth disease (peroneal muscular atrophy)

1. Causes and findings
   - Autosomal dominant sensory motor demyelinating neuropathy
   - Two forms are described: a hypertrophic form with onset during the second decade of life, and a neuronal form with onset during the third or fourth decade but with more extensive foot involvement.
   - Orthopaedic manifestations include **pes cavus,** hammer toes with frequent corns and calluses, peroneal weak-

Table 3-9 Major Hereditary Motor Sensory Neuropathies

Type	Terminology	Inheritance	Description
I	Charcot-Marie-Tooth syndrome (hypertrophic form)	Autosomal dominant	Peroneal weakness, slow nerve conduction, absence of reflexes
II	Charcot-Marie-Tooth syndrome (neuronal form)	Variable	Peroneal weakness, normal nerve conduction, and normal reflexes
III	Dejerine-Sottas disease	Autosomal recessive	Begins in infancy and more severe

ness, and muscular atrophy usually distal to the knees ("stork legs").
- Involves motor defects much more than sensory defects.
- Low nerve conduction velocities with prolonged distal latencies are noted in peroneal, ulnar, and median nerves.
- **Diagnosis is made most reliably by DNA testing for a duplication of a genomic fragment that encompasses the peripheral myelin protein-22 (PMP22) gene on chromosome 17.**
- Intrinsic wasting is noted in the hands.
- **The most severely affected muscles are the tibialis anterior, peroneus longus, and peroneus brevis.**
  - **Plantar flexion of the first ray is the foot deformity that occurs first, as a result of a weakened tibialis anterior muscle.**

2. Treatment for feet
   - **Plantar release, posterior tibial tendon transfer (if hindfoot varus is flexible)**
   - Triple arthrodesis (poor long-term results) versus calcaneal and metatarsal osteotomies (if heel varus is fixed and the foot not too short)
   - The Jones procedure for hammer toes, and intrinsic procedures for hand deformity
   - The Coleman block test, to help decide whether calcaneal osteotomy is needed

E. Dejerine-Sottas disease

1. Causes and findings
   - Autosomal recessive hypertrophic neuropathy of infancy
   - Delayed ambulation, pes cavus foot, footdrop, stocking-glove dysesthesia, and spinal deformities are common.
   - The patient is wheelchair dependent by the third or fourth decade.

F. Riley-Day syndrome (dysautonomia)

1. Causes and findings
   - One of five inherited (autosomal recessive) sensory and autonomic neuropathies
   - This disease is found only in patients of Ashkenazi Jewish ancestry.
   - Clinical presentation includes dysphagia, alacrima, pneumonia, excessive sweating, postural hypotension, and sensory loss.

VI. MYASTHENIA GRAVIS

A. Causes and findings

1. Chronic disease with insidious development of easy muscle fatigability after exercise
2. Caused by competitive inhibition of acetylcholine receptors at the motor end plate by antibodies produced in the thymus gland

B. Treatment consists of cyclosporin, anti-acetylcholinesterase agents, or thymectomy.

VII. ANTERIOR HORN CELL DISORDERS

A. Poliomyelitis

1. Causes and findings
   - Viral destruction of anterior horn cells in the spinal cord and brainstem motor nuclei
     - This disease all but disappeared in the United States after vaccine was developed. However, it is still common in underdeveloped countries and in locales where vaccination is unpopular.
   - Many surgical procedures in current use were originally developed for the treatment of polio.
   - The hallmark of polio is muscle weakness with normal sensation.

B. Spinal muscular atrophy

1. Causes and findings
   - **Autosomal recessive, associated with survival motor neuron gene (*SMN*)**
   - Loss of anterior horn cells from the spinal cord. There are three types (Table 3-10).
   - Patients have symmetric paresis with more involvement of the lower extremity and proximal muscles.
   - **Hip subluxation or dislocation is common and treated nonoperatively.**

Table 3-10 Spinal Muscular Atrophy

Type	Description	Age at Onset	Prognosis
I	Acute Werdnig-Hoffman disease	<6 mo	Poor
II	Chronic Werdnig-Hoffman disease	6-24 mo	May live into fifth decade
III	Kugelberg-Welander disease	2-10 yr	Good: may need respiratory support

2. **Scoliosis is treated surgically, like Duchenne muscular dystrophy curves, except that fusion may be required while patient is still ambulatory (may result in loss of ambulatory ability).**
   - **Upper extremity function may decrease after spinal fusion, but this decrease may be temporary.**
   - **Before fusion, ensure that the patient does not have lower extremity muscle contractures that could interfere with sitting balance.**

VIII. ACUTE IDIOPATHIC POSTINFECTIOUS POLYNEUROPATHY (GUILLAIN-BARRÉ SYNDROME)

A. Causes and findings

1. Symmetric ascending motor paresis caused by demyelination after viral infection
2. Cerebrospinal fluid protein level is typically elevated.
3. Usually self-limiting; better prognosis with the acute form

IX. OVERGROWTH SYNDROMES

A. Proteus syndrome

1. Causes and findings
   - An overgrowth of the hands and feet, with bizarre facial disfigurement
   - Scoliosis, genu valgum, hemangiomas, lipomas, and nevi are also common.
   - Must be differentiated from neurofibromatosis and McCune-Albright syndrome

B. Klippel-Trénaunay syndrome

1. Causes
   - Overgrowth caused by underlying arteriovenous malformations
   - Associated with cutaneous hemangiomas and varicosities
2. Treatment
   - Embolization of vascular abnormalities in selected patients
   - Severely hypertrophied extremities often must be amputated.
   - Epiphysiodesis is mainstay for treatment of deformities of limb length.

C. Hemihypertrophy

1. Causes
   - Can be caused by various syndromes, but most cases are idiopathic
   - The most commonly known cause is neurofibromatosis.
   - This disorder is often associated with renal abnormalities (especially Wilms tumor).
     - Best evaluated with serial ultrasonography until age 5 years
2. Treatment
   - Epiphysiodesis versus lengthening to correct leg-length discrepancies
   - Length can be manipulated, but the girth of the limb will always be asymmetric.

SECTION 8 CONGENITAL DISORDERS

For a description of genetic defects, see Table 3-1.

SECTION 9 PEDIATRIC SPINE

I. SCOLIOSIS

A. Definition: lateral deviation and rotational deformity of the spine with many known causes or related conditions

B. Most common type of scoliosis is idiopathic, which has no known cause.

C. Causes:

1. Neuropathic
2. Myelopathic
3. Miscellaneous

D. Idiopathic scoliosis may be classified by age:

1. Infantile: onset before 3 years of age
2. Juvenile: onset between 3 and 10 years of age
3. Adolescent: onset after 10 years of age

II. ADOLESCENT IDIOPATHIC SCOLIOSIS

A. Cause: unknown

1. May be related to a hormonal, brainstem, or proprioception disorder
2. Most patients have a positive family history, but variable expression

B. Diagnosis

1. Referral from two main sources: school screening and pediatrician
   - School screening: mandated by several states
2. Rotational deformities noted on the Adams forward bend test, with the use of a scoliometer
   - Threshold level of **7 degrees** is thought to be an acceptable compromise between overreferral and a false-negative diagnosis and is correlated best with a 20-degree coronal curve.
3. Physical findings
   - Shoulder elevation, waistline asymmetry, a trunk shift, limb-length inequality, rib rotational deformity (rib hump), and prominent scapula
   - Neurologic examination:
     - Findings should be normal.
     - Abnormal findings, especially asymmetric abdominal reflexes, should prompt an MRI study.
   - Examination of the lower extremities: look for cavus deformities; if present, obtain an MRI.
4. Imaging studies
   - Standing posteroanterior and lateral radiographs; the Cobb method is used to measure curves (Figure 3-16).
     - Posteroanterior radiograph; the Cobb method is used to measure curves (see Figure 3-16).
       - Assess Risser sign (ossification of the iliac crest apophysis and graded 0 to 5).
       - Assess trunk balance.
       - Look for congenital abnormalities.
       - Scoliotic curves are classified by type (Figure 3-17).

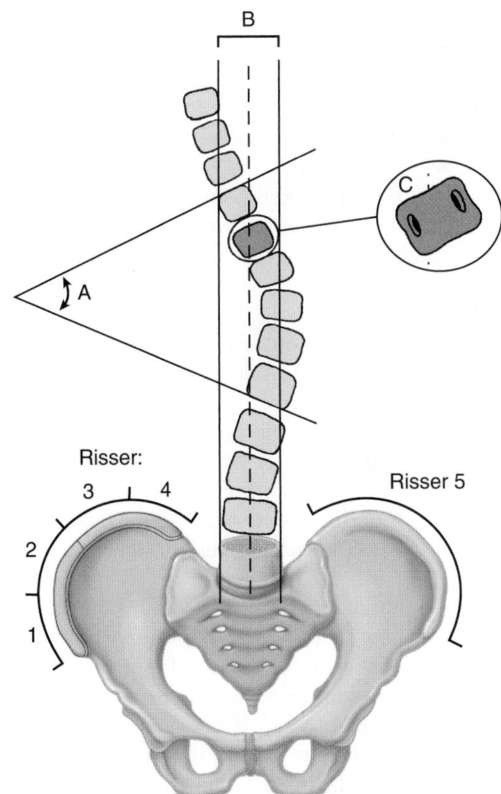

Figure 3-16 Measurements for idiopathic scoliosis: Cobb angle *(A)*; Harrington stable zone *(B)*; Moe neutral vertebra *(C)*; and grading of Risser sign (1 to 5). (Modified from Herring JA, editor: *Tachdjian's pediatric orthopaedics*, ed 4, Philadelphia, 2008, WB Saunders.)

- Lateral radiograph:
  - Hypokyphosis of the apical vertebrae in the sagittal plane is seen with idiopathic scoliosis. If hypokyphosis is absent, an MRI should be obtained.
  - Look for spondylolisthesis at the level of L5 to S1.
- **MRI scan:**
  - **Indications**
    - **Left thoracic curves**
    - **Painful scoliosis**
    - **Apical kyphosis of the thoracic curve**
    - **Juvenile-onset scoliosis (onset before age 11 years)**

Table 3-11 Incidence of Curve Progression as Related to the Magnitude of the Curve and Risser Stage

	PERCENTAGE OF CURVES THAT PROGRESSED	
Risser Stage	5 to 19 Degrees (Curves)	20 to 29 Degrees (Curves)
0, 1	22%	68%
2, 3, 4	1.6%	23%

From Lonstein JE, Carlson JM: The prediction of curve progression in untreated idiopathic scoliosis during growth, *J Bone Joint Surg Am* 66:1067, 1984.

- **Rapid curve progression**
- **Associated syndromes**
- **Neurologic signs and symptoms**
- **Congenital abnormalities**

5. Risk factors for curve progression (Table 3-11)
   - Curve magnitude (>20 degrees) in young patients and more than 45 degrees at skeletal maturity
   - Young age (<12 years)
   - **Skeletal immaturity (Risser stages 0 to 1)**
   - **Curve magnitude before or during peak height velocity**
     - **Peak height velocity is the best predictor of progression.**
     - **Occurs before the onset of menarche and during Risser stage 0**
     - Bone age films can assist in determining peak height velocity.
       - Digital skeletal age of 4-6 indicates peak height growth velocity.
6. Treatment: dependent on the likelihood of curve progression
   - **Observation**
     - **Skeletally immature: curves are less than 25 degrees**
     - **Skeletally mature (Risser stages 2 and higher): curves are less than 45 degrees**
   - Bracing
     - Goal: to halt or slow curve progression; however, does not reverse the magnitude of the deformity in skeletally immature patients (Risser stages 0 to 2)

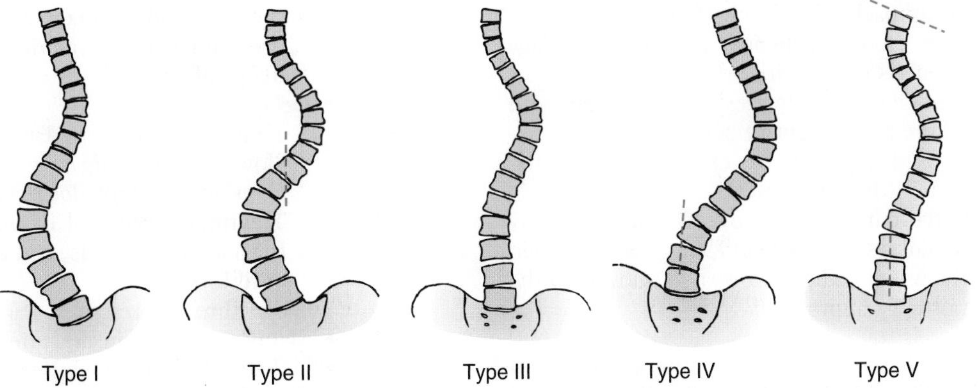

Figure 3-17 Five types of scoliotic curves. Type I: single thoracic curve; type II: double thoracic curve; type III: double major curve; type IV: triple major curve; type V: single thoracolumbar/lumbar curve. (Adapted from King HA, et al: The selection of fusion levels in thoracic idiopathic scoliosis, *J Bone Joint Surg Am* 65:1302–1313, 1983.)

- Indications: curve of more than 30 degrees (or progression of more than 25 degrees while under direct observation)
- Types of braces:
  - Milwaukee brace (cervicothoracolumbosacral orthosis); *rarely* used
  - Boston underarm thoracolumbosacral orthosis
    - For curves with the apex at T8 or below
    - Patients with thoracic lordosis or hypokyphosis are poor candidates.
    - Effectiveness of bracing patients with idiopathic scoliosis is "dose" related (the more the brace is worn each day, the more effective it is).

- Surgical options
  - Goals
    - To prevent curve progression
    - To obtain and maintain correction in the coronal, axial, and sagittal planes
  - Mechanisms of achieving goals
    - Instrumentation
      - Anchor points: pedicle screws (most common), hooks, wires, rods
    - Arthrodesis
      - Fusing the segments of the spine
      - Most common: using allograft to supplement fusion
    - Approach
      - Posterior: most common
        - Anchor points:
          - Thoracic: traditionally hooks, but screws becoming more common because they provide better fixation with three-column control
          - Lumbar: pedicle screws
        - Rod: various sizes; most common are 5.5 and 6.35 mm in diameter
        - Metal: stainless steel or titanium
      - Anterior
        - Uncommon as single approach but useful in two cases:
          - Single thoracic fusion: especially if hypokyphosis is present and if fusion levels can be saved
          - Single thoracolumbar/lumbar fusion
        - Indications for use in combination with posterior approach:
          - Very young patients: triradiate cartilage open; usually in girls younger than 10 to 11 years and in boys ages 11 to 12 years and before peak height velocity
            - Used to prevent the crankshaft phenomenon (described later)
          - Large curve: to improve flexibility, usually for curves of more than 75 degrees. However, the use of pedicle screws may allow only the posterior approach.
    - Fusion levels
      - Main goal: to minimize the number of fusion levels while achieving good coronal and sagittal balance
  - Definitions
    - Stable vertebra: most proximal vertebra that is the most closely bisected by the center sacral line
    - End vertebra: the most tilted vertebra
    - Neutral vertebra: the vertebra that has no rotation in the axial plane
  - Lenke classification: six curve types, three lumbar modifiers, three thoracic sagittal modifiers
    - Curve type:
      - Type I: single thoracic curve
      - Type II: double thoracic curve
      - Type III: double major curve
      - Type IV: triple major curve
      - Type V: single thoracolumbar/lumbar curve
      - Type VI: primary thoracolumbar/lumbar curve and compensatory thoracic curve
        - Structural curves: (1) the largest curve; (2) additional curves that fail to bend to less than 25 degrees
    - Lumbar modifier: based on position of the center sacral vertical line (CSVL) in relation to the apical vertebra of the thoracolumbar/lumbar curve
      - Type A: CSVL is between the pedicles of the apical vertebra.
      - Type B: CSVL touches between the concave pedicle and the lateral body.
      - Type C: CSVL is medial to the apical vertebra.
  - Level of proximal fusion
    - Anterior: proximal end vertebra
    - Posterior: proximal end vertebra
  - Level of distal fusion
    - Anterior approach: distal end vertebra
    - Posterior approach:
      - Lenke types I and II curves: last vertebra touched by CSVL.
      - Lenke types III to VI curves: usually distal end vertebra; in general, fusion levels for anterior spinal fusion surgery are to include the proximal and distal end vertebrae.
- Complications
  - Infection
    - **Acute**
      - ***S. aureus***
      - **Incision and drainage and antibiotic suppression usually required until fusion if deep infection**
    - Delayed
      - Typically occurs after 1 to 2 years
      - Slow-growing organisms: ***Propionibacterium acnes, Staphylococcus epidermidis***
      - **Treatment: removal of implants, a check for pseudoarthrosis, and a short course of antibiotics**
  - Pseudoarthrosis: present in 1% to 3% of cases
    - Manifests with pain, fractured rod
    - Difficult to visualize with imaging studies
    - Treatment: compression instrumentation over the pseudoarthrotic level and bone graft

- Neurologic deficits
  - Rare: present in 0.5% to 0.7% of cases
  - Implant related: with anchors placed in the canal; vascular related: during correction
  - Intraoperative spinal cord monitoring is crucial.
  - If changes occur intraoperatively: reverse steps of surgery and reassess.
    - If still neurologic responses still diminished: complete removal of implants
- Crankshaft phenomenon
  - Continued anterior spinal growth after posterior fusion in skeletally immature patients
  - Increased rotation and deformity of the spine
  - Can be avoided by anterior discectomy and fusion coupled with posterior spinal fusion

III. INFANTILE IDIOPATHIC SCOLIOSIS

A. Idiopathic scoliosis manifesting before the age of 3 years

B. Differences from adolescent idiopathic scoliosis:

1. Left curves more common
2. More common in boys
3. Plagiocephaly (skull flattening) often present
4. Other congenital defects

C. Risk for curve progression: in general, most curves resolve spontaneously.

1. Phase of the ribs: position of the medial rib relative to the apical vertebra
   - Phase I: *no* rib overlap
     - Measure the rib-vertebral angle difference with Mehta classification:
       - Twenty degrees or less: low risk for progression
       - More than 20 degrees: high risk for progression
   - Phase II: rib overlaps the apical vertebra
     - High risk for curve progression

D. Evaluation

1. Clinical: Look for plagiocephaly, neurologic examination, developmental milestones.
2. MRI: Progressive infantile idiopathic scoliosis should be evaluated with MRI of the spinal cord.
   - The incidence of neural axis abnormalities is 20%.

E. Treatment

1. Mehta casting
   - Indications: for young patients with relatively flexible curves
   - Serial casting
     - Goals
       - In very young patients: to force the spine to grow straight
       - Older patients: a stalling tactic to keep the curve relatively small for other treatment
2. Bracing
   - Indications
     - After Mehta casting for curves that are not grown straight
     - For later-presenting cases with relatively flexible curves
3. Surgery
   - Growing rods
     - Dual rods
     - Fusion at the proximal and distal anchors (foundations)
     - Serial lengthening every 6 to 8 months
     - Definitive fusion when patient is older than 10 years, if possible

IV. JUVENILE IDIOPATHIC SCOLIOSIS

A. Definition: idiopthiac scoliosis in children 3 to 10 years of age

B. Presentation: similar to that of adolescent scoliosis in terms of manifestations and treatment

C. Rate of spinal cord abnormality: 25%

1. **MRI should routinely be obtained.**
2. Chiari type I malformations with cervical syrinx, thoracic syrinx, brainstem tumor, dural ectasia, and low-lying conus

D. Risk for rrogression: relatively high

1. Of affected patients, 70% require treatment; of those, 50% need bracing and 50% require surgery

E. Treatment

1. Bracing: for curves of less than 45 degrees
2. Growing rods for patients younger than 8 to 10 years
3. Definitive fusion for patients older than 10 years
   - Anterior and posterior fusion often required

V. EARLY-ONSET SCOLIOSIS

A. Definition: spinal deformity occurring before the age of 6 years

1. Often associated with chest wall deformities
2. Concerns may be different than in other forms of scoliosis.
   - Spine deformity
   - Chest deformity
     - Associated pulmonary issues

B. Thoracic insufficiency syndrome

1. Inability of the thorax to support normal respiration or lung growth
2. Diagnosis
   - Clinical signs of respiratory insufficiency
   - Loss of chest wall mobility as demonstrated by the thumb excursion test
   - Worsening indices of three-dimensional thoracic deformity
     - Radiographic studies: measurement of T1-T12 height
     - CT scans: lung volumes
     - Relative decline in percentage of predicted vital capacity as a result of thoracic failure to thrive, as demonstrated by pulmonary function tests.
3. Treatment
   - Surgery to expand the chest and spine
     - Vertical Expandable Prosthetic Titanium Rib (VEPTR)
       - Can be placed on the rib (rib-to-rib device) or on spine and rib (rib-to-spine device)
     - Results are encouraging but preliminary.

VI. NEUROMUSCULAR SCOLIOSIS

A. Spine deformity is common with neuromuscular conditions.

B. Typical underlying neuromuscular conditions associated with scoliosis (in descending order of relative frequency):

1. Traumatic paralysis
2. Duchenne muscular dystrophy
3. Friedrich ataxia
4. Spinal muscular atrophy
5. Spina bifida (myelomeningocele)
6. Cerebral palsy
7. Neurofibromatosis
8. Arthrogryposis

C. Curve characteristics:

1. Long, sweeping C-shaped curves
2. Associated pelvic obliquity
3. Can be rapidly progressive, especially for patients who are in a wheelchair

D. Associated characteristics

1. Pulmonary issues
   - Most affected patients have some involvement secondary to the underlying condition (Duchenne muscular dystrophy) and detrimental contribution from the scoliosis.
2. Cardiac issues
   - Duchenne muscular dystrophy and other conditions

E. Evaluation

1. Pulmonary: Bilevel positive airway pressure (BiPAP) may be required before and after surgery.
2. Cardiac: for patients with Duchenne muscular dystrophy
3. Nutritional lab markers
   - More than 1500 leukocytes per microliter
   - Albumin level higher than 3.5 g/dL

F. Treatment

1. Wheelchair modifications
   - For patients in a wheelchair, the trunk support can be modified to provide better truncal balance.
2. Orthotics
   - Controversial and not typically used
   - May be used to delay surgical treatment
3. Surgical treatment
   - **Indications: vary with diagnosis**
     - **Duchenne muscular dystrophy**
       - **Curve exceeding 25 to 30 degrees, because curve progression is rapid and pulmonary and cardiac conditions worsen with time**
     - Cerebral palsy
       - Ambulatory patients: curve exceeding 50 degrees
       - Nonambulatory patients:
         - Dependent on sitting balance and whether there are challenges with caring for the child
         - Curve magnitudes may be very large before surgical treatment.
   - Fusion levels
     - Nonambulatory patients:
       - Usually from T2 to the pelvis
       - Pelvic fixation
         - Traditional:
           - Galveston technique with unit rod
           - Dunn-McCarthy rods: S-shaped hooks that travel over the sacral ala
         - Iliac screws:
           - Long screws placed beginning at the posterior superior iliac spine
           - Travel just anterior to the sciatic notch
         - Sacroiliac screws:
           - Begin just distal and lateral to the S1 neural foramina and travel in a similar direction as iliac screws
     - Segmental fixation
       - Traditional: sublaminar wires
       - Current: pedicle screws are more common
   - Goal of surgery
     - To center the trunk over the pelvis and to achieve a balanced spine
   - Complications
     - Infection: more common than in idiopathic scoliosis

VII. CONGENITAL SCOLIOSIS

A. Caused by a developmental defect in the formation of the mesenchymal anlage during the fourth to sixth week of gestation

B. Three basic types of defects

1. Failure of segmentation (i.e., vertebral bar)
2. Failure of formation (i.e., hemivertebrae)
3. Mixed

C. Evaluation

1. Plain radiographs
2. Three-dimensional CT scanning: helpful for defining the type of vertebral anomaly (Figure 3-18)
3. **Spinal MRI should be performed before any surgery to assess the patient for intraspinal anomalies (syringomyelia, diastematomyelia).**
4. **Renal ultrasonography to reveal genitourinary defects (25% of cases)**
5. **Assessment for cardiac anomalies (10% of cases)**

D. Risk for progression (Table 3-12)

1. Dependent on the morphologic characteristics of the vertebrae
   - A fully segmented hemivertebra is free, with normal disc spaces on both sides (higher risk for progression), whereas an unsegmented hemivertebra is fused above and below (lower risk; see Figure 3-18).
   - An incarcerated hemivertebra (within the lateral margins of the vertebrae above and below) confers a better prognosis than does an unincarcerated (laterally positioned) hemivertebra.
   - Unilateral, unsegmented bar is a common disorder and is likely to progress.
   - **Block vertebra (bilateral failure of segmentation) confers the best prognosis.**
   - **A unilateral, unsegmented bar with a contralateral, fully segmented hemivertebra confers the worst prognosis.**

E. Treatment

1. Bracing may be effective for compensatory curves or for smaller, supple curves above a vertebral anomaly, but it is ineffective for controlling congenital curves.
2. Surgical options
   - In situ posterior spinal fusion (older patients) or anterior/posterior spinal fusion (younger patients)

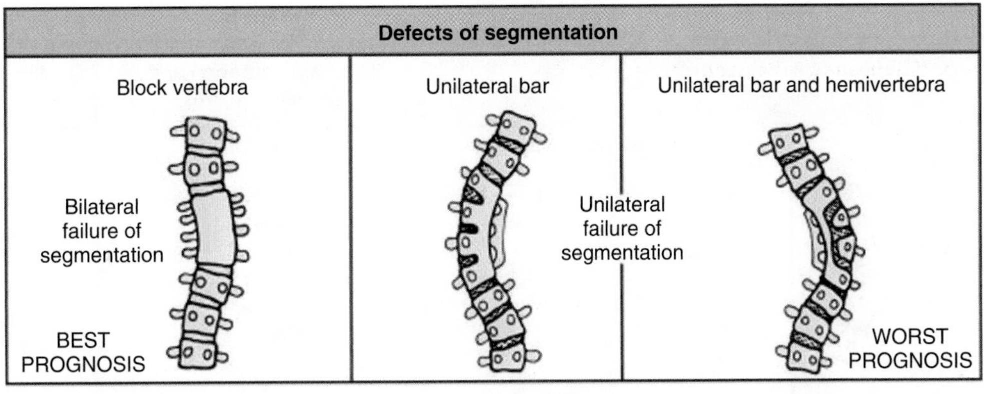

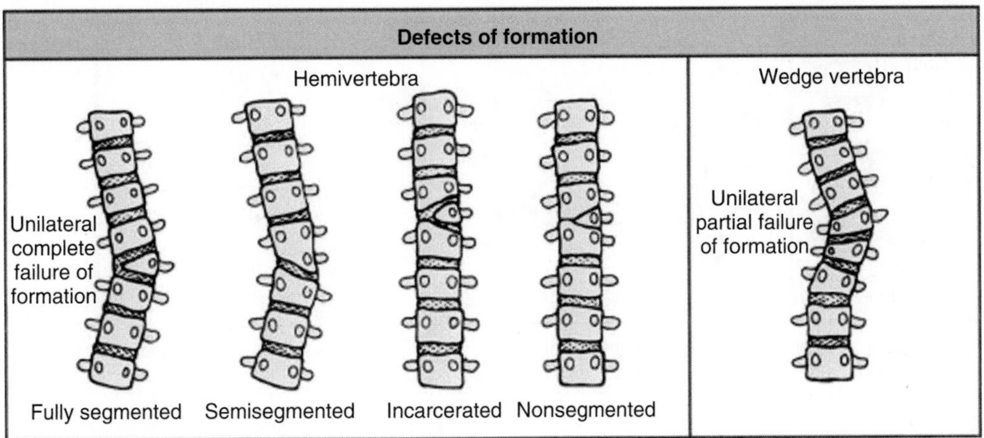

Figure 3-18 Vertebral anomalies that lead to congenital scoliosis. (Adapted from Herring JA, editor: *Tachdjian's pediatric orthopaedics,* ed 4, Philadelphia, 2008, WB Saunders, Figure 12-57.)

- Posterior fusion in situ
  - Crankshaft phenomenon may occur because of continued anterior spinal growth.
  - In such cases, anterior/posterior spinal fusion may be required.
- Convex anterior and posterior hemiepiphysiodesis (implants are necessary)
- **Resection of the hemivertebra if fully segmented**
  - Surgical options should not be considered until other deformities demonstrate progression.
  - Anterior and posterior hemivertebra excision may be indicated for lumbosacral hemivertebrae associated with progressive curves and an oblique takeoff (severe truncal imbalance).
  - Isolated hemivertebral excision should be accompanied by anterior/posterior arthrodesis with instrumentation to stabilize the adjacent vertebrae. A summary of treatment recommendations for congenital scoliosis is found in Table 3-11.

VIII. CONGENITAL KYPHOSIS

A. Causes (Figure 3-19)

1. Failure of formation (type I)
   - Most common
   - **Worse prognosis**
   - Highest risk for neurologic complications
   - When severe: immediate indication for surgery

Table 3-12 Progression of Congenital Scoliosis Patterns and Treatment Options

Risk for Progression (Highest to Lowest)	Character of Curve Progression	Treatment Options
Unilateral unsegmented bar with contralateral hemivertebra	Rapid and relentless	Posterior spinal fusion (add anterior fusion for girls younger than 10 yr, boys younger than 12 yr)
Unilateral unsegmented bar	Rapid	Posterior spinal fusion (add anterior fusion for girls younger than 10 yr, boys younger than 12 yr)
Fully segmented hemivertebra	Steady	Anterior spinal fusion Hemivertebra excision
Partially segmented hemivertebra	Less rapid; curve usually < 40 degrees at maturity	Observation, hemivertebra excision
Incarcerated hemivertebra	May slowly progress	Observation
Nonsegmented hemivertebra	Little progression	Observation

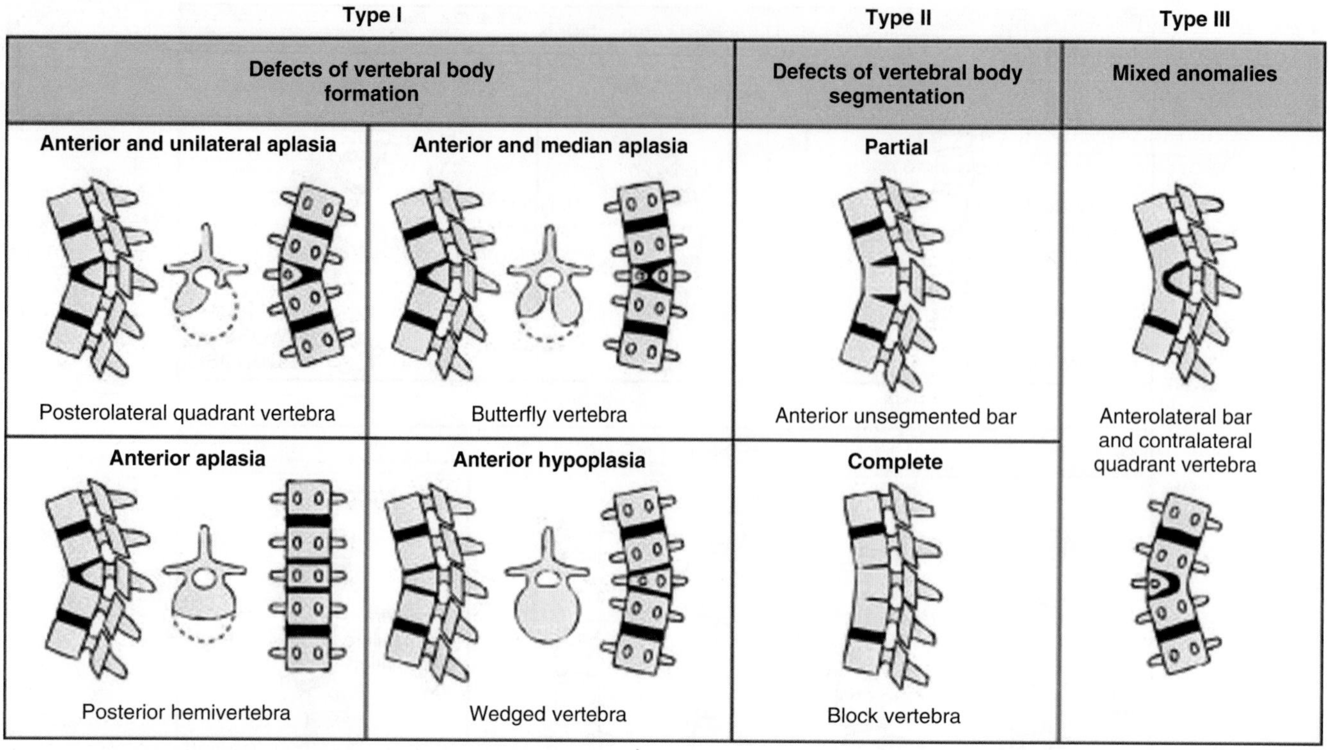

Type I		Type II	Type III
Defects of vertebral body formation		**Defects of vertebral body segmentation**	**Mixed anomalies**
Anterior and unilateral aplasia Posterolateral quadrant vertebra	**Anterior and median aplasia** Butterfly vertebra	**Partial** Anterior unsegmented bar	Anterolateral bar and contralateral quadrant vertebra
Anterior aplasia Posterior hemivertebra	**Anterior hypoplasia** Wedged vertebra	**Complete** Block vertebra	

Figure 3-19 Vertebral anomalies leading to congenital kyphosis. (Adapted from Herring JA, editor: *Tachdjian's pediatric orthopaedics,* ed 4, Philadelphia, 2008, WB Saunders, Figure 12-69.)

2. Failure of segmentation (type II)
3. Mixed abnormalities (type III)
4. The presence of significant congenital kyphosis: secondary to failure of formation.

B. Treatment

1. **Posterior fusion:**
   - **Favored in young children (<5 years old) with curves of less than 50 degrees and normal findings on neurologic examination**
   - Functions as a posterior (convex) hemiepiphysiodesis
2. Anterior/posterior fusion:
   - Reserved for older children or more severe curves
3. Anterior vertebrectomy, spinal cord decompression, and anterior fusion followed by posterior fusion are indicated for curves associated with neurologic deficits.
4. Vertebral column resection: hemi-vertebra causing coronal or saggital plane deformity and/or large fixed spinal deformity
5. A type II congenital kyphosis can be monitored to document progression, but progressive curves should be fused posteriorly.

IX. NEUROFIBROMATOSIS

A. Autosomal dominant disorder of neural crest origin, often associated with neoplasia and skeletal abnormalities

B. Diagnosis: characterized by neurofibromas and café au lait spots

C. The spine is the most common site of skeletal involvement.

D. Curve classification:

1. **Nondystrophic (similar to idiopathic scoliosis)**
2. **Dystrophic**
   - Characteristic radiographic abnormalities:
     - Short segment curves with tight apex
     - Vertebral scalloping
     - Enlarged foramina
     - Penciling of transverse processes
     - Penciling of ribs
     - Severe apical rotation
3. Spinal deformity secondary to neurofibromatosis is characteristically kyphoscoliosis in the thoracic region with dystrophic changes, but nondystrophic scoliosis or cervical involvement may also be noted.
4. Evaluation
   - Plain radiographic findings
     - **Penciling of three or more ribs is a prognostic factor for impending rapid progression of spinal deformity.**
   - MRI
     - Neurologic involvement is common in neurofibromatosis and may be caused by the deformity itself, an intraspinal tumor, a soft tissue mass, or dural ectasia.
   - CT scan
     - Especially when surgery is planned
     - To assess the bony anatomy
       - Pedicle sizes and posterior body are small and eroded secondary to the dural ectasia.
5. Treatment
   - Nondystrophic scoliosis: treatment is similar to that of idiopathic scoliosis.
   - Dystrophic deformities:
     - More aggressively treated, especially when kyphosis is present; surgical treatment is indicated for any progression and when curves reach 40 degrees.

- **Anterior/posterior surgery:**
  - **In young patients, especially when deformities are associated with kyphosis**
  - **To prevent crankshaft phenomenon**
  - **To improve fusion rates**
- Isolated kyphosis of the thoracic spine is treated with anterior decompression of the kyphotic angular cord compression, followed by anterior and posterior fusion or vertebral column resection from the posterior approach.
- Cervical spine involvement includes kyphosis or atlantoaxial instability.
  - Treatment: Posterior fusion with autologous grafting and halo immobilization is recommended for severe cervical spine deformity with instability.

X. OTHER SPINAL ABNORMALITIES

A. Diastematomyelia

1. Fibrous, cartilaginous, or osseous bar creating a longitudinal cleft in the spinal cord
2. More commonly occurs in the lumbar spine: can lead to tethering of the cord, with associated neurologic deficits
3. Intrapedicular widening on plain radiographs is suggestive of the diagnosis, and myelographic CT scan or MRI is necessary to fully define the disorder.
4. Must be resected before correction of a spinal deformity, but if it is otherwise asymptomatic and without neurologic sequelae, it may monitored without surgery

B. Sacral agenesis

1. Partial or complete absence of the sacrum and lower lumbar spine
2. **Strongly associated with maternal diabetes**
3. Often accompanied by gastrointestinal, genitourinary, and cardiovascular abnormalities
4. Clinically, affected children have a prominent lower lumbar spine and atrophic lower extremities; they may sit in a "Buddha" position. Motor impairment is at the level of the agenesis, but sensory innervation is largely spared. Management may include amputation of the legs or spinal-pelvic fusion.

C. Low-back pain (Table 3-13)

In children, complaints of low-back pain and especially painful scoliosis should be taken seriously. However, results of one study suggested that 75% of pediatric patients with low-back pain have no definitive diagnosis and that most of the diagnoses were made at the initial visit on the basis of findings on physical examination or plain radiographs.

1. Discitis and osteomyelitis
   - Manifestations
     - Acute back pain
     - Refusal to sit or walk
     - Increased ESR
   - Radiographic findings
     - **Loss of normal lumbar lordosis (the earliest radiographic finding)**
     - Disc space narrowing but preservation of end plates (develops over a period of 3 weeks after loss of lumbar lordosis)
   - Treatment
     - Antibiotics
2. Herniated nucleus pulposus
   - Uncommon in children
   - Manifestations
     - Back pain
     - Pain radiating down the leg
   - Treatment
     - Pain management
     - Rest in the acute period
     - PT when symptoms allow
3. Spondylolysis: stress fracture at the pars interarticularis
   - Common in athletes who use hyperextension (gymnasts, football lineman)
   - Imaging
     - Plain radiographs: oblique, to see "collar" in the Scotty dog appearance
     - CT scan: best image
   - Treatment
     - When asymptomatic and discovered incidentally: unilateral pars defects do not progress to spondylolisthesis, and patients do not require further monitoring.
     - Nonoperative for symptomatic spondylolysis:
       - **Bracing in the acute period with an antilordotic brace**
       - Physical therapy: core strengthening and hamstring stretch
     - Operative:
       - Undertaken if conservative treatment fails
       - Fusion of L5 to S1 most common if defect is at L5
       - If defect is at L4 or higher, then pars repair
         - Buck technique: lag screw across the defect
         - Scott technique:
           - Wiring technique from the spinous process to the transverse processes
           - Modified Scott technique: pedicle screw with wire around screw head across the spinous process
         - Pedicle screw and sublaminar hook at the same level
4. Spondylolisthesis: forward slippage of the proximal vertebra on the distal vertebra
   - Most commonly seen at L5 to S1
   - Types
     - Lytic (from spondylolysis)
     - Dysplastic (congenital absence or dysplasia of the facets)
       - Greater risk for progression

Table 3-13 Differential Diagnosis for Low-Back Pain in Children

Category	Disease
Mechanical	Muscle strain Herniated nucleus pulposis
Infection and tumor	Discitis osteomyelitis Eosinophilic granuloma Osteoid osteoma Osteoblastoma Ewing spinal cord tumor Metastatic disease
Developmental	Spondylosis Spondylolisthesis Syringomyelia Tethered cord

- Classification
  - Translation: Meyerding grading system (low: grades 1 and 2; high: grades 3 and 4)
    - Grade 1: 0% to 25% translation
    - Grade 2: 25% to 50% translation
    - Grade 3: 50% to 75% translation
    - Grade 4: 75% to 100% translation
      - The larger the slippage, the greater the chance of progression
  - Kyphosis:
    - Most important determinant for nonunion and pain
    - Slippage angle
      - Measured from the bottom end plate of L5 and a perpendicular to the line on the posterior sacrum
      - Curve of more than 25 degrees is a risk factor for nonunion, continued pain, and slippage.
- Clinical manifestation
  - Low-grade slippage may manifest with low-back pain and normal examination findings.
  - High-grade slippage (>50%) may be accompanied by a flexed hip and knee posture with equinus, sacral prominence, and proximal hyperlordosis.
- Treatment
  - **Low-grade (1 and 2) slippage:**
    - **Bracing in the acute period**
    - **Activity modification and physical therapy**
    - **If continued pain then arthrodesis with or without instrumentation**
  - **High-grade (3 and 4) slippage:**
    - **In general, surgery is indicated because slippage usually produces pain and has a high risk for progression.**
    - **Surgery:**
      - **In general, L4-S1 fusion required**
      - Decompression with high-grade slippage or neurologic symptoms
      - Anterior fusion through posterior approach should be considered.
      - Correction of slippage angle as reduction maneuver (controversial because it may increase risk of neurologic deficits)

5. Osteoma or spinal cord anomaly
   - Should be investigated aggressively. A bone scan is an excellent screening method for a child or adolescent with back pain.

XI. KYPHOSIS

A. Congenital kyphosis: See the previous discussion of congenital spinal disorders.

B. Scheuermann disease

1. Definition
   - Increased thoracic kyphosis (>45 degrees) with 5 degrees or more anterior wedging at three sequential vertebrae
   - Cause unknown
2. Other radiographic findings
   - Disc space narrowing
   - End plate irregularities
   - Spondylolysis (30% to 50% of cases)
   - Scoliosis (33% of cases)
   - Schmorl nodes (Figures 3-20 and 3-21).

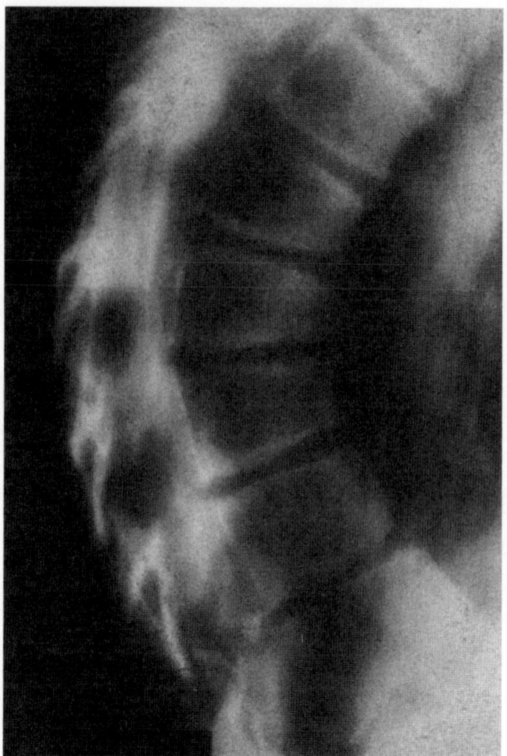

Figure 3-20 Scheuermann thoracic hyperkyphosis: lateral radiograph. Note the anterior wedging at three sequential vertebrae. (From Benson M, et al: *Children's orthopaedics and fractures,* New York, 1994, Churchill Livingstone, p 19.)

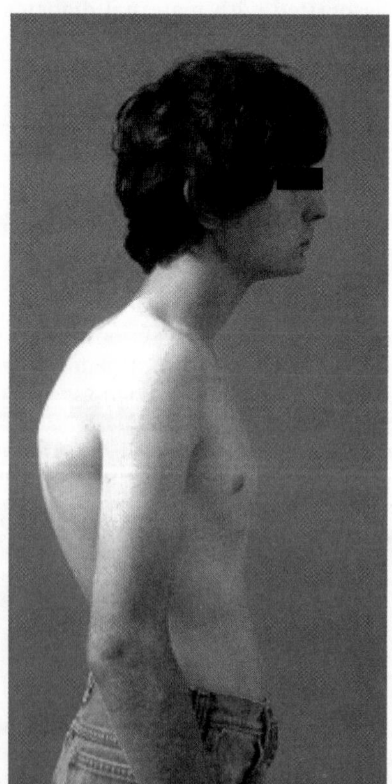

Figure 3-21 Scheuermann thoracic kyphosis: clinical photograph. (From Herring JA, editor: *Tachdjian's pediatric orthopaedics,* ed 4, Philadelphia, 2008, WB Saunders.)

3. Diagnosis
   - Radiographic findings
     - Excessive kyphosis
     - Three sequential vertebra with more than 5 degrees of wedge
   - Clinical characteristics
     - More common in boys
     - Affected patients usually overweight
     - Kyphosis is not postural: does not complete correct with hyperextension.
     - Neurologic changes are rare: MRI indicated if they are present.
   - **Treatment**
     - **Bracing**
       - **Progressive curve in a patient with 1 year or more of skeletal growth remaining (Risser stage 2 or below)**
       - **Indicated for kyphotic curvature of 50 to 75 degrees**
       - A modified Milwaukee brace is used but often not well tolerated
     - Surgery
       - Indications
         - Progressive curve
         - Continued pain despite physical therapy
         - Skeletal maturity
         - Severe kyphosis (curve >75 degrees)
         - Cosmesis (relative indication)
       - Technique
         - All posterior: nearly always enough
           - Multiple Ponte osteotomies to create wide facets
           - Fusion levels
             - Proximal: for thoracic Scheuermann disease, T2; for thoracolumbar Scheuermann disease, T3 or T4
             - Distal: always include the first lordotic disc and the vertebra touched by the posterior sacral vertical line (vertical line extending from the posterior edge of S1)
         - Anterior release is rare today.
       - Thoracolumbar or lumbar Scheuermann disease
         - Less common than thoracic form
         - Causes more back pain
         - End plates may be more irregular
         - Not associated with vertebral wedging

C. Postural round back: also associated with kyphosis but does not demonstrate vertebral body changes. Forward bending reveals kyphosis, but there is no sharp angulation as in Scheuermann disease. Correction with backward bending and prone hyperextension is typical. Treatment includes a hyperextension exercise program.

D. Other causes of kyphosis

1. Trauma
2. Infections
3. Spondylitis
4. Bone dysplasias (mucopolysaccharidoses, Kniest syndrome, diastrophic dysplasia), and neoplasms
5. Postlaminectomy kyphosis (most often for spinal cord abnormalities) can be severe and necessitates anterior and posterior fusion as soon as possible. The performance of total laminectomy in immature patients without stabilization is contraindicated.

XII. CERVICAL SPINE DISORDERS

A. Klippel-Feil syndrome

1. Abnormalities in multiple cervical segments as a result of failure of normal segmentation or formation of cervical somites at 3 to 8 weeks of gestation
2. Associations
   - Congenital scoliosis
   - Renal disease (aplasia: 33% of cases)
   - Synkinesis (mirror motions)
   - Sprengel deformity (30% of cases)
   - Congenital heart disease
   - Brainstem abnormalities
   - Congenital cervical stenosis
3. The classic triad (seen in <50% of cases)
   - Low posterior hairline
   - Short "webbed" neck
   - Limited cervical ROM
4. Disc degeneration: almost 100% of cases
5. Treatment
   - Avoid collision sports
   - Conservative (most commonly)
   - Surgery for chronic pain with myelopathy

B. Atlantoaxial instability

1. Anteroposterior instability
   - Associated with Down syndrome (trisomy 21)
     - If normal neurologic picture: avoid contact sports
     - If neurologic symptoms: posterior fusion (associated with high rate of complications)
   - Juvenile rheumatoid arthritis
   - Various osteochondrodystrophies
   - **Os odontoideum and other abnormalities**

C. Rotatory atlantoaxial subluxation

1. May manifest with torticollis
2. Causes
   - Retropharyngeal inflammation (Grisel disease)
     - Probably caused by secondary ligamentous laxity
     - **Treated with early traction and bracing**
     - Diagnosis:
       - CT scans at the C1-C2 level with the head straight forward, then in maximum rotation to the right, and then in maximum rotation to the left (Figure 3-22)
     - Late diagnosis may necessitate C1-C2 fusion.

D. Traumatic atlantoaxial subluxation

1. May manifest as torticollis
2. Treatment:
   - Initially with a soft collar for up to 1 week
   - If symptoms present, cervical traction is initiated.
   - If late presentation (>1 month), fusion required if fixed rotatory subluxation is present
3. Also seen in the following conditions:
   - Rheumatoid arthritis
   - Down syndrome
   - Congenital anomalies
   - Cervical tumors

E. Os odontoideum

1. Previously thought to result from the failure of fusion of the base of the odontoid

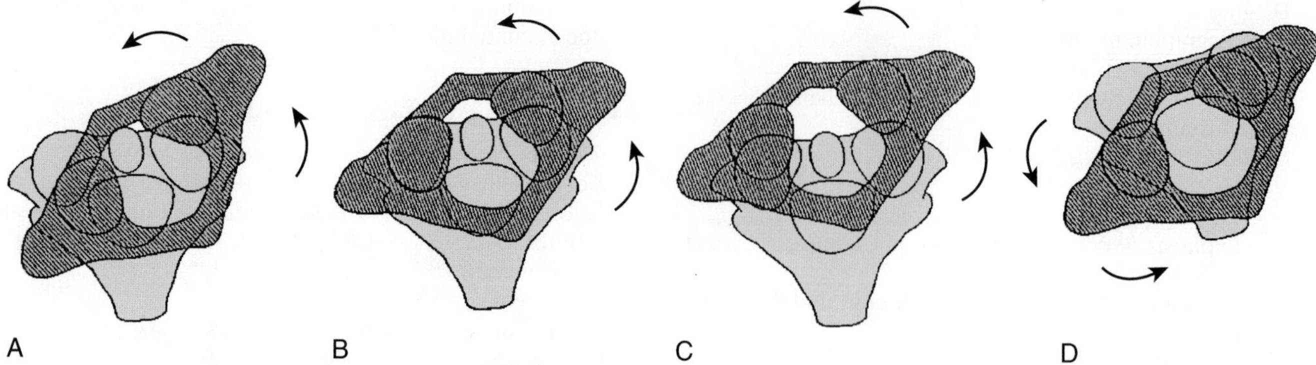

Figure 3-22 Four types of rotatory fixation. **A,** Type I: rotatory fixation with no anterior displacement and the odontoid acting as the pivot. **B,** Type II: rotatory fixation with anterior displacement of 3 to 5 mm, with one lateral process acting as the pivot. **C,** Type III: rotatory fixation with anterior displacement of more than 5 mm. **D,** Type IV: rotatory fixation with posterior displacement. (Adapted from Fielding JW, Hawkins RJ: Atlantoaxial rotatory fixation, *J Bone Joint Surg Am* 59:42, 1977.)

2. May represent the residue of an old traumatic process
3. Two types
   - Orthotopic type: in place of the normal odontoid process
   - Dystopic type: may fuse to the clivus (more often seen with neurologic compromise)
4. Treatment
   - Conservative except in the following cases:
     - Instability (>10 mm of the atlanto-dens interval or <13 mm space available for the cord)
     - Presence of neurologic symptoms, which necessitate a posterior C1-C2 fusion

F. Pseudosubluxation of the cervical spine

1. **Subluxation of C2 on C3 (and occasionally of C3 on C4) of up to 40%, or 4 mm**
2. Can be a normal finding in children younger than 8 years because of the orientation of the facets
3. Rapid resolution of pain, relatively minor trauma, lack of anterior swelling
4. **Continued alignment of the posterior interspinous distances and the posterior spinolaminar line (Swischuk line) on radiographs** (Figure 3-23)
5. The fact that the subluxation can be reduced with neck extension helps differentiate this entity from more serious disorders.

G. Intervertebral disc calcification syndrome

1. Pain, decreased ROM
2. Low-grade fevers
3. Increased ESR
4. Characteristic radiographic finding: disc calcification (within the annulus) without erosion
5. Usually involves the cervical spine
6. Conservative treatment indicated for this self-limiting condition

H. Basilar impression/invagination

1. Deformity at the base of the skull causes odontoid migration into the foramen magnum.
2. Sagittal MRI scan best demonstrates impingement of the dens on the brainstem.
3. Clinical presentation: Weakness, paresthesias, and hydrocephalus may result.
4. Treatment is often operative and may include transoral resection of the dens, occipital laminectomy, and occipitocervical fusion and wiring.

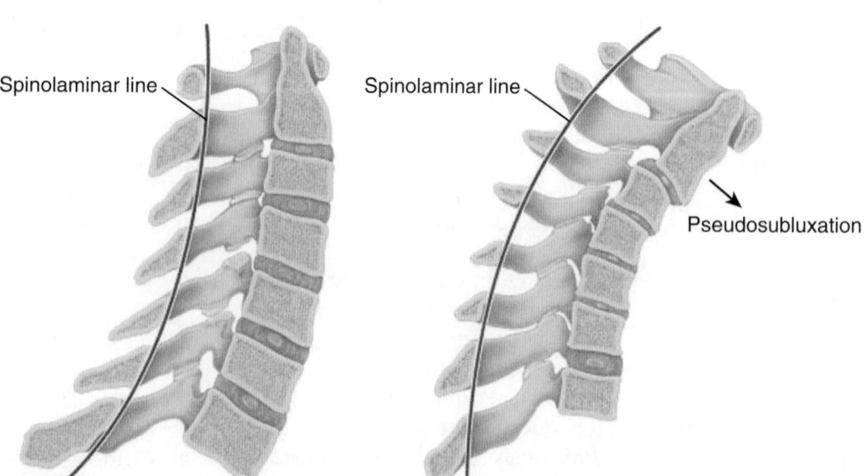

Figure 3-23 Pseudosubluxation of C2 to C3 (most common). Actual subluxation is not possible because of the intact spinolaminar line at C2 to C3. (From Herring JA, editor: *Tachdjian's pediatric orthopaedics,* ed 4, Philadelphia, 2008, WB Saunders, Figure 11-4.)

SECTION 10 UPPER EXTREMITY PROBLEMS*

I. SPRENGEL DEFORMITY

A. Clinical features

1. Undescended scapula often associated with winging, hypoplasia, and omovertebral connections (30% of cases; Figure 3-24)
2. The most common congenital anomaly of the shoulder in children
3. Affected scapulae are usually small, relatively wide, and medially rotated.
4. Increased association with Klippel-Feil syndrome, kidney disease, scoliosis, and diastematomyelia

B. Treatment

1. Surgery for cosmetic or functional deformities (decreased abduction) includes distal advancement of the associated muscles and scapula (Woodward procedure) or detachment and movement of the scapula (Schrock and Green procedures)
2. Clavicular osteotomy is often needed to avoid brachial plexus injury caused by stretch.
3. Surgery is best done when patients are 3 to 8 years of age.

II. FIBROTIC DELTOID PROBLEMS

A. Clinical features

1. Short, fibrous bands replace the deltoid muscle and cause abduction contractures at the shoulder, with elevation and winging of the scapula when the arms are adducted.

B. Treatment

1. Surgical resection of these bands is often required.

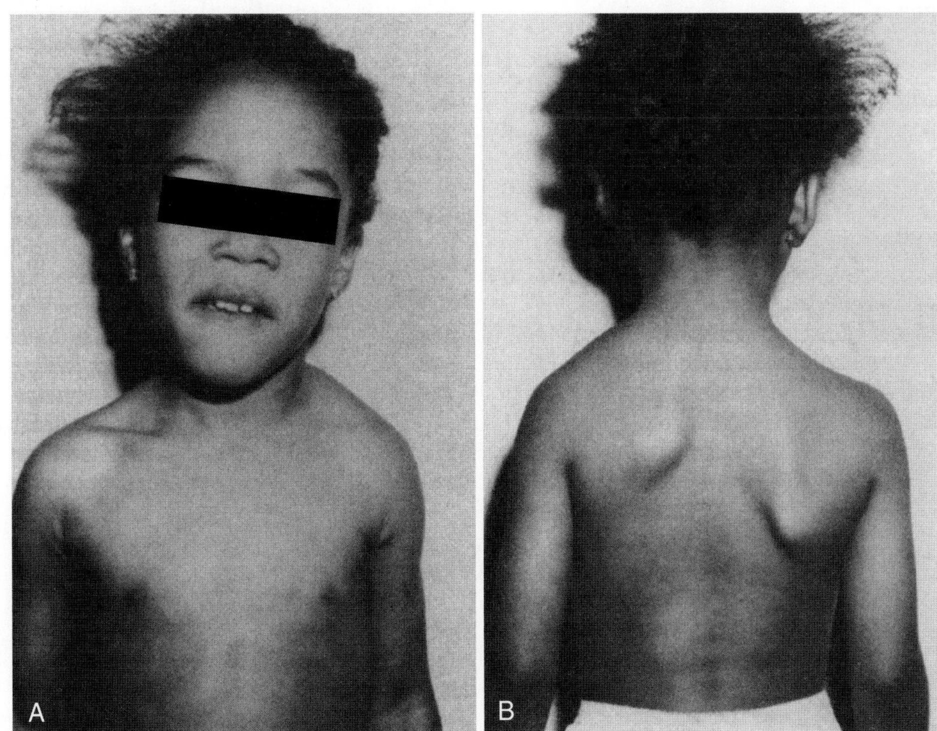

Figure 3-24 Sprengel shoulder: clinical photographs of a child affected on the left side. **A,** Anterior view. **B,** Posterior view. Note the elevation and rotation of the scapula. (From Benson M, et al: *Children's orthopaedics and fractures,* New York, 1994, Churchill Livingstone, p 365.)

SECTION 11 LOWER EXTREMITY PROBLEMS: GENERAL

I. INTRODUCTION

Lower extremity problems that are best considered as a whole are presented in this section to provide a basis for understanding and comparison.

*See Chapter 7, Hand, Upper Extremity, and Microvascular Surgery.

II. ROTATIONAL PROBLEMS OF THE LOWER EXTREMITIES

A. Introduction

1. **In-toeing is usually attributable to metatarsus adductus (in infants), internal tibial torsion (in toddlers) and femoral anteversion (in children younger than 10 years).**

Table 3-14 Evaluation of Rotational Problems of the Lower Extremities

Measurement	Technique	Normal Values (Degrees)	Significance
Foot-progression angle	Foot vs. straight line	−5 to +20	Nonspecific rotation
Medial rotation	Prone hip ROM	20-60	>70 Degrees: femoral anteversion
Lateral rotation	Prone hip ROM	30-60	<20 Degrees: femoral anteversion
Thigh-foot angle	Knee bent; foot up	0-20	<−10 Degrees: tibial torsion
Foot lateral border	Convex; medial crease	Straight; flexible	Metatarsus adductus

ROM, range of motion.

2. **Out-toeing is typically a result of an external rotation hip contracture (in infants), and external tibial torsion and external femoral torsion (in older children and adolescents).**
3. All of these problems may be a result of intrauterine positioning and commonly manifest with a pigeon-toed gait.
4. These deformities are usually bilateral, and the clinician should be wary of asymmetric findings.
5. Evaluation should include the measurements noted in Table 3-14 and illustrated in Figure 3-25.

B. **Metatarsus adductus**

1. Clinical features
   - The forefoot is adducted at the tarsal-metatarsal joint.
   - Usually seen during the first year of life
   - May be associated with hip dysplasia (10% to 15% of cases)
   - Approximately 85% of cases resolve spontaneously.
2. Treatment
   - Nonoperative
     - Feet that can be actively corrected to neutral position require no treatment.
     - Stretching exercises are used for feet that can be passively corrected to neutral position (heel bisector line aligns with the second metatarsal).
     - Feet that cannot be passively corrected (a rare situation) usually respond to serial casting.
   - Surgery
     - Cuneiform osteotomies and limited medial release are indicated in resistant cases.
     - The results with osteotomies are best when the surgery is performed after 5 years of age.

C. **Tibial torsion**

1. Clinical features
   - The most common cause of inward turning of toes
   - **Usually seen during the second year of life and can be associated with metatarsus adductus**
   - It is often bilateral and may be secondary to excessive medial ligamentous tightness.
   - Internal rotation of the tibia causes the pigeon-toed gait.
   - Transmalleolar axis is internal.
2. Treatment
   - **Resolves spontaneously with growth**
   - **Operative correction is rarely necessary except in severe cases, which are addressed with a supramalleolar osteotomy when child is between 7 and 10 years of age.**

D. **Femoral anteversion**

1. Clinical features
   - **Internal rotation of the femur, seen in 3- to 6-year-olds**
   - **Children with this problem classically sit with the legs in a W-shaped position.**

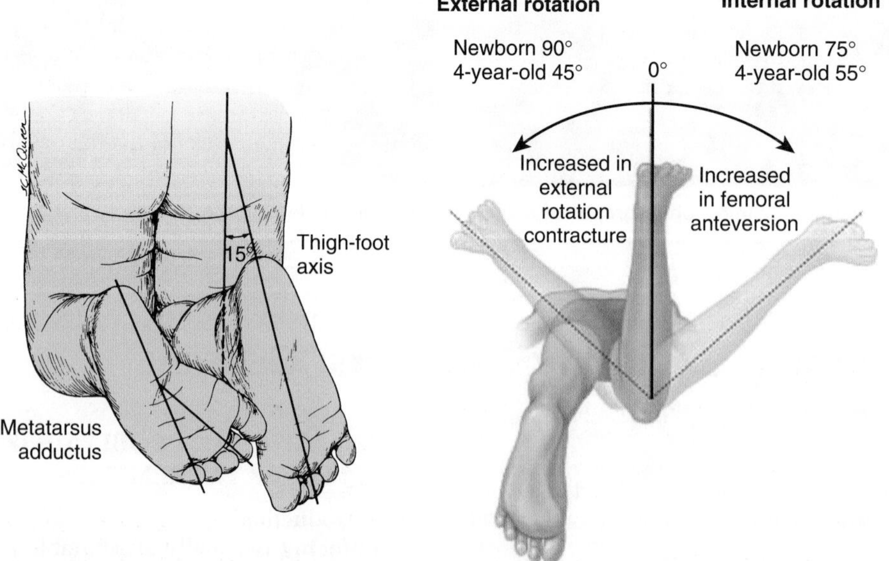

Figure 3-25 Deviation of the forefoot in metatarsus adductus. Note also the normal thigh-foot angle (15 degrees); negative thigh-foot angles (<−10 degrees) are seen in tibial torsion. (Adapted from Fitch RD: Introduction to pediatric orthopedics. In Sabiston DC Jr, editor: *Sabiston's essentials of surgery,* Philadelphia, 1987, WB Saunders.)

- If associated with tibial torsion, femoral anteversion may lead to patellofemoral problems.

2. Treatment
   - This disorder usually corrects spontaneously by age 10 years.
   - In older children with less than 10 degrees of external rotation, femoral derotational osteotomy (intertrochanteric is best) may be considered for cosmesis, although this is not a functional problem.

SECTION 12 HIP AND FEMUR

I. DEVELOPMENTAL DYSPLASIA OF THE HIP

A. Introduction

1. Previously called *congenital dysplasia of the hip,* this disorder represents abnormal development or dislocation of the hip secondary to capsular laxity and mechanical factors (e.g., intrauterine positioning).

B. Risk factors

1. **Breech positioning, positive family history, female sex, and being a firstborn child are risk factors (in that order).**
2. Less intrauterine space accounts for the increased incidence of DDH in firstborn children.
3. DDH is observed most often in the left hip (67% of cases), in girls (85%), in infants with a positive family history (≥20%), in the presence of increased maternal estrogens, and in breech births (30% to 50%).

C. Clinical features

1. Associated with other problems related to intrauterine positioning, such as torticollis (20% of cases) and metatarsus adductus (10%), it is partially characterized by increased amounts of type III collagen.
2. This disorder includes the spectrum of complete dislocation, subluxation, instability, and acetabular dysplasia.
3. If left untreated, muscles about the hip become contracted, and the acetabulum becomes more dysplastic and filled with fibrofatty tissue (pulvinar).
4. Potential obstructions to obtaining a concentric reduction in DDH are an iliopsoas tendon, pulvinar, a contracted inferomedial hip capsule, the transverse acetabular ligament, and an inverted labrum.
5. The teratologic form is most severe and usually necessitates early surgery.
   - In this form of DDH, a pseudoacetabulum is present at or near birth.
   - Teratologic hip dislocations commonly manifest in association with syndromes such as arthrogryposis and Larsen syndrome.

D. Diagnosis

1. Physical examination
   - **Early diagnosis is possible with the Ortolani test (elevation and abduction of femur relocates a dislocated hip) and the Barlow test (adduction and depression of femur dislocates a dislocatable hip).**
   - Three phases are commonly recognized: (1) *dislocated* (positive result of the Ortolani test, early; negative result of the Ortolani test, late, when femoral head cannot be reduced), (2) *dislocatable* (positive result of the Barlow test), and (3) *subluxatable* (suggestive result of the Barlow test).
   - **Subsequent diagnosis is made with limitation of hip abduction in the affected hip as the laxity resolves and stiffness becomes more clinically evident.**
     - Caution: Abduction may be decreased symmetrically with bilateral dislocations.
   - Another sign of dislocation includes the Galeazzi sign, demonstrated by the clinical appearance of foreshortening of the femur on the affected side.
     - This clinical test is performed with the feet held together and knees flexed (a congenitally short femur can also cause the Galeazzi sign).
   - Other clinical findings associated with DDH include asymmetric gluteal folds (less reliable) and Trendelenburg stance (in older children).
   - Repeated examination, especially in an infant, is important because a child's irritability can prevent proper evaluation.
2. Radiography
   - Dynamic ultrasonography is useful for making the diagnosis in young children before ossification of the femoral head **(which occurs at age 4 to 6 months)** (Figure 3-26).
     - It is also useful for assessing reduction in a Pavlik harness and diagnosing acetabular dysplasia or capsular laxity; however, its success is dependent on the operator's skill.
     - On the coronal view, the normal α angle is greater than 60 degrees, and the femoral head is bisected by the line drawn down the ilium.
   - Radiographic studies and findings
     - Used in older children (after age 3 months); measurement of the acetabular index (normal, <25 degrees), **measurement of the Perkins line (normally the ossific nucleus of the femoral head is medial to this line),** and evaluation of the Shenton line are useful (Figure 3-27).
     - Later, delayed ossification of the femoral head on the affected side may be visible.
     - Arthrography is helpful after closed reduction to determine concentric reduction.

E. Treatment (Figure 3-28)

Based on achieving and maintaining early "concentric reduction" in order to prevent future degenerative joint disease. **Specific therapy is based on the child's age.**

1. **Birth to 6 months:**
   - Pavlik harness
   - **Check reduction after 3 weeks on ultrasonography**
     - **Not reduced: closed reduction, arthrography, and spica casting**
     - **Reduced: continue harness until findings of examination and ultrasonography are normal**

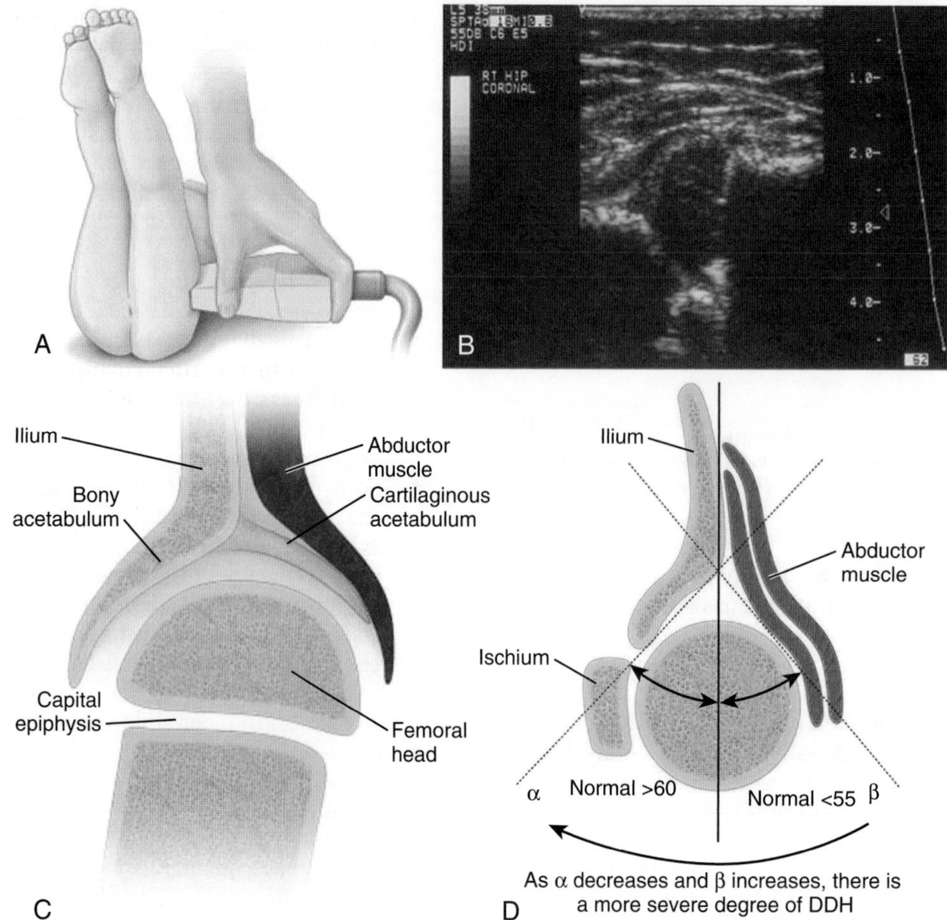

Figure 3-26 Ultrasound evaluation of the neonate's hip. **A,** Positioning of ultrasound transducer on a normal hip. **B,** Ultrasonogram. **C,** Illustration of ultrasound findings of a dislocated hip with poor bony roof. **D,** Graphic illustration of the dislocated hip. DDH, developmental dysplasia of the hip. (From Herring JA, editor: *Tachdjian's pediatric orthopaedics*, ed 4, Philadelphia, 2008, WB Saunders.)

2. **6 to 18 months:**
   - **Hip arthrography, percutaneous adductor tenotomy, closed reduction, and spica casting**
   - Postreduction CT scan used to confirm concentric reduction
   - If closed reduction fails: open reduction
3. 18 months to 3 years:
   - Open reduction
4. 3 to 8 years:
   - Osteotomy
     - Salter, Dega, Pemberton, or Staheli procedures
5. Older than 8 years:
   - Osteotomy
     - Growth plate open: triple (Steele), double pelvic (Southerland), Staheli procedure
     - Growth plate closed: Ganz and Chiari procedures
   - Wait until the child is an adult to perform total hip arthroplasty.

F. **Specific treatment modalities**

1. Pavlik harness
   - Designed to maintain reduction in infants (< 6 months) in about 100 degrees of flexion and mild abduction (the "human position" [Salter procedure])
   - The reduction should be confirmed by radiographs or ultrasound scans after placement in the harness and brace adjustment.
   - The position of the hip should be within the "safe zone" of Ramsey (between maximum adduction before redislocation and excessive abduction, which increases risk of avascular necrosis).
   - Impingement of the posterosuperior retinacular branch of the medial femoral circumflex artery has been implicated in osteonecrosis associated with DDH treated in an abduction orthosis.
   - Pavlik harness treatment is contraindicated in teratologic hip dislocations.
   - A patient with a narrow safe zone (less than 40 degrees) should be considered for an adductor tenotomy.
   - Excessive flexion may result in transient femoral nerve palsy.
   - **If attempts to reduce a hip do not succeed in 3 weeks, the Pavlik harness should be discontinued to prevent "Pavlik disease": erosion of the pelvis superior to the acetabulum and subsequent difficulty with closed reduction and casting.**

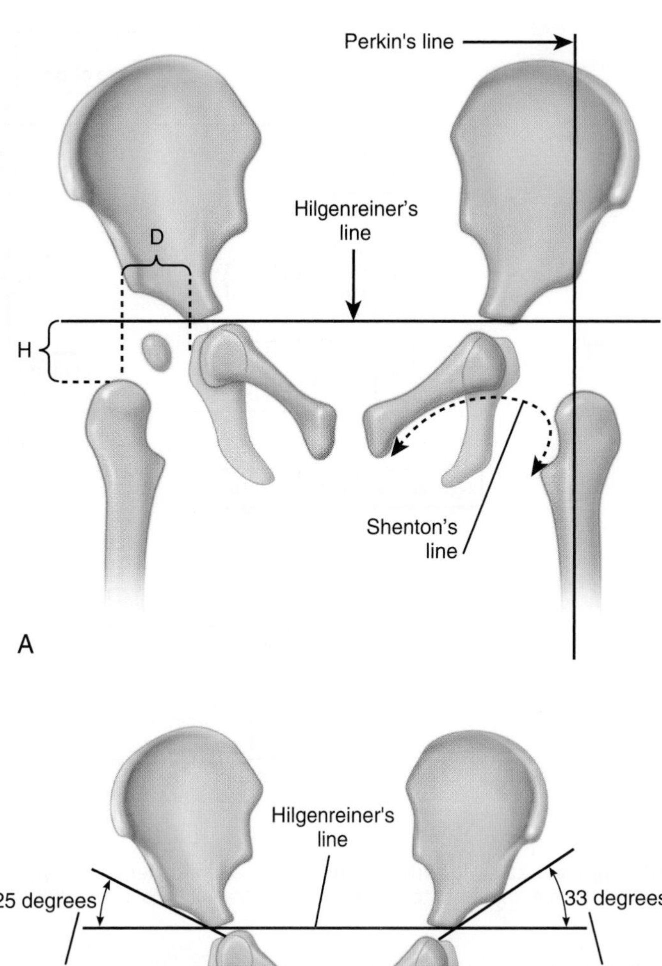

Figure 3-27 Common measurements used to evaluate developmental dysplasia of the hip, anterior view. Note the delayed ossification, disruption of the Shenton line, and increased acetabular index on the left hip, which is dislocated. (From Herring JA, editor: *Tachdjian's pediatric orthopaedics,* ed 4, Philadelphia, 2008, WB Saunders.)

- The Pavlik harness is usually worn 23 hours a day for at least 6 weeks after a reduction has been achieved and then an additional 6 to 8 weeks part time (nights and during naps).

2. Closed and open reduction
   - Closed reduction
     - In general, performed for patients for whom Pavlik treatment fails and for patients 6 to 18 months of age
     - This is performed with the patient under general anesthesia; the procedure includes a physical examination, arthrography to assess reduction (look for "thorn sign" on arthrogram, indicating normal labral position), and hip spica casting with the legs flexed to at least 90 degrees and in the stable zone of abduction.
     - CT scan is often performed to confirm that the hip is well reduced, especially in questionable cases.
   - Open reduction
     - Reserved for children 6 to 18 months old in whom closed reduction fails, who have an obstructive limbus, or have an unstable safe zone
     - Open reduction is also the initial treatment for children 18 months of age and older.
     - It is usually done through an anterior approach, especially for patients older than 12 months (less risk to the **medial femoral circumflex artery**) and includes capsulorrhaphy, adductor tenotomy, femoral shortening to take tension off the reduction, and an acetabular procedure if severe dysplasia is present.
     - The five obstacles to reduction are transverse acetabular ligament, pulvinar, in-folded labrum, inferior capsular restriction, and psoas tendon.
     - The medial open reduction can be performed in children up to 12 months of age, results in less blood loss, directly addresses the obstacles to reduction but does not provide access for a capsulorrhaphy, and is more often associated with osteonecrosis.
     - Surgical risks: The major risk associated with both open and closed reductions is osteonecrosis (caused by direct vascular injury or impingement vs. disruption of the circulation from osteotomies). Failure of open reduction is difficult to treat surgically because of the high complication rate of revision surgery (osteonecrosis in 50% and pain and stiffness in 33%, according to one study). Diagnosis after the age of

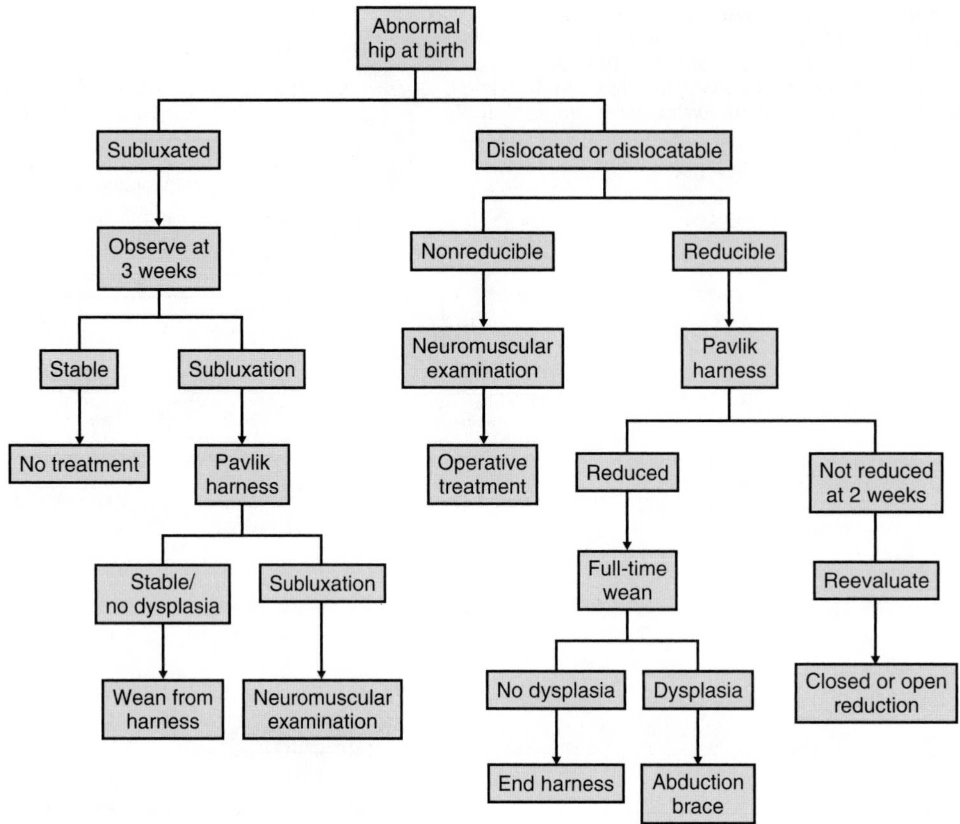

Figure 3-28 Algorithm for the treatment of developmental dysplasia of the hip. (Redrawn from Guille JT, et al: Developmental dysplasia of the hip from birth to 6 months, *J Am Acad Orthop Surg* 8:232–242, 2000.)

8 years (younger in patients with bilateral DDH) may contraindicate reduction because the acetabulum has little chance to remodel, although reduction may be indicated in conjunction with salvage procedures.

- Osteotomy
  - Indications
    - May be required in toddlers and school-age children, usually for residual and persistent acetabular dysplasia
    - **Osteotomies should be performed only after a congruent reduction is confirmed on an abduction–internal rotation view, with satisfactory ROM, and after reasonable femoral sphericity is achieved by closed or open methods.**
    - The choice of femoral versus pelvic osteotomy (Figure 3-29) is sometimes a matter of the surgeon's preference.
    - Some surgeons prefer to perform pelvic osteotomies in patients older than 4 years and femoral osteotomies in younger patients.
    - In general, pelvic osteotomies should be performed when severe dysplasia is accompanied by significant radiographic changes on the acetabular side (i.e., increased acetabular index, failure of lateral acetabular ossification), whereas changes on the femoral side (e.g., marked anteversion, coxa valga) are best treated by femoral osteotomies.
    - These osteotomies rarely correct hip dysplasia successfully after the age of 5 years. Table 3-15 lists common reconstructive osteotomies.

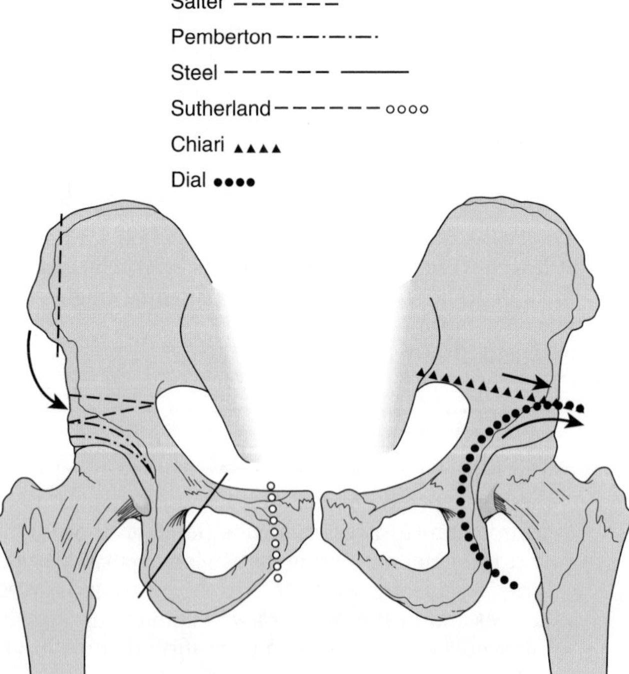

Figure 3-29 Common pelvic osteotomies for the treatment of developmental dysplasia of the hip.

Table 3-15 Common Pelvic Osteotomies, Procedures, Requirements, and Indications

Osteotomy	Procedure	Requirement	Indications
Femoral	Intertrochanteric osteotomy (VDRO)	Concentric reduction before the age of 8 years	High neck-shaft angle, hip subluxation; usually performed in patients with cerebral palsy
Salter	Open-wedge osteotomy through ileum	Concentric reduction before the age of 8 years	Acetabular dysplasia without posterior wall loss; redirection osteotomy
Pemberton	Through acetabular roof to triradiate cartilage	Concentric reduction before the age of 8 years	Acetabular dysplasia with a patulous cup; volume-reducing osteotomy
Sutherland (double)	Salter and pubic osteotomy	Concentric reduction Open triradiate cartilage	More severe acetabular dysplasia
Steel (triple)	Salter and osteotomy of both rami	Concentric reduction Open triradiate cartilage	Most severe acetabular dysplasia
Ganz	Periacetabular osteotomy	Surgeon's experience Closed triradiate cartilage	Acetabular dysplasia in a skeletally mature patient
Chiari	Through ilium above acetabulum (makes new roof)	Nonreconstructable acetabulum	Salvage procedure for asymmetric incongruity
Shelf	Slotted lateral acetabular augmentation	Nonreconstructable acetabulum	Salvage procedure for asymmetric incongruity

VDRO, varus derotation osteotomy.

- Procedures
  - Salter osteotomy: redirectional; may lengthen the affected leg up to 1 cm
  - Pemberton acetabuloplasty: volume reducing; a good choice for residual dysplasia (bends on triradiate cartilage)
  - Acetabular reorientation procedures in older patients: These include the triple innominate osteotomy (Steel or Tönnis procedure).
  - Dega-type osteotomies: volume reducing; often favored for paralytic dislocations and in patients with posterior acetabular deficiency.
  - Ganz periacetabular osteotomy: redirectional; provides improved three-dimensional correction because the cuts are close to the acetabulum, allow immediate weight bearing, spare stripping of the abductor muscles, allow for a capsulotomy to inspect the joint, and are performed through a single incision. However, the triradiate cartilage must be closed.
  - Chiari osteotomy: **salvage procedure when a concentric reduction of the femoral head within the acetabulum cannot be achieved.** This osteotomy shortens the affected leg and requires periarticular soft tissue metaplasia for success. It depends on metaplastic tissue (fibrocartilage) for a successful result.
  - Lateral shelf acetabular augmentation procedure: for patients older than 8 years with inadequate lateral coverage or trochanteric advancement and increased trochanteric overgrowth (improves hip abductor biomechanics). **It does not require concentric reduction.** Success of this procedure depends on metaplastic tissue (fibrocartilage).

II. CONGENITAL COXA VARA

A. Clinical features

1. It is bilateral in one third to half of cases.
2. Coxa vara can be congenital (noted at birth and differentiated from DDH by MRI), developmental (autosomal dominant, progressive), or acquired (e.g., trauma, Legg-Calvé-Perthes, SCFE).
3. May manifest with a waddling gait (bilateral) or a painless limp (unilateral)

B. Radiographic findings

1. Triangular ossification defect in the inferomedial femoral neck in developmental coxa vara is common.
2. Neck-shaft angle is decreased as a result of a defect in ossification of the femoral neck.
3. The evaluation of the **Hilgenreiner epiphyseal angle** (the angle between the Hilgenreiner line and a line through the proximal femoral physis) is the key to treatment (Figure 3-30).

C. Treatment

1. Based on the Hilgenreiner line
   - An angle of less than 45 degrees spontaneously corrects, whereas an angle of 45 to 60 degrees requires close observation, and an angle of more than 60 degrees (with a neck-shaft angle of less than 110 degrees) usually necessitates surgery.
2. The surgical treatment is a corrective valgus osteotomy of the proximal femur.
3. Proximal femoral (valgus) with or without derotation osteotomy (Pauwels) is indicated for a neck-shaft angle of less than 90 degrees, a vertically oriented physeal plate, progressive deformities, or significant gait abnormalities.
4. Concomitant distal/lateral transfer of the greater trochanter may also be indicated to restore more normal hip abductor mechanics.

III. LEGG-CALVÉ-PERTHES DISEASE (COXA PLANA)

A. Clinical features

1. Noninflammatory deformity of the proximal femur secondary to a vascular insult of unknown origin, leading to osteonecrosis of the proximal femoral epiphysis.
2. Pathologically, the osteonecrosis is followed by revascularization and resorption through creeping substitution that eventually allows remodeling and fragmentation.

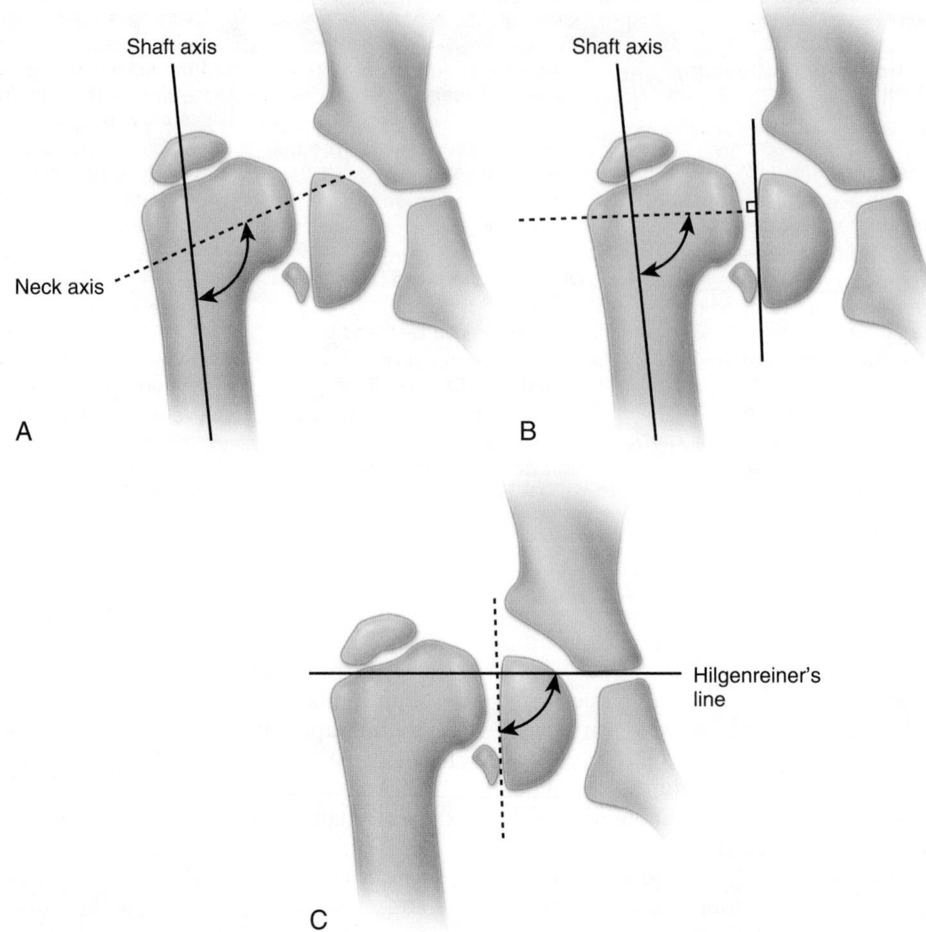

Figure 3-30 Quantification of the extent of radiographic deformity of the proximal femur in developmental coxa vara. **A,** The neck-shaft angle is the angle between the axis of the femoral shaft and the axis of the femoral neck. **B,** The head-shaft angle is the angle between the axis of the femoral shaft and an imaginary perpendicular line to the base of the capital femoral epiphysis. **C,** The Hilgenreiner–epiphyseal angle is the angle between the Hilgenreiner line and an imaginary line parallel to the capital femoral physis. (From Herring JA, editor: *Tachdjian's pediatric orthopaedics,* ed 3, Philadelphia, 2002, WB Saunders, p 767.)

3. Most common in boys 4 to 8 years of age with delayed skeletal maturation who are very active
4. There is an increased incidence with a positive family history, low birth weight, and abnormal birth presentation.
5. Symptoms include pain (often knee pain), effusion (from synovitis), and a limp.
6. Decreased hip ROM (especially abduction and internal rotation) and a Trendelenburg gait are also common.
7. Bilateral involvement may be seen in 12% to 15% of cases.
   - However, in bilateral cases the involvement is asymmetric and virtually never simultaneous.
   - **Bilateral involvement may mimic MED and warrants a skeletal survey.**
8. Differential diagnosis: includes septic arthritis, blood dyscrasias, hypothyroidism, and epiphyseal dysplasia

B. **Radiographic findings**
1. Vary with the stage of disease but include cessation of growth of the ossific nucleus, medial joint space widening, and development of a "crescent sign" that represents subchondral fracture.
2. Classification
   - The Waldenström classification determines the four stages that all cases follow: initial, fragmentation, reossification, and healed or reossified.
   - **The classification that is most prognostic is the Herring classification, or lateral pillar classification, which is based on the involvement of the lateral pillar of the capital femoral epiphysis during the fragmentation stage** (Table 3-16; Figure 3-31).

C. **Prognosis**
1. Maintaining the sphericity of the femoral head is the most important factor in achieving a good result.
2. The use of circular Mose templates is helpful for evaluating this parameter.
3. **Early degenerative hip joint disease results from aspherical femoral heads.**
4. **Poor prognosis is associated with older age at onset (bone age >6 years), female sex, lateral column C classification (regardless of age), and decreased hip ROM (decreased abduction).**
5. Radiographic findings associated with poor prognosis (Catterall "head at risk" signs) include (1) lateral

Table 3-16 Lateral Pillar Classification

Group	Pillar Involvement	Prognosis
A	Little or no involvement of the lateral pillar	Uniformly good outcome
B	>50% of lateral pillar height maintained	Good outcome in younger patients (bone age <6 yr) but poorer outcome in older patients
C	<50% of lateral pillar height maintained	Poor prognosis in all age groups

calcification, (2) Gage sign (V-shaped defect at lateral physis), (3) lateral subluxation, (4) metaphyseal cyst formation, and (5) a horizontal growth plate.

D. Treatment

1. In general, the goals of treatment are relief of symptoms, restoration of ROM, and containment of the hip.
2. **The use of outpatient or inpatient traction, anti-inflammatory medications, and partial weight bearing with crutches for periods of 1 to 2 days to several weeks is helpful for relieving symptoms.**
3. ROM is maintained with traction, muscle release, exercise, the use of a Petrie cast, or a combination of these measures.
4. Containment of the hip by use of traction, muscle release, abduction bracing, or varus femoral versus pelvic osteotomy is helpful for maintaining hip sphericity.
5. Herring described a treatment plan based on age and the lateral pillar classification of disease involvement
6. **Surgical treatment improves radiographic outcome at skeletal maturity for older patients (chronologic age >8 years or bone age >6 years) with lateral pillar groups B and B/C hips.**

IV. SLIPPED CAPITAL FEMORAL EPIPHYSIS

A. Clinical features

1. **Disorder of the proximal femoral epiphysis caused by weakness of the perichondrial ring and slippage through the hypertrophic zone of the growth plate.**
2. The femoral head remains in the acetabulum, and the neck is displaced anteriorly and rotates externally.
3. SCFE is seen most often in obese adolescent African American boys (10 to 16 years of age); occasional patients have a positive family history.
4. Up to 25% of cases are bilateral and related to puberty.
5. Patients presenting when younger than 10 years of age should have an endocrine workup.
6. **SCFE may be associated with hormonal disorders in young children, such as hypothyroidism (most common), growth hormone deficiency, or renal osteodystrophy.**
7. Patients present with a coxalgic, externally rotated gait; decreased internal rotation; thigh atrophy; and **hip, thigh, or knee pain.**
   - **The diagnosis is missed most often because patients present with knee pain.**
8. **In all patients, physical examination reveals obligate external rotation with flexion of the hip.**

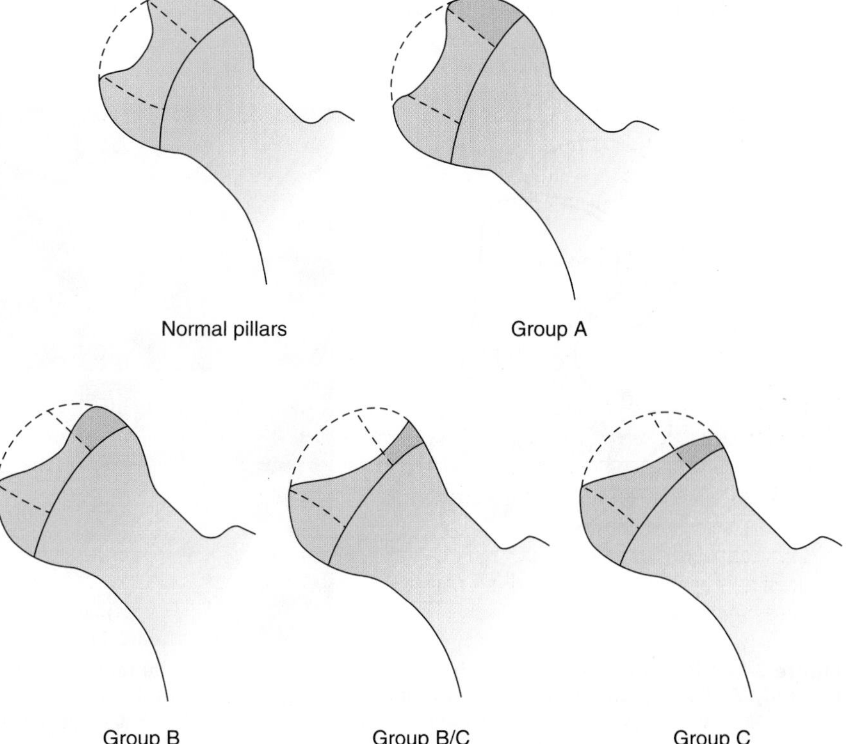

Figure 3-31 Lateral pillar classification of Legg-Calvé-Perthes disease. The definition of normal pillars was derived by noting the lines of demarcation between the central sequestrum and the remainder of the epiphysis on the anteroposterior radiograph. In group A, the normal height of lateral pillar is maintained. In group B, more than 50% of height of lateral pillar is maintained. In group B/C (borderline), lateral pillar is 50% or less in height, but (1) it is very narrow (2 to 3 mm wide), (2) it has very little ossification, or (3) it has depressions in comparison with the central pillar. In group C, less than 50% of height of lateral pillar is maintained. (Adapted from Herring JA, et al: The lateral pillar classification of Legg-Calvé-Perthes disease, *J Pediatr Orthop* 12:143–150, 1992.)

B. Classification

1. Stability
   - **The Loder classification of SCFE, which is based on the patient's ability to bear weight at the time of presentation, is prognostic for the severe complication of osteonecrosis of the femoral head.**
   - **In stable slippages, weight bearing with or without crutches is possible.**
   - **In unstable slippages, weight bearing is not possible because of severe pain.**
   - **No patients with stable slippages develop osteonecrosis, whereas 47% of the patients with unstable slips develop it.**

C. Radiographic studies

1. Anteroposterior and frog-leg pelvic views are needed for comparison.
2. If the slippage is unstable, a shoot-through lateral view is required.
3. SCFE can be graded on the basis of the percentage of slippage:
   - Grade I: 0% to 33% slippage
   - Grade II: 34% to 50% slippage
   - Grade III: more than 50% slippage
4. In mild cases, loss of the lateral overhang of the femoral ossific nucleus (Klein line) and blurring of the proximal femoral metaphysis may be all that is visible on the anteroposterior radiograph.

D. Treatment

1. **Recommended treatment for stable and unstable slippages is pinning in situ.**
2. Positioning on the table may partially reduce the acute component of an unstable slippage.
   - Forceful reduction before pinning is not indicated.
3. A single pin can be placed percutaneously (Figure 3-32).
4. The pin should be started anteriorly on the femoral neck, ending in the central portion of the femoral head.
5. The goal of treatment is to stabilize the epiphysis and promote closure of the proximal femoral physis.
6. **Prophylactic pinning of the opposite hip is controversial but is generally recommended in patients with an endocrinopathy or in young children (<10 years old) or with an open triradiate cartilage.**

E. Prognosis and complications

1. In severe SCFE, the residual proximal femoral deformity may partially remodel with the patient's remaining growth.
2. Intertrochanteric (Kramer) or subtrochanteric (Southwick) osteotomies may be useful in treating the deformities caused by SCFE that fail to remodel.
3. Cuneiform osteotomy at the femoral neck has the potential to correct severe deformity but remains controversial because of the high reported rates of osteonecrosis (37% of cases) and future osteoarthritis (37%).
4. Complications associated with SCFE include the following:
   - Osteonecrosis
     - Unstable slippage is the most accurate predictor.
   - Chondrolysis
     - Characterized by narrowed joint space, pain, and decreased motion
     - **Pin placement into the anterior superior quadrant of the femoral head has the highest rate of joint penetration.**
   - Degenerative joint disease
     - Pistol-grip deformity of the proximal femur

V. PROXIMAL FEMORAL FOCAL DEFICIENCY

A. Clinical features

1. Developmental defect of the proximal femur recognizable at birth
2. Clinically, patients with proximal femoral focal deficiency (PFFD) have a short, bulky thigh that is flexed, abducted, and externally rotated.

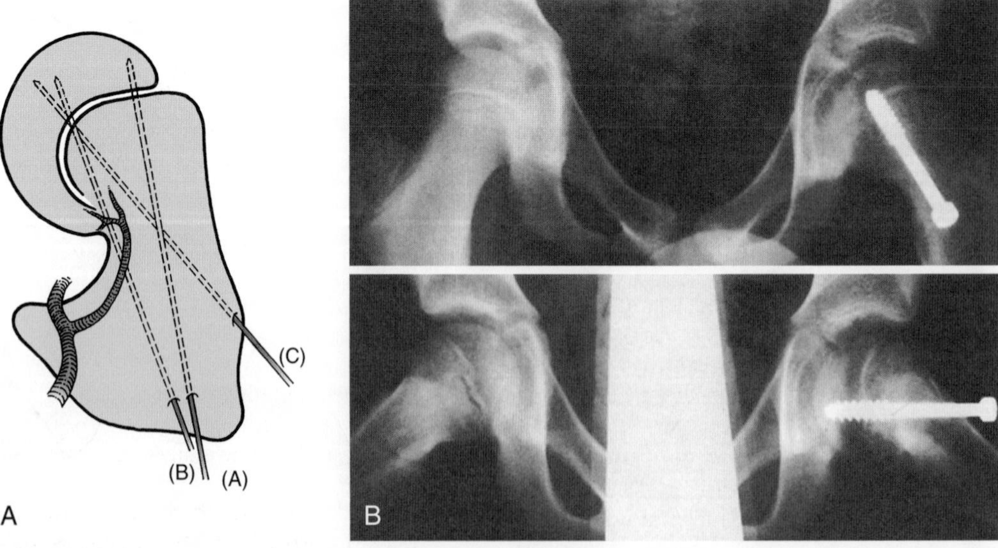

Figure 3-32 Percutaneous pinning or screw fixation for slipped capital femoral epiphysis. Note that the epiphysis slips posteriorly and inferiorly. **A,** The implant must be inserted into the anterior femoral neck and directed toward the center of the epiphysis. Pin C is optimally placed. **B,** Radiographs show satisfactory screw placement, with the screw entering the anterior femoral neck. (From Benson M, et al: *Children's orthopaedics and fractures,* New York, 1994, Churchill Livingstone, p 464.)

3. PFFD is often associated with coxa vara or fibular hemimelia (50% of cases).
4. Congenital knee ligamentous deficiency and contracture are also common.

B. Treatment

1. Individualized on the basis of leg-length discrepancy, adequacy of musculature, proximal joint stability, and the presence or absence of foot deformities.
2. In general, prosthetic management with foot amputation is used when the femoral length is less than 50% that of the opposite side, whereas lengthening with or without contralateral epiphysiodesis is used when the femoral length is more than 50% that of the opposite side.
3. The percentage of shortening remains constant during growth.
4. Aiken classification
   - In PFFD classes A and B, the femoral head is present, which potentially allows for reconstructive procedures that include limb lengthening.
   - In PFFD classes C and D, the femoral head is absent; treatment includes amputation, femoral-pelvic fusion (Brown procedure), Van Ness rotationplasty, and limb lengthening.

VI. LEG-LENGTH DISCREPANCY

A. Clinical features

1. There are many causes of leg-length discrepancy, such as congenital disorders (e.g., hemihypertrophy, dysplasias, PFFD, DDH), paralytic disorders (e.g., spasticity, polio), infection (pyogenic disruption of the physis), tumors, and trauma.
2. Long-term problems associated with leg-length discrepancy include an inefficient gait, equinus contractures of the ankle, postural scoliosis, and low-back pain.
3. The discrepancy must be measured accurately (e.g., with blocks of set height under the affected side; with scanography).
   - **A knee flexion contracture must be evaluated with lateral CT scanography.**
4. Can be tracked with the Green-Anderson or Moseley graph (with serial leg-length radiographs or CT scanograms and with bone age determinations)
5. **A gross estimation of leg-length discrepancy can be made under the following assumption of growth per year up to age 16 in boys and age 14 in girls** (Figure 3-33):
   - **Distal femur: ⅜ inch (9 mm) per year**
   - **Proximal tibia: ¼ inch (6 mm) per year**
   - **Proximal femur: ⅛ inch (3 mm) per year**
     - The Moseley data helps obtain more accurate results.

B. Treatment

1. In general, projected discrepancies at maturity of less than 2 cm are observed or treated with shoe lifts.
2. Discrepancies of 2 to 5 cm can be treated with epiphysiodesis of the long side, shortening of the long side (ostectomy), or lengthening of the short side.
3. Discrepancies of more than 5 cm are generally treated with lengthening.
4. Lengthening:
   - With the use of standard techniques, lengthening of 1 mm a day is typical.

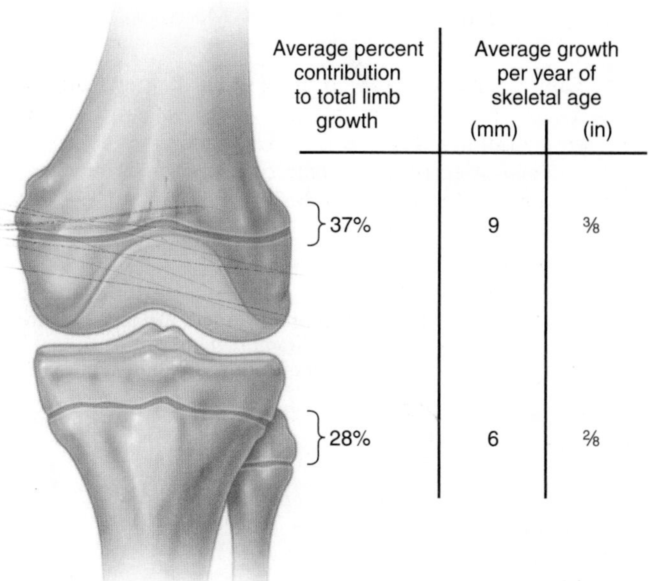

Average percent contribution to total limb growth
Average growth per year of skeletal age
(mm)
(in)
37%
9
⅜
28%
6
²⁄₈

Figure 3-33 Approximate percentage contribution to total leg-length increase and average growth per skeletal year of maturation (in millimeters and inches) of the distal femoral and proximal tibial physes. (From Herring JA, editor: *Tachdjian's pediatric orthopaedics,* ed 4, Philadelphia, 2008, WB Saunders, Figure 24-16.)

   - The Ilizarov principles are followed, including metaphyseal corticotomy (preserving the medullary canal and blood supply), followed by gradual distraction.
   - On rare occasions, physeal distraction (chondrodiastasis) can be considered.
     - This procedure must be performed in patients near skeletal maturity because the physis almost always closes after this type of limb lengthening.

VII. LOWER EXTREMITY INFLAMMATION AND INFECTION

See Chapter 1, Basic Sciences (Table 3-17).

A. Transient synovitis

1. Clinical features
   - Most common cause of pain in hips during childhood, but the diagnosis is one of exclusion.
   - Can be related to viral infection, allergic reaction, or trauma; however, the cause is unknown
   - The onset can be acute or insidious.
   - The symptoms, which are self-limiting, include muscle spasm and voluntary limitation of motion.
   - With transient synovitis, the ESR is usually less than 20 mm/hr.
2. Imaging studies
   - Entire limb
   - Consider spine radiographs.
   - Hip ultrasonography
   - Consider MRI to evaluate persistent pain.
3. Treatment
   - **Evaluate for septic hip with aspiration (especially in children with fever, leukocytosis, or elevated ESR); if findings are negative, observe the patient with a trial of NSAIDs.**
   - Symptoms should improve within 24 to 48 hours.

Table 3-17 Causative Organisms for Musculoskeletal Infections and Empirical Antibiotic Regimens Based on Patient Age and Risk Factors

Patient Characteristics	Causative Organisms	Empirical Antibiotics
Age Group		
Neonatal (birth to 8 wk)		
Nosocomial infection	*Staphylococcus aureus, Streptococcus* species, Enterobacteriaceae, *Candida* species	Nafcillin or oxacillin plus gentamicin *or* Cefotaxime (or ceftriaxone) plus gentamicin
Community-acquired infection	*S. aureus,* group B streptococci, *Escherichia coli, Klebsiella* species	Nafcillin or oxacillin plus gentamicin *or* Cefotaxime (or ceftriaxone) plus gentamicin
Infantile (2 to 18 mo)	*S. aureus, Kingella kingae, Streptococcus pneumoniae, Neisseria meningitidis*	Immunized: nafcillin, oxacillin, or cefazolin
	Haemophilus influenzae type b (nonimmunized)	Nonimmunized: nafcillin or oxacillin plus cefotaxime, or cefuroxime
Early childhood (18 mo to 3 yr)	*S. aureus, K. kingae, S. pneumoniae, N. meningitidis*	Immunized: nafcillin, oxacillin, or cefazolin
	H. influenzae type b (nonimmunized)	Nonimmunized: nafcillin or oxacillin plus cefotaxime, or cefuroxime
Childhood (3 to 12 yr)	*S. aureus,* GABHS	Nafcillin, oxacillin, or cefazolin
Adolescent (12 to 18 yr)	*S. aureus,* GABHS, *Neisseria gonorrhoeae*	Nafcillin, oxacillin, or cefazolin; ceftriaxone and doxycycline for disseminated gonococcal infection
Risk Factor		
Sickle cell disease	*Salmonella* species, *S. aureus, S. pneumoniae*	Ceftriaxone
Foot puncture wound	*Pseudomonas aeruginosa, S. aureus*	Ceftazidime or piperacillin-tazobactam and gentamicin
HIV	*S. aureus, Streptococcus* species, *Salmonella* species, *Nocardia asteroides, N. gonorrhoeae,* cytomegalovirus, *Aspergillus, Toxoplasma gondii, Torulopsis glabrata, Cryptococcus neoformans, Coccidioides immitis*	Broad-spectrum antibiotics per infectious disease recommendations
CGD	*Aspergillus* species, *Staphylococcus* species, *Burkholderia cepacia, Nocardia* species, *Mycobacterium* species	Nafcillin, oxacillin, or cefazolin

From Herring JA, editor: *Tachdjian's pediatric orthopaedics,* ed 4, Philadelphia, 2008, WB Saunders, Table 35-2.
CGD, chronic granulomatous disease; GABHS, group A beta-hemolytic streptococci; HIV, human immunodeficiency virus.

B. Osteomyelitis

1. Clinical features
   - Occurs more often in children because of their rich metaphyseal blood supply and thick periosteum
   - Pathology:
     - **Most common organism is *S. aureus***
     - With the advent of the *Haemophilus influenzae* vaccination, *H. influenzae* is now much less commonly found in musculoskeletal sepsis.
     - *Kingella kingae* infection is becoming more common in younger age groups.
   - A history of trauma is common in children with osteomyelitis.
   - Osteomyelitis in children usually begins through hematogenous seeding of a bony metaphysis in the small arterioles that bend just beyond the physis, where blood flow is sluggish and phagocytosis is poor; in this way, a bone abscess is created (Figure 3-34).
   - Pus lifts the thick periosteum and puts pressure on the cortex, causing coagulation.
   - Chronic bone abscesses may become surrounded by thick, fibrous tissue and sclerotic bone (Brodie abscess).
   - Manifests with a tender, warm, sometimes swollen area over a long-bone metaphysis
   - Fever may or may not be present.
   - **Methicillin-resistant *S. aureus* (MRSA) is associated with deep venous thrombosis and septic emboli.**
2. Diagnosis
   - Laboratory tests may be helpful (blood cultures, white blood cell [WBC] count, ESR, C-reactive protein).
   - Imaging studies
     - **Radiographs show soft tissue edema early, metaphyseal rarefaction late.** Periosteal new bone appears at 5 to 7 days; evidence of osteolysis—30% to 50% loss of bone mineral—may not appear until 10 to 14 days.
     - MRI examination is key to evaluate for pus accumuluation.
     - **Definitive diagnosis is made with aspiration (50% of affected patients have positive cultures).**
3. Treatment
   - **Intravenous antibiotics are the best initial treatment if osteomyelitis is diagnosed early,** before radiographic changes or the development of a subperiosteal abscess.
   - Broad-spectrum antibiotics are initially chosen, followed by antibiotics specific for the organism cultured.
     - **C-reactive protein measurements can be used to monitor the therapeutic response to antibiotics; failure to decline within 48 to 72 hours warrants alteration in treatment.**
   - **Failure to respond to antibiotics, appearance of frank pus on MRI, or the presence of a sequestered abscess (not accessible to antibiotics) necessitates operative drainage and débridement.**

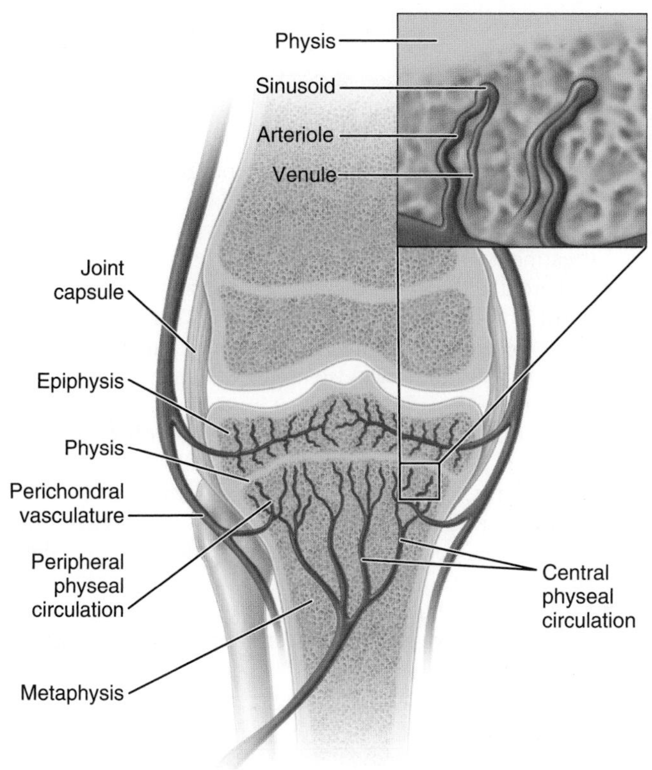

Figure 3-34 Metaphyseal sinusoids, where sluggish blood flow increases susceptibility to osteomyelitis. (From Herring JA, editor: *Tachdjian's pediatric orthopaedics,* ed 4, Philadelphia, 2008, WB Saunders.)

- Drilling the metaphysis can assist in draining some of the infection.
- Specimens should be sent for histologic study and culture.
- Antibiotics should be continued until the ESR (or C-reactive protein level) returns to normal, usually at 4 to 6 weeks.

C. **Septic arthritis**

1. Clinical features
   - **Can develop from osteomyelitis**
     - **Especially in neonates, in whom transphyseal vessels allow proximal spread into the joint in joints with an intraarticular metaphysis (hip, elbow, shoulder, and ankle)**
     - Septic arthritis can also occur as a result of hematogenous spread of infection.
     - **Because pus is chondrolytic, septic arthritis in children is an acute surgical emergency.**
     - **Most frequently occurs in children younger than 2 years**

Table 3-18 Common Organisms in Septic Arthritis, by Age

Age	Common Organisms	Empirical Antibiotics
<12 mo	*Staphylococcus* species, group B streptococci	First-generation cephalosporin
6 mo–5 yr	*Staphylococcus* species, *Haemophilus influenzae*	Second- or third-generation cephalosporin
5-12 yr	*Staphylococcus aureus*	First-generation cephalosporin
12-18 yr	*S. aureus, Neisseria gonorrhoeae*	Oxacillin/ cephalosporin

     - Infecting organisms vary with age (Table 3-18).
     - Septic arthritis manifests as a much more acute process than osteomyelitis. **Decreased ROM and severe pain with passive motion may be accompanied by systemic symptoms of infection.**
   - Diagnosis and radiographic findings
     - **Radiographs may show a widened joint space or even dislocation.**
     - Joint fluid aspirate shows a high WBC count (>50,000/mm^3); glucose level may be 50 mg/dL lower than in serum; and in patients with gram-positive cocci or gram-negative rods, lactic acid level may be high.
     - **Distinguishing septic arthritis of the hip from transient synovitis is a common problem; however, when three of four of the following criteria are present, the diagnosis of septic arthritis is made in more than 90% of cases: WBC count higher than 12,000 cells/mL; ESR higher than 40; inability to bear weight; and temperature higher than 101.5° F (38.6° C).**
     - Ultrasonography can be helpful in identifying the presence of an effusion.
     - Lumbar puncture should be considered in a joint when sepsis is caused by *H. influenzae,* because of the increased incidence of meningitis.
     - The prognosis is usually good except in patients with a delayed diagnosis.
     - *Neisseria gonorrhoeae* septic arthritis is usually preceded by migratory polyarthralgia, small red papules, and multiple joint involvement.
       - This organism typically elicits less WBC response (<50,000 cells/mL) and usually does not necessitate surgical drainage.
       - Large doses of penicillin are required to eliminate this organism.
   - **Treatment: Aspiration should be followed by irrigation and débridement in major joints (especially in the hip; a culture of synovium is also recommended).**

SECTION 13 KNEE AND LEG

I. LEG

A. Introduction
1. Genu varum (bowed legs) normally evolves naturally to genu valgum ("knock-knees") by age 2.5 years, with a gradual transition to physiologic valgus angulation by age 4 years.

B. Physiologic genu varum (bowed legs)
1. Normal in children younger than 2 years
2. Radiographs in physiologic bowing typically show flaring of the tibia and femur in a symmetric manner.
3. Pathologic conditions that can cause genu varum include osteogenesis imperfecta, osteochondromas, trauma, various dysplasias, and (most commonly) **Blount disease.**

C. Infantile Blount disease (ages 0 to 4 years)
1. Clinical features
   - Abnormal tibia vara
   - More common and usually affects both extremities
   - Classic presentation is in a child who is overweight and who begins walking before 1 year of age; disease is associated with internal tibial torsion.
2. Radiographic findings
   - Metaphyseal-diaphyseal angle abnormality and metaphyseal beaking
   - A Drennan metaphyseal-diaphyseal angle of more than 16 degrees is considered abnormal and is formed between the metaphyseal beaks (demonstrated in Figure 3-35).
   - The epiphyseal-metaphyseal angle is also useful (Figure 3-36).
   - Langenskiöld classification is based on the degree of metaphyseal-epiphyseal changes (Figure 3-37).
3. **Treatment**
   - **Based on age and correlated with the stage of disease**
   - **Stage I or stage II: bracing in patients younger than 3 years**
   - **Stage II (if patient is older than 3 years) and stage III: proximal osteotomy for tibia/fibula valgus angulation to overcorrect the deformity (because medial physeal growth abnormalities persist)**
   - Stages IV to VI are complex, and multiple procedures may be required. Epiphysiolysis is also needed for stages V and VI disease.

D. Adolescent Blount disease
1. Clinical features
   - Less severe than infantile forms and more often unilateral
   - The epiphysis appears relatively normal and does not have the beaking seen in infantile forms.
   - The most characteristic radiographic finding is widening of the proximal medial physeal plate.
2. Treatment
   - The initial treatment is proximal tibial and fibular lateral hemiepiphysiodesis when growth remains.
   - If residual deformity exists or the physes are closed proximally, tibial and fibular osteotomy is performed.
   - When significant leg-length discrepancy is present, the Ilizarov technique allows for deformity correction and lengthening.

E. Genu valgum ("knock-knees")
1. Clinical features
   - Up to 15 degrees at the knee is common in children 2 to 6 years of age.
   - Patients within this physiologic range do not require treatment.
   - Differential diagnosis includes renal osteodystrophy (the most common cause if condition is bilateral), tumors (e.g., osteochondromas), infections (may stimulate proximal asymmetrical tibial growth), and trauma.
2. Treatment
   - Conservative treatment is ineffective in pathologic genu valgum.
   - Consider surgery at the site of the deformity in children older than 10 years with more than 10 cm between the medial malleoli or more than 15 degrees of valgus angulation.
   - Hemiepiphysiodesis or physeal stapling of the medial side is effective before the end of growth for severe deformities.

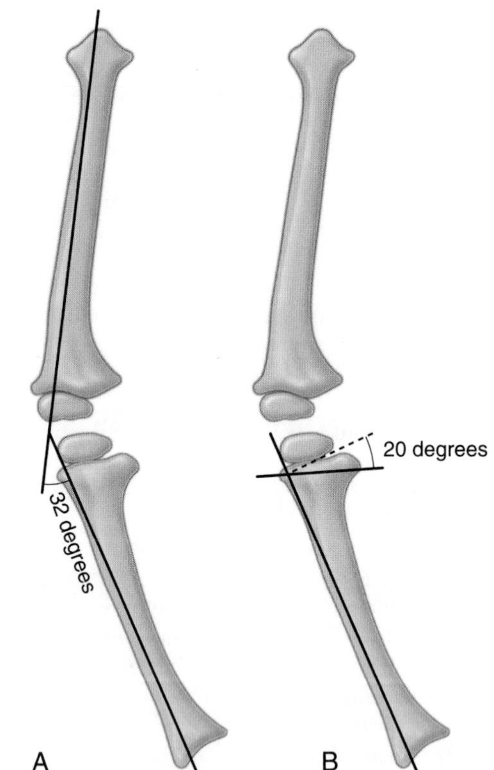

Figure 3-35 Comparison of tibiofemoral angle with the Drennan metaphyseal-diaphyseal angle in tibia vara. **A,** Lines are drawn along the longitudinal axes of the tibia and the femur; the angle between the lines is the tibiofemoral angle (32 degrees). **B,** The metaphyseal-diaphyseal angle method is used to determine the metaphyseal-diaphyseal angle in the same extremity. A line is drawn perpendicular to the longitudinal axis of the tibia, and another is drawn through the two beaks of the metaphysis to determine the transverse axis of the tibial metaphysis. The metaphyseal-diaphyseal angle (20 degrees) is the angle bisected by the two lines. (From Herring JA, editor: *Tachdjian's pediatric orthopaedics,* ed 4, Philadelphia, 2008, WB Saunders.)

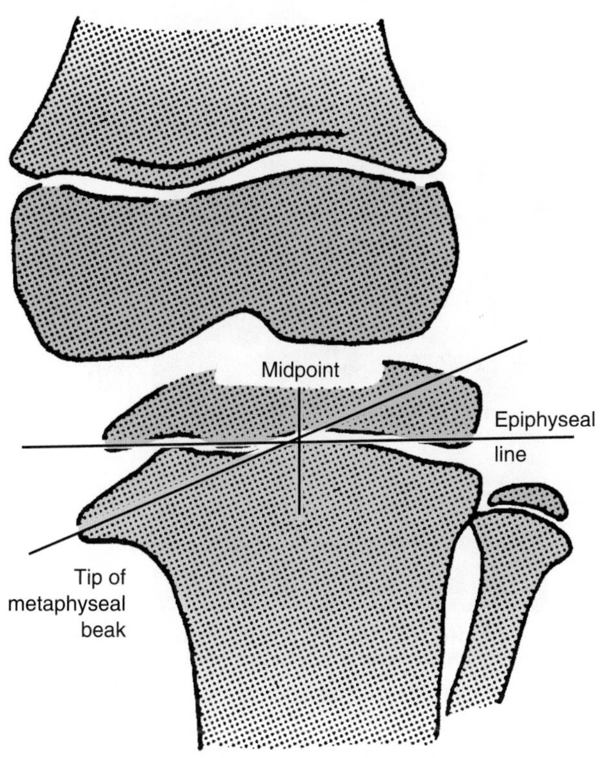

Figure 3-36 Measurement of the epiphyseal-metaphyseal angle in Blount disease. (Redrawn from Tachdjian MO: *Pediatric orthopaedics,* ed 2, Philadelphia, 1990, WB Saunders.)

II. TIBIAL BOWING

Tibial bowing is classified in three types (Table 3-19), on the basis of the apex of the curve.

A. **Posteromedial tibial bowing**

1. Physiologic

Table 3-19 Tibial Bowing

Type	Cause	Treatment
Posteromedial	Physiologic	Observation
Anteromedial	Fibular hemimelia	Bracing vs. amputation for severe deformities
Anterolateral	Congenital pseudarthrosis	Total-contact brace, intramedullary fixation, vascularized bone graft, or amputation of the leg and foot

2. Usually of the middle and distal thirds of the tibia and may be the result of abnormal intrauterine positioning (Figure 3-38).
3. **It is commonly associated with leg-length discrepancy, calcaneovalgus feet, and tight anterior structures.**
4. **Spontaneous correction is the rule, but the patient should be monitored to evaluate leg-length discrepancy.**
5. The most common sequela of posteromedial bowing is an average leg-length discrepancy of 3 to 4 cm, which may necessitate an age-appropriate epiphysiodesis of the long limb.
6. Tibial osteotomies are not indicated.

B. **Anteromedial tibial bowing**

1. Commonly caused by fibular hemimelia (a congenital longitudinal deficiency of the fibula, which is the most common long-bone deficiency)
2. It is usually associated with anteromedial bowing, ankle instability, equinovarus foot (with or without lateral rays), tarsal coalition, and femoral shortening. Significant leg-length discrepancy often results from this disorder.
3. Classically, skin dimpling is seen over the tibia.
4. The fibular deficiency can be intercalary, which involves the whole bone (fibula is absent), or terminal.
5. Fibular hemimelia is frequently associated with femoral abnormalities such as coxa vara and PFFD.

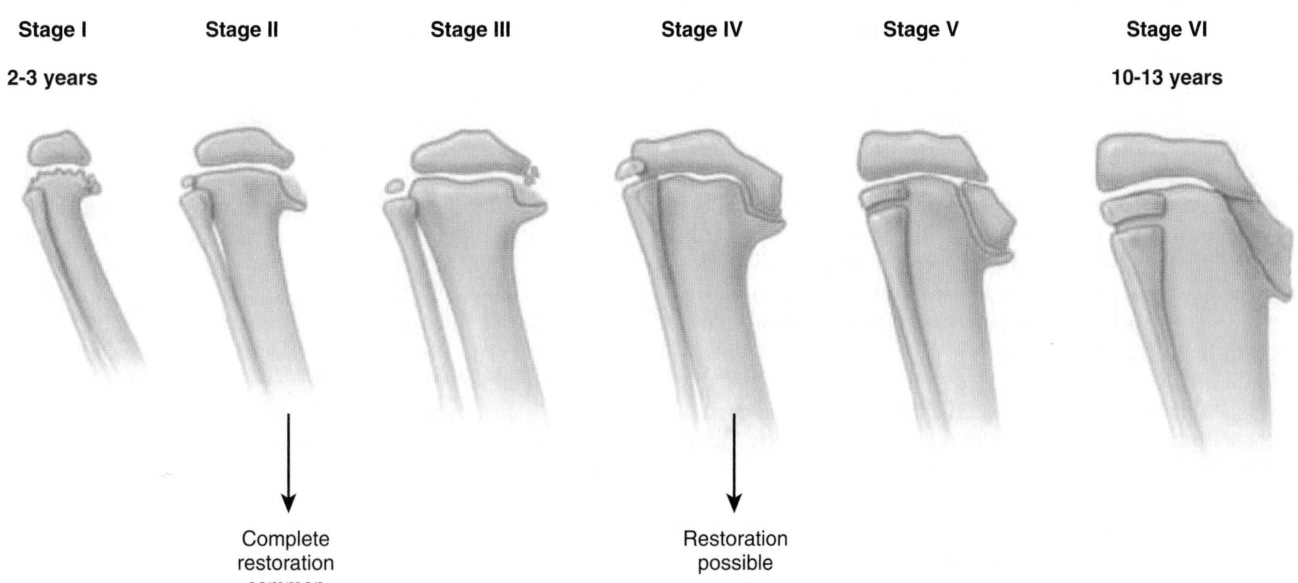

Figure 3-37 Langenskiöld classification of infantile tibia vara in six progressive stages with increasing age. (From Herring JA, editor: *Tachdjian's pediatric orthopaedics,* ed 4, Philadelphia, 2008, WB Saunders, Figure 22-8.)

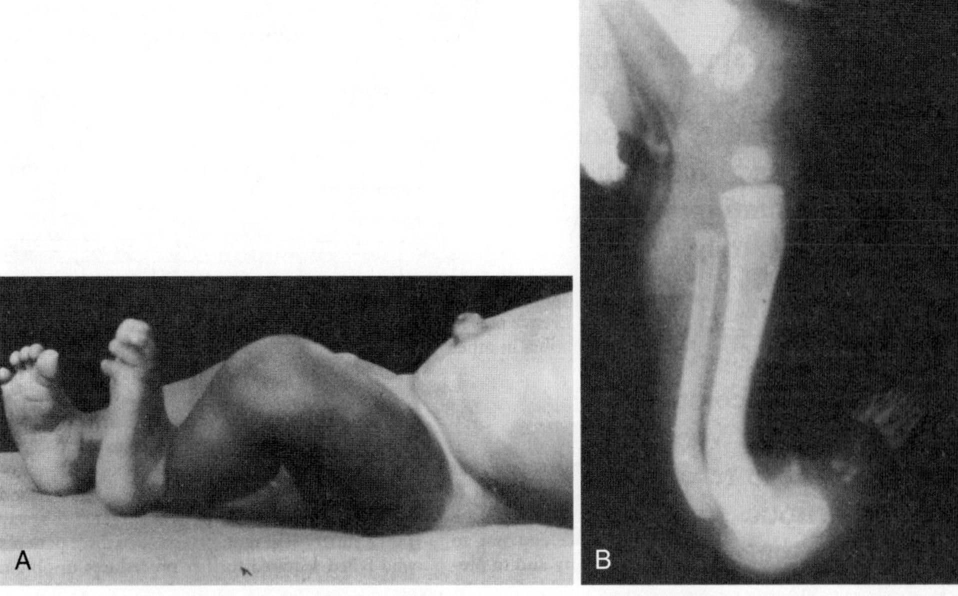

Figure 3-38 Posterior medial angulation of the tibia. **A,** Clinical photograph of an affected 5-month-old. **B,** Lateral radiograph of the same patient. The appearance is dramatic, but these deformities are best treated with stretching and splinting into equinus position. (From Benson M, et al: *Children's orthopaedics and fractures,* New York, 1994, Churchill Livingstone, p 408.)

6. Radiographic findings:
   - Complete or partial absence of the fibula, a ball-and-socket ankle joint (secondary to tarsal coalitions), and deficient lateral rays in the foot
7. Treatment:
   - Varies from a simple shoe lift or bracing to Syme amputation
   - Decisions are based on the degree of foot deformity, the number of rays, and the degree of shortening of the limb
   - Amputation is usually performed in limbs with severe shortening or a stiff, nonfunctional foot at about 10 months of age.
   - For less severe cases, reconstructive procedures, including lengthening, may be an alternative.
   - This procedure should include resection of the fibular anlage to avoid future foot problems.

C. Anterolateral tibial bowing

1. Clinical features
   - **Congenital pseudarthrosis of the tibia is the most common cause of anterolateral bowing.**
   - **It is often accompanied by neurofibromatosis (in 50% of patients with anterolateral tibial bowing; however, only 10% of patients with neurofibromatosis have the tibial bowing).**
2. Radiographic findings
   - Classification (Boyd) is based on bowing and the presence of cystic changes, sclerosis, or dysplasia; dysplasia and cystic changes are the most common.
3. Treatment
   - **Initial treatment includes a total-contact brace to protect the patient from fractures.**
   - Intramedullary fixation with excision of hamartomatous tissue and autogenous bone grafting are options for nonhealing fractures.
   - A vascularized fibular graft or the Ilizarov method should also be considered if bracing fails.
   - Osteotomies to correct the anterolateral bowing are contraindicated.
   - Amputation (Syme) and prosthetic fitting are indicated after two or three failed surgical attempts or as primary treatment.
     - Syme amputation is preferred to below-knee amputation in these patients because the soft tissue available at the heel pad is superior to that in the calf as a weight-bearing stump.
     - The soft tissue in the calf in these patients is often scarred and atrophic.

D. Other lower limb deficiencies

1. Tibial hemimelia
   - Congenital longitudinal deficiency of the tibia.
   - Tibial hemimelia is the only long-bone deficiency with a known inheritance pattern (autosomal dominant).
   - It is much less common than fibular hemimelia and is often associated with other bone abnormalities (especially a lobster-claw hand).
   - Clinically, the extremity is shortened and bowed anterolaterally with a prominent fibular head and an equinovarus foot, with the sole of the foot facing the perineum.
   - The treatment for severe deformities with an entirely absent tibia is a knee disarticulation.
   - Fibular transposition (Brown) has been unsuccessful, especially when quadriceps function is absent and when the proximal tibia is absent.
   - When the proximal tibia and quadriceps functions are present, the fibula can be transposed to the residual tibia and create a functional below-knee amputation.

III. OSTEOCHONDRITIS DISSECANS

A. Clinical features

1. An intraarticular condition common in children 10 to 15 years of age that can affect many joints, especially the knee and elbow (capitellum)
2. The lesion is thought to be secondary to trauma, ischemia, or abnormal epiphyseal ossification.
3. The lateral portion of the medial femoral condyle is most frequently involved.
4. Classified into three categories (Pappas classification) according to age at appearance
5. Symptoms include activity-related pain, localized tenderness, stiffness, and swelling, with or without mechanical symptoms.
6. Differential diagnosis includes anomalous ossification centers.

B. Radiographic studies

1. Tunnel (notch) view to evaluate the condyles
2. MRI can determine whether there is synovial fluid behind the lesion (the worst prognosis for nonoperative healing).

C. Treatment

1. **Nonoperative:**
   - **Bracing and restricted weight bearing if the potential for growth remains significant**
2. Operative:
   - Surgical therapy is reserved for the adolescent with minimal growth left or a loose lesion.
   - Operative treatment includes drilling with multiple holes, fixation of large fragments, and bone grafting of large lesions.
   - Osteochondritis dissecans is commonly treated arthroscopically.
   - Poor prognosis is associated with lesions in the lateral femoral condyle and patella.

IV. OSGOOD-SCHLATTER DISEASE

A. Clinical features

1. An osteochondrosis, or fatigue failure, of the tibial tubercle apophysis caused by stress from the extensor mechanism in a growing child (tibial tubercle apophysitis)
2. Pain over tibial tubercle, especially with direct pressure
3. Seen in active children

B. Radiographic findings

1. Irregularity and fragmentation of the tibial tubercle

C. Treatment

1. It is usually self-limiting; activity modification may be required.
2. Ice and quadriceps stretching also may alleviate symptoms.
3. The condition usually does not resolve until growth has halted.
4. Late excision of separate ossicles is rarely needed.

V. DISCOID MENISCUS

A. Clinical features

1. Abnormal development of the lateral meniscus leads to the formation of a disc-shaped (or hypertrophic) meniscus, rather than the normal crescent-shaped meniscus.
2. Symptoms include mechanical block and pain with catching and palpable click at knee.

B. Radiographic findings

1. Widening of the cartilage space on the affected side (up to 11 mm)
2. Squaring of condyles may be visible.
3. **MRI yields three successive sagittal images with the meniscal body present.**

C. Treatment

1. **If symptomatic and torn, the discoid meniscus can be arthroscopically débrided.**
2. If not torn, it should be observed.

SECTION 14 FOOT

Figure 3-39 depicts common childhood foot disorders.

I. CLUBFOOT (CONGENITAL TALIPES EQUINOVARUS)

A. Clinical features

1. Clubfoot is more common in boys, and half the cases are bilateral.
2. **Forefoot adductus and supination in combination with hindfoot equinus and varus.**
3. Talar neck deformity (medial and plantar deviation) with medial rotation of the calcaneus and medial displacement of the navicular and cuboid.
4. It is associated with shortening or contraction of muscles (intrinsic muscles, Achilles tendon, tibialis posterior, flexor hallucis longus, flexor digitorum longus), joint capsules, ligaments, and fascia, which leads to the associated deformities.
5. Can be associated with hand anomalies (Streeter dysplasia), diastrophic dwarfism, arthrogryposis, prune-belly syndrome, tibial hemimelia, and myelomeningocele

B. Causes

1. Genetic cause is strongly suggested.

C. Radiographic studies and findings

1. Radiographs should include the dorsiflexion lateral view (Turco), in which a talocalcaneal angle of greater than 35 degrees is normal; a smaller angle with a flat talar head is seen with clubfoot.
2. On the anteroposterior view a talocalcaneal (Kite) angle of 20 to 40 degrees is normal (is <20 degrees with clubfoot). The talus–first metatarsal angle is normally 0 to 20 degrees; a negative talus–first metatarsal angle is seen with clubfoot (Figure 3-40).
3. **"Parallelism" of the calcaneus and talus is seen on both views.**

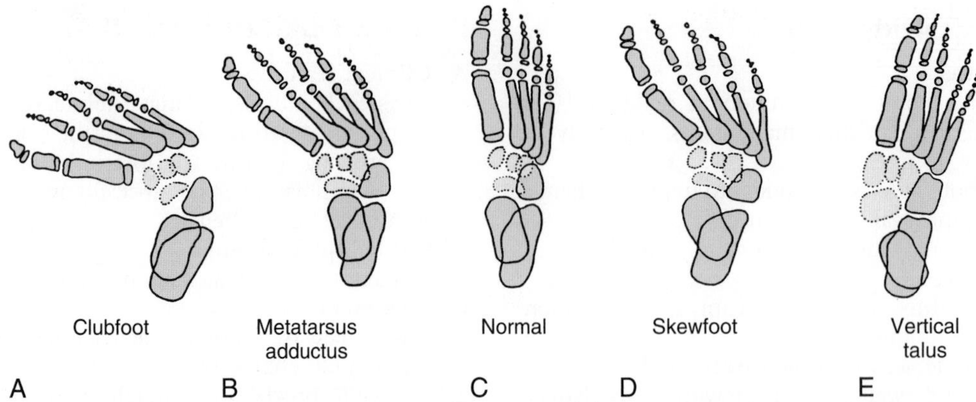

Figure 3-39 Skeletal illustrations of common childhood foot disorders: anteroposterior view. **A,** Varus position of hindfoot and adducted forefoot in clubfoot. **B,** Normal hindfoot and adducted forefoot in metatarsus adductus. **C,** Normal foot. **D,** Valgus hindfoot (with increased talocalcaneal angle) and adducted forefoot in skewfoot. **E,** Increased talocalcaneal angle and lateral deviation of the calcaneus in congenital vertical talus.

D. Treatment

1. Casting
   - Ponseti method of serial weekly casting has replaced primary surgery because it yields more favorable long-term results.
   - This method requires a series of long-leg plaster casts and most often an Achilles tendon release, and it is followed by external rotation of the feet in boots and bars for 2 to 3 years.
   - **To remember the sequence of correction, use the mnemonic "CAVE":**
     - ***Cavus***
     - ***Adductus***
     - ***Varus***
     - ***Equinus***
   - Casting begins with correction of the cavus angulation by aligning the first ray with the remaining metatarsals.
   - Subsequent manipulation and casting uses lateral pressure on the distal talar head as a fulcrum to correct the forefoot adduction and heel varus position.
   - All deformities are corrected gradually. Equinus angulation is corrected last; of the patients with residual equinus deformity, more than 90% require Achilles tendon release.
   - Overcorrection of the foot in all planes is necessary at the completion of casting, and compliance in wearing the brace is essential for a successful outcome.
   - **A common deformity after clubfoot treatment is persistent supination of the forefoot. Proposed causes include the following:**
     - **Overpull of the anterior tibialis with a weak peroneus longus**
     - **Undercorrection of forefoot supination**

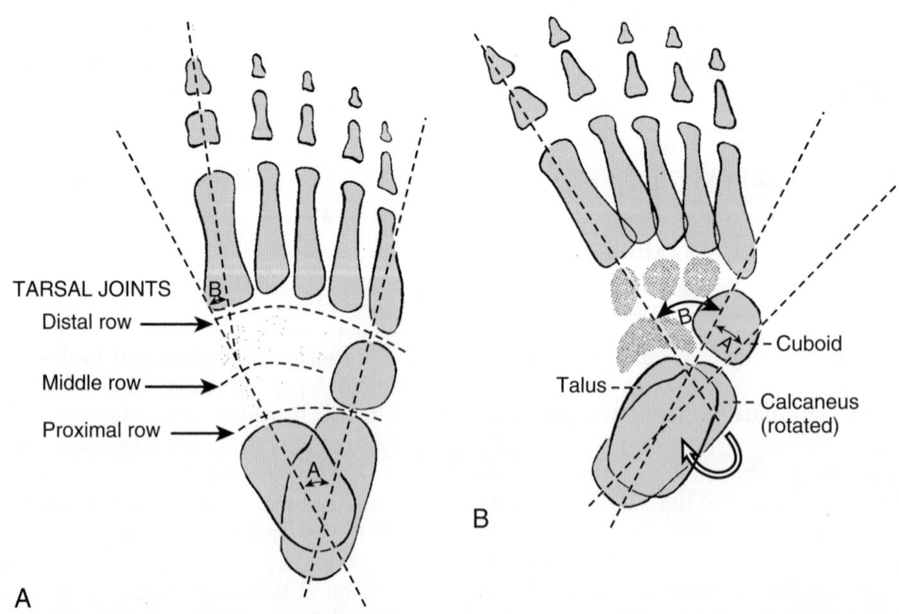

Figure 3-40 Skeletal illustrations of the radiographic evaluation of the foot. **A,** Normal foot. **B,** Clubfoot. Note the "parallelism" of the talus and calcaneus, with a talocalcaneal angle (angle A) of less than 20 degrees and a negative talus–first metatarsal angle (angle B) on the clubfoot side. (From Simons GW: Analytical radiology of club feet, *J Bone Joint Surg Br* 59:485–489, 1977.)

Table 3-20 Structures to Be Addressed in the Surgical Correction of Clubfoot

Structure	Procedure
Achilles tendon	Z-lengthening
Calcaneal-fibular ligament	Release
Posterior talofibular ligament	Release
Posterior tibialis tendon	Z-lengthening
Flexor digitorum longus tendon	Z-lengthening
Superficial deltoid	Release
Flexor hallucis longus tendon	Z-lengthening
Tibiotalar, subtalar capsule	Complete release
Talonavicular capsule	Release

- **This subsequent dynamic forefoot adduction/supination requires transfer of the anterior tibialis laterally in 15% to 20% of cases.**

2. Surgical release
   - Reserved for resistant or refractory clubfeet
   - Surgical soft tissue release with tendon lengthening is favored in resistant feet, usually at ages 6 to 9 months (Table 3-20).
   - The posterior tibial artery must be carefully protected. The dorsalis pedis artery is often insufficient.
   - Casting for several months is usually required postoperatively.
   - In older patients (3 to 10 years of age), a medial opening or lateral column–shortening osteotomy or cuboidal decancellation is recommended.
   - For children who present with refractory clubfoot late (8 to 10 years of age), triple arthrodesis is the only procedure possible for eliminating associated pain and deformity. Triple arthrodesis is contraindicated in patients with insensate feet because it causes rigidity of the foot, which may lead to ulceration.
   - Talectomy can be used in salvage operations.
   - **Development of a dorsal bunion can occur after clubfoot surgery. Flexor hallucis brevis and abductor hallucis overpull secondary to weak plantar flexion is thought to be responsible.**
     - **Treatment is with capsulotomy, flexor hallucis longus lengthening and transfer of the flexor hallucis brevis to become a metatarsophalangeal extensor**

Table 3-21 Metatarsus Adductus (MTA)

Type*	Features
Simple MTA	MTA alone
Complex MTA	MTA + lateral shift of midfoot
Skewfoot	MTA + valgus hindfoot
Complex skewfoot	MTA, lateral shift, valgus hindfoot

*Based on Berg Classification.

II. FOREFOOT ADDUCTION (FIGURE 3-41)

A. Metatarsus adductus: see the discussion on rotational problems of lower extremities earlier in Section 11, Lower Extremity Problems: General.

1. Clinical features: In general, adduction of the forefoot is commonly associated with DDH.
   - Grading: A simple clinical grading system (Bleck) is based on the heel bisector line (see Figure 3-41).
   - Normally, the heel bisector should align with the web space between the second and third toes.
   - Four subtypes (Berg) have been identified (Table 3-21).
2. Treatment
   - If peroneal muscle stimulation corrects metatarsus adductus, the condition usually responds to stretching.
   - Otherwise, manipulation and off-the-shelf orthoses or serial casting may be required.
   - Surgical options in refractory cases (usually those with a medial skin crease) include abductor hallucis longus recession (for an atavistic first toe), medial capsular release with Evans calcaneal osteotomy (lateral-column shortening), and medial-opening cuneiform and lateral-closing cuboid osteotomies with or without metatarsal osteotomies, according to the severity of deformity.

B. Medial deviation of the talar neck: benign disorder of the foot that generally corrects spontaneously

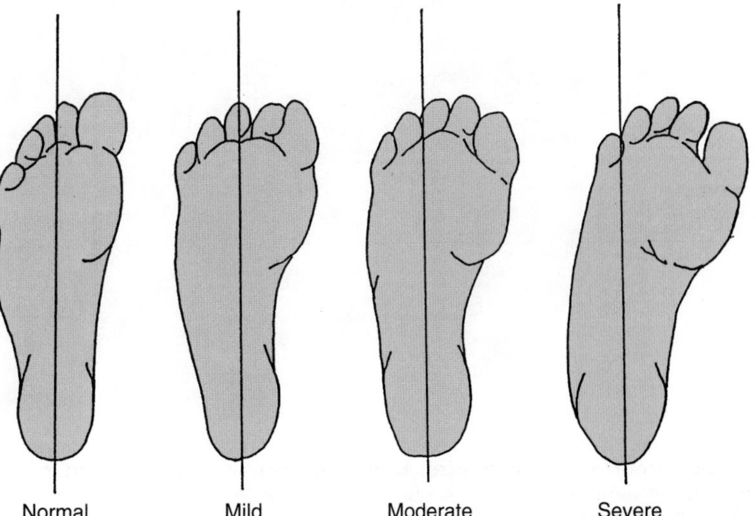

Figure 3-41 Classification of metatarsus adductus. (Adapted from Bleck EE: Metatarsus adductus: classification and relationship to all kinds of treatment, *J Pediatr Orthop* 3:2-9, 1983.)

C. Serpentine (Z) foot (complex skewfoot)

1. Clinical features
   - Residual tarsometatarsal adductus, talonavicular lateral subluxation, and valgus hindfoot
2. Treatment
   - Nonoperative treatment is ineffective in correcting the deformity.
   - Surgical treatment of this difficult problem is demanding and may include medial calcaneal sliding osteotomy (for valgus hindfoot), open-wedge cuboid osteotomy, and closed-wedge cuneiform osteotomy (to correct midfoot lateral subluxation), and metatarsal osteotomy (to correct forefoot adductus).
   - Most cases can be monitored with observation.

III. PES CAVUS

A. Clinical features

1. Causes
   - Cavus deformity of the foot (elevated longitudinal arch) caused by fixed plantar flexion of the forefoot
   - Commonly associated with neurologic disorders that include polio, cerebral palsy, Friedreich ataxia, and Charcot-Marie-Tooth disease (an imbalance between the tibialis anterior and peroneus longus muscles).
   - Full neurologic workup is mandatory.
2. Physical examination
   - The lateral block (Coleman) test is used to assess hindfoot flexibility of the cavovarus foot (a flexible hindfoot corrects to neutral, with a lift placed under the lateral aspect of the foot; Figure 3-42).

B. Treatment

1. Nonoperative management is rarely successful.
2. Soft tissue surgery:
   - Surgical options in supple deformities include plantar release, metatarsal osteotomies, and posterior tibial tendon transfers.
   - Only if varus hindfoot is not fixed
3. Bone surgery:
   - If results of the lateral block test are abnormal (rigid deformity), a calcaneal osteotomy is also performed.
   - Triple arthrodesis has been used for rigid deformity in skeletally mature patients.
   - Calcaneal sliding osteotomy, with multiple metatarsal extension osteotomies, may offer an alternative to subtalar fusion procedures.

IV. PES CALCANEOVALGUS

A. Congenital vertical talus (convex pes valgus)

1. Clinical features
   - Irreducible dorsal dislocation of the navicular bone on the talus, with a fixed equinus hindfoot deformity
   - Talar head is prominent medially, the sole is convex, the forefoot is abducted and in dorsiflexion, and the hindfoot is in equinovalgus (Persian slipper foot).
   - Patients may demonstrate a "peg-leg" gait (awkward gait with limited forefoot push-off).
   - Can be isolated or occur with chromosomal abnormalities, myeloarthropathies, or neurologic disorders
   - Differential diagnosis includes an oblique talus (corrects with plantar flexion), tarsal coalition, and paralytic pes valgus.
2. Radiographic findings (Figure 3-43)
   - **Plantar-flexion lateral radiographs show a line along the long axis of the talus that passes below the first metatarsal–cuneiform axis** (Meary line; tarsal–first metatarsal angle >20 degrees, whereas normal angle is 0 to 20 degrees of dorsal tilt).
   - Anteroposterior radiographs show a talocalcaneal angle of more than 40 degrees (normal, 20 to 40 degrees).
3. Treatment
   - Casting
     - Three months of corrective casting (foot plantar flexed/inverted) or manipulative stretching is tried initially.
   - **Surgery when the patient is 6 to 12 months old includes soft tissue release with lengthening of the extensor tendons, peroneal muscles, and Achilles tendon and reduction of the talonavicular joint with reconstruction of the spring ligament.**

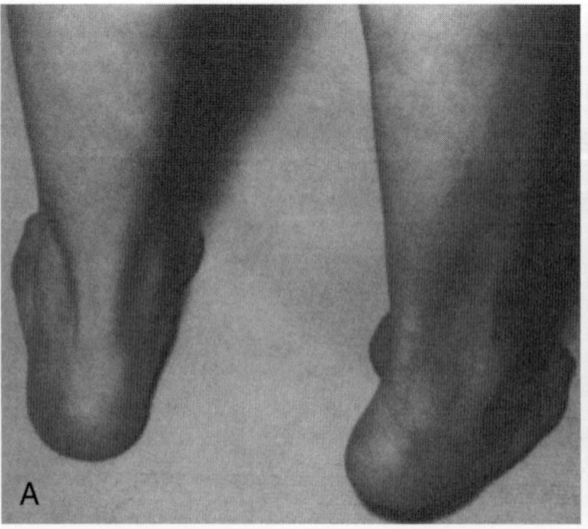

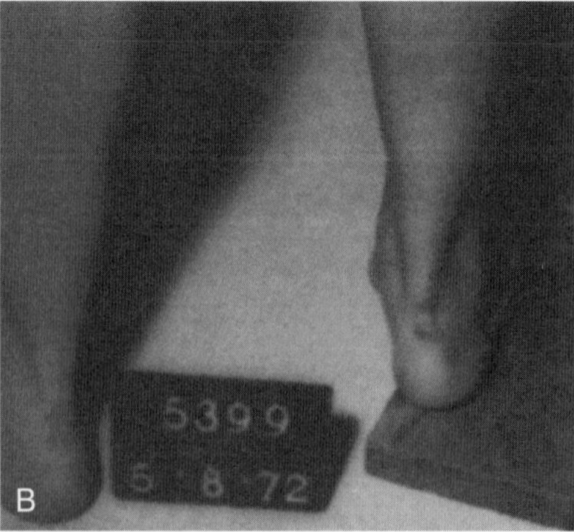

Figure 3-42 Coleman block test to document hindfoot flexibility in a cavovarus foot. Posterior views of the foot of a 9-year-old boy with Charcot-Marie-Tooth disease. **A,** Note the varus heel. **B,** Placed on a 3-cm block, the heel assumes a normal position; thus, the calcaneus can be spared from an osteotomy during surgical correction. (From Benson M, et al: *Children's orthopaedics and fractures,* New York, 1994, Churchill Livingstone, p 563.)

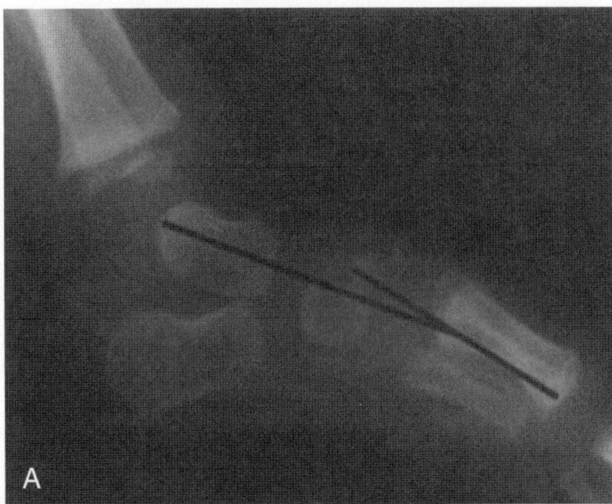

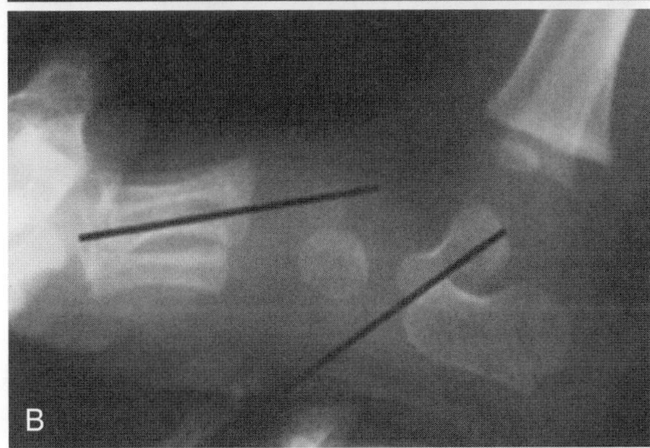

Figure 3-43 Lateral stress radiographs of plantar flexion in the diagnosis of congenital vertical talus. **A,** In the normal foot, the long axis of the first metatarsal passes in a plantar direction toward the long axis of the talus. **B,** In congenital vertical talus, the long axis of the first metatarsal remains dorsal to the long axis of talus, indicating dorsal dislocation of midfoot and forefoot. Note equinus deformity of calcaneus. (From Canale ST, Beaty JH, editors: *Campbell's operative orthopaedics,* ed 11, Philadelphia, 2008, Elsevier.)

B. **Oblique talus**
1. Clinical features
   - Talonavicular subluxation that reduces with plantar flexion of foot
2. Treatment consists of observation and sometimes a shoe insert (University of California, Biomechanics Laboratory [UCBL] heel cup).
3. Some patients require pinning of the talonavicular joint in the reduced position and Achilles tendon lengthening.

V. TARSAL COALITIONS (FIGURE 3-44)

A. **Clinical features**
1. A disorder of mesenchymal segmentation that leads to fusion of tarsal bones and rigid flatfoot
2. Occurs primarily as a talocalcaneal or calcaneonavicular coalition and is the leading cause of peroneal spastic flatfoot
3. The symptoms, which appear by age 10 to 12 years, include calf pain caused by peroneal spasticity, flatfoot, and limited subtalar motion.
4. Coalitions may be fibrous, cartilaginous, or osseous.
5. **Calcaneonavicular coalition** is most common in children 10 to 12 years of age, and **subtalar coalition** is more common in children 12 to 14 years of age.

B. **Radiographic findings**
1. Lateral radiographs may demonstrate an elongated anterior process of the calcaneus ("anteater" sign).
2. Talocalcaneal coalitions may demonstrate talar beaking on the lateral view (does not denote degenerative joint disease) or an **irregular middle facet on the Harris axial view.**
3. **The best study for identifying and measuring the cross-sectional area of a talocalcaneal coalition is a CT scan, which can also reveal multiple coalitions (seen in 20% of cases).**

C. **Treatment**
1. Nonoperative
   - **Initial treatment for either type involves immobilization (casting) or orthoses.**
   - Observation is reasonable for asymptomatic bars in young children.
2. Surgery
   - Resection is commonly successful in restoring motion.
   - **For subtalar coalition, a symptomatic bar involving less than 50% of the middle facet should be resected.**
     - **Origin of extensor digitorum brevis is placed into space between calcaneus and navicular.**
     - Less successful in alleviating pain
   - **If more than 50% of the middle facet is involved, then subtalar arthrodesis is preferred.**
   - In advanced cases and in cases in which attempts at resection fail, triple arthrodesis is often required.

VI. CALCANEOVALGUS FOOT

A. **Clinical features**
1. Neonatal condition associated with intrauterine positioning
2. It is common in firstborn children.
3. Manifests with a dorsiflexed hindfoot and eversion and abduction of the hindfoot that is passively correctable to neutral positioning
4. Also seen with myelomeningocele at the L5 level as a result of muscular imbalance between foot dorsiflexors/everters (L4 and L5 roots) and plantar flexors/inverters (S1 and S2 roots)

B. **Treatment**
1. Passive stretching and observation

VII. JUVENILE BUNIONS

A. **Clinical features**
1. Often bilateral and familial
2. Less common and usually less severe than the adult form
3. May be associated with ligamentous laxity, hypermobile first ray, and metatarsus primus varus
4. Usually occurs in adolescent girls

B. **Treatment**
1. Nonoperative
   - Modification of shoe wear with a wide toe box and arch supports

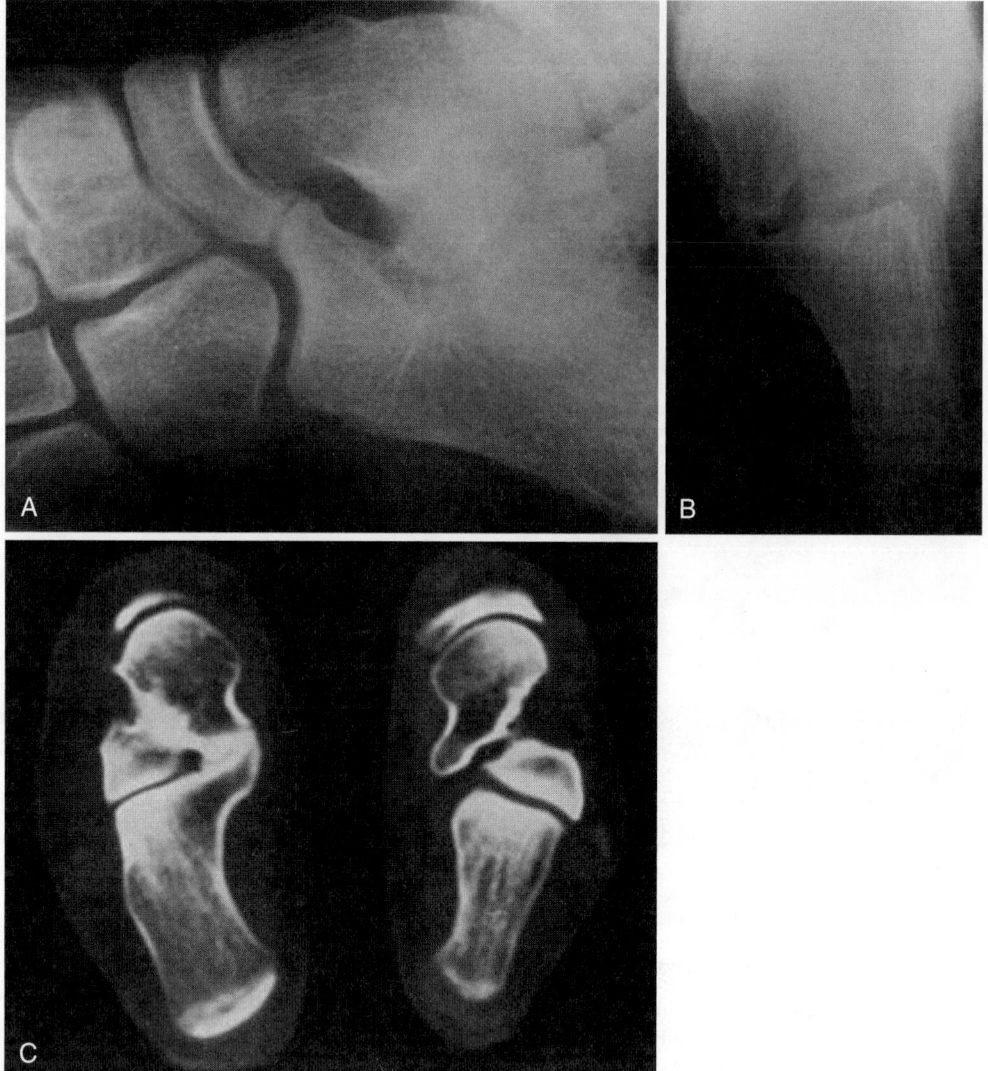

Figure 3-44 Tarsal coalition. **A,** Oblique radiograph demonstrating a calcaneonavicular coalition. **B,** Harris view, showing irregular surfaces and narrowing of the medial facet, suggestive of a talocalcaneal coalition. **C,** Computed tomographic scan, showing a large bar across the medial facet of the subtalar joint, which confirms the subtalar coalition. (From Herring JA, editor: *Tachdjian's pediatric orthopaedics,* ed 4, Philadelphia, 2008, WB Saunders, Figure 23-83.)

2. Surgical
   - Should be avoided because recurrence is frequent in growing patients
   - If surgery is performed, symptomatic patients with an intermetatarsal angle of more than 10 degrees (metatarsus primus varus) and a hallux valgus angle of more than 20 degrees may necessitate proximal metatarsal osteotomy, distal capsular reefing, and adductor tenotomy with a bunionectomy (modified McBride procedure).
   - Complications include recurrence, overcorrection, and hallux varus.

VIII. KOHLER DISEASE

A. Clinical features

1. Osteonecrosis of the tarsal navicular bone; usually manifests at the age of about 5 years
2. Pain is the typical presenting complaint.
3. **Radiographs show sclerosis of the navicular bone.**

B. Treatment

1. Resolves spontaneously with decreased activity, with or without immobilization

IX. FLEXIBLE PES PLANUS

A. Clinical features

1. Foot is flat only when standing and not with toe walking or foot hanging.
2. This condition is frequently familial and almost always bilateral.
3. It is commonly associated with minor lower extremity rotational problems and ligamentous laxity.
4. Symptoms can include an aching midfoot or pretibial pain.

B. Radiographic findings

1. Lateral radiographic findings mimic those of vertical talus, but a plantar-flexed lateral view demonstrates a line along the long axis of the talus that passes above the metatarsal-cuneiform axis. In addition, x-ray evaluation can

Table 3-22 Radiologic Views for Pes Planus

View	Assessment
Standing anteroposterior	Talar head coverage, talocalcaneal angle
Standing lateral	Calcaneal/talar equinus, talocalcaneal angle
Oblique	To rule out coalition

demonstrate talar head coverage and equinus hindfoot, which may be a portion of the deformity (Table 3-22).

C. Treatment
1. **Asymptomatic patients should be monitored with observation.**
2. When the patient is symptomatic, arch supports and shoes with stiffer soles may offer pain relief but do not result in deformity correction.
3. Thorough evaluation should be completed to rule out tight heel cords and decreased subtalar motion.
4. UCBL heel cups are sometimes indicated for advanced cases with pain (symptomatic treatment only).
5. **Calcaneal lengthening osteotomy with or without medial soft tissue tightening may provide pain relief at the expense of inversion/eversion in adolescents with disabling pain refractory to every means of conservative treatment.**

X. HABITUAL TOE WALKING

A. Clinical features
1. Can be associated with many neurologic diagnoses, such as autism
2. Other diagnoses (muscular dystrophy, cerebral palsy) must be ruled out with neurologic evaluation.
3. Contracture of the Achilles tendon may be present.

B. Treatment
1. Nonoperative
   - Stretching and night splints
   - Serial casting
   - Botox may play a role.
2. Operative treatment
   - Contracture of the Achilles tendon necessitates lengthening of the tendon.

XI. ACCESSORY NAVICULAR

A. Clinical features
1. Normal variant that is present in up to 12% of the general population.
2. The posterior tibial tendon typically inserts into the accessory navicular.
3. Commonly associated with flat feet
4. The symptoms usually include medial arch pain with overuse; they usually resolve with activity restriction or immobilization.

B. Radiographic studies
1. **External oblique radiographic views are often helpful in the diagnosis.**

C. Treatment
1. **Most cases resolve spontaneously and can be treated with activity restriction and shoe modification.**
2. **The accessory bone (with repair of the posterior tibial tendon) is occasionally excised, which can correct symptoms (but not flatfoot) in most patients.**

XII. BALL-AND-SOCKET ANKLE

A. Clinical features
1. Abnormal formation with a spherical talus (ball) and a cup-shaped tibiofibular articulation (socket)
2. It usually necessitates no treatment but should be recognized because of its high association with tarsal coalition (50% of cases), absence of lateral rays (50% of cases), fibular deficiency, and leg-length discrepancy.

XIII. CONGENITAL TOE DISORDERS

A. Syndactyly
1. Fusion of the soft tissues (simple) and sometimes bones (complex) of the toes
2. Simple syndactyly usually does not necessitate treatment; complex syndactyly is treated in the same way as it is in the hand.

B. Polydactyly (extra digits)
1. May be autosomal dominant and usually involves the lateral ray in patients with a positive family history
2. Treatment includes ablation of the extra digit and any bony protrusion of the common metatarsal (the border digit is typically excised; it is not the best formed digit).
3. The procedure is usually done at ages 9 to 12 months, but some rudimentary digits can be ligated in the newborn nursery.

C. Oligodactyly
1. Congenital absence of the toes
2. May be associated with more proximal agenesis (i.e., fibular hemimelia) and tarsal coalition
3. Usually necessitates no treatment

D. Atavistic great toe (congenital hallux varus)
1. Deformity involving great-toe adduction that is often associated with polydactyly. Must be differentiated from metatarsus adductus.
2. The deformity usually occurs at the metatarsophalangeal joint and includes a short, thick first metatarsal and a firm band (abductor hallucis longus muscle) that may be responsible for the disorder.
3. Surgery is sometimes required and includes release of the abductor hallucis longus muscle.

E. Overlapping toe
1. The fifth toe overlaps the fourth (usually bilaterally) and may cause problems with footwear.
2. Initial treatment includes passive stretching and "buddy" taping, but usually the overlapping toes resolve with time.
3. Surgical options include tenotomy, dorsal capsulotomy, and syndactylization to the fourth toe (McFarland procedure).

F. Underlapping toe (congenital curly toe)
1. **Usually involves the lateral three toes and is rarely symptomatic**
2. Surgery (flexor tenotomies) is occasionally indicated.

TESTABLE CONCEPTS

SECTION 1 BONE DYSPLASIAS (DWARFISM)

- Majority of dwarfisms not associated with mucopolysaccharidosis are autosomal dominant.
  - Autosomal recessive: diastrophic dysplasia, McKusick metaphyseal chondroplasia
  - X-linked recessive: spondyloepiphyseal dysplasia tarda
- Major mucopolysaccharidoses are autosomal recessive disorders, except Hunter syndrome, which is X-linked recessive.
- Common genetic associations:
  - Achondroplasia: FGFR3
  - Pseudoachondroplasia: COMP
  - Diastrophic dysplasia: sulfate transport protein
  - MED: type II collagen genes
  - Cleidocranial dysplasia: CBFA1
- Achondroplasia, the most common form of disproportional dwarfism, is autosomal dominant and caused by a mutation in FGFR3 that results in a failure in the proliferative zone of the physis.
  - Spine: lumbar stenosis; excessive lordosis (short pedicles with decreased interpedicular distances); foramen magnum stenosis
  - Pelvis: wider than it is deep ("champagne glass")
  - Legs: genu varum; tibia vara
  - Elbow: radial head subluxation
  - Growth plates: U- or V-shaped
- MED is characterized by irregular, delayed ossification at multiple epiphyses.
  - The proximal femoral involvement can be confused with Perthes disease. MED is bilateral and symmetric and is characterized by early acetabular changes and not by metaphyseal cysts. Perform a bone survey to differentiate between Perthes disease, spondyloepiphyseal dysplasia (MED plus spine involvement), and MED.
- Morquio syndrome is the most common form of mucopolysaccharidosis and is a proportionate dwarfism characterized by urinary excretion of keratan sulfate.
  - C1-C2 instability (resulting from odontoid hypoplasia) can be seen with Morquio syndrome, manifesting with myelopathy and necessitating decompression and cervical fusion.
- Diastrophic dysplasia is autosomal recessive disorder of the sulfate transport protein; it manifests with cauliflower ears, rigid clubfeet, hitchhiker's thumb, and cleft palate. Cervical kyphosis may be severe and necessitate early fusion to prevent quadriplegia.
- Cleidocranial dysplasia affects bone formed by intramembranous ossification. It is characterized by hypoplasia or aplasia of the clavicle with delayed ossification of the symphysis pubis.

SECTION 2 CHROMOSOMAL AND TERATOLOGIC DISORDERS

- Down syndrome (trisomy 21) is associated with atlantoaxial instability, hip instability, patellar dislocation, scoliosis, SCFE, and spondylolisthesis. The pathogenesis of generalized laxity is thought to be abnormal type VI collagen, whose genes *COL6A1* and *COL6A2* are located on chromosome 21.
  - Screening for cervical spine instability is somewhat controversial but is absolutely mandatory before induction of anesthesia.
  - Hip instability initially may be treated with closed reduction, but capsulorrhaphy, pelvis osteotomy, and femoral osteotomies may be required.

    Scoliosis: bracing for 25- to 30-degree curves, surgery for 50- to 60-degree curves.
- Beckwith-Wiedemann syndrome is associated with hemihypertrophy and spastic cerebral palsy. There is a predisposition to Wilms tumor (affected patients must be screened regularly by kidney ultrasonography).

SECTION 3 HEMATOPOIETIC DISORDERS

- Sickle cell anemia is a condition of hemolysis and microvascular occlusion. Consequently, bone infarction, osteomyelitis, osteonecrosis of the femoral and humeral heads and septic arthritis are common.
  - Bone infarction is differentiated from osteomyelitis with sequential bone marrow tests and bone scans within 24 hours, as well as gadolinium-enhanced T1-weighted MRI sequences.
  - *S. aureus* and *Salmonella* infections are the most common cause of osteomyelitis. Empirical antibiotic therapy is with ceftriaxone.
- Hemophilia is an X-linked recessive disorder. Orthopaedic manifestations are secondary to repeated episodes of hemorrhage.
  - Recurrent hemarthroses result in hemophilic arthropathy.
  - Synovectomy is indicated for hemarthroses that recur despite optimal medical management.
  - Iliacus hematoma can result in femoral nerve neurapraxia.
  - Factor VIII levels should be increased for prophylaxis in the following situations: vigorous physical therapy (20% of cases), treatment of hematoma (30%), acute hemarthrosis or soft tissue surgery (>50%), and skeletal surgery (approaching 100% of cases preoperatively and maintained in more than 50% for 10 days postoperatively).

SECTION 4 METABOLIC DISEASE/ARTHRITIDES

- Rickets manifests with physeal widening and metaphyseal cupping. Growth plate abnormalities include enlarged and distorted maturation zone (zone of hypertrophy) and a poorly defined zone of provisional calcification.
- Osteogenesis imperfecta is caused by a defect in type I collagen (*COL1A2* gene) that causes abnormal cross-linking and leads to decreased secretion of collagen.
  - Fractures are ubiquitous, with normal healing but abnormal remodeling.
  - Basilar invagination is common in more severe types.
  - Bisphosphonates have been shown to decrease the number of fractures in affected patients. Iatrogenic osteopetrosis can occur with long-term use of high-dose bisphosphonates.
  - Scoliosis is common; bracing is ineffective, and so segmental instrumentation is often necessary.

- Osteopetrosis is a failure of osteoclastic resorption, probably secondary to a defect in the thymus, and leads to dense bone.
  - Loss of the medullary canal can cause anemias and encroachment on the optic and oculomotor nerves, which lead to blindness.
  - Radiographic features include "marble bone," "rugger jersey spine," and an Erlenmeyer flask deformity of the proximal humerus and distal femur.
  - Bone marrow transplantation may be helpful in treating the malignant form.
- Marfan syndrome is an autosomal dominant disorder of fibrillin-1, an important component of elastic and nonelastic connective tissues.
  - Nonorthopaedic manifestations are most important; aortic dilation is the major cause of death.
  - Scoliosis is common; bracing is ineffective, and so both anterior and posterior fusion are often necessary.
  - Acetabular protusio rarely causes severe hip dysfunction, and prophylactic surgical closure of the triradiate cartilage is not recommended.
- Juvenile idiopathic arthritis typically manifests before the age of 4 years and commonly involves the knee, wrist, and hand. Cervical spine involvement can lead to kyphosis, facet ankylosis, and atlantoaxial subluxation.
  - Slit-lamp examination is required twice yearly, because progressive iridocyclitis can lead to rapid loss of vision if left untreated.
- Ankylosing spondylitis is associated with HLA-B27, but the HLA-B27 test is not useful as a screening tool. Limitation of chest wall expansion is more specific.

SECTION 5 BIRTH INJURIES

- Brachial plexus palsy can be classified on the basis of root involvement.
  - Erb-Duchenne palsy (C5, C6): "Waiter's tip" deformity with the shoulder adducted and internally rotated, the elbow extended, the forearm pronated, and the wrist and fingers flexed.
  - Klumpke palsy (C8, T1): elbow flexion and forearm supination contracture
  - Total plexus palsy (C5 to T1): complete sensory and motor deficits
  - Progressive glenoid dysplasia occurs in 70% of children with significant internal rotation contracture.
  - Lack of biceps function 6 months after injury and Horner syndrome carry a poor prognosis.
  - Treatment includes latissimus and teres major transfer to the shoulder external rotators.
- Torticollis is a symptom and a sign but not a disease. Congenital muscular torticollis is a diagnosis of exclusion, and the affected patient should be evaluated for infection, congenital spinal deformity, rotatory subluxation of cervical spine, hearing loss, and optic dysfunction.
  - Of patients with congenital muscular torticollis, 90% respond to passive stretching within the first year. The chin should be rotated toward the affected side with a lateral head tilt away from the affected side.
  - Ultrasound demonstration of severe fibrosis of the sternocleidomastoid muscle is associated with failure of nonoperative management.

SECTION 6 CEREBRAL PALSY

- Cerebral palsy can be classified on the basis of physiology, anatomy, or function.
  - Anatomic classification divides cerebral palsy into three types:
    Hemiplegia: one side of body, both upper and lower extremities
    Diplegia: lower half involved more than upper half
    Quadriplegia: both sides, both halves involved
  - A patient's locomotor profile is based on the persistence of primitive reflexes; the presence of two or more usually means that the child will be unable to walk.
    Moro startle reflex: normally disappears by age 6 months
    Parachute reflex: normally disappears by age 12 months
- The ability to sit independently by age 2 years is highly prognostic of walking.
- Intramuscular botulinum A toxin can temporarily decrease dynamic spasticity by means of a presynaptic blockade at the neuromuscular junction.
- Dorsal rhizotomy is primarily performed in ambulatory spastic diplegic patients to help reduce spasticity and complement orthopaedic management.
- Baclofen is used to control overall tone in the extremities by inhibiting signals through the GABA pathway.
- In general, surgery should be avoided in the first 3 years of life.
- The risk for scoliosis is highest in children with total body involvement (spastic quadriplegic). Surgical indications include curves greater than 45 to 50 degrees, worsening pelvic obliquity, and wheelchair seating problems.
- Hip subluxation and dislocation is a common problem, but in many children, hip disease is asymptomatic. Treatment can be based on four stages:
  - Hip at risk: significant adduction and flexion contractures but minimal subluxation. Adductor and psoas release should be performed before the child is 5 years of age.
  - Hip subluxation: adductor tenotomy in children with abduction of less than 20 degrees, sometimes with psoas release/recession. Femoral or pelvic osteotomies may be considered in femoral coxa valga and acetabular dysplasia.
  - Spastic dislocation: Patients may benefit from open reduction, femoral shortening, varus derotation osteotomy, Dega osteotomy, triple osteotomy, or Chiari osteotomy. Addressing both hips can prevent dislocation of the opposite hip.
  - Windswept hips: characterized by abduction of one hip and adduction of the contralateral hip. Bilateral femoral osteotomies to more varus positioning can assist in maintaining reduction.
- Equinovarus foot is more common in spastic hemiplegia and is caused by overpull of either the posterior or anterior tibialis tendon.
  - Split-muscle transfers are helpful when the affected muscle is spastic during both the stance and swing phases of gait. The split–posterior tibialis transfer (rerouting half of the tendon dorsally to the peroneus brevis) is used in cases of spasticity of the muscle, flexible varus foot, and weak peroneal muscles.

Continued

SECTION 7 NEUROMUSCULAR DISORDERS

- Arthrogryposis is a nonprogressive disorder in which multiple joints are congenitally rigid.
  - Active elbow flexion achieved via anterior triceps transfer and posterior soft tissue release
  - Hip dislocation, unilateral: medial open reduction with possible femoral shortening
  - Hip dislocation, bilateral: typically left unreduced because ambulation is often preserved
  - Knee: Contractures are treated with early (at ages 6 to 9 months) soft tissue releases (especially hamstrings). Knee contractures should be corrected before hip reduction in order to maintain the reduction.
  - Foot: Clubfoot and vertical talus are initially treated with a soft tissue release, but later recurrences may necessitate bone procedures (talectomy). The goal is for the foot to be stiff and plantigrade, in order to wear shoes and possibly ambulate.
- Myelodysplasia (spina bifida) is a spectrum of disorders caused by incomplete spinal cord closure or rupture of the developing cord secondary to hydrocephalus. In myelomeningocele, the sac with the neural elements protrudes through the skin.
  - It can be diagnosed in utero through increased levels of α-fetoprotein and is related to folate deficiency.
  - The myelodysplasia level is based on the lowest functional level. L4 is a key level because the quadriceps can function and allow independent ambulation in the community.
  - Fractures are common, occurring most often about the knee and hip in children 3 to 7 years of age, and can frequently be diagnosed only by noting redness, warmth, and swelling that is caused by pain insensitivity.
  - A significant proportion of patients with spina bifida have a serious allergy to latex. A latex-free environment is required in all cases involving spina bifida.
  - Hip dislocation: Treatment is controversial, but in general, containment is considered essential only in patients with functioning quadriceps. Redislocation may occur regardless of treatment type. The functional outcome of thoracic-level myelomeningocele is independent of whether the hips are located or dislocated. Management should focus on limiting soft tissue contractures.
  - Ankle and foot:
    Calcaneal deformity is most common. Treat with tibialis anterior transfer to the calcaneus.
    Valgus tibia or subtalar joint: Skeletally immature patients should have hemiepiphysiodesis or Achilles tendon–fibular tenodesis. Skeletally mature patients should undergo distal tibial osteotomy.
    Rigid clubfoot: Treatment consists of complete subtalar release through a transverse (Cincinnati) incision, lengthening of the tibialis posterior and Achilles tendons, and transfer of the tibialis anterior tendon to the dorsal midfoot.
- Myopathies (muscular dystrophies) are inherited disorders with progressive weakness. Several types exist and are classified on the basis of their inheritance patterns.
  - Duchenne: X-linked recessive; absence of dystrophin protein; proximal muscle groups weaker than distal groups
  - Becker: X-linked recessive; decreased dystrophin protein
- Hereditary sensory motor neuropathies are a group of inherited neuropathic disorders with similar characteristics. Charcot-Marie-Tooth disease is the most common.
  - Two types of Charcot-Marie-Tooth disease; type I shows autosomal dominant inheritance. Diagnosis is made most reliably by DNA testing for a duplication of a genomic fragment that encompasses the peripheral myelin protein-22 (PMP22) gene on chromosome 17.
  - The most severely affected muscles are the tibialis anterior, peroneus longus, and peroneus brevis. Plantar flexion of the first ray is the first foot deformity to appear as a result of a weakened tibialis anterior muscle.
  - If the varus limb is flexible, plantar release and posterior tibial tendon transfer is performed.
- Spinal muscular atrophy is an anterior horn cell disorder. It is caused by a loss of anterior horn cells from the spinal cord.
  - Characterized by autosomal recessive inheritance and associated with survival motor neuron gene (*SMN*)
  - Scoliosis should be treated early. Upper extremity function may decrease after spinal fusion, but this decrease may be temporary. Before fusion, ensure that the patient does not have lower extremity muscle contractures that could interfere with sitting balance.
  - Hip subluxation or dislocation is common and is treated nonoperatively.

SECTION 9 PEDIATRIC SPINE

II. Adolescent Idiopathic Scoliosis

- Indications for an MRI to rule out syringomyelia: left thoracic curves; painful scoliosis; apical kyphosis of the thoracic curve; juvenile-onset scoliosis (before the age of 11 years); rapid curve progression; associated syndromes; neurologic signs/symptoms; congenital abnormalities
- Risk factors for curve progression:
  - Skeletal immaturity (Risser stages 0 to 1)
  - Curve magnitude before or during peak height velocity. Peak height velocity is the best predictor of progression; it occurs before the onset of menarche and during Risser stage 0. (Modalities of treatment for idiopathic scoliosis are listed in Table 3-23.)

III. Infantile Idiopathic Scoliosis

- Manifests in children younger than 3 years
- Differences from adolescent idiopathic scoliosis: left curves, more common in boys, plagiocephaly (skull flattening), congenital defects
- In general, most curves resolve spontaneously.
  - Risk for progression is calculated according to rib-vertebral angle difference; 20 degrees is the cutoff between low and high risk for progression.

IV. Juvenile Idiopathic Scoliosis

- Manifestations are generally similar to those of adolescent idiopathic scoliosis, but risk for progression is higher:

Table 3-23 Guidelines for Treating Patients with Idiopathic Scoliosis

Curve Magnitude (Degrees)	RISSER SIGN Grade 0/ Premenarchal	Grade 1 or 2	Grade 3, 4, or 5
<25	Observation	Observation	Observation
25-45	Brace therapy (begin when curve is >25 degrees)	Brace therapy	Observation
>45	Surgery	Surgery	Surgery (when curve >50 degrees)

From Herring JA (editor): *Tachdjian's pediatric orthopaedics,* ed 4. Philadelphia, 2008, WB Saunders, Table 12-2.)

70% require treatment (of those who do, 50% need bracing and 50% require surgery).
- Rate of spinal cord abnormality is 25%, and MRI should be routinely obtained.

VI. Neuromuscular Scoliosis

- Scoliosis is caused by various neuromuscular conditions, including traumatic paralysis, Duchenne muscular dystrophy, Friedrich ataxia, spinal muscular atrophy, spina bifida (myelomeningocele), cerebral palsy, and neurofibromatosis. (Modalities of treatment for neuromuscular scoliosis are listed in Table 3-24.)

VII. Congenital Scoliosis

- Caused by a failure of segmentation (vertical bar) or formation (hemivertebra)
- A block vertebra has the best prognosis; a unilateral bar with hemivertebra has the worst prognosis.
- Associated abnormalities are common. MRI should be ordered (reveals abnormalities in 35% of cases), along with renal (25%) and cardiac (10%) ultrasonography.
- Fully segmented hemivertebra has a very high likelihood of progressive deformity, and resection should be performed before a fixed compensatory curve develops.

VIII. Congenital Kyphosis

- Three types of defects: failure of formation, failure of segmentation, mixed
- Failure of formation generally involves retained posterior elements and absence of anterior elements, resulting in relentless kyphosis. As such, it has the worst prognosis.
- Failure of formation and mixed defects should be surgically managed, generally around the time of diagnosis (even in infants). The goal is to prevent paraplegia.
- Posterior fusion is favored in young children (<5 years of age) with curves of less than 50 degrees and normal findings of neurologic examination. Such fusion functions as a posterior (convex) hemiepiphysiodesis.

IX. Neurofibromatosis

- Scoliosis is common and the curve can be classified as nondystrophic (similar to idiopathic scoliosis) and dystrophic. Dystrophic curves have a short segment with tight apex, vertebral scalloping, enlarged foramina, penciling of transverse processes, severe apical rotation, and penciling of ribs.
  - Penciling of three or more ribs is a prognostic factor for impending rapid progression of spinal deformity
- Anterior and posterior surgery is required in the majority of patients with dystrophic curves, especially when the curves are associated with kyphosis.

X. Other Spinal Abnormalities

- Discitis often manifests with vague signs and symptoms. The diagnosis should be considered in all patients with refusal to sit or walk. Loss of normal lumbar lordosis is the earliest radiographic finding; disc space narrowing with preservation of end plates is the classic finding (but takes 3 weeks). *S. aureus* is the most common cause, and treatment is with antistaphylococcal antibiotics.
- Spondylolysis that is symptomatic can be treated with an antilordotic brace.
- Spondylolisthesis is most commonly seen at the level of L5 to S1.
  - Risks for progression: dysplastic type, higher grade slippage, slippage angle

Table 3-24 Treatment in Neuromuscular Scoliosis

Condition	Bracing	Operative
Duchenne muscular dystrophy	Ineffective	Early; 25-30 degrees to delay pulmonary function deterioration
Friedrich ataxia	Ineffective	Fusion if >50 degrees or progressive
Spinal muscular atrophy	Useful to delay fusion in young patients with curves between 25 and 45 degrees	Fusion if >50 degrees or progressive
Spina bifida (myelomeningocele)	Useful to delay fusion in young patients with curves between 25 and 45 degrees	Fusion if >50 degrees or progressive
Cerebral palsy	Ineffective	>50 Degrees in ambulatory patients Progressive curves >50 degrees in communicative and aware patients Curve interfering with seating and nursing, with family desire for surgery
Neurofibromatosis	Nondystrophic curves between 25 and 40 degrees	Fusion if >40 degrees or progressive
Arthrogryposis	Ineffective	Fusion if >50 degrees or progressive

Continued

- Treatment for low-grade (1 and 2) slippage: bracing in the acute situation, physical therapy, arthrodesis if nonoperative treatment fails.
- Treatment for high-grade (3 and 4) slippage: typically, surgery is indicated and L4-S1 fusion required.

XI. Kyphosis

- Defined as increased thoracic kyphosis (>45 degrees curvature) with 5 degrees or more of anterior wedging at three sequential vertebrae
- Nonoperative treatment: bracing in a patient with relative skeletal immaturity (Risser stage 2 or below) and kyphotic curvature of 50 to 75 degrees. A Milwaukee brace is used.
- Operative indications: kyphotic curvature of more than 70 to 75 degrees, rigid deformity, progressive curve with failure of 6-month nonoperative management. Only posterior procedures are typically performed.

XII. Cervical Spine Disorders

- Rotatory atlantoaxial subluxation often manifests with torticollis. It is thought to be caused by retropharyngeal inflammation. Most cases are self-limited and necessitate no treatment.
  - Present less than 1 week: soft collar, heat, analgesics.
  - Present more than 1 week without resolution: Halter traction, muscle relaxants; halo traction may be required.
  - Present more than 1 month: attempt traction (typically halo); if no resolution after 1 week, closed versus open reduction and posterior C1-C2 fusion.
- Os odontoideum is either congenital or an unrecognized odontoid fracture that has resulted in nonunion. Instability or presence of neurologic symptoms necessitates posterior C1-C2 fusion.
- Pseudosubluxation of the cervical spine is most common at C2 on C3.
  - If the spinolaminar line remains intact, up to 4 mm of vertebral body subluxation can be accepted.

SECTION 11 LOWER EXTREMITY PROBLEMS: GENERAL

- In-toeing is usually attributable to metatarsus adductus (in infants), internal tibial torsion (in toddlers), and femoral anteversion (in children younger than 10 years).
  - Metatarsus adductus: inward deviation of lateral board of foot from base of fourth metatarsal
  - Internal tibial torsion: inward (negative) thigh-foot angle
  - Femoral anteversion: increased internal rotation and decreased external rotation
- Out-toeing is typically caused by external rotation hip contracture in infants.
- Most of these cases are treated nonoperatively.

SECTION 12 HIP AND FEMUR

I. Developmental Dysplasia of the Hip

- Risk factors (in order): breech positioning, positive family history, female sex, and being a firstborn child
- Early diagnosis is possible with the Ortolani test (elevation and abduction of femur relocates a dislocated hip) and the Barlow test (adduction and depression of femur dislocates a dislocatable hip).
- Subsequent diagnosis is made with limitation of hip abduction in the affected hip as the laxity resolves and stiffness becomes more clinically evident.
- Dynamic ultrasonography is used for diagnosis before ossification of the femoral head at ages 4 to 6 months.
  - Radiographic signs of DDH: broken Shenton line, metaphysis lateral to the Perkins line, increased acetabular index
- Therapy is based on the child's age:
  - Birth to 6 months: Pavlik harness
    Check reduction with ultrasonography after 3 weeks.
    Not reduced: closed reduction, arthrogram and spica casting
    Reduced: Continue harness until examination and ultrasound findings are normal.
  - Ages 6 to 18 months: hip arthrography, percutaneous adductor tenotomy, closed reduction and spica casting; if closed reduction fails, perform open reduction
  - Ages 18 months to 3 years: open reduction
  - Ages 3 to 8 years: osteotomy
- Pavlik harness complications include avascular necrosis (caused by excessive abduction) and femoral nerve palsy (hyperflexion). If attempts to reduce a hip in 3 weeks fail, the Pavlik harness should be discontinued to prevent "Pavlik disease" (erosion of the pelvis superior to the acetabulum) and subsequent difficulty with closed reduction and casting.
- Open reductions are typically performed through an anterior approach (less risk to the medial femoral circumflex artery than in the medial approach).
- Osteotomies should be performed only after a congruent reduction is confirmed on an abduction–internal rotation radiograph, with satisfactory ROM, and after reasonable femoral sphericity is achieved by closed- or open-reduction methods.
  - The Chiari osteotomy is a salvage procedure when a concentric reduction of the femoral head within the acetabulum cannot be achieved.
  - The lateral shelf acetabular augmentation procedure also does not require concentric reduction. A successful result depends on fibrocartilage.

II. Congenital Coxa Vara

- When to observe:
  - Bilateral arthrogryposis
  - Myelomeningocele if no functional quadriceps
  - Spinal muscular atrophy
- When to treat or operate:
  - Down syndrome
  - Cerebral palsy, unless chronic

III. Legg-Calvé-Perthes Disease

- Bilateral involvement occurs in 15% of cases, but it is virtually never synchronous and may mimic MED.
- The Herring lateral pillar classification, which is most prognostic, is based on involvement of the lateral pillar of the capital femoral epiphysis during the fragmentation stage.

- Group A has a uniformly good outcome.
- Group B and a bone age of less than 6 years has a good prognosis.
- Group C has a poor prognosis.
- Poor prognosis is also associated with older age (bone age >6), female sex, and decreased hip abduction.
- Early degenerative hip disease results from aspherical femoral heads.
- Treatment is somewhat controversial. Symptoms may be relieved with traction, anti-inflammatory medications, and partial weight bearing.
  - Surgical treatment improves radiographic outcome at skeletal maturity for older patients (chronologic age >8 years or bone age >6 years) with lateral pillar group B and B/C hips.

IV. Slipped Capital Femoral Epiphysis

- Disorder of the proximal femoral epiphysis caused by weakness of the perichondrial ring and slippage through the hypertrophic zone of the growth plate
- Associated with hormonal disorders in young children, such as hypothyroidism (most common), growth hormone deficiency, or renal osteodystrophy
- The diagnosis is missed most often because patients present with knee pain.
- On physical examination, all patients have obligate external rotation with flexion of the hip.
- Classification of SCFE is based on ability to bear weight at time of presentation.
  - Stable: weight bearing is possible; avascular necrosis is rare.
  - Unstable: weight bearing is not possible; rate of avascular necrosis is 50%.
- Treatment is with in situ pinning. Prophylactic pinning of the contralateral hip is controversial but generally recommended in patients with an endocrinopathy, those younger than 10 years, or those with open triradiate cartilage.
  - Pin placement into the anterior superior quadrant of the femoral head has the highest rate of joint penetration.

VI. Leg-Length Discrepancy

- A gross estimation of leg-length discrepancy can be made under the following assumption of growth per year up to age 16 in boys and age 14 in girls:
  - Distal femur: 9 mm
  - Proximal tibia: 6 mm
  - Proximal femur: 3 mm
- Discrepancies of 2 to 5 cm can be treated with epiphysiodesis of the long side, shortening of the long side (ostectomy), or lengthening of the short side. Discrepancies of more than 5 cm are generally treated with lengthening.

VII. Lower Extremity Inflammation and Infection

- Transient synovitis is the most common cause of painful hips during childhood. However, the patient must be evaluated for septic hip with aspiration (especially in children with fever, leukocytosis, or elevated ESR); if findings are negative, observe the patient with a trial of NSAIDs, and symptoms should improve within 24 to 48 hours.
- Acute hematogenous osteomyelitis is most commonly caused by *S. aureus,* regardless of age.
  - Methicillin-resistant *S. aureus* (MRSA) is associated with deep venous thrombosis and septic emboli.
  - Treatment is with intravenous antibiotics.
  - C-reactive protein measurements can be used to monitor the therapeutic response to antibiotics; failure to decline within 48 to 72 hours warrants alteration in treatment.
  - Failure to respond to antibiotics, frank pus on MRI, or the presence of a sequestered abscess (not accessible to antibiotics) necessitates operative drainage and débridement.
- Septic arthritis is most commonly caused by hematogenous seeding of the synovium. It also occurs through direct contact with osteomyelitis in joints with intracapsular metaphyses (hip, elbow, shoulder, ankle).
  - Distinguishing septic arthritis of the hip from transient synovitis is a common problem; however, when three of four of the following criteria are present, the diagnosis of septic arthritis is made in more than 90% of cases: WBC > 12,000 cells/mL, ESR > 40, inability to bear weight, and fever higher than 101.5°F.
  - Radiographs may show a widened joint space or even dislocation.
  - Because pus is chondrolytic, septic arthritis in children is an acute surgical emergency.

SECTION 13 KNEE AND LEG

- Blount disease occurs in infantile (more common) and adolescent forms.
  - Infantile Blount disease: Treatment is based on age and correlated with stage of disease.
    Stage I or stage II in children younger than 3 years: bracing
    Stage II (in children younger than 3 years) or stage III: proximal osteotomy with valgus overcorrection
    Stages IV to VI: multiple complex procedures. Epiphysiolysis may be required.
  - Adolescent Blount disease: Manifests with a relatively normal-appearing physis that shows widening of the proximal medial physeal plate. Beaking is not seen.
- Tibial bowing is classified into three types, according to the apex of the curve:
  - Posteromedial
    Physiologic; commonly associated with leg-length discrepancy, calcaneovalgus feet, and tight anterior structures. Spontaneous correction is the rule, but monitor the patient to evaluate leg-length discrepancy.
  - Anteromedial
    Fibular hemimelia
  - Anterolateral
    Congenital pseudarthrosis is the most common cause and often accompanied by neurofibromatosis.
    Initial treatment with total-contact brace to prevent fracture
- Osteochondritis dissecans most frequently involves the lateral portion of the medial femoral condyle. If growth plates are open, treat with bracing and restricted weight bearing.

Continued

- Discoid meniscus appears on MRI in three successive sagittal images with the meniscal body present. Saucerization or débridement should be performed.

SECTION 14 FOOT

- Clubfoot deformity is forefoot adductus and supination in combination with hindfoot equinus and varus.
  - Radiographs demonstrate "parallelism" of the calcaneus and talus.
  - Ponseti method is primarily used. A mnemonic for the sequence of correction is "CAVE": *c*avus, *a*dductus, *v*arus, *e*quinus.
  - A dynamic forefoot adduction/supination may develop after clubfoot treatment, as a result of overpull of the anterior tibialis. This necessitates transfer of the anterior tibialis tendon laterally.
  - Clubfoot surgery is reserved for resistant or refractory clubfeet.

    Development of a dorsal bunion can follow operative treatment. Treatment is with capsulotomy, flexor hallucis longus lengthening, and transfer of the flexor hallucis brevis to become a metatarsophalangeal extensor.
- Congenital vertical talus is an irreducible dorsal dislocation of the navicular bone on the talus, with a fixed equinus hindfoot deformity.
  - Plantar-flexion lateral radiographs show a line along the long axis of the talus that passes below the first metatarsal–cuneiform axis.
  - Initial treatment is with corrective casting. Surgery when the patient is 6 to 12 months of age includes soft tissue releases and reduction of the talonavicular joint with reconstruction of the spring ligament.
- Tarsal coalitions are most commonly calcaneonavicular (in children 10 to 12 years of age) and talocalcaneal (in children 12 to 14 years of age).
  - Radiographs may show talar beaking on the lateral view and an irregular middle facet on the Harris axial view.
  - CT scan reliably demonstrates the coalition.
  - Initial treatment is with immobilization.
  - Subtalar coalition involving less than 50% of the joint should be resected and the extensor digitorum brevis interposed. If involvement is more than 50%, performing a subtalar arthrodesis is recommended.
- Köhler disease manifests with sclerosis of the navicular. It is self-limiting.
- Flexible pes planus should be observed if asymptomatic. Surgical treatment is with calcaneal lengthening osteotomy.
- An accessory navicular manifests with medial arch pain and is typically self-limiting. Excision of the accessory bone with reconstruction of the posterior tibial tendon is performed in refractory cases. However, it does not correct the flatfoot.

SELECTED BIBLIOGRAPHY

The selected bibliography for this chapter can be found on www.expertconsult.com.

Chapter 4

SPORTS MEDICINE

Matthew D. Milewski, Jennifer A. Hart, and Mark D. Miller

CONTENTS

SECTION 1 KNEE

I. ANATOMY AND BIOMECHANICS

A. Anatomy

1. Hinge joint that also incorporates both gliding and rolling, which are essential to its kinematics
2. See Chapter 2, Anatomy, for a thorough discussion of knee anatomy.
3. Ligaments
   - Anterior cruciate ligament (ACL)
     - Despite intensive research, the function and anatomy of the ACL are still debated.
     - Femoral attachment: semicircular area on the posteromedial aspect of the lateral femoral condyle (Figure 4-1)
     - Tibial insertion: broad, irregular, oval area just anterior to and between the intercondylar eminences of the tibia
     - Length: 30 mm
     - Diameter: 11 mm
     - **Has two "bundles" named on the basis of tibial insertion:**
       - **Anteromedial: tight in flexion; primarily an anterior restraint; evaluated by Lachman and anterior drawer tests**
       - **Posterolateral: tight in extension; primarily a rotatory restraint; evaluated by pivot shift test**
     - Composition: 90% type I collagen and 10% type III collagen
     - Blood supply: Both cruciate ligaments receive their blood supply via branches of the middle geniculate artery and the fat pad.
     - Mechanoreceptor nerve fibers within the ACL have been found and may have a proprioceptive role.
   - Posterior cruciate ligament (PCL)
     - Femoral attachment: broad, crescent-shaped area on the anterolateral medial femoral condyle

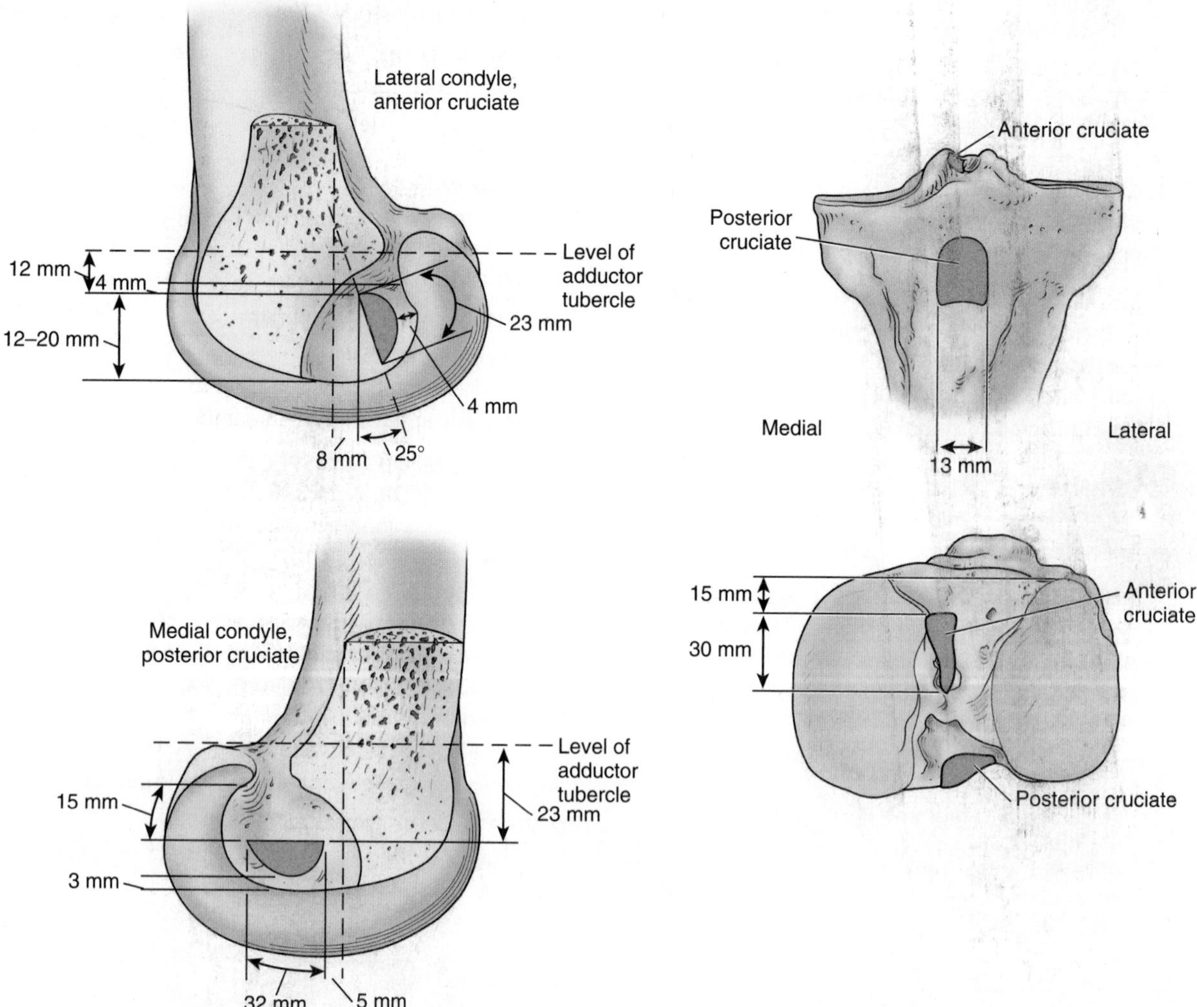

Figure 4-1 Origins and insertions of the anterior cruciate ligament and posterior cruciate ligament. (From Scott WN: *Insall & Scott surgery of the knee,* Philadelphia, 2006, Elsevier.)

- Tibial insertion: tibial sulcus below articular surface (see Figure 4-1)
- Length: 38 mm
- Diameter: 13 mm
- Two bundles:
  - Anterolateral: tight in flexion
  - Posteromedial: tight in extension
- Variable meniscofemoral ligaments originate from the posterior horn of the lateral meniscus and insert into the substance of the PCL.
  - Humphrey: anterior
  - Wrisberg: posterior
- Neurovascular supply is similar to that of the ACL.

- Medial collateral ligament (MCL)
  - Superficial and deep fibers
    - Superficial MCL (tibial collateral ligament)
      - Lies deep to the gracilis and semitendinosus tendons
      - Originates 3.2 mm proximal and 4.8 mm posterior from the medial femoral epicondyle
      - Inserts onto the periosteum of the proximal tibia, deep to the pes anserinus
      - Superficial fibers insert 61.2 mm distal to the knee joint.
      - Anterior fibers tighten during first 90 degrees of motion; posterior fibers tighten during extension.
    - Deep portion of the ligament (medial capsular ligament)
      - Capsular thickening that blends with superficial fibers
      - Intimately associated with the medial meniscus (coronary ligaments)
- Lateral collateral ligament (LCL); also known as the fibular collateral ligament
  - Cordlike structure
  - Origin: lateral femoral epicondyle
    - **Posterior and superior to the insertion of the popliteus tendon**
  - Insertion: anterolateral aspect of the fibular head
    - **Most anterior structure inserting on the proximal fibula**
  - Tight in extension and lax in flexion because of its location behind the axis of knee rotation
- Posteromedial corner
  - Deep and posterior to the superficial MCL, contiguous with the deep MCL
  - Important factor in rotary stability
  - The posteromedial corner has three components:
    - Capsular thickenings of the multiple insertions of the semimembranosus
    - Posterior oblique ligament, which originates on the adductor tubercle
    - Oblique popliteal ligament, or thickening of the posterior capsule
- Posterolateral corner (PLC)
  - Increasingly important factor in the treatment of the multiple ligament injured knee
  - The PLC has seven components:
    - Biceps femoris
    - Iliotibial band
    - Popliteus
      - Originates on the back of the tibia
      - **The femoral insertion is inferior, anterior, and deep to the LCL.**
      - Internally rotates the tibia
    - Popliteofibular ligament
    - Lateral capsule
    - Arcuate ligament (which is contiguous with the oblique popliteal ligament medially)
    - Fabellofibular ligament (lateral two are really just thickenings of the joint capsule)
  - **The PLC is the primary stabilizer of external tibial rotation.**

Table 4-1 Medial Structures of the Knee

Layer	Components
I	Sartorius and fascia
II	Superficial MCL, posterior oblique ligament, semimembranosus
III	Deep MCL, capsule

MCL, medial collateral ligament.
Note: The gracilis, semitendinosus, and saphenous nerves run between layers I and II.

4. Medial structures of the knee (three layers) (Table 4-1; Figure 4-2)
5. Lateral structures of the knee (three layers) (Table 4-2; see Figure 4-2)
   - **The order of insertion of structures on the proximal fibula is, from anterior to posterior, the LCL, the popliteofibular ligament, and the biceps femoris.**
6. Menisci
   - Crescent-shaped, fibrocartilagenous structures
   - Triangular in cross-section
   - Composed predominantly of type 1 collagen
   - Only the peripheral 20% to 30% of the medial meniscus and the peripheral 10% to 25% of the lateral meniscus are vascularized (medial and lateral genicular arteries, respectively; see Figure 4-1).
   - Medial meniscus is more C-shaped; lateral meniscus is more circular (see Figure 4-1).
   - Role: to deepen the articular surfaces of the tibial plateau and function in stability, lubrication, and joint nutrition
   - The two menisci are connected anteriorly by the transverse (intermeniscal) ligament.
   - They are attached peripherally by coronary ligaments.
   - The menisci move anteriorly in extension and posteriorly with flexion. **The lateral meniscus has fewer soft tissue attachments and is more mobile than the medial meniscus.**

Table 4-2 Lateral Structures of the Knee

Layer	Components
I	Iliotibial tract, biceps, fascia
II	Patellar retinaculum, patellofemoral ligament
III	Arcuate ligament, fabellofibular ligament, capsule, LCL

LCL, lateral collateral ligament.
Note: The inferior lateral geniculate artery is deep to the LCL and is at risk with aggressive meniscal resection.

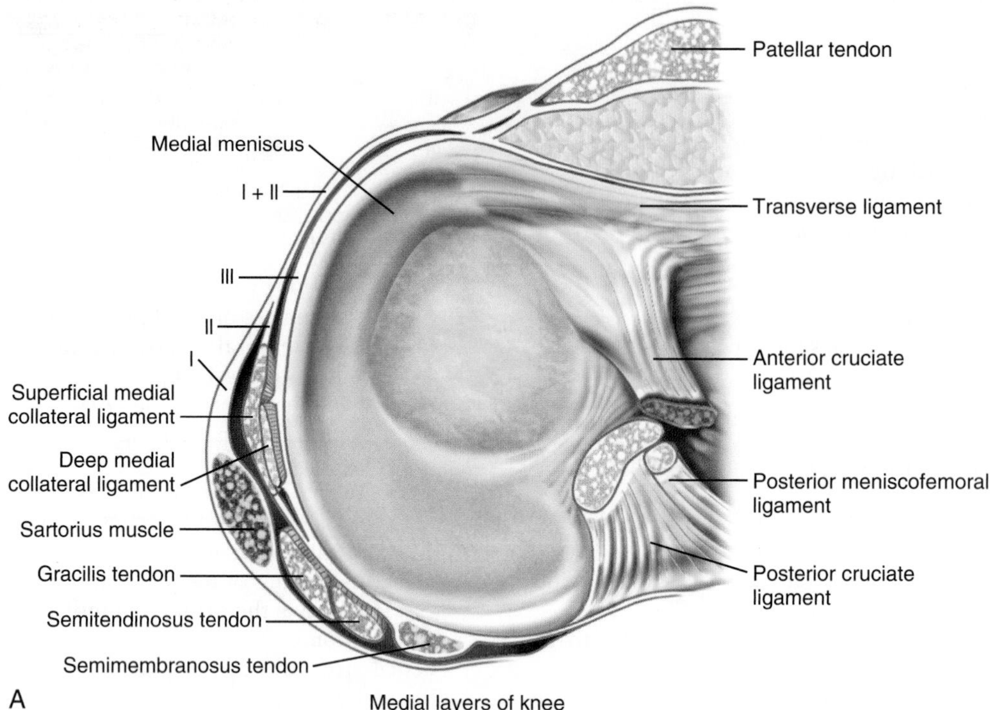

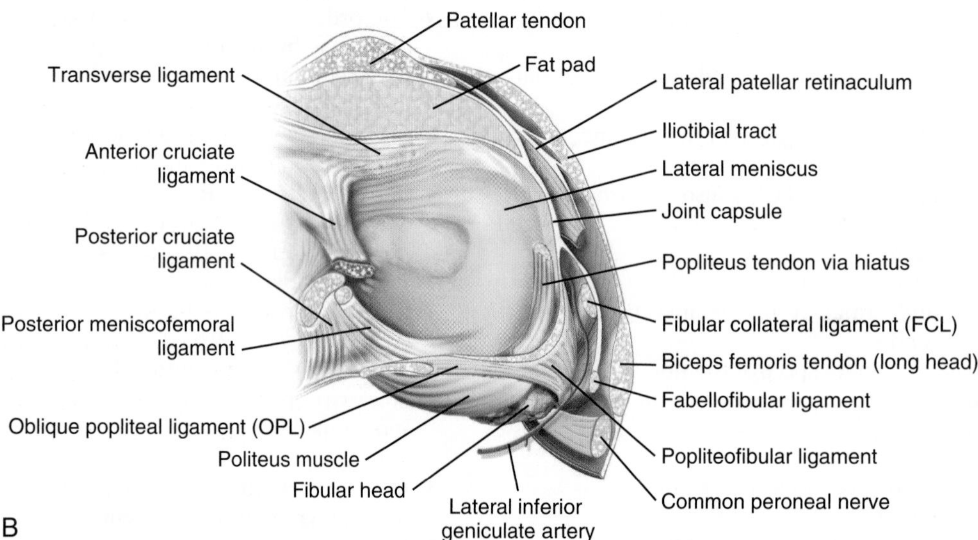

Figure 4-2 Medial and lateral supporting structures of the knee. **A,** Medial structures of the knee include the sartorius, its fascia, and the patellar retinaculum (layer I); the hamstring tendons and superficial medial collateral ligament (layer II); and the deep medial collateral ligament (layer III). **B,** Lateral structures of the knee include the iliotibial tract and biceps (layer I); the patellar retinaculum (layer II); and the capsule and lateral collateral ligament (layer III). (From Noyes FR: *Noyes' knee disorders,* Philadelphia, 2009, Elsevier.)

7. Joint relationships
   - Femoral condyles
     - Lateral
       - Greater anteroposterior dimensions than medial condyle
       - Relatively straight in comparison with medial condyle
       - Has a terminal sulcus and a groove of the popliteus insertion (Figure 4-3)
     - Medial
       - Anteroposterior dimensions are smaller than those of the lateral condyle.
       - Medial condyle is more curved (allowing medial tibial plateau to rotate externally in full extension: the "screw-home mechanism").
   - Patellofemoral joint
     - Articulation between the patella and femoral trochlea
     - Patella has variably sized medial and lateral facets.
     - Articular surface of the patella is the thickest in the body.

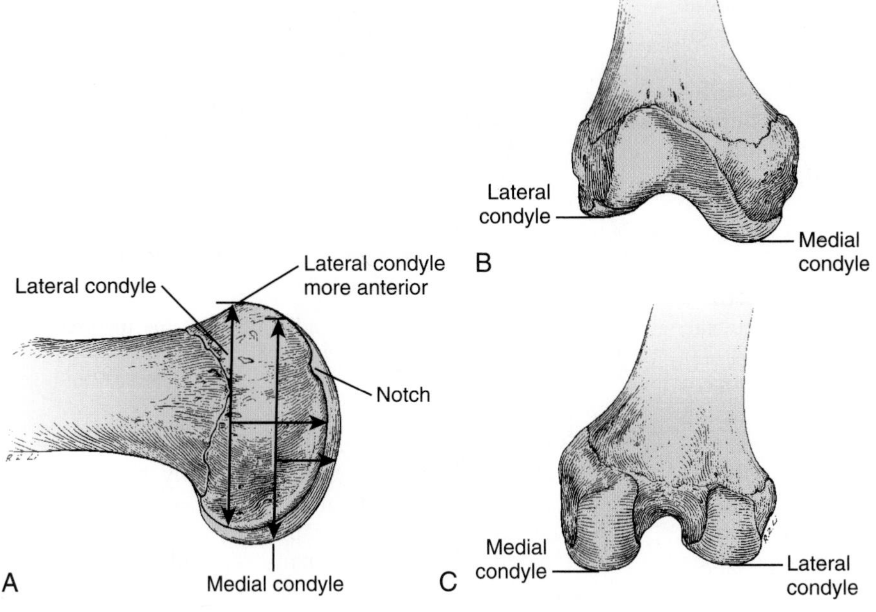

Figure 4-3 **Relationships of the femoral condyles. On the lateral projection (A), the lateral condyle projects more anteriorly and is notched. Anterior (B) and posterior (C) views demonstrate the difference in size and curvature of the medial femoral condyle.** (From Tria AJ, Klein KS: *An illustrated guide to the knee,* New York, 1992, Churchill Livingstone, p 5.)

- The patella can withstand forces several times those of body weight.
- The patella is restrained in trochlea by the valgus axis of the quadriceps mechanism (Q angle), the oblique fibers of the vastus medialis oblique and lateralis muscles (and their extensions, all of which constitute the patella retinaculum), the bony and cartilaginous anatomy of the trochlea, and the patellofemoral ligaments.
- The medial patellofemoral ligament is present in the second medial layer (Figure 4-4).

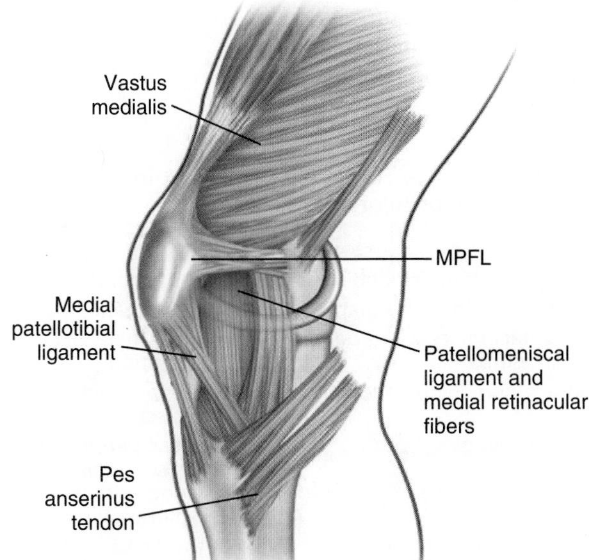

Figure 4-4 **Patellar restraints include the patellofemoral and patellotibial ligaments, as well as the oblique fibers of the vastus medialis oblique and lateralis muscles. MPFL, medial patellofemoral ligament.** (From Hunter RE, Sgaglione NA: *AANA advanced arthroscopy: the knee,* Philadelphia, 2010, Elsevier. Copyright © 2010 Arthroscopy Association of North America.)

  - Origin: **just anterior and distal to the adductor tubercle** or just superior to the origin of the superficial medial collateral ligament
  - Insertion: junction of proximal and middle third on the medial border of the patella as well as the undersurface of the vastus medialis oblique muscle
  - Role: to prevent lateral displacement of the patella, contributing more than 50% of the total medial restraint to lateral subluxation

B. Biomechanics

1. Ligamentous biomechanics: The role of the ligaments of the knee is to provide passive restraints against abnormal motion (Table 4-3).
2. Structural properties of ligaments: The **tensile strength** of a ligament, or maximal stress that a ligament can sustain before failure, has been characterized for all knee ligaments. However, it is important to consider age, ligament orientation, preparation of the specimen, and other factors before determining which graft to use.
   - ACL: approximately 2200 N and up to 2500 N in young individuals

Table 4-3 Biomechanics of Knee Ligaments

Ligament	Restraint
ACL	Minimizing anterior translation of the tibia in relation to the femur (85%)
PCL	Minimizing posterior tibial displacement (95%)
MCL	Minimizing valgus angulation
LCL	Minimizing varus angulation
MCL and LCL	Acting in concert with posterior structures to control axial rotation of the tibia on the femur
PCL and posterolateral corner	Acting synergistically to resist posterior translation and posterolateral rotary instability

ACL, anterior cruciate ligament; LCL, lateral collateral ligament; MCL, medial collateral ligament; PCL, posterior cruciate ligament.

- The tensile strength of a 10-mm patellar tendon graft (young specimen) is more than 2900 N and is about 30% stronger when it is rotated 90 degrees. However, this strength quickly diminishes in vivo.
- **Studies suggest that the quadrupled hamstring graft has even greater tensile strength but is dependent on graft fixation.**
- PCL: approximately 2500 to 3000 N, but this has been disputed
- MCL: approximately 5000 N
- LCL: approximately 750 N

3. Kinematics: The motion of the knee joint and interplay of ligaments have been described as a four-bar cruciate linkage system (Figure 4-5).
   - As the knee flexes, the center of joint rotation (intersection of the cruciate ligaments) moves posteriorly, causing rolling and gliding at the articulating surfaces.
   - The concept of ligament "isometry" remains controversial.
     - Reconstructed ligaments should approximate normal anatomy and lie within the flexion axis in all positions of knee motion.
     - As the joint flexes, ligaments anterior to the flexion axis stretch, and ligaments posterior to the axis shorten.
     - Although many instruments have been designed to achieve isometry, other considerations, such as graft impingement and avoiding flexion contractures, may be of more importance for ligament reconstructions.
4. Meniscal biomechanics:
   - The collagen fibers of the menisci are arranged radially and longitudinally (Figure 4-6).
     - The longitudinal fibers help dissipate the hoop stresses in the menisci.
     - The combination of fibers allows the meniscus to expand under compressive forces and increase the contact area of the joint.
   - The lateral meniscus has twice the excursion of the medial meniscus during range of motion (ROM) and rotation of the knee.

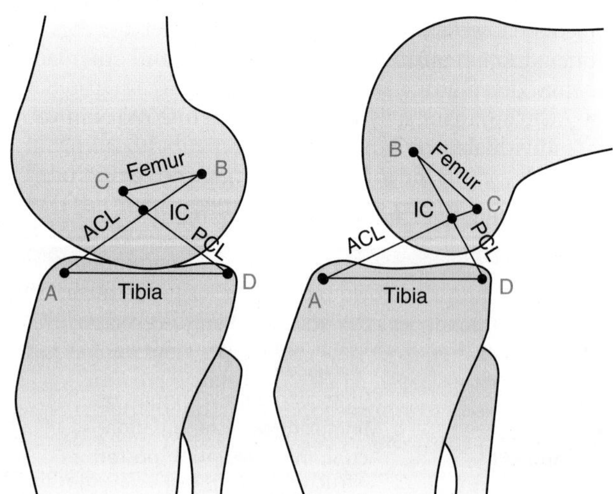

Figure 4-5 **The four-bar linkage system consists of the anterior cruciate ligament (ACL)** ***(bar AB),*** **the posterior cruciate ligament (PCL)** ***(bar CD),*** **the femoral link** ***(bar CB),*** **and the tibial link** ***(bar AD). IC*** **represents the intersection of the cruciate ligaments.** (From DeLee JC, Drez D Jr, Miller MD, editors: *DeLee and Drez's orthopaedic sports medicine: principles and practice,* ed 3, Philadelphia, 2009, WB Saunders.)

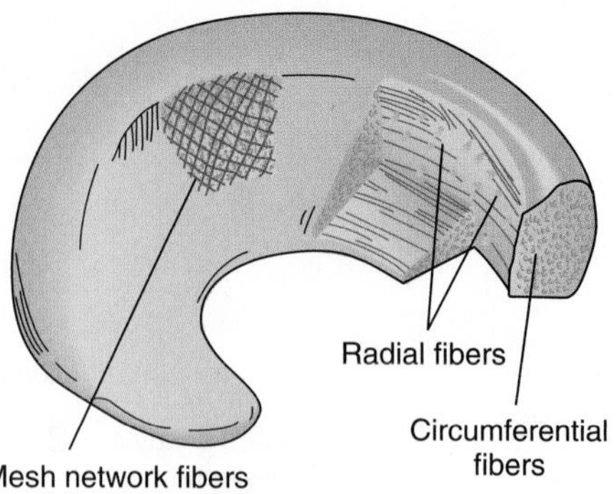

Figure 4-6 **Longitudinal and radial fibers of the menisci.** (From Bullough PG, et al: The strength of the menisci of the knee as it relates to their fine structure, *J Bone Joint Surg Br* 52:564–567, 1970.)

   - Studies have shown that an ACL deficiency may result in abnormal meniscal strain, particularly in the posterior horn of the medial meniscus (Figure 4-7).
   - Mensical root tears completely disrupt the circumferential fibers of the meniscus, leading to meniscal extrusion.
   - Biomechanical studies have shown similar load patterns between posterior root tear and complete meniscectomy.
5. Patellofemoral joint:
   - Must withstand forces more than three times those of body weight
   - Main restraint to lateral displacement is the medial patellofemoral ligament (50% of total restraint).

II. DIAGNOSTIC TECHNIQUES

A. History

1. Complete history of the injury
2. Clarification of mechanism of injury
3. Patient's age
4. Important key historical points (Table 4-4)

B. Physical examination

1. Key examination points are shown in Table 4-5.

Table 4-4 **Key Historical Points That Indicate Mechanism of Injury**

History	Significance
Pain after sitting or climbing stairs	Patellofemoral cause
Locking or pain with squatting	Meniscal tear
Noncontact injury with "popping" sound/sensation	ACL tear, patellar dislocation
Contact injury with "popping" sound	Collateral ligament tear, meniscal tear, fracture
Acute swelling	ACL tear, peripheral meniscal tear, osteochondral fracture, capsule tear
Knee "gives way"	Ligamentous laxity, patellar instability
Anterior force: **dorsiflexed foot**	Patellar injury
Anterior force: **plantar-flexed foot**	PCL injury
Dashboard injury	PCL or patellar injury
Hyperextension, varus angulation, and tibial external rotation	Posterolateral corner injury

ACL, anterior cruciate ligament; PCL, posterior cruciate ligament.

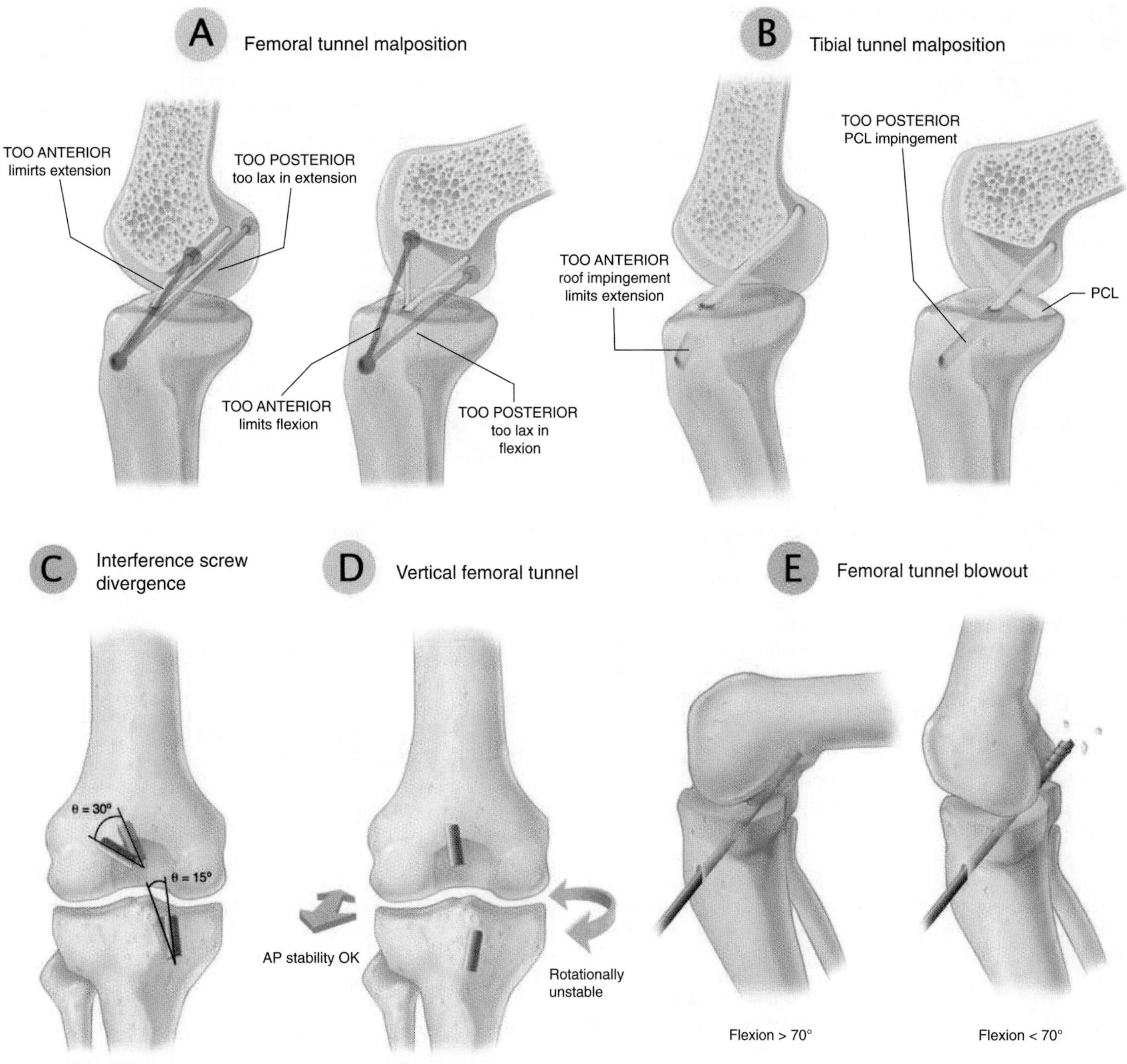

Figure 4-7 Common complications of ACL reconstruction. AP, anteroposterior.

- **Most common causes of an acute hemarthrosis: ACL tear (70%), patella dislocation, osteochondral fracture, and isolated meniscal tear**

2. Examination performed with the patient under anesthesia may be helpful in some cases.

C. **Instrumented measurement of knee laxity**

1. KT-1000 and KT-2000 Knee Ligament Arthrometers (MEDmetric, San Diego, California) are the devices most commonly used for standardized laxity measurement.
   - ACL laxity is measured with the knee in slight flexion (20 to 30 degrees) with the application of a standard force (30 pounds [13.6 kg]).
   - Values are reported as millimeters of anterior displacement, with comparisons with the opposite (normal) side.
   - A difference of more than 3 mm between sides is considered significant.
   - PCL laxity can also be measured with this device, although it is less accurate.

D. **Imaging the knee**

1. Standard radiographs:
   - Anteroposterior view
   - Weight-bearing 45-degree posteroanterior view
     - **Most sensitive view for revealing early osteoarthrosis**
   - Lateral view
   - Merchant or Laurin view of the patella
   - Additional views include long-cassette, lower extremity hip-to-ankle views; oblique views; stress radiographs.
   - Several findings and their significance are listed in Table 4-6.
   - Normal bony anatomy is demonstrated in Figure 4-8, *A*. Many of these findings are illustrated in Figure 4-8, *B*.
   - Evaluation of patella height is accomplished by one of three commonly used methods (see Figure 4-8, *C*).

Table 4-5 Knee: Key Examination Points

Examination or Test	Method or Appearance	Significance
Standing and gait deformity	Observe gait	Based on pathologic process
	Observe patient standing	Based on pathologic process; check valgus/varus deformity
Effusion	Patella: balloting/milking	Ligament/meniscal injury (acute), arthritis (chronic)
Point of maximal tenderness	Palpate for tenderness	Based on location (joint line tenderness indicates meniscal tear)
ROM	Active and passive	Block indicates meniscal (bucket handle) injury, loose body, impingement of ACL tear
Patellar crepitus	Passive ROM	Patellofemoral pathologic process
Patellar grind	Push patella with quadriceps contraction	Patellofemoral pathologic process
Patellar apprehension	Push patella laterally at 20 to 30 degrees of flexion	Patellar subluxation or dislocation
Q angle	ASIS–patella–tibial tubercle	Increased with patellar malalignment (normal <15 degrees); most pronounced in flexion
Flexion Q angle	ASIS–patella–tibial tubercle	Increased with patellar malalignment
J sign	Lateral deviation of the patella in extension	Patella instability
Patellar tilt	Tilt up laterally	>15 degrees indicates laxity; <0 degrees indicates tight lateral constraint
Patellar glide	Push patella laterally at 20 to 30 degrees of flexion	>50 degrees indicates increased medial constraint laxity
Active glide	Lateral excursion with quadriceps contraction	Lateral excursion > proximate excursion indicates increased functional Q angle of quadriceps
Quadriceps circumference	10 cm (VMO), 15 cm (quadriceps)	Atrophy from inactivity
Symmetric extension	Difference in distance of back of knee from ground or in prone heel height	Contracture, displaced meniscal tear, or other mechanical block
Varus/valgus stress	Laxity of 30 degrees	MCL/LCL laxity (grade I: opening = 1 to 5 mm; grade II: opening = 6 to 10 mm; grade III [complete]: opening >10 mm)
	Deformity of 0 degrees	MCL/LCL and PCL laxity
Apley	Prone-flexion compression	DJD, meniscal disease
Lachman	Tibia forward at 30 degrees of flexion	ACL injury (most sensitive test)
Finacetto	Lachman test with tibia subluxation beyond posterior horns of menisci	ACL injury (severe)
Anterior drawer	Tibia forward at 90 degrees of flexion	ACL injury
Internal-rotation drawer	Foot internally rotated with drawer	Tighter is normal; looser indicates ACL injury
External-rotation drawer	Foot externally rotated with drawer	Loose is normal; looser indicates ACL/MCL injury
McMurray	Internal and external tibial rotation while moving from a starting point of maximal flexion into extension of the knee	Meniscal pathologic process
Pivot shift*	Flexion with internal rotation and valgus angulation	ACL injury
Pivot jerk*	Extension with internal rotation and valgus angulation	ACL injury
Posterior drawer	Tibia backward at 90 degrees of flexion	PCL injury
Tibial sag	Flex 90 degrees, observe	PCL injury
90-degree quadriceps active test	Extend flexed knee	PCL injury
Asymmetric external rotation	"Dial" feet externally at 30 and 90 degrees of flexion	Asymmetric increased external rotation of >10 to 15 degrees indicates injury of posterolateral corner if difference is 30 degrees only; difference at both 30 and 90 degrees indicates injury of PCL and posterolateral corner
External rotation recurvatum	Pick up great toes	PCL injury
Reversed pivot	Extension with external rotation and valgus	PCL injury
Posterolateral drawer	Posterior drawer, lateral > medial	PCL injury

*Examination performed with the patient under anesthesia.

ACL, anterior cruciate ligament; ASIS, anterior superior iliac spine; DJD, degenerative joint disease; LCL, lateral collateral ligament; MCL, medial collateral ligament; PCL, posterior cruciate ligament; ROM; range of motion; VMO, vastus medialis oblique muscle.

Table 4-6 Knee Injuries: Radiographic Findings

View/Sign	Findings	Significance
Lateral-high patella	Patella alta	Patellofemoral pathologic process
Congruence angle	$\mu = -6$ degrees; SD = 11 degrees	Patellofemoral pathologic process
Tooth sign	Irregular anterior patella	Patellofemoral chondrosis
Varus/valgus stress view	Opening	Collateral ligament injury; Salter-Harris fracture
Lateral capsule (Segond) sign	Small tibial avulsion off lateral tibia	ACL tear
Pellegrini-Stieda lesion	Avulsion of medial femoral condyle	Chronic MCL injury
Lateral-stress view: stress to anterior tibia with knee flexed 70 degrees	Asymmetric posterior tibial displacement	PCL injury
Weight-bearing posteroanterior view flexion		Early DJD, OCD, notch evaluation
Fairbank changes	Square condyle, peak eminences, ridging, narrowing	Early DJD (postmeniscectomy)
Square lateral condyle	Thickened joint space	Discoid meniscus

ACL, anterior cruciate ligament; DJD, degenerative joint disease; MCL, medial collateral ligament; OCD, osteochondral dissecans; PCL, posterior cruciate ligament; SD, standard deviation.

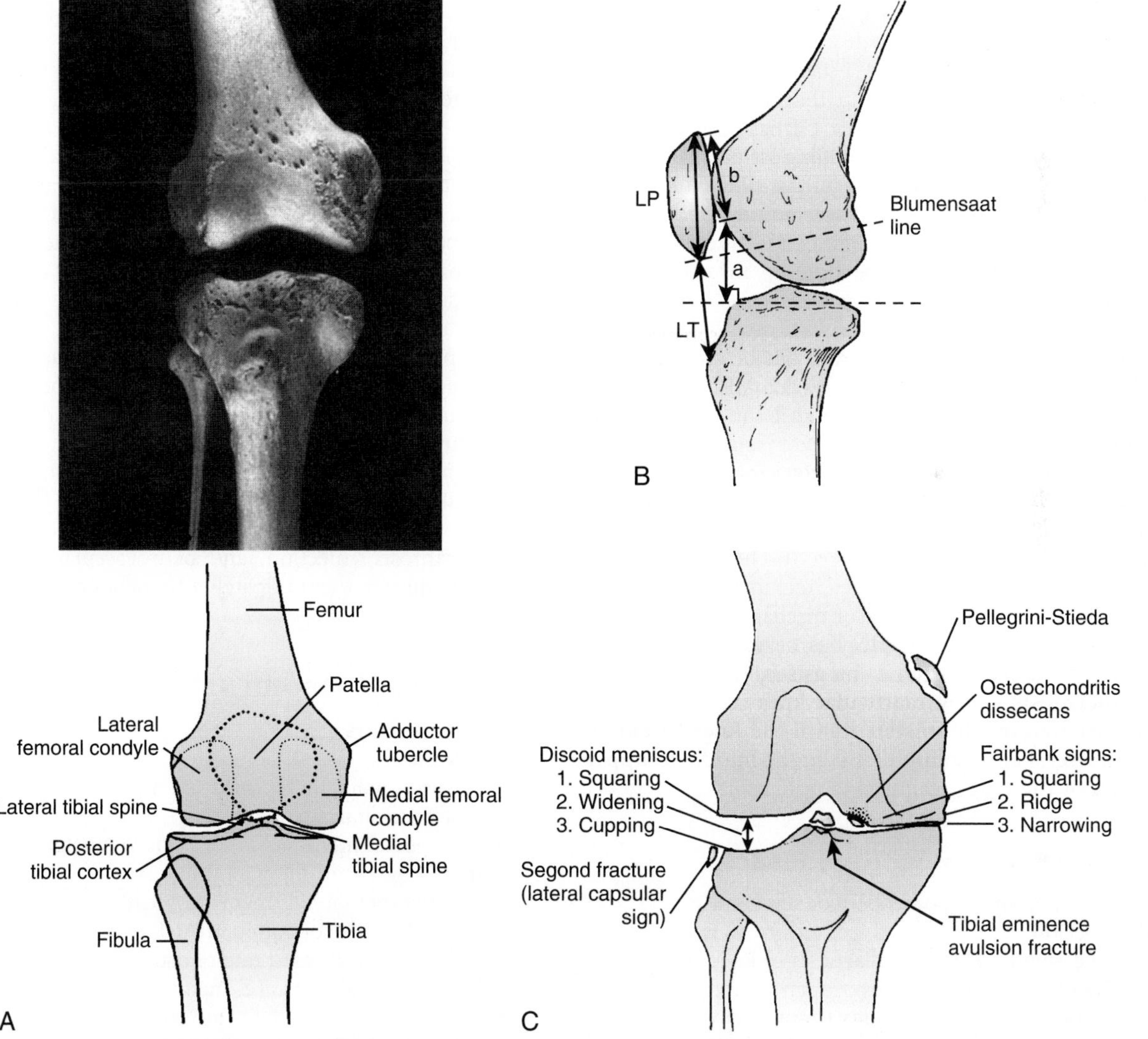

Figure 4-8 **A,** Anterior view *(top)* and drawing *(bottom)* demonstrating the bones of the knee. **B,** Three popular methods for evaluating patella alta and baja: *(1)* Blumensaat line: When the knee is flexed 30 degrees, the lower border of the patella should lie on a line extended from the intercondylar notch. *(2)* Insall-Salvati index: Ratio, or index, of patella tendon length *(LT)* to patella length *(LP)* should be 1.0. An index of 1.2 characterizes patella alta, and 0.8 characterizes patella baja. *(3)* Blackburne-Peel index: Ratio of the distance from the tibial plateau to the inferior articular surface of the patella *(a)* to the length of the articular surface of the patella *(b)* should be 0.8. An index of 1.0 characterizes alta patella. **C,** Common radiographic abnormalities. (**A** from Weissman BNW, Sledge CB: *Orthopedic radiology,* Philadelphia, 1986, WB Saunders, p 498. **B** from Harner CD, Miller MD, Irrgang JJ: Management of the stiff knee after trauma and ligament reconstruction. In Siliski JM, editor: *Traumatic disorders of the knee,* New York, 1994, Springer-Verlag, p 364.)

2. Stress radiographs: These are useful for evaluating injuries to the femoral physis (to differentiate from MCL injury) and are becoming the "gold standard" in diagnosing and quantifying PCL injury. They can also be used to evaluate LCL and PLC injuries.
3. Nuclear imaging: Technetium-99m bone scans are useful in diagnosing stress fractures, early degenerative joint disease, and complex regional pain syndrome.
4. Magnetic resonance imaging (MRI): This has become the imaging modality of choice for diagnosis of ligament injuries, meniscal disease, avascular necrosis, spontaneous osteonecrosis of the knee, and articular cartilage defects and has replaced the use of arthrography. On coronal MRI sequences, meniscal root tears are seen as a band of low-signal fibrocartilage. **Occult fractures of the knee can be identified by a double fluid-fluid layer, which signifies lipohemarthrosis.**
5. Magnetic resonance arthrography: Intraarticular magnetic resonance arthrography is the most accurate imaging method for confirming the diagnosis of repeated meniscal tears after repair.
6. Computed tomography (CT): CT has been replaced largely by MRI, but it is still useful in the evaluation of bony tumors, patellar tilt, and fractures. CT has been advocated as a tool to assist in operative planning for patellar realignment by allowing measurement of the tibial tuberosity–trochlear groove (TT-TG) distance; authors recommend distal realignment procedures for a TT-TG distance exceeding 20 mm. MRI can also be used to measure TT-TG distance.
7. Arthrography: This technique was useful historically for the diagnosis of MCL tears and has been supplanted by MRI. However, it can be useful when MRI is not available or tolerated by the patient, and it can be combined with CT.
8. Tomography: Tomograms are preferred to CT in the evaluation of tibial plateau fractures at some medical centers.
9. Ultrasonography: This technique is useful for detecting soft tissue lesions about the knee, including patellar tendinitis, hematomas, and extensor mechanism ruptures, in some centers. Ultrasonography has begun to be used to evaluate meniscal tears but is not as sensitive as MRI.

E. Arthrocentesis and intraarticular knee injection

1. **Most accurately administered with the knee in extension; a lateral entry point that is in the middle to upper portion of the patella is used**

III. KNEE ARTHROSCOPY

See Supplemental Images on expertconsult.com.

A. Introduction

1. The "gold standard" for the diagnosis of knee disease
2. The benefits of arthroscopic over open techniques include smaller incisions, less morbidity, improved visualization, and decreased recovery time.

B. Portals

1. Standard portals
   - Superomedial and superolateral outflow portals
     - Made with the knee in extension but may not be necessary with newer pump systems
   - Inferomedial and inferolateral portals
     - Made with the knee in flexion; for instrument placement and the arthroscope, respectively (Figure 4-9)
2. Accessory portals, sometimes helpful for visualizing the posterior horns of the menisci and PCL
   - Posteromedial portal: 1 cm above the joint line behind the MCL (be careful to avoid saphenous nerve branches)
   - Posterolateral portal: 1 cm above the joint line between the LCL and biceps tendon (avoiding the common peroneal nerve)
   - Transpatellar portal: 1 cm distal to the patella, splitting the patellar tendon fibers; can be used for central viewing or grabbing but should be avoided in patients who require subsequent harvesting of autogenous patellar tendon
3. Less commonly used portals
   - Medial and lateral midpatellar portals
   - Proximal superomedial and superolateral portals (4 cm proximal to the patella)
     - Used for patellofemoral compartment visualization
   - Far medial and far lateral portals
     - Used for accessory instrument placement (loose-body removal)

C. Technique

1. Each knee arthroscopy should include an evaluation of the suprapatellar pouch; patellofemoral joint and tracking; medial and lateral gutters; medial compartment, including the medial meniscus and the articular surface; the lateral compartment, including the lateral meniscus and the articular surface; and the intercondylar notch to visualize the ACL and PCL.
2. The posteromedial corner can be best visualized with a 70-degree arthroscope placed through the notch (modified Gillquist view) or a posteromedial portal.

D. Arthroscopic complications

1. The most common arthroscopic complication is iatrogenic articular cartilage damage.
2. Additional complications include instrument breakage, hemarthrosis, infection, and neurovascular injury, especially injury to the infrapatellar branches of the saphenous nerve.

IV. MENISCAL INJURIES

A. Meniscal tears

1. Overview
   - Meniscal tears are the most common injury to the knee that necessitates surgery.
   - The medial meniscus is torn approximately three times more often than the lateral meniscus.
     - However, lateral meniscus tears occur more commonly with concomitant ACL tear.
   - There is an increased rate of osteoarthritis in knees after both meniscal tears and meniscectomy.
   - Traumatic meniscal tears are common in young patients with sports-related injuries.
   - Degenerative tears usually occur in older patients and can have an insidious onset.
   - Meniscal tears can be classified according to their location in relation to the vascular supply, their position (anterior, middle, or posterior third), and their appearance and orientation (Figure 4-10).

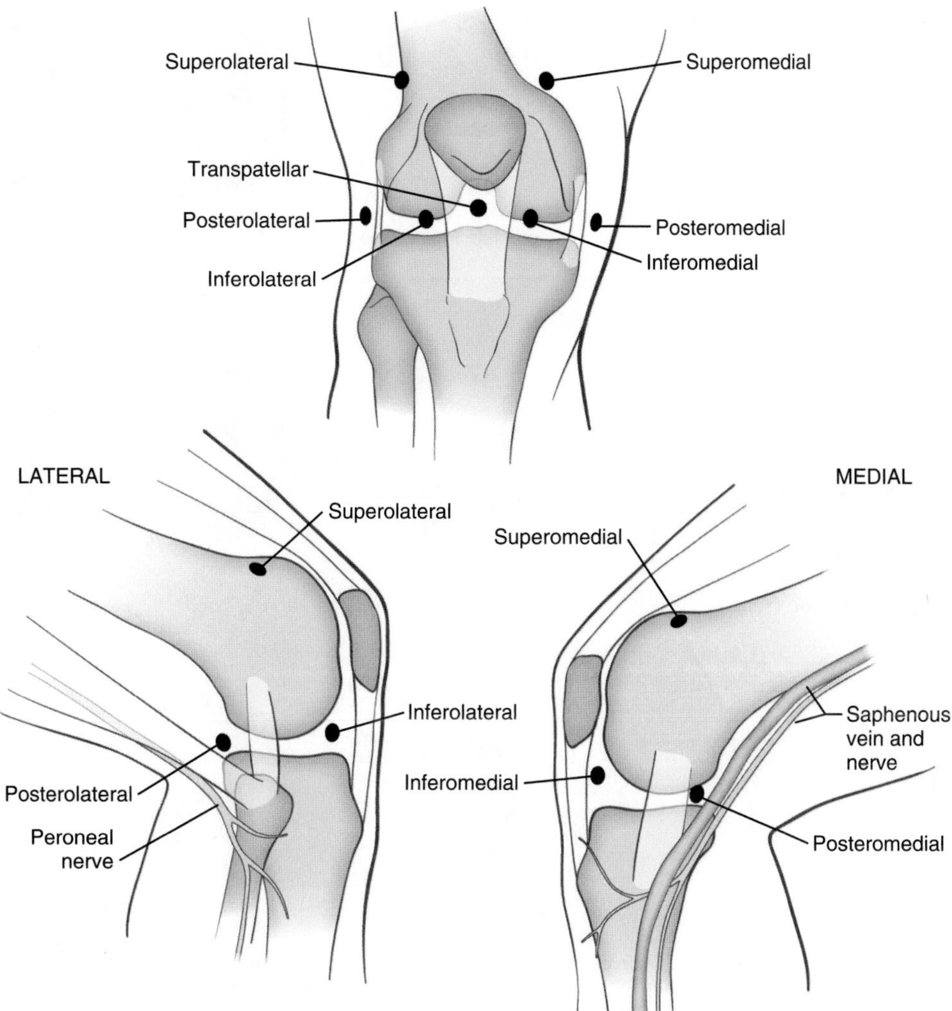

Figure 4-9 Knee arthroscopy portals. (From Miller MD, et al: *Orthopaedic surgical approaches,* Philadelphia, 2008, Elsevier.)

  - Meniscal root tears completely disrupt the circumferential fibers of the meniscus and can lead to meniscal extrusion.
- **The vascular supply of the meniscus is a primary determinant of healing potential.**
  - **Tears in the peripheral third have the highest potential for healing (Figure 4-11).**

2. Treatment
   - In the absence of intermittent swelling, catching, locking, or giving way, meniscal tears—particularly those degenerative in nature—may be treated conservatively.
   - Younger patients with acute tears, patients with tears causing mechanical symptoms, and patients with tears that fail to improve with conservative measures may benefit from operative treatment.
     - Partial meniscectomy:
       - Tears that are not amenable to repair (e.g., peripheral, longitudinal tears)—excluding those that do not necessitate any treatment (e.g., partial-thickness tears, those <5 to 10 mm in length, and those that cannot be displaced >1 to 2 mm)—are best treated by partial meniscectomy.
       - In general, complex, degenerative, and central/radial tears are treated with resection of a minimal amount of normal meniscus. A motorized shaver is helpful for creating a smooth transition zone.
       - The role of lasers or other devices for this purpose is still under investigation. There is concern about possible iatrogenic chondral injury caused by lasers and other thermal devices.
     - Meniscal repair:
       - Should be done for all peripheral longitudinal tears, especially in young patients and in conjunction with an ACL reconstruction
       - Augmentation techniques (fibrin clot, vascular access channels, synovial rasping) may extend the indications for repair.
       - Four techniques are commonly used: open, "outside-in," "inside-out," and "all-inside" (Figure 4-12).
       - Newer techniques for all-inside repairs (e.g., arrows, darts, staples, screws) are popular because of their ease of use; however, they are probably not as reliable as vertical mattress sutures.
       - The latest generation of "all-inside" devices allows tensioning of the construct.
       - **The "gold standard" for meniscal repair remains the inside-out technique with vertical mattress sutures.**

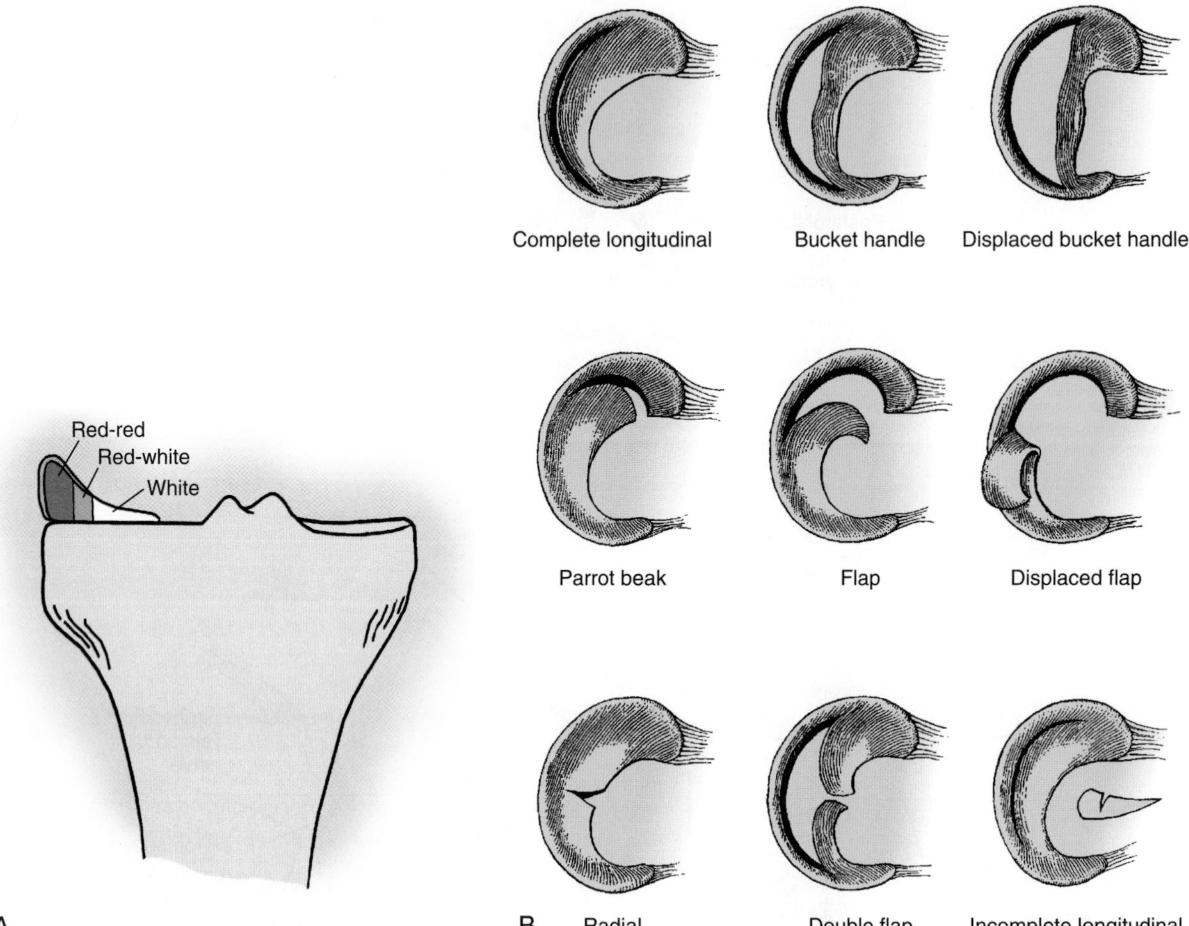

Figure 4-10 Classification of meniscal tears. **A,** Vascular zones. The red zone has the highest potential for meniscal healing, and the white zone has essentially no potential for healing without enhancement. **B,** Common appearances and orientations of meniscal tears. (**A** modified from Miller MD, Warner JJP, Harner CD: Meniscal repair. In Fu FH, Harner CD, Vince KG, editors: *Knee surgery,* Baltimore, 1994, Williams & Wilkins. **B** from Tria AJ, Klein KS: *An illustrated guide to the knee,* New York, 1992, Churchill Livingstone, p 616.)

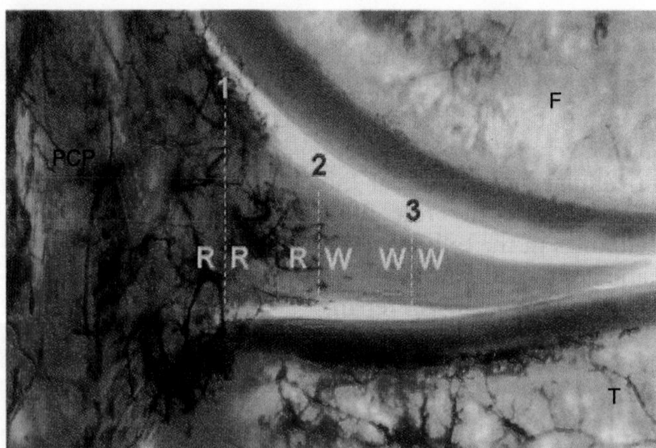

Figure 4-11 Three zones of meniscal vascularity are shown: *1,* RR (red-red) is fully within vascular area; *2,* RW (red-white) is at border of vascular area; and *3,* WW (white-white) is within avascular area. (From Canale ST, Beaty JH: *Campbell's operative orthopaedics,* ed 11, Philadelphia, 2008, Elsevier.)

- **Regardless of the technique used, it is essential to protect the saphenous nerve branches (anterior to both the semitendinosis and gracilis muscles and posterior to the inferior border of the sartorius muscle) during medial repairs and to protect the peroneal nerve (posterior to the biceps femoris) during lateral repairs (Figure 4-13).**

- Results of meniscal repair
  - In several studies, 80% to 90% success rates with meniscal repairs have been reported. However, success depends on location, type of tear, and chronicity.
  - It is generally accepted that the results of meniscal repair are best with acute peripheral tears in young patients with concurrent ACL reconstruction.
  - In general, success rates are 90% when meniscal repair is performed in conjunction with an ACL reconstruction, 60% with a repair in which the ACL is intact, and 30% with a repair in which the ACL is deficient.

B. **Meniscal cysts**

1. Occur primarily in conjunction with horizontal cleavage tears of the lateral meniscus (Figure 4-14)
2. Operative treatment consisting of arthroscopic partial meniscectomy and decompression through the tear (sometimes including "needling" of the cyst) has been shown to be effective.

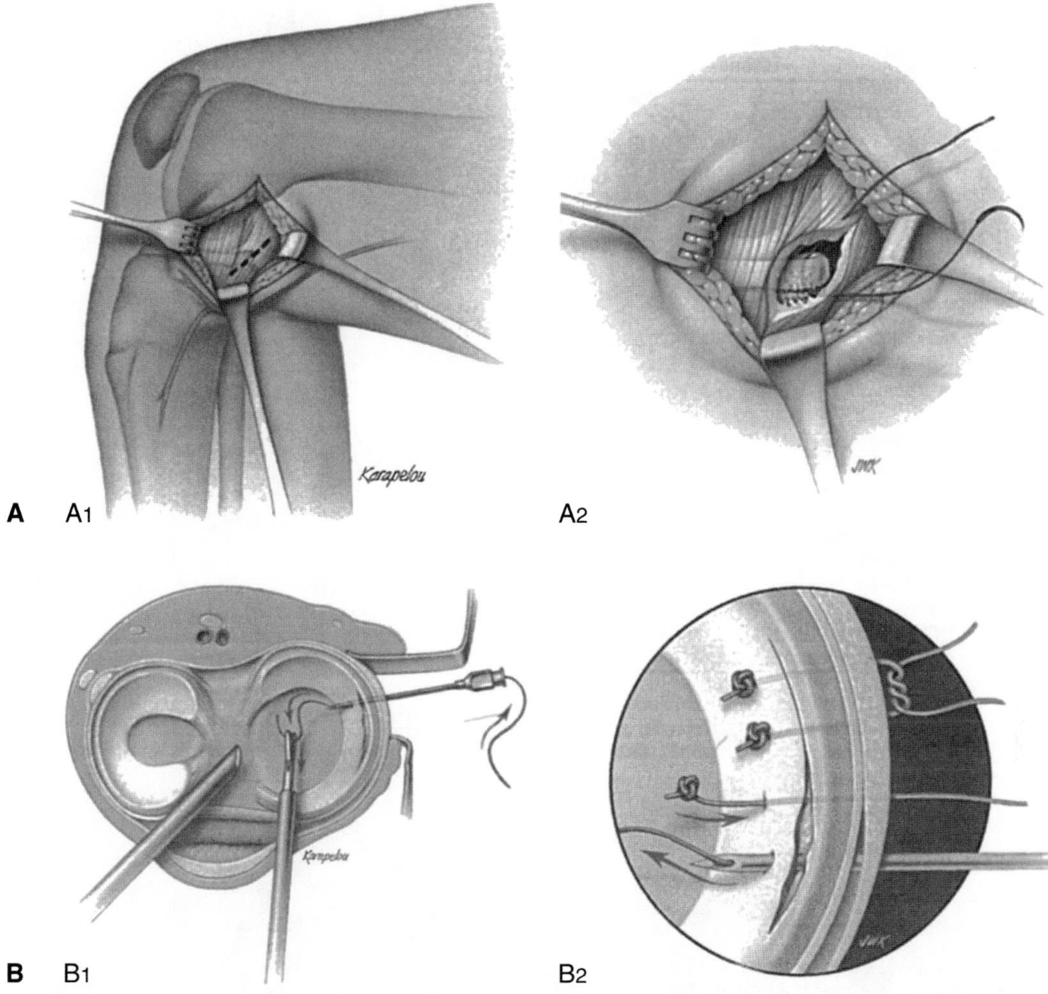

Figure 4-12 Meniscal repair techniques. **A,** Open repair of the medial meniscus (right knee). *A1* shows superficial dissection. *A2* shows suture passage. **B,** "Outside-in" repair of the medial meniscus (right knee). *B1* and *B2* show "outside-in" suture passage and knot tying.

Continued

3. En bloc excision is no longer favored for most meniscal cysts.
4. Popliteal (Baker) cysts are commonly related to meniscal disorders and usually resolve with treatment of the primary disorder.
   - Usually located between the semimembranosus and medial head of the gastrocnemius

C. **Discoid menisci ("popping knee syndrome")**

1. Can be classified as (I) incomplete, (II) complete, or (III) the Wrisberg variant (Figure 4-15).
2. Patients may develop mechanical symptoms, or "popping," with the knee in extension.
3. Plain radiographs may demonstrate a widened joint space, squaring of the lateral femoral condyle, cupping of the lateral tibial plateau, and a hypoplastic lateral intercondylar spine.
4. Appearance of a contiguous lateral meniscus on three consecutive sagittal images on MRI is diagnostic; MRI may also demonstrate associated tears. Treatment includes partial meniscectomy (saucerization) for tears, meniscal repair for peripheral detachments (Wrisberg variant), and simple observation for discoid menisci without tears.

D. **Meniscal transplantation**

1. Remains controversial but may be indicated for young patients who have had near-total meniscectomy (especially lateral meniscectomy) and who have early symptomatic chondrosis
2. **Relative contraindications include diffuse grades III and IV chondral lesions, so-called kissing lesions (chondral lesions adjacent to each other on the femur and tibia), advanced age of patient, and joint space narrowing.**
3. ACL deficiency, as well as limb alignment, must be addressed to increase the success rates of meniscal transplantation.
4. **Graft size accurate to within 5% of the native meniscus is crucial for success.**
5. Pain relief is the most consistent benefit; most studies have short-term to 5-year data available.
6. Three-phase bone scans can be used diagnostically in patients who fit inclusion criteria to help determine whether they are good surgical candidates. Allograft tissue needs to be appropriately sized and is typically harvested with a sterile technique, appropriately screened, and frozen.
7. Techniques for implantation include the use of individual bone plugs for the anterior and posterior horns and the use of a bone bridge, especially laterally.

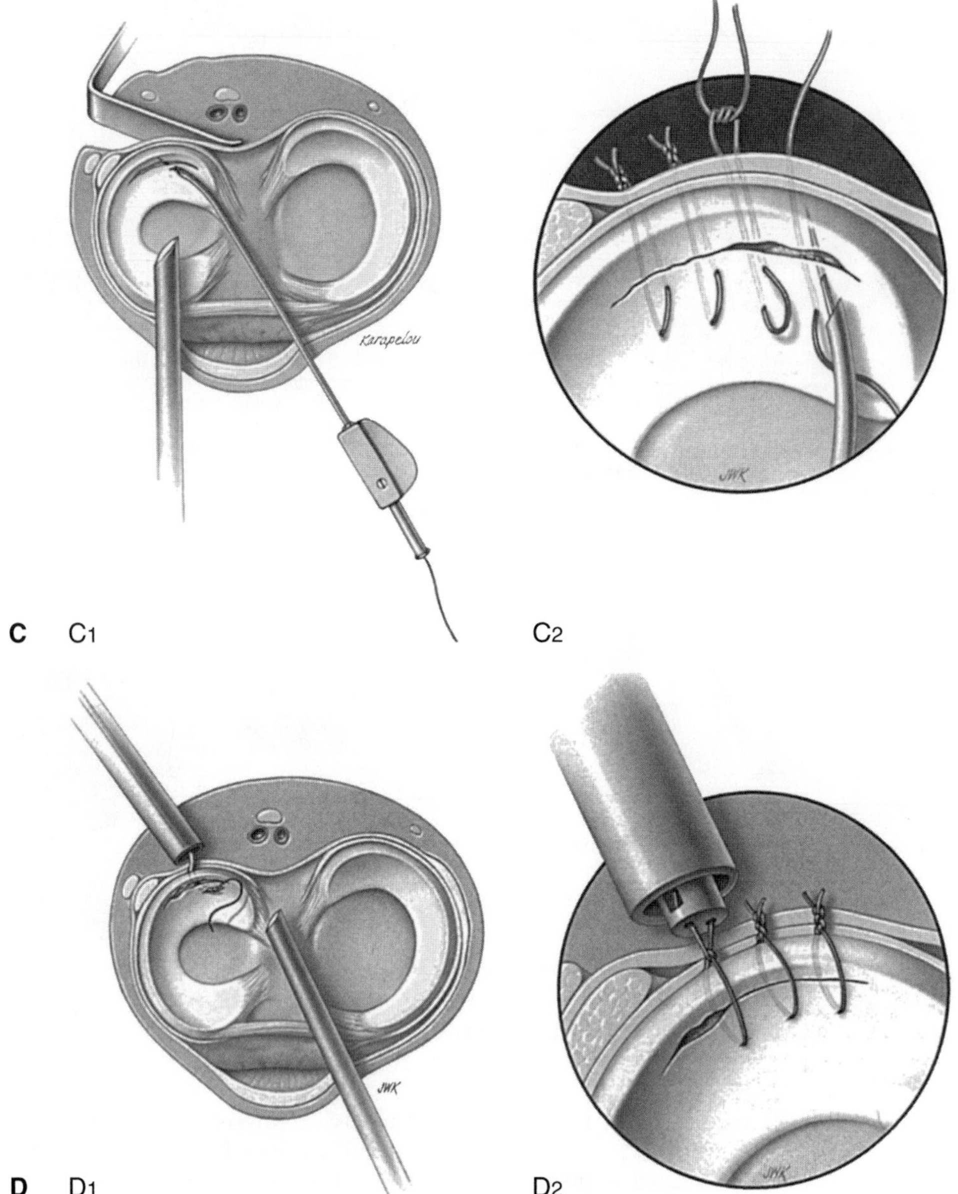

Figure 4-12, cont'd **C,** "Inside-out" repair of the lateral meniscus (right knee). *C1* shows "inside-out" repair of the lateral meniscus. *C2* shows a magnified view. **D,** Traditional "all-inside" repair of the lateral meniscus (right knee) (*D1* and *D2*). (From Miller MD: Atlas of meniscal repair, *Op Tech Orthop* 5:70–71, 1995.)

8. Collagen meniscal implantation has yielded promising initial results for irreparable medial meniscal tears with new meniscus-like matrix formation, in comparison with partial meniscectomy. However, long-term results, especially by independent sources, have not been reported.

V. LIGAMENT INJURIES

A. ACL injury

1. Introduction
   - Controversy continues with regard to the development of late arthritis in ACL-deficient versus reconstructed knees.
   - Chronic ACL deficiency is associated with a higher incidence of complex meniscal tears not amenable to repair and chondral injury.
   - **Bone bruises (trabecular microfractures) occur in more than half of acute ACL injuries.**
     - **Bone bruises are typically located near the sulcus terminalis on the lateral femoral condyle and the posterolateral aspect of the tibia.**
     - Although the long-term significance of these injuries is unknown, they may be related to late cartilage degeneration.
   - Treatment decisions should be individualized on the basis of age, activity level, instability, associated injuries, and other medical factors (Figure 4-16).
   - **The ACL injury rate is higher in women than in men.**
     - **This higher rate is thought to occur because women have smaller notches, smaller ligaments,**

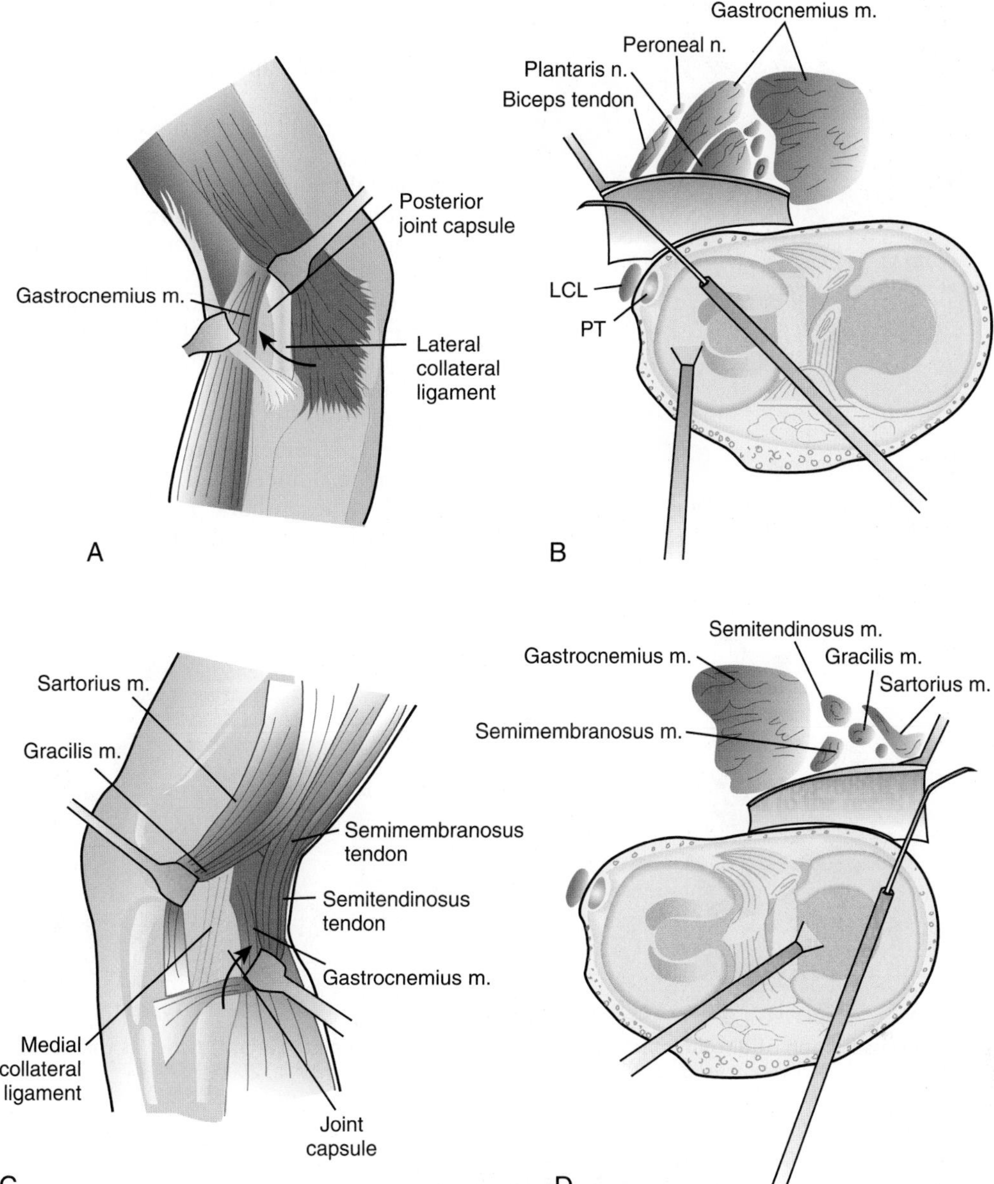

Figure 4-13 Incisions for meniscal repair must be planned to allow for retraction and protection of the saphenous nerve branches during medial meniscal repairs **(A, B)** and the peroneal nerve during lateral meniscal repairs **(C, D)**. LCL, lateral collateral ligament; PT, patellar tendon. (From DeLee JC, Drez D, Miller MD, editors: *DeLee and Drez's orthopaedic sports medicine,* ed 3, Philadelphia, 2009, Elsevier.)

increased generalized ligament laxity, increased knee laxity, and different landing biomechanics.
   - **In landing, women have a greater total valgus knee loading.**
- The in situ force of the ACL is highest at 30 degrees of flexion in response to anterior tibial load.
- **ACL injury prevention programs emphasize proprioceptive training and the strengthening of knee flexors.**

2. History and physical examination
   - ACL injuries are often the result of noncontact pivoting injuries.
   - They are commonly associated with an audible "pop" and an immediate hemarthrosis.
   - Associated injuries, including meniscal tears (75%), are common.
     - Acute lateral meniscal tears are more common than acute medial tears, whereas medial tears occur more often with chronic ACL deficiency.
   - **The Lachman test is the most sensitive examination for acute ACL injuries.**
   - **Performance on the pivot shift test is most closely correlated with outcome after ACL reconstruction.**
     - This test is also helpful in evaluating an ACL-deficient knee, especially in an examination with the patient under anesthesia.
   - The KT-1000 and KT-2000 Knee Ligament Arthrometers are useful in quantifying laxity.

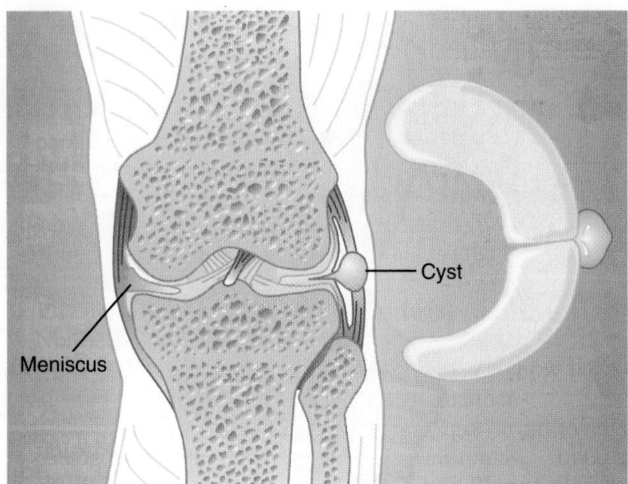

Figure 4-14 Meniscal cysts usually involve the lateral meniscus. (From Tria AJ, Klein KS: *An illustrated guide to the knee,* New York, 1992, Churchill Livingstone, p 101.)

- Plain radiographs are essential in evaluating ACL injuries.
  - **A lateral capsule sign or Segond fracture may be present.**
- MRI is useful in confirming the diagnosis.

3. Treatment
   - **Initial management consists of physical therapy for mobilization. Immobilization is avoided.**
   - Intraarticular reconstruction is currently favored for patients who meet the criteria indicated in Figure 4-15.
   - Graft selection depends on patient's factors and surgeon's preference and usually includes (1) a bone-patella, tendon-bone (BPTB) autograft; (2) a four-strand hamstring autograft, (3) a quadriceps tendon autograft, and (4) an allograft.
     - **BPTB demonstrates faster incorporation into the bone tunnels than does hamstring autograft and, for the authors, is often the graft of choice for patients who desire an early return to sports activity.**

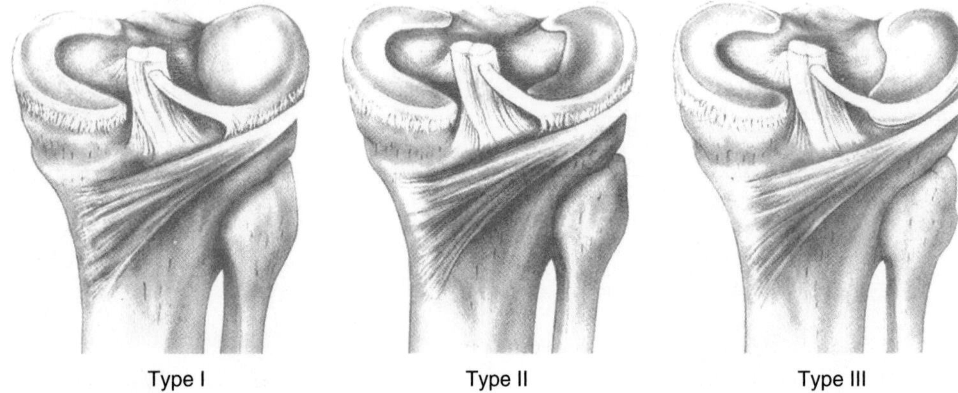

Figure 4-15 Watanabe classification of discoid lateral meniscus. *Type I* is the complete variant, *type II* is the partial variant, and *type III* is the Wrisberg variant. (From Scott WN: *Insall & Scott surgery of the knee,* ed 4, Philadelphia, 2006, Elsevier.)

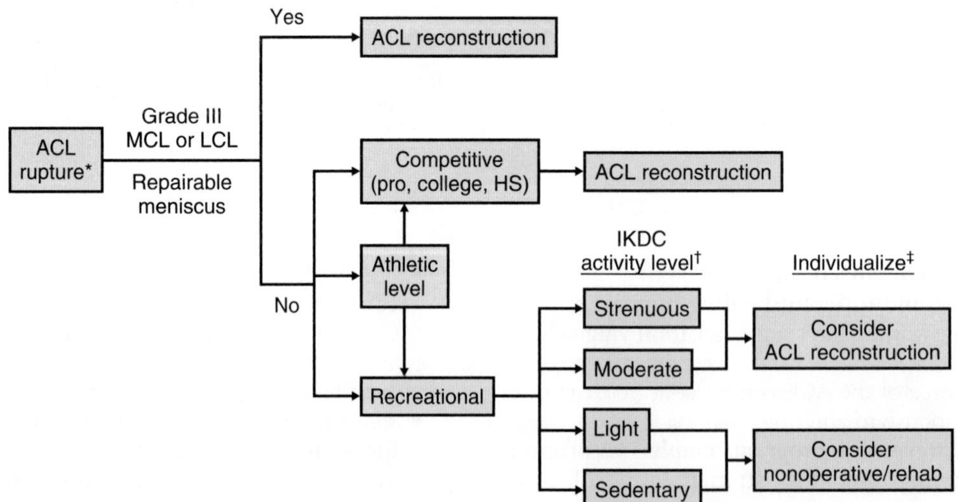

Figure 4-16 Algorithm for the treatment of ruptures of the anterior cruciate ligament. Midsubstance tears are denoted by *. †Strenuous activities: jumping/pivoting sports; moderate activities: heavy manual work, skiing; light activities: manual work, running; and sedentary activities: activities of daily living. ‡Individualize on the basis of age, arthritis, occupation, activity modification, and other medical conditions. ACL, anterior cruciate ligament; HS, high school; IKDC, International Knee Documentation Committee; LCL, lateral collateral ligament; MCL, medial collateral ligament. (From Spindler KP, Walker RN: General approach to ligament surgery. In Fu FH, Harner CD, Vince KG, editors: *Knee surgery,* Baltimore, 1994, Williams & Wilkins, p 652.)

- Several studies have, however, demonstrated a higher incidence of arthritis associated with the use of BPTB autograft than with hamstring autograft 5 to 7 years after ACL reconstruction.
- Primary repair of ACL tears is not currently recommended.
  - Myofibroblasts "coat" the end of the ACL stumps, making primary healing impossible.
- Significant controversy exists regarding the double-bundle ACL reconstruction.

4. Surgical technique
   - Single-bundle reconstruction is still the most commonly performed reconstruction.
   - Placement of a more horizontal femoral tunnel (10 or 2 o'clock position) to center the graft in the middle of the femoral ACL footprint has been the focus of newer anteromedial or "far medial" portal drilling techniques (in contrast to traditional transtibial-femoral drilling techniques).
     - A more horizontal graft position may reduce rotational instability.
5. Partial ACL tears
   - The existence and treatment of "partial" ACL tears are controversial, although clinical examination and functional stability remain the most important considerations in determining the need for reconstruction.
   - Single-bundle tears can occur and may be addressed with reconstruction of the injured bundle and preservation of the intact bundle.
6. Postoperative rehabilitation
   - Rehabilitation has evolved, and early motion (emphasis on extension) and weight bearing are encouraged in most protocols.
   - **Closed-chain rehabilitation (fixation of the terminal segment of extremity)** and compressive loading have been emphasized because they allow physiologic co-contraction of the muscles around the knee.
     - **Open-chain extension exercises place increased stress on the reconstructed ACL and should be avoided for the first 6 weeks.**
   - No difference in outcome has been found between accelerated and nonaccelerated rehabilitation programs.
   - Postoperative bracing has not proved beneficial after ACL reconstruction *except* in downhill skiers.
   - Early progressive eccentric exercise has yielded good initial results in terms of quadriceps and gluteus maximus muscle size and function after ACL reconstruction.
7. Complications
   - **Complications in ACL surgery are usually a result of aberrant tunnel placement.**
     - **The most common technical error is placement of the femoral tunnel too far anteriorly, which results in limited flexion.**
     - **Vertical graft placement results in decreased rotational stability.**
   - Arthrofibrosis often occurs with reconstruction for acute ACL tears.
   - **Aberrant hardware placement (interference screw divergence of >30 degrees [for endoscopic femoral tunnels] and >15 degrees [for tibial tunnels]) can also result in complications.**
   - BPTB autograft harvest carries the risk of anterior knee pain, pain with kneeling, loss of extension, and poorer recovery of quadriceps strength.
   - Hamstring autograft harvest carries the risk of weakness of knee flexion and internal rotation, along with injury to branches of the saphenous nerve.
     - **Use of a horizontal incision at the harvest site decreases the risk of damaging the infrapatellar branch of the saphenous nerve.**
   - The use of allograft with ACL reconstruction in younger, more active patients may be associated with a higher rate of rerupture.
     - Allograft risk also includes infection risk (e.g., with *Clostridium* species and human immunodeficiency virus [HIV]), although rates are low (1 : 1.6 million).

B. PCL injury

1. History
   - Injuries occur most commonly as a result of a direct blow to the anterior tibia with the knee flexed (the "dashboard injury"), with hyperflexion, or with hyperextension.
   - **A fall onto the ground with a plantar-flexed foot is also a mechanism of injury for PCL tears.**
2. Physical examination and classification
   - The key examination is the posterior drawer test; diagnostic results are an absent or posteriorly directed tibial step-off.
     - Grade I injury: an isolated PCL injury in which the tibia remains anterior to the femoral condyles
     - Grade II injury: an isolated, complete PCL injury in which the anterior tibia becomes flush with the femoral condyles
     - Grade III injury: an injury in which the tibia is posterior to the femoral condyles and is usually indicative of associated ACL or PLC injuries or both
3. Imaging
   - Plain radiographs should be obtained to evaluate for avulsion injuries (acute) and arthrosis of the medial and patellofemoral compartments (chronic).
   - Stress radiographs are becoming the standard for evaluation and grading of PCL injuries; side-to-side differences of more than 12 mm on stress radiographs are suggestive of a combined PCL and PLC injury.
   - MRI is a confirmatory study.
4. Treatment
   - Nonoperative treatment is favored for most grades I and II (isolated) PCL injuries.
     - **Rehabilitation should focus on strengthening the knee extensors.**
   - Grade III injuries are indicative of a combined injury, usually to the posterolateral corner.
   - Bony avulsion fractures can be repaired primarily with good results, although primary repair of midsubstance PCL (and ACL) injuries has not been successful.
   - Chronic PCL deficiency can result in late chondrosis of the patellofemoral compartment or medial femoral condyle, or both.
   - PCL reconstruction is recommended for functionally unstable or combined injuries (Figure 4-17).
     - In general, the results of PCL reconstruction are not as good as those of ACL reconstruction, and some residual posterior laxity often remains.

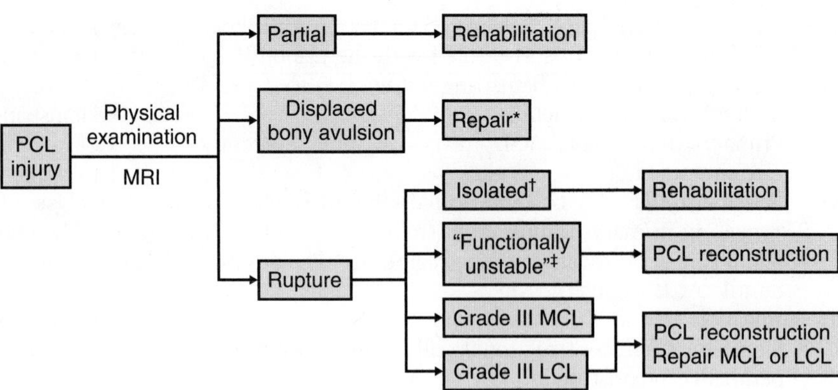

Figure 4-17 Algorithm for treatment of injuries to the posterior cruciate ligament. *Indicates an intact ligament; †indicates lack of posterolateral injury or combined ligamentous injury; ‡indicates failed rehabilitation or unstable/symptomatic in activities of daily living. LCL, lateral collateral ligament; MCL, medial collateral ligament; PCL, posterior cruciate ligament. (From Spindler KP, Walker RN: General approach to ligament surgery. In Fu FH, Harner CD, Vince KG, editors: *Knee surgery,* Baltimore, 1994, Williams & Wilkins, p 655.)

- For successful reconstruction, concomitant ligament injuries must be addressed.
- Many techniques for PCL reconstruction have been published, and they can generally be divided into tibial inlay versus transtibial methods and single-bundle versus double-bundle methods.
  - **Single-bundle reconstructions should be tensioned in 90 degrees of flexion.**
  - Tibial inlay has biomechanical advantages, such as a decrease in the "killer turn" and decreased attenuation of the graft.
  - **In the tibial inlay technique, the average distance from screws used for fixation to the popliteal artery is 20 mm.**
  - Double-bundle techniques may improve biomechanical function in both extension and flexion, but a clinical advantage to those techniques has not yet been shown.
    - The anterolateral bundle is the most important for posterior stability at 90 degrees of flexion and should be tensioned in flexion.
    - The posteromedial bundle has a reciprocal function and should be tensioned in extension.

C. Collateral ligament injury

1. MCL injury
   - History and physical examination
     - MCL injury occurs as a result of valgus stress to the knee.
     - Pain and instability with valgus stress testing at 30 degrees of flexion (and not in full extension) is diagnostic.
     - Opening in full extension usually signifies other concurrent injuries (ACL and PCL).
     - Injuries most commonly occur at the femoral insertion of the ligament.
   - Treatment
     - Nonoperative treatment (hinged knee brace) is highly successful in alleviating isolated MCL injuries.
     - Clinical work has shown the advantage of nonoperative treatment (bracing) of an associated MCL injury in patients receiving an ACL reconstruction.
     - **Distal injuries have less healing potential than do proximal injuries.**
     - **Prophylactic bracing may be helpful for football players, especially interior linemen.**
     - Advancement and reinforcement of the ligament are rarely necessary for chronic injuries that do not respond to conservative treatment (Figure 4-18).
     - In chronic injuries, calcification may be present at the medial femoral condyle insertion (Pellegrini-Stieda sign).
     - Pellegrini-Stieda syndrome, which can occur with chronic MCL injury, usually responds to a brief period of immobilization followed by progressive motion.
2. LCL injury

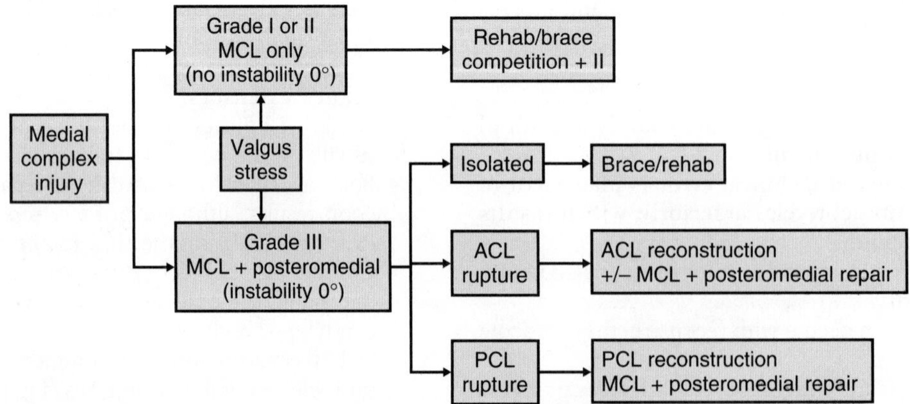

Figure 4-18 Algorithm for treatment of injuries to the medial collateral ligament (MCL). ACL, anterior cruciate ligament; PCL, posterior cruciate ligament. (From Spindler KP, Walker RN: General approach to ligament surgery. In Fu FH, Harner CD, Vince KG, editors: *Knee surgery,* Baltimore, 1994, Williams & Wilkins.)

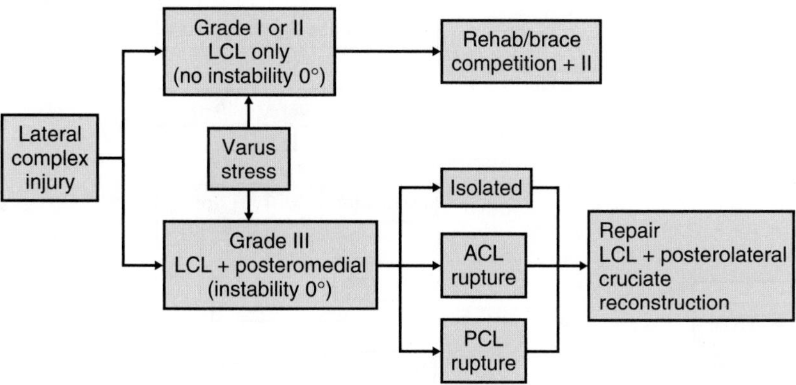

Figure 4-19 Algorithm for treatment of injuries to the lateral collateral ligament (LCL). ACL, anterior cruciate ligament; PCL, posterior cruciate ligament. (From Spindler KP, Walker RN: General approach to ligament surgery. In Fu FH, Harner CD, Vince KG, editors: *Knee surgery,* Baltimore, 1994, Williams & Wilkins.)

- Varus instability in 30 degrees of flexion is diagnostic only for an isolated LCL ligament injury.
- Isolated injuries to the LCL ligament are uncommon and should be managed nonoperatively if laxity is mild (Figure 4-19).

D. Posterolateral corner injury

1. History
   - Rarely isolated and are usually associated with other ligamentous injuries (especially those of the PCL)
   - Because of poor results with reconstructions with chronic injury, repair of acute injury combined with reconstruction is advocated.
   - **Examination for increased external rotation (dial test), the external rotation recurvatum test, the posterolateral drawer test, and the reverse pivot shift test are important (see Table 4-5).**
   - Long-leg standing radiographs are necessary, especially with chronic injuries, to determine mechanical axis and whether a proximal tibial osteotomy is necessary for varus correction.
     - **Varus alignment is associated with higher rates of PLC reconstruction failure.**
   - Evaluation for triple varus alignment should always be performed.
     - Primary varus alignment: tibiofemoral malalignment
     - Secondary varus alignment: LCL deficiency contributing to increased lateral opening
     - Triple varus alignment: deficiency of the remaining PLC with overall varus recurvatum alignment
2. Treatment
   - Early anatomic repair is often successful, but these injuries are frequently missed.
   - Procedures recommended for chronic injuries include posterolateral corner advancement (only if structures are attenuated but intact); popliteal bypass (not currently favored); two- and three-tailed reconstruction; biceps tenodesis; and (more recent) "split" grafts and anatomic reconstructions, which are used to reconstruct both the LCL and the popliteal/posterolateral corner (Figures 4-20 and 4-21).
   - **The treatment of choice for chronic PLC injuries is often a valgus opening wedge osteotomy.**

E. Multiple-ligament injury

1. History and physical examination
   - Combined ligamentous injuries (especially ACL-PCL injuries) can be a result of a knee dislocation, and neurovascular injury must be suspected (Table 4-7).
   - The incidence of vascular injury after anterior knee dislocation is 30% to 50%.
   - Liberal use of vascular studies is recommended early (Figure 4-22).
     - In one study by Stannard et al (2004) serial examinations—including ankle-brachial index exceeding 90% over 48 hours—were used to determine whether arteriography was necessary. The authors noted success with this technique and noted that a four-ligament injury was associated with a higher rate of vascular injury.

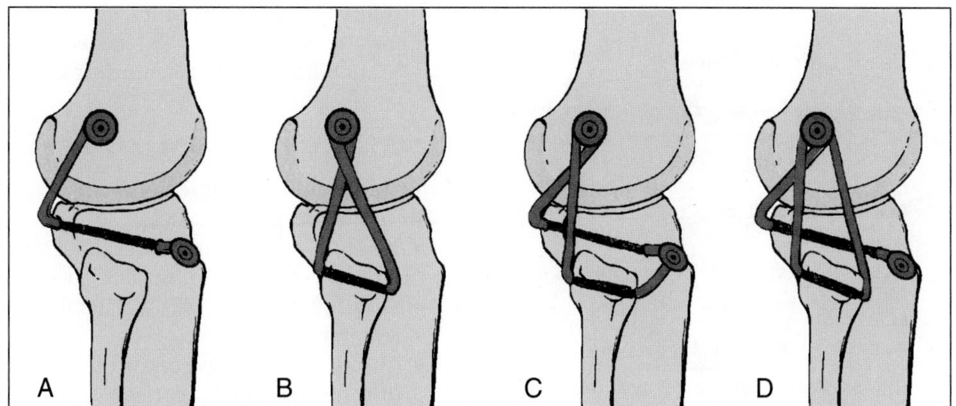

Figure 4-20 Techniques for posterolateral corner reconstruction. **A,** Popliteal bypass (Muller). **B,** Figure-eight (Larsen). **C,** Two-tailed (Warren). **D,** Three-tailed (Warren/Miller). (From Miller MD, Cooper DE, Warner JJP: *Review of sports medicine and arthroscopy,* ed 2, Philadelphia, 2002, WB Saunders.)

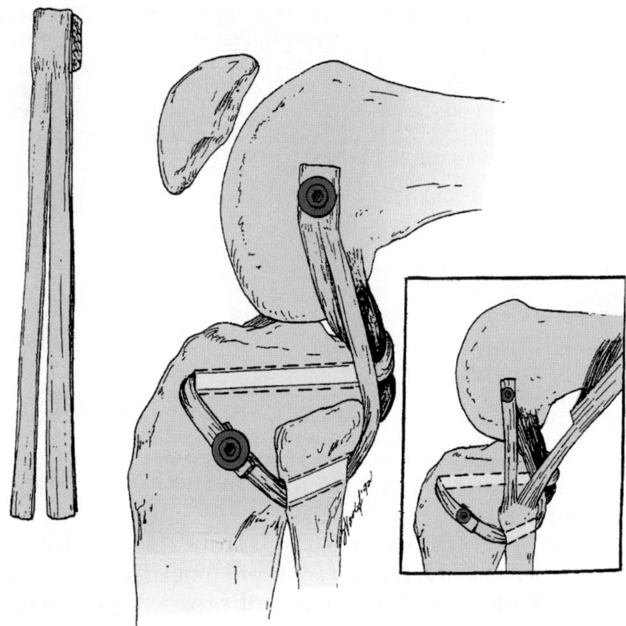

Figure 4-21 Split posterolateral corner graft. (From McKernan DJ, Paulos LE: Graft selection. In Fu FH, Harner CD, Vince KG, editors: *Knee surgery,* Baltimore, 1994, Williams & Wilkins, p 669.)

- Dislocations are classified on the basis of the direction of tibial displacement (Figure 4-23).

2. Treatment
   - Initial treatment involves immediate reduction and neurovascular examination.
   - Definitive treatment is usually operative.
   - Emergency surgical indications include popliteal artery injury, compartment syndrome, open dislocations, and irreducible dislocations.
   - Most surgeons recommend delaying surgery 1 to 2 weeks to ensure that no vascular injury occurs.
   - The use of the arthroscope, especially with a pump, must be limited during these procedures because of the risk of fluid extravasation. Avulsion injuries can be repaired primarily; however, interstitial injuries must be reconstructed.

Table 4-7 Schenck Classification of Knee Dislocations

Classification	Ligaments Affected
KDI	ACL + either MCL or LCL *or* PCL + either MCL or LCL
KDII	ACL + PCL
KDIII	ACL + PCL + one collateral ligament
KDIIIM	MCL
KDIIIL	LCL
KDIV	ACL + PCL + MCL + LCL

Data from SchenK RC, Jr: The dislocated knee, *Instr Course Lect* 43: 127–136, 1994.

ACL, anterior cruciate ligament; KD, knee dislocation; LCL, lateral collateral ligament; MCL, medial collateral ligament; PCL, posterior cruciate ligament.

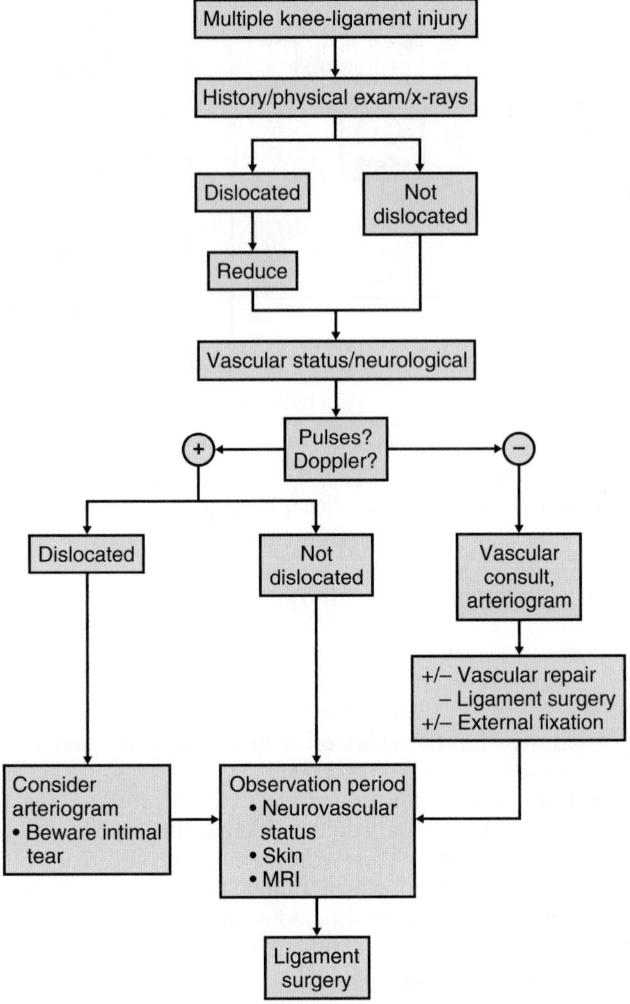

Figure 4-22 Algorithm for treatment of injuries to multiple knee ligaments. MRI, magnetic resonance imaging. (From Marks PH, Harner CD: The anterior cruciate ligament in the multiple ligament–injured knee, *Clin Sports Med* 12:825–838, 1993.)

- The incidence of stiff knee after these combined procedures is high; early motion is crucial for avoiding it.
- According to a meta-analysis, staged treatment might have produced better subjective outcomes but, like acute treatment, was associated with additional procedures to treat joint stiffness. Early mobility was associated with better subjective outcomes than was immobilization after acute surgical treatment.

VI. OSTEOCHONDRAL LESIONS

A. Osteochondritis dissecans

1. Introduction
   - Involves subchondral bone and overlying cartilage separation, probably as a result of occult trauma
   - Most often involves the lateral aspect of the medial femoral condyle
   - The lateral femoral condyle is involved in 15% to 20% of cases; the patella is rarely involved.
   - **The condition resolves spontaneously in the majority of the juvenile cases, in about 50% of adolescents, and rarely in adults.**

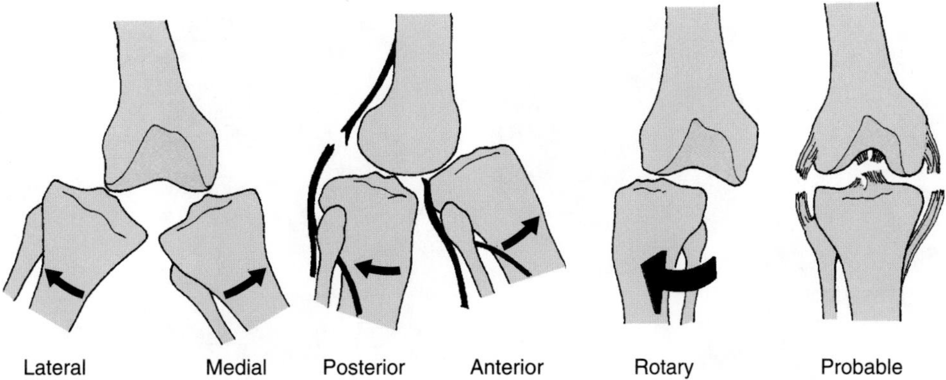

Figure 4-23 Classification of knee dislocations. (From Miller MD, Cooper DE, Warner JJP: *Review of sports medicine and arthroscopy,* Philadelphia, 1995, WB Saunders, p 51.)

2. Diagnosis
   - Patients usually have poorly localized, vague complaints. Radiographs, nuclear imaging, and MRI can be helpful in determining the size, location, and characteristics of the lesion.
3. Treatment and prognosis
   - **Children with open growth plates have the best prognosis, and often these lesions can be simply observed.**
   - In situ lesions can be treated with retrograde drilling.
   - Detached lesions may necessitate abrasion chondroplasty or newer, more aggressive techniques.
   - Osteochondritis dissecans in adults is usually symptomatic and leads to arthritis if left untreated.

B. **Articular cartilage injury**

1. Overview
   - The distinction between articular cartilage injury and osteochondritis dissecans is not often clear, but articular cartilage injury occurs as a result of rotational forces in direct trauma. It usually occurs on the medial femoral condyle. The lesions are classified according to their arthroscopic appearance.
2. Treatment
   - Débridement and chondroplasty are currently recommended for symptomatic lesions.
   - Displaced osteochondral fragments can sometimes be replaced and secured with small, recessed screws or absorbable pins.
   - For discrete, isolated, full-thickness cartilage injuries, several treatment options are in clinical use: microfracture, periosteal patches (chondrocyte implantation), and osteochondral transfer (plugs), including autograft and allograft options (Figure 4-24).
     - **Diffuse chondral damage is a relative contraindication to these procedures.**
   - Donor-site problems and the creation of true articular cartilage at the recipient site are still challenges.
   - Age, lesion size, patient's desired activity level, alignment, meniscal integrity, and ligamentous stability must all be taken into consideration in selecting the appropriate treatment option. An algorithm is presented in Figure 4-25.
     - **Marrow-stimulating techniques—including microfracture, drilling, and abrasion arthroplasty—involve perforation of the subchondral bone after removal of the "tidemark" cartilage with eventual clot formation and fibrocartilaginous repair tissue (type I collagen with inferior wear characteristics).** Good clinical results in small defects (<4 cm^2) are obtained in 60% to 80% patients.
     - Autologous chondrocyte implantation allows for the creation of type II–rich hyaline-like cartilage. It is indicated for medium-sized to larger chondral lesions without bony defects. Multiple surgical procedures are required for biopsy/harvest and then definitive repair. Complications related to autologous chondrocyte implantation include chondrocyte overgrowth and periosteal flap hypertrophy along with the morbidity of the second surgical procedure.
     - Osteochondral autografts (i.e., osteochondral autograft transplantation, mosaicplasty) can be used to address medium-sized lesions (3 cm^2) that include subchondral bone loss. Complications include donor site morbidity.
     - **Osteochondral allografts can be used for larger lesions, especially with bone loss.** The main concerns include the small risk of disease transmission and condrocyte viability, which has improved with graft preservation techniques (storage at 4° C).

C. **Degenerative joint disease**

1. Diffuse chondral damage is usually not considered "sports medicine," but treatment modalities include medications, nutritional supplements such as glucosamine with chondroitin sulfate, hyaluronic acid injections, arthroscopic débridement, osteotomies, and arthroplasty. These treatment modalities are addressed in detail in Chapter 5, Adult Reconstruction.

D. **Osteonecrosis**

1. Atraumatic osteonecrosis is similar to idiopathic osteonecrosis of the hip. Risk factors are similar to those of the hip and are common in elderly women.
2. Spontaneous osteonecrosis of the knee is thought to represent a subchondral insufficiency fracture and is typically a self-limiting condition. This condition can follow knee arthroscopy in middle-aged women. It should be treated with limited weight bearing until it resolves.
3. One hypothesis for the cause of spontaneous osteonecrosis of the knee involves a meniscal root tear.

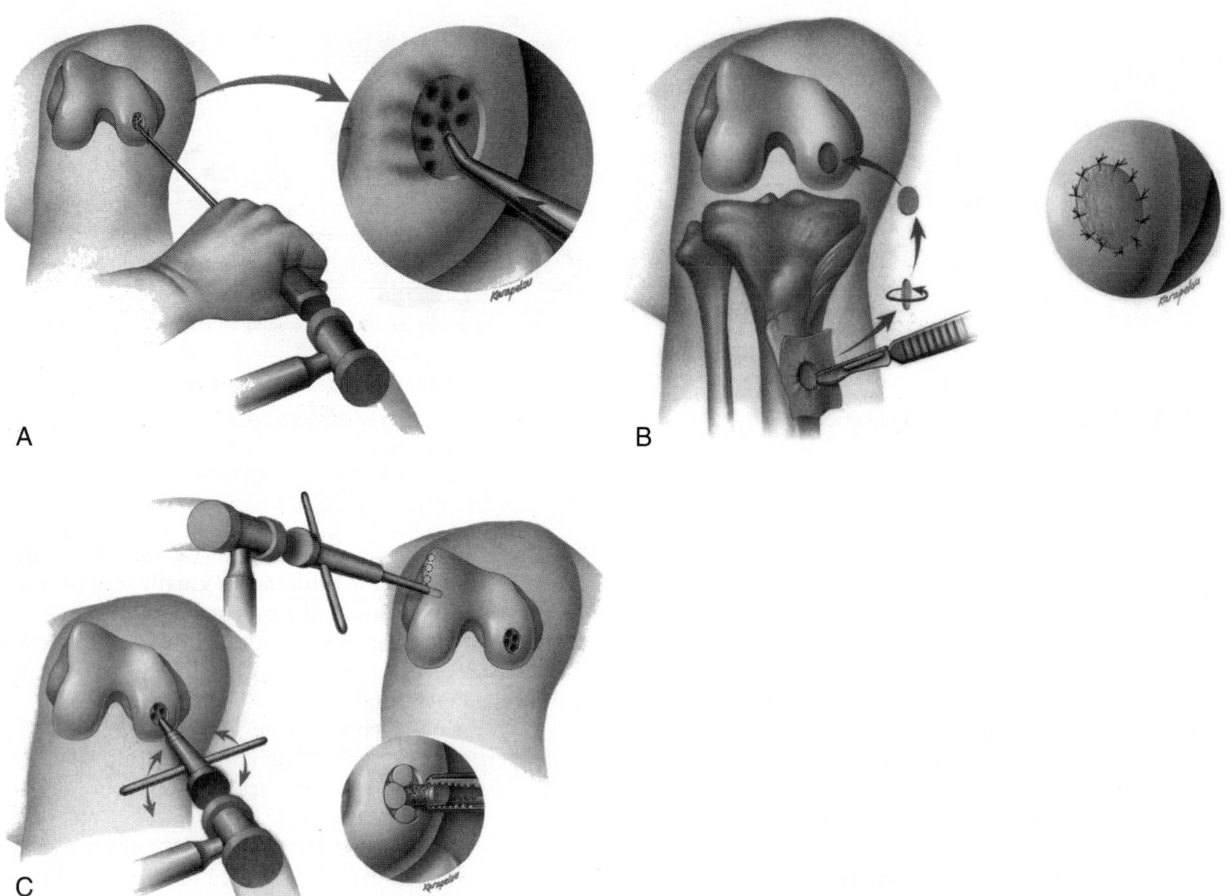

Figure 4-24 Treatment of chondral injuries. **A,** Microfracture. Awls, with various degrees of angulation, are introduced throughout the ipsilateral arthroscopic portal and used to penetrate the subchondral bone and encourage stem cell production of cartilage-like tissue. **B,** Periosteal graft. The periosteum is used as a patch. The inner cambium layer is rotated so that it is facing outward. The patch is carefully sewn in place, and cartilage-like tissue may grow out from the undifferentiated cambium layer of the graft. **C,** Osteochondral plugs. Cylindrical plugs of exposed bone are removed from the defect. Plugs of normal, non–weight-bearing cartilage and bone are harvested and placed into the defect. (From Miller MD: Atlas of chondral injury treatment, *Op Tech Orthop* 7:289–294, 1997.)

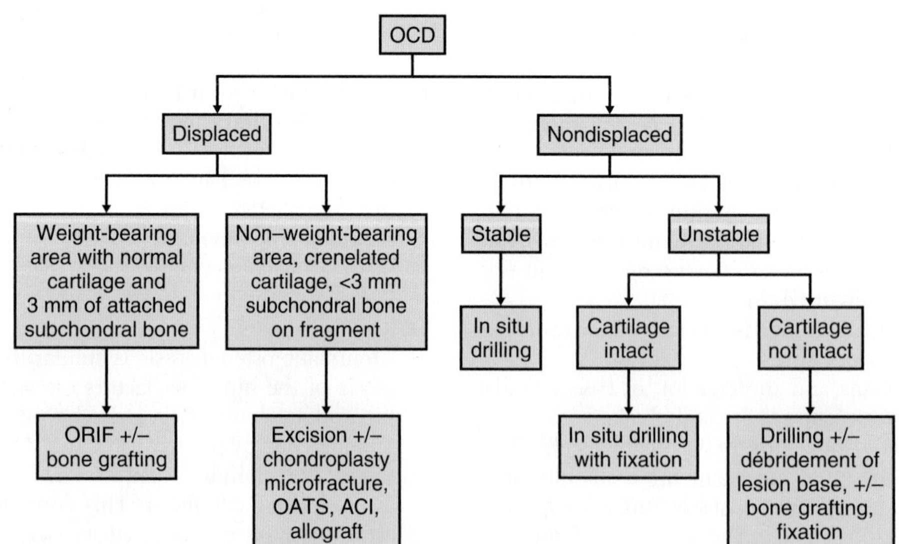

Figure 4-25 A treatment algorithm for stable and unstable osteochondritis dissecans (OCD) lesions. ACI, autologous chondrocyte implantation; OATS, osteochondral autograft transplantation; ORIF, open reduction with internal fixation. (From Miller M, Cole B: *Textbook of arthroscopy,* Philadelphia, 2004, WB Saunders.)

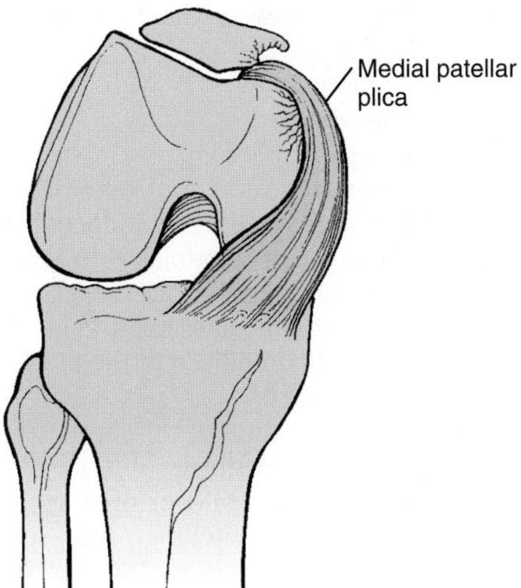

Figure 4-26 Medial patellar plica with associated chondromalacia of the medial femoral condyle and patella. (From Miller MD, Cooper DE, Warner JJP: *Review of sports medicine and arthroscopy,* ed 2, Philadelphia, 2002, WB Saunders.)

VII. SYNOVIAL LESIONS

A. Pigmented villonodular synovitis

1. Affected patients may present with pain and swelling and may have a palpable mass.
2. **MRI demonstrates intraarticular nodular masses of low signal intensity on T1- and T2-weighted images.**
3. There are nodular and diffuse types.
   - The diffuse type has a higher recurrence rate. Synovectomy is effective, but the recurrence rate is still high.
   - Arthroscopic techniques are as effective as traditional open procedures if a complete synovectomy with multiple portals is performed.

B. Synovial chondromatosis

1. This proliferative disease of the synovium is associated with cartilaginous metaplasia, which results in multiple intraarticular loose bodies.

C. Plicae

1. Synovial folds that are embryologic remnants
2. They are occasionally pathologic, particularly the medial patellar plica, which can cause abrasion of the medial femoral condyle and sometimes responds to arthroscopic excision (Figure 4-26).

D. Other synovial lesions that respond to synovectomy include chondromatosis, osteochondromatosis, pauciarticular juvenile rheumatoid arthritis, and hemophilia. Additional arthroscopic portals are required for complete synovectomy.

VIII. PATELLOFEMORAL DISORDERS

A. Introduction

1. Anterior knee pain is classified based on etiologic factors (Box 4-1). The term *chondromalacia* should be replaced with a specific diagnosis that is based on this classification.

B. Trauma

1. Includes fractures of the patella (discussed in Chapter 11, Trauma) and tendon injuries (Figure 4-27).

Box 4-1

Classification* of Patellofemoral Disorders

I. Trauma (conditions caused by trauma in the otherwise normal knee)
   A. Acute trauma
      1. Contusion (924.11)
      2. Fracture
         a. Patella (822)
         b. Femoral trochlea (821.2)
         c. Proximal tibial epiphysis (tubercle) (823.0)
      3. Dislocation (rare in the normal knee) (836.3)
      4. Rupture
         a. Quadriceps tendon (843.8)
         b. Patellar tendon (844.8)
   B. Repetitive trauma (overuse syndromes)
      1. Patellar tendinitis ("jumper's knee") (726.64)
      2. Quadriceps tendinitis (726.69)
      3. Peripatellar tendinitis (e.g., anterior knee pain of the adolescent caused by hamstring contracture) (726.699)
      4. Prepatellar bursitis ("housemaid's knee") (726.65)
      5. Apophysitis
         a. Osgood-Schlatter disease (732.43)
         b. Sinding-Larsen-Johansson disease (732.42)
   C. Late effects of trauma (905)
      1. Post-traumatic chondromalacia patellae
      2. Post-traumatic patellofemoral arthritis
      3. Anterior fat pad syndrome (post-traumatic fibrosis)
      4. Complex regional pain syndrome
      5. Patellar osseous dystrophy
      6. Acquired patella infera (719.366)
      7. Acquired quadriceps fibrosis
II. Patellofemoral dysplasia
   A. Lateral patellar compression syndrome (LPCS) (718.365)
      1. Secondary chondromalacia patellae (717.7)
      2. Secondary patellofemoral arthritis (715.289)
   B. Chronic subluxation of the patella (CSP) (718.364)
      1. Secondary chondromalacia patellae (717.7)
      2. Secondary patellofemoral arthritis (715.289)
   C. Recurrent dislocation of the patella (RDP) (718.361)
      1. Associated fractures (822)
         a. Osteochondral (intraarticular)
         b. Avulsion (extraarticular)
      2. Secondary chondromalacia patellae (717.7)
      3. Secondary patellofemoral arthritis (715.289)
   D. Chronic dislocation of the patella (718.362)
      1. Congenital
      2. Acquired
III. Idiopathic chondromalacia patellae (717.7)
IV. Osteochondritis dissecans
   A. Patella (732.704)
   B. Femoral trochlea (732.703)
V. Synovial plicae (727.8916) (anatomic variant made symptomatic by acute or repetitive trauma)
   A. Medial patellar ("shelf") (727.89161)
   B. Suprapatellar (727.89163)
   C. Lateral patellar (727.89165)

From Merchant AC: Classification of patellofemoral disorders, *Arthroscopy* 4:235, 1988.

*Orthopaedic ICD-9-CM (International Classification of Diseases [of the World Health Organization]–9-Master in Surgery) Expanded Diagnostic Codes are in parentheses.

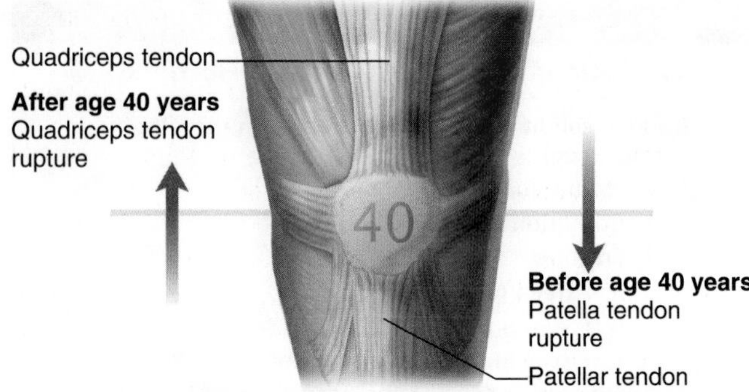

Figure 4-27 Patellar tendon ruptures are more common before the age of 40 and quadriceps tendon ruptures are more common after the age of 40.

2. Tendon ruptures
   - Quadriceps tendon ruptures are more common than patellar tendon ruptures and occur most often with indirect trauma in patients older than 40 years. In younger patients, patellar tendon ruptures occur with direct or indirect trauma.
   - Both types of tendon rupture are more common in patients with underlying disorders of the tendon.
   - A palpable defect and the inability to extend the knee are diagnostic signs.
   - **Patella alta is a consistent finding with patella tendon rupture.**
   - Primary repair with temporary stabilization (McLaughlin wire or suture) is indicated.
3. Repetitive trauma: overuse injuries
   - Patellar tendinitis (jumper's knee)
     - This condition is perhaps better termed *tendinosis.*
     - Most common in athletes who participate in sports such as basketball and volleyball
     - Associated with pain and tenderness near the inferior border of the patella (worse in extension than in flexion)
     - Treatment includes nonsteroidal anti-inflammatory drugs (NSAIDs), physical therapy (strengthening including eccentric exercise and ultrasonography), and orthoses (patella tendon strap).
     - **Surgery involving excision of necrotic tendon fibers is rarely indicated.**
   - Quadriceps tendinitis
     - Less common than patella tendinosis but just as painful
     - Patients may note painful clicking and localized pain at the superior border of the patella.
     - Operative treatment is occasionally necessary.
   - Prepatellar bursitis (housemaid's knee)
     - The most common form of bursitis of the knee and associated with a history of prolonged kneeling
     - Supportive treatment (knee pads, occasional steroid injections) and, in rare cases, bursal excision are recommended.
     - Aspiration is advocated in wrestlers to rule out infection because wrestling requires kneeling on the flexed knee.
   - Iliotibial band friction syndrome
     - Can occur in runners (especially those running hills) and cyclists
     - Result of abrasion between the iliotibial band and the lateral femoral condyle
     - Localized tenderness, worse with the knee flexed 30 degrees, is common.
     - The Ober test (patient lies in lateral decubitus position with hyperextension of the ipsilateral hip; the leg can be brought from abduction to adduction to demonstrate tightness of the iliotibial band) is helpful in making the diagnosis.
     - Rehabilitation is usually successful.
     - Surgical excision of an ellipse of the iliotibial band is occasionally necessary.
   - Semimembranosus tendinitis
     - Most common in male athletes in their early thirties
     - Can be diagnosed with MRI or nuclear imaging and often responds to stretching and strengthening exercises
     - A steroid injection may be added if no improvement occurs.
   - Pes anserinus bursitis
     - Characterized by localized pain, tenderness, and swelling over the proximal anteromedial tibia at the insertion site of the sartorius, gracilis, and semitendinosus (approximately 6 cm inferior to the joint line)
     - Treated conservatively with oral anti-inflammatory medication, localized corticosteroid injections, and activity modification

C. **Late effects of trauma**

1. Patellofemoral arthritis
   - Injury and malalignment can contribute to patellar degenerative joint disease.
   - Lateral release may be beneficial early only if there is objective evidence of patellar tilting.
   - Other procedures may be required for advanced patellar arthritis.
   - Options include anterior (Maquet) or anteromedial (Fulkerson) transfer of the tibial tubercle or patellectomy for severe cases.
   - Tibial rotational alignment and overall lower extremity alignment should always be assessed in evaluating the cause of patellofemoral disease. Patellofemoral arthroplasty has been introduced as another treatment option but remains controversial.
2. Anterior fat pad syndrome (Hoffa disease)
   - Trauma to the anterior fat pad can lead to fibrous changes and pinching of the fat pad, especially in patients with genu recurvatum.
   - Activity modification, ice, knee padding, and injection can be helpful.
   - Arthroscopic excision is occasionally beneficial.
3. **Complex regional pain syndrome** (formerly known as *reflex sympathetic dystrophy*)
   - Characterized by pain out of proportion to physical findings, this condition is an exaggerated response to injury.
   - Three stages are typical: (1) swelling, warmth, and hyperhidrosis; (2) brawny edema and trophic changes; and (3) glossy, cool, dry skin and stiffness.
   - Patellar osteopenia and a "flamingo gait" are also common.
   - Treatment includes nerve stimulation, NSAIDs, and sympathetic or epidural blocks—response to which can be diagnostic.

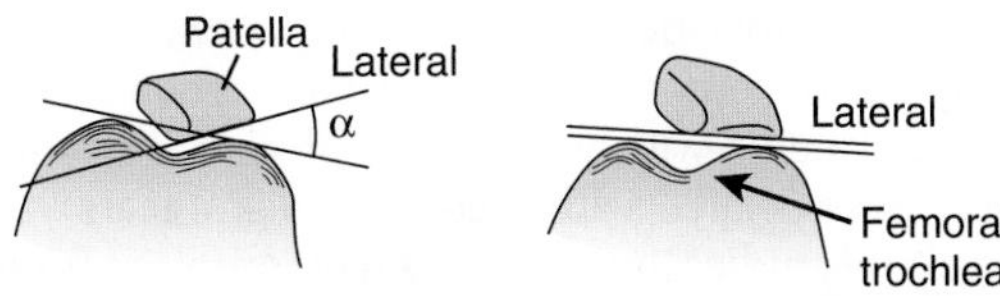

Figure 4-28 The measurement of the lateral patellofemoral angle. *One line* is drawn across the slope of the femoral condyles. A *second line* is drawn across the slope of the lateral patellar facet. A normal angle (α, shown on the left) opens laterally.

D. Patellofemoral dysplasia

1. Lateral patellar facet compression syndrome
   - This problem is associated with a tight lateral retinaculum and excessive lateral tilt without excessive patellar mobility.
   - Treatment includes activity modification, NSAIDs, and strengthening of the vastus medialis oblique muscle.
   - Arthroscopy and lateral release are occasionally required but indicated only in the setting of objective evidence of lateral tilt that has not responded to extensive nonoperative management.
     - **Lateral tilt is best evaluated by measurement of the lateral patellofemoral angle (Figure 4-28).**
     - The best candidates for arthroscopy and lateral release have a neutral or negative tilt with a medial patellar glide of less than one quadrant and a lateral patellar glide of less than three quadrants. Arthroscopic visualization through a superior portal demonstrates that the patella does not articulate medially with 40 degrees of knee flexion.
2. Patellar instability
   - Recurrent subluxation or dislocation of the patella can be characterized by lateral displacement of the patella, a shallow intercondylar sulcus, or patellar incongruence.
     - **The articular cartilage on the medial facet of the patella is most commonly injured after a patellar dislocation.**
   - If this injury is associated with femoral anteversion, genu valgum, and pronated feet, the symptoms can be exacerbated, especially in adolescents ("miserable malalignment syndrome").
   - **Extensive rehabilitation is often curative.**
   - **Girls and women with previous instability are at increased risk.**
   - Several radiographic findings are somewhat helpful in diagnosing patellar malalignment (see Figure 4-28). Tibial rotational alignment can also influence patellar alignment and tracking.
   - Surgical procedures include proximal and distal realignment.
   - Acute, first-time patella dislocations have traditionally been treated nonoperatively, but some surgeons advocate early surgical treatment with arthroscopic evaluation or débridement and acute repair of the medial patellofemoral ligament (usually at the medial epicondyle). This protocol is still somewhat controversial.
     - Affected patients should be evaluated with radiographs for an avulsion fracture of the medial patellofemoral ligament that occurs at the middle third of the patella.
     - The articular cartilage of the medial patellar facet is the most common donor site.
     - Distal realignment, typically tibial tubercle anterior medialization, is indicated for patients with an increased Q angle or a TT-TG distance exceeding 20 mm.
     - **Proximal arthrosis of the medial patellar facet is a contraindication to this procedure.**
   - Abnormalities of patellar height:
     - Patella alta (high-riding patella) and patella baja (low-riding patella) are determined on the basis of various measurements made on lateral radiographs of the knee (see Figure 4-8).
     - Patella alta can be associated with patellar instability because the patella may not articulate with the sulcus, which normally constrains the patella.
     - Patella baja is often the result of fat pad and tendon fibrosis, and proximal transfer of the tubercle may be required in refractory cases.

E. Idiopathic chondromalacia patellae

1. Articular damage and changes to the patella have traditionally been referred to as *idiopathic chondromalacia patellae*; however, this term has fallen into disfavor.
2. Treatment is usually symptomatic, and physical therapy is emphasized heavily.
3. Débridement procedures are of questionable benefit.
4. The Outerbridge classification system is still in common use today (Figure 4-29).

IX. PEDIATRIC KNEE DISORDERS

A. Physeal injuries

1. Most often involve Salter-Harris II fractures of the distal femoral physis
2. Pain, swelling, and an inability to ambulate are common.
3. Stress radiographs and/or MRI may be necessary to make the diagnosis.
4. Open reduction and internal fixation are indicated for displaced Salter-Harris II, III and IV fractures and Salter-Harris I that cannot be adequately reduced.

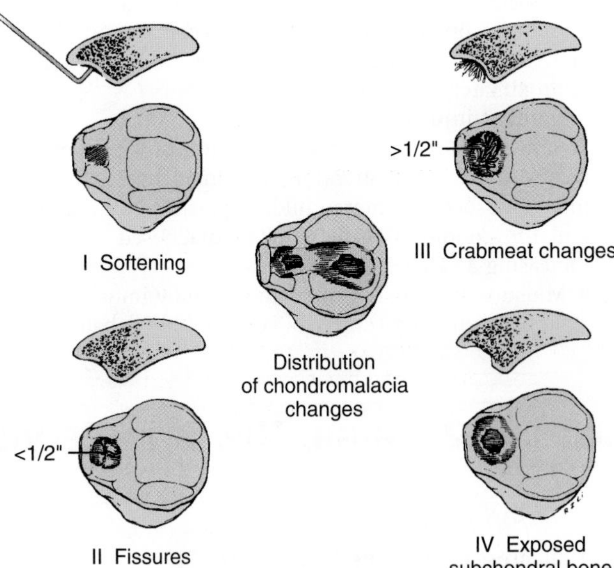

Figure 4-29 Outerbridge classification of chondromalacia. (From Tria AJ, Klein KS: *An illustrated guide to the knee,* New York, 1992, Churchill Livingstone.)

5. It is important to counsel the parents that knee physeal injuries, and particularly distal femoral physeal injuries, may have a worse prognosis than other physeal fractures.

B. **Tibial spine fractures**

1. Classification: Avulsion fractures of the intercondylar eminence of the tibia are described as types I through IV.
   - Type I: displacement of less than 3 mm
   - Type II: avulsion and elevation of the anterior third to half
   - Type III: displacement of entire fragment
   - Type IV: comminuted fracture
2. Types I and II avulsion fractures are usually amenable to closed treatment.
3. Types III and IV fractures, and types I and II fractures for which closed treatment fails, are amenable to open or arthroscopic reduction and fixation of the fragment.
4. The medial or lateral menisci may become trapped beneath the bony fragment and thus prevent reduction if not addressed. Medial meniscal entrapment is more common in the Kocher et al series (2003).

C. **Tibial tubercle fractures**

1. Classification: Ogden modification of the Watson-Jones classification
   - Type 1A: incomplete separation of fragment from metaphysis
   - Type 1B: compete separation through secondary ossification center
   - Type 2A: complete tubercle fracture through cartilaginous bridge between the proximal tibia epiphysis and tuberosity without displacement at articular surface proximally
   - Type 2B: same as type 2A fracture pattern plus comminution
   - Type 3A: compete tubercle fracture with displacement through the proximal tibial epiphysis and articular surface.
   - Type 3B: same as type 3A fracture pattern plus comminution
2. Treatment: Displaced (>5 mm) type 2 and 3 fractures necessitate open reduction with internal fixation. Postoperative care includes immobilization in extension for approximately 6 weeks.

D. **Ligament injuries**

1. Treatment: ACL injury in skeletally immature athletes has received increased attention; the incidence is probably increasing because more children participate in athletics, and the condition is more often diagnosed because of increasing awareness.
   - Midsubstance ACL injuries in skeletally immature individuals remain a subject of considerable debate.
   - Procedures that do not violate the growth plate, especially on the femoral side, are usually recommended for young patients with wide, open physes. Delay in treatment is associated with medial meniscal tears.
   - In several studies, investigators have reported no angular deformities or bony bridges in children at Tanner stages 2 to 4 after ACL reconstruction despite the use of multiple grafts and different techniques.
   - Techniques: Kocher and colleagues (2005, 2007) demonstrated good results with physeal sparing, combined intraarticular and extraarticular reconstruction in patients at Tanner stage 1 or 2, and transphyseal reconstruction with autologous quadrupled hamstring graft with metaphyseal fixation in patients at Tanner stage 3.
   - Other authors have recommended newer all-epiphyseal reconstruction techniques.
   - Other techniques that have been successful with no growth arrest include a central vertical tibial tunnel and "over-the-top" placement of the femoral side with a soft tissue graft.

E. **Traction apophysitis**

1. This condition is present in such disorders as Osgood-Schlatter disease and Sinding-Larsen-Johansson disease.
2. Usually treated symptomatically, with immobilization as needed.
3. Procedures such as ossicle excision are occasionally indicated for refractory cases (Figure 4-30).

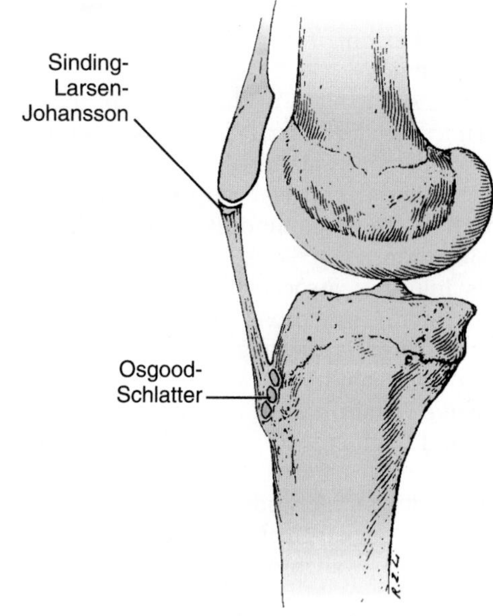

Figure 4-30 Two types of traction apophysitis affecting adolescent knees. (From Tria AJ, Klein KS: *An illustrated guide to the knee*, New York, 1992, Churchill Livingstone, p 140.)

SECTION 2 THIGH, HIP, AND PELVIS

I. CONTUSIONS

A. **Iliac crest contusions ("hip pointer")**

1. Direct trauma to this area can occur in contact sports.
2. An avulsion of the iliac apophysis should be confirmed or ruled out in adolescent athletes.
3. Treatment consists of ice, compression, pain control, and placing the affected leg on maximal stretch.
4. Corticosteroid injections have occasionally been advocated.
5. Additional padding is indicated after the acute phase.

B. Groin contusions

1. An avulsion fracture of the lesser trochanter, traumatic phlebitis, thrombosis, athletic pubalgia, or femoral neuropathy must be confirmed or ruled out before supportive treatment is initiated.

C. Quadriceps contusions

1. This can result in hemorrhage and late myositis ossificans.
2. **Acute management includes cold compression and overnight immobilization in 120 degrees of flexion.**
3. Close monitoring for compartment syndrome is indicated in the acute phase.

II. MUSCLE INJURIES

A. Hamstring strain

1. This common injury is often the result of sudden stretch on the musculotendinous junction during sprinting.
2. It can occur anywhere in the posterior thigh.
3. Treatment is supportive, followed by stretching and strengthening.
4. To prevent recurrence, return to play should be delayed until strength is approximately 90% that of the opposite side.

B. Athletic pubalgia ("sports hernia")

1. Common in sports such as soccer, these injuries must be differentiated from subtle hernias.
2. **Injury to the muscles of the abdominal wall or adductor longus produce anterior pelvis or groin pain, or both, without the classic physical findings of a true inguinal hernia.**
3. Can result from acute trauma or microtrauma associated with overuse of the affected muscle.
   - **Combination of abdominal hyperextension and thigh hyperabduction**
4. Confirm or rule out other causes of pain with radiography, bone scan, or MRI, or a combination of these.
5. Treat nonoperatively for 6 to 8 weeks with rest and therapy.
6. **Repair or reinforcement of the anterior abdominal wall is indicated after conservative measures have failed and after other causes have been excluded.**
7. Decompression of the genital branch of the genitofemoral nerve is also favored by some authors in patients presenting with athletic pubalgia.

C. Rectus femoris strain

1. Acute injuries are usually located more distally on the thigh, but chronic injuries are usually nearer the muscle origin.
2. Pain is elicited with resisted hip flexion or extension.
3. Treatment includes ice and stretching/strengthening exercises.

III. BURSITIS

A. Trochanteric bursitis

1. Occurs frequently in female runners and is associated with training on banked surfaces
2. Treatment includes oral anti-inflammatory drugs, stretching, and rest.
3. Corticosteroid injections are occasionally advocated.

B. Iliopsoas bursitis

1. A cause of anterior hip pain in athletes and often associated with mechanical irritation of the iliopsoas tendon
2. Also a cause of "snapping" or "clicking" symptoms associated with hip pain

C. Ischial bursitis

1. Caused by direct trauma or prolonged sitting and hard to distinguish from hamstring injuries

IV. NERVE ENTRAPMENT SYNDROMES

A. Ilioinguinal nerve entrapment

1. This nerve can be constricted by hypertrophied abdominal muscles as a result of intensive training.
2. Hyperextension of the hip may exacerbate the pain that patients experience, and hyperesthesia symptoms are common. Surgical release is occasionally necessary.

B. Obturator nerve entrapment

1. Can lead to chronic medial thigh pain, especially in athletes with well-developed hip adductor muscles (e.g., skaters)
2. Nerve conduction studies are helpful for establishing the diagnosis.
3. Treatment is usually supportive.

C. Lateral femoral cutaneous nerve entrapment

1. Can lead to meralgia paresthetica, a painful condition
2. Tight belts and prolonged hip flexion may exacerbate symptoms.
3. Release of compressive devices, postural exercises, and NSAIDs are usually curative.

D. Sciatic nerve entrapment

1. Can occur anywhere along the course of the nerve, but the two most common locations are at the level of the ischial tuberosity and by the piriformis muscle, known as *piriformis syndrome*

V. BONE DISORDERS

A. Stress fractures

1. A history of overuse, an insidious onset of pain, and localized tenderness and swelling are typical.
2. Stress fractures occur via propagation of a crack.
3. Bone scan can be diagnostic, even with normal plain radiographs.
4. **MRI is the most specific test for detecting stress fractures.**
5. **Treatment includes protected weight bearing, rest, cross-training, analgesics, and therapeutic modalities.**
6. There are several especially problematic stress fractures:
   - Anterior tibial stress fracture: This is especially worrisome with the appearance of the "dreaded black line" on imaging. Persistence of the "dreaded black line" for more than 6 months, especially with a positive bone scan, can be an indication for bone grafting, intramedullary nailing, or both.
   - Femoral neck stress fractures: Tension (transverse) fractures are more serious than compression fractures (on the medial side of the neck), and operative stabilization may be required.
   - Femoral shaft stress fractures: These usually respond to protected weight bearing but can progress to complete fractures if unrecognized. The fulcrum test may be helpful in making this diagnosis.

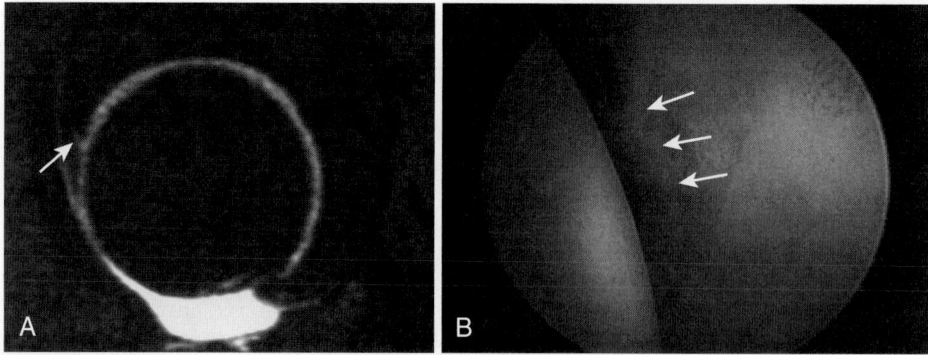

Figure 4-31 Labral tear in a 27-year-old with mechanical symptoms in the left hip. **A,** Sagittal magnetic resonance arthrogram with gadolinium enhancement reveals a tear of the anterior labrum *(arrow)*. **B,** Arthroscopic image shows the anterior labral tear *(arrows)*. (From Miller MD, Cooper DE, Warner JJP: *Review of sports medicine and arthroscopy,* ed 2, Philadelphia, 2002, WB Saunders.)

- Pelvic stress fractures: Stress fractures to the sacrum and pubis are rare but must be considered.
- Metatarsal stress fracture.

B. Proximal femoral fractures

1. Can occur in athletes, especially cross-country skiers (skier's hip)
2. Release bindings have reduced the incidence of these injuries.

C. Avascular necrosis

1. Traumatic hip subluxation can disrupt the arterial blood supply to the hip and result in avascular necrosis.
2. Early recognition of these injuries, which are seen in football players, is essential.
3. With posterior subluxation or dislocation, one study revealed a 25% incidence of avascular necrosis.
4. Obturator oblique radiographs (to determine the presence of an avulsion injury) and MRI are recommended.
5. Such imaging should be followed by aspiration of the hip if a large hemarthrosis is present, 6 weeks of minimal weight bearing, and a repeat MRI.
6. With atraumatic injuries, other causative factors (alcohol, catabolic steroids, and decompression sickness) should be sought.

D. Osteitis pubis

1. Repetitive trauma can cause an inflammation of the symphysis.
2. It occurs frequently in soccer players, hockey players, and runners.
3. Conservative management is usually curative.

E. Tumors

1. Because more than 10% of all musculoskeletal tumors occur in the hip and pelvis, they must be suspected in cases of unexplained pain.

VI. INTRAARTICULAR DISORDERS

A. Loose bodies

1. Often result from trauma or diseases such as synovial chondromatosis
2. Should be removed, either in an open procedure or arthroscopically, to prevent third-body wear

B. Labral tears

1. Often a cause of mechanical hip pain manifesting with vague symptoms
2. Magnetic resonance arthrography has greater than 90% sensitivity and is often used for diagnosis, but arthroscopy is the "gold standard" test (Figure 4-31).
3. The incidence of labral tears is highest in patients with acetabular dysplasia.
4. Underlying hip disease should be addressed in addition to the labral tear for the best results.
5. Arthroscopic labral débridement has yielded good short-term and midterm results.
6. Labral repair may yield better results than débridement, according to emerging data on new techniques.

C. Chondral injuries

1. Articular surface injury is often a cause of mechanical hip pain.
2. Microfracture is effective in the treatment of focal lesions.

D. Ruptured ligamentum teres

1. Associated with mechanical hip pain as the ruptured ligament catches within the joint after a hip dislocation.
2. Débridement is often necessary.
3. The viability of the femoral head is not in jeopardy with a ruptured ligamentum teres.

VII. FEMOROACETABULAR IMPINGEMENT

A. Definition

1. Abnormal contact between proximal femur and acetabulum that leads to chondral damage and symptoms.

B. Types

1. Cam, pincer, and a combination of cam and pincer
   - Cam impingement is a disorder of proximal femoral head and neck structure whereby the head loses sphericity and has decreased offset.
     - This results in abnormal loading of the cartilage on the femoral and acetabular sides along with the labrum.
   - Pincer impingement is a disorder of acetabular structure and can be caused by inadequate acetabular anteversion or acetabular protrusio.

C. Causes

1. Acetabular retroversion; an old slipped capital femoral epiphysis; a nonspherical head; decreased femoral offset or decreased head/neck ratio; overhang of the anterosuperior acetabular rim; protrusio; and a retroverted femoral neck (after fracture).

D. Evaluation
1. Groin or hip pain in association with limitation in ROM, especially in flexion, can be a symptom.
2. Patients generally have more passive external rotation than internal rotation.
3. **A positive result of an anterior impingement test is the reproduction of symptoms with passive flexion, adduction, and internal rotation.**

E. Imaging
1. Plain radiographs should include anteroposterior pelvis and true lateral views with hip in 15 degrees of internal rotation.
2. CT or MRI can give additional information about femoral-acetabular mismatch and chondral or labral lesions.
3. The false profile view **(faux profil)** was originally described by Lequesne to assist in the diagnosis of early osteoarthritis and developmental dysplasia of the hip. It is obtained by having the patient stand next to a vertical radiograph cassette. The hip of interest is closest to the cassette. The ipsilateral foot is parallel to the cassette also. The pelvis is rotated 25 degrees backward (the back of the patient is at a 65-degree angle with the cassette).

F. Treatment
1. Treatment options include open or arthroscopic procedures to trim the femoral head and neck or acetabular rim; periacetabular osteotomy; femoral osteotomy; a combinations of these procedures with labral débridement; and repair.
2. Total hip arthroplasty is reserved for patients with significant arthritic changes.

VIII. OTHER HIP DISORDERS

A. Snapping hip (coxa saltans)
1. Condition in which the **iliotibial band abruptly catches on the greater trochanter** or the iliopsoas impinges on the hip capsule.
2. The iliotibial condition *(external snapping hip)* is more common in women with wide pelvises and prominent trochanters and can be exacerbated by running on banked surfaces.
3. The snapping may be reproduced with passive hip flexion from an adducted position.
4. Stretching and strengthening exercises, modalities such as ultrasonography, and occasionally surgical release may relieve the snapping.
5. This condition must be differentiated from the less common snapping iliopsoas tendon *(internal snapping hip)*, which can be diagnosed with extension and internal rotation of the hip from a flexed and externally rotated position.
6. Dynamic ultrasonography, arthrography, and bursography may also be helpful in determining the diagnosis.

IX. HIP ARTHROSCOPY

See Supplemental Images on expertconsult.com.

A. Indications
1. As techniques improve, so do the indications. Hip arthroscopy is currently effective for the treatment of loose bodies, labral tears, chondral injuries, femoroacetabular impingement, avascular necrosis, synovial disease, ruptured ligamentum teres, impinging osteophytes, and unexplained mechanical symptoms.

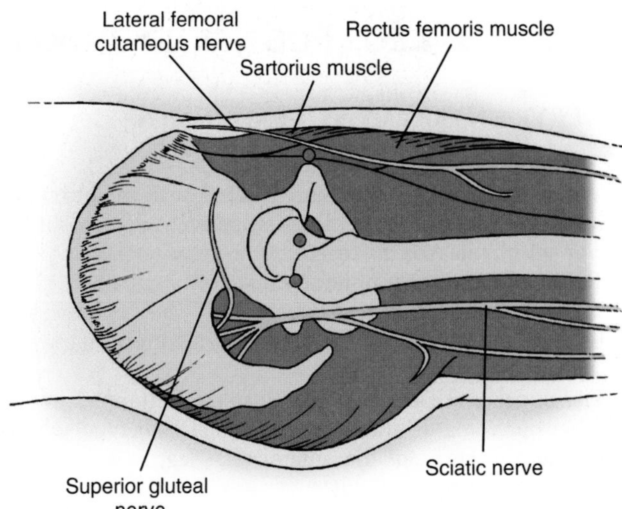

Figure 4-32 Portals *(red circles)* for hip arthroscopy are the anterior portal and two portals on either side of the greater trochanter. (From Canale ST, Beaty JH: *Campbell's operative orthopaedics,* ed 11, Philadelphia, 2008, Elsevier.)

B. Setup
1. Hip arthroscopy is typically performed with the patient in the supine or lateral position with approximately 50 lb (22.7 kg) of traction and a well-padded perineal post.

C. Portals
1. Three portals are commonly used for instrumentation: one on each side of the greater trochanter and an additional anterior portal (Figure 4-32).

D. Compartments
1. Three compartments are described:
   - The central compartment refers to the intraarticular portion of the hip joint between the cartilagenous portions of the proximal femur and acetabulum.
   - The peripheral compartment refers to the intraarticular portion of the hip joint along the neck of the femur and the edge of the acetabulum.
   - The lateral compartment refers to the extraarticular portion in the peritrochanteric region and trochanteric bursa.

E. Complications
1. **Complications, which are rare, are associated with traction injuries, iatrogenic chondral injuries, and neurovascular injury caused by aberrant portal placement.**
2. **The anterior portal puts the lateral femoral cutaneous nerve at risk.**
   - Also at risk are the ascending branch of the lateral femoral circumflex artery and the femoral neurovascular bundle.
3. The anterolateral portal is associated with injury to the superior gluteal nerve.
4. **The posterolateral portal places the sciatic nerve at risk, particularly when the hip is externally rotated.**

SECTION 3 LEG, FOOT, AND ANKLE

I. NERVE ENTRAPMENT SYNDROMES

A. Saphenous nerve entrapment

1. When compressed at the Hunter canal or in the proximal leg, the saphenous nerve can cause painful symptoms inferior and medial to the knee.

B. Peroneal nerve entrapment

1. The common peroneal nerve can be compressed behind the fibula or injured by a direct blow to this area.
2. The superficial peroneal nerve can be entrapped about 12 cm proximal to the tip of the lateral malleolus, where it exits the fascia of the anterolateral leg, as a result of inversion injuries.
   - Fascial defects can be present as well and contribute to the problem.
   - Compartment release is sometimes indicated.
3. **Superficial peroneal nerve entrapment manifests with numbness and tingling over the dorsum of the foot that worsens with plantar flexion and inversion of the foot.**
4. The deep peroneal nerve can be compressed by the inferior extensor retinaculum, which leads to anterior tarsal tunnel syndrome and sometimes necessitates release of this retinaculum.

C. Tibial nerve entrapment

1. Compression of the tibial nerve under the flexor retinaculum behind the medial malleolus may result in tarsal tunnel syndrome. Electromyography or nerve conduction evaluation is helpful, and surgical release is sometimes indicated.
2. **Distal entrapment of the first branch of the lateral plantar nerve (Baxter nerve) (to the adductor digiti quinti), between the fascia of the abductor hallucis and the medial side of the quadratus plantae, has also been described.**

D. Medial plantar nerve entrapment

1. Occurs at the point where the flexor digitorum longus and flexor hallucis longus cross (knot of Henry)
2. Most commonly caused by external compression from orthoses
3. Commonly called *jogger's foot,* this condition usually responds to conservative measures
4. Orthotics can exacerbate symptoms and should thus be avoided.

E. Sural nerve entrapment

1. Can occur anywhere along the course of the nerve, but the nerve is most vulnerable 12 to 15 mm distal to the tip of the fibula as the foot rests in equinus position
2. Surgical release is usually effective.

F. Interdigital nerve entrapment

1. Commonly called a *Morton neuroma*
2. Entrapment can occur during the push-off phase during running in athletes and with the demi-pointe position in dancers.
3. It usually occurs between the third and fourth metatarsals plantar to the transverse metatarsal ligament and responds to surgical resection if conservative measures fail.

II. MUSCLE INJURIES

A. Gastrocnemius-soleus strain

1. Nicknamed *tennis leg* because of its common association with tennis
2. Much more common than rupture of the plantaris tendon
3. Supportive treatment is indicated.

III. TENDON INJURIES

A. Peroneal tendon injuries

1. Subluxation and dislocation
   - Violent dorsiflexion of the inverted foot can result in injury of the fibroosseous peroneal tendon sheath.
   - **Diagnosis is confirmed by observing the subluxation or dislocation by means of eversion and dorsiflexion of the foot.**
   - Plain radiographs may demonstrate a rim fracture of the lateral aspect of the distal fibula.
   - **Treatment of acute injuries includes restoration of the normal anatomy (Figure 4-33).**
   - Chronic reconstruction involves direct repair, groove-deepening procedures, tissue transfers, or bone block techniques.
2. Tenosynovitis
   - These injuries, which are being recognized more frequently with MRI, often lead to tears of the peroneal tendons.
3. Longitudinal tears of the peroneal tendons (especially the peroneus brevis tendon)
   - These injuries are now recognized with increasing frequency.
   - Repair and decompression are generally recommended.

B. Posterior tibialis tendon injury

1. This injury often occurs in older athletes.
2. Patients complain of midarch foot pain, with difficulty pushing off.
3. Débridement of partial ruptures and flexor digitorum longus transfer for chronic injuries are recommended.

C. Anterior tibialis tendon injury

1. Rupture of this tendon is uncommon but has been reported in elderly athletes.
2. Repair is recommended.

D. Achilles tendon injuries

1. Tendinitis and tendinosis
   - Overuse injury to the Achilles tendon usually responds to rest and physical therapy, with an eccentric loading program and local modalities such as ultrasound. Progression to partial rupture may necessitate surgical excision of scar and granulation tissue.
2. Rupture
   - Complete rupture of the tendon is caused by maximal plantar flexion with the foot planted.
   - Patients may relate that they felt as if they were "shot."
   - The Thompson test (squeezing the calf should result in normal plantar flexion of the foot) is helpful for confirming the diagnosis.

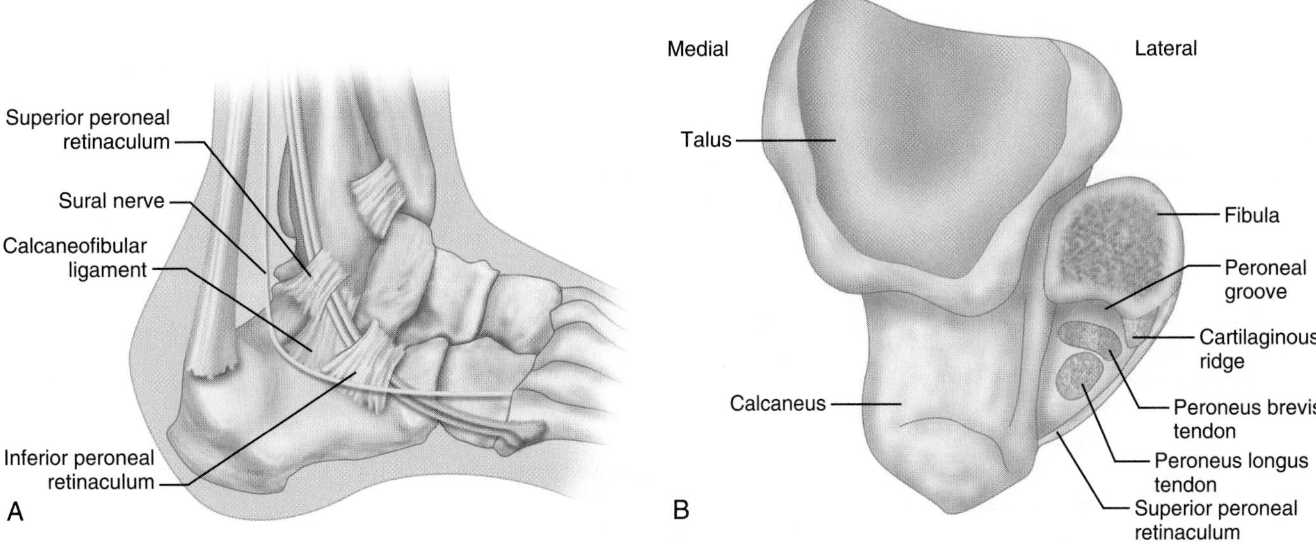

Figure 4-33 Normal relationship of the peroneal tendons. Note the superior and inferior retinacula and the cartilaginous ridge on the posterolateral fibula. **A,** Lateral view. **B,** Superior view. (From Miller MD, Cooper DE, Warner JJP: *Review of sports medicine and arthroscopy,* Philadelphia, 1995, WB Saunders, p 82.)

- **Treatment remains controversial; however, recurrence rates are reduced with primary repair, and other complications (i.e., wound problems) are increased with surgical repair.**
- Early weight bearing after repair has been advocated with improved subjective outcomes.

IV. CHRONIC EXERTIONAL COMPARTMENT SYNDROME

A. Although it is more commonly encountered with trauma, compartment syndrome is becoming more frequently diagnosed in athletes.

B. Athletes (especially runners and cyclists) may note pain that has a gradual onset during exercise, ultimately restricting their performance.

C. Compartment pressures should be measured before, during, and after exercise.

1. **Pressures higher than 20 mm Hg 5 minutes after exercise, absolute values higher than 15 mm Hg during rest, or pressures higher than 30 mm Hg 1 minute after exercise can help establish the diagnosis.**

D. The anterior compartment of the leg is the most frequently involved and has the best prognosis.

E. Fasciotomy is sometimes indicated for refractory cases (Figure 4-34).

F. Popliteal artery entrapment syndrome is often confused with chronic posterior compartment syndrome.

1. Patients present with intermittent claudication, including intermittent calf pain, cramping, coolness, and, at times, paresthesias into the foot.
2. **Provocative clinical tests for the syndrome of popliteal artery entrapment include obliteration of pedal pulses by active plantar flexion or passive dorsiflexion of the ankle as detected by Doppler recordings.**
3. Treatment is release and recession of the medial head of the gastrocnemius.

V. FRACTURES

A. Stress fractures

1. Common in athletes who have undergone a change in their training routines and in female endurance athletes (examiner must ask about the menstrual history).
2. Usually responds to rest and activity modification
3. Recalcitrant fractures may necessitate operative fixation.
   - Tibial shaft fractures
     - This is a complication of unrecognized tibial stress fractures and can be a difficult problem.
     - Persistence of the "dreaded black line" (Figure 4-35) for more than 6 months, especially with a positive bone scan, can be an indication for bone grafting or intramedullary nailing, or both.
   - Tarsal navicular fractures
     - This injury is often found in basketball players.
     - Immobilization and non–weight bearing are important during the early management of these stress fractures.
     - **Open reduction with internal fixation is occasionally indicated with linear fractures (as seen on CT).**
   - Freiberg infarction
     - Flattening of the second metatarsal head, usually as a result of stress overloading in a child's foot
     - Conservative management is indicated unless the patient is having mechanical symptoms (Figure 4-36).

B. Jones fractures

1. Fractures at the metaphyseal-diaphyseal junction of the fifth metatarsal in an athlete.
2. **Early intramedullary screw fixation allows for earlier healing and an earlier return to conditioning activities.**
3. A screw with a minimal diameter of 4 mm should be used (Figure 4-37).
4. **Returning to sports activity before radiographic union increases the risk of nonunion.**

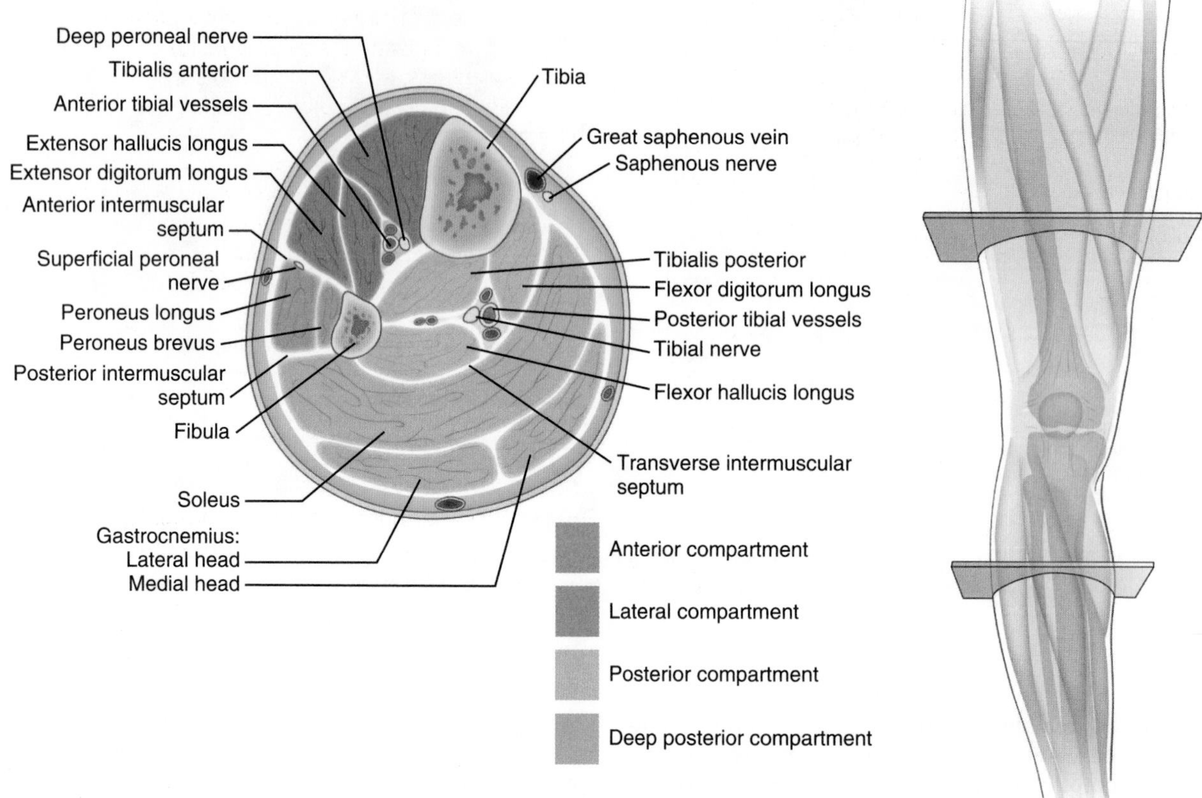

Figure 4-34 Anterior and lateral compartment release. (From DeLee JC, Drez D Jr: *Orthopaedic sports medicine: principles and practice,* Philadelphia, 1994, WB Saunders, p 1618.)

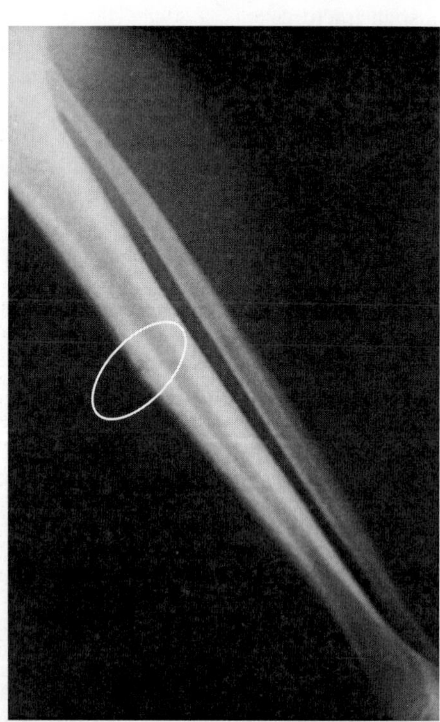

Figure 4-35 Radiograph demonstrating the "dreaded black line" *(circled area)* associated with an impending complete fracture of the tibial shaft. (From Miller MD, Cooper DE, Warner JJP: *Review of sports medicine and arthroscopy,* Philadelphia, 1995, WB Saunders, p 81.)

VI. OTHER FOOT AND ANKLE DISORDERS

A. Plantar fasciitis

1. **Inflammation of the plantar fascia, usually in the central to medial subcalcaneal region, is common in runners.**
2. **Plantar fasciitis is associated with a tight heel cord on physical examination.**

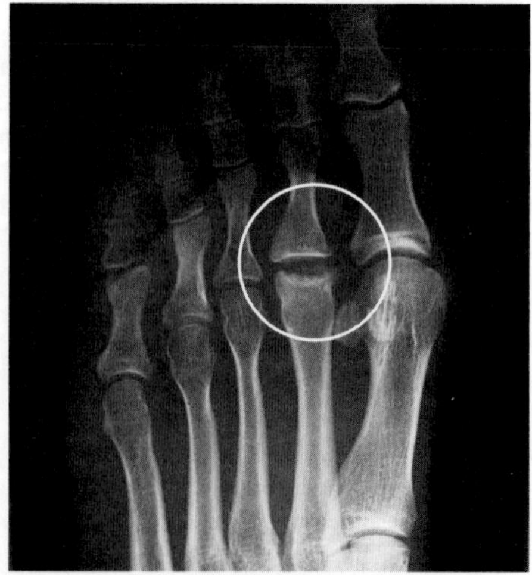

Figure 4-36 Radiographic appearance of Freiberg infarction *(circled area).*

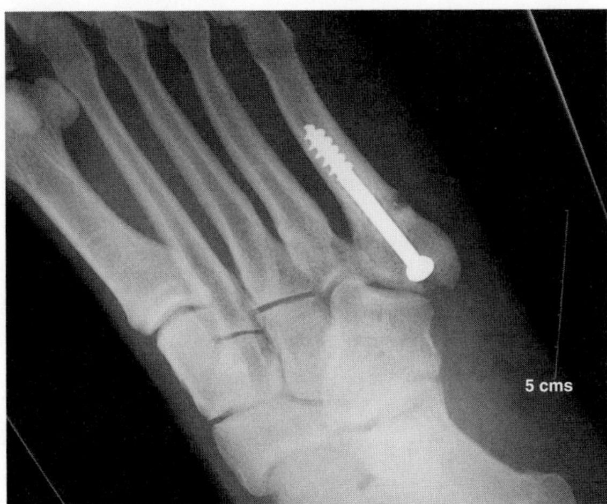

Figure 4-37 Radiographic appearance of Jones fracture after open reduction with internal fixation with a 6.5-mm screw.

3. Rest, orthoses, stretching, NSAIDs, and local steroid injections are helpful.
4. Partial plantar fasciotomy is occasionally necessary, but recovery can be protracted.
5. Refractory cases may be treated with extracorporeal shock wave therapy.

B. **Os trigonum (posterior impingement) syndrome**

1. Can cause impingement with plantar flexion of the foot, especially in ballet dancers
2. Treatment may include local anesthetic injection and other supportive measures.
3. **Surgical excision of the offending bone with or without release of the flexor hallucis longus is occasionally necessary,** and arthroscopic techniques have been described.

C. **Ankle sprains and instability**

1. Common in athletes and most often involve the anterior talofibular ligament and occasionally involve the calcaneofibular ligament
2. The posterior talofibular ligament is rarely involved.
3. The Ottawa ankle rules (Stiell et al, 1995) indicate that radiographs are required only in patients with tenderness at the distal (especially posterior) tibia or fibula, tenderness at the base of the fifth metatarsal or navicular, and an inability to bear weight.
4. Surgical treatment is reserved for recurrent, symptomatic ankle instability with excessive tilt and a positive finding of the anterior drawer test on examination or on stress radiographs that have not responded to orthoses and peroneal strengthening and proprioceptive exercises over an extended period.
5. Anatomic procedures (modified Broström procedure) are usually successful.
6. Involvement of the subtalar joint necessitates tendon rerouting procedures that include this joint.
7. Patients with "high" ankle sprains involving the syndesmosis require recovery periods almost twice as long as those for patients with common ankle sprains.
   - **Pain in the anterior syndesmosis in response to an external rotation stress test is suggestive of the diagnosis.**
   - **Tibiofibular synostosis may occur, and excision should be performed for persistent pain.**

D. **Turf toe**

1. Severe dorsiflexion of the metatarsophalangeal joint of the great toe (injuring the plantar plate) can result in tenderness, stiffness, and swelling of the toe.
2. Treatment includes physical therapy, ice, and taping in plantar flexion.
3. If symptoms persist, a stress fracture of the proximal phalanx should be ruled out with a bone scan or MRI.
4. Chronic turf toe can result in hallux rigidus.

E. **Snowboarder's foot and ankle**

1. Fracture of the lateral process of the talus (Figure 4-38).
2. The injury involves the leading leg on the board.
3. CT can help confirm the diagnosis.
4. Fracture with small fragments (<2 mm) can be treated in a short leg cast for 6 weeks, whereas a fracture with large fragments should should be treated with open reduction with internal fixation.

F. **Ankle impingement**

1. Soft tissue or bony conditions leading to decreased ROM, chronic pain around the ankle, or both
   - Anterior impingement
     - Common in ballet dancers and football, basketball, and soccer players
     - Pain with dorsiflexion along with cutting and pivoting maneuvers are common symptoms.
     - Lateral radiographs reveal a combination of anterior osteophyte formation on the distal anterior tibia and divot-like formation on the dorsal aspect of the talar neck.
     - Treatment may include arthroscopic bony resection.
   - Posterior impingement
     - Also common in ballet dancers, gymnasts, soccer players, and downhill runners
     - Known as *os trigonum syndrome* or *talar compression syndrome*
     - Pain is worse with plantar flexion and push-off maneuvers.
     - Soft tissue can become trapped between the distal posterior tibia and calcaneus during plantar flexion.

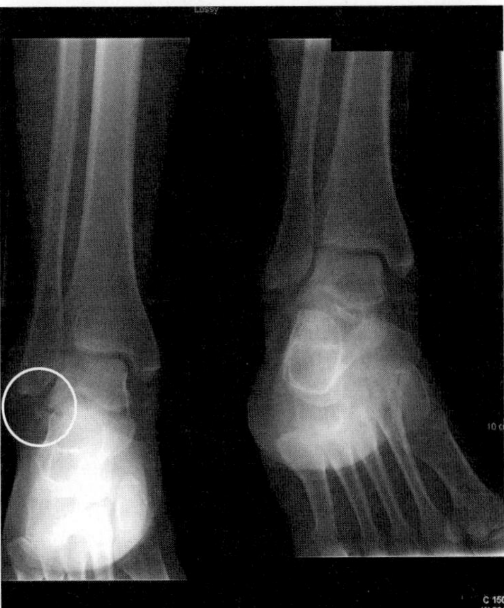

Figure 4-38 Radiographic appearance of snowboarder's ankle *(circled area).*

- Bony lesions that can contribute include os trigonum (present in 7% of adults), Stieda process (elongated lateral talar tubercle), and loose bodies.
- **Soft tissue causes include flexor hallucis longus synovitis** and posterior recesses of the subtalar and tibiotalar joints. Excision (open or arthroscopic) of the os trigonum is often effective.

VII. ANKLE ARTHROSCOPY

See Supplemental Images on expertconsult.com.

A. Indications

1. Include treatment of osteochondral injuries of the talus, débridement of post-traumatic synovitis, anterolateral impingement secondary to chronic pain from an ankle sprain, removal of anterior tibiotalar spurring, os trigonum excision, and cartilage débridement in conjunction with ankle fusions.
2. Osteochondral injuries of the talus
   - Treatment includes drilling of the base of these lesions and fixation of replaceable lesions.
3. Lateral lesions are usually traumatic, shallow, and anterior, whereas medial lesions are atraumatic, deeper, and posterior.
   - Lateral lesions are usually associated with inversion and dorsiflexion. Medial lesions are seen with inversion, plantar flexion, and rotation.
4. The modification to the Berndt and Harty classification scheme (Figure 4-39) by Loomer and coworkers (1993) is helpful in the management of these osteochondral lesions of the talus.

B. Technique

1. Supine positioning with the leg over a well-padded bolster and an external traction device are currently popular.
2. **Meticulous attention to portal placement is required because the most common complication of ankle arthroscopy is nerve injury.**

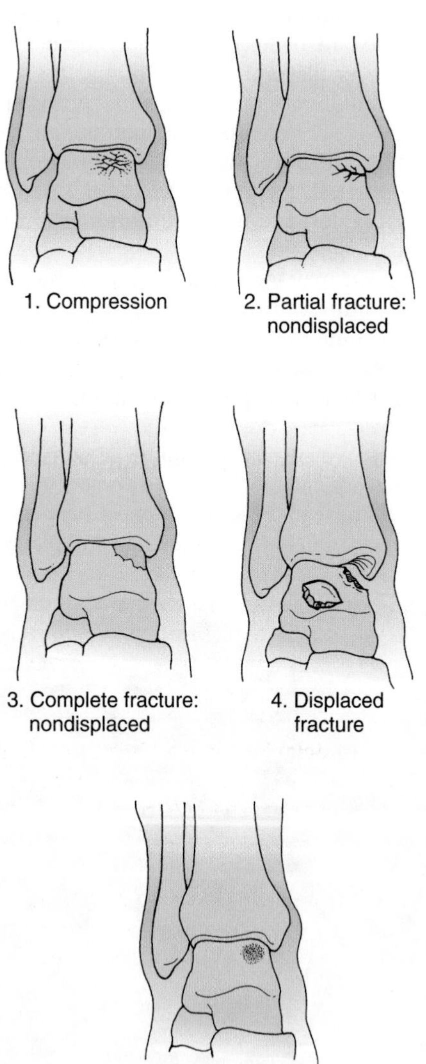

Figure 4-39 **Loomer and coworkers' (1993) modification of the Berndt and Harty classification of osteochondral lesions of the talus.** (From Miller MD, Cooper DE, Warner JJP: *Review of sports medicine and arthroscopy,* Philadelphia, 1995, WB Saunders, p 95.)

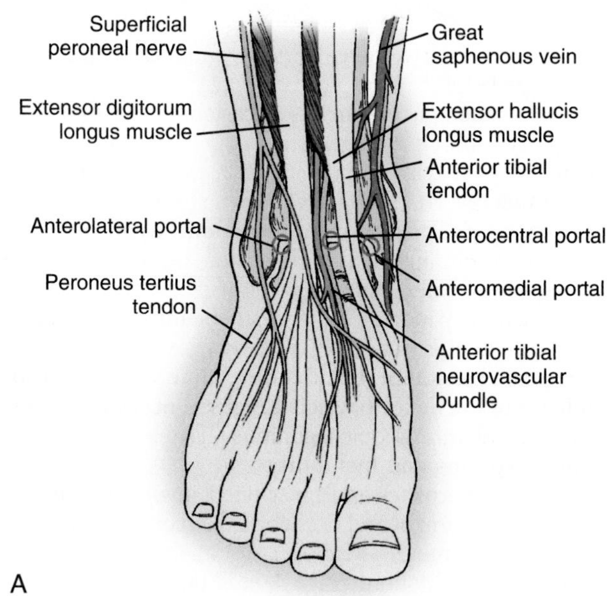

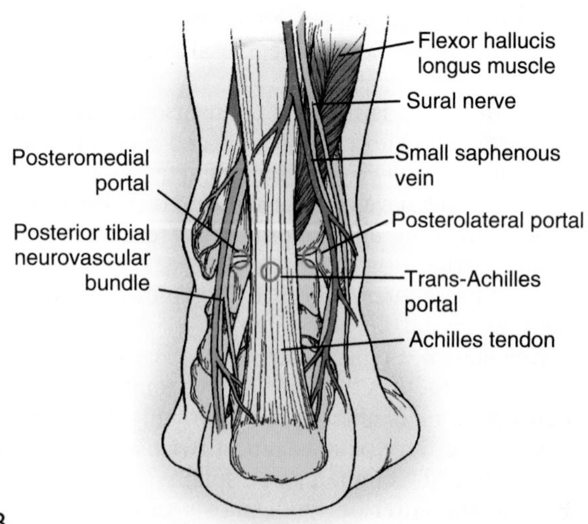

Figure 4-40 **Portals for ankle arthroscopy are the (A) anteromedial, anterolateral, and posterolateral (B).** (From Canale ST, Beaty JH: *Campbell's operative orthopaedics,* ed 11, Philadelphia, 2008, Elsevier.)

3. Five portals—anteromedial, anterolateral, posterolateral, posteromedial, and anterocentral—have been suggested (Figure 4-40), but most surgeons avoid both the posteromedial portal (because of the risk to the posterior tibial artery and tibial nerve) and the anterocentral portal (because of the risk to the dorsalis pedis and deep peroneal nerve).
4. The "nick and spread" method is advocated for the anterolateral portal (superficial peroneal nerve) and the anteromedial portal (saphenous vein).

SECTION 4 SHOULDER

I. ANATOMY AND BIOMECHANICS*

The shoulder consists of three bones and four joints.

A. Osteology

1. Clavicle
   - An S-shaped bone, it is the last to ossify (the medial growth plate fuses in the early 20s).
2. Scapula
   - Serves as the insertion site for 17 muscles.
   - Two important prominences: the coracoid process and the acromion
   - Os acromiale, an unfused secondary ossification center, occurs with a 3% incidence; in 60% of affected patients, it is bilateral.
     - The most common location is at the junction of the mesoacromion and meta-acromion.
     - **Persistent symptoms may be treated with open reduction and internal fixation.**
   - Glenoid
     - The shoulder "socket," or glenoid cavity, is a lateral projection of the scapula.
     - Rim is surrounded by fibrocartilaginous thickening (the labrum), which serves to both deepen the socket (acting as a chock block) and anchor the inferior glenohumeral ligament complex.
     - Surface is pear-shaped, with an average upward tilt of 5 degrees and an average range of 7 degrees of retroversion to 10 degrees of anteversion.
3. Humeral head
   - Is approximately spheroidal in 90% of individuals and has an average diameter of 43 mm
   - Normally retroverted an average of 30 degrees to the transepicondylar axis of the distal humerus
   - Articular surface inclined an average of 130 degrees superiorly in relation to the shaft.

B. Articulations

1. The four joints of the shoulder are the glenohumeral, sternoclavicular, acromioclavicular, and scapulothoracic.
   - Glenohumeral joint
     - Spheroidal (ball-and-socket) joint, it is the principal articulation of the shoulder and is stabilized by both static and dynamic restraints (see the following discussion on biomechanics).
     - Part of the static restraints, the glenohumeral ligaments are discrete capsular thickenings that act as a kind of rein to limit excessive rotation or translation of the humeral head.
     - The capsuloligamentous structures include the superior glenohumeral ligament (SGHL), coracohumeral ligament, middle glenohumeral ligament, and inferior glenohumeral ligament complex (Figure 4-41).
     - Additional capsular elements include the posterior capsule, which is the thinnest portion (<1 mm) of the shoulder capsule, and the rotator interval.
       - **The contents of the rotator interval include the coracohumeral ligament, SGHL, biceps tendon, and glenohumeral capsule.**
         - Bounded medially by the lateral coracoid base, superiorly by the anterior edge of the supraspinatus, and inferiorly by the superior border of the subscapularis
         - The transverse humeral ligament forms its apex laterally.
   - Sternoclavicular joint
     - Gliding joint with a disc that serves to anchor the shoulder girdle to the chest wall.
     - Elevation of the arm from 0 to 90 degrees produces clavicular rotation about its longitudinal axis and elevation at the sternoclavicular joint of 0 to 40 degrees. **The posterior capsule is the primary restraint of excessive anterior and posterior translation.**
   - Acromioclavicular joint
     - The articulation of the scapula with the clavicle occurs through a diarthrodial joint containing an incomplete intraarticular disc.
     - Stabilized by the acromioclavicular ligaments, which primarily resist anteroposterior translation and the coracoclavicular ligaments, which prevent inferior translation of the coracoid and acromion from the clavicle (Figure 4-42).
     - **The acromioclavicular joint is best evaluated in the Zanca view, in which the x-ray beam is directed 10 degrees cephalad at 50% of normal penetrance (see Table 4-10).**
   - Scapulothoracic joint
     - The medial border of the scapula articulates with the posterior aspect of the second to seventh ribs.
     - Angled 30 degrees anteriorly and has a 3-degree upward tilt
     - There are two major scapulothoracic bursae.
     - The ratio of glenohumeral to scapulothoracic motion during shoulder abduction is approximately 2 : 1.

C. Supporting structures

1. It is helpful to consider the shoulder in layers (Figure 4-43).
2. **The rotator cable is a thickening of the coracohumeral ligament that is present at the margin of the avascular**

*See Chapter 2, Anatomy, for a more detailed description of shoulder anatomy.

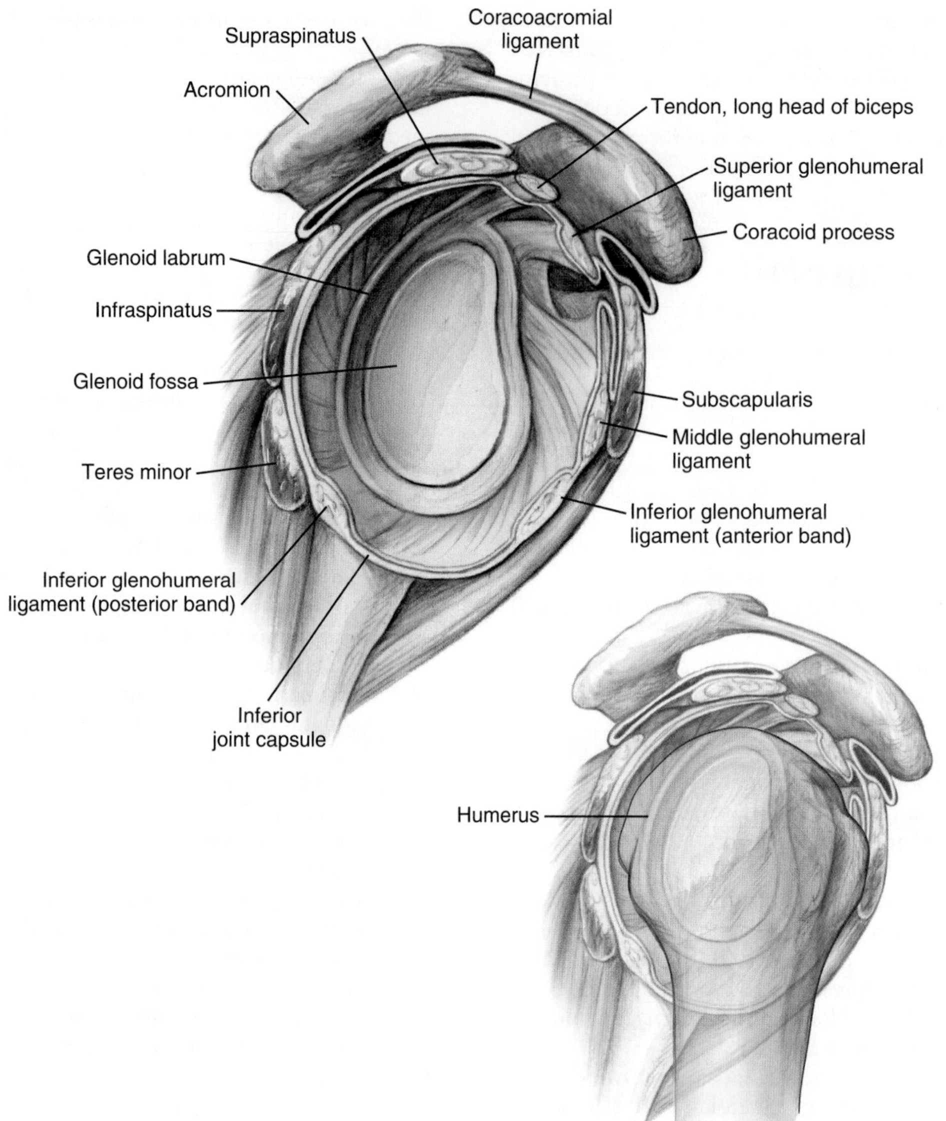

Figure 4-41 Important ligaments of the shoulder. (From Miller MD, et al: *Orthopaedic surgical approaches,* Philadelphia, 2008, Elsevier.)

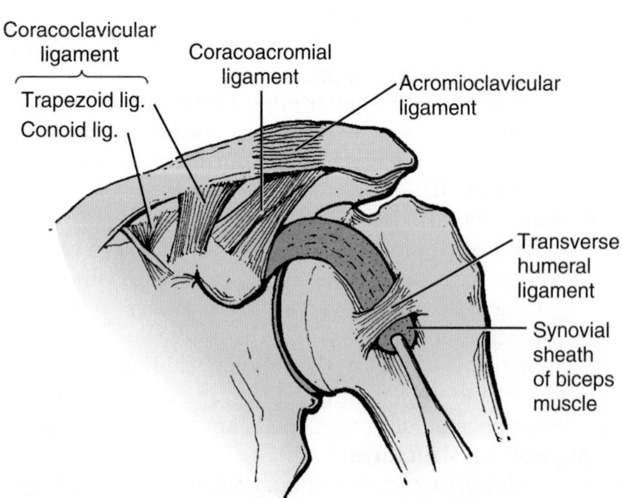

Figure 4-42 Acromioclavicular joint anatomy. (From Tibone J, et al: Functional anatomy, biomechanics, and kinesiology: the shoulder. In DeLee JC, Drez D Jr, editors: *Orthopaedic sports medicine: principles and practice,* Philadelphia, 1994, WB Saunders, p 465.)

zone. The rotator cable distributes stress away from the avascular portion of the rotator cuff.

D. Biomechanics

1. The shoulder is stabilized by both static and dynamic restraints.
   - Static restraints
     - These include the glenoid labrum, articular version, articular conformity, negative intraarticular pressure, capsule (posterior capsule and rotator interval), and capsuloligamentous structures.
     - Imbrication of the rotator interval decreases inferior and posterior translation, whereas its release produces increased forward flexion and external rotation.
     - **The SGHL and coracohumeral ligament are reinforcing structures of the rotator interval, limiting inferior translation and external rotation when the arm is adducted and posterior translation when the arm is flexed forward, adducted, and internally rotated.**
     - The middle glenohumeral ligament limits external rotation of the adducted humerus, inferior translation

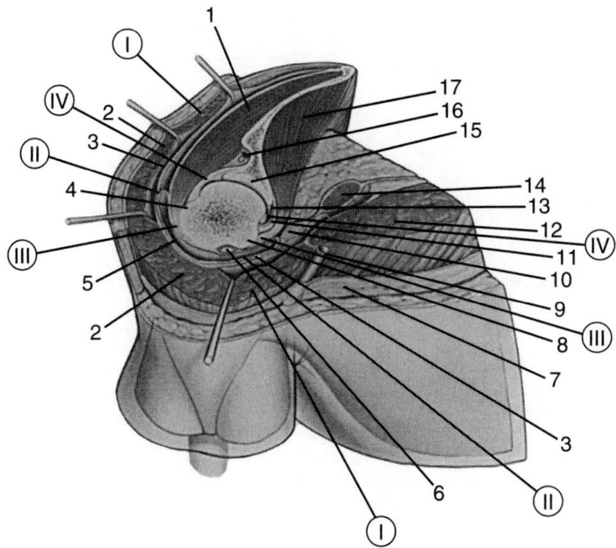

Figure 4-43 Cross-sectional view of the right shoulder at the level of the lesser tuberosity. Note the four layers of the shoulder and their components: Layer I consists of the deltoid (*2*), pectoralis major (*12*), and cephalic vein (*9*); layer II consists of the conjoined tendon (*10*), pectoralis minor (*14*), and clavipectoral fascia (*7*); layer III consists of the subdeltoid bursa (*5*), rotator cuff muscles (*1, 17*), glenohumeral capsule (*11*), greater tuberosity (*4*), long head of biceps (*6*), lesser tuberosity (*8*), fascia (*3*), synovium (*13*), glenoid (*15*) and suprascapular neurovascular nerve bundle (*16*); layer IV consists of the glenohumeral capsule (*11*), glenoid (*15*), synovium (*13*) and long head of the biceps (*6*). (From Cooper DE, O'Brien SJ, Warren RF: Supporting layers of the glenohumeral joint: an anatomic study, *Clin Orthop* 289:151, 1993.)

of the adducted and externally rotated humerus, and anterior and posterior translation of the partly abducted (at 45 degrees) and externally rotated arm.
   - **The inferior glenohumeral ligament complex serves as the primary restraint to anterior, posterior, and inferior glenohumeral translation at 45 to 90 degrees of glenohumeral elevation (Table 4-8).**
- Dynamic restraints
   - These include **joint concavity compression produced by synchronized contraction of the rotator cuff, acting to stabilize the humeral head within the glenoid;** increased capsular tension produced by direct attachments of the rotator cuff to the capsule; the scapular stabilizers that act to maintain a stable glenoid platform ("ball on a seal's nose"); and proprioception.

Table 4-8 Glenohumeral Ligaments

Structure	Arm Position	Resists
SGHL/CHL	Adduction	Inferior translation/external rotation
	Forward flexion/abduction/internal rotation	Posterior translation
MGHL	Adduction/external rotation	External rotation
	45-degree abduction/external rotation	Anterior/posterior translation
IGHL	45- to 90-degree glenohumeral elevation	Primary restraint to anterior/posterior/inferior glenohumeral translation

CHL, coracohumeral ligament; IGHL, inferior glenohumeral ligament; MGHL, middle glenohumeral ligament; SGHL, superior glenohumeral ligament.

E. Throwing

1. Significant forces are generated during throwing and can result in anatomic variation and injury.
2. **Typically, there is greater external rotation and a loss of internal rotation of the dominant shoulder in comparison with the nondominant shoulder; this condition is referred to as glenohumeral internal rotation deficit (GIRD).**
   - The anterior capsule is selectively stretched, whereas the posterior capsule is tightened. These developments can predispose to both instability and internal impingement.
   - Bony changes have also been observed in the dominant shoulder, including increased humeral head retroversion and glenoid retroversion.
3. The five phases of throwing are shown in Figure 4-44.
4. Maximal torque is generated during two actions: maximal external rotation (late cocking) and just after ball release (deceleration).

II. DIAGNOSTIC TECHNIQUES

A. History

1. Age and chief complaint are two important considerations.
2. Instability, acromioclavicular injuries, and distal clavicle osteolysis are more common in young patients.
3. Rotator cuff tears, arthritis, and proximal humeral fractures are more common in older patients.

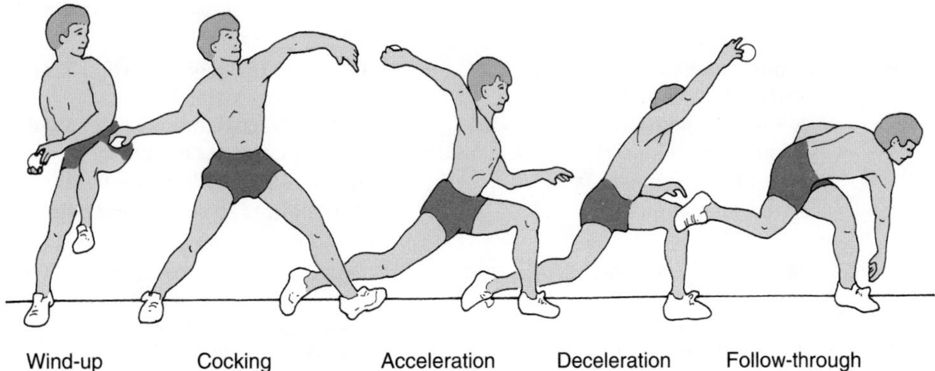

Figure 4-44 The five phases of throwing. (From Miller MD, Cooper DE, Warner JJP: *Review of sports medicine and arthroscopy,* Philadelphia, 1995, WB Saunders, p 123.)

4. Direct blows are usually responsible for acromioclavicular separations.
5. Instability occurs with injury to the abducted, externally rotated arm.
6. Chronic overhead pain and night pain are associated with rotator cuff tears.

B. Physical examination

1. Observation, palpation, and strength testing can provide important diagnostic clues.
2. Examination includes assessment of range and quality of motion (forward flexion of 150 to 180 degrees, external rotation with the arm adducted 30 to 60 degrees, and internal rotation reaching the level of T4 to T8 are considered normal), as well as specific muscle testing (Table 4-9; Figures 4-45 and 4-46).
3. Note that the scapula must be stabilized in order to evaluate true ROM of the glenohumeral joint.

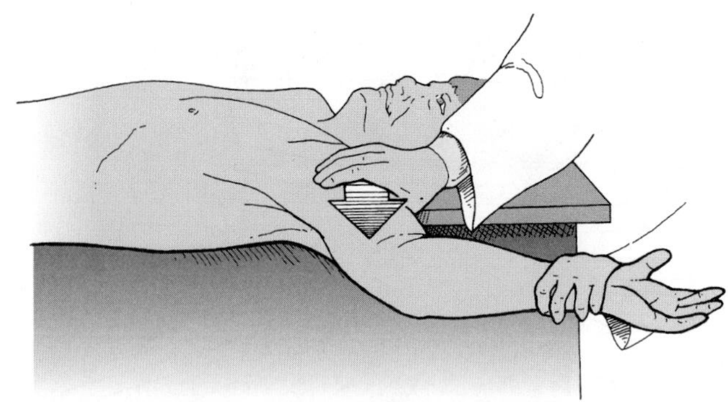

Figure 4-45 Relocation test. Anterior pressure on the proximal arm relocates the humerus and causes relief of apprehension. (From Miller MD, Cooper DE, Warner JJP: *Review of sports medicine and arthroscopy,* Philadelphia, 1995, WB Saunders, p 128.)

Table 4-9 Muscle Testing for Shoulder Injuries

Examination	Technique	Significance
Impingement/Rotator Cuff		
Impingement sign	Passive FF >90 degrees	Pain indicates impingement syndrome
Impingement test	Passive FF >90 degrees continues after subacromial injection	Relief of pain indicates impingement syndrome
Hawkins test	Passive FF of 90 degrees and IR	Pain indicates impingement syndrome
Jobe test	Resisted pronation/FF of 90 degrees	Pain indicates supraspinatus lesion
Drop-arm test	Maintaining FF in plane of scapula	Inability indicates supraspinatus lesion
Hornblower sign	Resisted maximal ER/abduction of 90 degrees	Pain indicates infraspinatus, supraspinatus, or post-supraspinatus lesion
Rubber band sign	Resisted maximal ER/slight abduction	Pain indicates infraspinatus lesion
Liftoff test	Arm in IR behind back	Inability to elevate from back indicates subscapularis lesion
Modified liftoff test	Resisted arm held off back	Inability to keep arm elevated when off back indicates subscapularis lesion
Belly-push test	Elbow held anterior with abduction pressure	Inability to hold elbow forward indicates subscapularis lesion
Instability		
Apprehension test	Supine abduction in 90 degrees and ER	Apprehension indicates anterior instability
Relocation test (see Figure 4-45)	Apprehension with posterior force	Relief of apprehension indicates anterior instability
Load-and-shift test	Anterior/posterior force on humeral head	Degree of translation reflects laxity or instability (see Table 4-11 for grading)
Modified load-and-shift test	Supine load/shift with elbow bending	Degree of translation reflects laxity or instability (see Table 4-11 for grading)
Jerk test	Post force with arm adduction and FF	A "clunk" sound indicates posterior subluxation
Sulcus sign	Inferior force with arm at side	Increased acromiohumeral interval reflects inferior laxity or instability (see Table 4-11 for sulcus grading)
Labrum/Biceps		
Active compression test	10 degrees adduction, 90 degrees FF, maximal pronation	Pain with resistance indicates SLAP lesion
Anterior slide test	Hand on hip, joint loading	Pain with resistance indicates SLAP lesion
Crank test	Full abduction, humeral loading, rotation	Pain indicates SLAP lesion
Speed test	Resisted FF in scapular plane	Pain indicates bicipital tendinitis
Yerguson test	Resisted supination	Pain indicates bicipital tendinitis
Miscellaneous		
Spurling maneuver (see Figure 4-46)	Lateral flexion, rotation, cervical loading	Cervical spine disease or injury
Wright test	Extension-abduction-ER of arm with neck rotated away	Loss of pulse and reproduction of symptoms indicates thoracic outlet syndrome

ER, external rotation; ext, extension; FF, forward flexion; IR, internal rotation; SLAP, superior labrum from anterior to posterior.

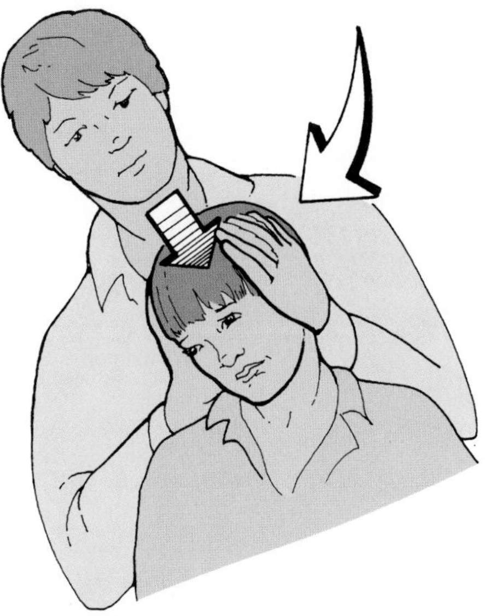

Figure 4-46 Spurling test. Lateral flexion and rotation with some compression may cause nerve root encroachment and pain on the ipsilateral side in patients with impingement of the cervical nerve root. (From Miller MD, Cooper DE, Warner JJP: *Review of sports medicine and arthroscopy,* Philadelphia, 1995, WB Saunders, p 129.)

C. **Imaging of the shoulder**

1. Trauma series
   - The trauma series of radiographs includes a "true" anteroposterior view (plate is placed parallel to the scapula, about 45 degrees from the plane of the thorax) and an **axillary lateral view.**
2. Other views
   - Other views that are sometimes helpful include a scapular Y or transscapular view and anteroposterior radiographs in internal and external rotation. Special radiographic views have also been developed for certain other abnormalities. For example, the supraspinatus outlet view is helpful in the evaluation of impingement (Figure 4-47; Table 4-10).

III. SHOULDER ARTHROSCOPY

See Supplemental Images on expertconsult.com.

A. **Portals**

1. Standard portals
   - Posterior portal (2 cm distal and medial to the posterolateral border of the acromion, used primarily for viewing)

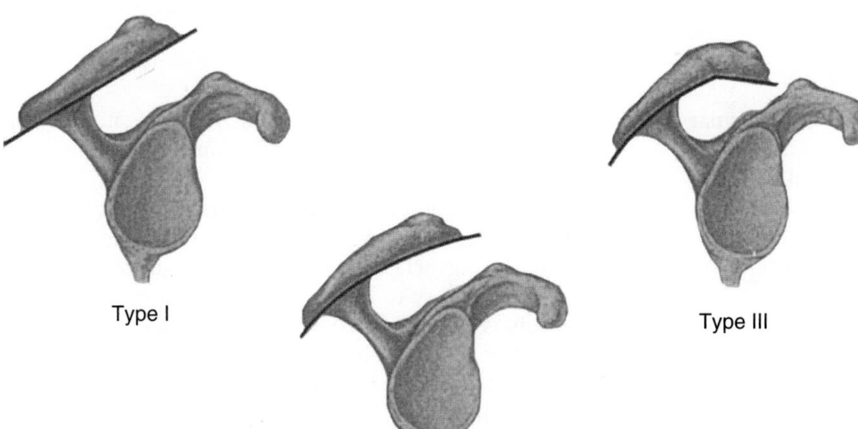

Figure 4-47 Acromion structure is classified on the basis of the supraspinatus outlet view as originally described by Bigliani. (From Esch JC: Shoulder arthroscopy in the older age group, *Op Tech Orthop* 1:200, 1991.)

Table 4-10 Radiographic Views of the Shoulder

View/Sign	Findings	Significance
View of supraspinatus outlet	Acromial structure (types I to III)	Type III acromion associated with impingement
View of 30-degree caudal tilt	Subacromial spurring	Area below level of clavicle is impingement area
Zanca 10-degree cephalic tilt	AC joint disease	AC DJD, distal clavicle osteolysis
West Point view	AI glenoid evaluation	Bony Bankart lesion seen with instability
Garth view	AI glenoid evaluation	Bony Bankart lesion seen with instability
Stryker notch	Humeral head evaluation	Hill-Sachs impression fracture
Anteroposterior internal rotation	Humeral head evaluation	Hill-Sachs defect
Hobbs view	SC injury	Anteroposterior dislocations
Serendipity view	SC injury	Anteroposterior dislocations
45-degree abduction, true anteroposterior view	Glenohumeral space	Subtle DJD
Arthrography	Rotator cuff injuries	Dye above cuff indicates tear
CT	Fractures	Classification is easier
MRI ± arthrography	Soft tissue evaluation	Labral, cuff, muscle tears

AC, acromioclavicular; AI, anteroinferior; CT, computed tomography; DJD, degenerative joint disease; MRI, magnetic resonance imaging; SC, sternoclavicular.

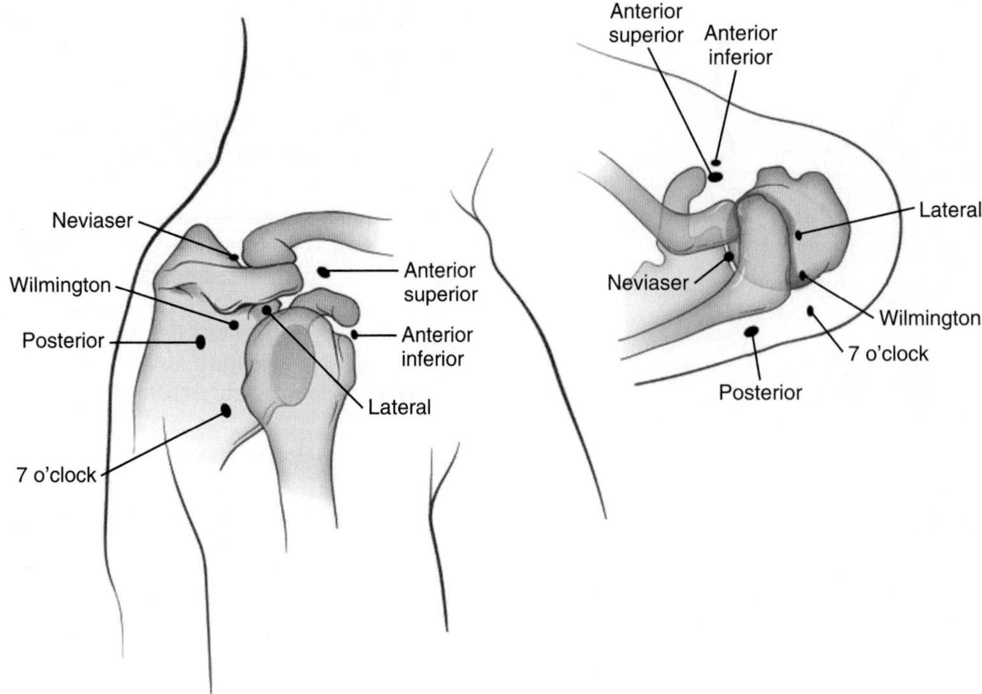

Figure 4-48 Arthroscopic portals of the shoulder. (From Miller MD, et al: *Orthopaedic surgical approaches,* Philadelphia, 2008, Elsevier.)

- Anterior portal (just anterior to the acromioclavicular joint)
- Lateral portal (1 to 2 cm distal to the lateral acromial edge)

2. Additional portals
   - Supraspinatus (Neviaser) portal for anterior glenoid visualization (through the supraspinatus fossa)
   - Anterolateral and posterolateral portals (Port of Wilmington, just anterior to the posterolateral corner of the acromion) are useful for labral tears or tears of the superior labrum from anterior to posterior (SLAP) and rotator cuff repair
   - Anteroinferior (5 o'clock position) portal for Bankart repair and stabilization procedures
   - Posteroinferior (7 o'clock position) portal for stabilization procedures (Figure 4-48)

B. **Technique**

1. Intraarticular structures should be systematically evaluated.
2. As the number and variety of arthroscopic procedures increase, so does the opportunity for iatrogenic injury.
3. Maintaining adequate visualization through hemostasis, avoiding chondral abrasion, maintaining adequate flow with thermal devices, and preventing fluid extravasation by preserving muscle fascial layers help minimize the risk.

IV. SHOULDER INSTABILITY

A. **Cause**

1. **Traumatic anterior shoulder dislocations typically result when the arm is abducted and in external rotation.**

B. **Diagnosis**

1. Because the shoulder has an extensive ROM, it is at risk for developing instability and is the joint most commonly dislocated in the body.
2. Instability is a pathologic condition manifesting as pain as a result of excessive translation of the humeral head on the glenoid during active shoulder motion; it represents a spectrum of injury to the shoulder stabilizers.
3. Diagnosis is based on history, physical examination findings, and imaging results.
   - **The axillary nerve is susceptible to injury after anterior dislocation because of its relatively fixed position.**
4. Clinical evidence of instability includes positive load-and-shift, modified load-and-shift, and apprehension-relocation testing, as well as a sulcus sign (see Table 4-9).
   - Instability is often associated with a Bankart lesion **(anteroinferior labral tear)** with disrupted medial scapular periosteum (Figure 4-49).
   - Variants include a bony or osseous Bankart lesion (glenoid rim fracture with functional labral detachment); Perthes lesion (nondisplaced labral tear with intact medial scapular periosteum); anterior labroligamentous periosteal sleeve avulsion (ALPSA, or "medialized Bankart" lesion: medial anterioinferior labral tear displaced medially by intact medial scapular periosteum); reverse Bankart lesion (posteroinferior labral tear); and glenolabral articular disruption (labral tear extending into glenoid cartilage).
   - **Humeral avulsion of the inferior glenohumeral ligament (HAGL) has typically necessitated open repair in the past, because of its inferior location, but newer arthroscopic techniques are being developed (Figure 4-50).**
   - Grading of instability is shown in Table 4-11.

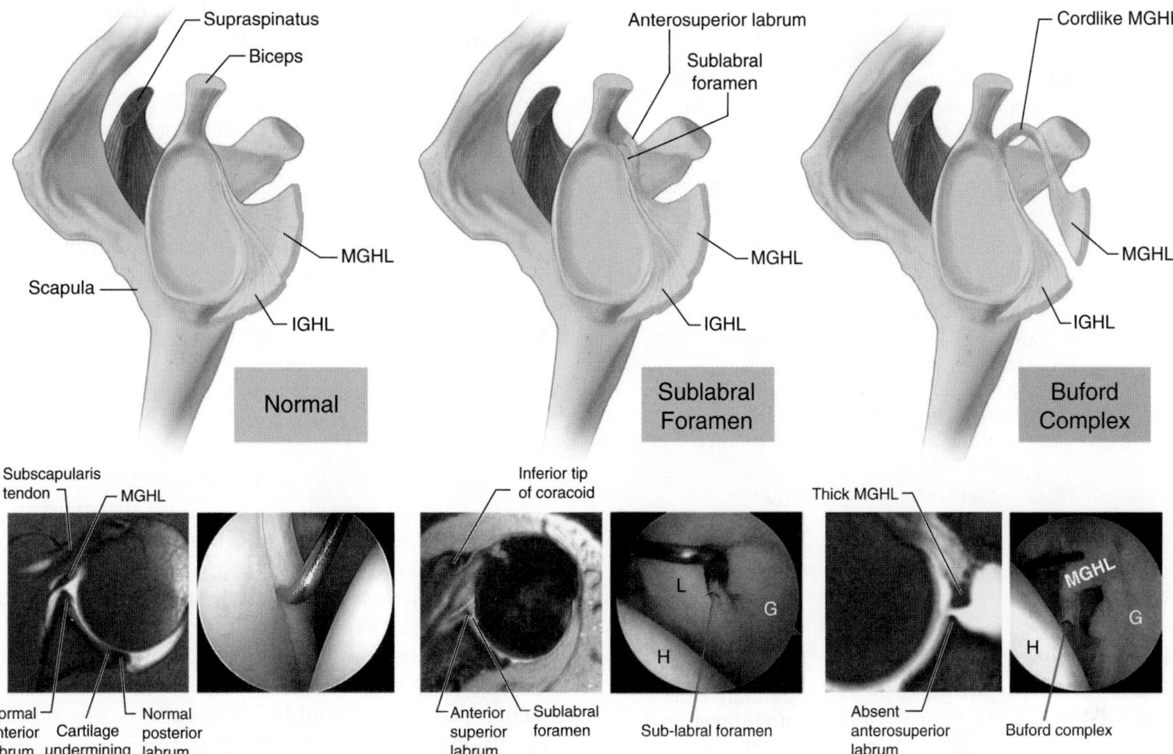

Figure 4-49 Common anterior labral variations with MRI and arthroscopic correlations. IGHL, inferior glenohumeral ligament; MGHL, middle glenohumeral ligament.

5. TUBS syndrome: *T*raumatic *u*nilateral dislocations with a *B*ankart lesion often necessitate *s*urgery because they typically occur in young patients and have recurrence rates of up to 90% with nonoperative management.
   - **Age at time of initial dislocation is an important risk factor for recurrent shoulder instability.**

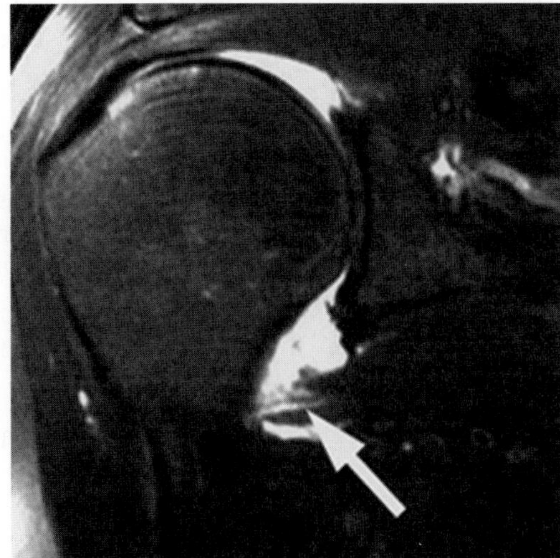

Figure 4-50 MRI appearance of a HAGL lesion.

6. AMBRI syndrome: *A*traumatic *m*ultidirectional *b*ilateral shoulder dislocation/subluxation often responds to *r*ehabilitation, and sometimes an *i*nferior capsular shift or plication is required.

C. Treatment

1. **Multidirectional instability should be treated with extended rehabilitation that focuses on scapular stabilization before operative intervention is considered. Closed kinetic chain exercises should be emphasized.**
2. Several open and arthroscopic techniques have been developed to address instability (Table 4-12).

Table 4-11 Grades of Instability

Grade	Anteroposterior Grading Scheme*	Sulcus Grading Scheme†
0	Normal small amount of humeral head translation	—
1	Humeral head translation to but not over the glenoid rim	Acromiohumeral interval <1 cm
2	Humeral head translation over the glenoid rim with spontaneous reduction when the applied force is withdrawn	Acromiohumeral interval 1 to 2 cm
3	Humeral head translation with locking over the glenoid rim	Acromiohumeral interval >2 cm

*Abnormal (vs. contralateral shoulder): anterior instability is ≥ grade 1; posterior instability is ≥ grade 3.

†Abnormal (vs. contralateral shoulder): ≥ grade 2.

Table 4-12 Treatment of Shoulder Instability

Procedure	Essential Features	Comments/ Complications
Bankart	Reattachment of labrum (and IGHLC) to glenoid	"Gold standard"
Staple capsulorrhaphy	Capsular reattachment and tightening	Staple migration/ articular injury
Putti-Platt	Subscapularis advancement capsular coverage	Decreased external rotation, DJD
Magnuson-Stack	Subscapularis transfer to greater tuberosity	Decreased external rotation
Boyd-Sisk	Transfer of biceps laterally and posteriorly	Nonanatomic, recurrence
Bristow/Latarjet	Coracoid transfer to inferior glenoid	Nonunion, migration, labral tears
Bone block osteotomy	Anterior bone block	Nonunion, migration, articular injury
Capsular shift	Inferior capsule shifted superiorly: "pants over vest"	Overtightening; "gold standard" for multidirectional instability

DJD, degenerative joint disease; IGHLC, inferior glenohumeral ligament complex.

- **Specific indications:**
  - **Glenoid deficiency greater than 25% of the humeral head: coracoid transfer (Latarjet procedure)**
  - **Failed rehab for multidirectional instability: capsular shift**
  - **Chronic dislocation with greater than 40% of articular surface deficit: allograft for young patients, prosthesis for older patients**

3. These procedures have been broadened to address both capsuloligamentous laxity (e.g., capsular plication, rotator interval closure) and labral disease with the use of various instruments, suture passage and knot-tying techniques, and fixation devices (both absorbable and nonabsorbable).
   - First-time dislocations: Debate still exists regarding treatment.
     - External rotation bracing for 3 to 6 weeks has been effective in decreasing the short-term rates of recurrent dislocation in an Asian population.
     - The rates of recurrent dislocation (generally <10%) are lowest after operative treatment, either open or arthroscopic.
     - The newest data show that outcomes with arthroscopic anterior stabilization are equivalent to those with open repairs.
     - Some authorities have advocated repair of first-time dislocations because of the decreased rate of dislocation 6 years after repair and the better quality of life associated with operative treatment; however, this is still controversial.
   - **Rotator interval closure results in decreased external rotation in shoulder adduction and posteroinferior translation.**
   - Complications of open procedures include subscapularis overtightening (Z-lengthening required) or rupture (repair or pectoralis transfer required) and hardware problems.
   - Instability: For injuries traditionally treated with open repair, arthroscopic repair—with improved surgical techniques, sutures and anchors, and postoperative rehabilitation—now yields equivalent outcomes.
   - The role of thermal capsular shrinkage is no longer recommended.
     - Good short-term results were initially reported, but newer long-term results have demonstrated worse outcomes.
     - Poor tissue quality and chondral damage at the time of revision have been noted after thermal shrinkage. Thus, it is no longer recommended.

D. Posterior instability

1. **Patients may exhibit positive results with load-and-shift and jerk testing.**
   - **A fixed posterior shoulder dislocation is diagnosed by lack of external rotation.**
2. **Acute posterior shoulder dislocations are most commonly caused by high-energy trauma, electric shocks, or epileptic seizures.**
3. Patients may present with their arms internally rotated and with observable coracoid and posterior prominence.
4. **Anteroposterior radiographs are unreliable but may demonstrate a "lightbulb" sign.** An axillary lateral radiograph is extremely helpful in making the diagnosis.
5. When they are recognized, posterior dislocations respond well to acute reduction and immobilization.
6. Rehabilitation focuses on rotator cuff and deltoid strengthening; surgical management (arthroscopic or open posterior Bankart repair, with or without capsular shift) is reserved for refractory cases.

E. Kim lesion

1. This is an incomplete and concealed avulsion of the posteroinferior labrum (Figure 4-51).
2. May be associated with posterior and multidirectional instability
3. The jerk (posterior lesion) and Kim (posteroinferior lesion) tests have been shown to be highly sensitive and specific.
4. Magnetic resonance arthrography can be helpful in establishing the diagnosis. However, the findings may be subtle or falsely negative.
5. After failure of conservative treatment, arthroscopic labroplasty (with a posterior capsular shift in primary posterior instability) or posterior labroplasty (with an inferior capsular shift and rotator interval closure when associated with multidirectional instability) has been effective.

V. IMPINGEMENT SYNDROME/ROTATOR CUFF DISEASE

A. Overview

1. Rotator cuff disease is a continuum beginning with mild impingement and progressing toward partial tear,

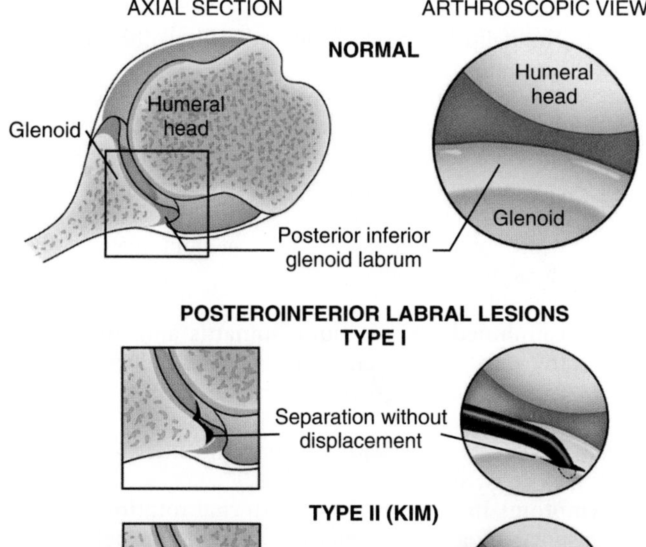

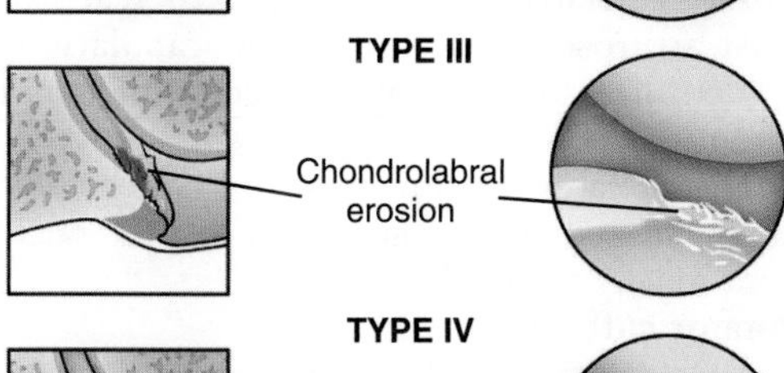

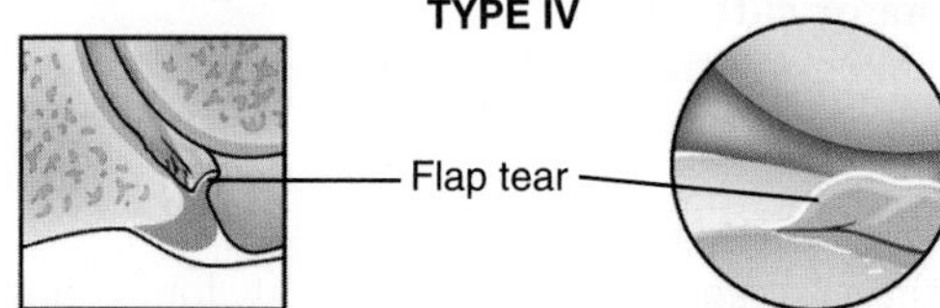

Figure 4-51 The Kim lesion is an incomplete and concealed avulsion of the posteroinferior labrum that may be associated with posterior and multidirectional instability and a spectrum of tear patterns as shown.

full-thickness tear, massive tear, and finally arthropathy of the rotator cuff.

2. Tears associated with chronic impingement syndrome typically begin on the bursal surface or within the tendon substance, in contrast to those that occur on the articular surface because of tension failure in younger athletes participating in overhead activities (Table 4-13).

B. **Epidemiology**

1. Millions of Americans have some aspect of rotator cuff disease.
2. **28% of those patients older than 60 years have a full-thickness tear, whereas 65% of those older than 70 years have a full-thickness tear.**
3. Patients older than 60 years with a tear have a 50% risk of having bilateral tears.
4. In those with a unilateral, painful, full-thickness tear, there is a 56% chance of having an asymptomatic, contralateral, full- or partial-thickness tear.
5. Of those with an asymptomatic tear, 50% will develop symptoms in 3 years, and of these patients, 40% may have progression of the tear.

C. **Diagnosis**

1. Physical examination
   - Patients typically present with an insidious onset of pain exacerbated by overhead activities.
   - Complaints of night discomfort, pain in the deltoid region, muscular weakness, and differences in active versus passive ROM are common; more significant weakness and loss of motion indicate a higher degree of cuff involvement.
   - Acute pain and weakness may be seen after traumatic rotator cuff rupture.
   - In young athletes, it is critical to confirm or exclude glenohumeral instability that causes a secondary impingement (nonoutlet impingement) from primary impingement syndrome (pathologic process within the subacromial space).
   - For specific testing, refer to Table 4-9.
2. Radiographs
   - May demonstrate classic changes within the acromion or coracoacromial ligament (spurring and calcification) in addition to cystic changes within the greater tuberosity
   - With chronic rotator cuff disease, superior migration of the humeral head with extensive degenerative change may be present.
3. Other imaging modalities
   - Ultrasonography: increasing in popularity as a tool both for diagnosis of rotator cuff disease and for confirmation of intraarticular or subacromial location of injections
   - MRI: used to assess for atrophy and retraction

D. **Treatment**

1. Nonoperative treatment
   - Initially indicated for impingement syndrome, chronic atraumatic cuff tears, noncompliant patients, medical contraindications to surgery, rotator cuff arthropathy, and athletes with a combined situation of instability and cuff tearing resulting from articular-side, partial thickness failure
   - Activity modification, avoiding repeated forward flexion beyond 90 degrees, and an aggressive program for strengthening the rotator cuff and stabilizing the scapula are initiated.
   - In addition, oral anti-inflammatory medications, therapeutic modalities, and judicious use of subacromial steroid injections may be implemented.
2. Chronic impingement syndrome

Table 4-13 Rotator Cuff Tears

Stage	Age (yr)	Pathologic Process	Clinical Course	Treatment
I	<25	Edema and hemorrhage	Reversible	Conservative
II	25-40	Fibrosis and tendinitis	Activity-related pain	Therapy/operative
III	>40	Acromioclavicular spur and cuff tear	Progressive disability	Acromioplasty/repair

- Symptoms that do not respond to a minimum of 4 to 6 months of nonoperative treatment may respond favorably to subacromial decompression. Similarly, of patients for whom rotator cuff repair is indicated, many require concomitant subacromial decompression at the time of repair.
- Exceptions include massive, irreparable rotator cuff tears that may benefit from débridement with preservation of the coracoacromial arch to prevent anterosuperior humeral migration.
- Additional exceptions include the acute, traumatic rotator cuff tear and injury in the overhead-movement athlete who may benefit from limited acromial smoothing and bursectomy, which is required for visualization and limiting postoperative irritation of the repair site.
- **Patients with workers' compensation claims have poor subjective outcomes after subacromial decompression.**

3. Rotator cuff surgery
   - Surgery reliably decreases pain and improves motion and function.
   - The operative approach has evolved from a classic open approach to a "mini-open" or deltoid-sparing approach and to an all-arthroscopic technique. Regardless of the technique, the rate-limiting step for recovery is the biologic healing of the rotator cuff tendon to the humerus, which is estimated to require a minimum of 8 to 12 weeks.
     - Classify tear size:
       - Small: less than 1 cm
       - Medium: 1 to 3 cm
       - Large: 3 to 5 cm
       - Massive: larger than 5 cm (two tendons)
     - **Acute rotator cuff tears: These should be repaired early because the disease process is accelerated in this setting.**
     - **Articular-side, partial-thickness tears (e.g., partial articular supraspinatus tendon avulsion [PASTA]): Treatment with débridement versus repair remains controversial. Tears in which more than 7 mm of bone lateral to the articular margin is exposed should be considered significant and represent 50% of the tendon insertion.**
     - Considerations include the depth of the tear, the pattern of the tear (avulsion versus degeneration), the amount of footprint uncovered, and the activity level of the patient.
     - Surgical techniques have evolved to include double-row and suture-bridge fixation techniques, which have improved biomechanical strength in vitro. Clinical correlation is still controversial.
   - Patients with a preponderance of impingement findings and a tear of less than 50% thickness may benefit from débridement and subacromial decompression.
   - Although excellent results have been reported with rotator cuff repair, a high percentage of such tears either do not heal or recur.
   - Despite this outcome, functional and subjective results remain excellent. A correlation appears to exist between younger age and repair success.
   - Large and massive tears:
     - Patch is not helpful.
     - The failure rate is higher; tissue failure is most common.
     - Irreparable tears are more likely to occur when the acromiohumeral distance appears shorter (<7 mm) on anteroposterior radiograph.
     - Larger, more retracted tears (>40 mm length/width) are characterized by fatty atrophy, supraspinatus width of less than 5 mm at glenoid margin, high signal in infraspinatus.
   - Irreparable tears:
     - **Combined tears of supraspinatus and infraspinatus may be treated with latissimus dorsi tendon transfer to the greater tuberosity.**

E. Subscapularis tears

1. May occur after anterior dislocation and anterior shoulder surgery (e.g., shoulder arthroplasty)
2. **Symptoms include increased external rotation and the presence of a liftoff, modified liftoff, or belly-press sign.**
3. **The appearance of an empty bicipital groove on axial MRI with tear of the transverse humeral ligament is often associated with subscapularis tear.**
   - **At arthroscopy, a chronic subscapularis tear can be identified by the comma sign, which represents an avulsed SGHL.**
4. Surgical treatment, either open or arthroscopic, is generally indicated; in chronic cases, a pectoralis transfer is occasionally required.

F. Rotator cuff arthropathy

1. Defined as a massive rotator cuff tear combined with fixed superior migration of the humeral head and severe glenohumeral arthrosis, presumably caused by chronic loss of the concavity-compression effect
2. Tendon transfer (latissimus/teres) for younger, active patients has been advocated.
3. Hemiarthroplasty might be helpful if the anterior deltoid is preserved.
   - This is a good option for patients whose predominant symptom is pain.
4. Use of a reverse shoulder prosthesis has become increasingly popular for treatment of rotator cuff arthropathy.
   - **It requires a competent deltoid and good glenoid bone stock.**
   - It is recommended only for older patients (typically older than 70 years) with low functional demands.
   - More predictable functional results are seen with the reverse prosthesis than with hemiarthroplasty, but a high rate of complications (40%) has been reported with its use.

G. Subcoracoid impingement

1. Patients with long or excessively laterally placed coracoid processes may have impingement of this process on the proximal humerus with forward flexion (120 to 130 degrees) and internal rotation of the arm.
2. It may occur after surgery that causes posterior capsular tightness and loss of internal rotation.
3. Local anesthetic injection should relieve these symptoms.
4. CT performed with the arms crossed on the chest is helpful in evaluating this problem.
5. A distance of less than 7 mm between the humerus and coracoid process is considered abnormal.

6. Treatment of chronic symptoms involves resection of the lateral aspect of the coracoid process and reattachment of the conjoined tendon to the remaining coracoid.
7. Arthroscopic coracoplasty has also been successful in treating this condition without detachment of the conjoined muscle group.

H. Internal impingement

1. **Impingement of the posterior-superior labrum and rotator cuff can occur in a throwing motions or overhead movements by athletes with external rotation and anterior translation (secondary impingement).**
2. Diagnosis can be aided with magnetic resonance arthrography.
3. An abduction–external rotation view sometimes shows the internal impingement and associated lesions.
4. **Bennett lesion (mineralization of the posterior inferior glenoid) is occasionally seen on radiographs or CT.**
5. **It is often associated with GIRD secondary to a tight posterioinferior capsule.**
6. **Alteration in glenohumeral kinematics leads to a posterosuperior shift of the humeral head; abduction and external rotation of the arm, in turn, lead to the internal impingement.**
7. This may cause pain associated with SLAP/biceps anchor disease, as well as undersurface rotator cuff tears of the posterior aspect of the supraspinatus and infraspinatus tendons.
8. A "peel-back" phenomenon of the superior labrum can be appreciated intraoperatively with abduction and external rotation of the arm.
9. Treatment
   - Primary treatment should include physical therapy and avoidance of aggravating activities.
   - **Patients with GIRD may benefit from posterior and posteroinferior capsular stretching exercises such as the sleeper stretch, as well as stretching of the pectoralis minor tendon.**
   - Operative treatment includes arthroscopic débridement or repair of the labrum, with débridement of the undersurface rotator cuff lesion.
   - Some authorities suggest repairing the rotator cuff if it is significantly thinned either by a transcuff technique or by taking down the remaining thinned cuff and advancing the unaffected normal tendon.
   - A posterior capsular release can be considered in patients who have GIRD and in whom nonoperative stretching has not caused improvement.

VI. SUPERIOR LABRAL AND BICEPS TENDON INJURIES

A. Superior labrum lesions

1. SLAP lesions have been classified into many varieties (Figure 4-52); specific types are associated with instability and rotator cuff disease.
   - Type II is the most common class (IIA is anterior, IIB is posterior, IIC is anterior and posterior).
2. In addition to biceps tenderness, patients may exhibit a positive result of the active compression (O'Brien) test, anterior slide, or crank test.
3. The dynamic labral shear test has a sensitivity of 86% and a specificity of 100% in diagnosing a SLAP tear (Table 4-14).
4. Treatment involves débridement (types I, III, and IV) with or without stabilization of the biceps anchor (types II, V, and VII) and repair vs. tenodesis of type IV.
5. In patients older than 40 years, biceps tenodesis or tenotomy can be considered instead of repair.

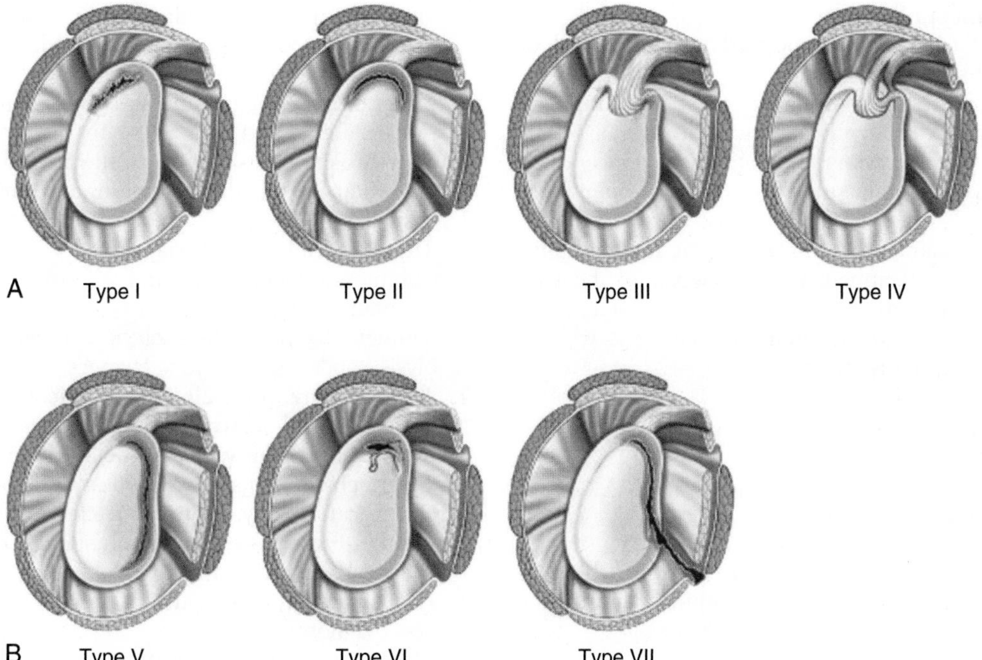

Figure 4-52 Anterior and posterior lesion types I to IV **(A)** and types V to VII **(B)** of the superior labrum. (From Kepler CK, et al: Superior labral tear. In Reider B, Terry M, Provencher MT, editors: *Operative techniques: sports medicine surgery,* Philadelphia, 2009, Elsevier.)

Table 4-14 Superior Labral and Biceps Tendon Injuries

Type	Description	Treatment
I	Biceps fraying, intact anchor on superior labrum	Arthroscopic débridement
II	Detachment of biceps anchor	Reattachment/stabilization
III	Bucket-handle superior labral tear; biceps intact	Arthroscopic débridement
IV	Bucket-handle tear of superior labrum into biceps	Repair or tenodesis of tendon based on symptoms and condition of remaining tendon
V	Labral tear + SLAP lesion	Stabilization of both
VI	Superior flap tear	Débridement
VII	Capsular injury + SLAP lesion	Repair and stabilization

SLAP, superior labrum from anterior to posterior.

B. Biceps tendinitis

1. Often associated with impingement, rotator cuff tears (subscapularis and leading-edge supraspinatus tears), and stenosis of the bicipital groove
2. Like most other cases of "tendinitis," this is probably best considered to be a "tendinosis."
3. Diagnosis is made by direct palpation, with the arm internally rotated 10 degrees, and confirmed with Speed and Yergason tests.
4. Initial management includes strengthening and local corticosteroid injection (around but not into the tendon).
5. Surgical release (with or without tenodesis) is usually reserved for refractory cases.
   - **Tenotomy without tenodesis is associated with subjective cramping and cosmetic deformity ("Popeye deformity").**

C. Biceps tendon subluxation

1. **This is most commonly associated with a partial or complete subscapularis tear.**
2. Tear of the coracohumeral ligament or transverse humeral ligament may produce tendon subluxation as well.
3. Arm abduction and external rotation may produce a palpable click as the tendon subluxates or dislocates outside of the groove.
4. Nonoperative treatment is similar to that for tendinitis, whereas operative treatment includes repair of the subscapularis and supporting structures of the bicipital groove but more often involves tenotomy or tenodesis with or without a subscapularis repair.

VII. ACROMIOCLAVICULAR AND STERNOCLAVICULAR INJURIES

A. Acromioclavicular separation

1. Overview
   - These injuries are typically caused by a direct blow to the shoulder, are common athletic injuries, and can be classified into six types (Figure 4-53).
2. Treatment of type III injuries
   - **Management of type III injuries is somewhat controversial; most authorities advocate conservative treatment, especially in elderly patients, inactive patients, or patients who do not perform manual labor. Some authorities advocate surgical reduction and repair or reconstruction.**
   - **The literature suggests that among patients treated immediately with surgery, the need for reoperation is higher that with primary surgery for those who are initially treated nonoperatively.**
3. Management of types IV through VI injuries
   - **These are typically treated surgically.**
   - Type V injury is defined by a coracoclavicular distance that is greater than 100% that of the opposite side (bilateral acromioclavicular views are required).
   - Type IV injury can be diagnosed on only an axillary lateral view.
4. Surgical treatment of failed, conservatively treated injuries or acute treatment
   - Reconstruction of the coracoclavicular ligament with a free soft tissue graft is becoming popular to allow for an anatomic reconstruction.
   - The distal clavicle is often resected in the chronic situation, and the coracoacromial ligament may then be transferred to the distal clavicle (modified Weaver-Dunn procedure).
   - Backup coracoclavicular stabilization is usually required for a successful outcome.

B. Acromioclavicular degenerative joint disease

1. As a result of the transmission of large loads through a small surface area, the acromioclavicular joint may begin to degenerate as early as the second decade of life.
2. In addition, direct blows or low-grade acromioclavicular separation may cause post-traumatic arthritis.
3. Diagnosed by direct palpation; other diagnostic features are pain elicited by crossed-chest adduction, radiographic evidence of osteophytes and joint-space narrowing, and pain relief with selective acromioclavicular joint injection.
4. Treatment includes both open and arthroscopic distal clavicle resections (Mumford procedure) with resection of less than 1 cm of the distal clavicle to preserve the posterior-superior capsule and avoid anterior and posterior instability and pain.
   - **Arthroscopic excision has the advantage of allowing evaluation of the glenohumeral joint at time of surgery.**

C. Distal clavicle osteolysis

1. Common in weightlifters and in persons with a history of traumatic injury
2. Radiographs of the distal clavicle reveal osteopenia, osteolysis, tapering, and cystic changes.
3. **After failure of selective corticosteroid injection, NSAIDs, and activity modification, this condition responds favorably to distal clavicle excision.**

D. Sternoclavicular subluxation and dislocation

1. **Often caused by motor vehicle accidents or direct trauma, but can be spontaneous and atraumatic during overhead elevation of the arm**
2. Plain imaging includes the Hobbs and Serendipity views; best diagnosed by CT.
3. Closed reduction is often successful.
4. **The posterior capsule is the most important anatomic restraint for anteroposterior translation.**

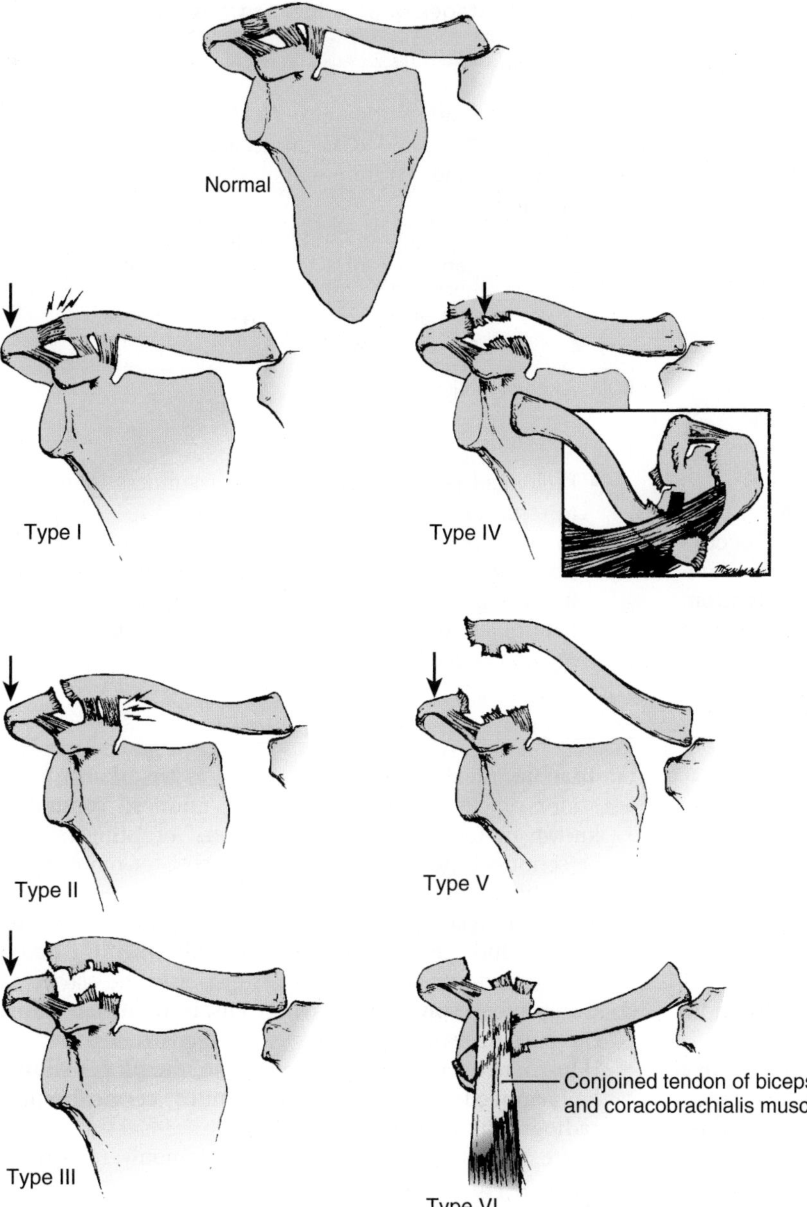

Figure 4-53 Classification of acromioclavicular (AC) separations. Type I injuries involve only an AC sprain. Type II injuries are characterized by a complete AC tear but intact coracoclavicular (CC) ligaments. Type III injuries involve both the AC and CC ligaments; the CC distance may be up to 100% of that in the opposite shoulder. Type IV injuries are associated with posterior displacement of the clavicle through the trapezius muscle. Type V injuries involve superior displacement; the CC distance is more than twice that of the opposite side. This injury is usually associated with rupture of the deltotrapezial fascia, leaving the distal end of the clavicle subcutaneous. Type VI injuries are rare and defined on the basis of inferior displacement of the clavicle below the coracoid. (From Rockwood CA Jr, Young DC: Disorders of the acromioclavicular joint. In Rockwood CA Jr, Matsen FA III, editors: *The shoulder,* ed 2, Philadelphia, 1998, WB Saunders, p 495.)

5. Anterior dislocation should be first treated with acute closed reduction.
6. Failures of reductions and chronic dislocations are treated conservatively.
7. Posterior dislocation should be treated with closed reduction and open reduction if necessary, particularly with compression of the posterior structures. Consultation with a cardiothoracic surgeon may be appropriate.
8. The use of hardware should be avoided whenever possible.

VIII. MUSCLE RUPTURES

A. Pectoralis major

1. Injury to this muscle is caused by excessive tension on a maximally eccentrically contracted muscle, often found in weightlifters.
2. **Most commonly results in a tendinous avulsion**
3. Localized swelling and ecchymosis, a palpable defect (axillary webbing), and **weakness with adduction and internal rotation are characteristic findings.** Surgical repair of bone is usually necessary.
4. Pectoralis major ruptures have not been reported in women.

B. Deltoid

1. Complete rupture of this muscle is unusual, and injuries are most often strains or partial tears.
2. Repair of bone is required for complete ruptures.
3. Iatrogenic injury occasionally occurs during open rotator cuff repair; some patients require deltoidplasty, which consists of mobilization and anterior transfer of the middle third of the deltoid. Unfortunately, this procedure is not always possible or successful.

C. Triceps

1. **Ruptures of the triceps are most often associated with systemic illness (e.g., renal osteodystrophy) or steroid use.**
2. Primary repair of avulsions is indicated.

D. Latissimus dorsi rupture

1. This is a very rare condition manifesting with local tenderness and pain with shoulder adduction and internal rotation.
2. Although nonoperative treatment may allow resumption of activities, operative repair has been described for high-demand athletes.

IX. CALCIFYING TENDINITIS AND SHOULDER STIFFNESS

A. Calcifying tendinitis

1. **A self-limiting condition of unknown origin that affects predominantly the supraspinatus tendon and occurs slightly more frequently in women. Radiographs demonstrate characteristic calcification within the tendon.**
2. Three stages have been elucidated: precalcific, calcific, and postcalcific.
3. Nonoperative treatment is the rule, consisting of physical therapy, modalities, and injections.
4. "Needling" of the lesion under image guidance has been described and is often successful.
5. Arthroscopic or open removal of the deposit is occasionally necessary.
6. The rotator cuff should be repaired if it is significantly involved.

B. Shoulder stiffness

1. Adhesive capsulitis
   - This disorder (also known as *frozen shoulder*) is characterized by pain and restricted glenohumeral joint motion, especially external rotation.
   - **Factors associated with the development of adhesive capsulitis include diabetes,** trauma after chest or breast surgery, prolonged immobilization, thyroid disease (cause is probably autoimmune), and other medical conditions.
   - The essential lesion involves the coracohumeral ligament and the rotator interval capsule.
   - Arthrography may demonstrate a loss of the normal axillary recess, revealing contracture of the joint capsule.
   - Three clinical and four arthroscopic stages have been defined (Table 4-15).
2. Post-traumatic shoulder stiffness
   - This is an asymmetric loss of glenohumeral motion secondary to a post-traumatic or postsurgical complication that results from excessive scar formation.
   - Motion loss is related to the area of surgery or trauma and may involve the humeroscapular motion interface between the proximal humerus and overlying deltoid and conjoined tendon, as well as contracture of the rotator cuff and capsule.
3. Treatment
   - **For idiopathic adhesive capsulitis, a supervised physical therapy program combined with anti-inflammatory medications or glenohumeral steroid injections, or both, is curative in the majority of patients within 12 weeks.**

Table 4-15 Stages of Shoulder Stiffness

Stage	Characteristics
Clinical	
Painful	Gradual onset of diffuse pain
Stiff	Decreased ROM; affects activities of daily living
Thawing	Gradual return of motion
Arthroscopic	
1	Patchy, fibrinous synovitis
2	Capsular contraction, fibrinous adhesions, synovitis
3	Increased contraction, resolving synovitis
4	Severe contracture

ROM, range of motion.

   - Prolonged post-traumatic shoulder stiffness is unlikely to respond to nonsurgical treatment.
   - If no improvement is seen after 12 to 16 weeks of nonsurgical treatment, operative intervention consisting of open or arthroscopic lysis of adhesions and manipulation with the patient under anesthesia is recommended.

X. NERVE DISORDERS

A. Brachial plexus injury

1. Minor traction and compression injuries, commonly known by football players as "burners" or "stingers," can be serious if they are recurrent or persist for more than a short time.
2. Results from compression of the plexus between the shoulder pad and the superior medial scapula when the pad is compressed into the Erb point (superior to the clavicle).
3. **Complete resolution of symptoms is required before the patient returns to play.**
4. **If burners occur more than one time, the player should be removed from competition until cervical spine radiographs can be obtained.**
5. Three grades of nerve injury are commonly recognized (Table 4-16).

B. Thoracic outlet syndrome

1. Results from compression of the nerves and vessels that pass through the scalene muscles and first rib.
2. This condition can be associated with cervical rib, scapular ptosis, or scalene muscle abnormalities.
3. Patients may note pain and ulnar paresthesias.
4. Positive findings with the Wright test (see Table 4-9) and on neurologic evaluation can be diagnostic.
5. First-rib resection is occasionally required.

C. Long thoracic nerve palsy

Table 4-16 Grades of Nerve Injury

Grade	Description	Pathophysiologic Process
1	Neurapraxia	Selective demyelination of the axon sheath
2	Axonotmesis	Disruption of axon and myelin sheath
3	Neurotmesis	Disruption of epineurium and endoneurium

1. **Injury to this nerve can result in medial scapular winging secondary to serratus anterior dysfunction.**
2. This condition can be caused by a compression injury (such as that occurring in backpackers) or a traction injury (as seen in weightlifters).
3. Simple observation is usually called for because many of these injuries spontaneously resolve within 18 months.
4. Treatment with a modified thoracolumbar brace may be beneficial, and in rare cases, pectoralis major transfer may be required for chronic palsies that do not improve.

D. Suprascapular nerve compression

1. This nerve may become compressed by various structures, including a ganglion in the spinoglenoid notch or suprascapular notch and a fracture callus in the area of the transverse scapular ligament.
2. **Weakness and atrophy of the supraspinatus (proximal lesions) and infraspinatus are present along with pain over the dorsal aspect of the shoulder.**
3. **Cysts within the spinoglenoid notch affect only the infraspinatus.**
4. Electrodiagnostic studies and MRI may confirm and elucidate the nature of the nerve compression.
5. **Compression caused by a cyst in association with a SLAP lesion may respond to arthroscopic decompression and labral repair.**
6. In the absence of a structural lesion, release of the transverse scapular ligament may provide relief.

E. Quadrilateral space syndrome

1. This condition is defined as axillary nerve or posterior humeral circumflex artery compression within the quadrilateral space.
2. Most commonly caused by a fibrous band between the teres major and the long head of the triceps
3. **Characterized by pain and paresthesias with overhead activity, as well as weakness or atrophy of the teres minor and deltoid**
4. **This is most often seen in athletes who participate in throwing activities and is associated with late cocking and acceleration with the abducted, extended, and externally rotated arm.** Diagnosis is confirmed by the arteriographic appearance of compression of the posterior humeral circumflex artery.

F. Other nerve injuries

1. Other injuries—including those of the axillary nerve, **the spinal accessory nerve (lateral scapular winging)**, and the musculocutaneous nerve—are usually the result of surgical injury to these structures.
2. Observation for several months is appropriate before exploration and repair of the affected nerve is considered.

XI. OTHER SHOULDER DISORDERS

A. Glenohumeral degenerative joint disease

1. Although it is more common in older patients, athletes who engage in throwing may develop arthritis at a younger age than usual.
2. **Osteoarthrosis typically results in posterior glenoid wear, whereas rheumatoid arthritis results in central glenoid wear.**
3. Arthritis may also be associated with other shoulder disorders, including instability and rotator cuff disease.
4. Certain iatrogenic factors may also contribute to the development of osteoarthritis of the shoulder, including the use of hardware in and around the shoulder and overtightening of the shoulder capsule during shoulder reconstruction.
   - Chondrolysis possibly secondary to thermal ablation or intraarticular pain pumps is another iatrogenic factor in degenerative joint disease.
5. Radiographs, including a true anteroposterior view taken in abduction, can be helpful in characterizing the amount of arthritis.
6. In some cases, arthroscopic débridement may be a temporizing measure before joint arthroplasty is considered.
7. Progressive pain, decreased ROM, and the inability to perform activities of daily living are reasonable indications for considering prosthetic replacement or humeral head resurfacing.
8. Complications of arthroplasty most commonly include glenoid loosening.

B. Scapulothoracic crepitus

1. Also known as *snapping scapula syndrome*
2. Manifestation: painful scapulothoracic crepitus in association with elevation of the arm
3. **Scapulothoracic dyskinesis may be present, and the pain is generally relieved with manual stabilization of the scapula.**
4. Many possible causes of symptomatic crepitus exist.
   - The differential diagnosis includes osteochondroma and elastofibroma dorsi.
5. Patients may respond to scapular strengthening exercises, local corticosteroid injections, or anti-inflammatory medications.
6. For more refractory cases, open or arthroscopic bursectomy and sometimes resection of the superomedial scapular border are necessary.

C. Scapular winging (Figure 4-54)

1. Can occur as a result of a nerve injury, bony abnormality, muscle contracture, intraarticular disease, or voluntarily
2. The description of the direction of the winging is based on the movement of the inferior border of the scapula.
3. Nerve injuries include injury to the spinal accessory nerve (trapezius palsy, lateral winging), the long thoracic nerve (serratus anterior palsy, medial winging), and the dorsal scapular nerve (rhomboid palsy).
4. Osseous causes include osteochondromas and fracture malunions.
5. Selective muscle strengthening may ameliorate winging.
6. **Surgical treatment includes lateral transfer of the levator scapulae and rhomboid muscles (Eden-Lange procedure) for lateral winging and pectoralis major transfer for medial winging.**

D. Complex regional pain syndrome (formerly known as *reflex sympathetic dystrophy*)

1. As in the knee, this condition responds poorly to both conservative and surgical treatments.
2. In a litigious medicolegal environment, it is often associated with malingering and issues of secondary gain.

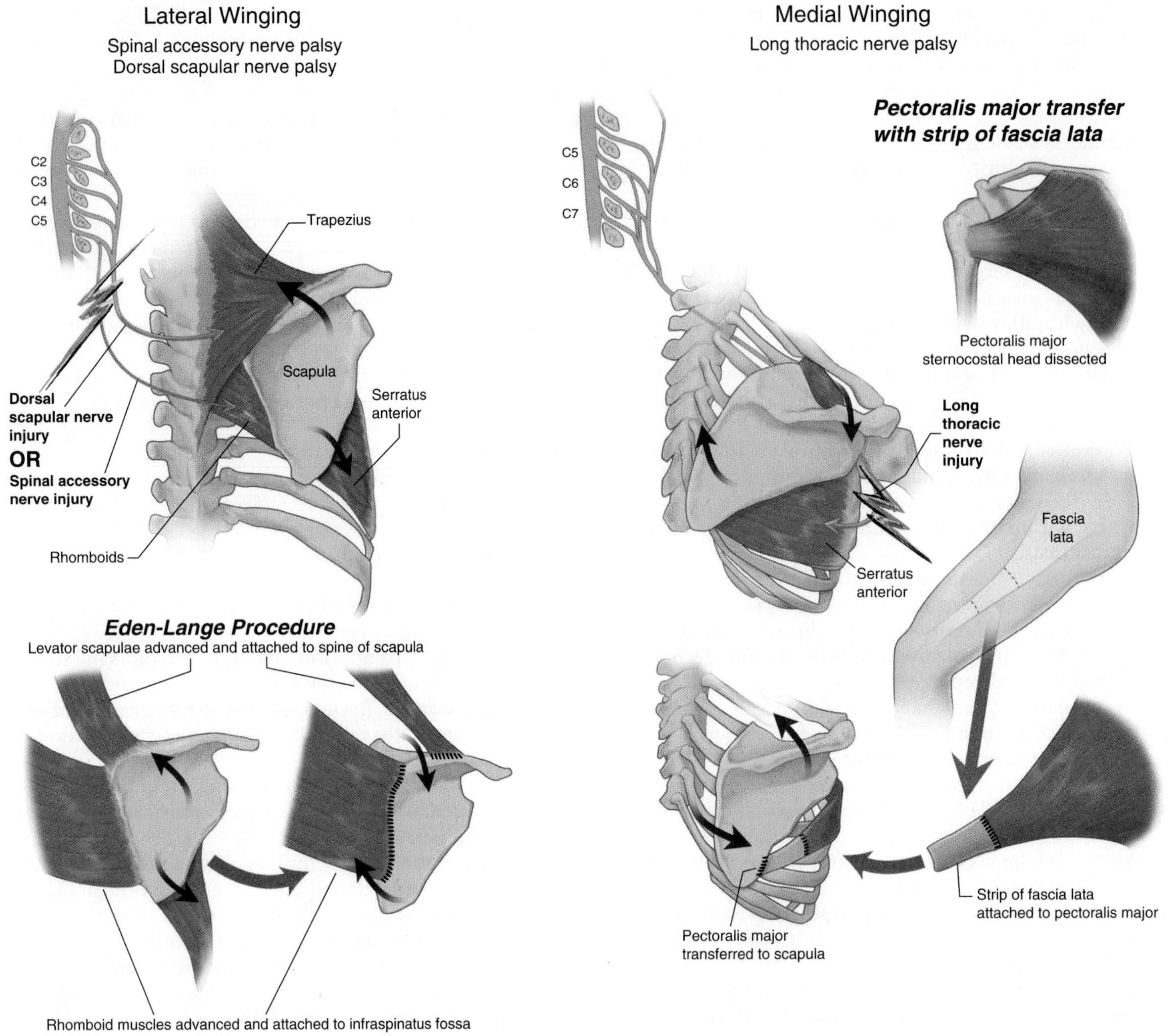

Lateral Winging
Spinal accessory nerve palsy
Dorsal scapular nerve palsy

Medial Winging
Long thoracic nerve palsy

Eden-Lange Procedure

Pectoralis major transfer with strip of fascia lata

Figure 4-54 Lateral and medial scapular winging. Lateral winging may be treated with the Eden-Lange procedure in which the levator scapulae and rhomboid are transferred laterally on the scapula. Medial winging may be treated with pectoarlis major transfer, supplemented with a strip of fascia late.

3. Diagnosis may be confirmed with a three-phase bone scan.
4. Treatment options are numerous and may include sympathetic nerve block.

E. **Little Leaguer's shoulder**

1. This disorder commonly occurs in young baseball players and is actually a Salter-Harris type I fracture or stress reaction of the proximal humerus.
2. Overuse of the shoulder as a result of failure to limit pitch count and provide periods of adequate rest are the key factors implicated in the development of this condition.
3. It has also been suggested that breaking pitches not be thrown until after skeletal maturity is reached.
4. **Radiographs may demonstrate widening of the proximal humeral physis in comparison with the contralateral proximal humerus.**
5. MRI can assist with the diagnosis if it is in question.
6. **The condition responds to rest and activity modification, with return to play allowed when symptoms have resolved completely.**
7. Recommendations regarding age and pitch counts have been made (Table 4-17).

Table 4-17 Pitch Count Recommendations for Youth Baseball

	PITCH COUNT			
Age	Per Game	Per Week	Per Season	Per Year
9-10	50	75	1000	2000
11-12	75	100	1000	3000
13-14	75	125	1000	3000

SECTION 5 ELBOW

I. TENDON INJURIES

A. Lateral epicondylitis (tennis elbow)

1. Causes and diagnosis
   - Commonly occurs with activities that involve repetitive pronation and supination of the forearm with the elbow in near extension (backhand in tennis)
   - **Initiated as a microtear at the origin of the extensor carpi radialis brevis (ECRB)**
   - May also involve the origin of the extensor carpi radialis longus (ECRL) and extensor carpi ulnaris
   - **Microscopic evaluation of this tissue shows angiofibroblastic hyperplasia.**
   - Diagnosis is clinical, with reproducible, localized tenderness at the extensor origin and reproduction of symptoms with resisted wrist extension.
2. Treatment
   - Treatment is predominantly nonoperative.
     - Activity modification (slower playing surfaces, more flexible racquet, lower string tension, larger grip), physical therapy (stretching, ultrasonography), anti-inflammatory medications, counterforce bracing, and up to three corticosteroid injections at the site of maximal tenderness, all achieving a success rate of up to 95%
     - In recalcitrant cases, open or arthroscopic débridement of the ECRB origin (Figure 4-55) is required.

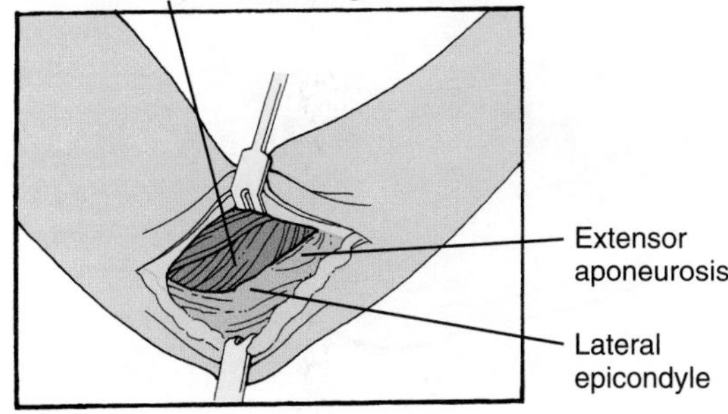

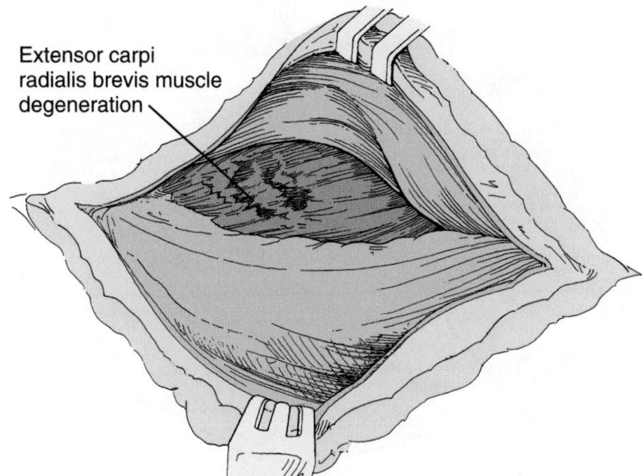

Figure 4-55 Operative exposure for lateral epicondylitis. (From Miller MD, Cooper DE, Warner JJP: *Review of sports medicine and arthroscopy,* Philadelphia, 1995, WB Saunders, p 178.)

     - **Excessive resection (beyond the equator of the radial head) can jeopardize the LCL and should be avoided.**

B. Medial epicondylitis (golfer's elbow)

1. This condition is classified as an overuse syndrome of the flexor/pronator mass.
2. Much less common and more difficult to treat than tennis elbow
3. Resisted forearm pronation and wrist flexion worsen the pain.
4. Treatment is similar to that for lateral epicondylitis.
5. Multiple corticosteroid injections and medial epicondylectomy should be avoided.

C. Distal biceps tendon rupture

1. Occurs almost exclusively in men after forceful, eccentric overload of the partially flexed elbow
2. **Up to 50% loss of supination power has been documented after rupture.**
3. Intraosseous tendon reattachment with the two-incision (Boyd-Anderson) technique has been traditionally favored.
   - However, this procedure is associated with increased rates of synostosis.
4. A one-incision technique is coming back into favor with some surgeons, who use a single-incision repair with an EndoButton fixation device, suture anchors, or an interference screw. In a cadaveric model, the EndoButton sustained the greatest load until failure in comparison with the standard suture technique, suture anchors, and interference screw fixation.
5. Among the fixation techniques, cyclic loading did not produce any statistically significant differences in gap formation.
6. Care must be taken not to disrupt the syndesmosis.
7. Complications include neurovascular injury (posterior interosseous nerve), loss of motion, and heterotopic ossification.
8. Neuropraxia of the lateral antebrachial cutaneous nerve is the most common nerve injury reported with repair of distal biceps tendon ruptures. This nerve pierces the fascia between the brachialis and biceps muscles at the level of the antecubital fossa and runs parallel to the cephalic vein within the subcutaneous fat.

D. Distal triceps tendon avulsion

1. This extremely uncommon injury results from a deceleration force to the outstretched elbow.
2. Associated with multiple corticosteroid injections or chronic olecranon bursitis
3. Repair with transosseous tunnels is mandatory for the restoration of extension power.

II. LIGAMENT INJURIES

A. Ulnar collateral ligament (UCL) injury

1. Causes and diagnosis
   - Repetitive, high-velocity valgus stress to the medial aspect of the elbow results in attenuation or rupture of the anterior band of the UCL

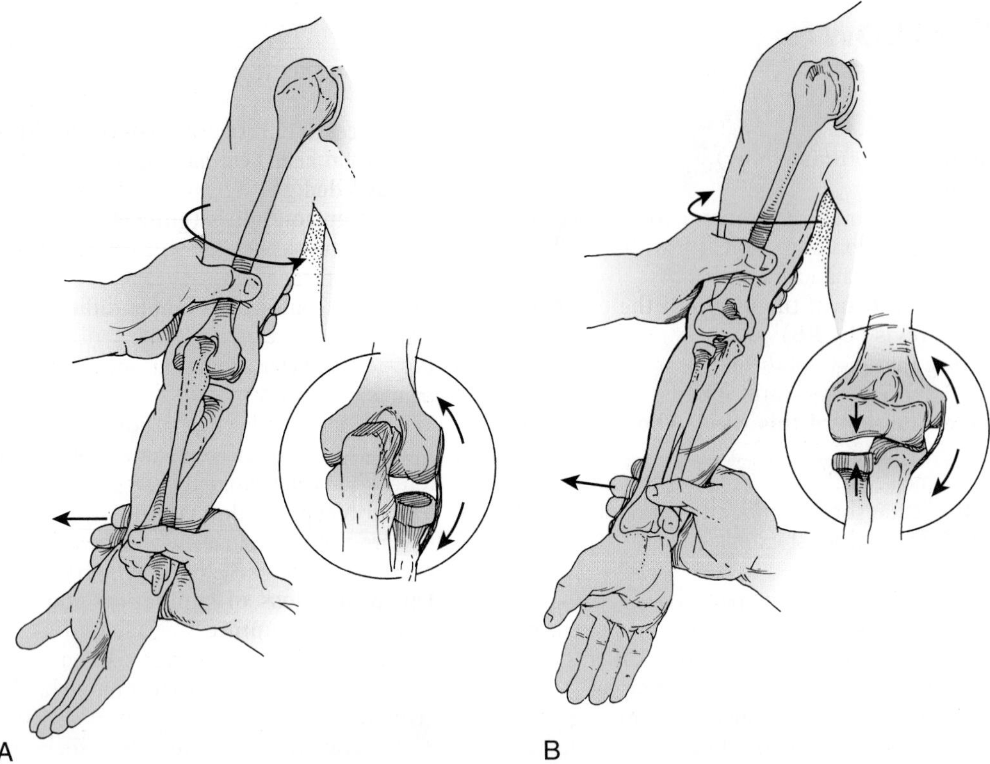

Figure 4-56 Varus **(A)** and valgus **(B)** instability testing of the elbow. Note the position and rotation of the arm. (From Morrey BF: *The elbow and its disorders,* ed 2, Philadelphia, 1994, WB Saunders, p 83.)

- **The anterior band of the UCL is the most important medial stabilizer of the elbow in flexion.**
- **The late-cocking and acceleration phases of throwing are periods of high stress generation.**
- Patients present with acute or chronic medial elbow tenderness and (frequently) associated ulnar nerve symptoms.
- The pain is localized to the course of the ligament from the medial epicondyle to the sublime tubercle.
- Valgus instability is demonstrated in only 50% of affected patients because it is usually a dynamic phenomenon involving the flexor digitorum superficialis and flexor carpi ulnaris origin (Figure 4-56). **The "moving valgus stress test" of O'Driscoll has been shown to have high sensitivity and specificity in detecting UCL injury.**
- Radiographs may demonstrate osteophyte formation at the posteromedial olecranon fossa.
- Magnetic resonance arthrography is useful for confirmation of the diagnosis.

2. Treatment
   - Initial treatment is with rest, physical therapy, and maintenance of joint motion.
   - **Surgery is required only in high-level athletes who desire a return to sports.**
   - Ligament reconstruction is favored over direct repair, and treatment of chronic injuries has demonstrated better results than that of acute injuries. The ligament is traditionally reconstructed with a palmaris tendon (or, more commonly now, a hamstring tendon) graft woven in a figure-eight manner (Tommy John procedure) (Figure 4-57). Ulnar transposition may accompany this

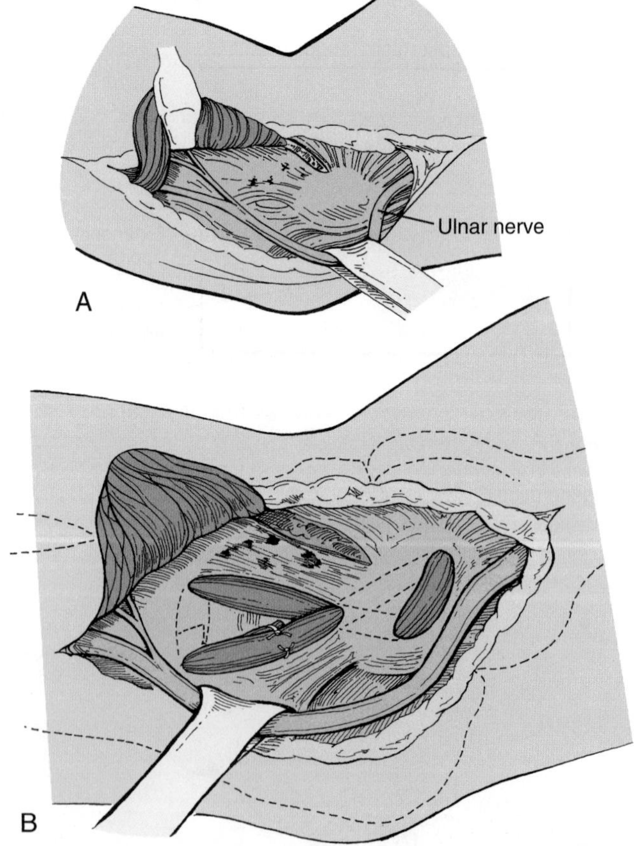

Figure 4-57 Reconstruction of the (medial) ulnar collateral ligament. **A,** Exposure with protection of the ulnar nerve. **B,** Figure-eight palmaris graft (Tommy John procedure). (From Miller MD, Cooper DE, Warner JJP: *Review of sports medicine and arthroscopy,* Philadelphia, 1995, WB Saunders, p 179.)

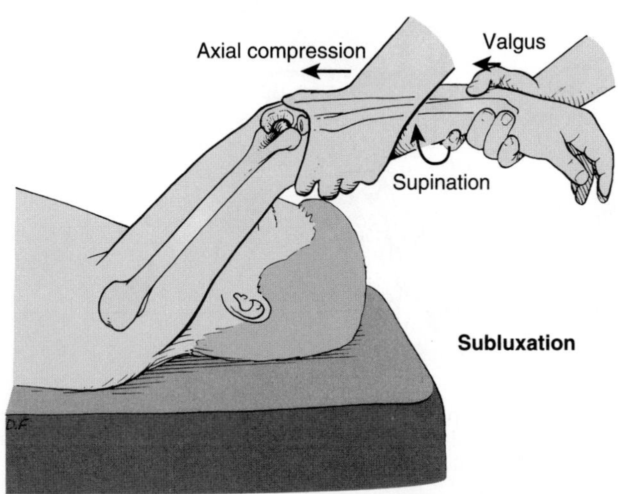

Figure 4-58 **Lateral pivot shift test of the elbow for posterolateral rotatory instability.** (Redrawn from O'Driscoll SW, Bell DF, Morrey BF: Posterolateral instability of the elbow, *J Bone Joint Surg Am* 73:404–446, 1991.)

procedure, depending on preoperative symptoms and surgeon's technique.

- Nearly 75% to 80% of patients return to sports at the same level or better 1 year after reconstruction.
- The docking procedure been used increasingly, with decreased rates of complications.
- Complications include loss of motion, graft site morbidity, and neurologic injury.

B. LCL injury

1. Typically, the first ligament is disrupted in elbow dislocation.
2. Patients with LCL insufficiency may complain of clicking or locking with elbow extension and often demonstrate posterolateral rotatory instability (Figure 4-58). Posterolateral rotatory elbow instability is caused by a deficiency in the ulnar portion of the lateral collateral ligament of the elbow. This can be tested by supinating the forearm and applying a valgus moment along with axial compression while the elbow is brought from extension to flexion. Flexion of more than 40 degrees reduces the radiocapitellar joint.
3. Surgical reconstruction with a palmaris longus autograft and capsular plication is indicated for patients with recurrent instability, pain, or mechanical symptoms (Figure 4-59).

III. ARTICULAR INJURIES

A. Osteochondritis dissecans

1. **Typically occurs in the capitellum of adolescent athletes engaged in repetitive overhead or upper-extremity weight-bearing activities**
2. Cause is thought to be related to vascular insufficiency and repetitive microtrauma.
3. Plain radiographs and improvement with activity modification confirm the diagnosis.
4. If the fragment is stable, this condition can be treated with activity modification and supportive methods.
5. Separated fragments may be arthroscopically reduced and stabilized or excised and the defects drilled.
6. Osteochondrosis of the capitellum is seen in younger patients (<12 years of age; Panner disease) and is associated with a more benign course.

B. Little Leaguer's elbow

1. This condition is defined as a stress fracture of the medial epicondyle in adolescents caused by repetitive valgus loading with throwing.
2. Rest and limitation of the number of innings pitched per week help to reduce the incidence of complete fracture (see Table 4-17).
3. Olecranon stress fractures also occur in this population.

C. Pitcher's elbow

1. Involves medial tension, lateral compression, and posterior extension overload
2. Adaptive changes common in this condition include increased valgus angulation, pronator mass hypertrophy, and loss of extension.
3. Radiographic changes include posteromedial olecranon osteophytes and chondromalacia of the medial wall of the olecranon fossa.

D. Osteoarthritis

1. Primary elbow osteoarthritis disproportionately affects football linemen, participants in racquet sports, and throwers.
2. Manifests with a decreased arc of motion and pain at the extremes of motion
3. Plain radiographs demonstrating joint space narrowing and osteophytic spurring confirm the diagnosis.
4. Surgical treatment consists of arthroscopic débridement, soft tissue release, and removal of loose bodies.
5. Persistent symptoms are treated with distraction/interposition arthroplasty, ulnohumeral arthroplasty, or total elbow arthroplasty.

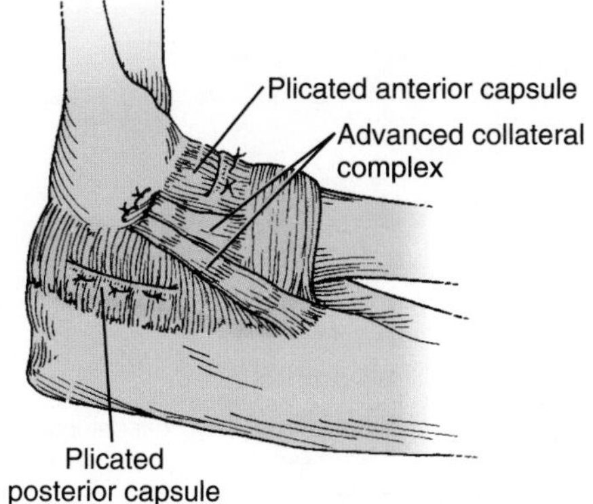

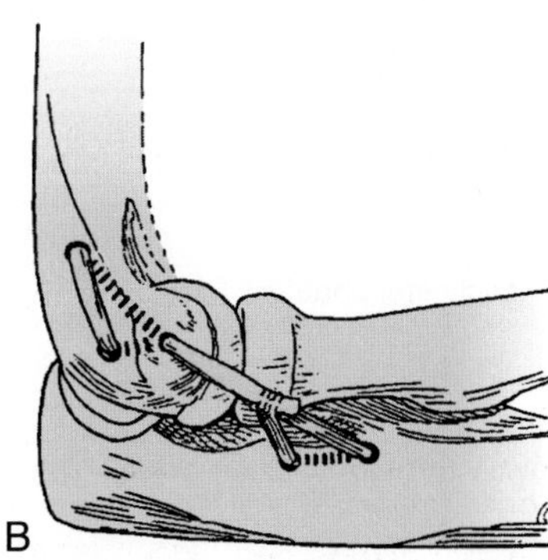

Figure 4-59 **A,** **Imbrication of the ulnar band and advancement of the radial part of the radial collateral ligament. B, Palmaris longus tendon through the ulnar and humeral tunnels and tied to itself.** (From Canale ST, editor: *Campbell's operative orthopaedics,* ed 9, St Louis, 1998, Mosby, p 1397.)

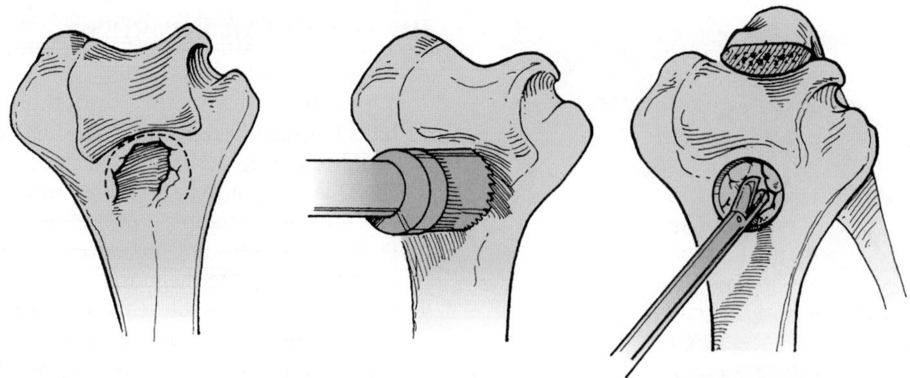

Figure 4-60 Outerbridge-Kashiwagi arthroplasty performed through a triceps-splitting approach. The coronoid is approached through a Cloward drill hole in the olecranon fossa. The olecranon can also be débrided with this approach. (From Miller MD, Cooper DE, Warner JJP: *Review of sports medicine and arthroscopy,* Philadelphia, 1995, WB Saunders, p 180.)

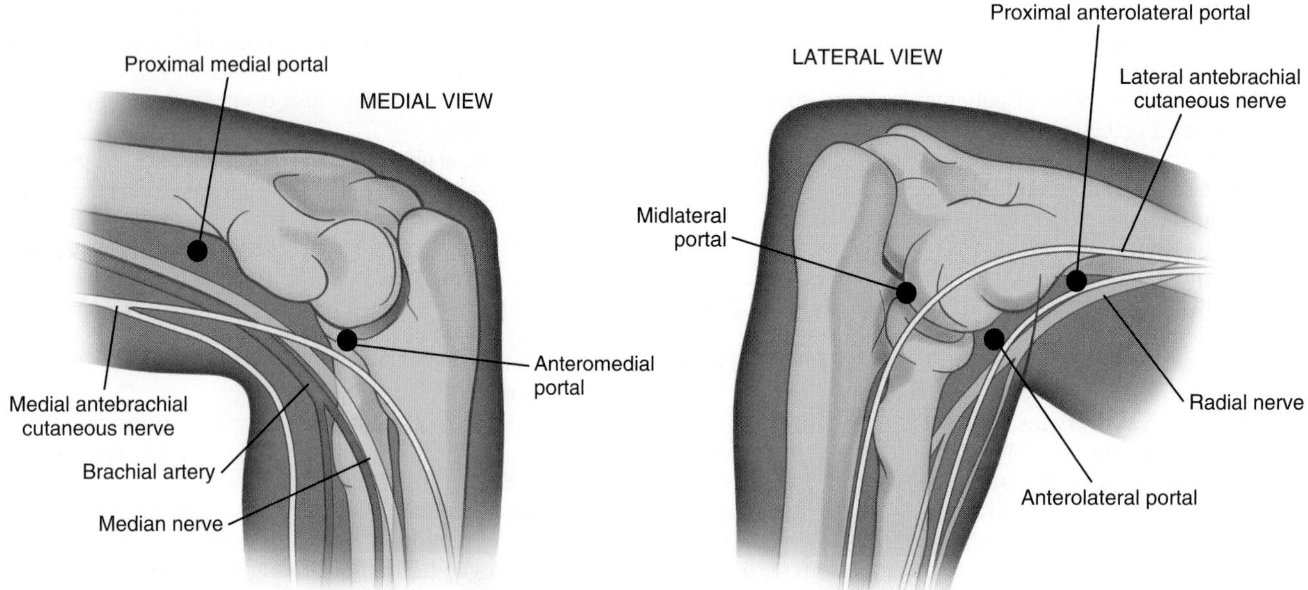

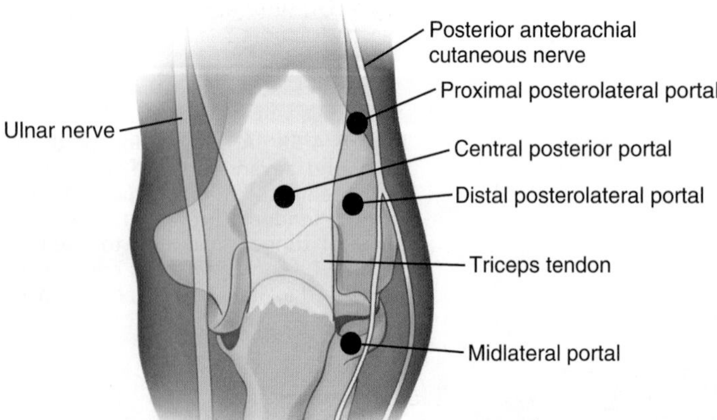

Figure 4-61 Arthroscopic portals for elbow arthroscopy. (From Miller MD, et al: *Orthopaedic surgical approaches,* Philadelphia, 2008, Elsevier.)

IV. ELBOW STIFFNESS

A. The loss of motion and function results from capsular contracture; from olecranon, coronoid, and radial fossa overgrowth; or from heterotopic ossification about the elbow after a single acute injury or because of degenerative disease.
B. Treatment involves open surgical débridement by means of a collateral ligament–sparing approach (Hastings-Cohen), olecranon fossa fenestration and débridement (Outerbridge-Kashiwagi procedure; Figure 4-60), or arthroscopic osteocapsular arthroplasty with resection of bone osteophytes and resection of the capsule.
C. Success is largely dependent the patient's compliance and participation in therapeutic exercise.
D. Loss of terminal extension is common after elbow dislocation and is usually managed with simple observation.

V. ELBOW ARTHROSCOPY

See Supplemental Images on expertconsult.com.

A. Indications

1. This procedure is typically indicated for diagnostic confirmation of suspected elbow pathology; removal of loose bodies; treatment of osteochondritis dissecans of the capitellum; osteophyte débridement (as seen with chronic valgus overload in pitchers); capsular release and débridement of the olecranon, radial, and coronoid fossa in the stiff elbow; and synovectomy.
2. Successful arthroscopic intervention depends on technical expertise in elbow arthroscopy and thorough anatomic familiarity because vital neurovascular structures are proximal to the intraarticular space and are thus prone to injury, particularly with overexuberant débridement.

B. Risks

1. The "nick and spread" method of portal placement is used to minimize inadvertent neurovascular injury.
2. The use of far-proximal portals may decrease these risks. **A posteromedial portal is least safe because of its proximity to the ulnar nerve.**
3. In patients with prior ulnar transposition and contractures, extra caution is needed.
4. Other risks include injury to the ulnar nerve (proximal medial and posteromedial portals) and brachial artery injury with removal of loose bodies (anteriorly).
5. The most common transient nerve palsy after elbow arthroscopy is an ulnar nerve palsy. Superficial radial nerve, posterior interosseous nerve, medial antebrachial cutaneous nerve, and anterior interosseous nerve palsies have also been reported.

C. Portals

1. Three portals are commonly used (Figure 4-61):
   - Anterolateral portal: placed after joint distension 1 cm distal and 1 cm anterior to the lateral epicondyle. The lateral antebrachial cutaneous and radial nerves are at risk.
   - Anteromedial portal: placed under direct visualization 2 cm distal and 2 cm anterior to the medial epicondyle. The medial antebrachial cutaneous and median nerves are at risk.
   - Posterolateral portal: placed 2 to 3 cm proximal to the olecranon and just lateral to the triceps tendon

SECTION 6 HAND AND WRIST

I. TENDON INJURIES

Common sites of wrist tendinitis are illustrated in Figure 4-62.

A. de Quervain disease

1. Stenosing tenosynovitis of the first dorsal wrist compartment **(abductor pollicis longus and extensor pollicis brevis)**
2. Typically occurs in participants in racquet sports and in golfers
3. Ulnar deviation of the wrist with the thumb in the palm (Finkelstein test) generally reproduces patient symptoms.
4. Treatment includes activity modification, splinting, local corticosteroid injection, and, on occasion, surgical release (Figure 4-63).
5. The abductor pollicis longus and extensor pollicis brevis may lie in separate sheaths in the first dorsal compartment, and care must be taken to release both of them.

B. Flexor carpi radialis/flexor carpi ulnaris tendinitis

1. Wrist flexor tendinitis is common and is associated with overuse, especially in golfers and in players of racquet sports.
2. Ulnar deviation and supination lead to dislocation.
3. Activity modification, splinting, and NSAIDs are generally effective.
4. Surgical tenolysis is rarely necessary.

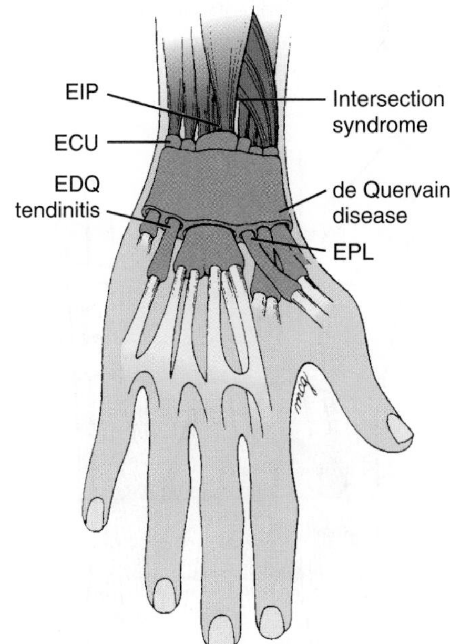

Figure 4-62 Location of common sites of tendinitis about the wrist. ECU, extensor carpi ulnaris; EDQ, extensor digiti quinti; EIP, extensor indicis proprius; EPL, extensor pollicis longus. (From Kiefhaber TR, Stern PJ: Upper extremity tendinitis and overuse syndromes in the athlete, *Clin Sports Med* 11:43, 1992.)

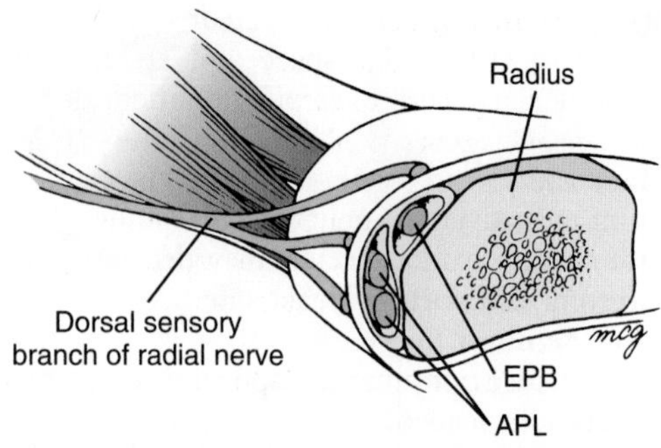

Figure 4-63 **Surgical release of the first compartment for refractory de Quervain syndrome should include preservation of the dorsal sensory branch of the radial nerve. APL, abductor pollicis longus; EPB, extensor pollicis brevis.** (From Kiefhaber TR, Stern PJ: Upper extremity tendinitis and overuse syndromes in the athlete, *Clin Sports Med* 11:44, 1992.)

C. Extensor carpi ulnaris tendinitis

1. Tendinitis or subluxation of the sixth dorsal compartment frequently occurs in tennis players and hockey players.
2. Patients experience painful snapping with forearm supination (tendon subluxates) and pronation (tendon reduces).
3. Must be distinguished from other ulnar wrist disorders
4. Long-arm cast immobilization in pronation may enable healing.
5. Surgical débridement of the sixth dorsal compartment and reconstruction of the fibroosseous tunnel with a slip of extensor retinaculum are occasionally necessary (Figure 4-64).

D. Intersection syndrome

1. Involves painful crepitus at the dorsal forearm caused by irritation and inflammation of the crossing point of the first (abductor pollicis longus and extensor pollicis brevis) with the second (ECRL and ECRB) dorsal compartments
2. Typically seen in rowers and weightlifters
3. Splinting and local corticosteroid injections are typically effective for this self-limiting condition.

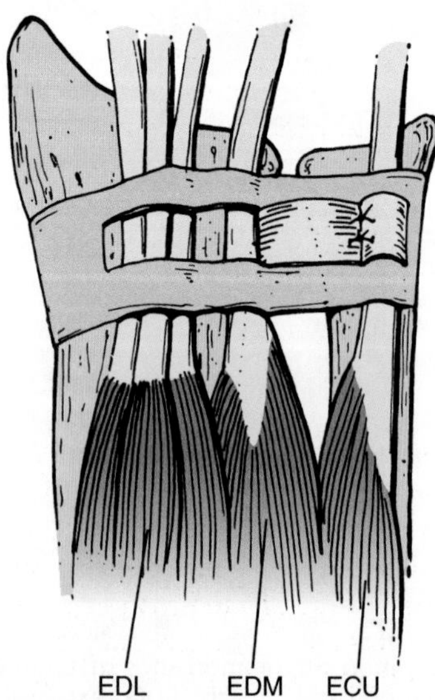

Figure 4-64 **Stabilization of the extensor carpi ulnaris (ECU) with a flap of the extensor retinaculum. EDL, extensor digitorum longus; EDM, extensor digiti minimi.** (From Spinner M, Kaplan EB: Extensor carpi ulnaris, *Clin Orthop* 68:124–129, 1970.)

4. Surgical decompression of the crossing point is rarely necessary.

E. Other extensor tendon tendinitis

1. May affect the extensor pollicis longus, extensor indicis proprius, or extensor digiti quinti
2. Usually responsive to local measures and surgical release, if indicated

F. "Jersey finger"

1. Avulsion injury of the flexor digitorum profundus tendon from its insertion at the base of the distal interphalangeal joint
2. The ring finger is the most commonly affected.
3. Avulsion occurs with sudden hyperextension during finger flexion and may be seen on plain radiographs.
4. Leddy classification describes three types: Type I is retraction of the tendon into the palm; type II is retraction to the proximal interphalangeal (PIP) joint; and type III is associated with a large, bony articular fragment, usually without significant retraction because of the A4 pulley.
5. These injuries necessitate retrieval of the retracted tendon and reattachment to the base of the PIP joint.
6. Type I injuries must be repaired early (within 1 week) because of loss of blood supply to the tendon.
7. Arthrodesis is generally favored over late (>3 months) repair because finger stiffness occurs after tendon grafting.

G. "Mallet finger"

1. Avulsion of the terminal extensor tendon
2. Radiography is used to rule out fracture.
3. **These injuries are typically treated with prolonged (>6 weeks) extension splinting.**
4. Results are almost uniformly good.
5. Chronic injuries may result in significant swan-neck deformities because of chronic overpull of the extensor tendon at the PIP joint with flexion of the distal interphalangeal joint.
6. Chronic deformities in young patients with preserved passive finger motion may be corrected by restoring the balance between extensors and flexors.

H. Sagittal band rupture ("boxer's knuckle")

1. Typically occurs in pugilists as a result of forceful subluxation of the extensor tendon
2. Usually involves the index and long fingers in professionals and the ring and small fingers in amateurs
3. Acute injuries are treated with extension splinting for 4 weeks.
4. Chronic injury leads to persistent extensor tendon subluxation and should be repaired or reconstructed with a slip of extensor tendon looped around the collateral ligament.

II. LIGAMENT INJURIES

A. Scapholunate ligament injury

1. Diagnosis
   - Most common wrist ligament injury
   - Patients experience snuffbox tenderness after hyperextension of a pronated wrist, such as that occurring after a fall.
   - Radial deviation of the hand with volar stabilization of the scaphoid (Watson test) may reproduce pain.
   - **Radiographic hallmarks include an increased scapholunate interval (>3 mm), a cortical ring sign (proximal and distal poles of scaphoid overlap on**

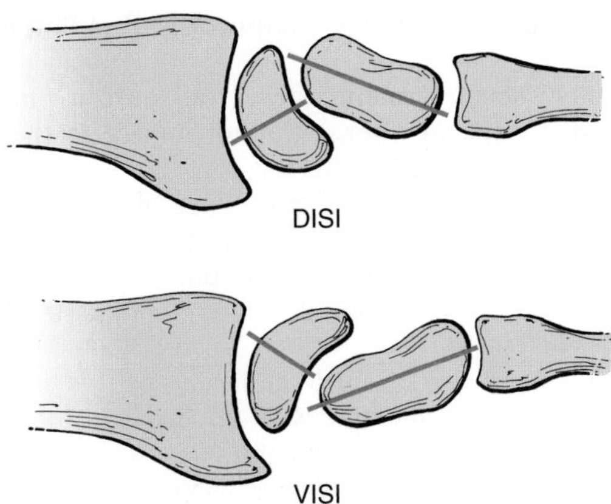

Figure 4-65 Scapholunate instability is associated with a dorsal intercalated instability pattern (dorsal intercalated segmental instability [DISI]). Triquetrum-lunate instability may have a volar intercalated instability pattern (volar intercalated segmental instability [VISI]). Note the increased scapholunate angle (>60 degrees) with the DISI pattern (normal, 30 degrees). (From McCue FC, Bruce JF: The wrist. In DeLee JC, Drez D Jr, editors: *Orthopaedic sports medicine: principles and practice,* Philadelphia, 1994, WB Saunders, p 918.)

posteroanterior projection), and an increased scapholunate angle (>70 degrees) on lateral projection.

- Persistent scapholunate dissociation with attenuation of extrinsic structures leads to an extended posture of the lunate (dorsal intercalated segment instability; Figure 4-65) that unloads its articulation with the radius and increases contact forces at the radioscaphoid articulation, which lead to progressive arthrosis.
- Diagnosis may be made with magnetic resonance arthrography, which may help to increase the sensitivity and specificity as opposed to MRI without arthrography.

2. Treatment
   - **Treatment involves either closed reduction with percutaneous pinning of the scapholunate joint for 8 to 10 weeks or open reduction with internal fixation of the articulation, combined with a capsulodesis.**
   - Partial tears can be treated with débridement or thermal modulation.

B. Lunotriquetral ligament injury

1. Lunotriquetral ligament injury is less common than scapholunate ligament injury.
2. Patients describe ulnar-sided wrist pain after a fall; this pain is worse with pronation and ulnar deviation (power grip).
3. Examination conducted to distinguish lunotriquetral injuries from the spectrum of injuries that usually accompany them (chondral lesions, triangular fibrocartilage complex [TFCC] tears)
4. Pain is reproduced with ballottement or shuck of the lunotriquetral articulation.
5. Radiographic hallmarks include widening of the lunotriquetral interval, volar flexion of the lunate, an increase in the capitolunate angle, and a decrease in the scapholunate angle. Magnetic resonance arthrography may help confirm the diagnosis.
6. Treatment after failure of conservative care is through débridement of the lunotriquetral ligament, with or without ulnar shortening.
7. Arthrodesis is useful in refractory cases.

C. Hand ligament injury

1. Digital collateral ligament injury
   - Often the result of a "jammed finger"
   - Management consists of buddy-taping: 3 weeks for simple tears, 6 weeks for complete tears.
   - Radial collateral ligament injury of the PIP joint of the index finger should be surgically repaired because of the need for pinch stability of this joint.
2. PIP joint dislocation
   - Typically occurs in a dorsal direction and results in a volar plate injury
   - Reduction is usually accomplished by the athlete, and incomplete reduction may result from volar plate interposition.
   - After reduction, the finger is buddy-taped to the adjacent digit for 3 to 6 weeks.
   - ROM exercises should begin early.
   - Flexion contracture of the PIP joint (pseudo-boutonnière deformity) may develop late but generally resolves with therapy and appropriate splinting.
   - Volar PIP joint dislocation (central slip injury) is unusual and generally results in a tear of the central slip insertion.
   - Treatment includes immobilization for 6 to 8 weeks with the PIP joint in extension.
3. Collateral ligament injury of the thumb
   - Includes radial and UCL injuries; "gamekeeper's or skier's thumb"
   - Instability should be examined in extension and at 30 degrees.
   - Instability in full extension is indicative of injury to the accessory UCL, whereas opening at 30 degrees is suggestive of proper UCL injury.
   - Radiographs are helpful in ruling out fracture; stress radiographs and MRI also play a role in confirming the diagnosis.
   - Nondisplaced, bony avulsions should not be subjected to stress radiography because of the risk of displacement.
   - Incomplete ulnar injuries may be immobilized.
   - For injuries with a side-to-side difference of more than 15 degrees or with opening of more than 45 degrees, operative intervention is required because the aponeurosis of the adductor becomes interposed between the ends of the torn ligament (Stener lesion; Figure 4-66).
   - Aponeurotic interposition does not occur on the radial side. These rare injuries are often treated with closed procedures.

III. FRACTURES

A. Scaphoid fracture

1. Scaphoid fractures occur frequently in contact sports.
2. Because the vascular supply enters distally, proximal fractures have a high rate of nonunion and avascular necrosis.
3. CT can be used to assess displacement; MRI is helpful in ruling out occult fracture and assessing vascularity.
4. Acute and subacute, nondisplaced fractures that have occurred less than 8 weeks previously may be treated in a thumb-spica cast.
5. Percutaneous fixation of nondisplaced fractures leads to earlier union, ROM, return to work, and possibly return to play.

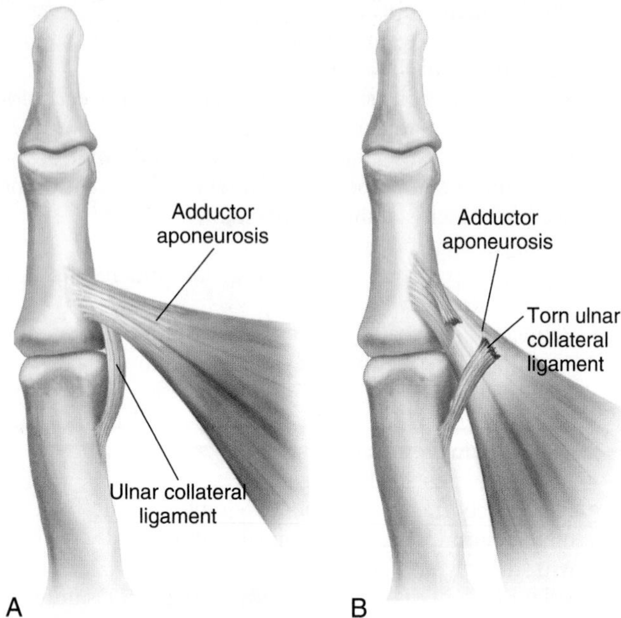

Figure 4-66 Stener lesion. The adductor aponeurosis separates the two ends of the ulnar collateral ligament, and the aponeurosis must be incised to repair the ligament. (From Morrison WB, Sanders TG: *Problem solving in musculoskeletal imaging,* Philadelphia, 2008, Elsevier.)

6. Displaced fractures should be managed operatively with either percutaneous or limited open fixation.
7. Nonunion may be managed with a local vascularized bone graft and internal fixation.

B. **Hamate fracture**

1. Hook-of-hamate fractures typically occur in a golfer or a baseball batter after repeated direct contact.
2. **Diagnosis is confirmed by a carpal tunnel view or CT.**
3. Treatment is either cast immobilization or excision of the hook. The latter enables more rapid return to play.

C. **Metacarpal and phalanx fractures**

1. Many of these fractures heal with closed reduction and immobilization.
2. Fourth and fifth metacarpal fractures can accept greater angulation than the index and long fingers.
3. Displaced fractures, those involving the joints, and those resulting in rotational malalignment should be treated surgically.
4. Early motion is the key to successful rehabilitation.
5. Fractures involving the base of the thumb carpometacarpal joint (Bennett fracture, Rolando fracture) often necessitate operative reduction and stabilization.

IV. ULNAR WRIST PAIN

A. **Differential diagnosis**

1. The differential diagnosis of ulnar-sided wrist pain in athletes includes TFCC tear, pisotriquetral arthritis, fracture (ulnar styloid, hook-of-hamate injury), lunotriquetral ligament injury, extensor carpi ulnaris subluxation or tendinitis, ulnar nerve entrapment at the Guyon canal, ulnar artery thrombosis (hypothenar hammer syndrome), chondral lesions, and wrist ganglia.

B. **Triangular fibrocartilage complex/distal radioulnar joint**

1. **Patients seek treatment after a fall onto a pronated, extended wrist or after a traction injury to the ulnar aspect of the wrist.**
2. Point tenderness is present at the base of the ulnar snuffbox, which is between the triquetrum and ulnar styloid.
3. Symptoms are reproduced with ulnar deviation (compresses TFCC) or radial deviation (applies tension to peripheral tear).
4. Diagnosis can also be made clinically; pain is associated with wrist extension and with applied axial load with resisted pronation and supination.
5. Arthrography and MRI may help diagnosis a tear, but both are highly user dependent and have a high rate of false-positive results (Table 4-18).
6. Arthroscopy is the diagnostic "gold standard."
7. Treatment (Figure 4-67) is based on tear type, the presence of instability or arthritis in the distal radioulnar joint, and ulnar variance.
8. A study of athletes with arthroscopic treatment of TFCC injuries revealed that 14 of 16 patients were able to return to play at 3 months and had improvement in subjective outcome scores.

C. **Ulnocarpal abutment syndrome**

1. Typically occurs in patients with ulnar-positive variance
2. Pain is exacerbated with rotation or ulnar loading of the wrist.
3. Sclerotic and cystic changes may be seen in the lunate and distal ulna.
4. If supportive measures fail, ulnar shortening (wafer procedure, ulnar-shortening osteotomy) provides predictable pain relief.

Table 4-18 Classification of Injuries to the Triangular Fibrocartilage Complex

Class*	Description	Treatment
1A	Horizontal tear adjacent to sigmoid notch	Débridement
1B	Avulsion from ulna with or without ulnar styloid fracture	Suture repair
1C	Avulsion from carpus; exposes pisiform	Débridement
1D	Avulsion from sigmoid notch	Débridement
2A	Thinning of triangular fibrocartilage complex without perforation	Débridement
2B	Thinning of disc with chondromalacia	Débridement
2C	Perforation of disc with chondromalacia	Débridement
2D	Perforation of disc, chondromalacia, partial tear of lunotriquetral ligament	Débridement
2E	Perforation of disc, chondromalacia, complete tear of lunotriquetral ligament, ulnocarpal degenerative joint disease	Débridement

From Miller MD, Cooper DE, Warner JJP: *Review of sports medicine and arthroscopy,* Philadelphia, 1995, WB Saunders, p 188.

*Class 1, traumatic lesions; class 2, degenerative lesions. Treatment for degenerative lesions includes débridement of loose, degenerated discs; intraarticular resection of the ulnar head; and débridement of lunotriquetral ligament tears with percutaneous pinning of the lunotriquetral joint, depending on the pathologic process present.

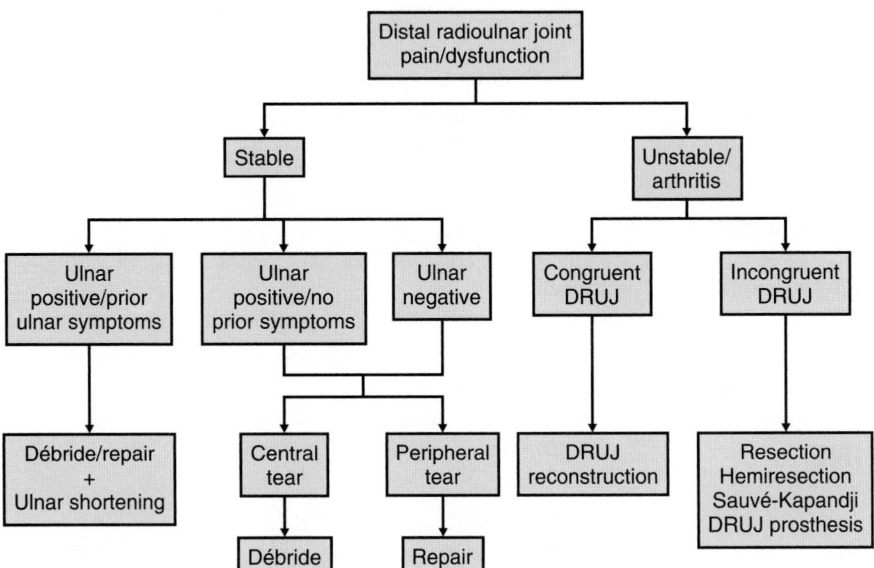

Figure 4-67 Algorithmic approach to treatment of injuries to the triangular fibrocartilage complex. DRUJ, distal radioulnar joint.

5. Ulnar head resection (Darrach), hemiresection with interpositional arthroplasty, the Sauvé-Kapandji procedure, and prosthetic ulnar head replacement are useful if significant arthritis is present.

D. Hypothenar hammer syndrome

1. Involves ulnar artery constriction, which can occur in baseball pitchers
2. Allen test reveals decreased ulnar filling.
3. Doppler evaluation and vascular referral may be necessary.

E. Guyon canal syndrome (handlebar palsy)

1. Characterized by pain and ulnar paresthesias, with weakness of the intrinsic hand muscles
2. Treatment includes modification of the cyclist's grip and, on occasion, ulnar nerve decompression.

V. POST-TRAUMATIC DYSFUNCTION OF THE WRIST AND HAND

A. Scaphoid avascular necrosis

1. Complication that is common because of the tenuous blood supply of this bone
2. Bone grafting and internal fixation are usually curative.
3. Unrecognized injuries may lead to the development of scaphoid nonunion–advanced collapse, which in turn may necessitate radial styloid excision, scaphoid excision and partial wrist arthrodesis (four-corner fusion), proximal row carpectomy, total wrist fusion, or a combination of these measures.

B. Osteochondrosis of the capitate

1. Most often found in gymnasts
2. May respond to débridement or limited wrist fusions

C. Kienbock disease

1. Avascular necrosis and collapse of the lunate
2. Probably related to overuse and ulnar negative wrist variance
3. Early in the disease process, ulnar lengthening or radial shortening may be helpful in arresting progression to collapse.
4. Limited wrist fusions may be necessary for cases of advanced collapse.

VI. WRIST ARTHROSCOPY

A. Introduction

1. This procedure serves as a useful diagnostic and staging adjunct and as an alternative to arthrotomy for the manipulation of intraarticular structures.

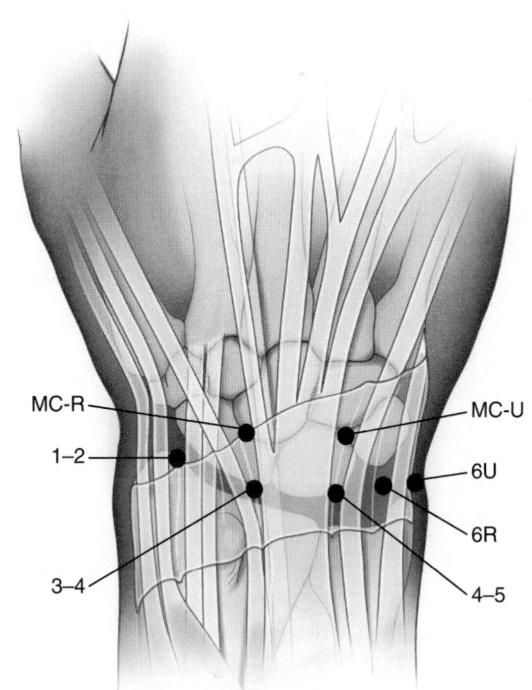

Figure 4-68 Arthroscopic wrist portals. Numbers indicate wrist extensor compartments and associated portals. MC-R, midcarpal radial; MC-U, midcarpal ulnar; R, radial; U, ulnar. (From Miller MD, Chhabra AB, Hurwitz S, et al: *Orthopaedic surgical approaches,* Philadelphia, 2008, Elsevier.)

2. Indicated for the establishment of a diagnosis for unexplained wrist pain, treatment of mechanical symptoms secondary to interosseous ligament injuries or TFCC tears, assistance in the anatomic reduction and fixation of intraarticular fractures, débridement of chondral lesions, removal of loose bodies, and synovectomy.

B. **Technique**

1. The wrist is placed in a traction apparatus, and a 2.5- or 3.0-mm arthroscope is used.
2. Portals are named in relation to the dorsal wrist compartments (Figure 4-68).
3. The 3-4 portal is established first; the 4-5 portal is used for instrumentation.
4. The 6R portal serves as a useful adjunct for visualization and instrumentation.
5. Midcarpal portals are necessary for complete carpal visualization, and the radiocarpal portals often help confirm the pathologic process.
6. The scaphotrapeziotrapezoid portal is typically used by experienced arthroscopists to evaluate localized pathologic processes.

SECTION 7 HEAD AND SPINE

I. HEAD INJURIES

A. **Diffuse brain injuries**

1. These include mild and "classical" cerebral concussions and diffuse axonal injury.
2. Mild concussions occur without loss of consciousness, which has relevance to management and return to play.

B. **Postconcussion syndrome**

1. Manifestation
   - Characterized by persistent headaches, irritability, confusion, and difficulty concentrating and can occur with after mild or severe concussions. If consciousness is lost for more than 5 minutes, a head CT should be performed.
2. Evaluations
   - Can be made with the standard assessment of concussion, neuropsychologic testing, memory testing, and the balance error scoring system
3. Return to play
   - According to newer guidelines that follow the lead of the National Collegiate Athletic Association (NCAA) guidelines, any athlete found or suspected to have suffered a concussion should not return to athletics the same day. Before an athlete can return to athletic activity, he or she must be evaluated by a physician with resolution of symptoms and must pass neurocognitive testing milestones. The athlete can return to play 1 week to 1 month after the first episode; after a second episode, the athlete should consider not participating for the entire season.
   - Diffuse axonal injury occurs with loss of consciousness lasting more than 6 hours; athletes who suffer this injury should consider total avoidance of contact sports in the future.
   - **Return to play on the same day should be prohibited if there is any sign of concussion.**

C. **Second-impact syndrome**

1. May occur with a second minor blow before initial symptoms have resolved
2. Leads to loss of autoregulation of the brain's blood supply and potential herniation
3. Second-impact syndrome is associated with a mortality rate of 50%.

D. **Focal brain syndromes**

1. Include contusions, intracranial hematomas, epidural hematomas, and subdural hematomas
2. CT is helpful for distinguishing these entities (Figure 4-69).
3. Although epidural hematomas are classically said to be characterized by a period of lucidity followed by loss of consciousness, this sequence may not occur. Neurosurgical consultation and monitoring in an intensive care unit are necessary.

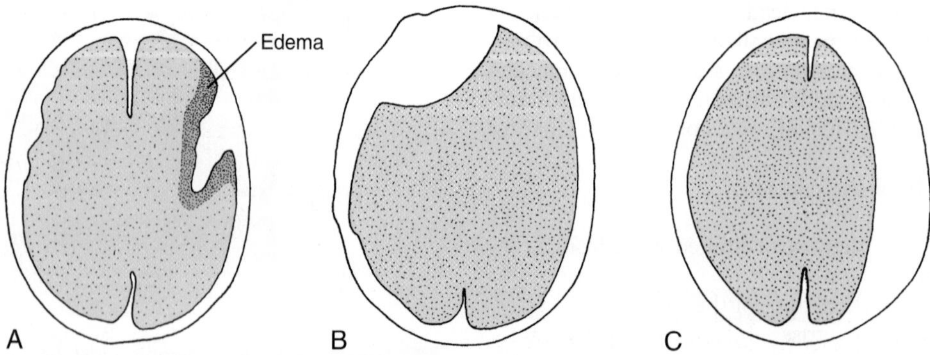

Figure 4-69 Drawing of computed tomographic findings in brain injury. **A,** Contusion includes a hemorrhagic area and surrounding edema. **B,** Epidural hematomas typically have a biconvex appearance. **C,** Subdural hematomas have a concave or crescentic appearance. (From Miller MD, Cooper DE, Warner JJP: *Review of sports medicine and arthroscopy,* Philadelphia, 1995, WB Saunders, p 204.)

4. Surgical treatment of intracranial hematomas may be indicated and are followed by seizure prophylaxis.

E. Prevention

1. Head protection—especially in contact sports, equestrian events, hockey, boxing, skating, and skiing—should be encouraged.
2. Strict adherence to guidelines for return to play after these injuries can minimize the risk of second-impact syndrome.

II. CERVICAL SPINE INJURIES

A. Introduction

1. Catastrophic injury to the cervical spine is unfortunately all too common in contact sports (especially football and rugby).
2. Soft tissue injuries of the cervical spine, as well as fractures and dislocations in athletes, are treated in the same manner other traumatic injuries to the spine (see Chapter 8, Spine).
3. Underlying cervical stenosis, or narrowing of the anteroposterior diameter of the spine (<13 mm), can make these injuries worse (Figure 4-70). Recommendations for return to play for athletes with cervical stenosis and transient symptoms are controversial (see the following entries).
4. Congenital conditions of the odontoid are usually contraindications to participation in contact sports.
5. Football players who repeatedly use poor tackling techniques can develop a condition known as "spear tackler's spine," which includes developmental cervical stenosis, loss of lordosis, and other radiographic abnormalities.
   - Return to contact sports should be avoided.
6. Spinal cord injury may lead to thermoregulatory problems.

B. On-field management

1. As with any trauma victim, careful handling and immobilization of the patient are crucial.

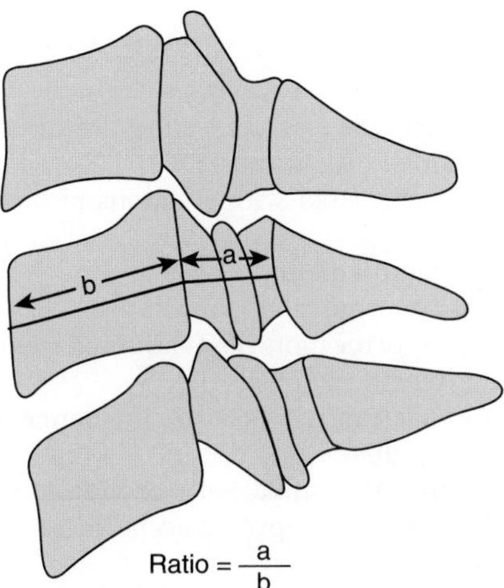

Figure 4-70 Pavlov ratio (a/b) of 0.8 is consistent with cervical stenosis. (Note that this ratio may not apply to larger individuals.) (From Pavlov H, Porter IS: Criteria for cervical instability and stenosis, *Op Tech Sports Med* 1:170, 1993.)

2. The mechanism of injury usually involves an axial load with flexion and compression of the spine.
3. **For a football player, the helmet and shoulder pads should not be removed. However, the facemask should be removed in the event that an emergency airway is needed.**
   - **The sequence for proper cervical spine stabilization is as follows:**
     - **Stabilize the head.**
     - **Log-roll the individual to the supine position.**
     - **Take off the facemask (not helmet).**
     - **Administer cardiopulmonary resuscitation if necessary.**
     - **Apply a backboard.**
     - **Transport the individual to an emergency department.**

C. No return to play

1. Criteria include transient quadriplegia with severe stenosis; cervical neurapraxia with ligamentous instability; congenital anomalies, with failure of fusion (os odontoideum, odontoid agenesis, odontoid hypoplasia); and spear tackler's spine.

III. THORACIC AND LUMBAR SPINE INJURIES*

A. Overview

1. Injuries commonly associated with sports include muscle injury, fractures, disc disease, and spondylolysis and spondylolisthesis.

B. Spondylolysis and spondylolisthesis

1. Diagnosis
   - This condition is common in football interior line positions and in gymnasts because of the repetitive hyperextension of the spine involved in these sports. Oblique radiographs (only 32% sensitive), bone scanning with **single-photon emission computed tomography** (SPECT; the most sensitive and effective imaging modality in the acute setting), and CT (useful in assessing healing) are all helpful for establishing the diagnosis.
2. Treatment
   - Treatment includes activity modification, bracing, and fusion for high-grade slips.
   - Individuals with grade I or II injuries may play if the injuries are asymptomatic.
   - For those with grades III, IV, or V injuries who are experiencing intractable pain or a progressive slip, a posterolateral fusion should be considered.

C. Herniated nucleus pulposus

1. Adolescent athletes may have a variety of findings that contribute to this diagnosis.
2. Typical among these are pain that is worse in flexion, sitting intolerance, the presence of radicular symptoms, and a positive result of the **straight-leg raise** test.
3. Treatment depends on the degree of herniation and may range from core muscle strengthening and injections to surgical decompression with or without fusion.

*See Chapter 8, Spine, for a more complete description of these injuries.

SECTION 8 MEDICAL ASPECTS OF SPORTS MEDICINE

I. PREPARTICIPATION PHYSICAL EXAMINATION

A. The orthopaedic history questionnaire is the most helpful for identifying musculoskeletal problems.
B. Family history of sudden cardiac death or any personal history of exertional chest pain or dyspnea necessitates further evaluation and cardiac workup.

II. MUSCLE PHYSIOLOGY

A. There are three types of muscle: I, IIA, and IIB.
B. Type I muscle is slow twitching/aerobic and is helpful in endurance sports.
1. Training can increase the number of mitochondria and increase capillary density.

C. Types IIA and IIB muscles are fast twitching/anaerobic and are helpful for sprinters.
D. These muscles have high contraction speeds, quick relaxation, and low triglyceride stores.
E. The mode of energy utilization differentiates type IIA from type IIB muscle: IIA has both aerobic and anaerobic capabilities, whereas IIB is primarily anaerobic.
F. Immobilization of muscle results in a shorter position with a decreased ability to generate tension.

III. EXERCISE

A. Benefits
1. Done on a regular basis, exercise can decrease heart rate and blood pressure (hypertension), decrease insulin requirements in diabetic patients, decrease cardiovascular risk, and increase lean body mass.
2. Also been shown to reduce risk of cancer, osteoporosis, and hypercholesterolemia

B. Aerobic threshold and conditioning
1. The aerobic threshold can be determined by measuring oxygen consumption and is useful for evaluating endurance athletes.
2. Sports-specific conditioning involves aerobic and anaerobic conditioning in different proportions, in accordance with the season and the sport.
3. In the off-season, long-distance runs can enable sprinters to increase aerobic recovery capability after sprints.
4. Several exercise categories have been described. Stretching has also been shown to have a beneficial effect (Table 4-19).

IV. DELAYED-ONSET MUSCLE SORENESS

A. This condition often follows unaccustomed eccentric exercise, usually appearing 24 to 48 hours after the activity.
B. Cause involves inflammation and edema of the connective tissue, with elevated creatine kinase levels.

Table 4-19 Exercise Types

Exercise	Description	Benefit
Isometric	Muscle tension without change in unit length	Muscle hypertrophy; not endurance
Isotonic	Weight training with a constant resistance through arc of motion	Improved motor performance
Isokinetic	Weight training with a constant velocity, variable resistance	Increased strength; less time consuming but more expensive
Plyometric	Rapid shortening	Power generation
Functional	Aerobic fitness	Easily performed

V. CARDIAC ABNORMALITIES IN ATHLETES

A. Sudden cardiac death
1. Usually related to an underlying heart condition
2. **Hypertrophic cardiomyopathy is the most common cause of sudden death in young athletes.**
3. Screening that includes electrocardiography can identify this problem early.

B. Commotio cordis
1. **Cardiac contusion from a direct blow to the chest (e.g., in Little League baseball) has a poor prognosis, even when immediately recognized and treated with immediate defibrillation.**

C. Hypertrophic cardiomyopathy and cardiac murmurs
1. Diastolic murmurs found on routine examination warrant further cardiac evaluation.
2. Murmurs that increase in intensity with Valsalva maneuvers are consistent with hypertrophic cardiomyopathy.
3. **Sports participation is contraindicated in cases of outflow obstruction.**

VI. METABOLIC ISSUES IN ATHLETES

A. Dehydration
1. Fluid and electrolyte loss can lead to decreased cardiovascular function and work capacity.
2. Absorption is increased with solutions of low osmolarity (<10%).

B. Nutritional supplements
1. Continue to be a source of controversy
   - Creatine, one of the more popular supplements, increases the water retention in cells.
   - **In-season use can increase the incidence of dehydration and cramps.**
   - The use of glucosamine with chondroitin sulfate has yielded improvement over placebo in some studies of knee arthritis.

VII. ERGOGENIC DRUGS

A. Anabolic steroids
1. Derivatives of testosterone are abused by athletes attempting to increase muscle mass and strength and increase erythropoiesis.

2. **Adverse effects include liver dysfunction, hypercholesterolemia, cardiomyopathy, testicular atrophy, gynecomastia, acne, mood disturbances (particularly increased aggression), and irreversible alopecia.**
   - **Heart disease can result from increased plasma levels of low-density lipoprotein and decreased levels of high-density lipoprotein**
3. Urine sampling has been the standard for evaluation by the International Olympic Committee.

B. Human growth hormone (HGH)

1. Made from recombinant DNA; illegal use of this drug is common
2. Athletes attempting to increase muscle size and weight abuse this drug, which has side effects similar to those of steroids, as well as hypertension and gigantism.
3. **Difficult to detect if suspected**
4. **Insulin-like growth factor-1** has effects similar to those of HGHs.

C. Prohormones

1. Derivatives of testosterone, **dehydroepiandrosterone** (DHEA) and androstenedione, have been used as anabolic agents.
2. However, their effects are controversial.

D. Other commonly abused drugs

1. Amphetamines, blood doping, diuretics, and laxatives

VIII. FEMALE ATHLETE–RELATED ISSUES

A. Physiologic differences

1. Women are typically smaller and lighter and have higher percentages of body fat.
2. Lower maximal oxygen consumption, cardiac output, hemoglobin, and muscular mass and strength are also important considerations.
3. Other differences contribute to the increased incidence of patellofemoral disorders, stress fractures, and knee ACL injuries in girls and women (especially in basketball, soccer, and rugby).

B. Amenorrhea

1. Secondary amenorrhea is common in female athletes.
2. Defined as the absence of normal menstruation for 6 months (not as a result of pregnancy)
3. **Insufficient caloric intake is the most common cause of amenorrhea in female athletes.** A low percentage of body fat may also play a role.
4. **Incidence in elite runners approaches 50% and is related to stress fractures (osteopenia) and eating disorders. The "female athlete triad" consists of amenorrhea, stress fractures, and eating disorders.**
5. Dietary management and birth control pills are helpful in treating this problem.

IX. OTHER SPORTS-RELATED INJURIES AND ISSUES

A. Blunt trauma

1. Can cause injury to solid organs
2. These injuries may be subtle, and diagnosing them requires a high index of suspicion.
3. **The kidney is the most commonly injured organ (especially in boxing), followed by the spleen (injured in football).**

B. Chest injuries

1. Can be serious and necessitates immediate on-field action
2. **Decreased breath sounds, deviated trachea, and hypotension may signify a tension pneumothorax.**
   - Treatment entails placing a 14-gauge intravenous needle in the second intercostal space at the midclavicular line, followed by the placement of a chest tube.
3. Airway obstructions must also be anticipated and treated.
4. Rib fractures may also occur in contact sports.
5. The player usually has "had the air knocked out" of him or her, which can be related to a problem with the diaphragm.

C. Eye injuries

1. These injuries are best avoided with proper protection.
2. A hyphema (blood in the eye) is associated with a vitreous or retinal injury in more than 50% of cases.

D. Ear injuries

1. Auricular hematomas ("cauliflower ear"), common in wrestlers, should be treated with aspiration and wrapping.

E. Tooth injuries

1. **The tooth or teeth should be replaced immediately but may be temporarily placed in the buccal fold or in milk if necessary.**
2. Crown fractures is the most common maxillofacial injury in ice hockey.

F. Heat illness

1. Heat stroke, common during the football preseason, is characterized by **collapse, with neurologic deficits, tachycardia, tachypnea, hypotension, and anhidrosis.**
2. Treatment involves rapidly cooling the body's core temperature.
3. Heat stroke is the second leading cause of death in football players.

G. Cold injury

1. Treatment involves rewarming the patient in a warm-water bath (110° to 112° F).

H. Exercise-induced bronchospasm

1. Involves transient airway obstruction that results from exertion
2. Symptoms include the triad of coughing, shortness of breath, and wheezing.
3. Commonly occurs in cold-weather sports, and the diagnosis is confirmed by a low forced expiratory volume.
4. Inhaled β_2 agonists are the first-line treatment.

I. Pneumothorax

1. A chest tube or large-bore angiocatheter must be inserted at the second intercostal space for tension pneumothorax.

J. Deep venous thrombosis (DVT) after knee arthroscopy

1. The incidence of DVT after knee arthroscopy is 10%; 2% of the cases are proximal without prophylaxis.
2. For patients at high risk for DVT (older age, personal or family history of DVT, concomitant medical illness), it is prudent to treat with prophylaxis against DVT.

K. On-field bleeding

1. The affected player must be immediately removed from play and may not return until the bleeding has stopped and the wound has been covered with an occlusive dressing.

L. Infectious disease in athletes

1. **Methicillin-resistant *Staphylococcus aureus*** (MRSA)
   - **Transmission occurs by means of direct person-to-person contact through disruptions in skin integrity.**
     - Inanimate object and airborne droplet transmission occurs infrequently.
   - Typically occurs around the area of previous skin trauma and is characterized by pustules on an erythematous base
   - Treated with trimethoprim-sulfamethoxazole (Bactrim) and rifampin
2. Human immunodeficiency virus
   - An athlete's HIV status is confidential; by itself, HIV infection is insufficient reason to restrict athletic participation.
   - Wound care in this population is the same as that for all athletes, with the use of universal precautions, application of compressive dressing, and waiting until the bleeding has stopped before a return to play.
3. Infectious mononucleosis
   - **The primary concern for athletic participation when this condition is diagnosed is the associated risk of spleen rupture.**
   - **Participation in contact sports should be restricted for 3 to 5 weeks, and splenomegaly must have resolved before a return to play.**
4. Meningitis
   - A concern in athletes because of the ease of spread from the "close quarters" environment of the training room
   - Symptoms include fever, headache, and nuchal rigidity.
   - The evaluation of **cerebrospinal fluid** is important for identifying cases of bacterial meningitis.
5. Other skin infections
   - Conditions such as tinea corporis ("ringworm"), herpes simplex, herpes gladiatorum, and impetigo are common in sports such as wrestling that involve close contact among athletes.
   - Treatment is administered with antifungal and antiviral medications, as appropriate.
   - Athletic participation should be restricted until all skin lesions have resolved.
   - Athletes with herpes zoster must have no new lesions for 72 hours before they resume participation.

M. Special athletes

1. Special considerations may be necessary for patients with congenital heart disease and Down syndrome.
2. Patients with Down syndrome may have congenital cervical instability, which should be assessed radiographically before sports participation.
3. An atlanto-dens interval of more than 9 mm on flexion and extension views is an indication for surgical fusion.

TESTABLE CONCEPTS

SECTION 1 KNEE

- The most common causes of an acute hemarthrosis: ACL tear (70%), isolated meniscus tear (15%), osteochondral fracture, patellar dislocation.
- The vascular supply of the meniscus is a primary determinant of healing potential; tears in the peripheral third have the highest potential for healing.
- The "gold standard" for meniscal repair is the inside-out technique with vertical mattress sutures. The saphenous nerve is at risk in medial repairs; the peroneal nerve is at risk in lateral repairs.
- The ACL injury rate is higher in female athletes than in male athletes because of smaller notches, smaller ligaments, increased generalized ligament laxity, increased knee laxity, and different landing biomechanics in women and girls.
- The Lachman test is the most sensitive examination for acute ACL injuries, whereas results of the pivot shift test are correlated most closely with outcome after ACL reconstruction.
- MRI evaluation of ACL injuries demonstrates characteristic "bone bruises" in more than half of cases; these bruises are typically located near the sulcus terminalis on the lateral femoral condyle and the posterolateral aspect of the tibia.
- BPTB autografts demonstrate faster incorporation into the bone tunnels than do hamstring autografts and are often the graft of choice for patients desiring an early return to sports activity.
- The most common technical error in ACL surgery is placement of the femoral tunnel too far anteriorly, which results in limited flexion. Vertical graft placement results in decreased rotational stability.
- PCL injuries often result from a fall onto the ground with a plantar-flexed foot.
- PCL reconstruction should be reserved for functionally unstable knees or combined injuries. Single-bundle reconstructions should be tensioned in 90 degrees of flexion.
- Chronic grade III posterolateral corner injuries often necessitate a valgus opening wedge osteotomy.
- Osteochondritis dissecans should be monitored in children with open physes. Adult lesions do not resolve and should be treated.
- Marrow-stimulating techniques, including microfracture, drilling, and abrasion arthroplasty, involve perforation of the subchondral bone after removal of the "tidemark" cartilage with eventual clot formation and fibrocartilaginous repair tissue (type I collagen with inferior wear characteristics).
- Lateral patellar facet compression syndrome should be treated with a lateral release only in the setting of objective evidence of lateral tilt that has not responded to extensive nonoperative management. Lateral tilt is best evaluated by measurement of the lateral patellofemoral angle.

SECTION 2 THIGH, HIP, AND PELVIS

- Quadriceps contusions are acutely managed with overnight immobilization in hyperflexion.
- Athletic pubalgia (sports hernia) is the result of abdominal hyperextension and thigh hyperabduction, which result in injury to the muscles of the abdominal wall and adductor longus. Treatment is primarily nonoperative.
- MRI is the most specific test for detecting stress fractures. Treatment typically includes protected weight bearing, rest, cross-training, analgesics, and therapeutic modalities.
- External snapping hip occurs when the iliotibial band abruptly catches on the greater trochanter, whereas internal snapping hip occurs when the iliopsoas impinges on the hip capsule.
- Complications of hip arthroscopy typically result from traction injuries or iatrogenic neurovascular injury from aberrant portal placement. Use of an anterior portal places the lateral femoral cutaneous nerve at risk. Use of an anterolateral portal places the superior gluteal nerve at risk. Use of a posterolateral portal places the sciatic nerve at risk, especially when the hip is externally rotated.

SECTION 3 LEG, FOOT, AND ANKLE

- Superficial peroneal nerve entrapment manifests with numbness and tingling over the dorsum of the foot that worsens with plantar flexion and inversion of the foot.
- Peroneal tendon subluxation is confirmed by observing the subluxation or dislocation by means of eversion and dorsiflexion of the foot.
- Treatment of Achilles tendon rupture is controversial. Recurrence rates are reduced with primary repair, but wound problems are increased with surgical repair.
- Chronic exertional compartment syndrome is characterized by pressures higher than 20 mm Hg 5 minutes after exercise, absolute values higher than 15 mm Hg during resting, and pressures higher than 30 mm Hg 1 minute after exercise.
- Popliteal artery entrapment syndrome manifests with obliteration of pedal pulses by active plantar flexion or passive dorsiflexion of the ankle during Doppler recordings.
- Tarsal navicular fractures should be treated with open reduction with internal fixation if linear fractures are seen on CT.
- Treatment of Jones fracture with early intramedullary screw fixation allows for earlier healing and an earlier return to conditioning activities. Returning to sports activity before radiographic union increases the risk of nonunion.
- Plantar fasciitis occurs in the central to medial subcalcaneal region and is common in runners. It is associated with a tight heel cord on physical examination.
- Syndesmotic ankle injury can be diagnosed with the external rotation stress test, which reproduces pain in the anterior syndesmosis. Tibiofibular synostosis may occur afterwards, and excision should be performed for persistent pain.
- Complications of ankle arthroscopy typically result from iatrogenic nerve injury. Avoid the posteromedial portal, which puts the posterior tibial artery and tibial nerve at risk. Avoid the anterocentral portal, which puts the

Continued

dorsalis pedis and deep peroneal nerve at risk. Use of the anterolateral portal puts the superficial peroneal nerve at risk. Use of the anteromedial portal puts the saphenous vein at risk.

SECTION 4 SHOULDER

- The most common location for an os acromiale is at the junction of the mesoacromion and meta-acromion.
- The contents of the rotator interval include the coracohumeral ligament, SGHL, biceps tendon, and glenohumeral capsule. The SGHL and coracohumeral ligament limit inferior translation and external rotation when the arm is adducted and posterior translation when the arm is flexed forward, adducted, and internally rotated. Rotator interval closure results in decreased external rotation in shoulder adduction and posteroinferior translation.
- The inferior glenohumeral ligament complex serves as the primary restraint to anterior, posterior, and inferior glenohumeral translation at 45 to 90 degrees of glenohumeral elevation.
- Traumatic anterior shoulder dislocations typically result when the arm is abducted and in external rotation. The axillary nerve is susceptible to injury.
- Instability is often associated with a Bankart lesion (anteroinferior labral tear) with disrupted medial scapular periosteum.
- Age at time of initial dislocation is an important risk factor for recurrent shoulder instability.
- Several open and arthroscopic techniques have been developed to address instability. Glenoid deficiency greater than 25% of the humeral head is a specific indication for coracoid transfer (Latarjet procedure). Failure of rehabilitation for multidirectional instability is an indication for capsular shift. Chronic dislocation with greater than 40% of articular surface deficit is an indication for allograft in young patients and for prosthesis in older patients.
- Physical examination for posterior instability includes load-and-shift and jerk testing.
- Multidirectional instability should be treated with extended rehabilitation that focuses on scapular stabilization before operative intervention is considered. Closed kinetic chain exercises should be emphasized.
- A fixed posterior shoulder dislocation is diagnosed by lack of external rotation. Anteroposterior radiographs are unreliable but may demonstrate a “lightbulb” sign.
- The prevalence of asymptomatic rotator cuff tears increases with age: 28% of those older than 60 years have a full-thickness tear, whereas 65% of those older than 70 years have a full-thickness tear.
- Acute rotator cuff tears should be repaired early because the disease process is accelerated in this setting. Combined tears of the supraspinatus and infraspinatus may be treated with latissimus dorsi tendon transfer to the greater tuberosity.
- Signs of a subscapularis tear include increased external rotation and the presence of a liftoff, modified liftoff, or belly-press sign. The appearance of an empty bicipital groove on axial MRI with tear of the transverse humeral ligament is often associated with subscapularis tear. At arthroscopy, a chronic subscapularis tear can be identified by the comma sign, which represents an avulsed SGHL.
- In athletes who participate in throwing activities, there is greater external rotation and a loss of internal rotation of the dominant shoulder than in the nondominant shoulder (GIRD). Initial treatment is posterior and posteroinferior capsular stretching exercises such as the sleeper stretch, as well as stretching of the pectoralis minor tendon.
- Internal impingement is between the posterior-superior labrum and rotator cuff. Alteration of the glenohumeral kinematics leads to a posterosuperior shift of the humeral head; abduction and external rotation of the arm, in turn, lead to the internal impingement.
- For type III acromioclavicular separations, recommended management is conservative in elderly patients, inactive patients, and patients who do not perform manual labor.
- Calcifying tendinitis is self-limiting condition of unknown origin that affects predominantly the supraspinatus tendon. Radiographs demonstrate characteristic calcification within the tendon.
- Adhesive capsulitis is associated with diabetes, thyroid disease, and trauma. Treat with physical therapy for 12 to 16 weeks, and if no improvement occurs, perform lysis of adhesions and manipulation with the patient under anesthesia.
- Suprascapular nerve compression by a ganglion in the spinoglenoid notch affects only the infraspinatus. Compression caused by a cyst in association with a SLAP lesion may respond to arthroscopic decompression and labral repair.
- Quadrilateral space syndrome is defined as axillary nerve or posterior humeral circumflex artery compression within the quadrilateral space, which results in pain and paresthesias with overhead activity, as well as weakness or atrophy of the teres minor and deltoid. This is most often seen in athletes who participate in throwing activities and is associated with late cocking and acceleration with the abducted, extended, and externally rotated arm.
- Medial scapular winging is caused by damage to the long thoracic nerve. Lateral scapular winging is caused by damage to the spinal accessory nerve.

SECTION 5 ELBOW

- Lateral epicondylitis is initiated as a microtear at the origin of the ECRB. Microscopic evaluation reveals angiofibroblastic hyperplasia.
- In distal biceps tendon ruptures, up to 50% loss of supination power has been documented.
- The anterior band of the UCL is the most important stabilizer of the elbow in flexion. In athletes who participate in throwing activities, the late-cocking and acceleration phases of throwing are periods of high stress generation. UCL injury is diagnosed with the moving valgus stress test.
- Treatment of UCL injury is nonoperative except in high-level athletes, who should have ligament reconstruction with a palmaris tendon graft.
- Osteochondritis dissecans typically occurs in the capitellum of the adolescent athlete engaged in repetitive overhead or upper-extremity weight-bearing activities.

- Complications of elbow arthroscopy typically result from iatrogenic nerve injury. The use of far-proximal portals may decrease these risks. A posteromedial portal is least safe because of its proximity to the ulnar nerve. Use of an anterolateral portal puts the lateral antebrachial cutaneous and radial nerves at risk. Use of an anteromedial portal puts the medial antebrachial cutaneous and median nerves at risk.

SECTION 6 HAND AND WRIST

- Mallet finger is treated with prolonged extension splinting. Open reduction with internal fixation is indicated for volar subluxation.
- Scapholunate ligament injury can be diagnosed by widening of the scapholunate interval, a cortical ring sign, and increased scapholunate angle. Treatment is with closed reduction and percutaneous pinning or with open reduction with internal fixation and capsulodesis.
- Hook-of-hamate fractures are confirmed by radiographic carpal tunnel view or CT. Treatment is cast immobilization or excision.

SECTION 7 HEAD AND SPINE

- Same-day return to play should be prohibited if concussion is suspected.
- For a football player, the helmet and shoulder pads should not be removed if a cervical spine injury is suspected. However, the facemask should be removed in case an emergency airway is needed.
- Minor traction or compression injuries to the brachial plexus are often termed "burners" or "stingers." Complete resolution of symptoms is required before the patient may return to play. More than one occurrence is a game requires removal from play and cervical spine radiographs.

SECTION 8 MEDICAL ASPECTS OF SPORTS MEDICINE

- The orthopaedic history questionnaire is the most helpful measure for identifying musculoskeletal problems.
- Hypertrophic cardiomyopathy is the most common cause of sudden death in young athletes. Sports participation is contraindicated in such cases of outflow obstruction.
- Adverse effects of anabolic steroids include liver dysfunction, hypercholesterolemia, cardiomyopathy, testicular atrophy, gynecomastia, acne, mood disturbances (particularly increased aggression), and irreversible alopecia. Heart disease results from increased plasma levels of low-density lipoprotein and decreased levels of high-density lipoprotein.
- The "female athlete triad" consists of secondary amenorrhea, stress fractures, and eating disorders. Insufficient caloric intake is the most common cause of secondary amenorrhea.
- Decreased breath sounds, deviated trachea, and hypotension may signify a tension pneumothorax. Emergency treatment is with needle thoracostomy.
- Heat stroke is characterized by collapse, with neurologic deficits, tachycardia, tachypnea, hypotension, and anhidrosis.
- MRSA transmission occurs by direct person-to-person contact through disruptions in skin integrity.
- Athletes with infectious mononucleosis should be restricted from contact sports participation for 3 to 5 weeks, and splenomegaly must have resolved before they return to play.

SELECTED BIBLIOGRAPHY

The selected bibliography for this chapter can be found on www.expertconsult.com.

Chapter 5

ADULT RECONSTRUCTION

Edward J. McPherson

CONTENTS

CONTENTS—cont'd

SECTION 1 Hip Dysplasia—Adult Presentation

I. NATURAL HISTORY

A. Hip pain in adults under the age of 50 years usually is a result of hip dysplasia.
B. Untreated dysplasia leads to degenerative joint disease in greater than 50% of patients by age 50 years.
C. Initial presentation of symptoms is soon followed by degeneration.
1. Do not wait to treat surgically if osteotomy is being considered.

II. SPECTRUM OF PRESENTATION

A. Subtle
1. Femoral acetabular impingement

B. Advanced morphologic changes with significant arthritis

III. CLASSIFICATION OF ADULT HIP DYSPLASIA

A. Acetabular dysplasia
1. **Too little coverage—classical**
2. Too much coverage
3. Malaligned coverage

B. Proximal femoral dysplasia
1. Altered head-neck offset
2. Altered neck version

IV. ACETABULAR DYSPLASIA (BOX 5-1 AND FIGURE 5-1)

A. Classical (too little coverage)
1. Deficient head coverage
   - Lack of anterior and lateral coverage
2. Decreased acetabular depth
   - Socket is less than a hemisphere.

B. Acetabular retroversion
1. **Acetabular socket faces backward. (Normal socket faces forward, i.e., anteversion.)**
   - Anterior wall is rotated forward.
   - Posterior wall is rotated backward.
2. Radiographic findings (Figure 5-2)
   - Crossover sign is pathognomonic (on anteroposterior pelvis).
     - Frequently will see ischial spine on anteroposterior radiograph

Box 5-1

Acetabular Dysplasia Classical Definitions

Lateral CE angle <20 degrees
- CE angle = head center to acetabular edge angle
- Measured on anteroposterior pelvis radiograph

Anterior CE angle <20 degrees
- Measured on standing lateral (false profile) view

Acetabular index >5 degrees
- Measured on anteroposterior pelvis radiograph

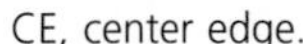
CE, center edge.

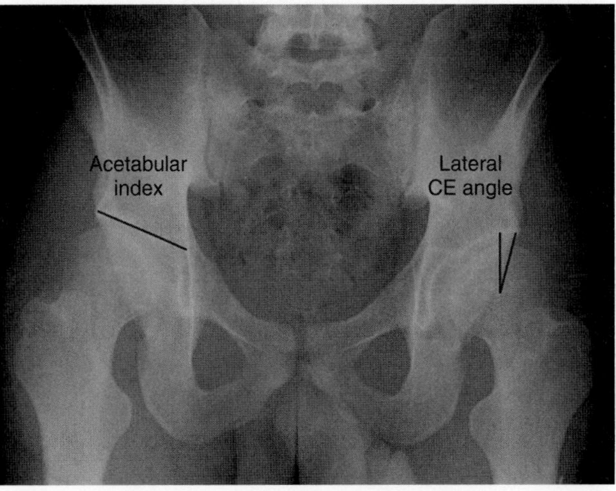

Figure 5-1 Anteroposterior pelvis radiograph displaying lateral center edge (CE) angle and acetabular index. Both hips in this case show a shallow socket dysplasia. The acetabular index should normally be horizontal, and the lateral CE angle should be 30 degrees.

C. Acetabular overcoverage
1. Excess anterior and lateral wall coverage of the femoral head
2. Defined radiographically with downsloping acetabular index (>5 degrees *downward*)
3. Frequently associated with retroversion dysplasia

V. PROXIMAL FEMORAL DYSPLASIA

A. Head-neck dysplasia (Figure 5-3)
1. Offset between edge of femoral head and edge of femoral neck is reduced (i.e., head/neck ratios reduced).
2. Radiographically this gives the appearance of a *pistol grip* deformity.
3. Head-neck offset is defined on the anteroposterior and lateral radiograph by the α-angle (Figure 5-4).
   - α-Angle is normally 40 degrees or less.

B. Altered neck version
1. Excess neck anteversion
2. Neck retroversion

VI. CLINICAL SYNDROME ASSOCIATED WITH DYSPLASIA

A. Femoral acetabular impingement
1. Abnormal impingement between femoral neck and anterior acetabular rim
   - Contact is *anterosuperior zone* of acetabulum.

B. Clinical progression
1. Impingement pain and hip inflammation
2. Labral degeneration leading to tears
3. Chondral surface degeneration and chondral flap tears
4. Degenerative joint disease is end result.

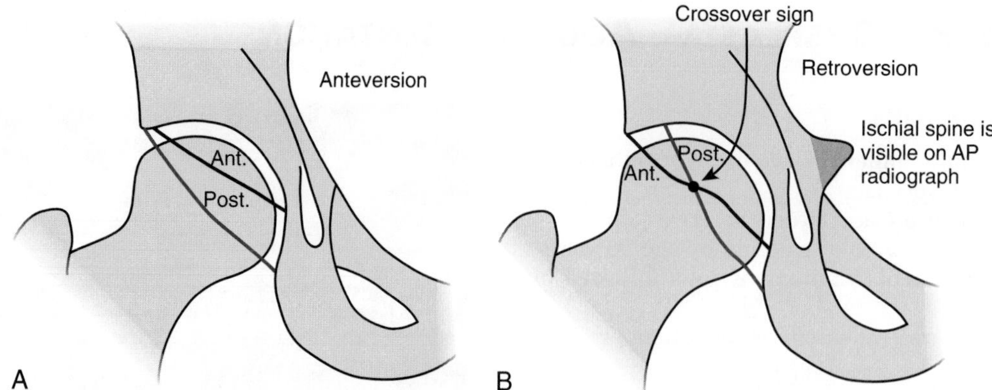

Figure 5-2 **A,** Diagram of acetabulum on anteroposterior radiograph. In a normal acetabulum, the socket is anteverted. On the anteroposterior radiograph, the anterior acetabular rim is above posterior rim. Three dimensionally, the acetabular socket is *open* and faces in an anterior direction. **B,** Diagram of acetabular retroversion. On the anteroposterior radiograph, the anterior rim is in a lower position, whereas the posterior rim is higher. Radiographically, the two rim lines cross, creating the *crossover* sign. Frequently with acetabular retroversion, the ischial spine is prominently seen. Three dimensionally, the acetabular socket is *closed* and faces in a posterior direction. Ant., anterior; AP, anteroposterior; Post., posterior.

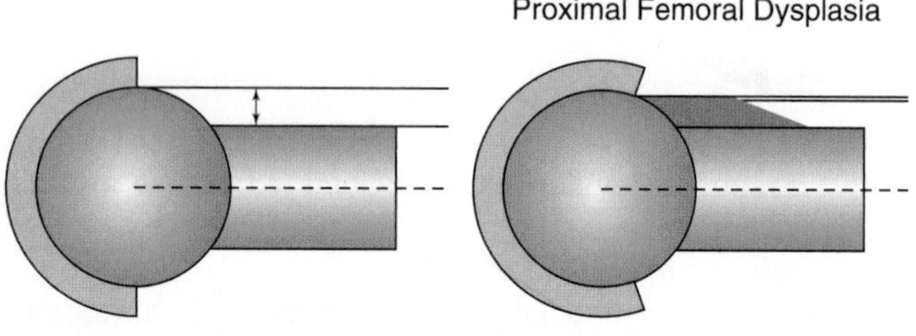

Figure 5-3 **A,** Diagram demonstrating normal head-neck offset. Offset is measured using lines parallel to the line defining the femoral head center and neck midline. **B,** In femoral neck dysplasia, the offset between the femoral head and neck is significantly reduced. A reduced head-neck offset increases the risk for neck impingement upon the acetabular rim.

C. Clinical presentation

1. Impingement test—positive
2. Significant restriction of hip internal rotation (tested with the hip at 90 degrees of flexion)

D. Causes of femoral acetabular impingement

1. Acetabular based
   - Retroversion and/or overcoverage
2. Femoral based
   - Reduced head-neck offset
3. Combination

E. Femoral acetabular impingement—two types

1. Pincer impingement (Figure 5-5)
   - **Anatomic aberration between socket and femoral neck that creates a mechanical block preventing further hip flexion**
   - The soft tissues between the bony mechanical block are *pinched.*

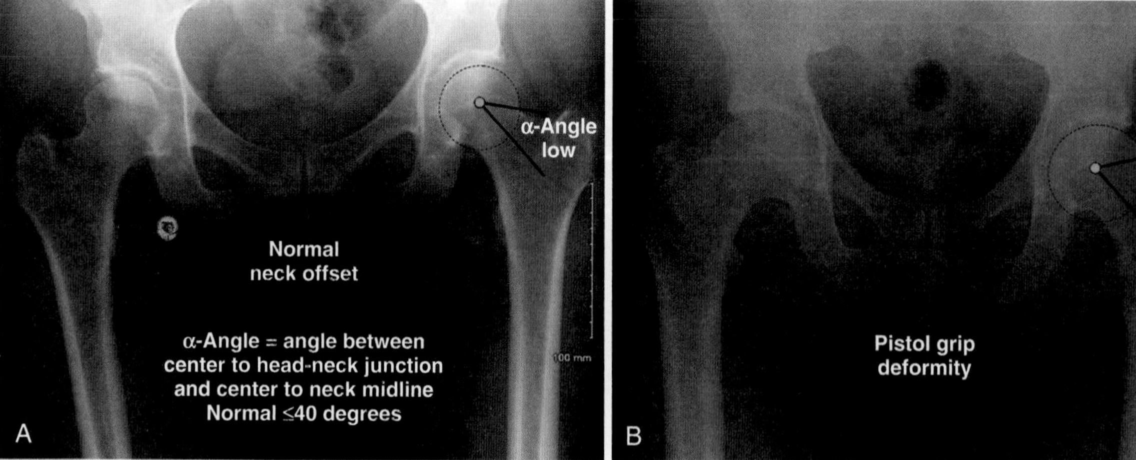

Figure 5-4 **A,** Anteroposterior radiograph measuring α-angle. The α-angle is a method to evaluate head-neck dysplasia. The α-angle is formed between the lines of femoral head center and neck midline, and femoral head center and head-neck junction. Normal α-angle typically is less than or equal to 40 degrees. **B,** Anteroposterior radiograph measuring α-angle in a dysplastic proximal femur. α-Angle is increased.

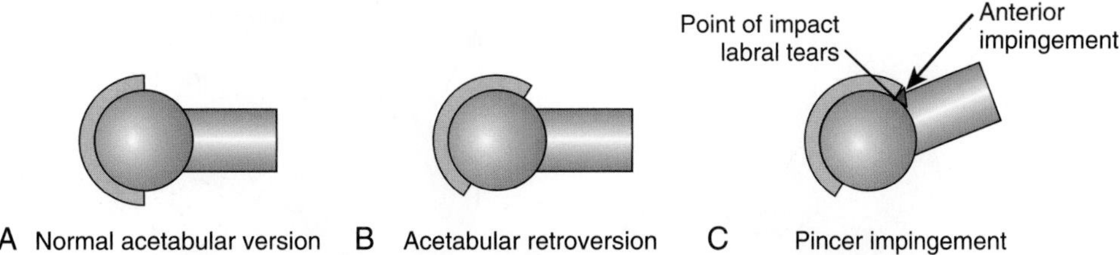

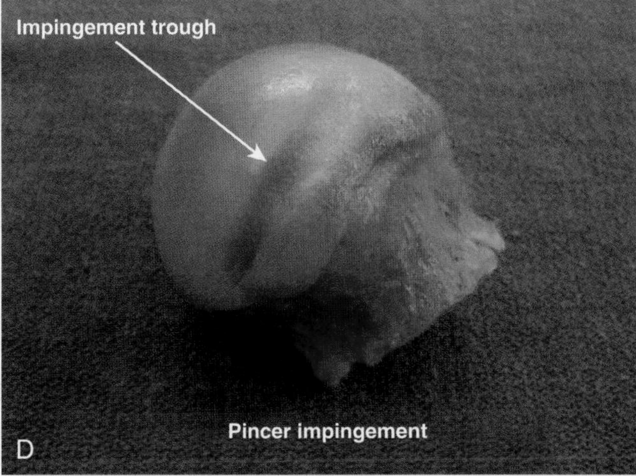

Figure 5-5 Pincer type of femoral acetabular impingement. **A,** Diagram showing normal acetabulum and proximal femur. **B,** Diagram depicting acetabular retroversion. Retroverted acetabulum will limit functional hip flexion. **C,** Mechanics of pincer impingement. In hip flexion, the femoral neck abuts acetabular rim. Typically, this results in localized damage to the labrum. **D,** Ex vivo demonstration of pincer impingement. In this case, repetitive pincer impingement created a bony indentation trough on the femoral head at the site of flexion impingement.

- Typically the soft tissues damaged in pincer impingement are the acetabular labral complex.

2. Cam impingement (Figure 5-6)
   - **Anatomic aberration in the proximal femoral neck creates a raised area (cam). The neck cam impinges upon the articular surface of the acetabulum in hip flexion.**
   - Compared to pincer impingement, the femoral neck is allowed to travel underneath the labrum a short distance, thus impinging more upon the articular surface.
   - Typically, the area of soft tissue damage in cam impingement is the chondral surface of the acetabulum.

VII. DYSPLASIA TREATMENT

A. Treatment depends upon the extent of deformity and location.

B. Surgical correction goals are to relieve pain and to correct anatomic deformity. Long-term goal is to reduce the occurrence of degenerative joint disease.

C. Surgical correction addresses the main anatomic deformity: shallow socket, retroverted socket, reduced femoral neck offset (i.e., fat neck), abnormal femoral neck version.

D. Main surgical options

1. Periacetabular osteotomy
2. Anterior hip decompression
3. Proximal hip osteotomy

E. Periacetabular osteotomy (Figure 5-7)

1. Allows large degree of socket correction
   - Correction of tilt and version
2. Permits joint *medialization* (i.e., center of hip rotation is positioned medial)
   - Lowers joint reactive forces
3. Technique advantages
   - Does not violate abductor complex
   - Does not violate posterior column
   - Allows early weight bearing
   - Low complication and morbidity rate
4. Technique goals
   - Acetabular roof index to zero
   - Head coverage: lateral center edge (CE) angle into normal range
   - Restored socket anteversion: no crossover sign

F. Anterior hip decompression (Figure 5-8)

1. Technique is *not* used for shallow-socket dysplasia.
2. Technique incorporates three main steps.
   - Femoral neck osteoplasty (removal of cam bump)
   - Anterior acetabular rim osteoplasty (reduction)
   - Repair of soft tissue tears
     - Acetabular labrum
     - Acetabular chondral flap tears
3. Surgical approach
   - Trochanteric slide (vastas lateralis and gluteus medius both kept attached to greater trochanter)
   - Anterior dislocation of femoral head
   - Anterior *Z-capsulotomy* preserves posterior vessels to femoral neck. This minimizes risk for head osteonecrosis.

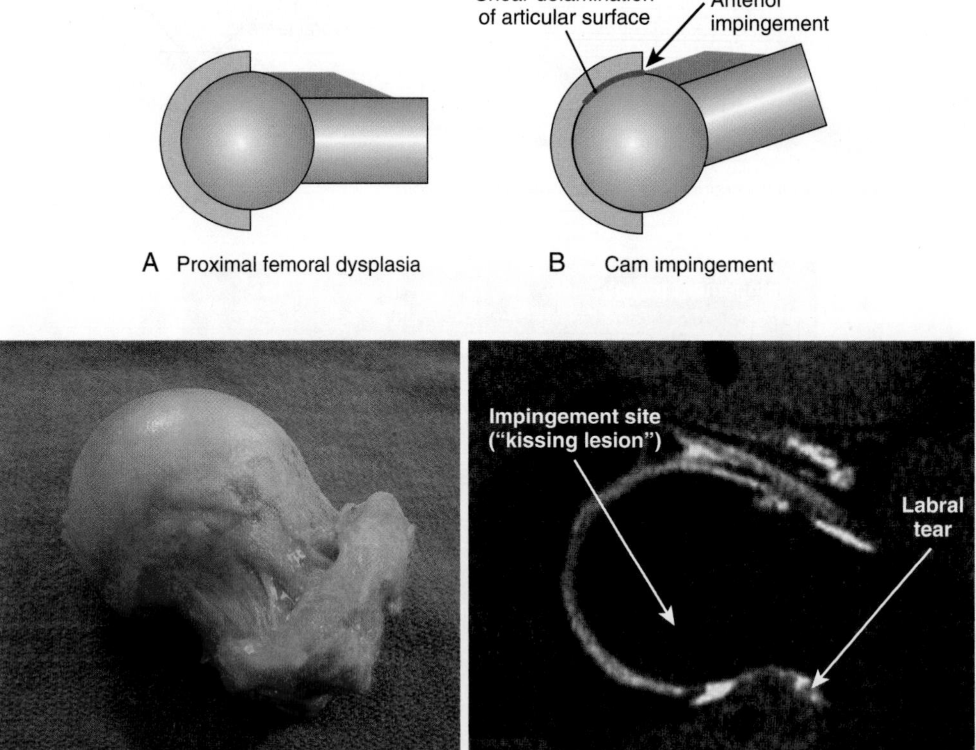

Figure 5-6 Cam type of femoral acetabular impingement. **A,** Diagram depicting proximal femoral neck dysplasia with reduced head-neck offset. The "fat" femoral neck still is able to travel into acetabular socket a short distance. **B,** Mechanics of cam impingement. In hip flexion, the *fat* femoral neck acts as a cam (a raised area) that abrades the anterior-superior region of the acetabulum. Typically this results in shear delamination of the chondral surfaces of the acetabulum. **C,** Ex vivo demonstration of cam impingement. Notice how superior femoral neck is almost up to the level of the superior-lateral femoral head. This region (the cam) is what impinges upon the articular surfaces of the acetabulum in flexion. **D,** Magnetic resonance image of femoral acetabular impingement. In this case, there is a combination of cam and pincer impingement. There is an enlarged femoral neck (reduced head-neck offset), but clinically there is also pincer impingement upon the anterior acetabulum.

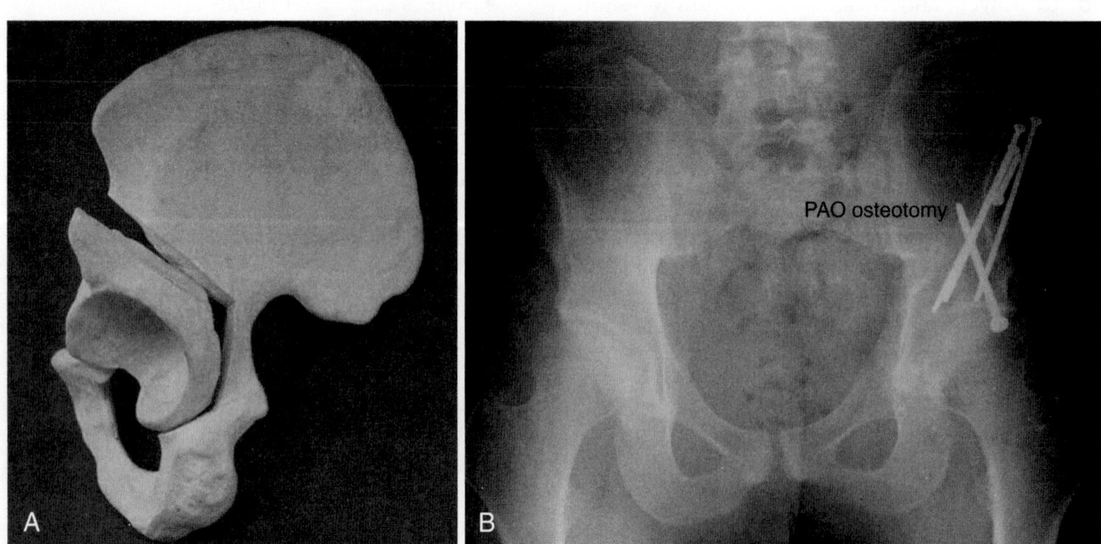

Figure 5-7 **A,** Model demonstrating periacetabular osteotomy (PAO). In the PAO technique, the posterior column is preserved. This maintains pelvic stability and allows for significant correction of acetabular tilt and version. **B,** Five-year postoperative radiograph of PAO. Notice acetabular index restored to horizontal and improved lateral center edge angle.

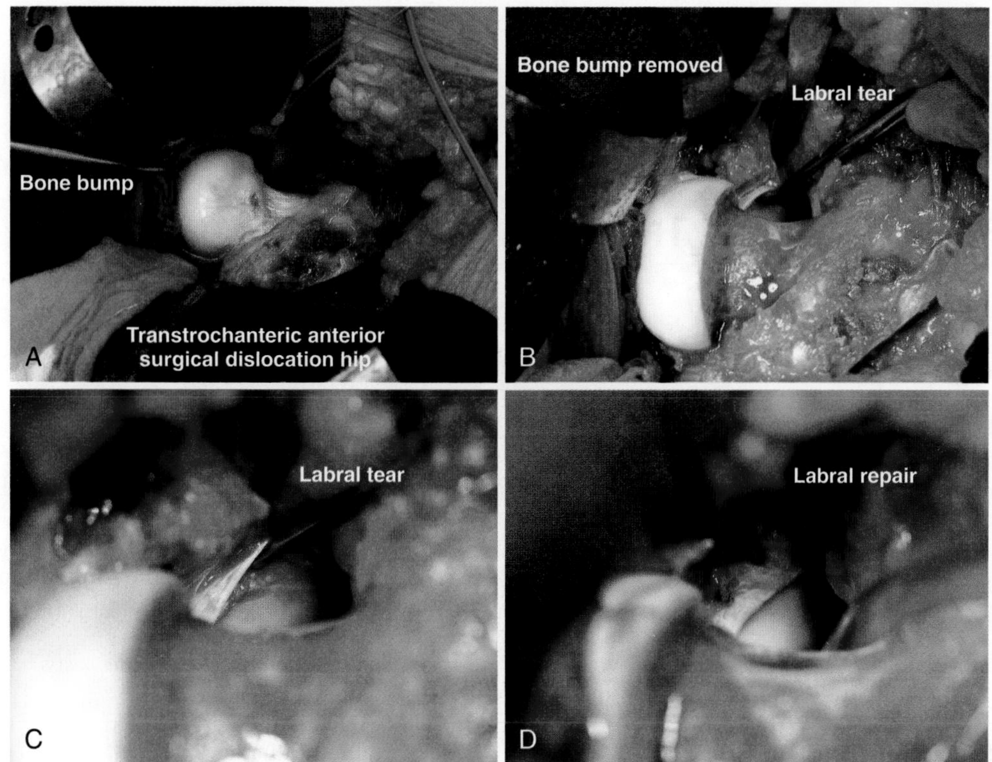

Figure 5-8 Intraoperative photographs demonstrating anterior hip decompression procedure. **A,** Lateral approach of right hip, using a greater trochanteric slide. The greater trochanter is retracted anteriorly. A Z-capsulotomy is performed, and the hip is dislocated anteriorly. **B,** Femoral osteoplasty. The excess bone in the anterior-superior femoral neck is removed. This improves head-neck offset. **C,** Labral tear identified in the anterior impingement zone of the acetabulum. **D,** Labral repair with suture anchor technique.

4. Hip arthroscopy for anterior hip decompression
   - Arthroscopy can be used for *mild* hip deformities with associated labral tears.
   - Arthroscopy can correct femoral deformity (i.e., femoral cam) better than acetabular retroversion.

G. **Proximal hip osteotomy**

1. Main indications for proximal hip osteotomy
   - Correction of proximal femoral retroversion or excessive anteversion
   - Significant coxa valga with decreased lateral offset

SECTION 2 HIP ARTHRITIS ASSESSMENT

Patient assessment of hip pain includes a physical examination and diagnostic radiographic modalities.

I. PHYSICAL EXAMINATION TESTS FOR HIP IRRITABILITY

A. **Impingement test**

1. Hip flexion to 90 degrees
2. Hip adduction and internal rotation yield pain response.
3. Hip internal rotation only yields pain response.
4. Pain located in area of anterior hip with pain radiating to either posterior hip or lateral hip

B. **Roll test**

1. Patient is positioned supine. Finger rolling of leg (at calf level) into internal rotation and external rotation
2. Leg will feel stiff or will occasionally grab.

C. **Stinchfield test**

1. Patient is positioned supine. Active straight leg raise of approximately 20 cm against mild resistance by examiner
2. Patient will feel pain in anterior hip against resistance.

D. **Patrick test**

1. Patient is positioned supine. Leg is positioned in figure-four position.
2. Pain will be elicited in area of anterior hip region or posterior hip region.
3. Be careful with interpretation of test. If pain is located over posterior pelvis, this indicates referred pain from L5-S1 facets or sacroiliac joint and not hip joint.

II. STUDIES

A. **Radiographs**

1. Still the standard imaging modality for initial evaluation of hip pain

B. Computed tomographic (CT) scan

1. Three-dimensional CT with pelvic remodeling used for preoperative planning for reconstruction associated with dysplasia planning, post-trauma planning, and complex revision total hip arthroplasty (THA) planning

C. Magnetic resonance imaging (MRI)

1. Used when osteonecrosis suspected
2. Gadolinium MRI arthrogram useful when labral pathology suspected, especially when associated with femoral acetabular impingement

SECTION 3 HIP ARTHRITIS TREATMENT

I. NONOPERATIVE

A. Activity modification

1. Reduce impact-loading exercises
2. Reduce weight
3. Avoid stairs, inclines, squatting.

B. Nonsteroidal anti-inflammatory drugs

1. Cyclooxygenase-2 inhibition

C. Joint injections

1. Corticosteroid—anti-inflammatory treatment
2. Hyaluronate
   - Backbone of proteoglycan chain of articular cartilage
   - Improves joint rheology
3. Approved by Food and Drug Administration for knee use only in United States

D. Assist device (cane or crutch)

1. Opposite hand of affected hip

II. OPERATIVE

A. Arthroscopy

1. Best indication
   - Traumatic labral tear *not* associated with dysplasia
   - Hip joint shows mechanical signs of locking, catching, and clicking.
2. Beware of labral resection in dysplasia.
   - Acetabular labrum provides stability in a shallow acetabular socket (labrum usually is hypertrophic).
   - Isolated removal of labrum will typically result in rapid progression of joint degeneration and pain.
   - In cases of significant dysplasia, arthroscopic débridement is *not* recommended.
3. Other indications
   - Loose body removal
   - Débridement of chondral flap tears
   - Synovitis
     - Diagnostic biopsy and therapeutic lavage
   - Diagnostic procedure
     - Undiagnosed mechanical hip pain
   - Degenerative arthritis
     - Therapeutic effect inversely related to severity of arthritis
     - Not helpful in moderate to advanced disease
     - Generally, will help only mechanical symptoms, not arthritic ache
4. Arthroscopy technique
   - Traction required
   - Fluoroscopy required
   - Long cannulated trochars that are designed for hip joint
5. Arthroscopy complications
   - Nerve injury—most frequent
     - Pudendal—due to traction post
     - Lateral femoral cutaneous—due to portal placement
     - Femoral—due to portal placement
   - Instrument breakage
   - Portal hematoma

B. Osteotomy (adult)

1. Salvage osteotomy
   - Abandoned in favor of THA for degenerative hip arthritis
2. Reconstructive osteotomy
   - Periacetabular osteotomy is preferred procedure to correct early hip degeneration in the adult due to dysplasia.
   - See the section Hip Dysplasia.

C. THA

1. See the section Total Hip Arthroplasty.

D. Hip fusion

1. Less frequently used as THA technology advances
2. Classical indication
   - Very young male laborer
   - *Unilateral* hip arthritis
3. Energy expenditure
   - Approximately 30% increase in energy output during ambulation
4. Collateral arthritis
   - Abnormal gait causes arthritis in these adjacent joints in 60% of patients.
     - Lumbar spine
     - Contralateral hip
     - Ipsilateral knee
   - Symptoms of pain typically start within 25 years of hip fusion.
5. Hip fusion technique
   - Preserve abductor complex.
     - Many fusions are taken down for disabling pain in adjacent joints.
     - Select fusion technique that allows successful conversion to THA.
     - Greater trochanteric osteotomy with lateral plate fixation is preferred technique.
     - Be careful not to injure superior gluteal nerve, which innervates abductor complex.
6. Fusion position
   - 20 to 25 degrees of flexion
   - *Neutral abduction*
     - Increased back and knee pain when fusion is in abduction
   - Neutral or slight external rotation of 10 degrees
7. **Fusion conversion to THA**
   - **Indications**
     - **Disabling back pain—most common**
     - Disabling ipsilateral knee pain with instability
       - Excess knee stress will cause knee ligament stretch-out if fusion position is incorrect.
     - Disabling contralateral hip pain

8. Function after conversion to THA
   - Hip function and clinical results directly related to integrity of abductor complex
     - Preoperative electromyogram of gluteus medius required
   - When hip abductor complex nonfunctional
     - Severe lurching gait will result.
     - THA will require *constrained* acetabular component.

E. Resection arthroplasty

1. Usually last step before hip disarticulation in a frustrating downward clinical course
2. Indications
   - Incurable infection
     - Patients are most often immune compromised.
     - Recurrent periprosthetic THA infection
     - Failed hip fusion with infection
     - Chronic destructive septic arthritis
   - Noncompliant patient with recurrent THA dislocation
     - Usually multiply revised patient
     - Psychiatric condition
     - Profound dementia
     - Limb paresis or paralysis
     - Drug-seeking behavior
   - Nonambulator
     - Intractable pain from arthritis
     - Hip fracture with open decubitus ulcers
     - Significant contracture interfering with hygiene and posture
   - Failed hip fusion in patient with prior major trauma to hip and/or pelvis
     - Soft tissue loss to hip region precludes successful placement of THA.
     - Neurologic injury to extremity precludes successful function of THA.

F. Hemiarthroplasty

1. Relegated to specific limited role
   - Fracture treatment in low-demand elderly patient
     - Best indication—displaced subcapital hip fracture with little or no prior history of symptomatic hip arthritis
   - Patient not able to comply with standard THA precautions
   - Best indication for THA for hip fracture
     - High activity level
     - Subcapital or high neck fracture
     - Older population (age ≥70 years)
     - Low risk for dislocation (no dementia or Parkinson disease)
2. Hemiarthroplasty advantage
   - Stability
     - Maximize head/neck ratio.
     - Large-diameter ball requires more distance to travel before dislocation.
     - Suction fit provided by labrum
       - Enhanced stability negated if labrum and capsule resected
3. Hemiarthroplasty disadvantage
   - Groin pain in active individuals
   - Increased osteolysis (compared to THA) in active individual
   - Protrusio deformity if ball not sized well and osteoporosis present (Figure 5-9)

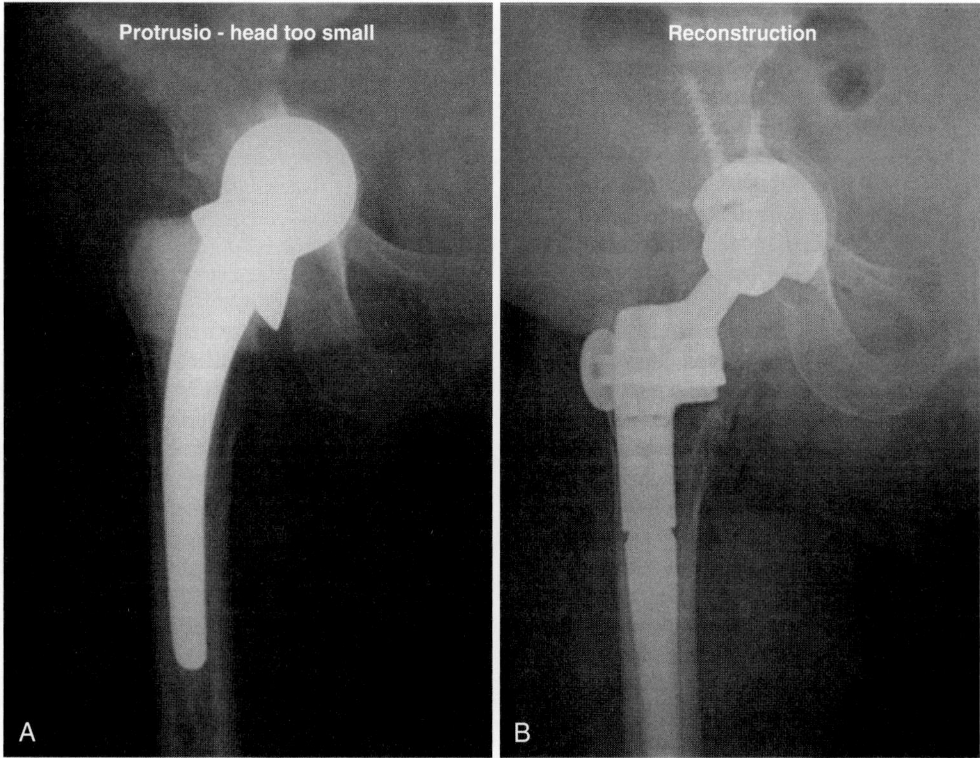

Figure 5-9 Protrusio deformity. **A,** Anteroposterior radiograph demonstrating protrusio deformity of cemented hip hemiarthroplasty. This patient suffers from osteoporosis. **B,** Conversion to total hip arthroplasty. Hip successfully reconstructed with protrusio revision cup with screws. Bone graft is placed into protrusio deformity.

SECTION 4 OSTEONECROSIS OF THE HIP

I. OCCURRENCE

A. Incidence not precisely known
B. No comprehensive information on number of asymptomatic cases
C. More common in males
D. Typically affects patients in late 30s or early 40s

II. ETIOLOGY (SEE CHAPTER 1, BASIC SCIENCE)

A. Hypercoagulable states may explain many *idiopathic* cases of osteonecrosis of the hip.
B. In all cases, end-stage result is vascular occlusion in the juxtaarticular sinusoids adjacent to joint.

III. CLINICAL PRESENTATION

A. Initial pain with sit to stand, stairs, inclines, and impact loading
B. Pain location tends to be most noticeable in anterior hip.
C. Can be acute in onset (acute infarct phenomenon), which can mimic an acute injury

IV. IMAGING

A. Start first with radiographs.
1. Pelvis, anteroposterior, and lateral radiographs
2. If osteonecrosis detected, must image contralateral hip
   - Fifty percent of osteonecrosis cases have bilateral involvement.

B. MRI is the standard imaging modality when radiographs are negative and osteonecrosis is suspected.

V. STAGING (TABLE 5-1)

A. Modified Ficat system (incorporates MRI information)

VI. TREATMENT

A. Nonsurgical
1. **Bisphosphonate treatment will decrease risk for head collapse.**

Table 5-1 Modified Ficat Staging System for Osteonecrosis of the Hip

Stage	MRI	Bone Scan	Radiographs	Patient Status
0	Positive	Positive	Negative	Asymptomatic
1	Positive	Positive	Negative	Symptomatic
2	Positive	Positive	Positive—no crescent	Symptomatic
3	Positive	Positive	Positive—crescent	Symptomatic
4	Positive	Positive	Positive—head flattening, DJD	Symptomatic

DJD, degenerative joint disease; MRI, magnetic resonance imaging.

2. **Must start *before* crescent sign**

B. Surgical treatment
1. Surgical treatment depends on these major variables.
   - Head collapse (i.e., crescent)
     - Yes or no
   - Age
     - 40 or younger
   - Irreversible etiology
     - Yes or no
     - Examples of irreversible etiology
       - Continued steroid use
       - Idiopathic
       - Hypercoagulable state
   - Extent of head involvement (by osteonecrosis)
     - Described as *volume* head involvement
     - Volume head involvement equals percent head involved on anteroposterior image multiplied by percent head involved on lateral image (e.g., 50% × 50% = 25% volume head involvement).
     - A—small lesion: less than 15% head involvement
     - B—medium lesion: 15% to 30% head involvement
     - C—large lesion: greater than 30% head involvement
2. **Younger age and crescent (or worse)**
   - **THA is recommended treatment.**
     - Cementless cup and stem
     - Improved bearing technology
     - Good pain relief and function
3. Younger age and no crescent
   - Common treatments
     - Core decompression
       - Treatment principles
         - Core decompression relieves pressure buildup within the femoral head by the inflammatory process.
         - Pressure relief translates to pain relief.
         - Stimulates a healing response
           - Bone and vascular neogenesis
       - Indications
         - No crescent
         - *Reversible etiology*
           - Patients on chronic steroids have poor results with core decompression.
         - Small head lesion (A lesion)
           - Patients with medium and large head lesions frequently collapse.
     - Vascularized fibular strut (Figure 5-10)
       - Treatment principles
         - Surgical removal of necrotic segment
         - Large core hole is needed.
         - Vascularized fibular strut is placed up against subchondral plate of femoral head to prevent collapse.
         - Particulate bone grafting of adjacent resected bone
       - Indications
         - Medium (B) and large (C) lesions
         - No crescent (preferred)
           - Reasonable success with crescent and minimal head collapse
         - Reversible etiology

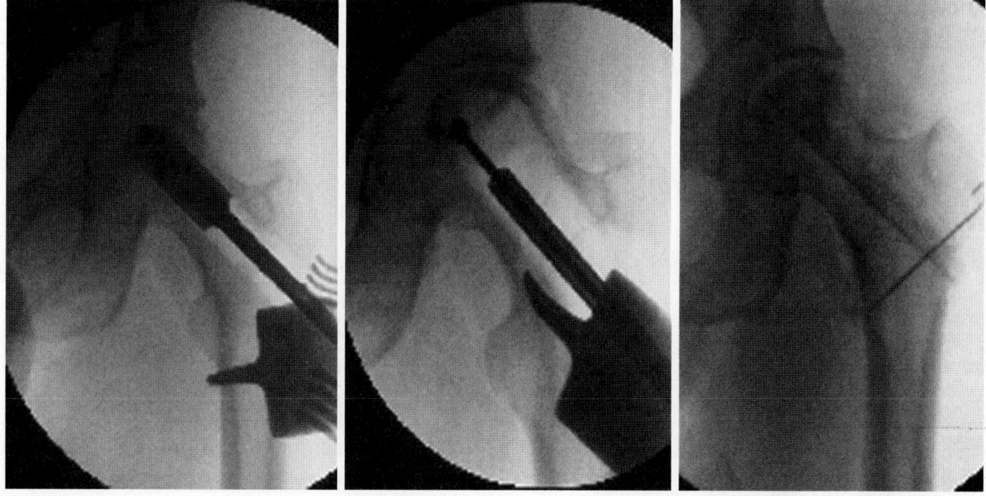

Figure 5-10 Fluoroscopic images of vascularized fibular strut technique. *Left,* Fluoroscopic image showing core reamer introduced to subchondral plate of femoral head. *Center,* Burr is introduced to remove remaining necrotic segment. *Right,* Vascularized fibular strut is placed up against subchondral plate of femoral head. Base of strut is secured with a K wire. Particulate bone graft has been impacted around fibular strut.

- Less-common treatments
  - Curettage of necrotic bone and bone grafting through femoral neck trap door
  - Rotational proximal femoral osteotomy
    - Must be able to rotate osteonecrotic segment out of weight-bearing zone and maintain good hip function

4. Age 40 years or older and medium (B) or large (C) lesion
   - Best option is total hip replacement.
   - Medium to large lesions prone to collapse
5. Older than 40 years and small (A) lesion
   - Best option is core decompression.
     - Patient must have reversible etiology.
     - Core decompression again is contraindicated if on chronic steroid treatment.
     - Result of vascularized fibular graft less predictable in older population

SECTION 5 TOTAL HIP ARTHROPLASTY

I. INDICATIONS

A. Debilitating pain affecting activities of daily living
B. Pain not well controlled by conservative measures
C. Medically fit for surgery
D. No active infection—anywhere

II. IMPLANT FIXATION

A. Methods of fixation

1. Cement
   - Polymethylmethacrylate (PMMA)
2. Cementless
   - Biologic fixation—bone growth into the prosthesis secures implant
   - Two methods
     - Bone *ingrowth*—porous coating
     - Bone *ongrowth*—grit coating

B. Cement fixation

1. Microinterlock with endosteal bone
2. Cement will fatigue with cyclic loading.
   - Fatigue starts at stress points within the cement mantle.
   - A *mantle defect* is an area where the prosthesis touches bone. This is an area of significant stress concentration (Figure 5-11).
3. Cemented cups fail at a higher rate than cemented stems.
   - Acetabular cup is positioned at an angle (i.e., theta (θ)-angle) relative to longitudinal axis of leg. This creates shear and tension forces at cement-bone interface.
   - Cement is strongest in *compression* and weaker in tension.
   - Cemented stems fail at a lower rate than cups because stems see primarily a compression force.

C. Cemented stem failure

1. Young, active patients have increased risk for failure.
2. Men are twice as likely to fail as women.
3. Young, active male is best candidate for cementless femoral stem.

D. Cement technique—success

1. *Porosity reduction* during mixing
   - Decreased porosity reduces stress points in cement.
   - Vacuum mixing is most common method to reduce cement porosity.
2. *Pressurization* of cement before component insertion
   - Enhances cement interdigitation with bone
3. *Pulsatile lavage* of bone before cementing
   - Clean, dry bone allows better cement interdigitation.
4. *Stem centralization* with distal stem centralizer
   - Maintains uniform cement mantle (i.e., no mantle defects)
5. *Stiff stem* lessens bending stress upon cement mantle.

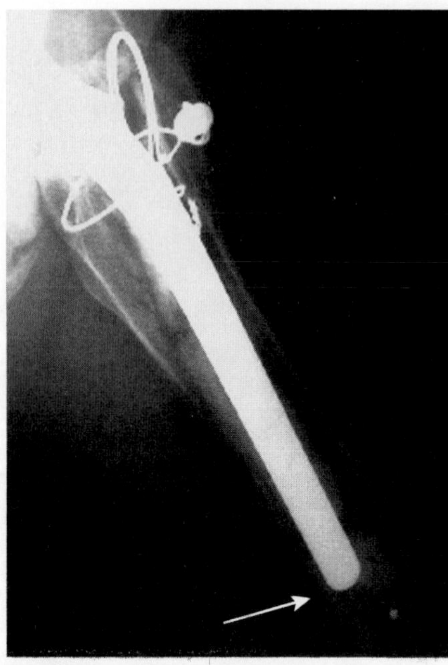

Figure 5-11 Lateral radiograph of cemented femoral stem with mantle defect. Note distal stem tip that touches bone.

E. Biologic fixation

1. Bone ingrowth (Figure 5-12)
   - Prosthesis is fabricated with metal pores into metallic alloy. Bone grows into the porous structure, stabilizing the prosthesis to bone.
   - **Successful bone ingrowth is based upon following factors.**
     - **Optimal pore size**
       - **Between 50 and 150 μm**
     - Pore depth (i.e., deeper distance into metal) is directly related to increased fixation strength.
     - Optimal metal porosity
       - **Porosity of 40% to 50% is best.**
     - Minimize gap distance between prosthesis and bone.
       - Gaps between metal and bone must be less than 50 μm.
       - Bone will not grow across anything wider than this.
     - Minimal implant micromotion
       - Implant must have an ***initial rigid fixation*** for bone to grow into prosthesis.
         - Bone fixation less than 30 μm
         - Fibrous fixation greater than 150 μm
         - Fibrous encapsulation—gross macromotion
     - Cortical contact with bone
       - Cancellous bone is not weight bearing.
       - Implants must be placed upon cortical bone to allow physiologic load transfer to weight-bearing regions of bone.
       - Shear and torsional strength stronger when implant is adjacent to cortical bone as opposed to cancellous bone
     - Viable bone
       - Prior irradiation to pelvis and hip increases risk for aseptic loosening of bone ingrowth/ongrowth implants.

F. Initial rigid fixation for cementless hip implants

1. Initial rigid implant fixation to host bone is required for long-term osteointegration. There are two techniques used. They are the *press fit* technique and the *line-to-line* technique.
2. Press fit technique (Figure 5-13)
   - Bone is prepared such that a slightly oversized implant (relative to bone contour) is wedged into position.
     - Femoral stem typically has a gradual taper design to allow press fit into bone. Stem is typically 0.5 to 1 μm larger in size.
     - Acetabular cup is a hemispheric design. Cup is typically 1 μm larger in size. Press fit is against the acetabular rim. Screws are *not* required.
3. **Complication of press fit technique**
   - **Fracture is the most common complication.**

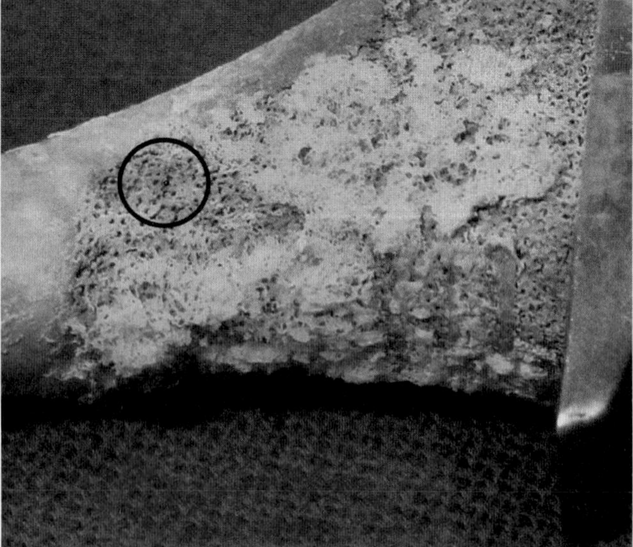

Figure 5-12 Ex vivo retrieval of bone ingrowth femoral stem. Notice metallic pores *(circle)* that allow bone to grow into prosthesis and osteointegrate.

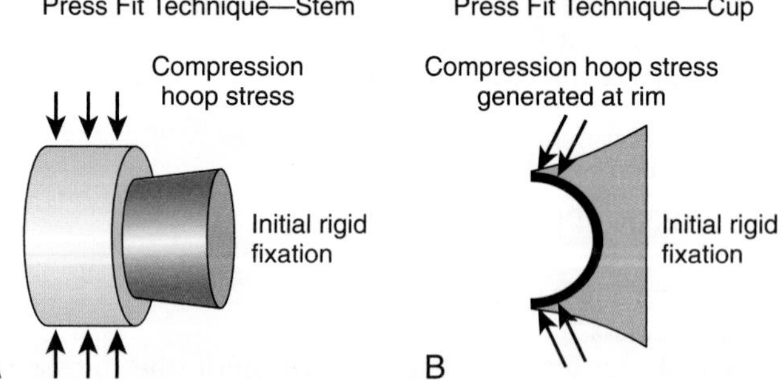

Figure 5-13 Diagram of press fit technique for cementless hip fixation. **A,** The canal of the femur is prepared with serial reaming and/or broaching to achieve desired implant size (remember that cortical contact is preferred). An implant of slightly larger size is impacted into position. The stem usually has a gradual wedge taper. The wedging effect generates compression hoop stresses that hold the implant still to allow bone to grow into implant interface. **B,** The acetabulum is prepared with serial hemispheric reamers to achieve desired implant size (ream to cortical margin of acetabular rim). An implant of slightly larger size is impacted into position. The wedge effect occurs at the rim of the acetabulum. The compression hoop stress generated at the rim holds the implant still to allow bone to grow into the implant interface.

- **The main reason for fracture is *underreaming*.**
- **Acetabular fracture**
  - **If cup is stable, add screws.**
  - **If cup is unstable, remove cup and stabilize fracture. Reinsert cup with screws.**
- Femur fracture
  - Femur fractures are *proximal* due to wedge splitting of bone.
  - **If crack is small and stem is stable, limit weight bearing and do not change stem.**
  - If stem is unstable, remove stem and stabilize fracture. Reinsert stem, or insert revision stem.

4. Line-to-line technique
   - Bone is prepared such that contour of bone is same size as implant.
     - Femoral stem has an *extensive porous coating*. The extensive coating provides an initial *frictional fit*. The rough surface provides enough resistance to motion that the implant is stable once impacted into final position. The frictional fit is also known as *scratch fit* or *interference fit*.
     - Acetabular cup is placed into position. Cup is a hemispheric design. Cup is secured with multiple screws placed into bone.
5. Complication of line-to-line technique
   - Fracture is complication seen with femoral stem insertion. The fracture typically occurs at the distal stem tip.
     - The force required to insert a straight stem into a bowed femur with a frictional fit can exceed the strength of the bone. The area of stress concentration is at the stem tip due to the modulus mismatch (bone/implant proximal versus hollow bone distal).

III. BONE ONGROWTH FIXATION

A. Description

1. Prosthetic surface is prepared by blasting surface with an abrasive grit material. Nickname is *grit blast fixation.*
2. Implant material for grit blast fixation is always titanium alloy.
3. Grit blasting process creates microdivots—no pores, just divots. Divot diameter approximately the same size as pore hole for a porous-coated implant
4. Bone grows *onto* rough surface, stabilizing prosthesis.

B. Surface roughness (R_a) (Figure 5-14)

1. R_a is defined as average peak to valley on the surface of the implant.
2. Implant roughness determines strength of biologic fixation.
   - Linear relation of R_a to fixation strength

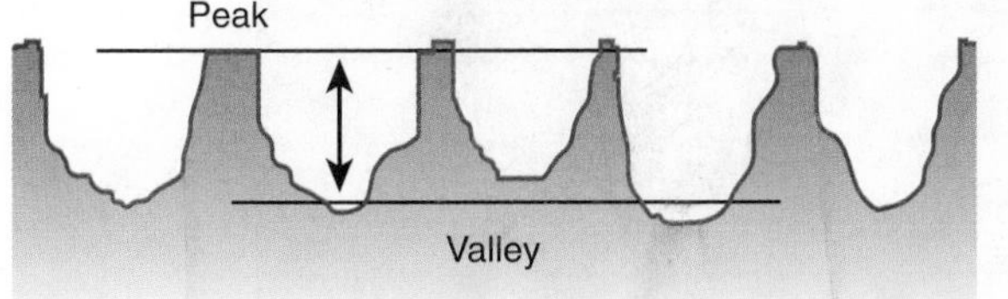

Figure 5-14 Surface roughness (R_a) of bone ongrowth prosthesis. R_a is defined as the average peak to valley on the surface of the implant. The value is typically in micrometers (μm).

Bone Ongrowth

Technique
- Always press fit technique
- Design typically a high-angle wedge taper design
- Long-term fixation biologic

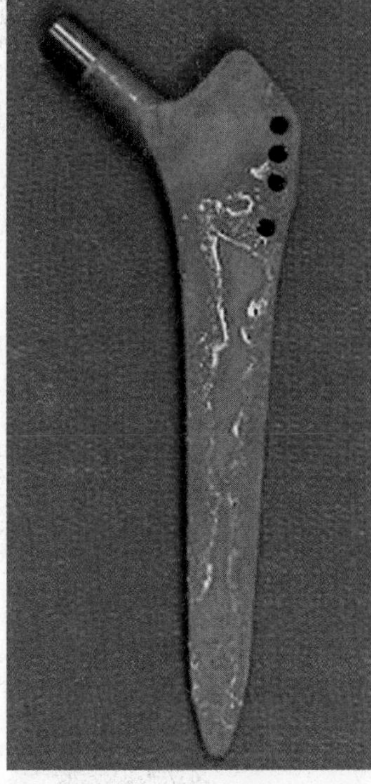

Figure 5-15 Photograph of bone ongrowth stem retrieval. The design of the stem has a sharp angle wedge design in two planes. The edges of the implant are sharp to provide rotational stability. Notice the rather scant amount of bone on the surface of this prosthesis. Implant was found biologically stable at the time of removal.

C. Technique

1. Initial rigid fixation of implant is always a *press fit* technique.
2. Femoral stem design is typically a high-angle double-wedge taper (wedge in both coronal and sagittal planes) (Figure 5-15).
3. Grit surface is extensile. The fixation strength with grit blast fixation is significantly lower than porous coating. Therefore the area of surface coating is greater.
4. There are very few cups designed with bone ongrowth surface coating.

D. Complication of bone ongrowth

1. Fracture
   - Bone ongrowth stem requires a very tight press fit to maintain initial rigid fixation. The double-wedge taper design is prone to proximal fracture.
2. Aseptic loosening
   - Stem settling occurs when initial rigid fixation is not good enough to allow osteointegration.

IV. HYDROXYAPATITE

A. Formula is $Ca_{10}(PO_4)_6\,(OH)_2$.

B. *Osteoconductive* only

C. Effect—allows more rapid closure of gaps between bone and prosthesis

1. Bidirectional closure of space between prosthesis and bone
2. Osteoblasts adhere to hydroxyapatite surface during implantation and then grow toward bone.
3. Clinically shortens time to biologic fixation

D. Success requires
1. High crystallinity—Amorphous areas of hydroxyapatite will dissolve.
2. Optimal thickness—A thick coating will crack and shear off.
   - Thickness under 50 to 70 μm preferred
3. Surface roughness
   - Higher implant R_a provides increased metal-hydroxyapatite interface fracture toughness.

V. PRIMARY THA—FIXATION SELECTION

A. Cup
1. Porous-coated cementless cup is preferred choice.
2. Porous-coated hemispheric cementless cups have reliable long-term results.

B. Stem
1. Both cementless and cemented fixation are acceptable techniques in primary THA.
2. Cementless stem indications
   - High–activity-level patient (cement would cyclically fatigue over time)
   - Young male patient (higher loading stress would cause cement cracks at stress points)

VI. FEMORAL STEM LOADING

A. Proximal porous coating (Figure 5-16)
1. Mechanical load is transferred to metaphysis and proximal diaphysis. This is termed *proximal bone loading.*
2. Proximal bone density is better maintained with proximal porous-coated implants.

B. Extensive porous coating (Figure 5-17)
1. More of the mechanical load bypasses the proximal femur because porous ingrowth is present throughout the diaphysis. This is termed *distal bone loading.*
2. In a well-fixed extensively porous-coated femoral stem there will be endosteal consolidation of bone near the end of the stem. This is called a *spot weld* (Figure 5-18).

C. Cemented stem
1. In a well-fixed cemented stem, the mechanical load is distributed throughout the cement mantle. Similar to an extensively porous-coated stem, more of the load bypasses the proximal femur. A cemented femoral stem is considered *distal bone loading.*

VII. FEMORAL STRESS SHIELDING

A. Description
1. Proximal femoral bone density loss observed over time in the presence of a solidly fixed implant; typically refers to cementless implants

B. Etiology
1. *Stem stiffness* is main factor.
   - Problem is modulus mismatch between stem and femoral cortex.
   - Hoek's law—When two springs are placed next to each other and loaded, more force is transmitted through the stiff spring and less through the flexible spring. Thus a cementless femoral stem that has a higher modulus than bone (i.e., stiff spring) sees much more loading stress than the surrounding proximal femur.
2. Extent of porous coating is less important.

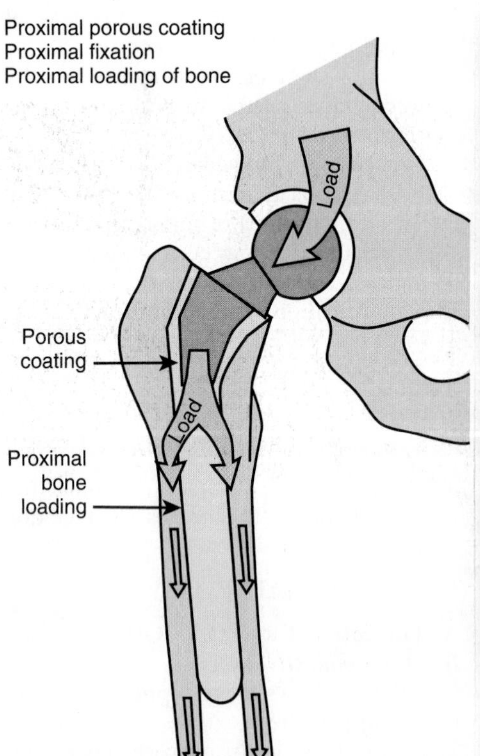

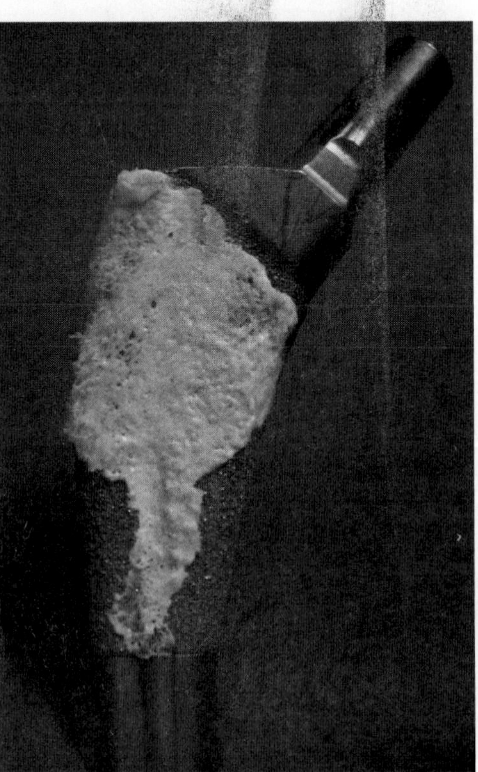

Figure 5-16 Diagram and retrieval photograph of proximal bone loading in a proximal porous-coated implant. With proximal porous coating, loading forces are transferred through the porous coating into the metaphysis and proximal diaphysis. This helps to maintain proximal bone density.

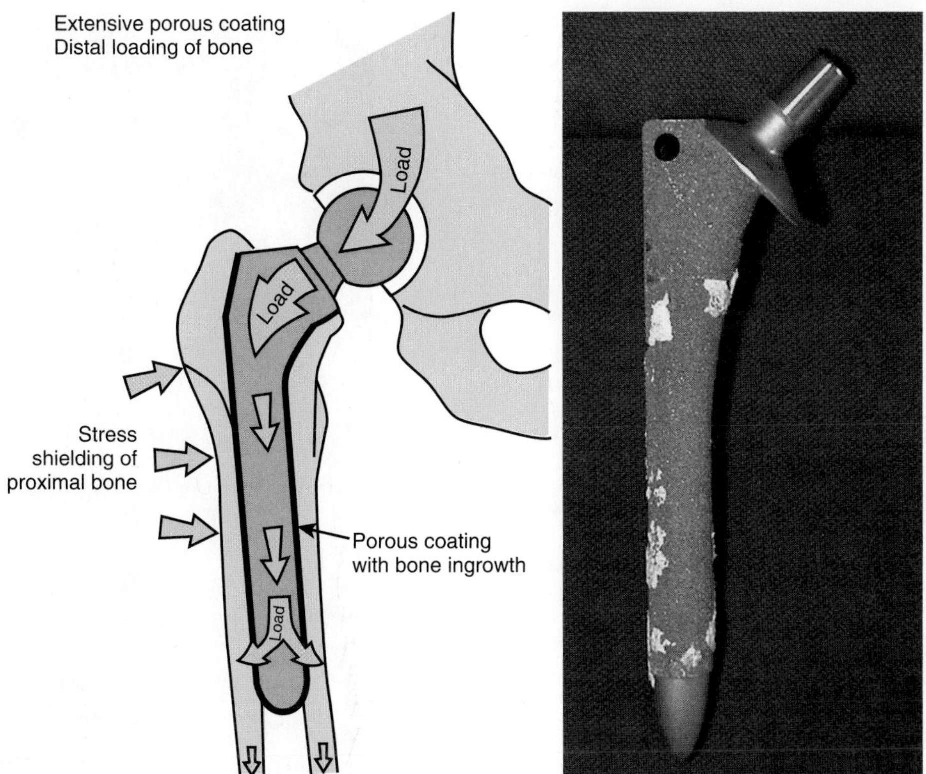

Figure 5-17 Diagram and retrieval photograph of distal bone loading in a extensively porous-coated prosthesis. With extensive porous coating, a majority of bone ingrowth occurs in the femoral diaphysis. Loading forces are transferred through the porous coating into the more distal diaphysis. As a result, bone density in the proximal femur is reduced because it does not see as much load.

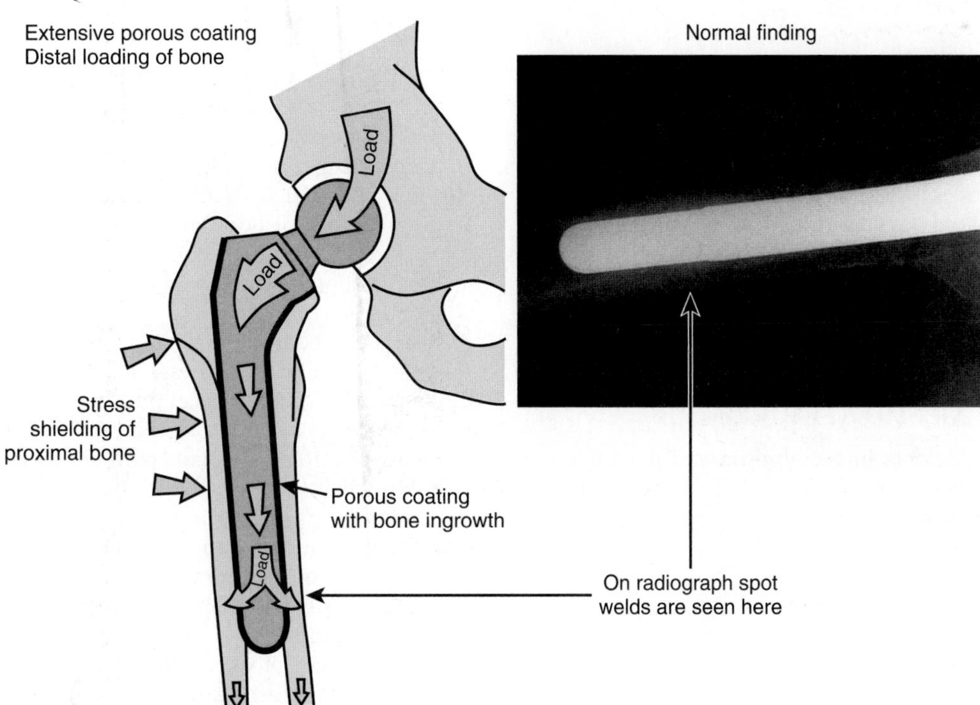

Figure 5-18 Diagram and radiograph of *spot weld*. A spot weld indicates stable osteointegration of an extensively porous-coated implant. In contrast, a *bony pedestal* is bone accumulation within the medullary canal below the tip of a mechanically loose stem. The bony pedestal seeks to keep the stem from sinking further down the medullary canal.

C. **Factors affecting stem stiffness**
1. Stem diameter is most important.
   - Stem stiffness approximates *radius*^{4} of stem.
   - Larger diameter stems are exponentially stiffer.
2. Metallurgy
   - Cobalt-chromium (Co-Cr) alloy is stiffer than titanium alloy.
3. Stem geometry
   - More stiff
     - Solid and round stems
   - Less stiff
     - Hollow, slots, flutes, taper designs

D. **Archetypical scenario creating stress shielding**
1. Large-diameter stem of 16 mm or greater
2. Co-Cr alloy stem
3. Round, solid cylindrical stem shaft
4. Extensive porous coating
   - Distal bone loading

VIII. FEMORAL STEM BREAKAGE (FIGURE 5-19)

A. **Failure mode is *cantilever bending*.**
1. Seen with smaller-diameter stems (cemented or cementless)

B. **Clinical scenario**
1. Stem is fixed distally and loose on top.
2. Loading of stem creates cyclic bending stress.
3. Fracture occurs generally in middle portion where stems taper and become thin.

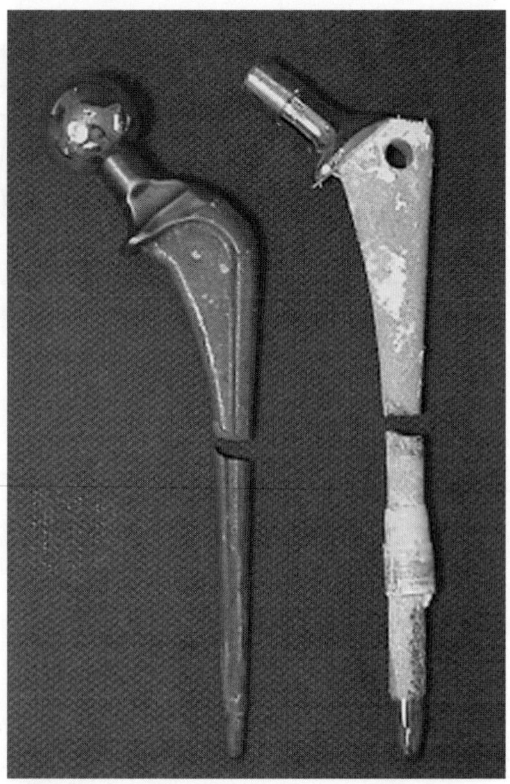

Figure 5-19 Photograph of stem retrievals due to stem fracture. Stem on the *left* was cemented. Stem on the *right* was cementless. Both stems have narrow-diameter stems. Both stems fractured in typical region, which is the transition region to narrow part of the stem.

SECTION 6 REVISION THA

I. PRESENTATION

A. ***Start-up pain* is the most common initial presentation.**
1. Groin pain indicates a loose acetabular cup.
2. Thigh pain indicates a loose femoral stem.

B. **Infection must always be ruled out as a cause of pain.**

C. **Anterior iliopsoas impingement and tendinitis is poorly understood and may be the cause of a painful THA when a prominent or malpositioned cup is present and no other causes can be found.**

II. ACETABULAR SIDE (FIGURE 5-20)

A. **Identify bone defects in acetabulum and pelvis.**
1. *Cavitary deficiency* is a loss of cancellous bone without compromise of main structural bone support.
2. *Segmental deficiency* is loss of main bony support structures.
   - Acetabular rim
   - Acetabular column
   - Medial wall
3. Combined deficiencies

B. **Well-fixed cementless implant with osteolytic defect**
1. **Can be treated with débridement, bone grafting, and bearing component exchange**
2. Contraindications to this are a poorly positioned cup, poor implant design, an ongrowth fixation surface, or damaged locking mechanism.

C. **Cementing a polyethylene (PE) liner into a damaged cup is associated with an increased rate of dislocation.**

D. **Significance of bone defects**
1. Major segmental bone deficiencies require a reconstruction cage and/or a structural bone graft. This is the recommended technique.
2. A structure bone graft (a graft that reconstructs a segmental defect) alone without a cage has a high loosening rate.

E. **Fixation revision of acetabulum**
1. Cementless porous biologic fixation is preferred.
2. **Hemispheric porous cup with screw is standard.**
   - Must have at least two thirds of rim and a reasonable initial press fit to work
   - **Recommended cup replacement is to recreate the native center of rotation.**
     - Cup placement should be inferior and medial (i.e., low and in).
       - Lowest joint reactive forces
     - Cup placement superior and lateral (i.e., up and out) is not recommended.
       - Highest joint reactive forces
       - Higher wear and component loosening

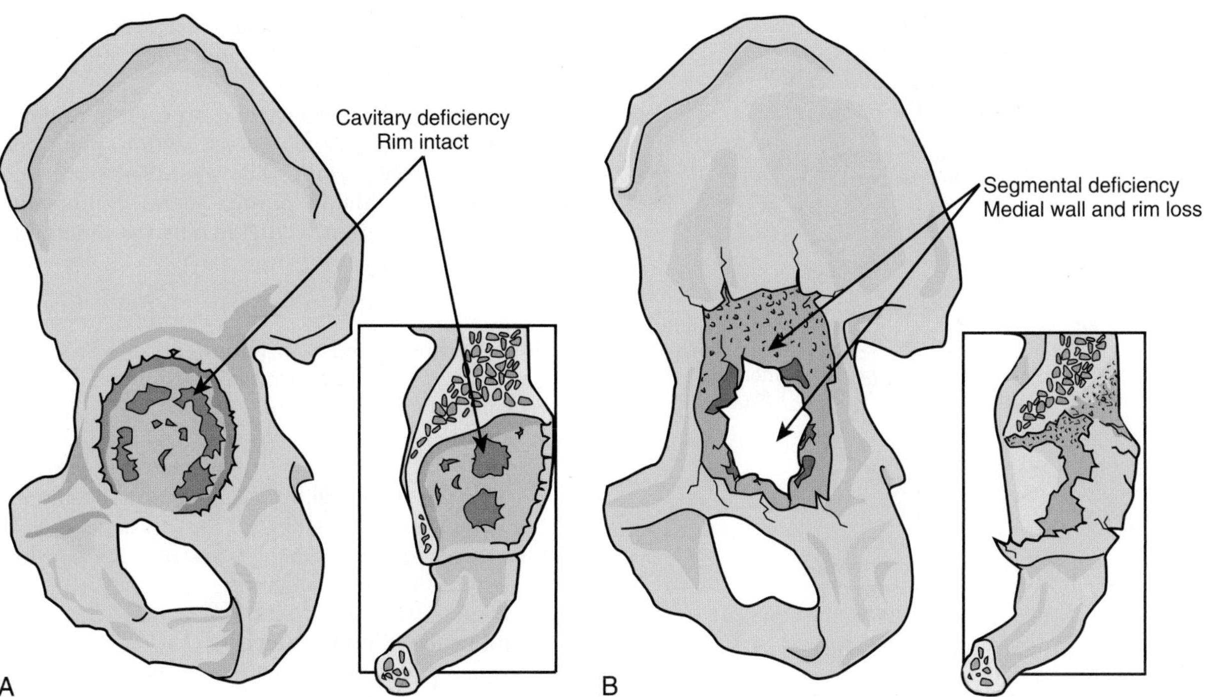

Figure 5-20 Diagrams of pelvis demonstrating cavitary and segmental deficiency. **A,** Cavitary deficiency. Bone loss involves cancellous bone. Main support structures are intact. **B,** Segmental deficiency. In this diagram there is structural loss of the medial wall and superior acetabular rim. Segmental defects are more difficult to reconstruct.

- Fill cavitary deficiencies with particulate bone graft.
- Acetabular metallic wedge augmentation is an acceptable adjuvent to hemispheric cup provided that cup is placed in good position and initial rigid fixation is achieved.

3. **Reconstruction cage** (Figure 5-21)
   - **Recommended when segmental bone deficiencies prevent initial rigid fixation of a hemispheric porous cup in desired position**
   - Bone graft
     - Cage placement is against acetabulum and pelvis. Bone graft is placed behind cage.
       - Particulate graft preferred
       - Bulk support allograft when needed
   - Acetabular cup insertion
     - Acetabular cup is cemented into reconstruction cage.
4. Acetabular screw placement (Figure 5-22)
   - *Posterior-superior* quadrant is the safe zone for acetabular screw placement. This is preferred zone for screw placement.
   - *Anterior-superior* quadrant is considered the zone of death. Screws and/or drill that penetrate too far risk laceration to the external iliac artery and veins.

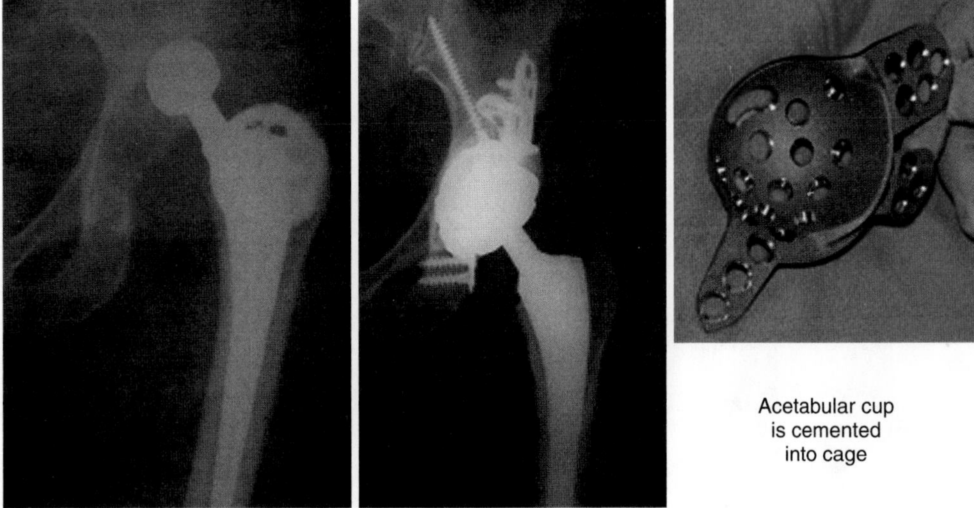

Figure 5-21 Reconstruction cage for segmental acetabular deficiency. *Left,* Displaced acetabular cup. Note segmental bone loss of posterior acetabulum. *Center,* Pelvic reconstruction with a triflange cage. The cage is secured to bone with screws. Acetabular cup is cemented into the cage. *Right,* Triflange cage before insertion.

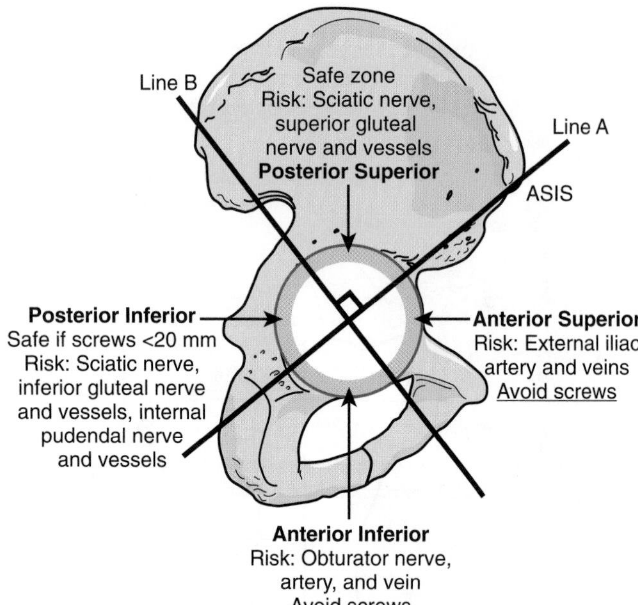

Figure 5-22 Diagram showing four quadrants for acetabular screw placement. *Line A* is formed by drawing a line from the anterior superior iliac spine (ASIS) to the center of the acetabular socket. *Line B* is then drawn perpendicular to *line A,* also passing through center of socket.

- ▫ Should a major vessel injury occur during screw placement, the hip wound should be immediately packed tight. Without closing the hip wound, an anterior pelvic incision is made to gain proximal control of the bleeding artery. Repair of the bleeding source is then addressed.

5. Pelvic dissociation
   - Defined as separation of the superior aspect of the pelvis from the inferior aspect by fracture and/or osteolysis
     - ▫ Risk factors are female sex, massive pelvic bone loss (osteolysis), and rheumatoid arthritis.
     - ▫ **Treatment/Options**
       - **Multiflange reconstruction cage is preferred.**
       - **Posterior pelvic reconstruction plate to ilium and ischium followed by hemispheric cup, jumbo cup, or highly porous metal component with augmentation, as dictated by the remaining bone**

III. FEMORAL SIDE (FIGURE 5-23)

A. Identify bone defects in femur.

1. *Cavitary deficiency* is loss of endosteal bone. Cortical tube remains intact.
   - Endosteal ectasia is a form of cavitary deficiency in which the outer cortex has increased in diameter as a result of mechanical irritation by a loose femoral stem.
2. Segmental bone deficiency is a loss of part of the cortical tube either in the form of holes or complete loss of a portion of the proximal femur.
3. Combined deficiencies

B. Significance of bone defects

1. Revision femoral stem must bypass the most distal defect.
   - New implant must bypass most distal cortical defect by a minimum of *two cortical diameters*. Otherwise, there is an increased risk for fracture at the tip of the stem.
     - ▫ The revision stem must prevent bending movements from passing **through the region of the cortical hole, which is a weak point.**

C. Fixation revision of femur

1. **Cementless porous biologic fixation is preferred.**
2. **Extensive porous-coated long-stem prosthesis is standard.**
   - An extensive grit-blasted stem with splines is also an accepted solution.
   - Cemented revision stem
     - ▫ High failure rate at intermediate term

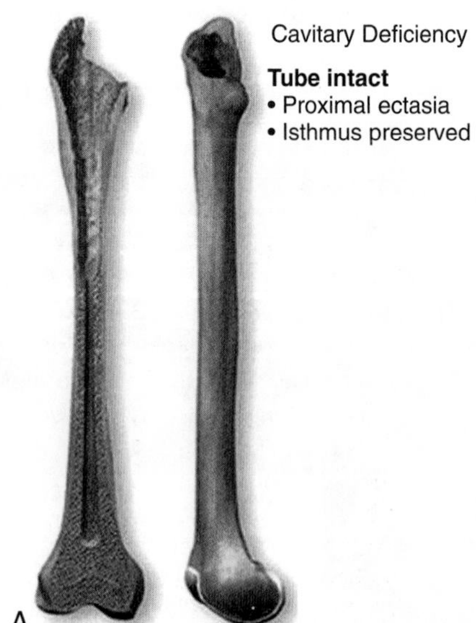

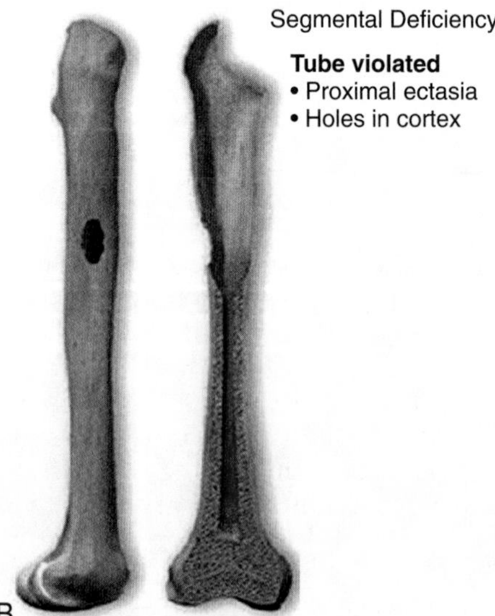

Figure 5-23 Diagrams of proximal femur demonstrating cavitary and segmental deficiencies. **A,** Cavitary deficiency. Bone loss involves cancellous bone and endosteal cortical bone within the femur. The outer cortical tube remains intact. The overall strength of the tube is diminished. **B,** Segmental deficiency. In this diagram the segmental defect is the hole in the diaphysis. A proximal cortical ectasia is also present (cavitary defect).

- Recommended in patients with irradiated bone
- Acceptable use in very elderly or very low demand patient when immediate full weight bearing is needed

3. **Longer stem than previous stem is recommended.**
   - **Resistance to torsion increases as length of stem increases.**
   - **Provides better initial rigid fixation**
4. Impaction grafting technique
   - Acceptable revision technique with limited indication
   - Surgical technique
     - Place distal PE restrictor into diaphysis.
     - Impact particulate allograft bone (fresh frozen bone recommended) into endosteal canal. Bone is impacted around a femoral stem trial.
     - Cement polished tapered stem into impacted allograft bone.
     - Polished tapered stem is allowed to settle slightly within cement. Mechanical load forces are transmitted as compression forces upon allograft bone.
     - Allograft heals to endosteal bone.
     - Cement stays interdigitated with allograft.
     - Endosteal bone is restored.
   - Indication
     - Used to reconstitute cortical bone when there is significant cortical ectasia
     - Must have intact cortical tube. Small cortical defects can be covered with an external mesh or allograft strut.
       - Must not devascularize bone in process of covering hole
   - Complication of impaction grafting
     - Most common complication is *subsidence.*
     - Choice of allograft and morcellization technique are important factors affecting success.
5. Segmental bone deficiency of femur
   - Cortical holes are reinforced with allograft cortical struts secured with cerclage cables (or wires).
   - Proximal cortical deficiencies may be restored with modular metallic endoprosthetic segments or with a bulk support allograft.
   - Proximal allograft technique
     - Cement revision stem into proximal allograft.
     - Connect allograft to host femur with a *step cut.*
     - Hold allograft to native femur with cables, plate, and/or allograft cortical strut.
     - Revision stem must have rigid fixation in native distal femur.

D. Modular bearing change

1. Indications
   - Significant linear PE wear associated with progressive radiographic osteolysis and/or mechanical symptoms of subluxation
   - Implants must be well fixed to bone.
2. Complications
   - **Most common complication is *dislocation.***
     - **Patients generally feel well and fail to allow adequate soft tissue healing.**
3. Technique
   - Must exchange both liner and head
   - Bone graft osteolytic lesions behind cup with particulate graft through cup holes or small iliac trap door
4. Cementing PE bearing into fixed porous cup
   - Indicated when there is a damaged/worn locking mechanism or replacement PE bearing is not available
   - Technique requirements
     - Optimize PE cup position to avoid neck impingement.
       - This reduces chance of hip instability.
     - Deep seating of PE liner into metal cup
       - This maximizes surface contact with cement and minimizes risk for PE cup debonding from cement.
     - Roughen back side of PE liner insert.
       - This increases surface area for bonding with cement.
     - Roughen inside surface of metal cup shell.
       - This also increases surface area for bonding with cement.
     - Close matching of PE liner to metal shell is *not important.*

SECTION 7 OSTEOLYSIS IN THA

I. INTRODUCTION

A. PE wear debris is the main culprit (when using traditional PE cup bearing). PE wear comes from two sources.

1. PE bearing wear—head-cup articulation
2. *Backside wear*—This occurs when the PE insert rubs against the metal shell, creating PE debris. This occurs because the PE locking mechanism does not completely inhibit PE micromotion against the metal shell. The more backside micromotion allowed, the more PE debris generated

B. *Submicron*-sized particles shed by the PE bearing are responsible for eliciting the osteolysis reaction.

1. Billions of particles are generated.
   - Osteolysis more likely when the number of PE particles exceeds 10 billion particles per gram of tissue.

C. *Adhesive* bearing wear is the most important process that generates submicron-sized PE particles.

1. Types of PE bearing wear
   - Adhesive wear (Figure 5-24)—This is most important mechanism in osteolysis process.
   - Abrasive wear—A rough femoral head surface causes mechanical scratching of PE surface with loss of PE material (*cheese grater* effect).
   - Third-body particles—Particles within the joint space get between head and PE cup, causing abrasion. These particles cause PE to be removed from cup surface. Third-body particle sources include
     - Cement debris
     - Metal debris shed from cup or stem
     - Metal debris from metal corrosion at modular metal-metal interfaces (i.e., modular junctions)
     - Hydroxyapatite debris shed from implant surfaces

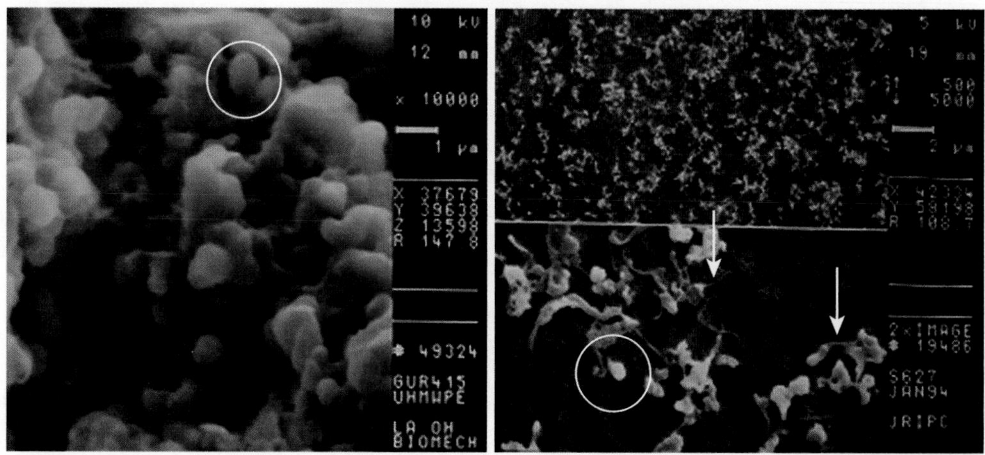

Primary articulation
PE beads being pulled off with each cycle

Figure 5-24 Scanning electron microscope photographs demonstrating *adhesive* wear in a polyethylene (PE) cup bearing. *Left,* Surface profile of a PE cup. Note submicron-sized beads that are melted together. *Top right,* PE particles collected after a bearing simulator test. *Bottom right,* Magnified view reveals that the particles collected *(circle)* are actually the beads pulled off the surface of the cup. *Arrows* point to the tails on the beads indicating the beads are individually pulled off as the femoral head moves against the PE cup.

- Abrasive material introduced at time of prosthetic joint implantation (i.e., metal debris from drill bit)

II. OSTEOLYSIS PROCESS

A. Phagocytes of submicron-sized PE particles by macrophage; macrophage becomes activated

B. Additional macrophage recruitment via cytokines released by activated macrophage

C. Release of osteolytic factors (cytokines) by the activated macrophage; these factors include

1. Tumor necrosis factor-α—interleukin-1-β
2. Transforming growth factor-β—interleukin-6
3. Platelet-derived growth factor—receptor activator of nuclear factor κB ligand (RANKL)

D. Bone resorption mediated via RANKL

E. Mechanism of bone resorption mediated by osteoblast/RANKL (Figure 5-25)

1. RANKL is produced by the osteoblast.
2. RANKL attaches to RANK receptor on osteoclast, which activates bone resorption process.
3. Osteoprotegerin, produced by many cell lines, blocks RANKL and mitigates bone resorption.
4. The only cell that resorbs bone is the osteoclast.
5. The RANKL/osteoprotegerin ratio in the bone microenvironment determines overall bone homeostasis.

III. OSTEOLYSIS AROUND THA PROSTHESIS—EFFECTIVE JOINT SPACE

A. The intraarticular generation by PE particles elicits an inflammatory response that results in a *hydrostatic pressure buildup* within the joint.

B. PE particles are then disseminated throughout the *effective joint space* (Figure 5-26).

1. Effective joint space is defined as any contiguous area around the joint where the implant touches bone. The effective joint space includes the area around the cup, stem, and screws.

C. Osteolysis can occur anywhere within the effective joint space (Figure 5-27).

1. Fluid moves in the path of *least resistance.*
   - Areas well sealed by biologic integration will inhibit particle dissemination.
   - Areas that are vulnerable to particulate debris dissemination include
     - Smooth areas next to porous areas
     - **Screw holes in cup**
     - Surface area around screws
     - Debonded cement-bone interfaces
     - Cement mantle defects
   - **With an extensively porous-coated stem, most osteolysis is seen at the greater trochanter and proximal femur. This can lead to late insufficiency fracture of the greater trochanter.**

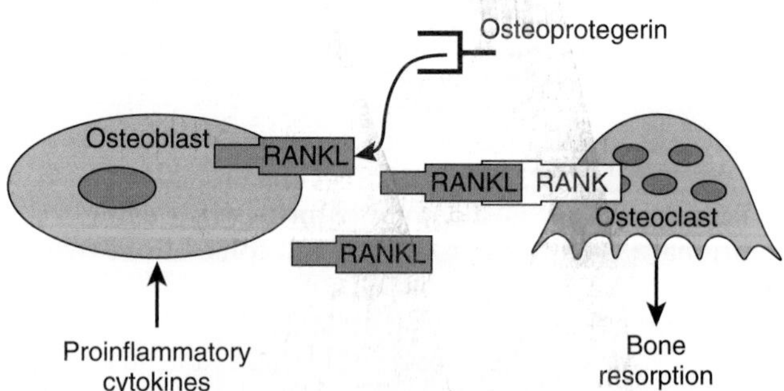

Figure 5-25 Diagrammatic representation of osteolysis-induced resorption of bone. Proinflammatory cytokines released by the activated macrophage reach the osteoblast, which in turn upregulates the production of receptor activator of nuclear factor κB ligand (RANKL). RANKL is produced on the surface of the osteoblast but is also released by the osteoblast in a soluble form. RANKL attaches to RANK receptor on the osteoclast surface. This induces osteoclastogenesis, resulting in bone resorption. RANKL is blocked by osteoprotegerin (expressed by osteoblasts and many other cell lines). The RANKL/osteoprotegerin ratio in the bone microenvironment determines overall bone homeostasis.

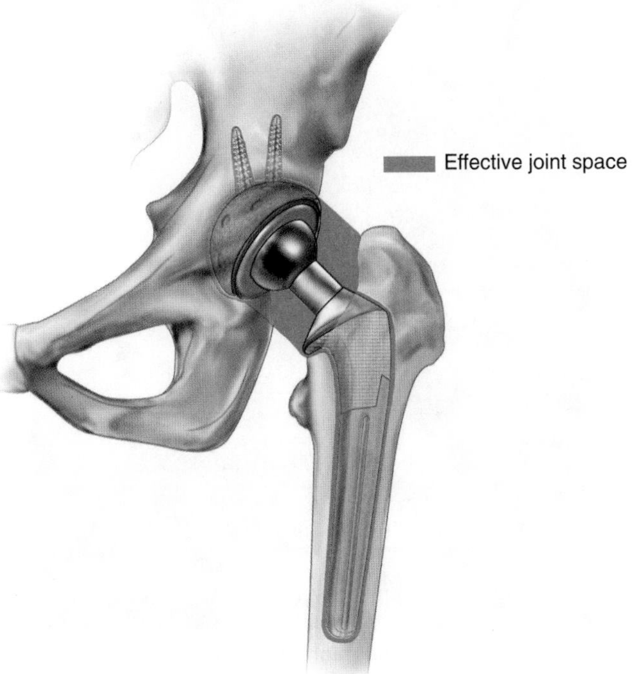

Figure 5-26 Effective joint space and osteolysis. Diagram of total hip arthroplasty depicts area of effective joint space. The effective joint space includes any area where the prosthesis touches bone. Polyethylene (PE) particulate debris can be pumped anywhere within the effective joint space if there is a path for PE particles to be pumped.

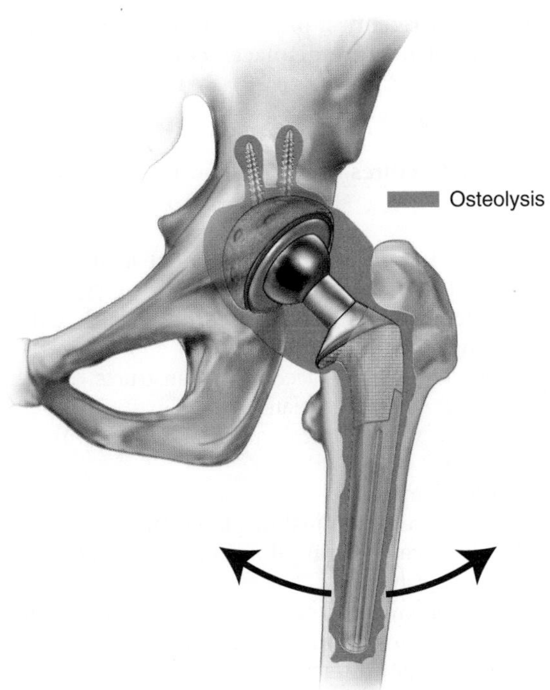

Figure 5-27 Diagram shows osteolysis around total hip arthroplasty prosthesis. Remember that fluid (and polyethylene particles) will move in path of least resistance. Prosthetic design, therefore, influences where osteolysis is likely to occur.

- **Proximal porous-coated femoral stems that do not have circumferential porous coating allow particles to be pumped toward distal stem region.**
  - **More osteolysis is seen at stem tip.**

IV. PARTICLE DEBRIS FORMATION—LINEAR VERSUS VOLUMETRIC WEAR

A. *Volumetric wear* is main determinant of the number of PE particles generated.

B. Volumetric wear is directly related to the square of the radius of the head (Figure 5-28).

1. The wear track generated *approximates* a cylinder. The volume of a cylinder, and hence the amount of PE debris generated, is formulated as follows:

$$V = 3.14\ r^2w$$

   where *V* is the volumetric wear of the PE cup, *r* is the radius of the femoral head, and *w* is the linear head wear (i.e., the distance the head has penetrated into the cup).
2. *Head size* is most important factor in predicting the amount of PE particles generated.
3. **Linear wear rates in excess of 0.1 mm/yr are associated with osteolysis.**

C. Volumetric wear versus linear—the trade off

1. The following comparison is for *traditional* PE cup (i.e., does not include improved bearing technology).
2. Small head—22 mm
   - Will have higher linear wear than 32-mm head
   - Will have lower volumetric wear than 32-mm head
   - Failure is more likely to result from wear through PE cup.
3. Large head—32 mm
   - Will have lower linear wear than 22-mm head
   - Will have higher volumetric wear than 22-mm head
   - Failure is more likely to result from osteolysis.
4. Compromise head—28 mm
   - Less volumetric wear than 32-mm head
   - Less linear wear than 22-mm head
   - Better stability than 22-mm head
   - Thus most hip systems use 28-mm head size.

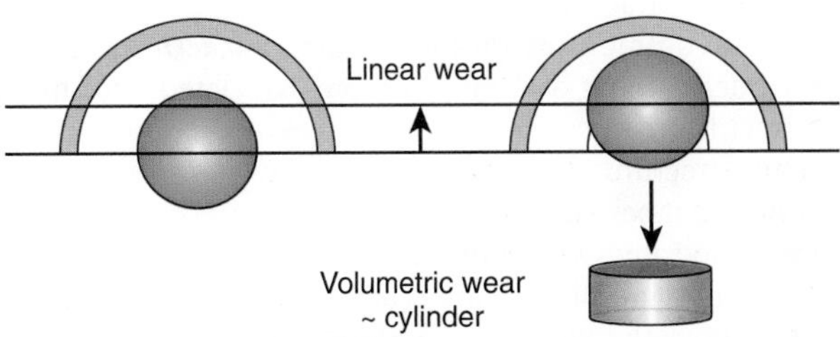

Figure 5-28 Diagram of polyethylene (PE) wear in total hip arthroplasty. As the head wears through the PE cup, a wear track is generated. Liner wear is measured where femoral head has penetrated into the PE cup. The wear track generated approximates a cylinder.

V. OSTEOLYSIS—RADIOGRAPHIC FINDINGS IN THA

A. *Endosteal scalloping* in femoral endosteal canal is hallmark finding (Figure 5-29).
B. Round lytic lesions behind acetabular cup with screw holes is common finding.
C. Round lytic lesion surrounding acetabular screw is also a typical finding.
D. Osteolytic lesions develop later in prosthetic life cycle (usually starting after 10 years). Osteolytic lesions spotted within the first 2 to 3 years of the prosthetic life cycle are most likely a result of infection.

VI. OSTEOLYSIS REDUCTION

A. Alternative bearing surfaces
1. Goal is to reduce macrophage-induced reaction.
   - Eliminate PE in hip system.
   - Less PE particles
   - Smaller PE particles that do not activate macrophage

B. Bisphosphonates
1. Inhibit osteoclast activity

C. Osteoprotegerin
1. Blocks RANKL activity, inhibiting osteoclastogenesis

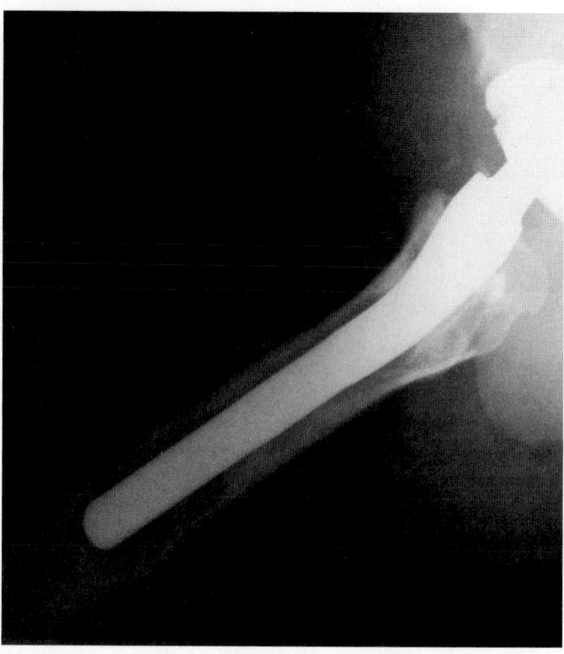

Figure 5-29 Lateral radiograph of femoral stem demonstrating osteolysis in total hip arthroplasty. The classical finding is *endosteal scalloping* of femoral cortex.

SECTION 8 PERIPROSTHETIC THA FRACTURE

I. TIME OF FRACTURE

A. Perioperative
1. Relates to surgical technique and implant design

B. Late
1. Associated with low-level trauma plus concomitant risk factors
   - Osteolysis
   - Stem loosening with bone abrasion
   - Segmental bone defect (i.e., hole in bone)
2. Most late fractures occur at *stem tip.*
   - This is area of *greatest modulus mismatch.*
     - Bone and stem—stiff
     - Hollow bone distal—flexible

II. PERIOPERATIVE FRACTURE

A. Highest risk is with *cementless* implants.
1. Acetabular fracture
   - Most common reason for fracture is *underreaming.*
   - Underreaming of 2 mm or more associated with higher fracture risk
2. Femur fracture
   - Wedge taper cementless stems
     - Associated with *proximal* femur fractures
   - Cylindrical fully porous-coated stems
     - Associated with *distal* femoral cracks

B. Treatment
1. If implant is loose and unstable
   - Open reduction with internal fixation (ORIF) and stem revision
2. **If implant still maintains initial rigid fixation**
   - **Observation and limited weight bearing if just a crack**
   - **Prosthetic retention plus ORIF of fracture if there is significant fracture displacement**

III. LATE FRACTURE

A. Most late fractures occur at stem tip.
B. Treatment
1. **Rule 1**
   - **If femoral stem is loose, treatment is stem revision and ORIF of femur fracture.**
     - **Cementless long-stem prosthesis with extensive biologic coating preferred**
     - Fracture fixation—acceptable constructs
       - ORIF with cable plate
       - ORIF with cortical allograft struts with cables/wires
2. Greater trochanter
   - Nonoperative if minimal displacement
   - ORIF with cable/wiring if significant displacement and *minimal osteolysis*
     - ORIF of greater trochanter in presence of massive osteolysis is not recommended. There is no good surface area for fracture healing and union.
3. Proximal metaphysis or diaphysis
   - Uncommon
   - Nonoperative treatment if minimal displacement
   - ORIF if significant displacement and stem stable

4. Stem tip fracture
   - For stem tip fracture that involves less than 25% of stem (cement and cementless stems) treatment options allowed are
     - Stem revision and ORIF
     - ORIF with cable plate
     - ORIF with cortical allograft struts and cables/wires
     - Choice for fixation depends upon construct that can provide stability for healing yet not compromise stem fixation.
   - For stem tip fracture that involves more than 25% of *cemented stem* (cement mantle is compromised), there is *only one* recommended treatment.
     - Stem revision and ORIF
       - Cementless long-stem prosthesis with extensive biologic coating preferred
       - Fracture fixation—acceptable constructs
         - ORIF with cable plate
         - ORIF with cortical allograft struts with cables/wires
   - For stem tip fracture that involves more than 25% of *cementless stem* (stem fixation biologically remains intact) treatment options allowed are
     - Stem revision and ORIF
     - ORIF with cable plate
     - ORIF with cortical allograft struts and cables/wires
     - Choice of fixation depends upon which construct can provide stability for healing yet not compromise stem fixation.
5. Supracondylar fracture distant to stem tip
   - Stem is not a major factor in fixation planning.
   - ORIF with lateral reconstruction plate is preferred treatment.
6. Supracondylar fracture at tip of long-stem revision prosthesis
   - Nonoperative treatment if fracture stable (i.e., crack)
     - Limit weight bearing during healing phase.
   - ORIF with lateral cable plate preferred if fracture is unstable

SECTION 9 TOTAL ARTICULAR RESURFACING

I. ADVANTAGE

A. Better stability compared to *standard THA* with small heads (22- to 32-mm)

II. RELATIVE CONTRAINDICATION

A. Coxa vara—increased risk for neck fracture

1. Vertical shear force on neck

III. COMPLICATION

A. Most common early complication (within the first 3 years) is *head failure* due to fracture.

1. Risk factors—female sex, poor bone quality, varus implant position, disruption of the extraosseous blood supply, notching of superior neck
2. Presents with groin pain
3. **Treatment is to convert to THA.**

SECTION 10 THA—MISCELLANEOUS

I. THA—NERVE INJURY

A. Eighty percent of injuries are to sciatic nerve; 20% involve femoral nerve.

B. *Compression* is most common pathologic mechanism of injury.

1. **In patients who have a nerve injury after primary THA, only 35% to 40% will recover to normal strength.**

C. Sciatic nerve travels closest to acetabulum at the level of *ischium*.

1. During surgery, the most common reason for sciatic nerve injury is errant retractor placement causing excess compression to nerve.
2. Peroneal nerve division is most often involved because this part of nerve is closest to acetabulum.

D. Risk factors for nerve injury

1. **Female**
2. **Post-traumatic arthritis**
3. **Revision surgery**
4. **Developmental dysplasia of the hip**

E. Developmental dysplasia of the hip

1. **Risk for nerve palsy increases with lengthening of leg over 3.5 cm.**

F. Postoperative functional footdrop

1. **Clinical scenario—Patient sits in chair after surgery and develops footdrop.**
   - **With hip flexed 90 degrees in chair, there is too much tension on sciatic nerve.**
   - **Treatment—Place patient back into bed.**
     - **Hip placed in extension (bed flat)**
     - **Knee flexed on one to two pillows**
     - **This position provides least tension on sciatic nerve.**

G. Postoperative hematoma

1. A hip hematoma from anticoagulation can cause sciatic nerve palsy.
   - Compression is mechanism of injury.
   - Treatment is immediate evacuation of hematoma.

II. THA—ANATOMY

A. Medial femoral circumflex artery
1. Located underneath quadratus femoris muscle or gluteus maximus tendon
2. Cutting deep to this area risks laceration to vessel.
   - Treatment is ligation/cauterization.

B. Transverse acetabular ligament and obturator vessels
1. Transverse acetabular ligament extends between the two cotyloid pads at the inferior aspect of the acetabulum.
2. Errant retractor placement inferior to the ligament can cause damage to *obturator artery* and vein.
   - Treatment is ligation/cauterization.

III. THA—SPECIFIC COMPLICATIONS

A. Sickle cell disease
1. Associated with early prosthetic loosening
   - Mechanism is extended bone infarct disease.

B. Psoriatic arthritis
1. Associated with higher periprosthetic infection rate

C. Ankylosing spondylitis
1. Associated with higher risk for heterotopic ossification
2. **Hip hyperextension due to fixed pelvic deformity can lead to a higher anterior dislocation rate.**

D. Parkinson disease
1. Higher dislocation rate
2. Higher perioperative mortality
3. Higher perioperative medical complications
4. Higher reoperation rate

E. Fat emboli syndrome
1. Occurs with *femoral stem* insertion
2. Fat and bone marrow emboli are pressurized into bloodstream.
3. **Intraoperative hypotension, hypoxia, mental status changes, and petechial rash are hallmark findings.**
4. Treatment is volume and respiratory support.

IV. VENOUS THROMBOSIS IN THA

A. Activation of clotting cascade begins *during surgery*.
1. Greatest risk for activation occurs during insertion of femoral component. Applies to both cemented and cementless implants
2. Mechanism for thrombogenesis
   - Femoral venous *occlusion* during preparation and insertion of femoral component
   - Typically, leg is twisted and mechanically levered during femoral stem preparation and insertion.

V. THA—SURGICAL APPROACH

A. Posterolateral
1. Dislocate posterior
2. **Rehabilitation—Limit flexion, adduction, and internal rotation.**

B. Direct lateral (Hardinge)
1. **Dislocate anterior**
2. Rehabilitation—Limit external rotation and extension.
3. **This approach is more commonly associated with *gluteus medius lurch*.**
4. Abductor dysfunction caused by excessive proximal splitting of gluteus medius muscle and damage to *superior gluteal nerve*
   - Gluteus medius muscle is denervated, resulting in gluteus lurch.
   - Superior gluteal nerve is located 5 cm superior to tip of the greater trochanter. Avoid splitting muscle above this level.
   - Abductor dysfunction is noted on CT scan or MRI.
     - Will see significant muscle atrophy
     - Muscle is replaced with fat.
     - Confirmation of abductor dysfunction is via electromyographic testing of abductor complex.

C. Anterior (Smith-Peterson)
1. Only approach with internervous plan
2. Interval
   - Sartorius (femoral nerve)
   - Tensor fascia (superior gluteal nerve)
3. **Dislocate anterior**
4. **Rehabilitation—Limit external rotation and extension.**

VI. THA—IMPLANT FACTS

A. THA biomaterials—Young's Modulus Relative Values (Table 5-2)

B. THA bearing friction—Relative values (Table 5-3)

Table 5-2 Total Hip Arthroplasty—Implant Facts

Implant Material	Young's Modulus (Material Stiffness) Relative Value Rating
Alumina ceramic	Highest Young's Modulus
Zirconia-reinforced alumina ceramic	↓
Zirconia ceramic	
Cobalt-chrome alloy	
Stainless steel	
Titanium alloy	
Cortical bone	
Cement (PMMA)	
Polyethylene (UHMWPE)	
Cancellous bone	
Tendon/ligament	
Cartilage	Lowest Young's Modulus

PMMA, polymethylmethacrylate; UHMWPE, ultra-high–molecular-weight polyethylene.

Table 5-3 Bearing Friction

Bearing Material	Coefficient of Friction Relative Value Rating
Articular cartilage	Lowest coefficient of friction
Al_2O_3 on Al_2O_3 (alumina on alumina)	↓
Co-Cr alloy on Co-Cr alloy	
Metal on PE	
Ice on ice	
Steel on steel	Highest coefficient of friction

Co-Cr, cobalt-chrome; PE, polyethylene.

SECTION 11 THA—JOINT STABILITY

Dislocation in THA frequently is a multifactorial issue. Treatment is patient specific, and the solution depends on the problem.

I. INCIDENCE OF THA DISLOCATION

A. Primary THA—typically 1% to 2%
B. Revision THA—typically 5% to 7%
C. Highest incidence of dislocation
1. THA in the elderly patient (age >80 years) for failed ORIF of femoral neck fracture—reasons
   - Muscular weakness
   - Mental compromise
   - Loss of balance and coordination

II. RISK FACTORS FOR DISLOCATION

A. Female
B. THA for osteonecrosis
C. Posterolateral approach
D. Smaller head size
E. Greater trochanteric nonunion
F. Revision THA
G. Obesity
H. Alcoholism
I. Neuromuscular conditions

III. DISLOCATING THA—ASSESSMENT

A. Component design
B. Component alignment
C. Soft tissue tension
D. Soft tissue function

IV. COMPONENT DESIGN

A. Prosthetic range of motion consists of two parts.
1. Primary arc range (Figure 5-30)
2. Lever range (Figure 5-31)
   - The range allowed as the hip starts to lever out of socket

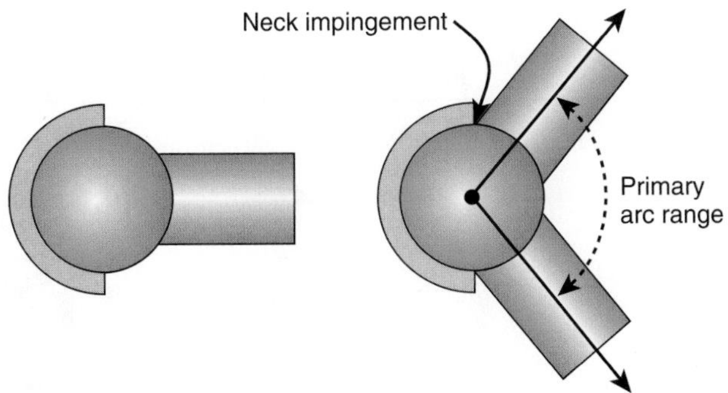

Figure 5-30 Diagram demonstrating primary arc range in total hip arthroplasty. At the end of hip range, neck impingement occurs, limiting motion. Primary arc range is the arc of motion allowed between the two ends of impingement.

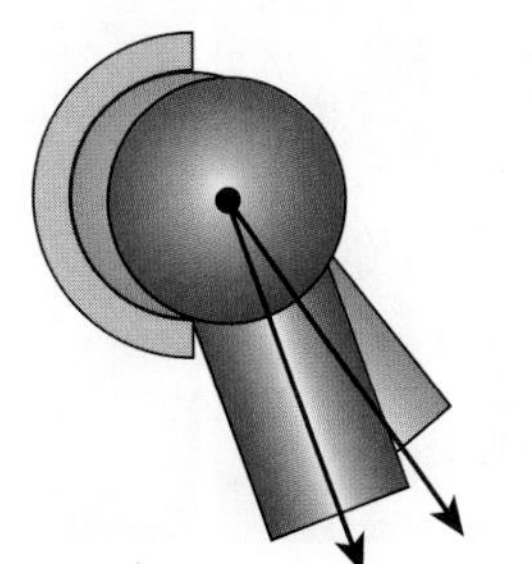
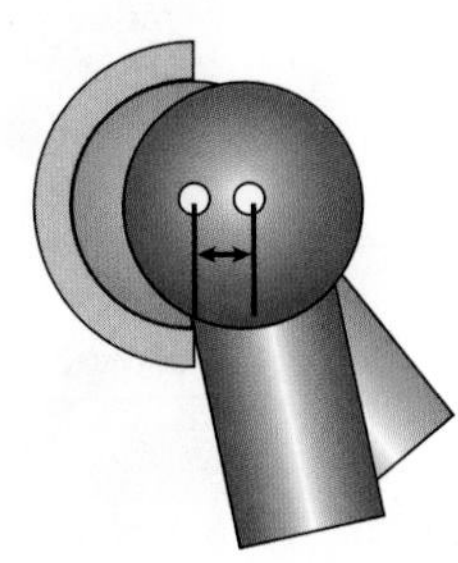

Figure 5-31 Diagram demonstrating lever range and excursion distance. **A,** Diagram showing lever range. When the femoral neck impinges on the acetabular cup, it begins to lever out of socket. The range of motion allowed before the hip dislocates is termed the lever range. **B,** Excursion distance. As the hip begins to lever, the femoral head is lifted out of socket. The excursion distance is the distance the head must travel to dislocate. The excursion distance is equal to the radius of the femoral head

V. PRIMARY ARC RANGE

A. Primary arc range is controlled by the head/neck ratio (Figure 5-32).
1. **Head diameter/neck diameter is head/neck ratio.**
2. **Best stability is achieved by *maximizing* head/neck ratio** (Figure 5-33).

B. Additions to acetabulum and/or femoral neck *decrease* primary arc range.
1. Neck skirt (also known as femoral head collar on femoral stem)
   - Decreases head/neck ratio
2. Acetabular hoods
   - Decrease primary arc range (Figure 5-34)
3. Acetabular constrained cups
   - *Markedly* decrease primary arc range (Figure 5-35)

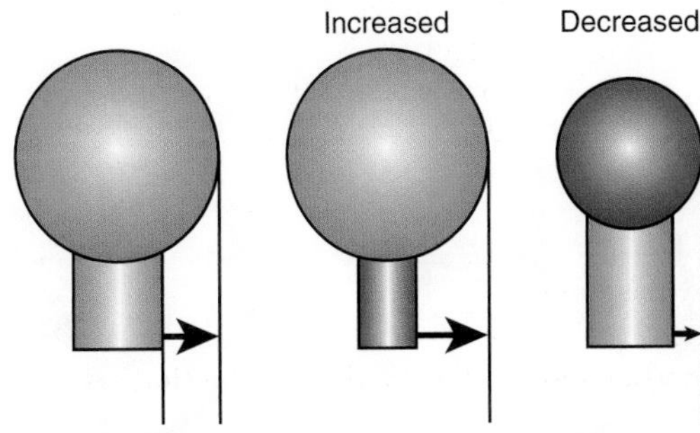

Figure 5-32 Diagram demonstrating head/neck ratio. Diagram on *left* defines head diameter/neck diameter as head/neck ratio. *Center* diagram shows an increased head/neck ratio when, in this example, the femoral neck diameter is decreased. Diagram on *right* shows a decreased head/neck ratio when, in this example, the femoral head diameter is decreased.

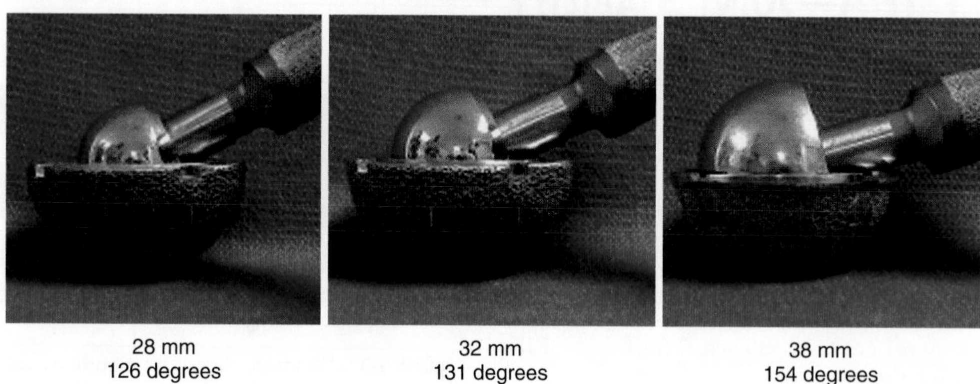

Figure 5-33 Photographs showing how increasing head/neck ratio increases primary arc range. In this demonstration, the neck diameter remains constant. As the head diameter increases, the head/neck ratio increases, and primary arc range increases as well.

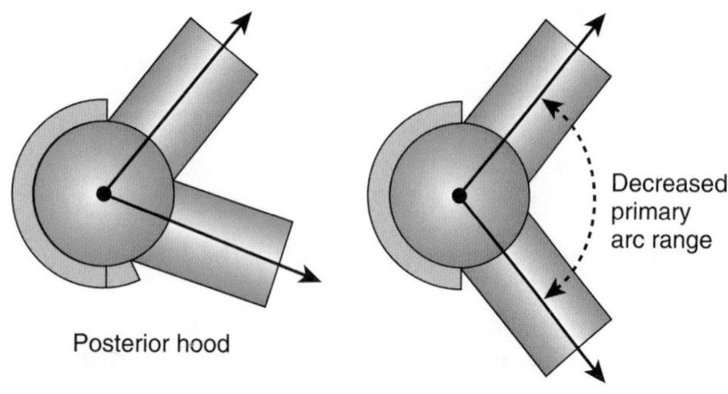

Figure 5-34 Diagram showing the addition of an acetabular posterior hood. The addition of an acetabular hood significantly reduces primary arc range.

- Rule—Constrained cups should be avoided as much as possible.

VI. LEVER RANGE

A. Lever range is controlled by head radius (Figure 5-36).
1. A large head has higher excursion distance and is more stable.
2. Most stable construct is a *bipolar* hemiarthroplasty (two pivot points).

VII. COMPONENT DESIGN—BEST RANGE IN THA

A. High primary arc range
1. Maximize head/neck ratio
2. No additions to cup or neck

B. High excursion distance
1. Large diameter head

VIII. COMPONENT ALIGNMENT

A. Primary arc range must be centered within patient's functional hip range (Figure 5-37).
B. Component malalignment does not decrease primary arc range.
C. Placement of components in a malaligned position results in a *stable side* and *unstable side* of the functional hip range.
D. Implant positioning in THA
1. **Cup anteversion—20 to 30 degrees** (Figure 5-38)
2. **Cup theta (θ)-angle (also known as coronal tilt)—35 to 40 degrees** (Figure 5-39)
3. **Stem anteversion—10 to 15 degrees** (Figure 5-40)

E. Cup malposition
1. **Retroversion—Risk is posterior dislocation.**
2. **Excess anteversion—Risk is anterior dislocation.**

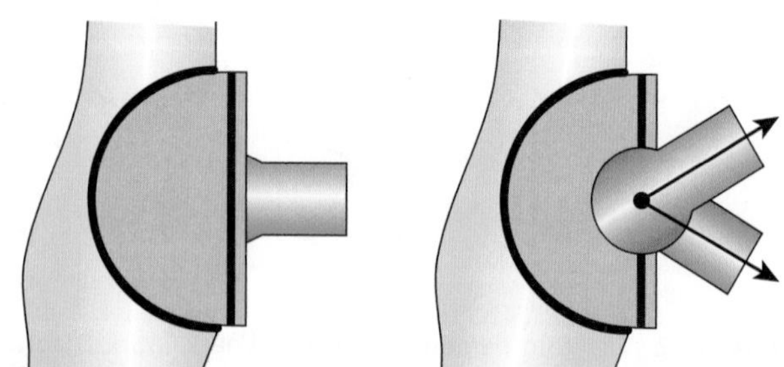

Figure 5-35 Diagram of constrained acetabular cup. A constrained liner covers the femoral head past its equator. This keeps the ball from coming out of socket. This has the adverse effect of severely restricting primary arc range.

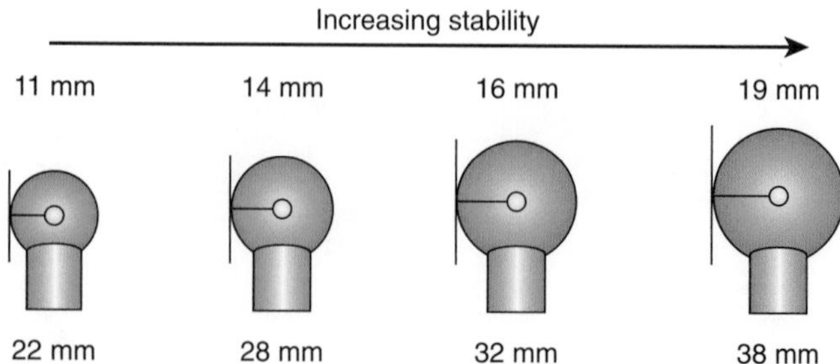

Figure 5-36 Diagram demonstrating excursion distance and effect on hip stability. Excursion distance is equal to the radius of the femoral head. By increasing femoral head diameter, excursion distance is increased. This increases hip stability.

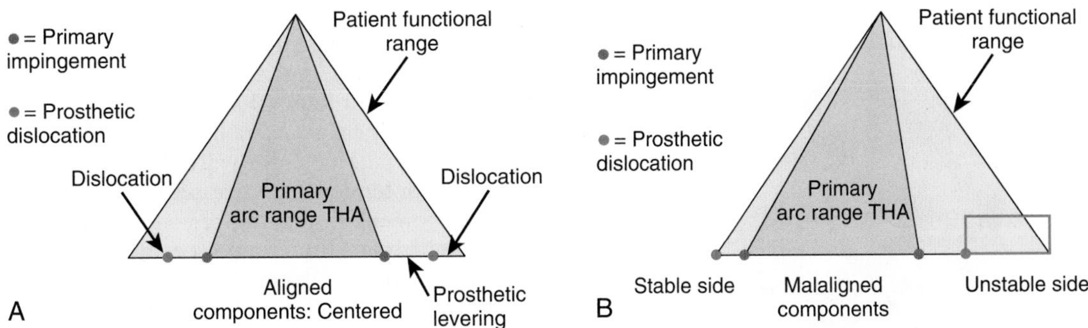

Figure 5-37 Diagrammatic representation of component malposition showing its effect on hip stability. **A,** Primary total hip arthroplasty (THA) arc range centered within patient's functional hip range. Generally, THA arc range is less than patient's hip range because of smaller head size. **B,** Component malalignment. Note that THA arc range has not changed. Instead, malposition allows the patient to exceed primary arc range and lever range. This in effect creates a stable side and an unstable side.

Figure 5-38 Diagram of acetabular cup version. **A,** In this figure, cup anteversion is referenced relative to the ilioischial line. The cup should be placed at 20 to 30 degrees of anteversion. **B,** With a retroverted cup, the femur impinges and levers in flexion, which can result in posterior hip dislocation.

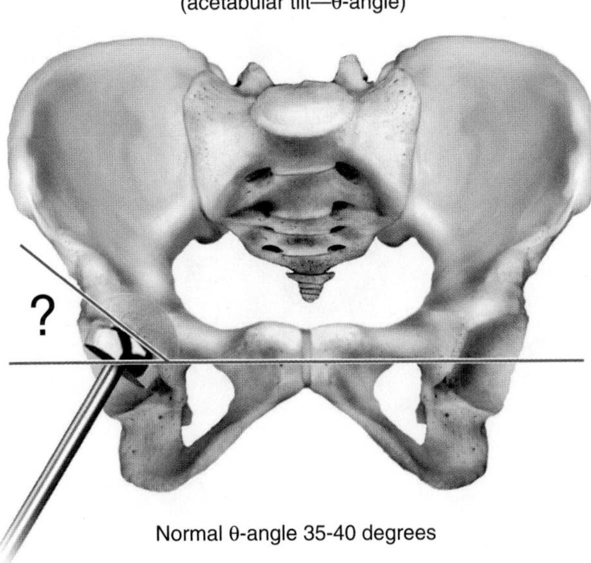

Figure 5-39 Diagram of theta (θ)-angle. In the coronal plane, the cup should be placed at a θ-angle of 35 to 40 degrees. A low θ-angle cup is a risk for abduction impingement. A high θ-angle cup increases risk for posterior-superior dislocation.

3. High θ-angle (vertical cup)—Risk is posterior-superior dislocation.
4. Low θ-angle (horizontal cup)—Risk is inferior dislocation.

F. Stem malposition

1. Retroversion—Risk is posterior dislocation.
2. Excess anteversion—Risk is anterior dislocation.

IX. SOFT TISSUE TENSION

A. Abductor complex is *key* to hip stability.

1. Consists primarily of gluteus medius muscle and gluteus minimus muscle

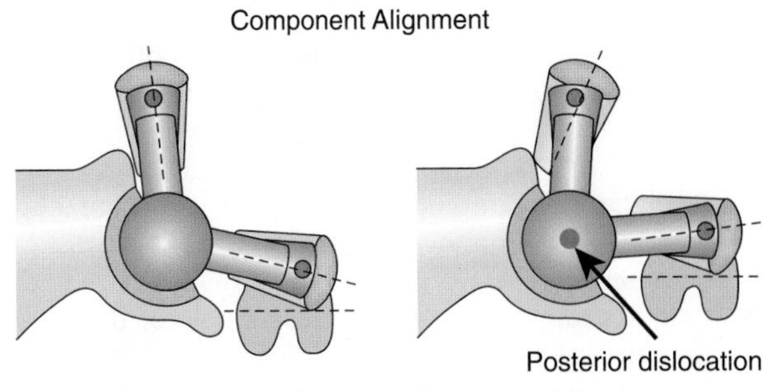

Figure 5-40 Diagram of stem anteversion. **A,** Normal stem anteversion of 10 to 15 degrees. This allows functional hip flexion without impingement. **B,** Stem retroversion. With a retroverted stem, the proximal femur impinges early against pelvis. This can result in levering and posterior dislocation.

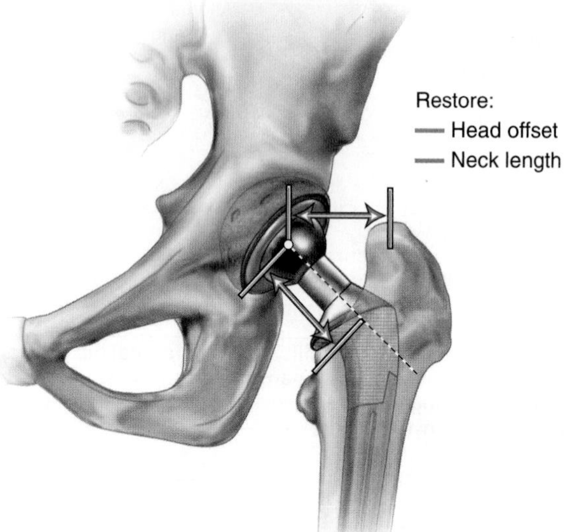

Figure 5-41 Diagram demonstrating head offset and femoral neck length. Head offset is the distance from the hip head center to the lateral femur (either the greater trochanteric tip or a line that is centered within the femoral medullary canal). Femoral neck length is the distance from femoral head center to the base of the femoral neck (usually the top of the lesser trochanter is used as the reference mark). Preoperative hip templating is used to make sure that the appropriate implant design and femoral neck osteotomy level are chosen to restore preoperative values.

2. Prosthetic implant design and positioning must maintain/restore proper abductor hip tension.

B. Restoration of abductor tension achieved by the following (Figure 5-41):

1. Restored normal hip center of rotation
2. Restored head offset
3. Restored femoral neck length

C. Reduced hip offset—problems

1. **Weakened abductor complex**
2. **Increased joint reaction force (decreased abductor lever arm)**
3. **Positive Trendelenburg sign**
4. **Gluteus medius lurch with walking**
5. **Increased risk for dislocation**

D. Short neck length—problems

1. Short neck length occurs by making a low neck cut or using a short prosthetic neck length (or both).
2. Shortens abductor muscle length, resulting in abductor weakness
3. Decreases hip offset, which also weakens abductor complex
4. Results in bony impingement of greater trochanter against pelvis during hip range (Figure 5-42)
   - Causes pain
   - Allows hip levering and increases risk for dislocation
5. Shortens leg length

E. Restored neck length using long head—problems

1. A short femoral neck cut can be compensated with an extralong prosthetic neck length. However, a long neck length requires a *skirt* (Figure 5-43).
   - A skirt decreases primary arc range.
   - Increases risk for dislocation
   - If the prosthetic neck-shaft angle is lower than the native hip, the addition of neck length will *excessively* increase neck offset.
     - This can cause trochanteric bursitis and chronic lateral hip pain (Figure 5-44).

F. Narrow-offset femoral stem design

1. A femoral stem with an offset designed with more narrow angle than the native hip will reduce hip offset. This reduces abductor tension and increases risk for hip dislocation.
2. A narrow-offset stem can be compensated by employing a longer femoral head length (i.e., neck length). This creates two potential problems.
   - The addition of neck length to restore offset will excessively lengthen the leg.
   - The addition of a long neck requires a *skirt,* which decreases primary arc range and increases risk for dislocation.

G. Greater trochanteric escape (Figure 5-45)

1. Greater trochanteric escape occurs when the greater trochanter pulls away from the proximal femur.
   - Usually a result of failed trochanter fixation after revision THA
     - Can also occur from trauma (usually associated with osteolysis in greater trochanter)
     - Successful reattachment is difficult and often fails.
   - Problems
     - Because the hip abductor complex attaches to the greater trochanter, trochanteric escape results in a loss of hip compression and increases risk for hip dislocation.
     - There is increased external and internal hip rotation because the greater trochanter no longer restricts rotation range. This also increases the risk for dislocation

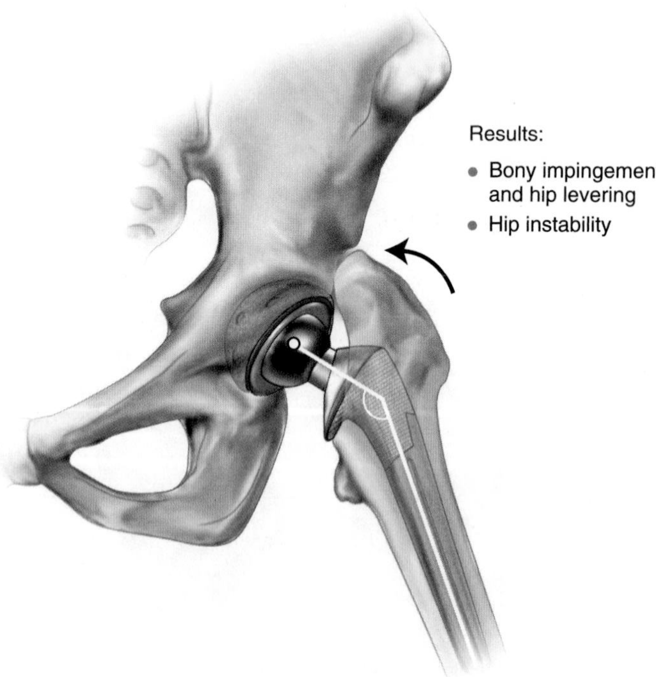

Figure 5-42 Diagram showing effect of decreased neck length. A decreased neck length brings the proximal femur closer to the pelvis. As the hip is ranged, the greater trochanter is more likely to abut the pelvis. This causes hip levering and increases risk for hip instability.

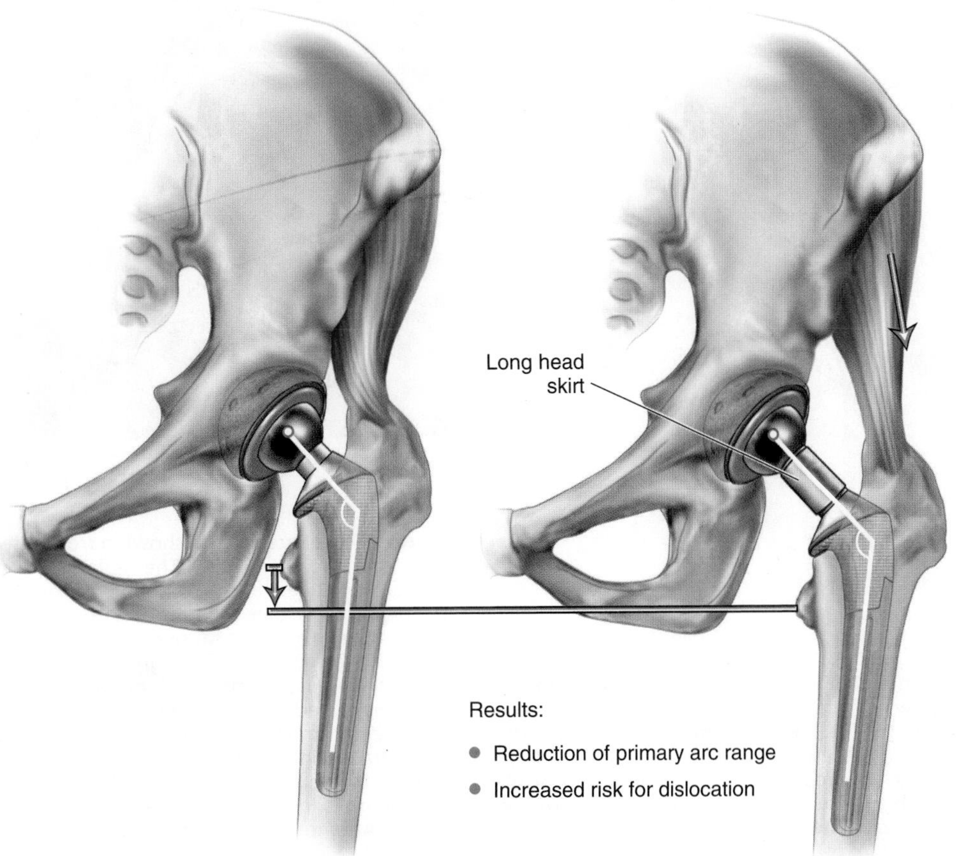
Long Femoral Neck with Skirt
(improved bending strength)
Long head
skirt
Results:
Reduction of primary arc range
Increased risk for dislocation

Figure 5-43 Diagram demonstrating the problem of using a long femoral head. A low neck cut is compensated by employing a long femoral neck (typically 9 mm or longer). When using a long head, a metal skirt is added to improve bending strength (to prevent metal fatigue and failure). The thick metal skirt can significantly reduce primary arc range, resulting in an increased risk for dislocation.

because the hip can more easily approach and exceed lever range.
  - The greater trochanter fragment can impinge between the hip and pelvis, causing hip levering.

1. Treatment
   - Maximize head/neck ratio.
     - No neck shirts and no acetabular hoods
   - Resect greater trochanter fragment to prevent impingement levering.
   - Constrained acetabular cup is last resort.

X. SOFT TISSUE FUNCTION

A. The soft tissues about the hip are controlled by several body systems. All are integrated together to provide hip stability. The three main factors controlling soft tissue function include

1. Central nervous system (CNS)
2. Peripheral nervous system
3. Local soft tissue integrity (surrounding hip region)

B. CNS mechanisms causing disruption to hip function and increasing risk for dislocation

1. Muscle dysfunction
2. Sensory impairment
3. Impaired coordination
4. Impaired balance
5. Cognitive loss of restraint (i.e., compliance/memory)

C. CNS conditions affecting hip function

1. Cerebral dysfunction
   - Stroke, seizure, CNS disease
2. Cerebellar dysfunction
   - Balance/coordination
3. Delirium
   - Medications, withdrawal phenomenon
4. Dementia
5. Psychiatric
   - Psychosis, addiction

D. Peripheral nervous system mechanisms causing disruption to hip function, increasing risk for dislocation

1. Muscle dysfunction
2. Sensory impairment
3. Pain

E. Peripheral nervous system conditions affecting hip

1. Spinal stenosis
2. Radiculopathy
3. Neuropathy
4. Paralysis/paresis

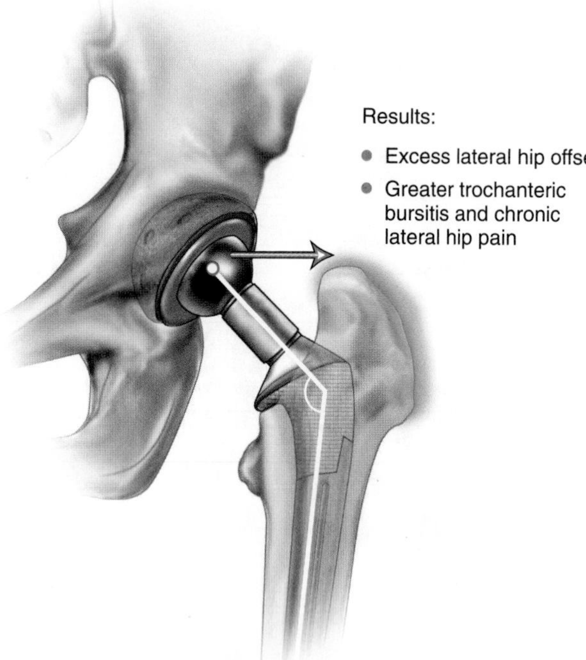
Low Neck-Shaft Angle
(more varus)
Results:
Excess lateral hip offset
Greater trochanteric bursitis and chronic lateral hip pain

Figure 5-44 Diagram demonstrating the problem of excess lateral hip offset. A low neck cut is compensated by employing a longer femoral head length (i.e., neck length). However, when the neck-shaft angle of the prosthesis is lower (i.e., more varus) than the native femoral neck, the addition of neck length excessively increases hip offset. This causes excess tension of the iliotibial band over the greater trochanter, which causes chronic pain and bursitis.

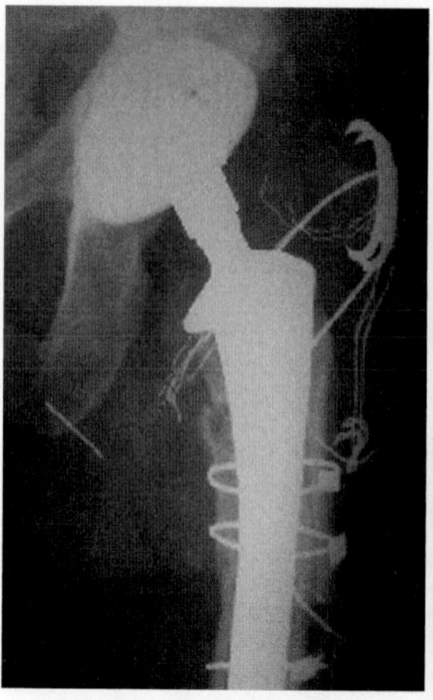
Note large skirt
Trochanteric escape
Dislocation after débridement
Revised to constrained
polyethylene insert

Figure 5-45 Radiographs showing trochanteric escape after revision total hip arthroplasty. The radiograph on *left* shows greater trochanter pulled away from the proximal femur. The greater trochanter was damaged from osteolysis, leaving little surface area for healing. Cyclic fatigue eventually resulted in cable breakage and detachment of the greater trochanter from the femur. When the greater trochanter is not attached to the vastus lateralis, it will be pulled cephalad toward the joint region. In this region, the greater trochanteric fragment is an impingement source. Radiograph on *right* shows subsequent dislocation. When the greater trochanter is not attached to the femur, prosthetic rotation range is increased and the hip is more likely to lever out of socket. Also note head skirt *(arrow)*, which diminishes primary arc range.

F. Local soft tissue integrity mechanisms causing disruption to hip function and increasing risk for dislocation

1. Muscle dysfunction
2. Soft tissue dysfunction (other than muscle)
3. Soft tissue loss
4. Skeletal deformity
   - Example—Patients with ankylosing spondylitis have increased risk for *anterior* dislocation.

G. Local soft tissue conditions affecting hip function

1. Trauma
   - Soft tissue loss
   - Myoligamentous disruption
2. Deconditioning
   - Poor health
   - Aging process
3. Irradiation
   - Radiation fibrosis with soft tissue contraction
4. Dysplasia
   - Musculoskeletal hypoplasia
5. Osteolysis
   - Bone loss
   - Myotendonous disruption
6. Collagen abnormalities
   - Clinical hyperelasticity
7. Myopathy
8. Malignancy
9. Infection

XI. DISLOCATING THA—TREATMENT

A. Each case of hip dislocation is unique. There is not one common treatment.

B. In each case assess

1. Component design
2. Component alignment
3. Soft tissue tension
4. Soft tissue function

C. Clinical review of dislocating event important

1. Was dislocation at extreme end range or within usual activities of daily living?
2. Patient's cognition—impaired versus normal
3. Clinical examination
   - Determine where THA starts to lever and sublux.

D. Radiographic review

1. **Scrutinize implant design and position.**

E. Initial treatment for dislocated THA

1. *Two thirds* of patients with a first-time THA dislocation can be successfully treated with closed measures.
2. Closed reduction
   - Sedation or anesthesia preferred to minimize soft tissue trauma
   - During closed reduction, take hip through full range and assess position of dislocation.
     - Determine if subluxation is within patient's activities of daily living or at extreme end range.
   - *Posterior* hip dislocation

- In supine position, the leg will lie in *internal* rotation, adduction, and shortened position.
- Reduction maneuver for posterior hip dislocation
  - Flexion to 80 to 90 degrees
  - Internal rotation
  - Adduction
  - Distraction
- **Anterior hip dislocation**
  - **In supine position, the leg will lie in external rotation, slight abduction, and slightly shortened position.**
  - Reduction maneuver for anterior hip dislocation
    - Extension
    - External rotation
    - Slight abduction
    - Distraction
- Postreduction treatment
  - Education—hip precautions
  - Immobilization of joint—(usually 6 weeks)
    - Spica brace/cast
    - Knee immobilizer—this will keep patient from putting hip in a compromised position
  - Physical therapy
    - Focus on strength, balance, agility, coordination
  - Optimization of medical conditions

F. Surgical treatment

1. Surgical options
   - Implant revision
   - Greater trochanteric advancement
   - Constrained acetabular socket
   - Conversion to bipolar hemiarthroplasty
   - Resection arthroplasty
2. **Rule 1—surgical treatment**
   - **If any implant component is malaligned, it needs to be changed.**
     - **May require complete hip revision**
3. Component revision—goals
   - Maximize head/neck ratio to increase primary arc range.
     - No neck skirts or acetabular hoods
   - Accurate component alignment
   - Recreate center of hip rotation and head offset.
   - Stabilize greater trochanter (if possible) if it is detached.
4. Greater trochanter advancement (also known as *Charnley tensioning*) (Figure 5-46)
   - Technique is to perform trochanteric osteotomy, advance greater trochanter distally on lateral femur, and resecure with claw, cables, and/or wires.
   - By advancing greater trochanter distally, the abductor complex is tensioned tighter, which increases hip compression forces.

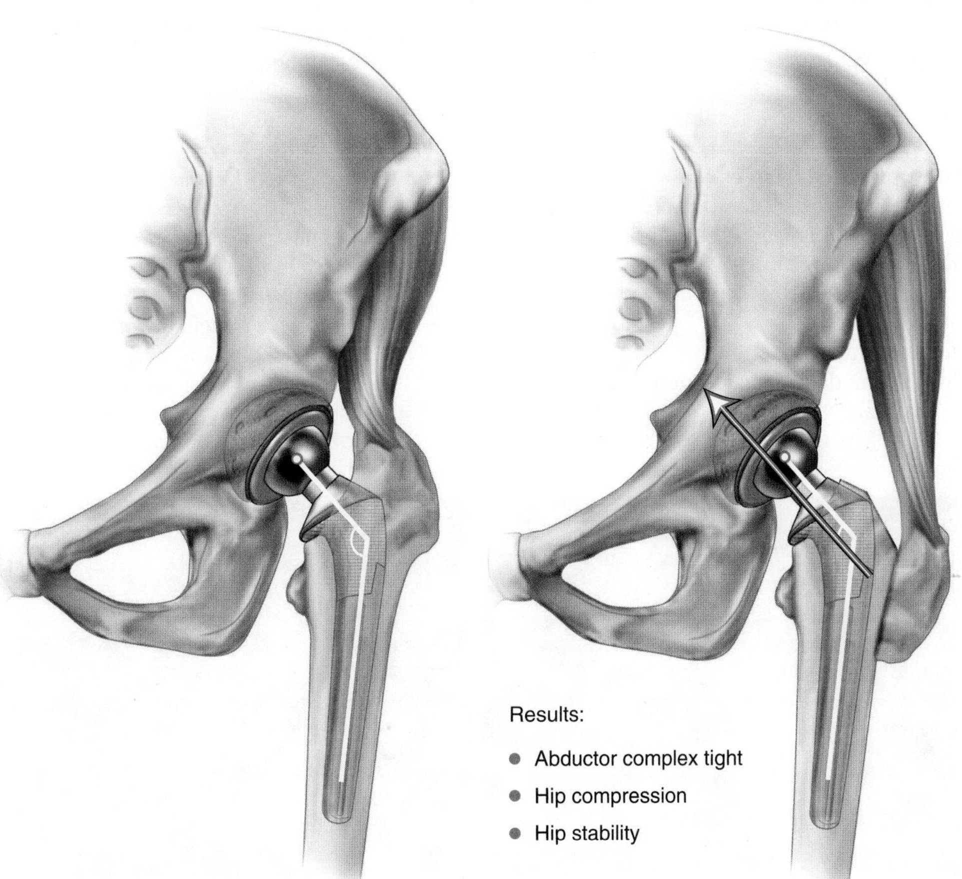
Trochanter Advancement
(adductors are retensioned)
Results:
Abductor complex tight
Hip compression
Hip stability

Figure 5-46 Example of greater trochanteric advancement. Diagram on the *left* shows implants in good alignment, but the abductor sleeve is lax in tension. When the greater trochanter is distally advanced *(right),* the abductor tension is improved, resulting in increased hip compression forces. This improves hip stability.

- Requirements
  - No component malalignment
  - Adequate distal bone surface for bony fixation and bone healing
  - Intact superior gluteal nerve

5. Constrained PE socket
   - A constrained PE socket encloses the femoral head and *mechanically* prevents hip from distracting out of socket.
   - Reserved for the multiple dislocator with *soft tissue dysfunction*
   - **Best indications**
     - **Elderly patient (i.e., low demand) with *normal* component alignment**
     - **Abductor deficiency/dysfunction**
     - **Central neurologic decline**
     - **Revision THA with reconstruction cage** (Figure 5-47)
       - Significant soft tissue dissection and potential muscle dysfunction with cage placement
   - **Contraindication**
     - **Cup malposition**
   - Constrained cup—failure mechanisms
     - Because a constrained cup significantly reduces primary arc range (as low as 60- to 70-degree arc range), the cup is exposed to more frequent and more intense lever range forces. With repetitive loading, the constrained cup will fail via two different mechanisms.
       - The PE deforms at the edges of the socket, and the hip dislocates.
       - The PE does not deform. In this case the levering forces are then transmitted to the acetabular prosthetic-bone interface, resulting in mechanical cup loosening.

6. Bipolar hemiarthroplasty conversion
   - Technique—Remove acetabular component. Ream remaining bone to a hemisphere. Press fit bipolar ball to rim of acetabulum (minimizes risk for medial migration of head).
   - Requirements
     - Fully intact acetabular bone
       - No segmental rim deficiencies, otherwise the bipolar ball will dislocate

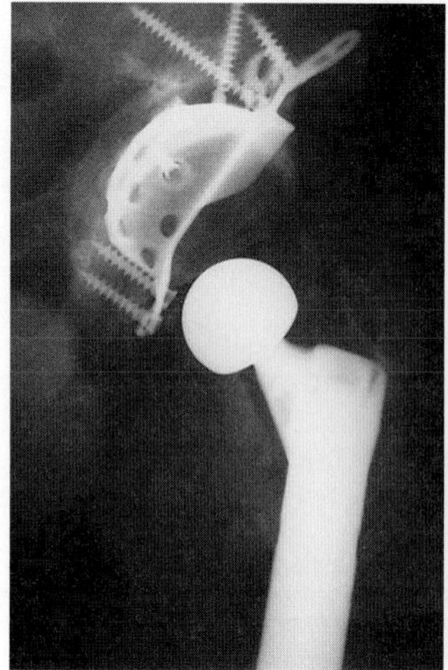

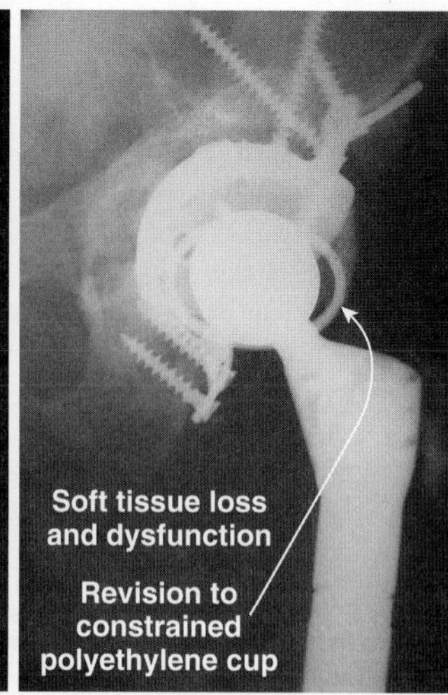

Figure 5-47 Radiographs showing dislocation in a multiply revised total hip arthroplasty. In this example the patient had multiple risk factors for dislocation: cage revision, greater trochanteric escape, spinal stenosis, and peripheral neuropathy. Note the loss of soft tissue tension as the hip has literally dropped out of socket *(left)*. Stability was achieved with placement of a constrained polyethylene socket *(right)*.

     - Good bone density
     - Rim fit technique
   - Advantage
     - Maximize fully head/neck ratio.
     - Bipolar construct has a little more inherent stability than monopolar ball.
   - Disadvantages
     - Groin pain—metal articulating on bone (Figure 5-48)
     - Medial migration of head developing into protrusio deformity
     - Accelerated PE wear
       - Larger overall PE wear surface area

7. Resection arthroplasty
   - Indications
     - Nonambulator
     - Neurologic deficits where stability cannot be achieved
     - Recurrent/ongoing periprosthetic infection
     - Drug-seeking behavior with purposeful voluntary dislocations

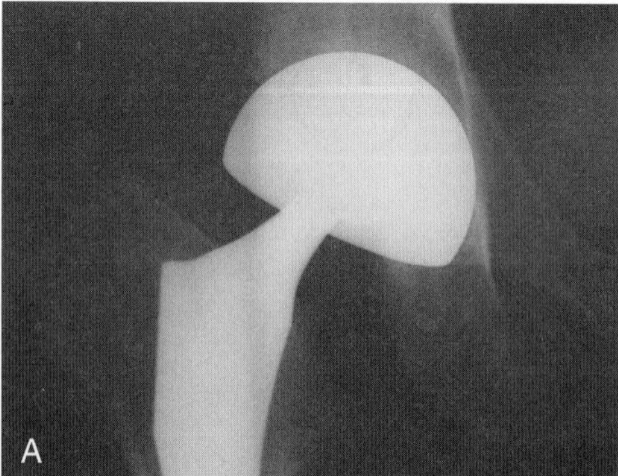

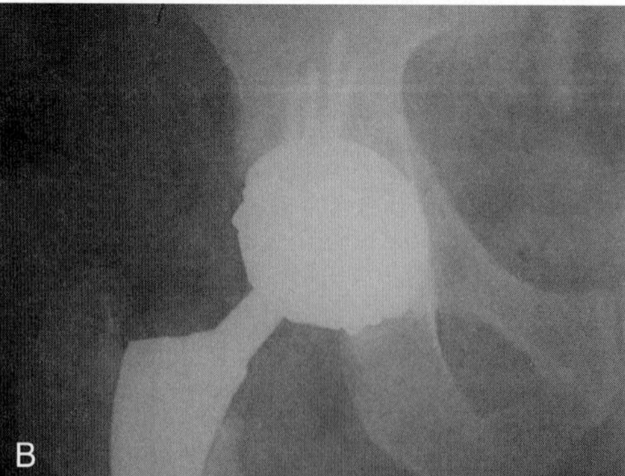

Figure 5-48 Example of hemiarthroplasty for recurrent total hip arthroplasty (THA) dislocation. This 66-year-old man was revised for recurrent THA dislocation. **A,** Bipolar ball articulating on bone. Although hip was stable, this active patient experienced significant groin pain. **B,** The acetabular socket was revised to a fixed acetabular socket with revision of femoral component to provide proper acetabular and femoral component alignment. This patient remains stable with current construct.

SECTION 12 THA—Articular Bearing Technology

I. BEARING TYPES

A. Hard on soft (traditional)
1. Metal on PE
2. Ceramic on PE

B. Hard on hard (alternative)
1. Metal on metal
2. Ceramic on ceramic
3. Metal-ceramic

II. HARD-ON-SOFT BEARING

A. Lubrication mechanism
1. **Boundary lubrication**
   - Asperities (surface rough points) on each surface make contact with each other—always.
   - Boundary lubricant (i.e., synovial fluid) separates surfaces just enough to prevent severe wear.

B. Bearing couples
1. Alumina ceramic on PE—good
2. Co-Cr alloy on PE—good
3. Zirconia ceramic on PE—not good
4. Stainless steel on PE—fair
5. Titanium alloy on PE—bad

C. Zirconia ceramic on PE—problem
1. Zirconia ceramic in vivo undergoes *phase transformation*. This means surface architecture changes over time, making the surface more rough.
   - Yttrium-stabilized *tetragonal* crystal phase changes to *monoclinic* crystal phase.
   - Monoclinic phase has increased surface roughness—increased PE wear

D. Titanium alloy on PE—avoid
1. Titanium alloy head is easily scratched (Figure 5-49).
   - Results in increased *abrasive* wear
   - Causes rapid PE wear

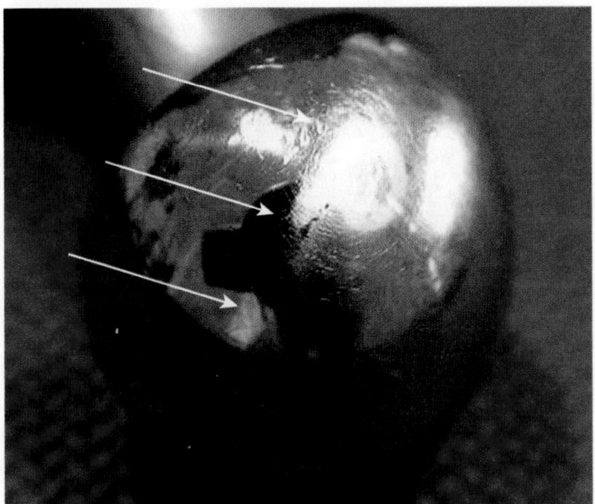

Figure 5-49 Femoral head retrieval of cemented femoral stem with nonmodular titanium femoral head. *Arrows* point to *hemisphere of abrasive wear*. This area articulates with the polyethylene (PE) cup. It has become scratched by third-body particles that have entered the joint-bearing region. This roughened surface greatly increases PE wear.

E. Factors affecting wear
1. Surface roughness of head
2. Sphericity of head
3. PE manufacturing process
4. PE sterilization process
5. PE irradiation modification
6. PE shelf life

F. Surface roughness of head
1. Co-Cr head (Figure 5-50)
   - Carbide asperities stick up and cause scratching.
2. Ceramic head (Figure 5-51)
   - Residual pits on surface create roughness.
3. Metal smearing—ceramic heads (Figure 5-52)
   - Metal smearing—transfer of metal to surface of ceramic head (ceramic head is not scratched)
   - Source of metal smear is hip subluxation with subsequent metal transfer from acetabular cup.
   - There is increased surface roughness in metal smear region.
   - Increased roughness causes increased wear.

G. Sphericity of head
1. Areas out of round are high stress points. These areas increase PE wear.

H. PE manufacturing process—four methods
1. Ram bar extrusion—machine component
2. Sheet molding—machine component
3. Compression molding—machine component
4. **Direct compression molding—no machining—*best wear***

I. Ram bar extrusion process—problem (Figure 5-53)
1. With ram bar extrusion process, calcium stearate is added to keep PE from binding up during extrusion process.
2. The addition of calcium stearate to PE *adversely* affects PE wear rates.
3. Calcium stearate in PE causes the following problems:
   - Inconsistent PE consolidation
   - Results in *unfused* PE resin particles
   - Increased PE oxidation potential
   - Reduced mechanical properties of PE
4. Calcium stearate *should not* be added to PE.

J. Direct compression molding
1. **Implant is made directly from the mold. There is no secondary machining of the bearing surface.**
2. **Bearing surface is less rough.**
3. ***Best wear* of the four manufacturing techniques**

K. PE sterilization process—three methods
1. Ethylene oxide gas
2. Gas plasma spray (peroxide)
3. Low-dose irradiation (generally between 2.5 and 4.5 mrad)

L. Irradiation of PE (Figure 5-54)
1. **Major key point—Irradiation of PE in air is bad.**
2. **Irradiation of PE—sequence of events**
   - **Irradiation of PE ruptures PE bond, creating *free radicals*.**
   - **Free radicals can rebond via two different pathways.**
     - **In presence of oxygen (i.e., air), the free radical can bond with oxygen, resulting in PE *chain scission*. This is termed *oxidized* polyethylene.**

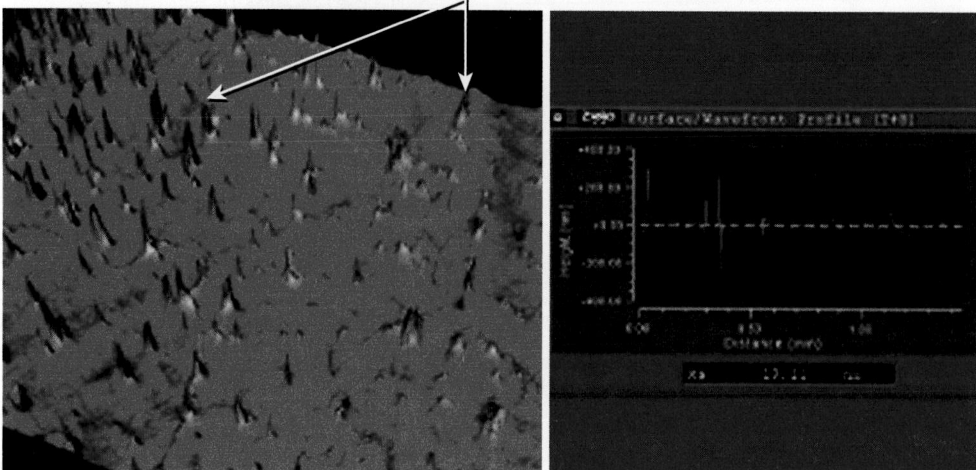

Figure 5-50 Scanning photomicrograph of cobalt chrome (Co-Cr) alloy head. The sharp peaks emanating from the surface are carbide asperities that protrude from the surface. (Courtesy of Ian Clarke, PhD, and Donaldson Arthritis Research Foundation.)

- **In absence of oxygen, the free radical will bond with an adjacent chain to create a *cross-link*. This is termed *cross-linked* polyethylene.**

3. Oxidized PE—main problem
   - Oxidation of PE results in *greatly reduced* mechanical properties.
   - Reduced mechanical properties cause accelerated PE wear and can also lead to catastrophic PE wear.
4. Cross-linked PE—advantage
   - Improved resistance to adhesive and abrasive wear
   - Improved wear compared to non–cross-linked PE
   - Irradiation of PE in an oxygen-free environment is the preferred process.
   - Methods to maintain the PE implant in an oxygen-free environment
     - Vacuum packaging
     - Oxygen-free gas packaging: argon or nitrogen

M. PE sterilization methods—comparison

1. Ethylene oxide and gas plasma
   - No cross-linking of PE
   - Generally *higher* wear rate for same product compared to oxygen-free irradiation cross-linking process

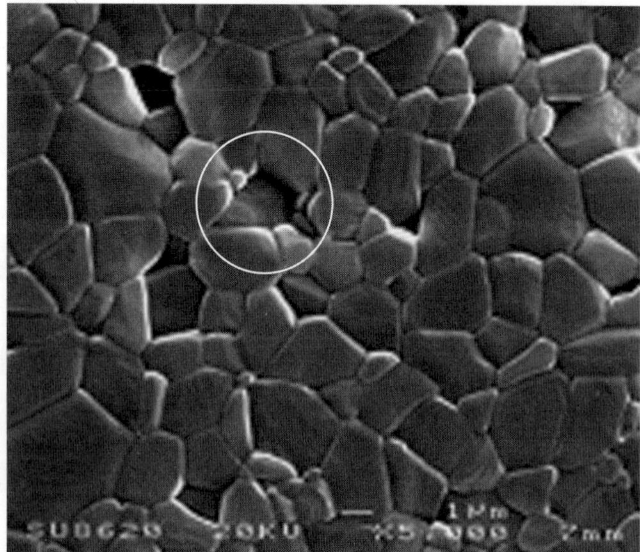

Hard on Soft
Surface roughness of head
• Ceramic head
+ Residual pits on surface create roughness

Figure 5-51 Scanning micrograph of surface of a ceramic head. Note residual pits *(circle)* on surface. These small areas create the roughness of a ceramic surface.

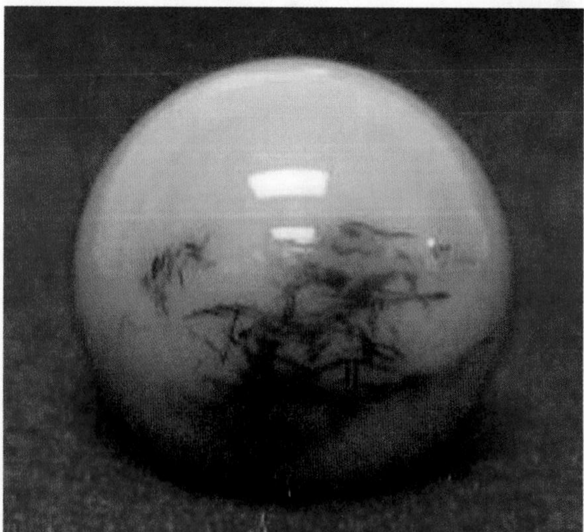

Figure 5-52 Photograph of a ceramic head retrieval demonstrating metal smear. With repetitive hip subluxation, metal from the acetabular cup is transferred to the ceramic head. The greater the smear area, the higher the rate of polyethylene wear.

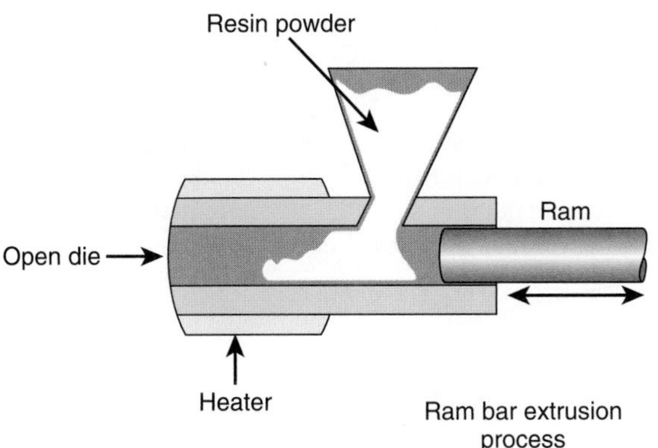

Figure 5-53 Diagram of ram bar extrusion process. Polyethylene (PE) powder is poured into chamber. The chamber is heated, and the bar of melted PE is pushed out the end of the die. Calcium stearate is added to the PE power to prevent it from sticking to surfaces of the die.

2. Low-dose irradiation in oxygen-free environment
   - Cross-linking of PE

N. PE irradiation modification

1. This is not a sterilization process.
2. Involves *high-dose irradiation*
   - 5 to 15 mrad (10 mrad = 100 kGy)
3. Product produced is *highly cross-linked PE* (HCLPE)

O. HCLPE

1. **Advantages compared to standard PE**
   - **Better wear resistance**
   - **PE wear particles tend to be *smaller* in size.**
     - **Potentially less osteolysis reaction**
   - **Generally, decreased number of particles generated (this is process dependent)**
2. **Disadvantages compared to standard PE**
   - **Decreased tensile strength**
     - **Pulling force to break**
   - **Decreased fatigue strength**
     - **Maximum cyclic stress the material can withstand**
   - **Decreased fracture toughness**
     - **Force to propagate a crack**
   - **Decreased ductility**
     - **Elongation without fracture**

P. HCLPE manufacturing process

1. There are several different methods to produce HCLPE.
   - The processes produce HCLPE products that are *not equivalent*.
2. First-generation HCLPE process consists of
   - High-dose irradiation
   - Heating of PE
   - Sterile packaging
3. The major factors important to HCLPE production include
   - High-dose irradiation
   - PE microstructure
   - PE crystallinity
   - PE heating process
4. **High-dose irradiation**
   - **The higher the dose of irradiation, the greater amount of free radicals generated.**
   - ***The problem*—Residual free radicals after cross-linking do remain.**
     - **This is an oxidation risk.**
5. PE (officially ultra-high–molecular-weight PE [UHMWPE]) microstructure
   - PE in a manufactured implant exists in two forms (i.e., phases; Figure 5-55).
     - Crystalline phase
       - Provides mechanical strength to PE
     - Amorphous phase
       - Only amorphous regions of PE cross-link.
6. PE properties—crystallinity
   - Optimum crystallinity 45% to 65%
   - Decreased crystallinity less than 45%
     - Decreases mechanical properties
     - PE more prone to macroscopic failure (i.e., cracks)
   - Increased crystallinity greater than 65%
     - The large crystalline phase leaves a very small amorphous phase.

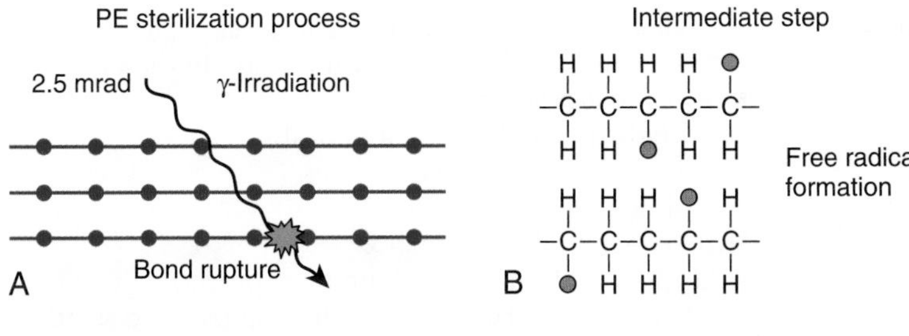

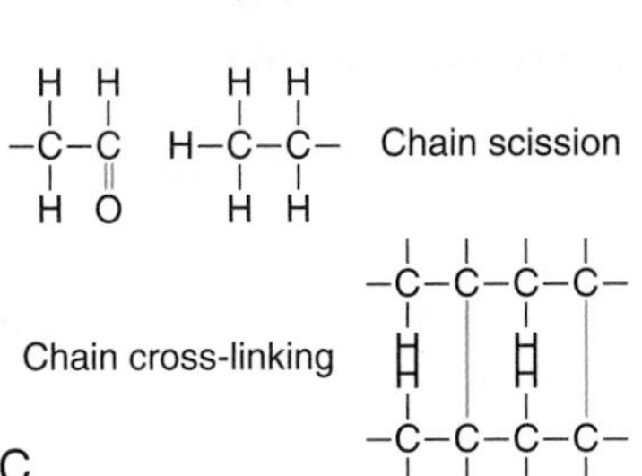

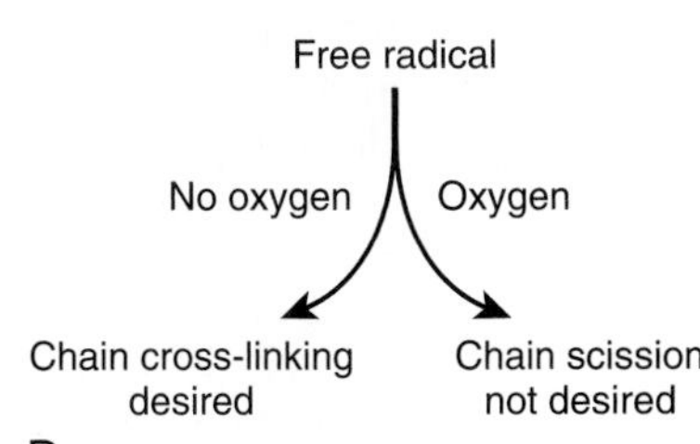

Figure 5-54 Diagram depicting irradiation process of polyethylene (PE). Irradiation of PE causes bond rupture **(A)**, which creates free radicals **(B)**. Free radicals can combine with oxygen to create an oxidized form of PE, which results in chair scission, or, in the absence of oxygen, the PE chains can form cross-links **(C)**. The presence or absence of oxygen determines the pathway that the PE free radicals will take **(D)**. Cross-linking is the desired pathway.

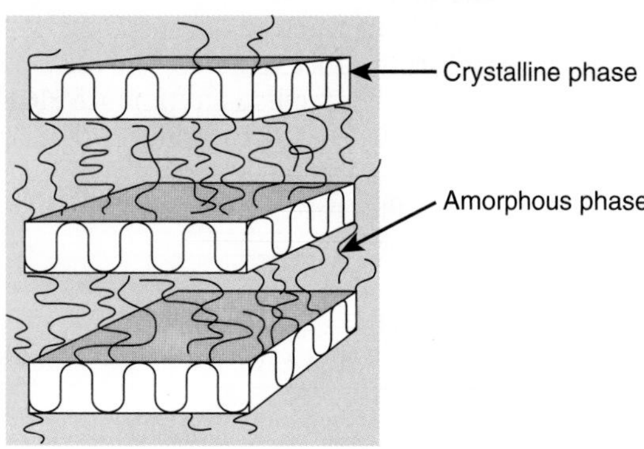

Figure 5-55 Diagram of ultra–high-molecular-weight polyethylene (UHMWPE) phases. The UHMWPE in an implant exists in two forms (phases). They are the crystalline phase and the amorphous phase. The crystalline phase provides the mechanical properties to the polyethylene (PE). When the PE is irradiated, only the amorphous areas cross-link. HCLPE, highly cross-linked polyethylene.

- □ The greatly reduced amorphous region is more susceptible to chain scission oxidation.
- □ Creates significant increase in particulate debris

7. PE heating during HCLPE process
   - There are two techniques of heating PE.
     - □ Annealing—Heat PE to a level *below* melting point.
     - □ Melting—Heat *above* PE melting point.
     - □ UHMWPE melting point—140° C (284° F)
   - Reason for PE heating
     - □ Postirradiation heating eliminates free radicals.
     - □ Melting terminates *all* free radicals.
     - □ Annealing eliminates some but not all free radicals.
       - Risk—potential for in vivo oxidation of PE, resulting in PE debris formation
   - **Melting of HCLPE—problem**
     - □ **Melting of PE reduces *mechanical properties.***
     - □ **Reason—cross-linking of free radicals occurs during melting, which prevents recrystallization.**
     - □ Result—lowered crystallinity with lowered mechanical properties
     - □ Clinical relevance
       - Cracking of PE cup may occur at edges of plastic with *neck impingement.*
       - In the knee—Edge loading or excess PE post loading may cause macroscopic cracks.
   - Annealing of HCLPE—problem
     - □ Annealing of PE increases oxidation potential.
     - □ Reason—Crystalline areas maintain free radicals.
       - During annealing, crystalline areas do not unravel and eliminate free radicals.
       - Crystalline areas do not cross-link, so free radicals remain, leading to oxidation risk.
   - Melted versus annealed HCLPE properties (Table 5-4)
     - □ There are several different methods to produce HCLPE.
       - The processes that produce HCLPE are *not equivalent.*

Table 5-4 Comparison of Melted versus Annealed HCLPE First-Generation Properties

Irradiated and Melted	Irradiated and Annealed
Low crystallinity (<50%)	Good crystallinity (>55%)
Low strength (<40 MPa)	Good strength (>45 MPa)
No oxidation potential	Potential for oxidation
Potential for macroscopic failure	Potential for osteolysis

HCLPE, highly cross-linked polyethylene.

     - □ Each process attempts to
       - Decrease the amount of free radicals
       - Improve oxidation resistance
       - Minimize adverse mechanical properties

8. Second-generation HCLPE processing
   - Similar to first generation, but with additional PE processing to further reduce free radicals
   - Second-generation process
     - □ High-dose irradiation
     - □ Processing of PE—combination of
       - Heating
       - PE treatment
     - □ Sterile packaging
   - Second-generation PE treatments
     - □ Mechanical compression
     - □ Vitamin E impregnation
     - □ Sequential processing
   - Mechanical compression technique
     - □ Heat anneal, then compress rod of plastic down to a smaller-diameter rod.
     - □ Mechanical compression allows PE chains to be closer aligned.
     - □ Free radicals are more likely to be recombined.
     - □ Mechanical compression creates *anisotropic* properties on surface of bearing.
       - This means the PE wear properties vary according to the main orientation of the PE chains.
   - Vitamin E enrichment of PE
     - □ Heat anneal PE
     - □ PE is soaked in vitamin E bath.
     - □ Vitamin E serves as a free-radical scavenger.
       - Vitamin E donates a hydrogen ion to the PE chain.
   - Sequential processing
     - □ Irradiation and low-heat anneal
     - □ Repeat sequence several times.
     - □ More reduction of free radicals
9. HCLPE—clinical performance
   - At this time, there is no long-term proven reduction in osteolysis and THA revision rates compared to standard UHMWPE implants.

Q. PE shelf life

1. Irradiated PE packed in oxygen-free environment minimizes oxidation.
2. However, any remaining free radicals stay in the PE indefinitely.
   - Any remaining free radicals are an oxidation risk.
   - When PE is oxidized, chain scission occurs, which results in increased PE particle debris.
3. Remaining free radicals in PE—relative rank
   - Ethylene oxide and gas plasma—low

- Irradiation (gamma irradiation) plus heat treatment—some
- Irradiation alone—a lot

4. **PE product storage**
   - **Depending on packaging technique, oxygen can diffuse back into PE product.**
   - **Result—*on-the-shelf* oxidation**
5. PE packaging
   - The amount of oxygen that diffuses back into the package depends on two main variables.
     - Packaging material—*most important* factor
       - Defined as diffusion capability
     - Time on shelf
6. **On-shelf oxidation—worst-case scenario**
   - **Gamma irradiation**
   - **Product packaging in air (i.e., oxygen)**
   - **Long shelf life of 5 years or more**
   - **Result is rapid PE wear.**
7. On-shelf oxidation—worrisome scenario
   - High-dose γ-irradiation—HCLPE
   - Heat anneal
   - Permeable oxygen packing
   - Long shelf life of 5 years or more
8. **On-shelf oxidation—Worry about these products.**
   - **Jumbo or extra small implants that are rarely used**
   - **Less frequent procedures—examples**
     - **Unicompartmental replacement**
     - **Elbow/ankle replacement**

III. HARD-ON-HARD BEARING

A. Lubrication mechanism

1. ***Boundary lubrication* when hip at rest or slow motion**
2. ***Hydrodynamic* (also known as *fluid film*) lubrication while walking**

B. Hydrodynamic lubrication

1. Asperities on each surface are small (i.e., highly polished surfaces) and do not make contact.
2. Fluid film lubrication *always* requires angular velocity.
   - Ball must be moving at significant speed.
3. **Factors affecting fluid film state**
   - **Radial clearance**
   - **R_a (Surface roughness)**
   - **Bearing size**
   - **Sphericity**
   - **Bearing material**
4. Radial clearance (Figure 5-56)
   - Radial clearance is defined as
     - Radius of cup minus radius of head
   - Radial clearance defines *contact area* of bearing.
     - Best radial clearance (value depends on biomaterial used) provides *polar contact* with *high conformity*. This value will provide best bearing wear rate.
5. R_a
   - The smoother the bearing surfaces, the better the chance for fluid film lubrication.
   - Supersmooth surfaces are used for hard-on-hard THA alternative bearings.
   - Hard-on-hard bearings—surface roughness
     - Metal (Co-Cr)—R_a 0.01 μm
     - Ceramics—R_a 0.006 μm
   - Comparison

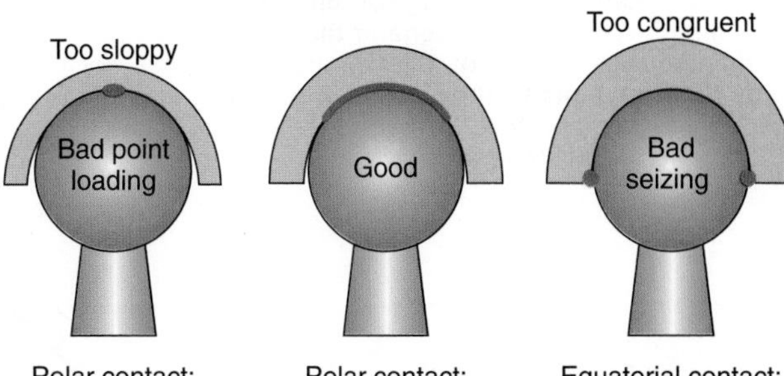

Figure 5-56 Diagram showing effect of radial clearance and surface contact area of alternative hard-on-hard total hip arthroplasty bearing. *Left,* A relatively high radial clearance. With a high radial clearance, hip loading is concentrated in a small polar contact region. This is disadvantageous and causes higher wear rates. *Right,* A relatively low radial clearance. With a low radial clearance, fluid is not able to effectively ingress and egress the bearing region. This creates a fluid *lockout* state, which causes high friction and wear. *Center,* Ideal radial clearance, which allows adequate fluid flow within the bearing, but also provides optimum surface contact area for best wear.

     - Red blood cell diameter—R_a 100s μm
     - Machined PE—R_a 7.0 μm

6. Bearing size
   - The greater the head radius, the better the chance for fluid film lubrication.
     - Head radius is *directly* related to the lambda (λ)-ratio (a formula defining fluid film mechanics). The higher the λ-ratio, the better the chance for fluid film mechanics.
7. Sphericity
   - Desired goal is perfectly round.
     - Sphericity depends on manufacturing technique and good quality assurance.
     - Goal is to keep sphericity less than 7 μm.
     - High points cause localized stress points that increase friction.
8. Bearing material
   - Metal (Co-Cr alloy)—High carbide (i.e., high carbon content alloy) content is better. A high carbide content creates a harder bearing surface, which provides better bearing wear.
   - Ceramics—generally smoother than superpolished Co-Cr alloy

C. The stripe line

1. Primarily described on ceramic-ceramic bearings, but similar effect can occur on metal-metal bearings
2. **Defined as an area of roughness created on the head and cup as a result of *repetitive subclinical subluxation;* hip is in *lever range*** (Figure 5-57)
   - Subluxation with sit to stand
   - Repetitive end-range activities
   - **Subluxation as head distracts out of socket during end swing phase**
   - Stripe line is detected microscopically. It is not caused by metal smear effect.
3. **Stripe line indicates abnormal bearing wear mechanics.**

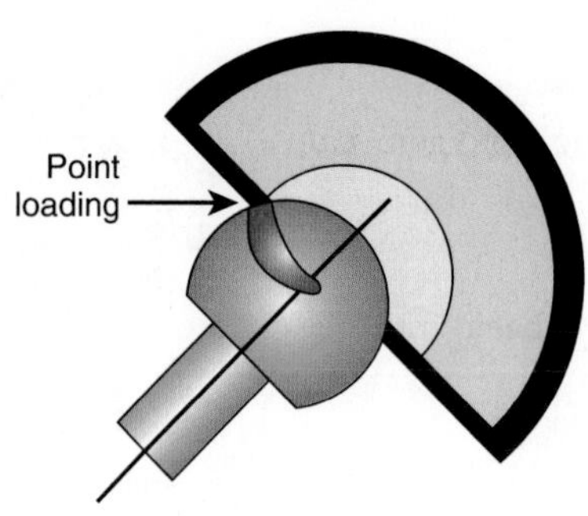

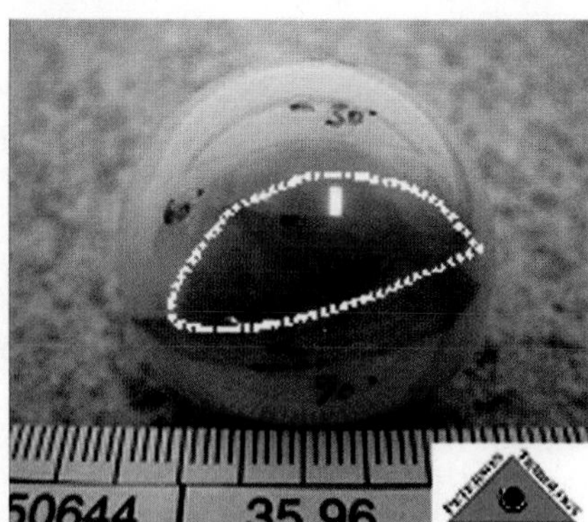

Figure 5-57 *Left,* Diagram depicting stripe line. With repetitive subclinical subluxation, the prosthetic head rotates upon the edge of cup bearing. This is a high-contact-stress scenario that roughens the articular surface of the femoral head. *Right,* Slide attempts to show stripe line, which is highlighted on the ball. Stripe line detection requires microscopic review.

- Technical goals surgically are to reduce lever range subluxation with better component design, positioning, and offset.

D. Metal-metal wear

1. **Very small particles generated**
   - **0.015- to 0.12-μm particles (i.e., nanometer-sized particles)**
2. **Very low linear wear**
3. **Very low volumetric wear**
4. **However, *absolute* number of particles generated is significantly *greater* than comparable PE bearing.**
5. *Run-in wear*
   - Described mainly for metal-metal bearing
   - Run-in wear is the higher wear rate seen within the first 1 million cycles (approximately 1 year of high activity).
   - Etiology—in vivo polishing of the two new round bearing surfaces
     - Polish out *high points*
       - Areas out of round
       - Areas of prominent carbide asperities
     - Very small changes occur in diameters with polishing.
   - After run-in wear, the wear rate reduces to a lower *steady state* rate.

E. Metal-metal debris response

1. Very small nanometer particles can dissolve to generate cobalt and low-valence (Cr^{3+}) chromium ions.
2. With normal bearing wear, there will be detectable cobalt and chromium levels in urine and blood.
3. Serum and urine levels *correlate* to bearing wear rate.
   - High blood levels of cobalt and chromium (after run-in phrase) correlate to abnormal bearing wear.
     - Usually a result of repetitive subclinical subluxation and poor prosthetic mating
4. **Biologic response to wear debris**
   - **Metal debris from metal-metal bearing processed by the *T-cell lymphocyte***
   - There are two distinct responses:
     - Hypersensitivity reaction
       - Seen immediately after implantation
     - Particulate-induced T-cell response (PITR)
       - Seen later (3 to 5 years)
6. Hypersensitivity response
   - Generally rare
   - Almost always associated with nickel (Ni^{2+}) ion
   - Reaction starts after placement of implant in vivo
     - Pain and ache start soon after postoperative recovery.
   - Persistent dull ache (24/7 characteristic)
   - Fluid aspiration—low white blood cell (WBC) count
   - Treatment is replacement with nickel-free implant (i.e., remove Co-Cr alloy metal).
7. **PITR**
   - **Related to continued debris formation at a *high rate***
   - **Involves a highly activated RANKL system**
   - Ultimate response is *pseudotumor formation.*
     - Cobalt and chromium particles combine with a serum protein, which is then recognized by the T cell.
   - The activated T-cell response has many associated cytokines, including
     - Interleukin-2, interleukin-6
     - Interferon-γ
     - RANKL (which stimulates osteoclastogenesis)
   - RANKL and RANK are partly controlled by sex hormones.
     - This is why *women* are more likely to be affected by the PITR reaction.
8. PITR/pseudotumor response—clinical presentation
   - Pain and ache about hip starts first (3 to 5 years after joint replacement).
   - Effusion develops around hip.
     - Detectable by ultrasonography and/or MRI
   - Osteolysis around implants
   - Pseudotumor formation (Figure 5-58)
     - MRI shows large inflammatory mass around hip that extends into pelvis and/or thigh.
     - Tissues show inflammatory mass primarily of lymphocytes.
       - Also known as *aseptic lymphocytic- and vasculitic-associated lesion (ALVAL)*
     - Regional tissues around hip show necrosis.
       - Cobalt and chrome toxicity
9. PITR/pseudotumor—treatment
   - Remove Co-Cr bearing.
   - Revise loose implants.
     - Use titanium alloy implants for revision.
   - Radical soft tissue débridement
     - Debulk toxic tissues.
   - Use ceramic-PE bearing or ceramic-ceramic bearing (no Co-Cr heads).

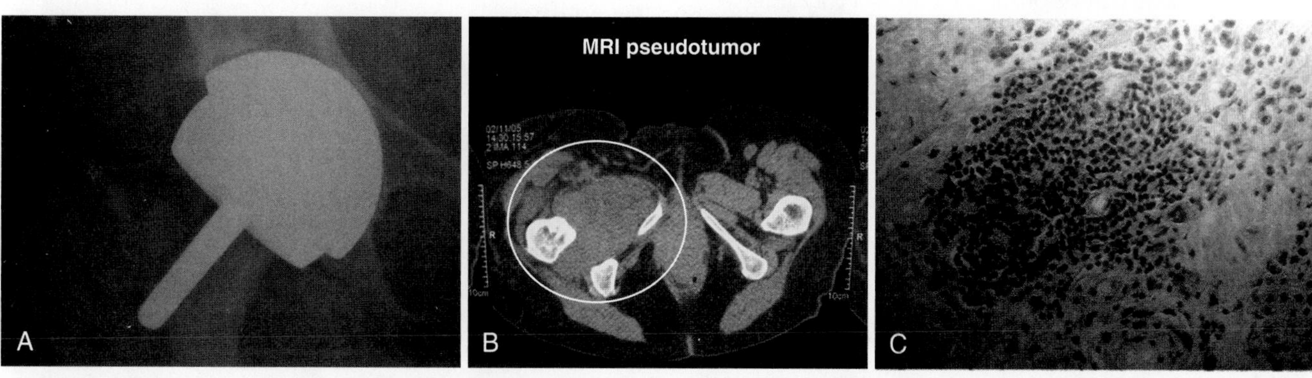

Figure 5-58 Case example of pseudotumor following metal-metal resurfacing arthroplasty. **A,** Radiograph of total articular resurfacing (TAR) implant with osteolysis in superior cup region and around superior femoral neck region. **B,** Magnetic resonance image (MRI) of local hip region showing large mass that extends into pelvis *(circle)*. **C,** At surgery, the large inflammatory mass shows aggregates of T cells surrounding vascular structures. Special staining will also reveal metal debris particles in these regions as well. PITR, particulate-induced T-cell response.

F. Metal-metal—specific conditions

1. **Avoid metal-metal bearing in a woman of childbearing age.**
   - **Metal ions do cross placenta.**
2. **Avoid in renal failure.**
   - **Metal ions no longer eliminated.**

G. Metal-metal—cancer risk

1. To date, with metal-metal bearing use, there has been *no increased* risk for cancer compared with standardized populations.
2. However, with high-bearing-wear scenarios, the local tissues are subject to potential metaplasia/dysplasia from metal ions.

H. Ceramic-ceramic bearing

1. **First-generation alumina—high head fracture rate (up to 13.4%)**—reasons
   - More related to *neck impingement* (Figure 5-59)
     - Adverse head/neck ratio
     - Ceramic heads with thick skirts
   - Poor manufacturing technique

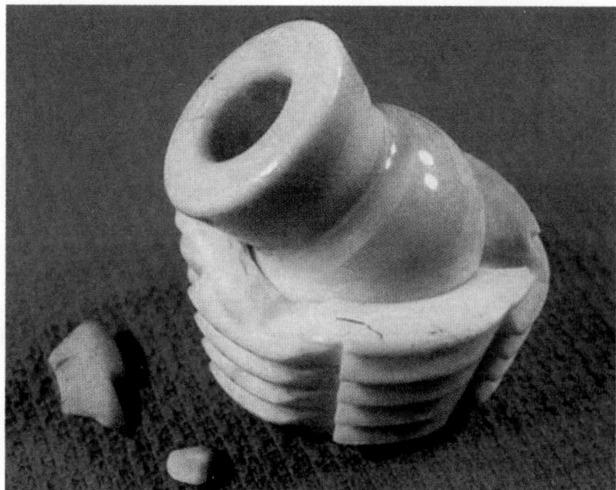

Figure 5-59 Photograph of retrieved first-generation ceramic-ceramic total hip arthroplasty. Notice very thick neck, which was required for strength in first-generation systems. The enlarged neck adversely reduced head/neck ratio. Also note acetabular fracture resulting from neck impingement.

   - Low ceramic density
   - Coarse microstructure
2. **Third-generation alumina results in lower fracture rate.**
   - Improved manufacturing technique
   - Hot isostatic pressed technique
   - High ceramic density
   - Finer microstructure
   - Skirt elimination results in better head/neck ratio.
3. Advantage
   - *Lowest wear*
     - Generally less wear (both linear and volumetric) than metal-metal
     - Fewer particles generated than with metal-metal
   - Bioinert debris
     - No ionization of particles
     - No cancer risk
     - No dysplasia/metaplasia effects on local soft tissues
4. Disadvantage
   - Head size limitation
     - Ceramic socket must be placed within a metal acetabular shell. Also, ceramic socket must have a minimum thickness to limit fracture. These factors limit ultimate ceramic head size.
     - Stability is less than large-diameter metal-metal bearing.
     - Fluid film mechanics less optimal with smaller head radius.
   - Head length limitation
     - No skirts allowed
     - Can potentially limit hip offset, leading to hip impingement and instability
   - Hip squeak
     - Psychologically affects patients with daily audible squeak
     - Etiology—perfect storm consisting of
       - Implant malpositioning
       - Lever range wear
         - Stripe line formation, which creates an arcuate rough area on head
       - Implant resonance—vibratory resonance created by lever range over rough region is amplified by

prosthetic construct, which is audible in ear frequency range
- Treatment is revision of the cup to PE bearing with head change (head is damaged by squeak).
- Fracture
  - The Achilles' heel of this material when used for hip bearing
  - Fracture is due to *low toughness* of material.
  - Fracture treatment
    - Must replace with another ceramic-ceramic bearing
    - After fracture, microscopic shards of ceramic remain and are *severely abrasive.*
    - If a PE bearing is placed after ceramic bearing fracture, there will be rapid PE wear.

5. Head change
   - Any ceramic head placed on a used femoral neck must have an internal metal jacket (Figure 5-60).
   - A used femoral neck is roughened by wear and corrosion.
   - A new ceramic head (without a metal jacket) placed on a roughened neck can fracture with repetitive hip loading. High points on roughened neck cause a *burst fracture.*

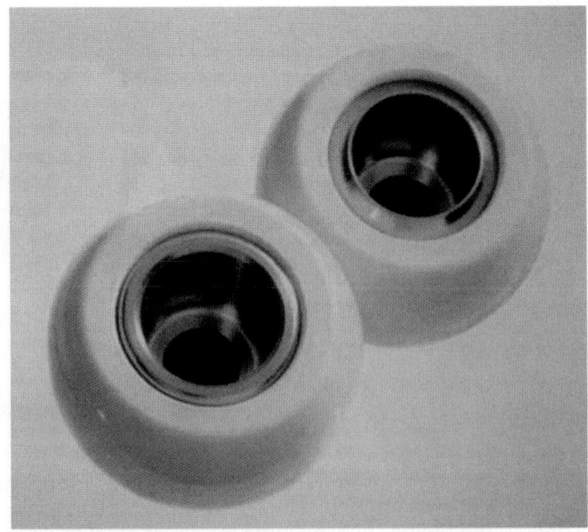

Figure 5-60 Photograph of internal metal jacket in ceramic head. This internal metal sleeve protects the head from burst fracture when placed onto a used femoral neck that has been roughened by use.

SECTION 13 KNEE ARTHRITIS ASSESSMENT

Patient assessment of knee pain includes a physical examination and diagnostic radiographic modalities.

I. CLINICAL PRESENTATION

A. Pain with weight bearing
1. Aggravated by stairs, hills, sit to stand

B. Bowing deformity and instability
1. Seen later in presentation

II. IMAGING STUDIES

A. Radiographs are still the standard for initial evaluation. Images should include
1. Weight-bearing anteroposterior and lateral
2. Weight-bearing 45-degree bent knee, imaged posterior to anterior
   - X-ray plate is positioned parallel to tibia.
3. Sunrise view (i.e., merchant view)
4. Extension and flexion lateral

B. MRI
1. Grossly overused in the arthritic patient population
2. If the joint space is significantly narrowed on radiograph, then MRI is *not* indicated.
3. Used when osteonecrosis is suspected

C. CT scan
1. Three-dimensional CT with remodeling used for preoperative planning for reconstruction associated with dysplasia planning, post-trauma planning, and complex total knee arthroplasty (TKA) planning

SECTION 14 KNEE ARTHRITIS TREATMENT

I. NONOPERATIVE

A. Activity modification
1. Reduce impact-loading exercises
2. Reduce weight
3. Avoid stairs, inclines, squatting

B. Nonsteroidal anti-inflammatory drugs
1. Cyclooxygenase-2 inhibition

C. Joint injections
1. Corticosteroid–anti-inflammatory treatment
2. Hyaluronate
   - Backbone of proteoglycan chain of articular cartilage
   - Improves joint rheology

D. Unloading brace
1. Helpful but compliance low
2. Best suited for exercise activity

E. Assist device (cane or crutch)
1. Opposite hand of affected knee

II. OPERATIVE

A. Arthroscopy
1. Palliative treatment only
2. Use selectively
   - Overaggressive articular shaving accelerates natural course of degeneration.

3. Success *directly* related to degree of *mechanical* symptoms noted preoperatively
   - Meniscal tears with catching and locking
   - Loose bodies
   - Unstable cartilaginous flaps
4. Success *inversely* related to the severity of arthritis
   - Not helpful in moderate to advanced disease
   - Will not take away toothache pain caused by reactive bone edema from mechanical overload
5. Palliative results less effective in the presence of knee malalignment (varus or excess valgus)
   - Malalignment causes mechanical overload and bone pain.

B. Osteotomy

1. **Best indication**
   - **Young active patient generally under the age of 50 years**
2. Most likely to succeed when disease affects predominantly one compartment
3. **For *varus* knee malalignment**
   - **Treatment is valgus-producing proximal tibial osteotomy.**
   - Reason—Problem typically is result of proximal tibial varus. (Surgery goal is to correct the deforming problem.)
   - Osteotomy goal—Maintain joint line of knee perpendicular to the *mechanical* axis of the leg.
     - Mechanical axis of leg defined as center of hip through center of knee to center of ankle
4. **For *valgus* knee malalignment**
   - **Treatment is varus-producing supracondylar femoral osteotomy.**
   - Reason—Problem typically is result of lateral femoral condylar hypoplasia. (Surgery goal is to correct the deforming problem.)
   - Osteotomy goal—Maintain joint line of knee perpendicular to the mechanical axis of the leg.
5. Valgus-producing tibial osteotomy (for varus knee deformity)
   - Selection criteria
     - Clinical examination and radiographs show other two compartments are free of arthritis.
   - **Contraindications**
     - **Inflammatory arthritis**
     - **Lack of flexion—minimum of 90 degrees needed**
     - Flexion contracture over 10 degrees
     - Ligament instability
       - Especially varus thrust gait
       - ***Not* contraindicated in cruciate-ligament insufficiency**
     - Lateral tibial subluxation greater than 1 cm
     - Medial compartment bone loss
     - Lateral compartment joint narrowing
       - Detected by valgus stress radiograph
   - Osteotomy less successful when
     - Smoking
     - Age 60 years or older
     - Varus deformity of 10 degrees or more
       - There is just not enough bone to remove to correct deformity.
     - Concomitant arthritis in other compartments
   - Main problems
     - Closed-wedge technique
       - Patella baja deformity
       - Loss of tibial posterior slope
     - Open-wedge technique
       - Nonunion
       - Loss of valgus correction (i.e., collapse of open wedge)
6. Varus-producing femoral osteotomy (for valgus knee deformity)
   - Selection criteria
     - Clinical examination and radiographs show other two compartments are free of arthritis.
   - **Contraindications**
     - **Inflammatory arthritis**
     - **Prior medial meniscectomy**
     - **Deformity over 15 degrees valgus**
       - There is just not enough bone to remove to correct deformity.
     - Flexion contracture over 10 degrees

C. Unicompartmental arthroplasty

1. Used for patients in whom arthritis predominantly affects one compartment
   - Most common is medical compartment replacement.
2. **Advantage**
   - **Quicker recovery compared to TKA and osteotomy**
   - Fewer short-term complications
   - Better knee function
     - Anterior cruciate ligament (ACL) is not sacrificed as it is in TKA.
   - **Smaller incision**
     - **Shorter hospital stay with less postoperative pain**
3. **Results**
   - High rate of short-term to midterm satisfaction
   - However, long-term survivorship is *not comparable* to TKA when measured by revision rates.
4. **Contraindications**
   - **Inflammatory arthritis**
   - **Significant fixed deformity**
     - **Must be able to correct deformity on clinical examination (e.g., must correct resting varus attitude to normal valgus)**
   - **Previous meniscectomy in *opposite* compartment**
   - **ACL deficiency—key**
     - **ACL deficiency is an *absolute* contraindication for a mobile-bearing unicompartmental replacement.**
   - **Flexion contracture greater than 10 degrees**
   - **Tricompartmental arthritis**
5. Selection criteria—important
   - Pain must be localized to the compartment being replaced.
   - Anterior knee pain means significant patellofemoral disease.
   - Diffuse or global pain means tricompartmental disease.
6. Technique
   - Do not overcorrect.
     - Overcorrection places increased load to unresurfaced compartment.
     - Can cause early failure due to arthritis
   - For varus deformity
     - Correct to 1 to 5 degrees of valgus
7. **Complication**
   - **Stress fracture**
     - **Always involves tibial side**

- **Associated with heavy weight and high activity level**
- **Clinically, pain-free interval, then spontaneous onset of pain with activity**
- Aspiration of knee shows blood.

8. Failure mechanisms
   - Overcorrection at time of surgery
     - Risk is disease progression in opposite compartment.
   - Undercorrection at time of surgery
     - Risk is implant overload with subsequent failure.
   - Fixed-bearing implants
     - More likely to fail from mechanical loosening
   - Mobile-bearing implants
     - More likely to fail from disease progression
   - Patellar impingement upon femoral implant
     - Patellar pain requiring revision to TKA

D. Isolated patellofemoral arthritis

1. TKA (not patellofemoral arthroplasty) is recommended choice in older patients.
   - Superior functional results compared to patellectomy or patellofemoral arthroplasty.
2. **Lateral retinacular release commonly seen with isolated patellofemoral arthritis.**
   - Maltracking is usually the cause of isolated patellofemoral arthritis.
3. Patellofemoral replacement procedure
   - Precise soft tissue balancing required for successful result
     - Residual maltracking causes pain.
     - Must restore a patellofemoral alignment to a normal Q angle

E. Total knee arthroplasty: See next section.

SECTION 15 TOTAL KNEE ARTHROPLASTY

I. INDICATIONS

A. Debilitating pain affecting activities of daily living
B. Pain not well controlled by conservative measures
C. Medically fit for surgery
D. No active infection—anywhere

II. TKA SURVIVAL

A. Best survival

1. Well-balanced knee
2. Neutral *mechanical* alignment

B. Decreased survivorship

1. Young age—55 years or less
2. Osteoarthritis
3. Reason—high activity level

C. Increased survivorship

1. Old age—70 years or older
2. Rheumatoid arthritis
3. Cemented fixation (all components)
4. Reason—low activity level

III. TECHNICAL GOALS OF TKA

A. Restore neutral *mechanical* alignment of limb
B. Restore joint line
C. Balanced ligaments
D. Normal Q angle

IV. PREOPERATIVE PLANNING FOR TKA

A. Preoperative radiographs should include

1. *Standing* bilateral anteroposterior knees
2. Extension and flexion lateral
3. Sunrise (merchant view)
4. Standing *full-length* anteroposterior hip to ankle when
   - Bony angular deformity present
   - Very short stature
     - Below 60 inches (152 cm)
   - Very tall stature
     - Above 75 inches (190 cm)

B. Radiographic analysis

1. Determine *end cuts*—femur and tibia.
2. Determine position of femoral canal entry site at the knee.
3. Identify bone defects.
4. Identify joint subluxation.
5. Identify ligament stretch-out.
   - If *varus thrust* gait is evident, then standing single-leg anteroposterior radiographs are recommended (Figure 5-61).
6. Determine anticipated ligament releases.
7. Anticipate extent of constraint needed from preoperative review of radiographs.

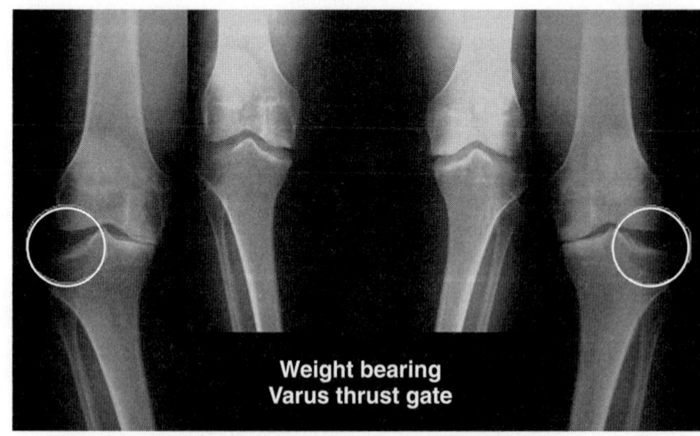

Figure 5-61 Preoperative review of patient in preparation of total knee arthroplasty. Standing anteroposterior (middle radiograph) shows varus attitude of knees. Patient clinically had significant varus thrust bilaterally. Standing single-leg-stance radiographs (*left* and *right* radiographs) demonstrate severity of lateral ligament stretch-out. In this case, a revision knee system was ordered to accommodate potential instability problems that may be encountered during balancing and trialing.

C. End cuts—distal femur and proximal tibia

1. Goal with end cuts is to restore neutral *mechanical* alignment of the limb.
   - Neutral mechanical alignment is defined as a line from hip head center, through knee center, to ankle center.
2. Preoperative analysis of femur (review of full-length radiographs) is used to determine the following (Figure 5-62).
   - Anatomic axis of femur (AAF)
     - □ A line that bisects the medullary canal of the femur
     - □ The AAF, drawn to the distal end of the femur, determines *entry point* for the femoral medullary guide rod for the cutting jigs.
   - Mechanical axis of femur (MAF)
     - □ A line from center of distal femur to center of femoral head
     - □ Significance—The distal femur is cut *perpendicular* to MAF.
       - This allows even mechanical loading to knee implant.
   - Valgus cut angle
     - □ Defined as angle between AAF and MAF
     - □ Intramedullary guide rod is placed into femur (this defines AAF).
     - □ Distal femoral cut jig is assembled to intramedullary guide rod.
     - □ Surgeon selects valgus cut angle (typically between 4 and 7 degrees).
     - □ Distal femur should end up being *perpendicular* to MAF.
     - □ Always measure valgus cut angle in tall and short patients (Figure 5-63).
       - Hip offset remains relatively constant.
       - Femur length, therefore, has more influence upon valgus cut angle.

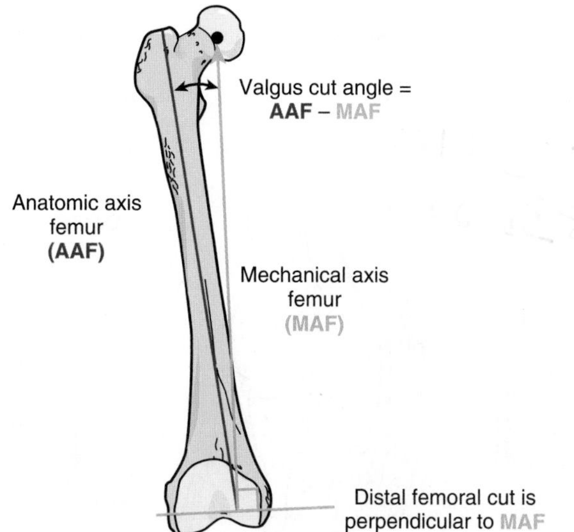

Figure 5-62 Diagram showing preoperative measurements of femur to make distal femoral end cut. The distal femur is cut perpendicular to the mechanical axis of the femur. The anatomic axis of the femur (AAF) is defined clinically by the intramedullary guide that is placed into the canal. A cutting jig is placed onto the medullary guide rod. The distal valgus cut angle is the value set into the cutting jig to make the distal femoral cut perpendicular to the mechanical axis. Also, note the location where the AAF exits the distal femur. This is the position to open the distal femur to insert the medullary guide rod.

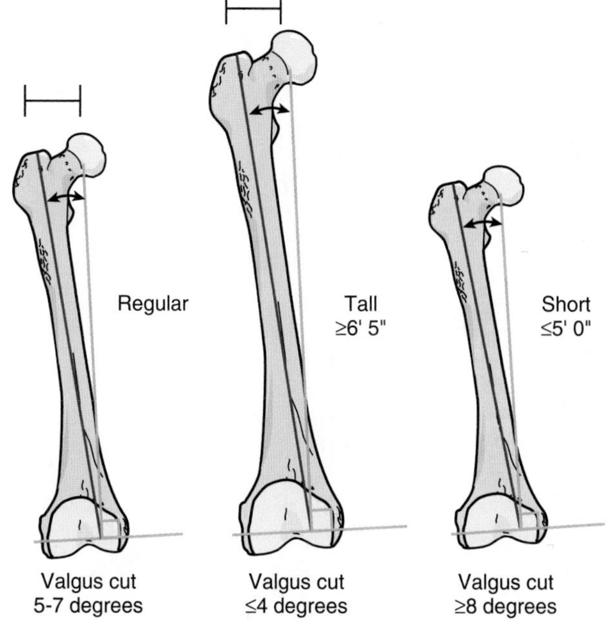

Figure 5-63 Effect of femoral length on valgus cut angle. Hip offset does not vary widely. Therefore valgus cut angle is more influenced by femoral length. Tall patients will have lower valgus cut angle, whereas short patients will have higher valgus cut angle.

3. Preoperative analysis tibia (review of full-length radiograph) is used to determine the following (Figure 5-64).
   - Anatomic axis of tibia (AAT)
     - □ A line that bisects the medullary canal of the tibia
     - □ The AAT, drawn through the proximal tibia, determines the entry point for the tibial medullary guide.
       - Both intramedullary and extramedullary cutting jigs for the proximal tibial end cut are acceptable techniques.
   - Mechanical axis of tibia (MAT)
     - □ A line from center of proximal tibia to the center of ankle
     - □ Significance—The proximal tibia is cut *perpendicular* to MAT.
       - This allows even mechanical loading to knee implant.
   - Tibial cut angle
     - □ Defined as angle between AAT and MAT
     - □ Intramedullary guide technique
       - Intramedullary guide is placed into tibia.
       - Proximal tibia cut jig is assembled to intramedullary guide.
       - Surgeon selects tibial cut angle (usually 0 degrees).
       - Proximal tibia should end up being cut *perpendicular* to MAT.
     - □ Extramedullary guide technique
       - The extramedullary guide technique is placed over the anterior tibia. A jig distally holds guide centered over ankle. A proximal jig holds guide centered over proximal tibia (landmark is medial one-third region of tibial tubercle).
       - Surgeon selects tibial cut angle.

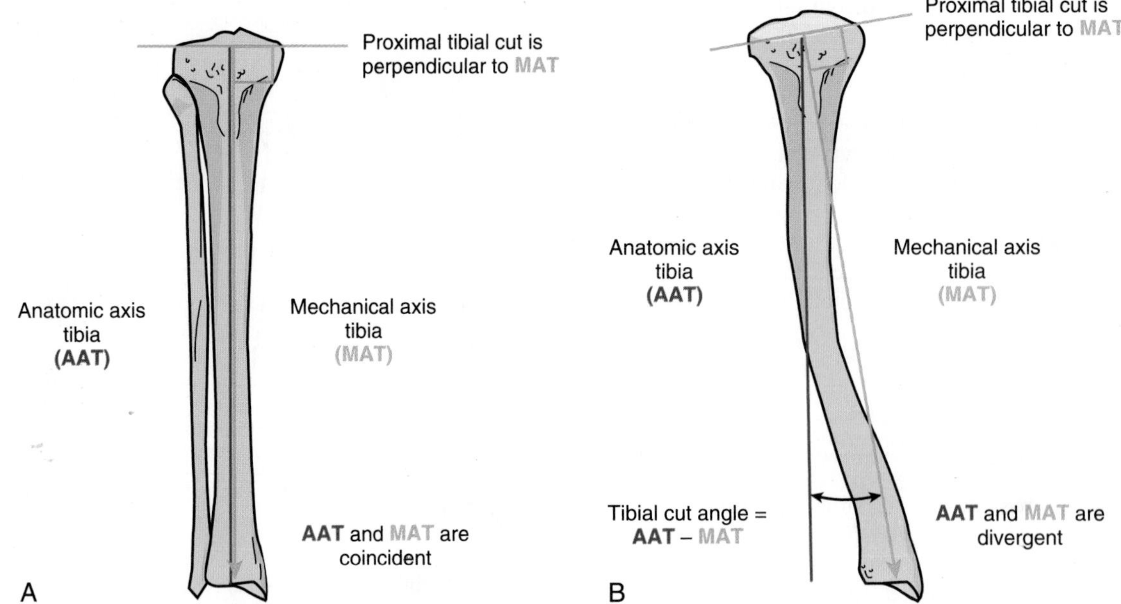

Figure 5-64 Diagrams showing preoperative measurements of tibia to make proximal tibial end cut. The proximal tibia is cut perpendicular to the mechanical axis of the tibia (MAT). **A,** Usually the anatomic axis of the tibia (AAT) and MAT are coincident. In this situation the tibial end cut is zero. **B,** In the situation where a tibial angular deformity is present, the AAT and MAT are divergent. The tibial cut angle is carefully measured to make a tibia end cut perpendicular to the MAT.

- In most cases the AAT and MAT are coincident. Therefore tibial cut angle is zero.
- When there is a tibial deformity (such as a fracture), the AAT and MAT are divergent. The tibial cut angle is then carefully measured and selected to provide a proximal tibial end cut perpendicular to MAT.

V. BONE CUTS IN TKA—GOALS

A. *Measured resection*—Replace bone and cartilage with implants that are of the same thickness.

1. Maintains joint line, which is important for proper ligament function
2. Maintains ligament tension
3. Accurate bone cuts are accomplished with cutting jigs.

VI. CORONAL PLANE LIGAMENT BALANCING IN TKA

A. Correction of varus or valgus deformity

B. Balancing goals

1. Equal ligament tension in medial and lateral compartments tested in extension and in flexion

C. Principle (Figure 5-65)

1. Release concave side—tight side
2. Retension convex side—loose side

D. Varus deformity

1. Convex side is lateral—loose
2. Concave side is medial—medial compartment release needed
3. **Medial compartment release in sequence**
   - **Osteophytes**
   - **Deep medial collateral ligament (MCL; also known as meniscal tibial ligament)**
     - Includes medial knee capsule
   - **Posterior medial corner**
     - Capsule
     - Semimembranosus
   - **Superficial MCL—key structure** (Figure 5-66)
     - ***Posterior oblique portion* tight in extension**
       - **Release for medial extension tightness.**
     - ***Anterior portion* tight in flexion**
       - **Release for medial flexion tightness.**

E. Valgus deformity

1. Convex side is medial side—loose
2. Concave side is lateral side—lateral compartment release needed
3. **Lateral compartment release in sequence**
   - **Osteophytes**

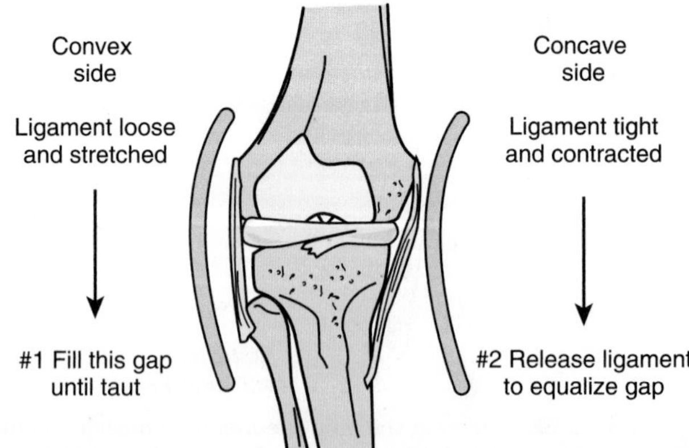

Figure 5-65 Diagram demonstrating principle of coronal plane balance in total knee arthroplasty. The knee in this example has a varus deformity. The lateral side of the knee is the convex side where the ligaments have been stretched from the deformity. On this side, the lateral joint space is filled with the prosthesis until the ligament is once again under normal tension. The concave side is the medial side where the ligament is tight and contracted. The medial ligament complex is released until there is equal tension between the medial and lateral compartments.

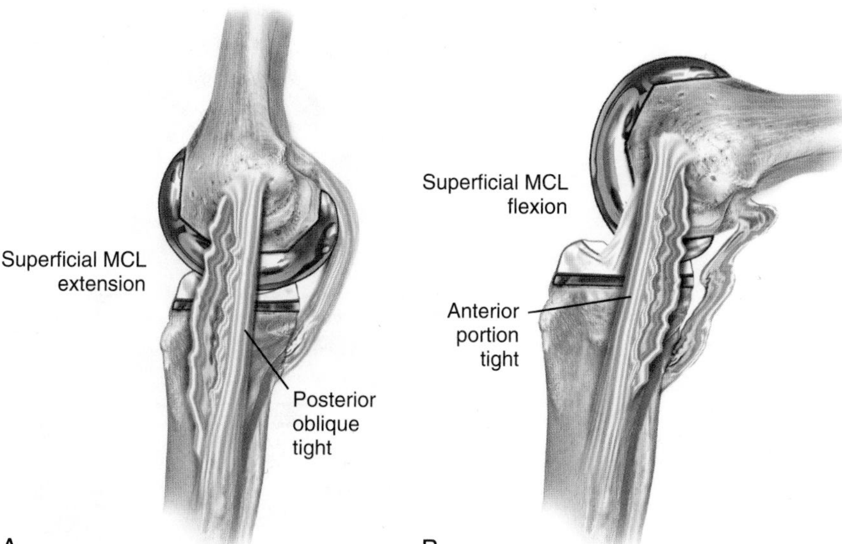

Figure 5-66 Diagram showing the two major portions of superficial medial collateral ligament (MCL). **A,** In extension, the posterior oblique portion of the ligament is taut. The posterior oblique portion is released for medial extension ligament contracture. **B,** In flexion, the anterior portion is tight. The anterior portion is released for medial flexion ligament contracture. (Courtesy of Leo Whiteside, MD.)

- **Lateral capsule**
- **Iliotibial band—key structure**
  - Tight in extension
    - Release for lateral extension tightness.
- **Popliteus—key structure**
  - Tight in flexion
    - Release for lateral flexion tightness.
  - Release popliteus off *anterior* portion of lateral epicondyle (Figure 5-67).
- **Lateral collateral ligament—last**

VII. FLEXION DEFORMITY (I.E., FLEXION CONTRACTURE)

A. **Concave side is posterior—posterior knee release required**

B. **Posterior knee release—in sequence**

1. **Osteophytes**
2. **Posterior capsule**
3. **Gastrocnemius muscle origin**

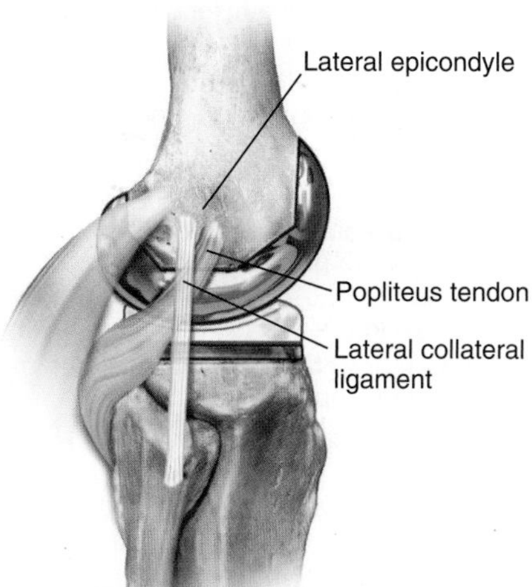

Figure 5-67 Anatomic relationship of popliteus tendon to lateral collateral ligament (LCL). The popliteal tendon inserts onto lateral epicondyle just in front of (distal and anterior to) lateral collateral ligament.

C. **Posterior releases are performed with the knee *flexed* (generally at 90 degrees of flexion).**

1. Less danger to popliteal artery

VIII. SAGITTAL PLANE BALANCING IN TKA

A. **Also known as *balancing the gaps***

B. **Balancing goal**

1. **Full extension and full flexion**

C. **Importance**

1. **Full functional knee range**
2. **Stability**
3. **Pain relief**
   Unbalanced gaps cause pain from tightness or pain from instability.

D. **Flexion gap—controlled by (Figure 5-68)**

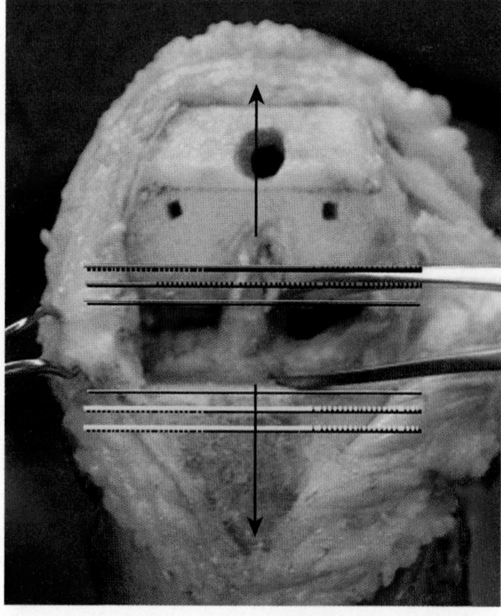

Figure 5-68 Intraoperative photo of knee showing structures that control flexion gap space. The flexion gap is controlled by the posterior cut of the femur, the tibial cut, and the posterior cruciate ligament (PCL).

1. *Posterior* cut of femur
2. Tibial cut
3. Posterior cruciate ligament (PCL)

E. Extension gap—controlled by (Figure 5-69)
1. *Distal* cut of femur
2. Tibial cut
3. Posterior capsule

F. Balancing the gaps
1. *McPherson's* rule
   - *Symmetric* gap problem—Adjust *tibia* first.
   - *Asymmetric* gap problem—Adjust *femur* first.
2. Table 5-5 reviews all sagittal plane gap scenarios. Follow above rule, and this will guide you to a solution.
   - For some gap imbalance scenarios, there is more than one possible solution.

IX. TKA—COMPLICATIONS

A. Femoral notch
1. Occurs when making anterior femoral bone cut, and saw cuts into femoral cortex
   - This happens when cutting jig is placed a little too low on distal femur.
2. An anterior femoral notch
   - Lessens load needed to cause fracture
   - In torsional load, there is no change in fracture location.

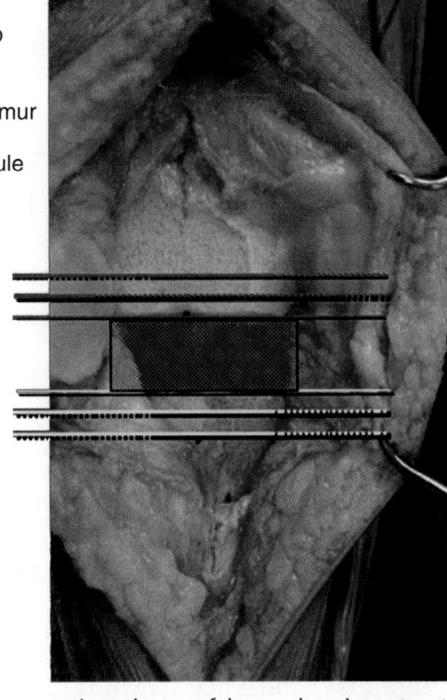
Extension Gap
Controlled by
• ***Distal*** cut of femur
• Tibial cut
• Posterior capsule

Figure 5-69 Intraoperative photo of knee showing structures that control extension gap space. The extension gap is controlled by the distal cut of the femur, the tibial cut, and the posterior capsule.

Table 5-5 Review of Sagittal Plane TKA Gap Scenarios Sagittal Plane Balancing—Total Knee Replacement

Scenario	Problem	Solutions
Tight in extension (contracture) Tight in flexion (will not bend fully)	Symmetric gap • Did not cut enough tibial bone	1. Cut more proximal tibia
Loose in extension (recurvatum) Loose in flexion (large drawer test)	Symmetric gap • Cut too much tibial bone	1. Use thicker polyethylene insert 2. Metallic tibial augmentation
Extension good Loose in flexion (large drawer test)	Asymmetric gap • Cut too much posterior femur	1. Increase size of femoral component from anterior to posterior (i.e., go up to next size). Fill posterior gap with either cement or metal augmentation. 2. Translate femoral component posteriorly (femur size unchanged). Fill posterior gap with either cement or metal augmentation. 3. Use thicker polyethylene insert and readdress as tight extension gap.
Tight in extension (contracture) Flexion good	Asymmetric gap • Did not release enough posterior capsule or • Did not cut enough distal femur	1. Release posterior capsule. 2. Take off more distal femur bone (1-2 mm at a time).
Extension good Tight in flexion (will not bend fully)	Asymmetric gap • Did not cut enough posterior bone or • PCL scarred and too tight (assuming use of a PCL-retaining knee system) • No posterior slope in tibial bone cut (i.e., anterior slope)	1. Decrease size of femoral component from anterior to posterior (i.e., recut to next smaller size). 2. Recess PCL 3. Check posterior slope of tibia, and recut if anterior slope is present.
Loose in extension (recurvatum) Flexion good	Asymmetric gap • Cut too much distal femur or • Anteroposterior size too big	1. Distal femoral augmentation 2. Use thicker tibial polyethylene inset, and readdress as tight flexion gap. 3. Decrease size of femoral component from anterior to posterior (i.e., recut to next smaller size), and readdress as symmetric gap problem.

PCL, posterior cruciate ligament; TKA, total knee arthroplasty.

- **In *bending*, fracture starts at notch, creating a short oblique fracture.**
- Caution—Do not manipulate a TKA with a notch.

B. Peroneal nerve palsy

1. **Deformity most likely to cause nerve palsy with TKA is *valgus flexion deformity.***
   - **Valgus deformity plus**
   - **Flexion contracture**
2. **When peroneal palsy is identified postoperatively, the *first* treatment is**
   - **Remove compressive wraps and**
   - **Flex the knee**
3. If the nerve is not cut, most palsies will resolve within 3 months.
4. If nerve palsy does not resolve after 3 months and nerve has not been cut (test by electromyogram/nerve conduction velocity)
   - Recommendation is to explore and decompress the peroneal nerve.

C. Lateral retinacular release

1. **The artery at risk for transection is the lateral superior genicular artery.**
   - **Transection of this artery increases risk for osteonecrosis of the patella.**

D. Patella fracture

1. Causes
   - Overresection of patella bone
     - □ Minimum thickness is *13 mm.*
   - Compromised circulation
     - □ Big lateral retinacular release (transection of lateral superior geniculate)
     - □ Osteonecrosis with fracture and fragmentation
   - Patellofemoral maltracking
   - Direct trauma
2. Treatment
   - Patella component solid and minimal lag
     - □ Controlled motion brace is initially locked in extension. Slowly increase flexion in increments.
   - Loose patella component
     - □ Component revision if there is enough remaining bone; remove smaller fragments
     - □ Component resection if there is not enough remaining bone to support resurfacing
   - Significant extensor lag
     - □ Extensor reconstruction

E. Intraoperative MCL injury

1. Recommended treatment is to convert to revision prosthesis with high post for varus/valgus support (i.e., constrained post, not a posterior stabilized post).
2. Primary repair of MCL is acceptable.
   - Postoperative brace with full knee range for 6 weeks

F. Extensor disruption

1. **Almost always occurs at patellar tendon attachment to tibial tubercle**
2. **Direct repair and nonsurgical treatment do not work.**
3. **Extensor allograft reconstruction provides best chance for successful salvage.**
   - ***Fresh frozen* allograft preferred**
     - □ Better healing compared to irradiated allografts
   - When allograft is used, the allograft is tensioned as tight as possible with the knee in full extension.
     - □ This gives best chance to minimize residual knee lag.

G. Arthrofibrosis

1. Manipulation of postoperative knee should be between 4 and 6 weeks.
   - Late manipulation has high rate of fracture.
2. Late stiffness—a big problem
   - Arthrotomy with scar resection and reduction of modular PE thickness is *not recommended.*
     - □ Very high failure rate with recurrent pain and stiffness
   - Revision TKA is recommended if preoperatively a problem with alignment, sizing, or component positioning can be identified.

H. Postoperative flexion contracture

1. **In a well-balanced TKA (with full range of motion) a postoperative flexion contracture is due to *hamstring tightness* and spasm.**
   - Treatment is therapy.
   - Keep knee straight at rest.
     - □ No pillows under knee

I. Postoperative TKA range

1. The most important predictor of postoperative knee range is *preoperative* knee range.

J. Severe extraarticular femoral deformity

1. A *severe* deformity is an angular deformity in the coronal plane (severe varus or valgus) where the correction of the deformity (at the knee) to a neutral mechanical axis would require radical bone cuts and radical ligament releases. This may compromise knee stability and function.
2. Treatment is *simultaneous*
   - Distal femoral extraarticular osteotomy and
   - TKA
     - □ A femoral stem is used to pass through the osteotomy site.

K. Osteolysis

1. Presentation in TKA
   - Starts later in life of implant—8 to 12 years
   - Gradual increase in effusion and weight-bearing pain
   - Mild warmth in knee
     - □ Not hot
     - □ No erythema
   - Normal infection laboratory results
     - □ Normal quantitative C-reactive protein (CRP)
   - Aspiration negative
     - □ Normal WBC count
       - A WBC count greater than 2500 cells/μL is suspicious for infection.
     - □ No crystals
     - □ Cultures are negative.
   - Radiographs show round lytic lesions behind implant (Figure 5-70).
     - □ Most common site is behind *posterior femoral condyle.*

L. Treatment

1. Revision TKA
2. Radical débridement of osteolytic bone lesions
3. Fill segmental defects with bone graft or metal augmentation.

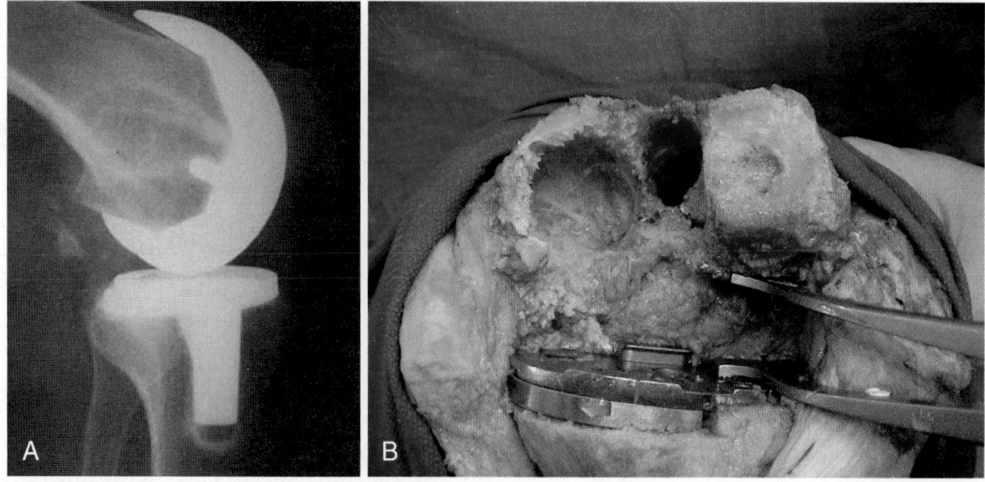
A
B

Figure 5-70 Osteolysis in total knee arthroplasty (TKA). **A,** Classical radiographic appearance of osteolysis in a TKA that is 10 years old. Note large round lytic lesions behind the posterior femoral condyle. **B,** Intraoperative photograph of same knee. Note severe bone loss in medial femoral condyle. This lesion required structural bone allograft. Knee was revised using a constrained revision knee system because the medial collateral ligament attachment onto the medial femoral condyle was compromised from osteolytic bone loss.

SECTION 16 TKA DESIGN

I. DESIGN CATEGORIES

A. Designs are categorized based upon an increasing level of mechanical constraint in knee system.

1. Least constrained
   - Cruciate-retaining TKA—keep PCL
   - Cruciate-sacrificing TKA
   - Both used for straightforward primary TKA
2. Constrained
   - Constrained nonhinge TKA
   - Used for complex primary or revision TKA
3. Highly constrained
   - Hinge TKA
   - Used for complex revision TKA

II. CRUCIATE-RETAINING PRIMARY TKA DESIGN

A. Description (Figure 5-71)

1. PCL helps regulate flexion stability.
2. **PCL tension influences femoral rollback.**
   - **Rollback is defined as the progressive posterior change in femoral-tibial contract point as the knee moves into flexion.**
3. Generally, cruciate-retaining implants have more flat PE inserts to accommodate for flexion rollback.

B. PCL retention—advantages

1. Bone conserving
2. More consistent joint line restoration
   - Keeping PCL keeps flexion gap smaller.
3. More proprioceptive feedback by keeping PCL

C. PCL retention—disadvantages

1. Harder to balance with severe deformities
   - *Avoid* cruciate-retaining implants when
     - Varus greater than 10 degrees
     - Valgus greater than 15 degrees
2. PCL balance is critical for long-term bearing wear.
   - A tight PCL in flexion causes PE wear.
     - Must balance PCL in flexion.
     - Avoid *lift-off* (Figure 5-72).
     - PCL can be released off femur or tibia.
     - PCL balance is sometimes hard to assess intraoperatively.
   - **Excess recession (i.e., release) can result in late failure caused by flexion instability and repetitive subluxation.**

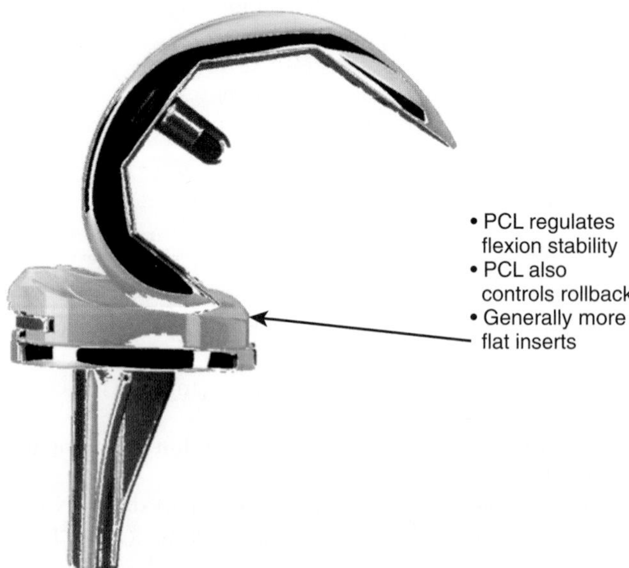
• PCL regulates flexion stability
• PCL also controls rollback
• Generally more flat inserts

Figure 5-71 Lateral view of cruciate-retaining (CR) total knee arthroplasty implant. This is the typical profile of femoral component. In this design the posterior cruciate ligament (PCL) is retained. The polyethylene insert is generally more flat to allow the femur to roll back onto the posterior part of bearing.

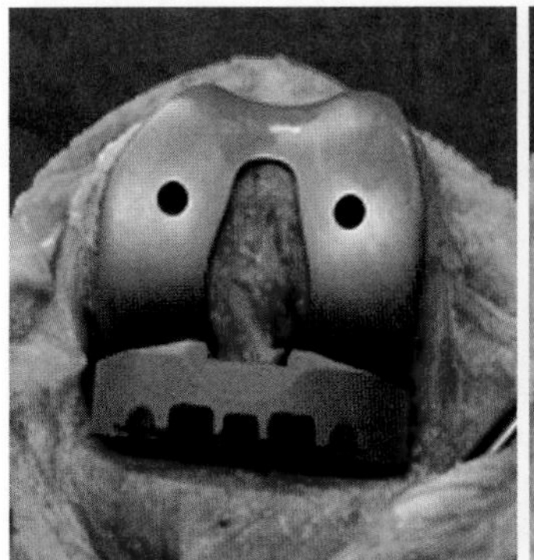
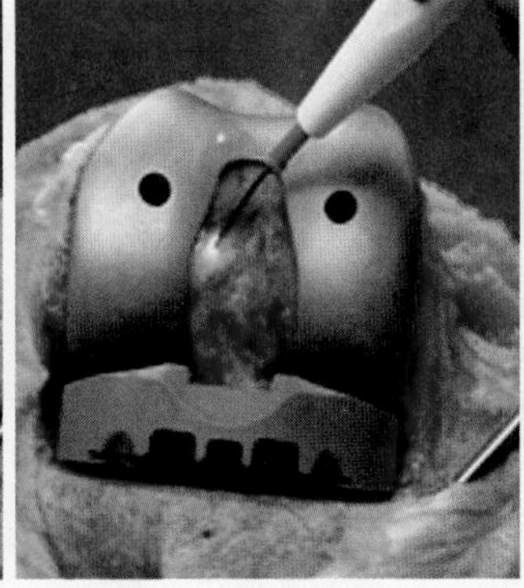
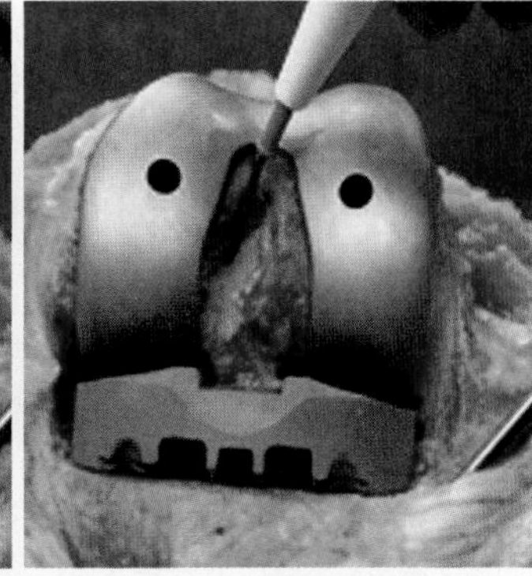

Figure 5-72 Intraoperative demonstration of posterior cruciate ligament (PCL) recession. PCL release off intercondylar notch allows flexion gap to increase in increments. Photograph on left shows classical presentation of tight PCL. With the knee in flexion, the tight PCL levers the anterior portion of the tibial insert upward creating *lift-off*. Sequential photographs show release of PCL just enough to allow tibial insert to lie back onto tibial. This sequence is termed *balancing the PCL*.

- **Instability is characterized by knee effusion, pain during weight bearing on flexed knee, and knee buckling.**

3. Late rupture of PCL with resultant instability
   - PE particle debris can cause osteolysis and result in disruption of PCL.
   - Traumatic fall onto flexed knee can cause rupture.
4. Paradoxical *forward sliding* as knee flexes
   - With ACL removed, knee kinematics are drastically altered.
   - As knee flexes, there is paradoxical sliding movement, which causes sliding wear on PE insert.
     - Sliding wear causes significant PE wear.

III. CRUCIATE-SACRIFICING PRIMARY TKA DESIGN

A. There are two options.

1. A spine and cam mechanism in the posterior aspect of the knee
   - Also called *posterior stabilized* knee
2. An extended anterior PE lip
   - Also called *anterior stabilized* knee

IV. POSTERIOR STABILIZED PRIMARY TKA DESIGN

A. Description (Figure 5-73)

1. A cam connects between the two posterior femoral condyles.
2. The cam engages a tibial PE post during flexion.
3. The cam and post control rollback.
4. Generally, posterior stabilized implants have more dished (i.e., congruent) PE inserts.

B. Posterior stabilized knee—advantages

1. Easier balancing in severe coronal deformities (i.e., varus/valgus)
2. Controlled flexion kinematics with spine and cam, less sliding wear

C. Posterior stabilized knee—disadvantages

1. *Femoral cam jump* (Figure 5-74)
   - Occurs when flexion gap is left too loose
   - Mechanism of cam jump
     - Varus or valgus stress when knee is flexed
     - Patient usually lying in bed or sitting on floor
     - Flexion gap opens up, and femoral cam then rotates in front of post and then comes to rest in front of tibial post.
   - Closed reduction maneuver
     - Knee is positioned at 90 degrees of flexion off the table (dependent dangle) under anesthesia.
     - An anterior drawer maneuver is performed.
       - Will feel clunk as knee is reduced
   - Ultimate solution requires knee revision to address loose flexion gap.

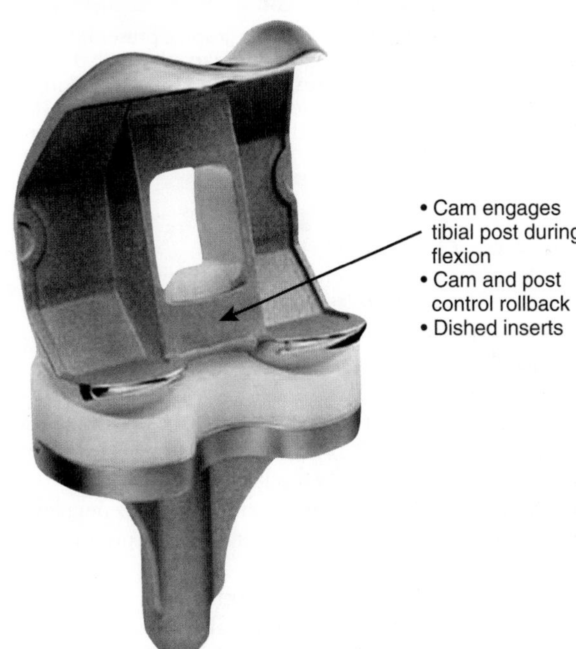
• Cam engages tibial post during flexion
• Cam and post control rollback
• Dished inserts

Figure 5-73 Posterior-lateral view of posterior stabilized (PS) implant. This is the typical profile of the femoral and tibial component. The cam on the femur engages a tibial post when the knee moves into flexion. This prevents anterior translation of the femur on the tibia, which *stabilizes* the knee in flexion in the absence of a posterior cruciate ligament.

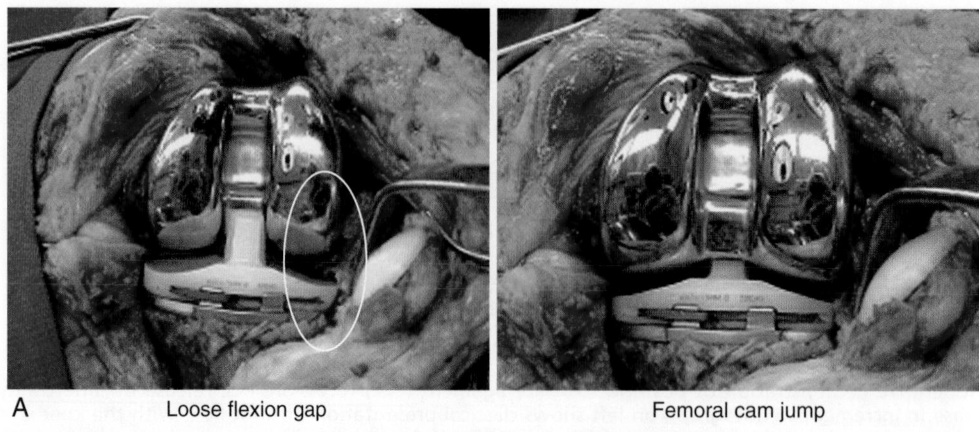

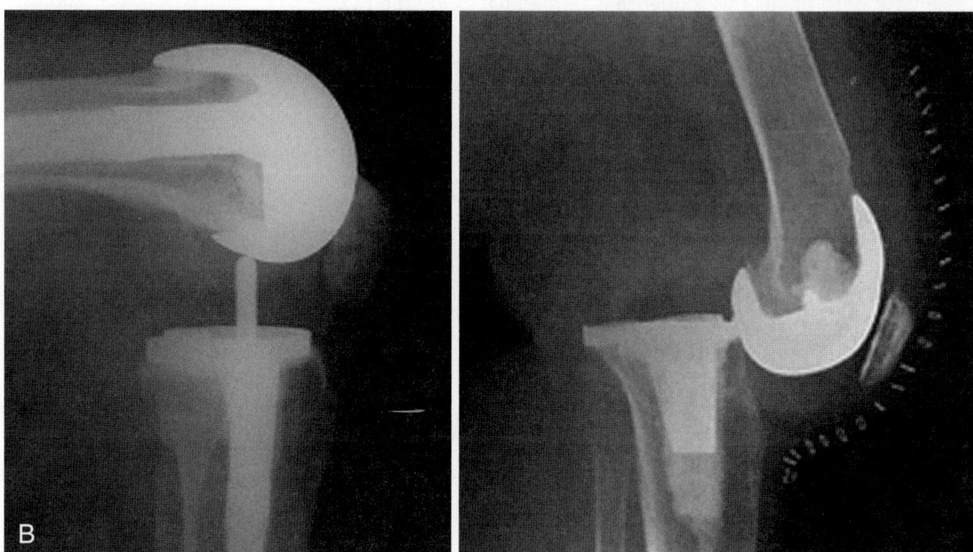

Figure 5-74 Intraoperative and radiographic presentation of femoral cam jump in posterior stabilized total knee arthroplasty. **A,** The photograph on left shows loose flexion gap. The circled area highlights loose lateral flexion gap caused by popliteal tendon deficiency. As the knee is stressed into varus, the tibia then rotates out in front of the tibial post. The cam then comes to rest in front of the tibial post. **B,** Two different presentations of femoral cam jump. Radiograph on *left* shows femur perched in front of tibial post (reinforced in this case with a metal post). Radiograph on *right* shows femur completely dislocated anteriorly when knee is brought into extension after cam jump.

- Causes of loose flexion gap
  - Overrelease of popliteus
    - Inadvertently occurs also with saw blade
  - Overrelease of *anterior portion* of superficial MCL
  - Anterior translation of femoral component

2. Patella clunk syndrome
   - Scar tissue (descriptively, a nodule of scar) superior to patella gets caught in box as knee moves from flexion into extension.
   - Scar catches in box, then releases with a clunk.
   - Clunk occurs in range between 30 and 45 degrees.
   - Treatment is removal of suprapatellar scar nodule (Figure 5-75).
     - Arthroscopic removal is acceptable.
     - Miniarthrotomy is also acceptable.
   - Preventive treatment (Figure 5-76)
     - Synovectomy and débridement of all scar from quadriceps tendon at time of TKA
3. Tibial post wear and breakage
   - Tibial post is an additional PE surface that can cause wear and osteolysis.
   - Aseptic loosening and osteolysis are *correlated* with tibial post wear and damage.
   - If the knee *hyperextends*, the edge of the femoral box can impinge on the *anterior* tibial post (Figure 5-77).
     - Causes anterior post damage and fatigue
     - Causes increased PE wear and osteolysis
   - Anterior tibial post wear occurs when TKA components are in *net hyperextension*. This includes
     - Flexion of femoral component on distal femur
     - Excess tibial posterior slope
     - Knee hyperextension (i.e., loose extension gap)
     - Anterior translation of tibial component on tibia
     - Note: Anterior translation of femoral component has *no effect* on anterior tibial post impingement.
4. Additional bone is removed from middle of distal femur.
   - Bone removed can be substantial in a small knee.
5. Flexion gap is bigger.
   - Flexion gap opens up when PCL is removed.
   - **To balance the extension gap, additional distal femur bone is removed in a posterior stabilized TKA.**

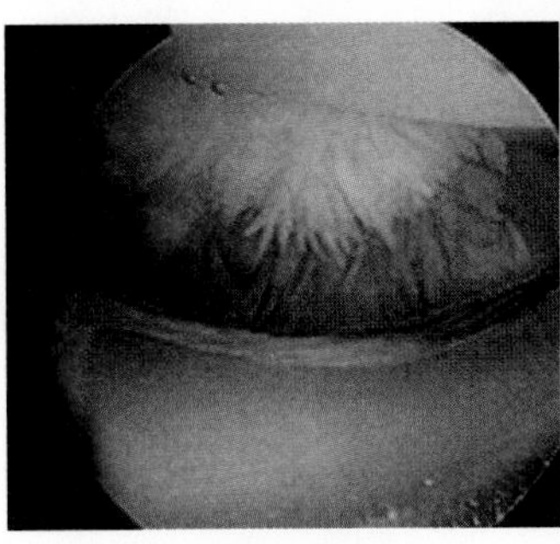
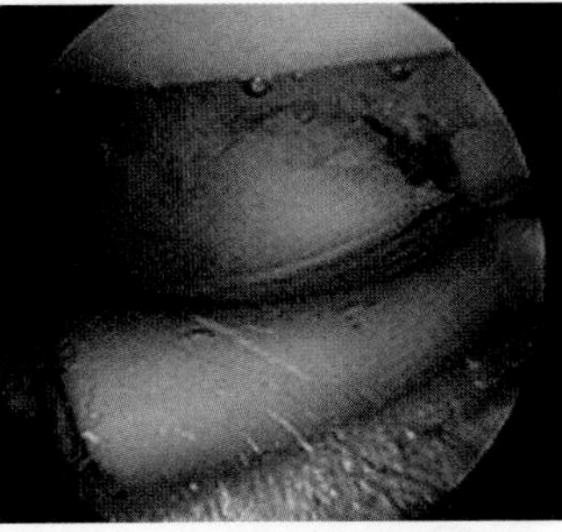
Treatment — Arthroscopy
Nodule superior to patella
Incarceration of nodule in box with flexion
Scar débridement with scope

Figure 5-75 Arthroscopic photographs demonstrating patella clunk syndrome. Classical appearance of fibrotic scar nodule in suprapatellar region *(left)*. Incarceration of scar in posterior stabilized box as knee is brought from flexion into extension *(center)*. Arthroscopic removal of nodule *(right)*.

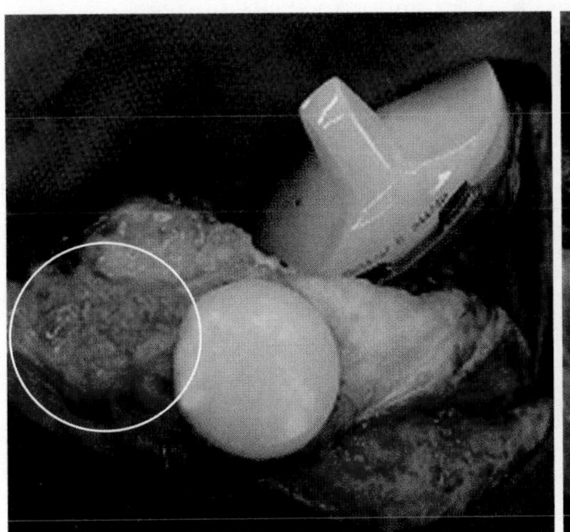
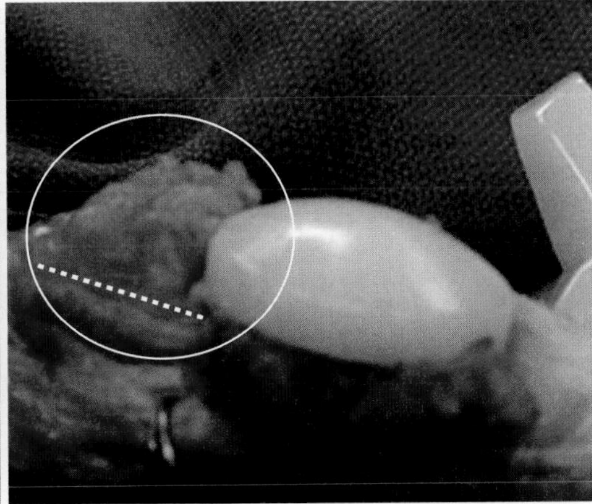
Preventative treatment
Remove tissue down to quadriceps tendon

Figure 5-76 Inflammatory tissue *(circle)* around arthritic patella at time of primary total knee arthroplasty *(left)*. This tissue, if not removed, will cause patellar clunk syndrome. This tissue should be aggressively débrided to level of quadriceps tendon *(dotted line; right)*.

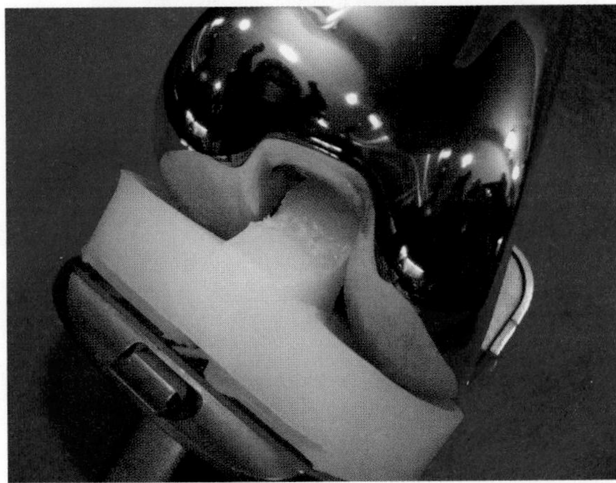

Figure 5-77 Photograph of posterior stabilized implant with anterior tibial post wear. Note indentation on anterior post where the edge of femoral box impinges upon anterior tibial post. This occurs when the knee moves into hyperextension.

- □ Consequence of additional distal femoral bone removal
  - ▪ Joint line elevation with possible baja deformity
- □ The maximum joint line elevation allowed in primary TKA is 8 mm.
  - ▪ This ensures proper kinematic function and stability of collateral ligaments.

D. Posterior stabilized TKA—indications

1. Patellectomy
   - ▪ Cruciate-retaining knee with a flat PE is prone to anterior subluxation when patella is absent.
2. Inflammatory arthritis
   - ▪ PCL is at risk for rupture with erosive disease process.
3. Trauma with PCL rupture or attenuation

V. ANTERIOR STABILIZED PRIMARY TKA DESIGN

A. Description (Figure 5-78)

1. A cruciate-retaining femoral component is used.
2. The PCL is removed (or highly recessed).

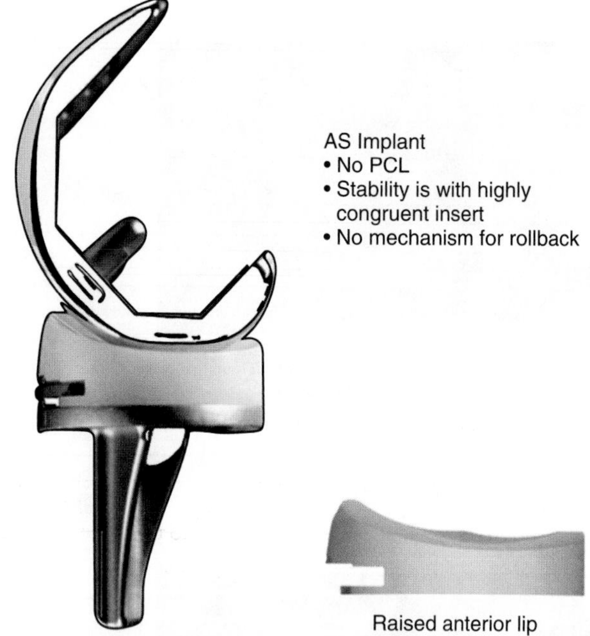
AS Implant
• No PCL
• Stability is with highly congruent insert
• No mechanism for rollback
Raised anterior lip

Figure 5-78 Lateral view of anterior stabilized (AS) total knee arthroplasty design. This is the typical profile of the femoral and tibial component. The tibial polyethylene (PE) bearing is highly congruent and also has a raised anterior PE lip to resist anterior translation. In this design there is minimal rollback. PCL, posterior cruciate ligament.

3. Tibial insert is a highly congruent bearing with a raised anterior PE lip.
4. No mechanism for rollback
5. Anterior lip resists anterior translation.

B. **Anterior stabilized knee—advantages**

1. Easier balancing in severe deformities (i.e., varus/valgus)
2. Bone conserving
3. Operative versatility
   - Do not have to switch to posterior stabilized system when PCL is lost or overreleased
4. Regulated flexion kinematics
   - High congruency limits sliding wear.
   - Knee flexion is achieved by placing knee flexion center in posterior part of tibia (i.e., posterior offset center of rotation).

C. **Anterior stabilized knee—disadvantages**

1. Increased PE surface area
   - This increases risk for increased PE wear debris and osteolysis.
2. Minimal rollback
   - Must adjust surgical technique to attain high flexion
     - Posterior translation of tibial component
     - Recreate native tibial posterior slope
3. Flexion gap laxity causes rotational instability and pain.
   - Similar to posterior stabilized design, a loose flexion gap will cause instability usually in mid-flexion.
   - Mechanism of mid-flexion instability
     - Varus or valgus stress when knee is flexed (between 50 and 90 degrees)
     - Patient usually lying in bed or sitting on floor
     - Flexion gap opens up, and tibia rotates anteriorly. This creates a subluxing event, but knee usually does not lock up.
     - Treatment requires revision to address loose flexion gap.

VI. TIBIAL ROTATING PLATFORM IN PRIMARY TKA

A. **Description** (Figure 5-79)

1. The tibial PE bearing rotates on a polished metal tibial baseplate.
2. The rotating platform can be used with both anterior stabilized (high congruent) and posterior stabilized TKA designs.
3. The PCL is removed when using a tibial rotating platform.

B. **Rotating platform knee—advantages**

1. Better articular conformity through entire knee range
   - Theoretically less PE wear
2. *Equivalent* survivorship to fixed-bearing knee, but *not superior*
   - Wear and osteolysis still seen

C. **Rotating platform knee—disadvantages**

1. Bearing *spinout* (Figure 5-80)
   - Occurs when flexion gap is left too loose
   - Mechanism of spinout
     - Varus or valgus stress when knee is flexed
     - Patient usually lying in bed or sitting on floor
     - Flexion gap opens up, and tibia rotates behind femur.
     - Femur then comes to rest in front of tibial PE bearing and locks into spinout position.
   - Closed reduction maneuver
     - Knee is positioned at 90 degrees of flexion off the side of the table (dependent dangle) under anesthesia.
     - Tibial bearing is manipulated by digital palpation and pressure into reduced position.
   - Ultimate solution requires knee revision to address loose flexion gap.

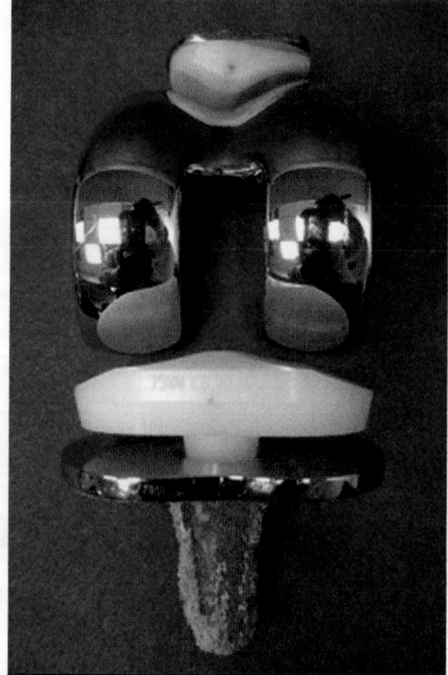

Figure 5-79 Retrieval of a primary total knee arthroplasty with a tibial rotating platform. Tibial polyethylene (PE) component has a yoke that inserts into tibial baseplate. The tibial PE bearing rotates on a polished tibial baseplate.

Rotating Platform

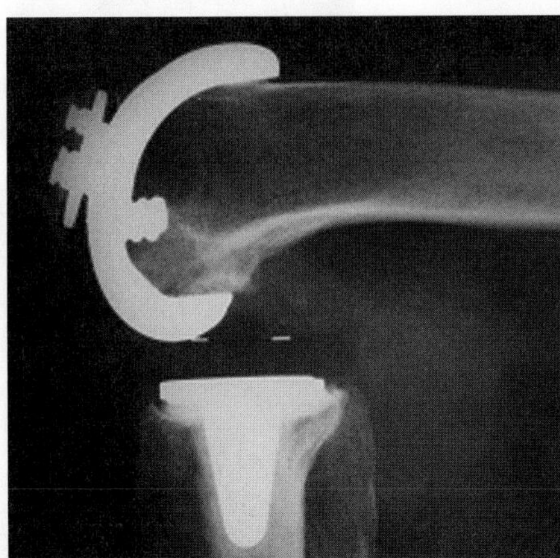

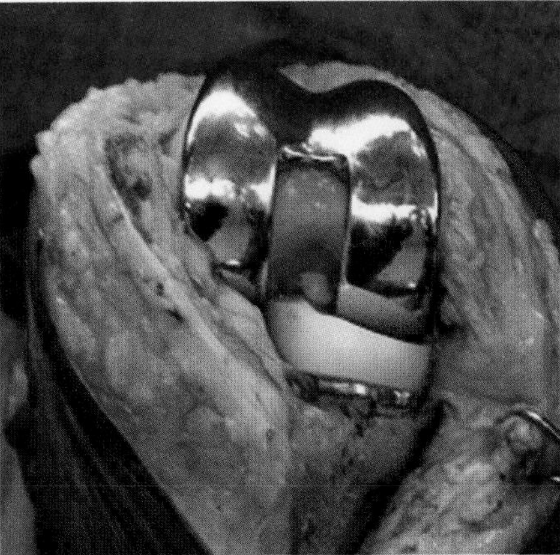

Figure 5-80 Demonstration of bearing spinout. Radiograph on *left* shows classical appearance of bearing spinout. Note that femur profile has no central box. Therefore this radiograph is not of a posterior stabilized knee with cam jump. Photograph on *right* is intraoperative appearance of same patient. Note that the lateral tibial polyethylene component is completely posterior to the lateral femoral condyle.

VII. MODULARITY IN PRIMARY TKA

A. Modular tibial component is now standard.

1. Metal baseplate
2. Modular PE insert
3. Stems can be attached to tibia and/or femur.

B. Modularity—advantages

1. Greater intraoperative flexibility
2. Modular bearing change for worn PE in well-fixed implants; major revision is avoided

C. Modularity—disadvantages

1. ***Backside*** **PE wear**
   - **Backside wear occurs when the tibial locking mechanism allows micromotion to occur between tibial baseplate and backside surface of tibial PE bearing.**
   - More osteolysis with modular designs
   - Locking mechanisms for tibial PE inserts do not completely eliminate micromotion.
   - **Backside wear is *not* a problem with a *monoblock* design.**
     - **With monoblock design, the tibial PE bearing is pressed onto metal baseplate at the factory.**
     - There is no backside wear with monoblock designs.
2. Backside wear—reduction
   - Polished tibial baseplate
   - Tighter locking mechanisms

VIII. CONSTRAINT IN TKA

A. Reason

1. **Soft tissues about knee will not support prosthesis.**
   - **Loss of key vital support structures**
2. Prosthesis must then accommodate for loss of soft tissue support.

B. Constraint options

1. High tibial post nonhinged
2. Hinge with rotating tibial platform
3. Hinge with no rotating tibial platform
   - Rarely used

C. Constrained nonhinged TKA

1. **Definition** (Figure 5-81)
   - **High central post that *substitutes for* MCL and** lateral collateral ligament **function**
   - **A standard posterior stabilized post *is not* constrained.**
2. **Indications**
   - Residual flexion gap laxity
     - Due to soft tissue weakness, the extension and flexion gaps cannot be completely balanced.
   - MCL attenuation
   - Lateral collateral ligament deficiency
   - MCL complete deficiency
     - Relative (still debatable)
   - **Charcot arthropathy**
     - **Relative (still debatable)**
3. Disadvantages
   - More constraint upon implant places more forces through implant and implant-bone interface. This causes
     - More PE wear/damage to PE post
     - Higher rate of aseptic loosening
   - Constrained high-post knee system *requires* medullary stem support in femur and tibia to help distribute increased load forces through implant.

D. Hinge TKA

1. Definition (Figure 5-82)
   - Femoral and tibial components are linked with a connecting bar and bearings.
   - There is a fixed extension stop.
   - Most designs incorporate a tibial rotating platform.
     - This reduces torque stress to implant bone interface.
2. Indications
   - Global instability
     - Due to trauma or infection
   - Hyperextension instability (Figure 5-83)
     - This is *absolute* indication for hinge.
     - Seen with postpolio knee conditions
   - Knee removal
     - Tumor
     - High-energy fracture with communication
     - Massive infection

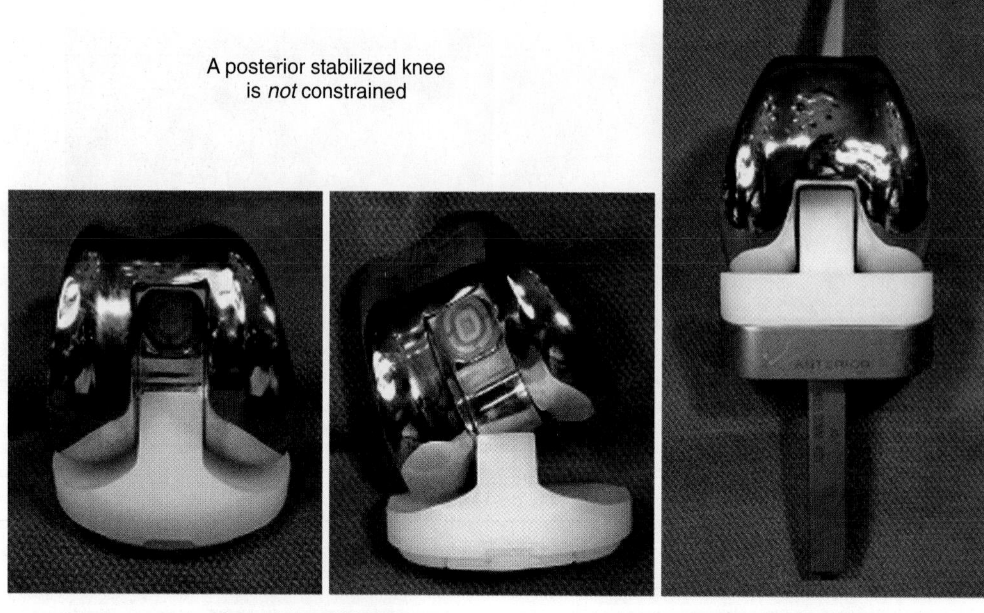

Figure 5-81 Diagram showing high-post constrained total knee arthroplasty (TKA). Photographs on *left* show a typical posterior stabilized TKA. If medial collateral ligament or lateral collateral ligament function is lost, the posterior stabilized post will not resist varus or valgus forces and the knee will be unstable. The photograph on the *right* shows a constrained high-post design. This polyethylene post is very tall and will not allow varus or valgus opening of the knee.

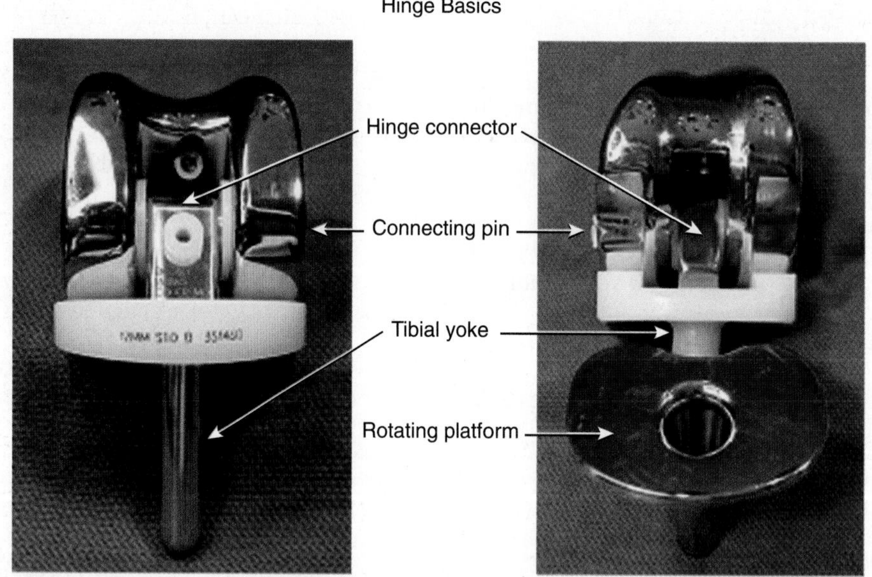

Figure 5-82 Diagram showing basic components of hinge total knee arthroplasty. In all hinge systems, the femur is connected to the tibia via a connecting post placed into the middle of the knee. A connecting pin of metal is placed through femur and tibial post. A locking pin keeps connecting pin in position. A tibial yoke rests in the tibial component. This allows rotation of the tibia.

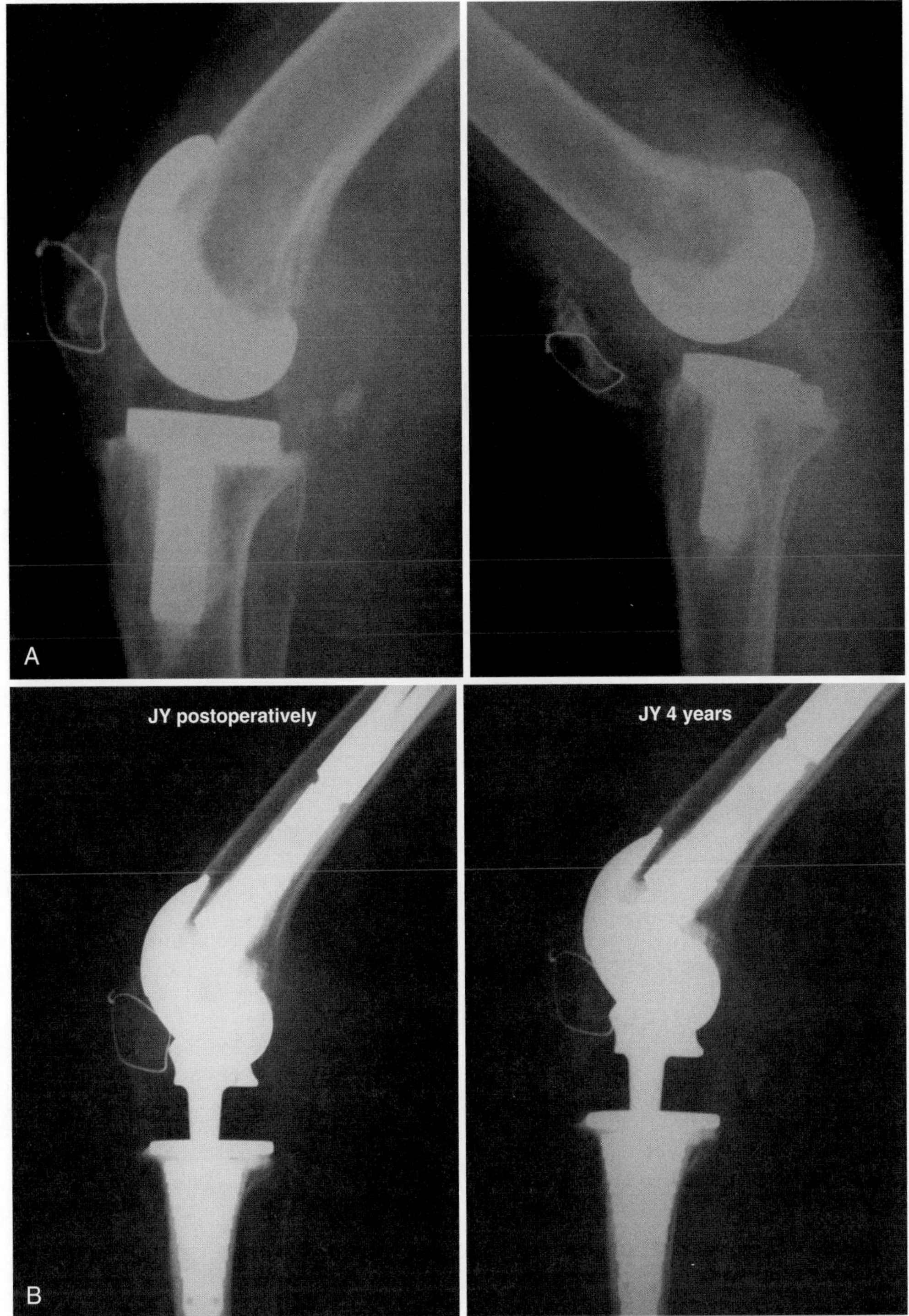

Figure 5-83 Case showing hyperextension instability. **A,** Total knee arthroplasty (TKA) in a patient with postpolio syndrome. Extension lateral shows severe hyperextension, which on presentation was only mildly painful. However, the patient had significant difficulty with walking. **B,** Revision to a hinge TKA.

SECTION 17 REVISION TKA

I. PREOPERATIVE EVALUATION

A. Revision of a painful TKA without an identified specific cause for pain is likely to have a *poor* outcome.

B. Must first identify intrinsic intraarticular source of pain versus extrinsic source of pain

C. Extrinsic sources of knee pain

1. Referred pain from the hip
   - Most common missed diagnosis
2. Referred pain from the spine
   - Typically L4 nerve root
3. Extraarticular at the knee
   - Allodynia—chronic regional pain syndrome
   - Local superficial neuroma

D. Intrinsic sources of knee pain

1. Mechanical loosening
2. Osteolysis with PE debris synovitis
3. Malposition and/or malalignment of implants
4. Instability
5. Infection
   - Typically, *constant global* pain with abnormal infection laboratory results and positive aspiration studies
6. Hypersensitivity
   - Typically, *constant global* pain with normal infection laboratory results and negative aspiration studies
   - Most common metal ion involved in knee hypersensitivity is *nickel.*
   - Diagnosis made by serum lymphocyte T-cell proliferation test (LTT), *not* skin patch test

E. Intraarticular aspiration

1. WBC count greater than 2500/μL raises suspicion for low-grade infection.

F. Intraarticular lidocaine challenge

1. Administer at least 15 mL of lidocaine or 50/50 mixture of lidocaine/Marcaine.
2. A positive test should take away over 90% of pain.

II. SURGICAL APPROACH

A. Use prior incisions.

B. Avoid making skin bridges with a new incision.

C. Lifting a subcutaneous soft tissue flap is much safer than a second incision with a skin bridge.

III. IMPLANT SYSTEM

A. Have comprehensive revision system available.

1. Revision surgery is often unpredictable.
2. Constrained tibial insert option is a must.
3. Stems and metallic augmentations

IV. MODULAR BEARING CHANGE FOR *PREMATURE* EXCESSIVE WEAR

A. Failure rate of isolated modular bearing change for excessive premature PE failure is 30% to 40%.

B. Reason for premature failure

1. Unappreciated malalignment
2. Poor knee balancing in either coronal or sagittal plane

C. Isolated modular bearing change in this scenario is not recommended.

V. REVISION TKA—TECHNIQUE

A. Implant removal

B. Joint line restoration with tibia first

1. **Joint line is generally 1.5 cm superior to top of fibular head.**
2. **Failure to restore joint line will result in decreased flexion.**

C. Femur restoration

1. Gap balancing
2. Adjust for patellar positioning.
   - Avoid baja impingement.

VI. REVISION TKA—PATELLA

A. Isolated patella component failure usually indicates subtle malalignment in patellar tracking.

1. Higher failure rate for isolated patellar revision
2. Consider full revision.

B. A mechanically loose patellar component can cause significant patellar bone loss.

1. For *revision* to another patellar component, bone thickness must be at least 12 mm, and there must be enough bone to support PE pegs within bone.
2. If bone is inadequate for revision resurfacing
   - Débridement of patella with bone retention is acceptable.
   - Patellectomy is recommended for bony fragmentation.

SECTION 18 PATELLAR TRACKING IN TKA

I. INTRODUCTION

A. The *most common* complications in TKA involve abnormalities in patellar tracking.

B. Preoperative maltracking is the only predictor of postoperative maltracking.

C. Most important factors for successful patellar tracking

1. Maintaining normal Q angle
2. Proper component rotation
3. Maintaining normal patellofemoral tension

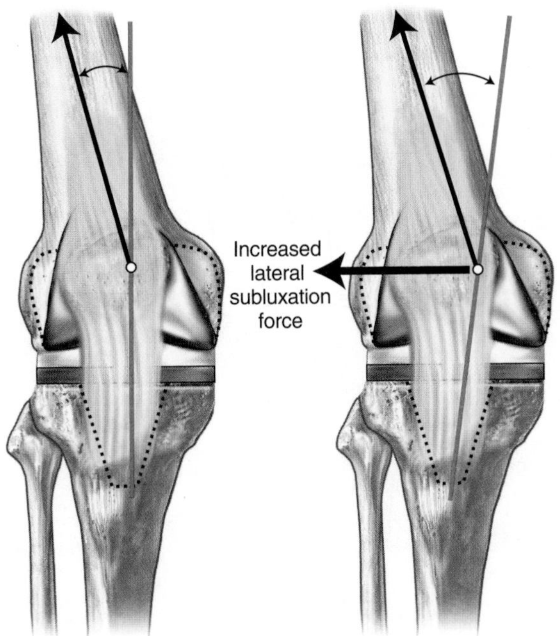

Figure 5-84 Diagram depicting effect of an increased Q angle in TKA. As the Q angle increases, so does the resultant lateral subluxation force. Because the shape of the resurfaced patella is a dome, this design is less able to resist the lateral pull effect. The result is an increased risk for patellar subluxation.

II. Q ANGLE IN TKA

A. Q angle definition—the *angle* between

1. A line defining the axial pull of the quadriceps tendon and a line bisecting the patellar tendon

B. Reasons an increased Q angle in TKA is bad (Figure 5-84)

1. An increased Q angle increases the resultant lateral subluxation force (i.e., lateral pull effect).
2. Prosthetic patellar replacements are *less restrained* than native patella.
3. Prosthetic patellar replacements are therefore more likely to sublux with increased Q angle forces.

C. Q angle goal in TKA

1. Restore proper Q angle with techniques that do not compromise mechanical alignment or stability of the knee.

III. TKA TECHNIQUES TO OPTIMIZE PATELLAR TRACKING

A. Reduce excess valgus.

1. Valgus deformity must be corrected to a *neutral* mechanical alignment—*always.*
2. Severe valgus deformities that require radical ligamentous releases can be adequately managed with sophisticated revision style of prosthetic systems.

B. Component positioning

1. **Patellar maltracking—causes**
   - **Internal rotation of**
     - **Femoral component**
     - **Tibial component**
   - **Medialization of**
     - **Femoral component**
     - **Tibial component**

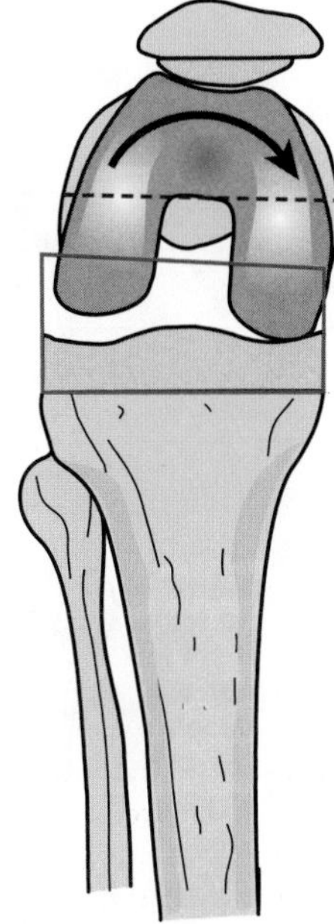

Figure 5-85 Diagram showing adverse effect of internal rotation of femoral component. Diagram depicts total knee arthroplasty at 90 degrees of flexion. With internal rotation of femur, the patellar groove faces inward and the flexion gap becomes asymmetric. Patellar tracking and flexion kinematics are both adversely affected.

C. Femoral component rotation

1. **Do not internally rotate femoral component.**
2. Internal rotation of femur—resultant problems (Figure 5-85)
   - **Relative lateral tilt of patella**
     - **Patellar groove faces inward.**
   - Trapezoidal flexion gap
     - Unbalanced flexion gap
3. Technique goal is slight *external rotation* of femur (Figure 5-86).

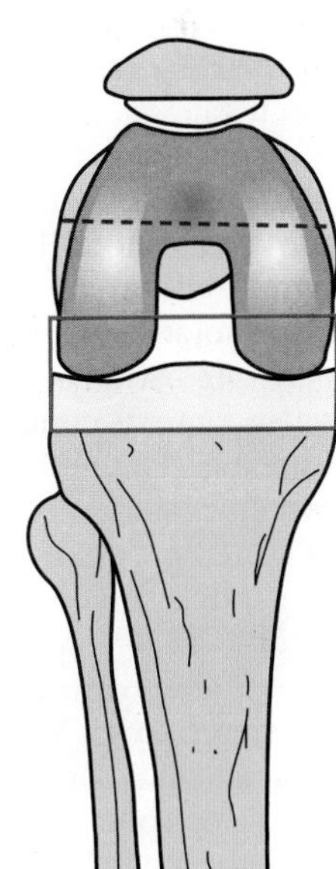

Figure 5-86 Diagram showing proper positioning of femoral component in slight external rotation. With slight external rotation, the patellar groove is centered under the patella and the flexion gap is balanced, which optimizes flexion kinematics.

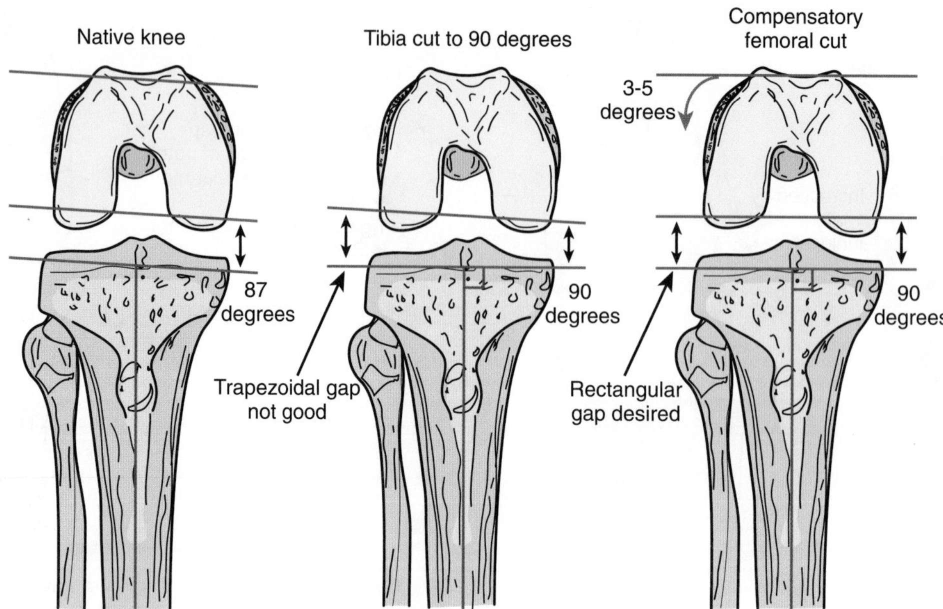

Figure 5-87 Diagrams demonstrating proper component rotation during total knee arthroplasty (TKA). *Left,* Native knee in flexion. In many instances, the native proximal tibia is actually in slight varus (average is 3 degrees). *Center,* In TKA procedure, the proximal tibia is cut perpendicular to mechanical axis. This leaves the flexion gap asymmetric and unbalanced. *Right,* Compensatory cut on femur, which is externally rotated to create a rectangular (i.e., balanced) flexion gap and to optimize patellar tracking.

- Patellar groove is centered under patella.
- Rectangular flexion gap
  - Balanced flexion gap

4. **External rotation of femoral component** (Figure 5-87)—Why?
   - **Commonly, the proximal tibia is actually in slight varus.**
     - **Average is 3 degrees varus.**
   - During TKA, the proximal tibia is cut perpendicular to mechanical axis.
   - This results in trapezoidal flexion gap (i.e., unbalanced flexion gap).
   - To compensate, the femoral component is externally rotated a similar amount to obtain a rectangular flexion gap (i.e., balanced flexion gap) and also optimize patellar tracking.
5. **External rotation of femoral component—techniques**
   - There are five established techniques to determine proper femoral component rotation. All methods are acceptable (Figure 5-88).
     - Anteroposterior axis method
       - Anteroposterior axis is defined as line from intercondylar notch (specifically the most lateral border of PCL) to center of trochlear groove.
       - A line drawn perpendicular to anteroposterior axis is used to set femoral rotation.
     - Epicondylar axis method
       - The epicondylar axis is a line drawn from the center of the medial epicondyle to the center of the lateral epicondyle.
       - Femoral rotation is set along this line.
     - **Posterior condylar axis method**
       - **The posterior condylar axis is a line connecting the apex of the medial femoral condyle and lateral femoral condyle measured at 90 degrees of flexion.**
       - **The femoral rotation line is mechanically chosen along a line that is 3 degrees externally rotated to this line (acceptable range is 3 to 5 degrees of external rotation).**
     - Tibial alignment axis method
       - The proximal tibial cut is with a cutting jig set 90 degrees to the mechanical axis of the tibia.
       - With the knee at 90 degrees of flexion, the same guide is used to set femoral component rotation by drawing rotation line on the femur.
     - Gap balance axis method
       - The proximal tibia is cut first.
       - With the knee at 90 degrees of flexion, tension devices are placed under the medial and lateral femoral condyles. A set tension is then applied to the flexion gap.
       - The femoral rotation line is drawn to create a *rectangular* flexion gap.
6. Beware of lateral femoral condylar hypoplasia.
   - In this condition the lateral femoral condyle is small.
     - Clinically, a knee with lateral femoral condylar hypoplasia presents with a prominent **valgus deformity.** With the knee viewed in flexion, the lateral femoral condyle looks small relative to the medial femoral condyle.
   - **In lateral femoral condylar hypoplasia the posterior axis *cannot* be used.**
     - **If the posterior condylar axis is used as the rotation reference, the femur will be placed in internal rotation.**

D. **Tibial component rotation**

1. **Do not internally rotate tibial component.**

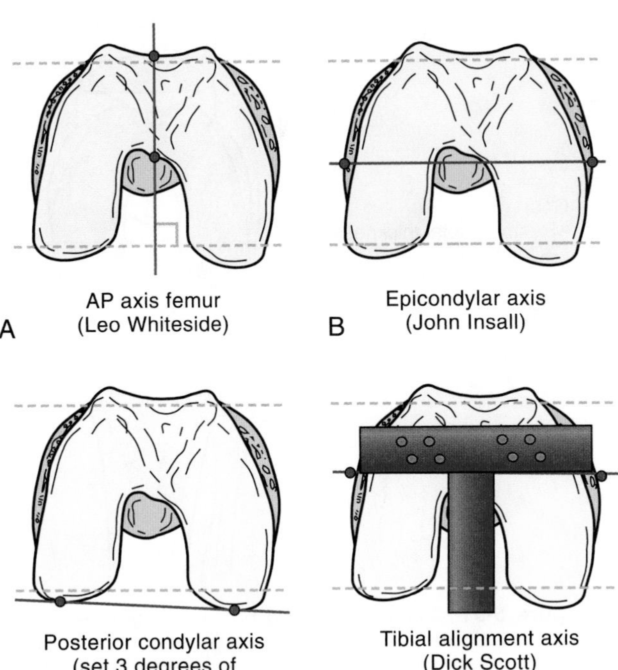

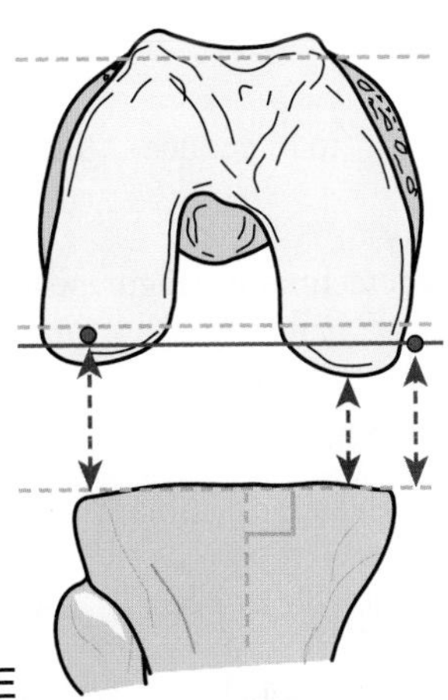

Figure 5-88 Diagrams showing methods to determine femoral component rotation. **A,** In the anteroposterior (AP) axis method, the AP line is drawn from the center of the intercondylar notch to the center of the trochlear groove. The femoral rotation is set along a line perpendicular to the AP axis. **B,** The epicondylar axis is a line drawn from the center of the medial and lateral epicondyles. Femoral rotation is set parallel to this line. **C,** Posterior condylar axis. The posterior condylar line is drawn between the two femoral condyles (at 90 degrees of flexion). Femoral rotation is set at 3 degrees of external rotation relative to this line. **D,** Tibial alignment axis. The tibial jig, used to cut the tibia at 90 degrees to the tibial mechanical axis, is also used to set femoral rotation. Either the jig is raised or a block is placed upon the jig to draw the femoral rotation line. **E,** Gap balance axis method. Tensiometers are placed into the flexion gap, and tension is applied to the flexion gap. The femoral rotation line is drawn to create a rectangular flexion gap with the knee ligaments under tension. LFC, lateral femoral condyle; MFC, medial femoral condyle.

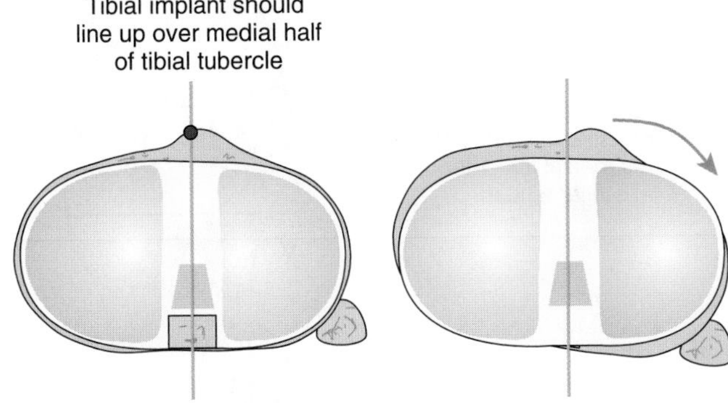

Figure 5-89 Diagram showing tibial component rotation in total knee arthroplasty. For optimal patellar tracking, the tibial component should be rotated over the medial half of the tibial tubercle *(left).* Avoid internally rotating tibia *(right).* When tibial component is internally rotated, the tibial tubercle is positioned in external rotation relative to the knee flexion plane. This increases the Q angle, which increases lateral subluxation forces.

2. **Internal rotation of tibia—resultant problem** (Figure 5-89)
   - **Increases Q angle**
   - **Increases lateral subluxation force**
3. Tibial component positioning should lie over medial half of tibial tubercle.

E. **Implant medialization**

1. **Do not medialize femoral component.**
   - Reason—Medialization of femur moves patellar groove medial relative to tibial tubercle. Result is net increase in Q angle.
   - Lateralization is acceptable.
2. **Do not medialize tibial component.**
   - Reason—Medialization moves knee articulation medial relative to tibial tubercle. Result is net increase in Q angle.
   - Lateralization is acceptable.
3. **Patellar component medialization is acceptable** (Figure 5-90).
   - Reason—The center of the patellar component is placed medial to the center of the patellar tendon. Result is net decrease in Q angle.
   - Avoid lateralization of patellar component.

F. **Patellofemoral tensioning (also called *third-gap balancing*)**

1. Restoring normal patellar height maintains normal retinacular tension (Figure 5-91).
   - Increasing net patellar height increases retinacular tension.
   - Increased retinacular tension will increase lateral pull forces upon patella, causing maltracking.
2. Patellofemoral height (i.e., patellofemoral gap) is controlled by sum of total of
   - Patella bone thickness
   - Patella implant thickness
   - Trochlea bone thickness
   - Trochlea implant thickness

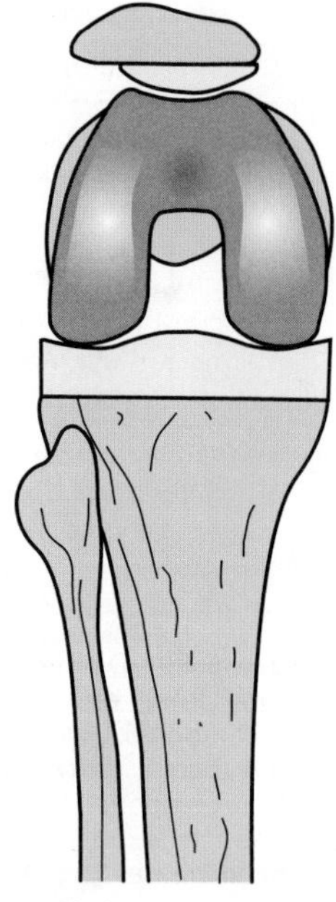
Result
• Net decrease in Q angle
✦ Center of patellar dome is medial to center of patellar tendon

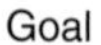

Figure 5-90 Diagram showing medialized patellar component. In this technique, a small patellar dome is used. It is placed in a medialized position. The center of the patellar dome, being medial to the center of the patellar tendon, reduces net Q angle.

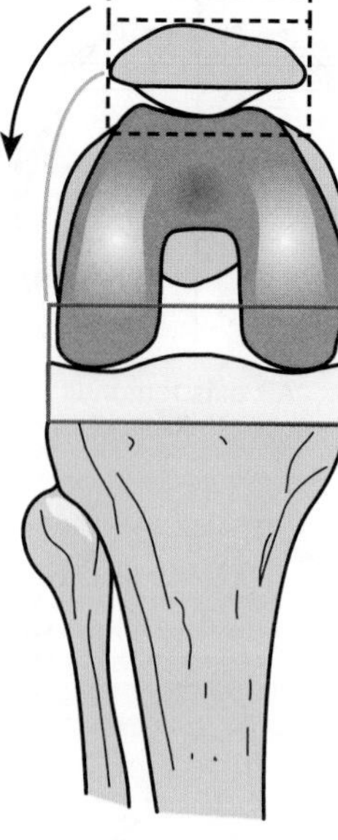
Goal
• Restored total thickness
✦ Must measure
• Normal retinacular tension
• No lateral overpull

Figure 5-91 Diagram showing patellar height. Measuring patellar height before and after patellofemoral resurfacing is important in maintaining normal retinacular tension. Increasing patellar height *(upper box, arrow)* increases retinacular tension. This increases lateral pulling forces on patella.

3. Increased patellofemoral gap—worst case
   - Thin bone cut on patella
   - Thick PE implant
   - Thin bone cut on trochlea
   - Thick femoral trochlear implant

IV. INTRAOPERATIVE ASSESSMENT OF MALTRACKING

A. If maltracking is seen with TKA implants in place, *first* release tourniquet, then reevaluate before making any changes.

B. The tourniquet can alter extensor tension and falsely create increased lateral pull forces.

V. POSTOPERATIVE ASSESSMENT OF MALTRACKING

A. If physical examination and plain radiographs do not reveal the cause of postoperative patellar maltracking, a CT scan can be used to determine rotational alignment of femoral and tibial components.

VI. PATELLA BAJA

A. Frequently seen after

1. **Proximal tibial closed-wedge osteotomy**
2. Tibial tubercle transfer/slide
3. Trauma

B. Baja in TKA will cause (Figure 5-92)

1. **Loss of knee flexion**
2. **Impingement pain**

C. Operative solutions to reduce baja in TKA

1. Superior placement of patellar component
   - Use smaller patellar dome placed superiorly on patella.
   - Trim/taper inferior bone to reduce flexion impingement.
   - Useful for mild baja deformity
2. Lower joint line—sophisticated technique (Figures 5-93 and 5-94)
   - Make a lower tibial bone cut.
   - Add distal femoral metallic augmentation.
   - Requires revision knee system
3. Cephalad transfer of tibial tubercle/anterior tibia
   - Procedure is risky.
     - Bone healing not always predictable (especially around a cemented tibial component)
     - Clinically, patient may have functional extensor lag.
4. Patellectomy for extreme cases
   - Patellectomy alters anterior knee tension.
     - Need to use cruciate substituting knee system

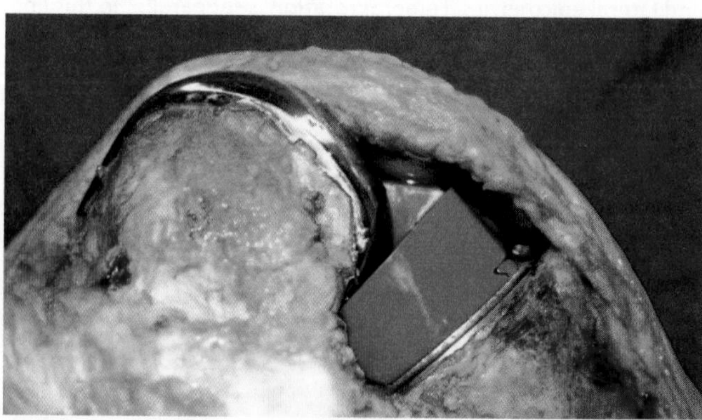

Figure 5-92 Intraoperative photograph of total knee arthroplasty with patella baja. With baja deformity, the patella component impinges upon the tibial component, limiting flexion and causing pain.

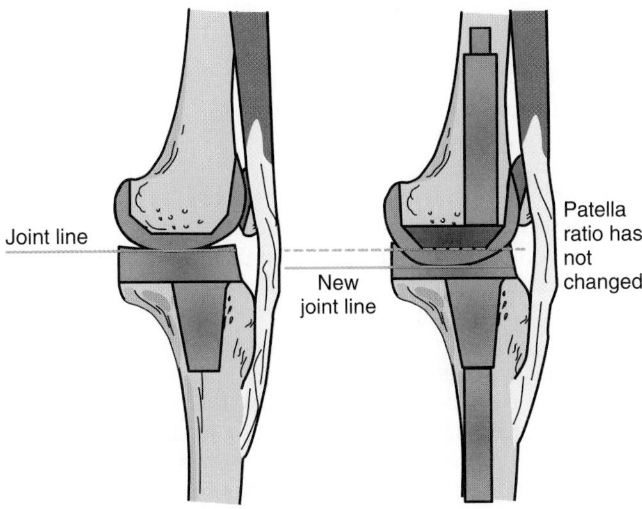

Figure 5-93 Technique to reduce patella baja impingement in total knee arthroplasty. *Left,* Patella baja and starting joint line. *Right,* Lowered joint line achieved by cutting more tibial bone and adding distal femoral augmentation.

VII. PATELLAR RESURFACING VERSUS NONRESURFACING

A. Between the two techniques, there is not an established superior method.

B. Patellar resurfacing—problems

1. Patella component loosening
   - Due to maltracking
   - Due to osteolysis
2. Patella *clunk* and *crunch*
   - Clunk occurs when suprapatellar scar tissue gets entrapped within the posterior stabilized box as the knee comes from flexion into extension.
   - Clunk is unique to posterior stabilized design.
   - Patellar crunch occurs when scar accumulates around patellar component, creating a crunching noise as the knee comes from flexion to extension.
3. Patella fracture
   - Reason—bone cut too thin
   - Minimum thickness for patella is 13 mm.
4. Avascular necrosis of patella with fragmentation
   - Reason—peripatellar devascularization

C. Unresurfaced patella problems

1. Anterior knee pain
   - Incidence increases over time.
   - Results of secondary resurfacing are variable.
     - Pain relief not predictable

D. Patella nonresurfacing—indications

1. Noninflammatory arthritis
2. Lower activity level
3. No dysplasia or maltracking
4. No baja

E. Patella nonresurfacing—requirements

1. Need anatomic femoral component
   - V-shape trochlea groove to match native patella
   - Deep insert groove to prevent overstuffing of patellar gap
2. Circumferential denervation of patella with electrocautery

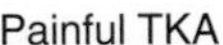

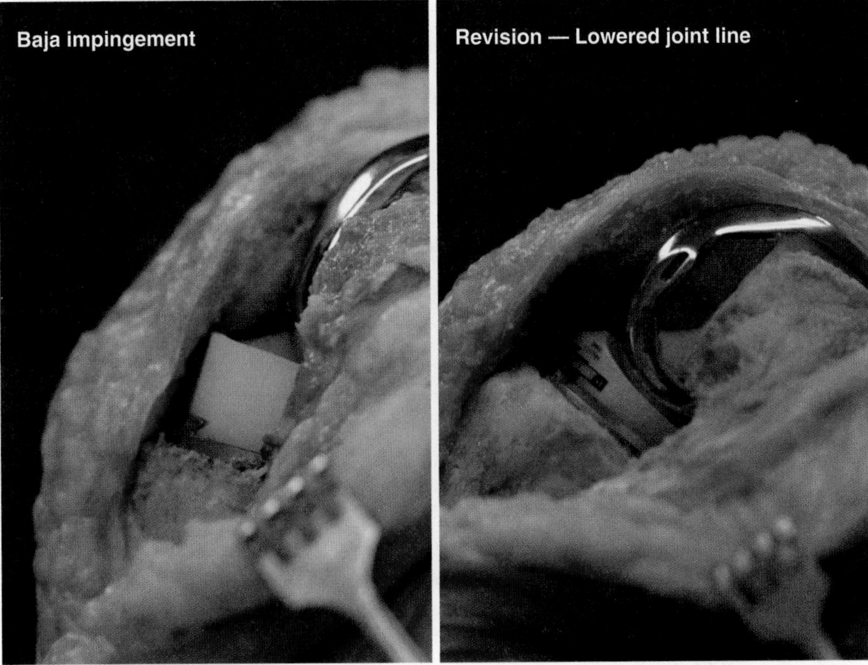

Figure 5-94 Intraoperative demonstration of lowering joint line to correct patella baja. *Left,* Baja impingement in flexion. *Right,* Same knee after revision total knee arthroplasty (TKA). The joint line was lowered by making a lower tibial bone cut and reducing tibial component thickness. Notice distal femoral augmentation used to bring femur distal.

SECTION 19 CATASTROPHIC WEAR IN TKA

I. PREMATURE FAILURE OF TKA IMPLANT

A. Etiology is *macroscopic* PE failure.

1. Problem is not a microscopic PE wear problem.

B. Clinically, patient presents with a large knee effusion that may or may not be painful.

C. Osteolysis is present but is a secondary problem.

D. Multiple factors are involved to create the *perfect storm* of catastrophic wear.

II. FACTORS INVOLVED IN CATASTROPHIC WEAR

A. PE thickness

B. Articular geometry

C. Knee kinematics

D. Surgical technique

E. PE processing

III. POLYETHYLENE THICKNESS

A. Thin PE breaks.

B. To keep knee bearing contact stress below the yield strength of UHMWPE (12 to 20 mPA), the PE must be at least 8 mm.

C. Many second-generation knee systems had PE knee inserts that had a PE thickness of 4 to 5 mm.

D. Current designs ensure that PE thickness in the thinnest areas of the insert is at least 8 mm.

IV. ARTICULAR GEOMETRY (FIGURE 5-95)

A. Avoid flat PE.

B. Knee loads will exceed yield strength of UHMWPE.

1. Thin line of joint contact during loading in flat PE insert
2. Results in high contact loads to PE
3. Goals of articulation
   - Maximize contact area.
   - Minimize contact loads (i.e., force/area).
   - Best design is biplanar congruency (Figure 5-96).
     - Congruent design in coronal plane and
     - Congruent design in sagittal plane

V. KNEE KINEMATICS

A. Sliding wear is bad for PE.

B. Sliding wear occurs when the ACL is sacrificed.

1. When the ACL is removed, and the PCL remains, the femur slides across the tibial PE during flexion and extension.
2. Sliding movements are *most* pronounced in a cruciate-retaining knee with a flat PE insert.
3. Sliding movements are *least* pronounced in a posterior stabilized knee with a congruent PE insert.
4. Sliding wear across the tibia in laboratory testing creates severe surface and subsurface cracking with high wear.

C. Current knee prosthetic systems are designed to minimize tibial sliding wear.

VI. SURGICAL TECHNIQUE

A. A tight flexion gap hastens sliding-wear effect.

1. Stress is amplified with
   - Tight PCL
   - Anterior tibial slope (Figure 5-97)

VII. POLYETHYLENE PROCESSING (REVIEW SECTION XII)

A. Fabrication

1. Ram bar extruded PE is not good.
   - Variation in PE quality within the bar

Articular Geometry

Low contact area

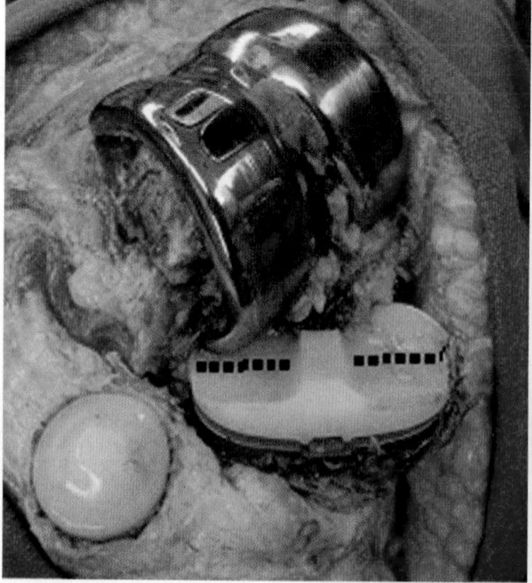

High contact load

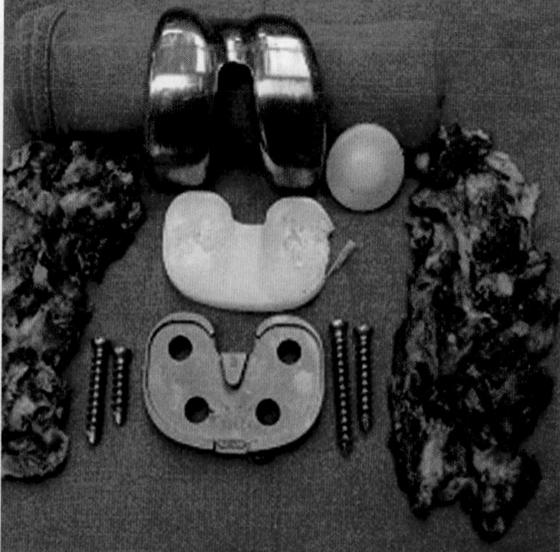

Figure 5-95 Intraoperative photograph of total knee arthroplasty with catastrophic wear after 9 years. *Left,* Flat polyethylene (PE) bearing articulating with a *flat* style femoral component. This allows for only a thin line of contact *(dotted line)* during knee load. The stresses generated upon the PE are excessive, and the PE fails macroscopically. *Right,* Inflammatory debris removed at the time of revision.

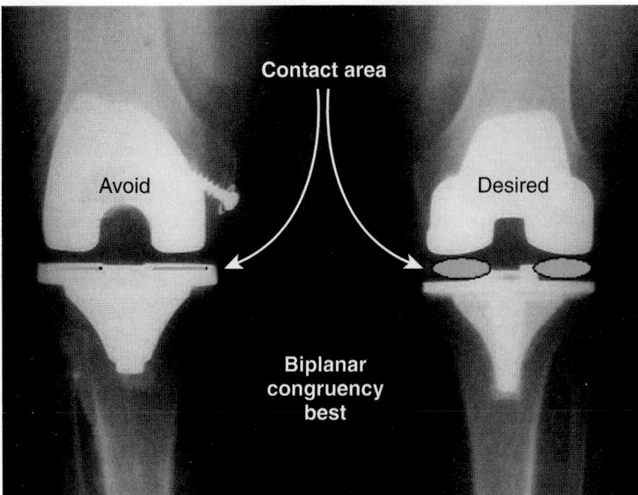

Figure 5-96 Radiograph showing two different articular bearing designs in total knee arthroplasty. *Left knee* has a *flat* bearing design in the coronal plane. The contact area is a line, and contact loads are high. *Right knee* has a congruent design in the coronal plane. The contact area of this design is an ellipse, and the contact loads are low.

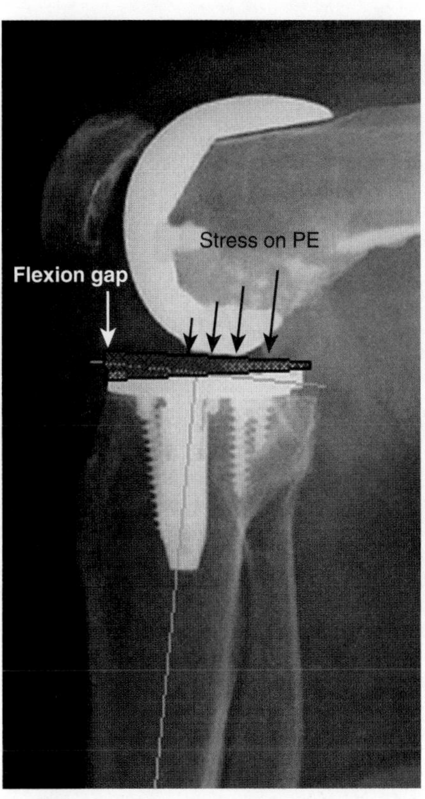

Figure 5-97 Radiograph demonstrating effect of anterior slope on polyethylene (PE) stress loads. In this radiograph, the *lines* define a neutral tibial slope. Compared to the neutral slope line, the tibial component is positioned with an anterior slope. As the knee flexes, the flexion gap *(triangle)* becomes smaller. Consequently, at end flexion, the contact stresses on the PE become excessively high *(arrows).*

2. Calcium stearate additive is bad.
   - Causes fusion defects in PE
3. ***Best* PE fabrication process is direct compression molding.**

B. **Sterilization**

1. Irradiated PE in air is bad.
   - Oxidized PE chains
   - Reduced *mechanical strength* of PE

C. **Machining (cutting-tool effect)**

1. The cutting tool used to machine PE microscopically *stretches* PE chains (Figure 5-98).
   - Amorphous areas are stretched.

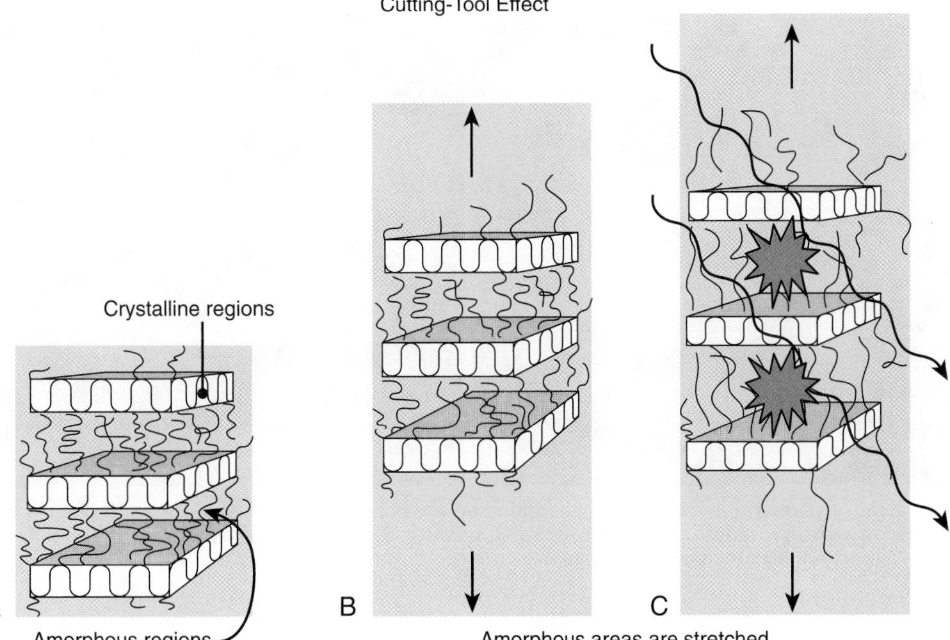

Figure 5-98 Diagram depicting the effect of machining upon polyethylene (PE). As the high-speed cutting tool removes the PE, the remaining nearby PE has stretched. Stretching occurs in the amorphous areas. The stretch effect is most pronounced in the PE 1 to 2 mm below the surface of the cut PE. The stretched PE chains are more susceptible to radiation, resulting in greater oxidation in this region.

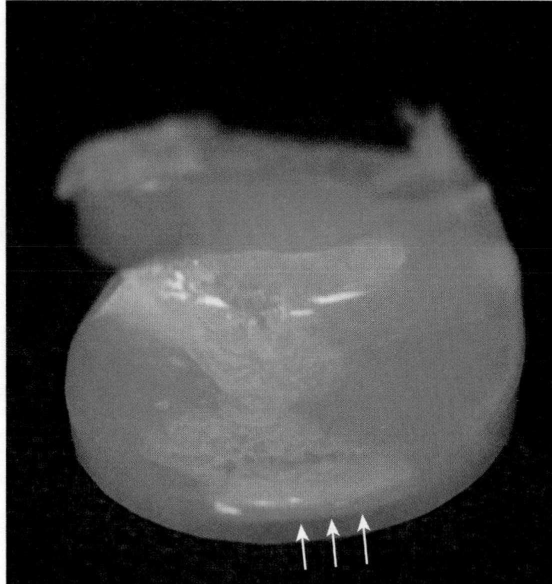

Figure 5-99 Retrieval polyethylene (PE) knee insert after 9 years in vivo. Note classical white band of oxidation located 1 to 2 mm below machined surface of PE *(arrows)*. The knee was revised for catastrophic wear.

2. The cutting-tool stretch effect is most pronounced 1 to 2 mm *below* the cut surface of the PE.
3. The stretched PE chains are more susceptible to radiation, resulting in greater oxidation in this region.
4. The clinical finding of the PE stretch/oxidation effect is the classical *white band* of oxidation in the subsurface of the PE (Figure 5-99).

VIII. PERFECT STORM SCENARIO FOR CATASTROPHIC WEAR (FIGURE 5-100)

A. Metal-backed tibial baseplate with bone-conserving tibial bone cut
1. Thin PE of 5 mm

B. Flat bearing design in coronal plane
1. Low contact area (a line)
2. High contact load

C. PCL retention with flat PE insert
1. High sliding wear

D. Ram bar PE with calcium stearate
1. Fusion defects in PE

E. γ-Irradiation sterilization in air (i.e., oxygen)
1. Weakened mechanical properties of PE

F. Machined PE surface
1. Cutting-tool stretch effect upon PE

IX. MEASURES TO MITIGATE CATASTROPHIC PE WEAR

A. PE thickness at least 8 mm

B. Congruent bearing design
1. High contact area
2. Low contact load

C. Sliding wear on tibia minimized
1. PCL substitution or
2. PCL *accepting* prosthesis
   - PCL is used as a static stabilizer only.

D. Direct compression molded PE bearing
1. No machining of articular surface

E. Inert PE irradiation
1. γ-Irradiation sterilization in oxygen-free environment
2. Quality packaging to minimize on-the-shelf oxidation

Catastrophic PE Failure

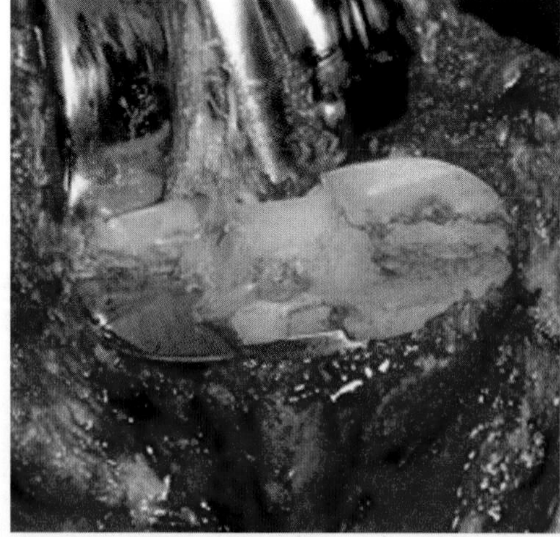

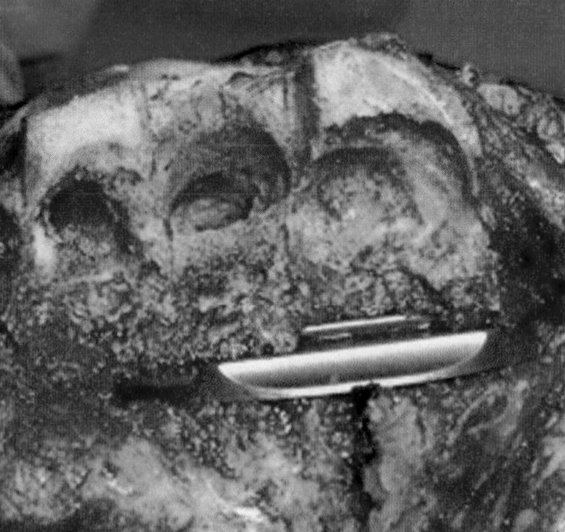

Figure 5-100 Intraoperative photographs of 8-year-old total knee arthroplasty in 58-year-old man. Patient presented with painless effusion. *Left,* Complete macroscopic failure of polyethylene (PE) bearing. *Right,* Effect of osteolysis in femur. Reconstruction required extensive bone allografts and complex revision knee system.

SECTION 20 SHOULDER ARTHROPLASTY

I. GLENOHUMERAL ARTHRITIS AND GLENOID WEAR (FIGURE 5-101)

A. Normal glenoid version is neutral to slight anteversion.

B. In osteoarthritis, glenoid orientation becomes *retroverted.*

1. **Retroversion due to the mechanical wear of bone**
2. **Results in posterior displacement of humeral head**

C. In juvenile idiopathic arthritis (also known as JRA) there is *central* glenoid bone loss.

1. **Clinically and radiographically, humeral head is medialized.**
   - **Also called *loss of humeral head offset***
   - Mechanically, reduced fulcrum for deltoid and weak elevation power with a medialized humeral head

D. Wear pattern on glenoid is posterior after anterior stabilization procedures.

1. Anterior stabilization results in relative internal rotation contracture.
   - Humeral head rests more in internal rotation, placing more wear forces on posterior glenoid.
2. Wear pattern on glenoid is *posterior,* resulting in glenoid retroversion.

II. SHOULDER ARTHROPLASTY—CONTRAINDICATIONS

A. Nonfunctioning deltoid and rotator cuff—both out

B. Active infection

C. Charcot arthroplasty

D. Intractable instability

E. Lack of patient compliance

III. CHARCOT ARTHROPATHY (FIGURE 5-102)

A. Severe destructive arthropathy

B. Etiology—neurologic in origin

C. Clinical presentation—*painless* loss of active motion

D. Neurologic evaluation—essential

1. Look for syrinx.
2. Rule out infection.

IV. SHOULDER HEMIARTHROPLASTY

A. Involves replacing only the humeral head

B. More limited indications for hemiarthroplasty because of improvement in long-term results of total shoulder replacement

C. Best indication—early-stage avascular necrosis of humerus (i.e., before degenerative changes occur on glenoid side) with normal glenoid articular cartilage in a young patient; older patients should have a total shoulder replacement

1. A *bipolar* hemiarthroplasty is not recommended in a young patient because this construct introduces PE debris into joint and risks osteolysis. Instead, a fixed humeral is advocated.

D. Requirements

1. Need normal glenoid bone stock and anatomy—no bone deficiencies
2. Normal chondral surface

E. Complications

1. Late glenoid pain—As glenoid surface wears, pain increases.
2. Conversion from hemiarthroplasty to total shoulder is sometimes difficult, and pain relief is not always predictable.

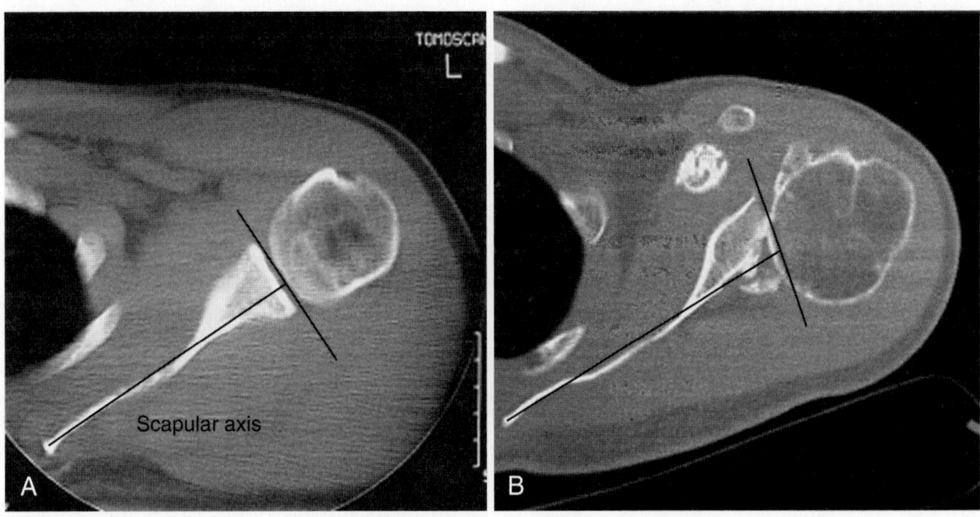

Figure 5-101 Computed tomographic scans demonstrating glenoid version. **A,** Neutral glenoid version. Version is determined by drawing a line along the scapular axis and a line from anterior glenoid to posterior glenoid. Normal version is neutral to slight anteversion. **B,** Glenoid retroversion in a patient with osteoarthritis. Note the significant amount of posterior glenoid wear and the posterior displacement of humeral head.

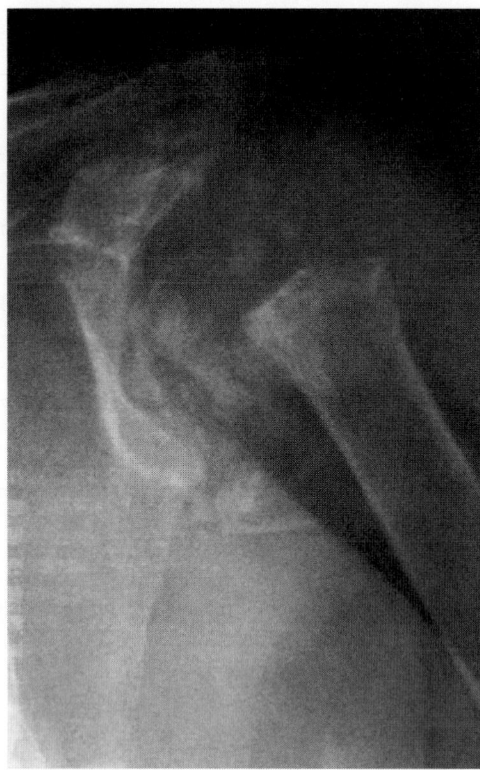

Figure 5-102 Radiograph of shoulder afflicted by Charcot arthropathy. This is a classical presenting radiograph showing advanced destructive arthroplasty. Note severe bone loss of glenoid and humeral head.

3. Abnormal shoulder balance causes eccentric glenoid bone loads, leading to glenoid bone loss, which can be significant.

V. TOTAL SHOULDER ARTHROPLASTY

A. Involves glenoid resurfacing and humeral head replacement

B. Clinically indicated when the glenoid chondral surface is worn to bone and pain limits activities of daily living

1. Clinically, glenoid pain from arthritis is felt anterior to posterior.

C. Requirements

1. **Rotator cuff must be intact and functional.**
   - **Isolated supraspinatus tear without retraction is acceptable condition to proceed with total shoulder arthroplasty (TSA).**
2. **Remember, incidence of *full-thickness* rotator cuff tears in patients undergoing TSA is 5% to 10%.**
   - Evaluate patient preoperatively with MRI if patient demonstrates positive shoulder impingement signs.

D. Preferred procedure for osteoarthritis of the shoulder

1. **Superior pain relief in long-term follow-up over hemiarthroplasty**
2. Results of hemiarthroplasty conversion to TSA show variable satisfaction.
3. Problems with hemiarthroplasty conversion to TSA
   - Severe glenoid bone loss from mechanical wear significantly compromises glenoid component fixation.
   - Pain relief is not predictable.
   - Many times, ultimate shoulder range of motion remains very limited.

E. Preferred procedure for inflammatory arthritis of the shoulder

1. Pain relief in long-term follow-up is superior to hemiarthroplasty.
2. Glenoid wear pattern in rheumatoid arthritis is *central.*

F. Approach

1. Approach for TSA is deltopectoral.
2. In deltopectoral approach, deep approach involves detachment of subscapularis muscle and capsule from anterior humerus.
3. Shoulder is dislocated anteriorly.
4. Most common complication is damage to the *axillary nerve.*
   - In shoulder region, axillary nerve and posterior humeral circumflex artery pass beneath glenohumeral joint in the quadrilateral space.
   - Quadrilateral space consists of the borders of
     - Teres minor
     - Teres major
     - Long head triceps
     - Humerus
5. Pectoralis tendon passes *on top* of biceps tendon to attach to humerus (Figure 5-103).
   - In a tight contracted shoulder, release of the upper half of the pectoralis tendon aids in exposure and dislocation.

G. Component position

1. Humeral stem is positioned in *retroversion.*
   - 25 to 45 degrees retroversion is accepted range.
2. Glenoid position should recreate *neutral* version.
   - Avoid glenoid retroversion.

H. Rehabilitation

1. **Avoid excessive *passive* external rotation exercises.**
2. **Excessive passive external rotation results in tear and pull-off of subscapularis tendon from anterior shoulder.**
   - Typical scenario
     - Subscapularis tendon and anterior capsule contracted from degenerative joint disease
     - Subscapularis tendon lengthened to rebalance
     - Reattachment to humerus pulled off with forced passive external rotation
3. Pull-off of subscapularis and anterior capsule results in *anterior* shoulder instability.
   - This is *most common* instability pattern after TSA.
4. Treatment of subscapularis pull-off is *early* surgical exploration and repair of the detached subscapularis tendon.
5. Test for subscapularis pull-off.
   - Weak *belly-press* test
     - In this test, patient has weakness in internal rotation arm toward chest against mild resistance.
   - Clinically, patient is unable to
     - Put hand into back pocket of pants
     - Tuck shirt behind the back
     - Hold dorsum of hand away from back
6. During postoperative rehabilitation phase of TSA, patient must avoid pushing self up from a low chair.
   - This places too much force on subscapularis, which may pull off and rupture.

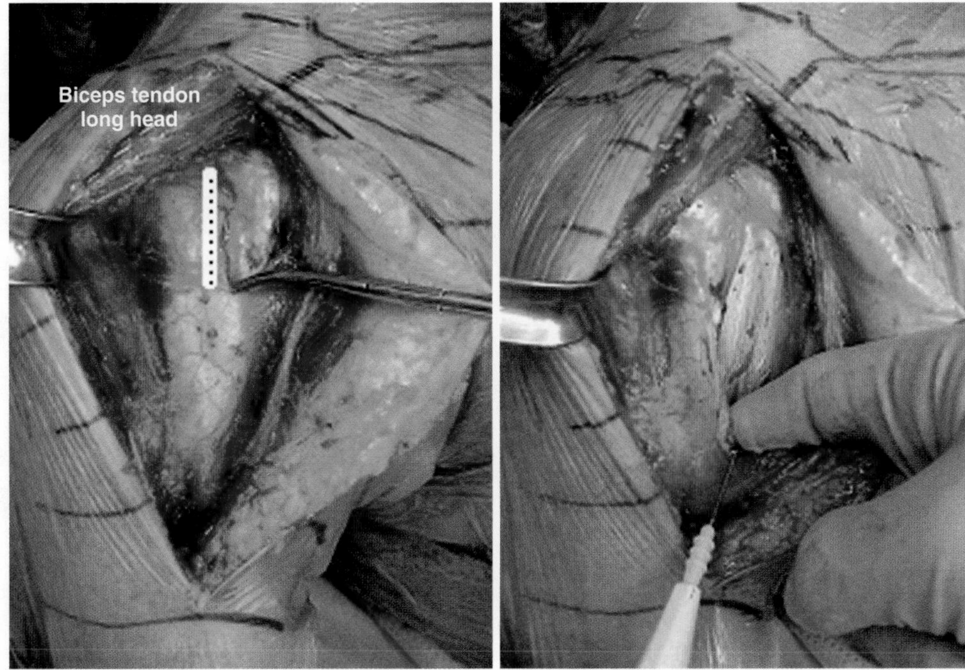
Biceps tendon
long head
• Pectoralis major tendon
• Crosses over biceps tendon
• If shoulder is tight and contracted, release
of upper half of tendon for exposure is okay

Figure 5-103 Intraoperative photographs of right shoulder with deltoid-pectoral approach. *Left,* Deltoid is reflected laterally, showing biceps tendon *(dotted line)* and pectoralis major tendon. The pectoralis tendon extends over the biceps tendon to attach to the humerus. *Right,* Release of the upper half of the tendon. This release aids in exposure and humeral component positioning.

VI. ROTATOR CUFF ARTHROPATHY

A. In this clinical condition there is complete loss of the supraspinatus and infraspinatus tendon, which is not repairable.

B. Clinically, humeral head is pulled superiorly by deltoid muscle, and the humeral head articulates with the undersurface of the acromion. This creates pain. Elevation strength and active motion are limited.

C. Radiographic finding is classical and must be recognized (Figure 5-104).

D. In rotator cuff arthropathy (RTCA), glenoid resurfacing is *contraindicated* using standard TSA implants (reverse TSA is acceptable).

1. **Glenoid resurfacing in presence of RTCA results in *rapid* glenoid failure due to eccentric loading on *superior* glenoid** (Figure 5-105).
2. A reverse TSA (when indicated) is best treatment for RTCA.
   - Better functional range of motion compared to hemiarthroplasty
   - Better pain relief compared to hemiarthroplasty
3. In RTCA, hemiarthroplasty is recommended if not using a reverse TSA (see indications for reverse TSA).
   - If hemiarthroplasty technique is used, *anatomic* head sizing is recommended.
     - Overstuffing with a large ball is associated with more pain.
   - In the hemiarthroplasty technique, the *coracoacromial ligament* must be preserved.
     - If the coracoacromial ligament is removed, the anterior acromial arch is disrupted.
     - The humeral head can escape and dislocate anterosuperiorly (Figure 5-106).

VII. REVERSE TOTAL SHOULDER ARTHROPLASTY

A. Involves insertion of following implants (Figure 5-107)

1. A porous-coated baseplate is secured to the glenoid with a central screw and multiple peripheral screws. Fixation is cementless.

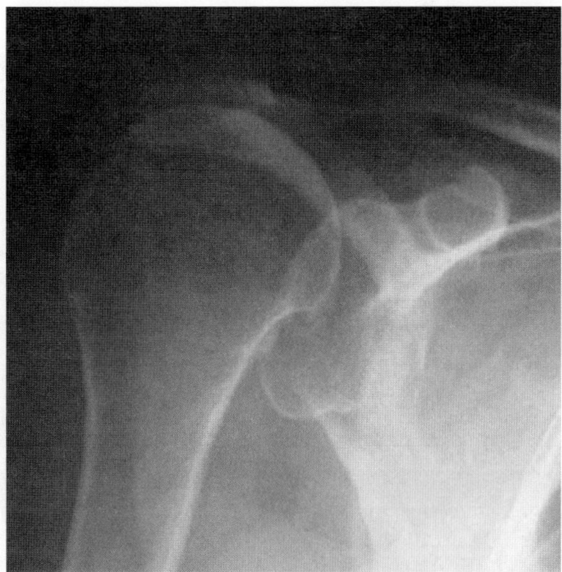

Figure 5-104 Anteroposterior radiograph showing classical radiographic appearance of rotator cuff arthropathy. Note that the humeral head articulates with the undersurface of the acromion. In this case, the undersurface of the acromion has been rounded out by the humeral head from mechanical abrasion. Also note that the humeral head is no longer centered within the glenoid.

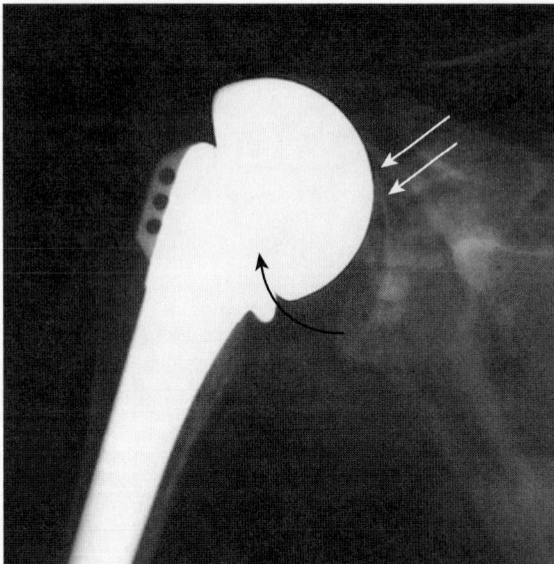

Figure 5-105 Anteroposterior radiograph of total shoulder arthroplasty (TSA) with a rotator cuff arthropathy. Patient had a fall 5 years after successful TSA. The superior rotator cuff completely ruptured, and now the humeral head articulates with the acromion superiorly. This position places high loads upon the superior glenoid *(white arrow),* and eventually the glenoid will loosen by repetitive levering (rocking-horse phenomenon; *black arrow*)

2. A glenosphere (i.e., ball) is assembled to baseplate.
3. A humeral stem is inserted into canal (cemented or cementless technique).
4. A humeral PE socket is assembled to the humeral stem.
5. Soft tissue tension is adjusted by varying the length of the glenosphere and humeral socket.

B. Resolves problem of superior migration of humeral head with RTCA

C. As deltoid contracts, the humerus rotates around glenosphere. Elevation power is provided by the deltoid muscle.

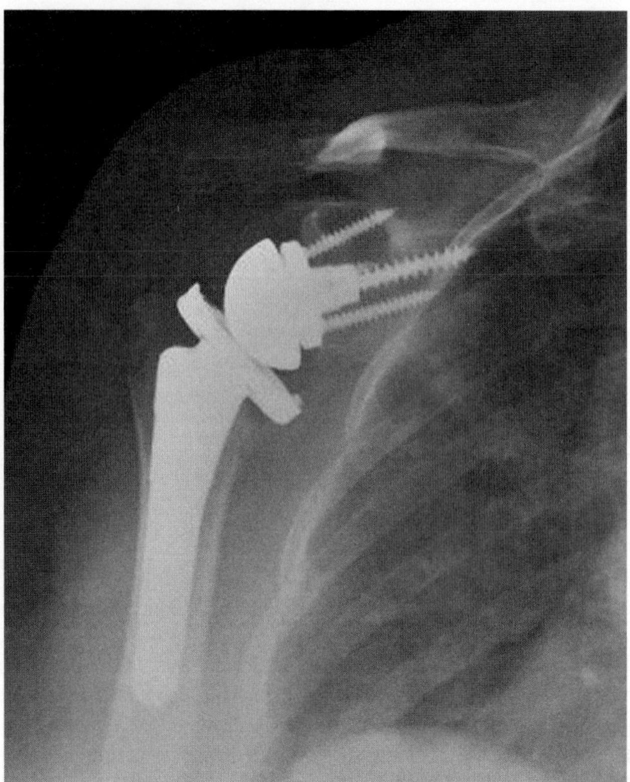

Figure 5-107 Radiograph of a reverse total shoulder arthroplasty (TSA). In the reverse TSA system, a porous-coated glenoid baseplate is inserted into the glenoid and secured with a central screw and peripheral screws. A glenosphere (i.e., ball) is attached to the baseplate. A humeral stem is placed into the humerus. A polyethylene cup is then assembled to the proximal humeral stem via a Morse taper junction. Note inferior tilt of glenoid component, which aids in deltoid tensioning.

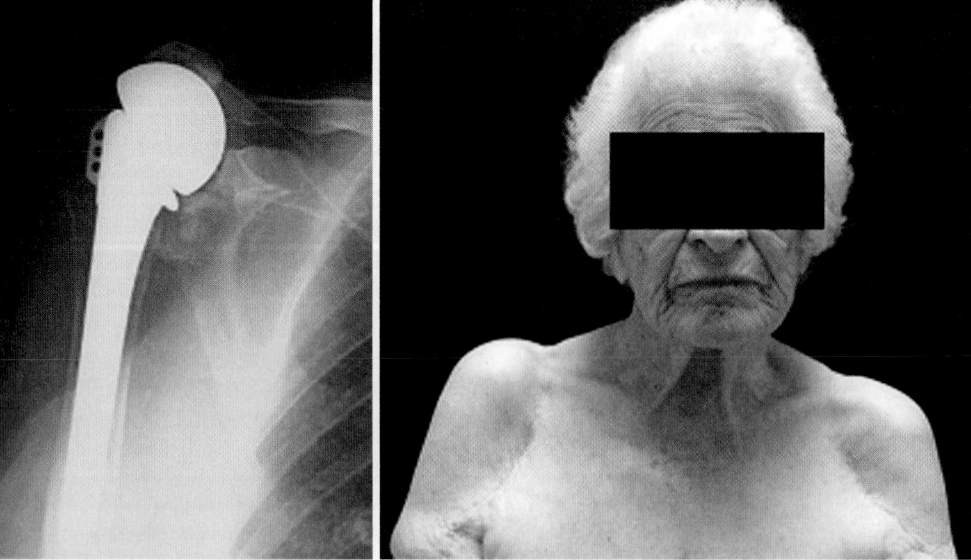

Figure 5-106 Rotator cuff arthropathy with anterosuperior dislocation. This patient has a rotator cuff arthropathy. *Left,* Superior positioning of the humeral head without the supraspinatus and infraspinatus tendon. In addition, the coracoacromial ligament has been removed. The humeral head has escaped anterosuperiorly. *Right,* Anterosuperior dislocation of humeral head. This patient was successfully treated with revision to a reverse total shoulder arthroplasty.

D. Deltoid power and efficiency are improved by *increasing* humeral offset via medialization of the center of rotation.

E. Stability of reverse TSA provided by

1. Deltoid tensioning
   - Adjust humeral offset.
   - Glenoid tilt
2. Head diameter
   - Larger diameter is more stable.
3. Component positioning
4. Dislocation of a reverse TSA most commonly is *anterior.*
   - Mechanism of dislocation is shoulder hyperextension and external rotation. In this position, the humeral socket levers posteriorly and dislocates.

F. Component positioning

1. **Glenosphere must be positioned as low as possible on the glenoid.**
   - This minimizes risk for scapular notching by humeral socket.
2. Glenoid baseplate (and glenosphere) should be *tilted inferiorly* 10 to 15 degrees. This is key to enhancing deltoid tensioning and thus providing implant stability.
3. Humeral stem is positioned in retroversion.
   - Twenty-five to 40 degrees retroversion preferred

G. Criteria for reverse TSA

1. **Intact axillary nerve**
2. **Full function of deltoid muscle**
3. **Adequate glenoid bone stock**
4. **Normal bone density**
5. **Light patient activity needs**
6. **Limited repetitive active elevation needs**

H. Exclusion criteria for reverse TSA

1. **Young active laborer**

I. Complications

1. Scapular notching
   - With the arm at the side and in adduction, the humeral socket can impinge upon scapular bone creating a bony defect (i.e., notch).
     - Notching causes pain.
     - Notching can lead to fracture.
     - Notching can cause levering and dislocation.
   - Minimize notching by
     - Positioning glenoid baseplate (and glenosphere) as low as possible on glenoid bone
     - Optimize glenosphere head length. This pushes humeral socket away from scapula.
2. Dislocation
   - Mechanism is hyperextension and external rotation.
   - In a reverse TSA the anterior repair of the subscapularis and anterior capsule is not as important, as in a standard TSA. In fact, in some contracted shoulders, with a reverse TSA the anterior subscapularis cannot be repaired to the humerus.

SECTION 21 PERIPROSTHETIC JOINT INFECTION

I. RISK FACTORS

A. Immune suppression

1. Drugs—especially
   - Anti–tumor necrosis factor agents
   - Antimetabolites such as methotrexate, leflunomide (Arava)
   - Corticosteroids
2. Immune system disorders, including dysplasia/neoplasia of immune system

B. Diabetes

C. Smoking

D. Obesity

II. BIOFILM (FIGURE 5-108)

A. The most important factor influencing periprosthetic infection treatment

B. All bacteria make biofilm.

C. Biofilm consists of approximately 15% cells and 85% *polysaccharide* matrix.

D. Biofilm forms on

1. All foreign materials
2. Devitalized tissues
   - Soft tissue and bone

E. Biofilm, once established, matures into sophisticated microenvironment.

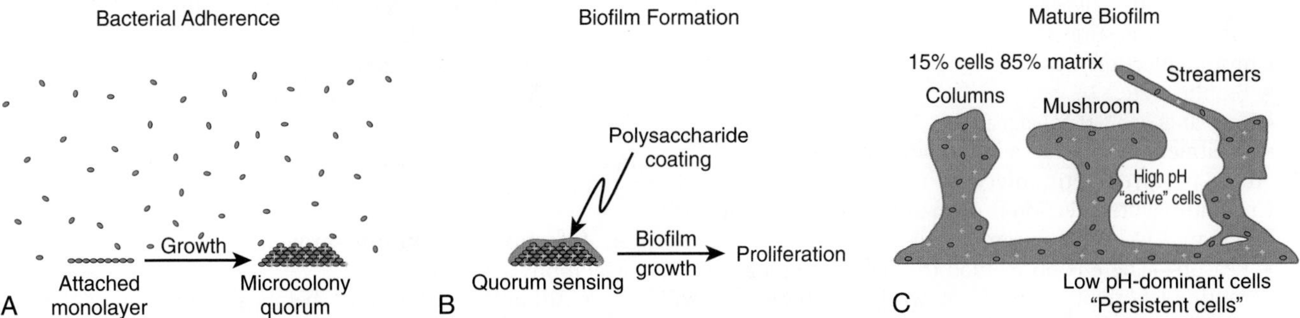

Figure 5-108 Diagram depicting biofilm formation on a prosthetic implant. **A,** Bacteria within the joint space adhere to implant (via adhesins) and multiply. Once the population of bacteria reaches a predetermined concentration (defined as a quorum), the colony expresses the biofilm. **B,** The biofilm under ideal conditions can rapidly proliferate and develop into mature biofilm. **C,** Mature biofilm state, in which bacteria interact with each other with signaling molecules and nanowires.

1. Bacteria communicate with signaling molecules and nanowires.

F. **Clinical importance of biofilm state**

1. Bacteria become 1000 to 1500 times more resistant to antibiotics.
   - Essentially, bacteria within a biofilm state cannot be killed with standard dosing regimens of antibiotics.
2. In vivo, biofilm can colonize, grow, and cover a surface within 4 to 8 days.
3. Effective treatment for established biofilm infection requires
   - Implant and foreign body removal
   - Removal of all devitalized bone and soft tissue
4. *Inadequate débridement* of biofilm material is the reason for treatment failure and infection recurrence.

III. DIAGNOSIS

A. **No current gold standard**

1. Draining sinus, intraoperative purulence, or positive culture results following joint aspiration are typically diagnostic.
2. Serologic tests, including erythrocyte sedimentation rate (ESR) and CRP, have low specificity but are utilized in periprosthetic infection detection and management.
3. **Synovial fluid cell count analysis values may be combined with the ESR and CRP to achieve a diagnosis.**
   - **Acute infection (within 2 to 4 weeks)**
     - **Three of the following**
       - **ESR greater than 30 mm/hr**
       - **CRP greater than 1 mg/dL**
       - **Fluid WBC greater than 10,700 cells/μL**
       - **Polymorphonuclear neutrophil percentage greater than 89%**
   - **Chronic infection (biofilm state)**
     - **Three of the following**
       - **ESR greater than 30 mm/hr**
       - **CRP greater than 1 mg/dL**
       - **Fluid WBC greater than 1760 cells/μL**
       - **Polymorphonuclear neutrophil percentage greater than 73%**

IV. TREATMENT ALGORITHM

A. **Classification**

1. Acute infection (less than 3 weeks known duration)
   - Nonbiofilm state
   - Implants are salvageable.
   - Treatment is surgical.
2. Chronic infection
   - Biofilm state
   - Implants are not salvageable.
   - Treatment is surgical, and implants are removed.

B. **Acute periprosthetic infection**

1. Currently, acute infection is defined as known infection of less than 3 weeks' duration.
   - Reason—There is no method to identify a biofilm with routine laboratory tests. Three weeks has been selected as a reasonable time frame to treat as acute.
2. **Treatment**
   - **Radical débridement surgery, including synovectomy and lavage**
   - **Modular bearings are exchanged.**
     - **Must access all prosthetic spaces and flush bacteria**
   - **Intravenous antibiotic therapy for 4 to 6 weeks**
   - Arthroscopic lavage of an acutely infected joint replacement is *not acceptable* treatment.
3. Failure
   - If infection recurs, treat as a chronic infection. Do not attempt second débridement surgery.

C. **Chronic periprosthetic infection**

1. **Currently, chronic infection is defined as known infection for more than 3 weeks' duration.**
2. **Treatment**
   - **Implant removal**
   - **Radial débridement, including synovectomy, removal of necrotic bone, and all devitalized soft tissue; copious lavage**
   - **Stabilization of joint with high-dose-antibiotic–loaded methylmethacrylate spacer**
     - Static spacer is used if joint stability is compromised by soft tissue and/or bone loss.
     - Articulated spacer is used if joint stability preserved.
       - Types of spacers
         - Antibiotic-loaded acrylic cement (ALAC)
           - Construct consists primarily of high-dose-antibiotic–loaded methylmethacrylate cement.
         - Prostalac (prosthesis and ALAC)
           - Construct that contains temporary metal and plastic prosthesis along with ALAC
         - Both constructs are acceptable for treatment. There is no proven superiority of ALAC versus Prostalac.
   - **Four to 6 weeks of intravenous antibiotic therapy**
   - **Second-stage reconstruction**
3. Second stage reconstruction—options
   - Reimplant joint arthroplasty
     - Most common treatment
     - Requires revision/salvage system to accommodate bone and soft tissue loss from infection débridement surgery
   - Arthrodesis
     - Used when there is significant loss of functional tissues
     - Must have adequate bone stock for fusion
   - Amputation—indications
     - Neuropathy and chronic pain are too debilitating to consider reimplantation.
     - Recurrent infection after resection arthroplasty
       - Patient is too medically compromised to help combat infection.
   - Permanent resection
     - Patient is unfit for surgery.

V. INFECTION PREVENTION—TOTAL JOINT REPLACEMENT

A. **Infection prevention—proven**

1. Prophylactic antibiotics
   - Administer 30 minutes before skin incision.
   - Continue for 24 hours after surgery.
2. Vertical laminar air flow
   - Vertical flow systems are *superior* to horizontal flow systems.

3. **Antibiotic-impregnated cement**
   - No more than 1 g of antibiotic per 40-g packet of cement (do not want to reduce mechanical properties of cement)
   - Indicated for higher-risk patients
   - **Use may be associated with increased rates of aseptic loosening.**

VI. WOUND COVERAGE IN TKA

A. Medial gastrocnemius rotational flap

1. The *workhorse* for deficiencies about the knee
2. Blood supply—medial sural artery.
3. Used to cover medial and anterior deficiencies
4. Good excursion

B. Lateral gastrocnemius rotational flap

1. Blood supply—lateral sural artery
2. Used to cover lateral soft tissue deficiencies
3. Little excursion
4. Risk—peroneal nerve palsy from traction of the flap as it is pulled anteriorly to lateral side of knee

TESTABLE CONCEPTS

SECTION 1 HIP DYSPLASIA—ADULT PRESENTATION

- The anatomic changes in adults with hip dysplasia are
  - Acetabulum: deficient anterior and lateral coverage; acetabular retroversion
  - Femur: reduced head/neck ratio (pistol grip deformity); excess neck anteversion
  - Treatment must address these four changes via periacetabular osteotomy, anterior hip decompression, and/or proximal hip osteotomy.
- Femoral acetabular impingement is defined as abnormal contact between the femoral neck and anterior acetabular rim.
  - Pincer: retroverted acetabulum results in block; more common in middle-age active women
  - Cam: nonspherical portion of femoral head abuts acetabulum; more common in young men

SECTION 4 OSTEONECROSIS OF THE HIP

- Risk factors
  - Most common: post-traumatic
  - Others: excessive alcohol, corticosteroid use, systemic lupus erythematosus, renal failure/transplant, human immunodeficiency virus, sickle cell disease, radiation, Gaucher disease, Caisson disease
  - Fifty percent rate of bilateral involvement—always image other hip
- Treatment
  - Based on age and whether the head is collapsed
  - Precollapse—bisphosphonates may decrease risk for head collapse
    - Less than 40 years of age
      - Core decompression, vascularized fibular strut, rotational proximal femoral osteotomy
    - Greater than 40 years of age
      - Small lesion—core decompression
      - Medium to large lesion—total hip arthroplasty (THA)
    - Core decompression is contraindicated if on chronic steroids.
  - Collapsed—THA

SECTION 5 TOTAL HIP ARTHROPLASTY

- Primary THA fixation selection
  - Cup—porous-coated cementless
  - Stem—cementless (high activity or young male) or cemented are acceptable
- Bone ingrowth optimal values—“Rule of 50s”
  - Pore size: 50 to 150 μm
  - Porosity: 40% to 50%
  - Gap distance: less than 50 μm
  - Initial rigid fixation and minimized implant micromotion
    - Fibrous fixation if greater than 150 μm
  - Must have cortical contact with bone, and bone must be viable (avoid in prior irradiation)

SECTION 6 REVISION THA

- In revision THA, infection must always be ruled out as a cause of pain.
- Acetabular revision
  - Recommended cup replacement
    - Cementless porous-coated hemispherical cup with screws
      - Posterior-superior quadrant is safe zone for screws
      - Anterior-superior quadrant is the zone of death due to risking the external iliac artery/vein.
    - Recreate the native center of rotation by placing inferior and medial to minimize joint reactive forces.
  - Well-fixed cementless implant with contained osteolytic defect—débridement, bone grafting, and bearing component exchange. Contraindicated if cup is malpositioned, has ongrowth fixation surface, or damaged locking mechanism
    - Cementing polyethylene (PE) liner into a damaged cup is associated with a increased rate of dislocation.
  - Major bone deficiency—reconstruction cage and/or a structural bone graft
  - Pelvic dissociation—separation of superior aspect of pelvis from inferior aspect. Treat with multiflange reconstruction cage or posterior pelvic reconstruction plate to ilium and ischium followed by cup, jumbo cup, or mental component, and augment as dictated by bone loss.
- Femoral revision—cementless extensively porous-coated long stem that is longer than the previous stem

SECTION 7 OSTEOLYSIS IN THA

- PE wear debris is the major cause of osteolysis. Adhesive wear is the most important process that generates these submicron particles.
- The osteolysis process begins with phagocytosis of PE particles by macrophages, which become activated and release cytokines. Bone resorption is mediated by osteoblasts and receptor activator of nuclear factor κB ligand (RANKL).
- Osteolysis can occur anywhere within the effective joint space. Particularly affected areas are screw holes in cup, surface area around screws, debonded cement-bone interfaces, and cement mantle defects.
  - Extensively porous-coated stem—osteolysis at greater trochanter and proximal femur; risk for greater trochanter fracture
  - Proximal porous noncircumferentially coated stem—osteolysis at stem tip
- Volumetric wear is the main determinant of PE particles and is directly related to the square of the head radius.
  - Linear wear rates in excess of 0.1 mm/yr are associated with osteolysis.

SECTION 8 PERIPROSTHETIC THA FRACTURE

- Perioperative fracture
  - If implant is loose and unstable—open reduction with internal fixation (ORIF) and revision

- If implant maintains initial rigid fixation and limited fracture—observe and protect weight bearing
  - If significant fracture displacement—ORIF
- Late fracture
  - Key rule: If femoral stem is loose, treatment is stem revision and ORIF of femur fracture.
    - Use cementless long-stem prosthesis with extensive biologic coating.
  - Stem tip fracture less than 25% of stem—various options
  - Stem tip fracture greater than 25% of *cemented* stem—ORIF and revision
  - Stem tip fracture greater than 25% of *cementless* stem but stem stable—various options
  - Fracture distal to stem tip—ORIF

SECTION 9 TOTAL ARTICULAR RESURFACING

- Advantages—better stability to standard THA; bone preserving
- Most common early complication is femoral neck fracture. Risk factors include female sex, poor bone quality, varus implant position, notching the superior neck, and disruption of the extraosseous blood supply.
  - Treat with conversion to THA.
- Relatively contraindicated in coxa vara because of vertical shear force on neck

SECTION 10 THA—MISCELLANEOUS

- Most common nerve injury—peroneal nerve division of sciatic nerve
  - Risk factors: female sex, post-traumatic arthritis, developmental dysplasia of the hip, revision surgery
  - Developmental dysplasia of the hip—lengthening greater than 3.5 cm increases risk
- Disease-associated complications
  - Sickle cell—early loosening
  - Psoriatic arthritis—high infection rate
  - Ankylosing spondylitis—high heterotopic ossification risk, increased anterior dislocation rate
  - Parkinson—high dislocation rate, perioperative mortality, medical complications, reoperation rate
- Surgical approaches
  - Posterolateral—limit flexion, adduction, and internal rotation postoperatively
  - Direct lateral—gluteus medius lurch; typically dislocate anterior
  - Anterior—limit external rotation and extension postoperatively; dislocate anterior
- Implants
  - Young's modulus relative values should be memorized. Ceramics have the highest, cartilage has the lowest. PMMA and UHMWPE separate cortical bone and cancellous bone in relative material stiffness.
  - The lowest coefficient of friction is articular cartilage, followed by ceramic on ceramic, metal on metal, metal on PE.

SECTION 11 THA—JOINT STABILITY

- Risk factors for dislocation after THA include female sex, preoperative diagnosis of osteonecrosis, use of a posterolateral approach, small head size, greater trochanteric nonunion
- The primary arc range is controlled by the head/neck ratio. Stability is best achieved by maximizing the head/neck ratio. Neck skirt, acetabular hoods, and constrained cups decrease the primary arc range.
- Implant positioning is critical to recognize on radiographs. The cup should be anteverted 20 to 30 degrees, abducted 30 to 40 degrees, and the stem anteverted 10 to 15 degrees.
  - Retroverted cup or stem—posterior dislocation
  - Anteverted cup or stem—anterior dislocation
  - Vertical cup—posterior superior dislocation
  - Horizontal cup—posterior inferior dislocation
- Abductor complex is key to hip stability, and the prosthetic implant design and positioning must maintain or restore proper abductor tension.
  - Reduced hip offset results in a weakened abductor complex, increased joint reaction force, positive Trendelenburg sign, gluteus medius lurch with walking, and increased risk for dislocation.
- In a dislocated THA, scrutinize implant design and position. If any implant component is malaligned, it needs to be changed.
- A constrained PE socket is best indicated in elderly patients, abductor deficiency, central nervous system decline and in revision THA with a reconstruction cage.
  - It is contraindicated if the acetabular cup is malpositioned.

SECTION 12 THA—ARTICULAR BEARING TECHNOLOGY

- Lubrication mechanisms
  - Hard on soft—boundary; synovial fluid separates surfaces just enough to prevent severe wear
  - Hard on hard—boundary when hip at rest or in slow motion; hydrodynamic when walking
    - Factors affecting the fluid film state include radial clearance, surface roughness, bearing size, sphericity, and the bearing material.

II. Hard-on-Soft Bearing

- Direct compression molding has the best wear of the four PE manufacturing techniques.
- Irradiation of PE should be performed in an oxygen-free environment.
  - In the presence of oxygen, free radicals within the PE cause chain scission, resulting in greatly reduced mechanical properties and accelerated PE wear.
- Highly cross-linked PE (HCLPE) has advantages and disadvantages compared to standard PE.
  - Advantages: better wear resistance; smaller PE wear particles; and decreased number of particles generated
  - Disadvantages: decreased tensile strength, fatigue strength, fracture toughness, and ductility (elongation without fracture)
- Melting of HCLPE reduces mechanical properties. Annealing of HCLPE increases oxidation potential.
- On-shelf oxidation can result from oxygen diffusing back into PE. Worst-case scenario is PE that is γ-irradiated, packed in air, and on the shelf for more than 5 years. Rarely used implants are subject to long shelf lives.

Continued

III. Hard-on-Hard Bearing

- The stripe line is typically described for ceramic-ceramic bearings but can be seen in metal-metal bearings. It is an area of roughness created on the head and cup because of repetitive subclinical subluxation. It indicates abnormal bearing wear mechanics.
- Metal-metal wear generates very small (nanometer) particles. There is very low linear and volumetric wear, but the absolute number of particles generated is significantly greater than comparable PE bearings.
- There are two distinct biologic responses to wear debris: hypersensitivity (immediate) and particulate-induced T-cell response (3 to 5 years later).
  - A persistent dull ache soon after postoperative recovery is characteristic of a hypersensitivity response. Treat with nickel-free implant.
  - Particulate-induced T-cell response involves metal debris being processed by the T-cell lymphocyte. It involves a highly activated RANKL system, and the ultimate response is a pseudotumor formation.
- Metal-metal bearings are contraindicated in women of childbearing age and in patients with renal failure. There is no increased risk for cancer.
- Ceramic-ceramic bearings
  - Advantages: lowest wear and bioinert debris
  - Disadvantages: head size and length limitation, hip squeak, bearing fracture risk
    - Fractured ceramic bearings must be replaced with another ceramic-ceramic bearing, because microscopic shards are severely abrasive and PE bearings would rapidly wear.

SECTION 14 KNEE ARTHRITIS TREATMENT

- Knee osteotomy is typically indicated in the active patient under 50 years of age.
  - Varus knee—valgus-producing high tibial osteotomy
  - Valgus knee—varus-producing supracondylar femoral osteotomy
  - Contraindications: inflammatory arthritis, less than 90 degrees of knee flexion, collateral ligament insufficiency
- Unicompartmental arthroplasty
  - Advantages: quicker recovery, smaller incision, better knee function
  - Disadvantages: long-term survivorship not as good as total knee arthroplasty (TKA)
  - Contraindications: inflammatory arthritis, greater than 10 degrees of flexion contracture, fixed varus/valgus deformity, anterior cruciate ligament deficiency, tricompartmental arthritis
  - Complications: stress fracture of tibia, patellar impingement

SECTION 15 TOTAL KNEE ARTHROPLASTY

- Varus knee balancing
  - Medial compartment release needed
  - Osteophytes, deep medial collateral ligament (MCL), posteromedial corner (capsule and semimembranosus), superficial MCL (posterior oblique tight in extension, anterior tight in flexion)
- Valgus knee balancing
  - Lateral compartment release needed
  - Osteophytes, lateral capsule, iliotibial band (tight in extension), popliteus (tight in flexion), lateral collateral ligament
- Flexion deformity balancing
  - Osteophytes, posterior capsule, gastrocnemius muscle origin
- Sagittal plane balancing
  - Flexion gap—*posterior* cut of femur, tibial cut, and posterior cruciate ligament (PCL)
  - Extension gap—*distal* cut of femur, tibial cut, posterior capsule
  - For some gap imbalance scenarios, there is more than one possible solution.
  - McPherson's rule
    - Symmetrical gap problem—adjust tibia first
    - Asymmetrical gap problem—adjust femur first
- TKA complications
  - Femoral notching—lessens load needed to cause fracture; suspect in supracondylar periprosthetic femur fracture with short oblique fracture
  - Peroneal nerve palsy—valgus knee with flexion contracture most at risk. Initial treatment is remove compressive dressing and flex knee.
    - Most recover within 3 months if nerve is not cut. If nerve palsy does not resolve, explore and decompress peroneal nerve.
  - Patella osteonecrosis—lateral retinacular release transects the lateral superior genicular artery.
  - Extensor disruption—*cannot repair*; must use allograft reconstruction

SECTION 16 TKA DESIGN

- PCL tension influences femoral rollback. Femoral rollback is defined as progressive posterior change in femoral-tibial contact point as knee moves into flexion.
- PCL retention
  - Advantages: bone conserving, consistent joint line restoration, improved proprioception
  - Disadvantages: harder to balance, excess recession can result in late failure caused by flexion instability
- Posterior stabilized TKA must be used if patellectomy, inflammatory arthritis, or PCL previously ruptured.
- Maximum joint line elevation is 8 mm to avoid patella baja deformity and decreased knee flexion.
- Modular tibial components can have backside PE wear from micromotion between tibial baseplate and tibial PE bearing.
- A constrained TKA must be used if the soft tissues will not support a standard prosthesis.
  - Indicated for residual flexion gap laxity, MCL or lateral collateral ligament deficiency, and Charcot arthropathy.

SECTION 18 PATELLAR TRACKING IN TKA

- Femoral and tibial components—do not internally rotate or medialize
  - In a valgus knee, the lateral condyle is frequently hypoplastic and the posterior condylar axis cannot be used.

- Patellar component medialization is acceptable because it decreases the Q angle.
- Maltracking
  - Intraoperatively—first release the tourniquet and reassess
  - Postoperatively—if examination and radiographs are acceptable, a computed tomographic scan can be used to determine rotational alignment of components
- Patella baja results in loss of knee flexion and impingement pain. Seen after proximal tibial closed-wedge osteotomy, tibial tubercle osteotomy, and trauma

SECTION 19 CATASTROPHIC WEAR IN TKA

- Five key fractures involved in catastrophic wear
  - PE thickness—greater than 8 mm
  - Articular geometry—avoid flat PE
  - Knee kinematics—minimize tibial sliding wear
  - Surgical technique—avoid tight flexion gap
  - PE processing—use direct compression molding and inert PE irradiation

SECTION 20 SHOULDER ARTHROPLASTY

- Glenoid wear patterns
  - Osteoarthritis—posterior wear and retroversion of glenoid
  - Juvenile idiopathic arthritis (also known as JRA)—central wear
  - Anterior stabilization procedure—posterior wear and retroversion
- Shoulder hemiarthroplasty typically indicated in early-stage avascular necrosis with normal glenoid articular cartilage in a young patient
- Total shoulder arthroplasty (TSA) requires a functional and intact rotator cuff.
  - Isolated supraspinatus tear without retraction is acceptable, however. Five percent to 10% of patients undergoing a TSA have a full-thickness tear.
  - Excessive passive external rotation exercises must be avoided postoperatively to protect the subscapularis tendon.
- Reverse TSA is indicated in patients with rotator cuff arthropathy. Patients must have an intact axillary nerve, fully functional deltoid, and adequate glenoid bone stock.
  - Radiographic findings of rotator cuff arthropathy include superior migration of the humerus with acromiohumeral distance less than 7 mm, acetabularization of the acromion, rounding of the greater tuberosity, and loss of joint space.
  - A reverse TSA improves deltoid power and efficiency by medialization of the center of rotation.
  - The glenosphere must be positioned as low as possible to minimize the risk for scapular notching.
  - The ideal patient is an elderly, low-demand person. Reverse TSA is generally avoided in young active laborers.

SECTION 21 PERIPROSTHETIC JOINT INFECTION

- There is currently no gold standard for diagnosis of a periprosthetic joint infection. Any painful arthroplasty should have infection excluded.
- Recent literature indicates that acute infection is suggested with an erythrocyte sedimentation rate (ESR) greater than 30 mm/hr, C-reactive protein (CRP) greater than 1 mg/dL, synovial fluid greater than 10,700 cells/μL, and polymorphonuclear neutrophil percentage greater than 89%. Chronic infection is suggested by ESR greater than 30 mm/hr, CRP greater than 1 mg/dL, synovial fluid greater than 1,760 cells/μL, and polymorphonuclear neutrophil percentage greater than 73%.
- The biofilm is the most important factor influencing periprosthetic infection treatment.
  - All bacteria make biofilm.
  - A biofilm, once established, cannot be erradicated with any current treatment regimen.
  - Once a biofilm is established, effective treatment requires prosthetic removal and radical soft-tissue débridement.
- Infection treatment
  - Acute (known infection <3 weeks)—irrigation and débridement, exchange of modular bearings, retention of components, and intravenous antibiotics
  - Chronic (biofilmstate)—implant removal, irrigation and débridement, stabilization of joint with antibiotic cement spacer, intravenous antibiotics, and second-stage reconstruction

SELECTED BIBLIOGRAPHY

The selected bibliography for this chapter can be found on www.expertconsult.com.

Chapter 6

DISORDERS OF THE FOOT AND ANKLE

Anish R. Kadakia and Todd A. Irwin

CONTENTS

CONTENTS—cont'd

This chapter provides a review of adult foot and ankle disorders and deformities. Pediatric and congenital deformities are covered in Chapter 3, Pediatric Orthopaedics.

SECTION 1 BIOMECHANICS OF THE FOOT AND ANKLE

The primary functions of the foot and ankle are to provide support and forward ambulation.

I. ANATOMY

A. Ankle

1. Ankle mortise is formed by the tibial plafond, medial malleolus, and lateral malleolus (Figure 6-1).
2. Mortise articulates with the dome of the talus.
3. Mortise widens and ankle becomes more stable in dorsiflexion due to shape of talar dome (wider anteriorly).
4. A simplified model of the ankle joint has a horizontal axis from anteromedial to posterolateral and a coronal axis from superomedial directed distally and laterally to the tip of the fibula (between the malleoli) (Figure 6-2).
5. Responsible for most sagittal plane motion of the foot and ankle
6. 23 to 48 degrees plantar flexion
7. 10 to 23 degrees dorsiflexion
8. Also contributes to inversion/eversion and rotation

B. Distal tibiofibular joint

1. Distal fibula—convex medial surface
2. Incisura fibularis—concave surface of distal lateral tibia
3. **Fibula rotates (~2 degrees) within incisura during ankle motion and ambulation. Ankle dorsiflexion results in external rotation and proximal translation of the fibula.**
4. Mortise widens 1 to 1.5 mm during motion from plantar flexion to dorsiflexion.

C. Ligamentous anatomy (Figure 6-3)

1. The lateral ankle ligaments function as a restraint to varus forces at the ankle.
   - The anterior talofibular ligament originates from the anteroinferior aspect of the lateral malleolus, 1 cm proximal to its tip, and extends to the lateral aspect of the talar neck.
   - The calcaneofibular ligament extends from the tip of the lateral malleolus to the lateral aspect of the calcaneus.

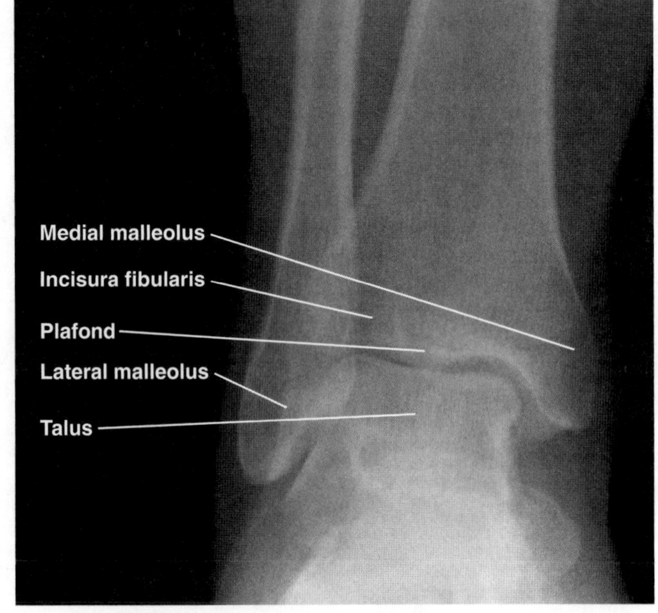

Figure 6-1 Anteroposterior radiograph of the ankle.

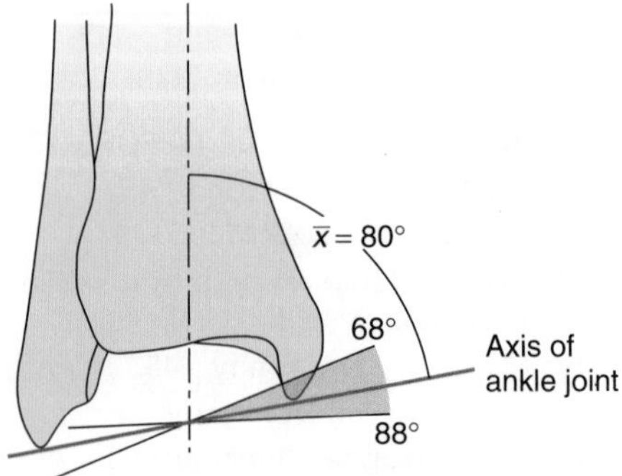

Figure 6-2 Angle between the axis of the ankle joint and the long axis of the tibia. (From Hsu J, et al: *AAOS atlas of orthoses and assistive devices,* Philadelphia, 2008, Elsevier.)

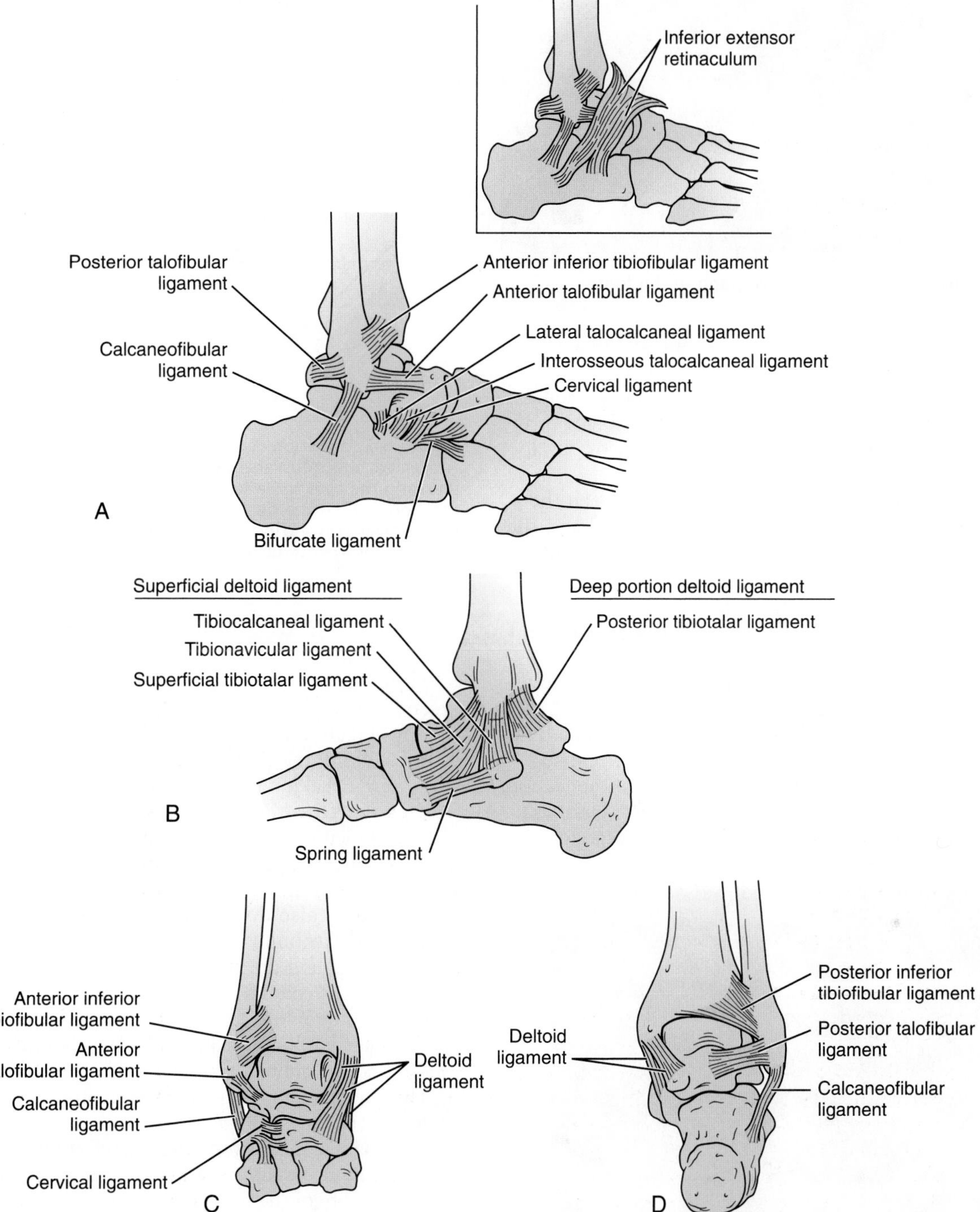

Figure 6-3 **Ligaments of the ankle and subtalar joint. A, Lateral view. B, Medial view. C, Anterior view. D, Posterior view.** (From Miller M: *Core knowledge in orthopaedics—sports medicine,* Philadelphia, 2006, Elsevier.)

- The posterior talofibular ligament extends from the posterior lateral malleolus to the posterolateral talus.
- The anterior talofibular ligament is the weakest ankle ligament, and the posterior talofibular ligament is the strongest.

2. The distal tibiofibular joint (ankle syndesmosis) and fibula provide stability against lateral talar translation.
   - Approximately 2 degrees of normal fibular rotation occurs at the syndesmosis during ambulation.
3. Deltoid ligament complex—main stabilizer of the ankle during stance
   - The deep deltoid ligament extends from the apex of the medial malleolus to the medial talar body. It functions primarily to resist lateral talar translation.
   - The superficial deltoid ligament extends from the distal medial malleolus to the navicular bone, sustentaculum tali of the calcaneus, medial talus, and spring ligament. It functions primarily to resist valgus ankle force (i.e., talar tilt).

D. Hindfoot and midfoot

1. The hindfoot includes the talus, calcaneus, and cuboid. The subtalar, calcaneocuboid (CC), and talonavicular (TN)

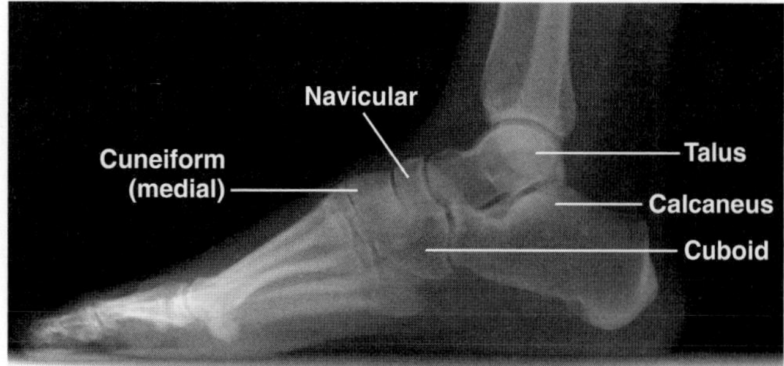

Figure 6-4 Lateral radiograph of the foot.

joints are included (Figure 6-4). The hindfoot functions in inversion and eversion.

- Inversion motion is normally greater than eversion.
    - Limited eversion accommodation contributes to the disability derived from even a mild cavovarus foot deformity.

E. The midfoot begins at the articulation between the navicular and the cuneiforms along with cuboid and the fourth and fifth metatarsals. The midfoot also includes the tarsometatarsal (TMT) joints.

1. The midfoot functions in adduction and abduction.

F. The forefoot includes all structures distal to the TMT joints (Figure 6-5).

G. The CC and TN joints are collectively referred to as the midtarsal, transverse tarsal, or Chopart joint.

1. This joint is important for providing stability of the hindfoot and midfoot to produce a rigid lever at heel-rise.
2. During heel-strike (hindfoot valgus, forefoot abduction, and dorsiflexion of the ankle), the transverse tarsal joints are parallel and supple, adapting to the uneven ground.

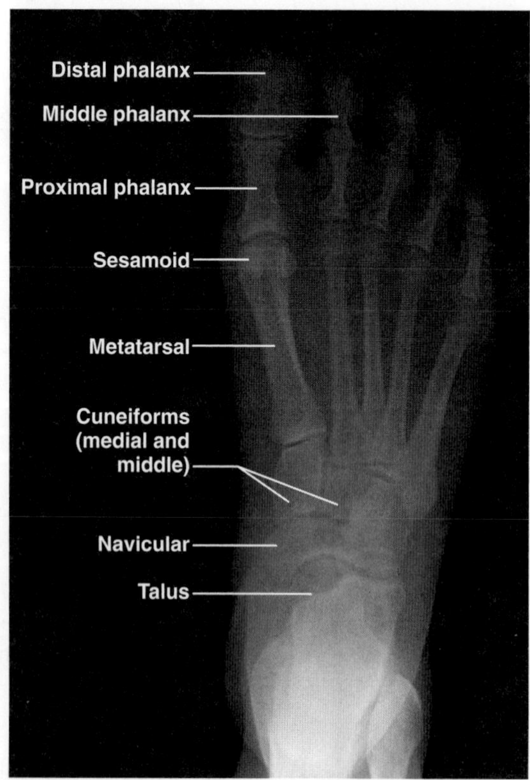

Figure 6-5 Anteroposterior radiograph of the foot.

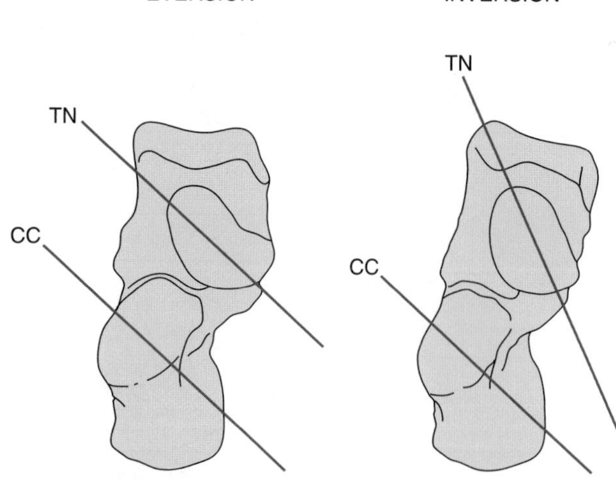

Figure 6-6 Function of the transverse tarsal joint. When the heel is everted, the transverse tarsal joints are parallel and unlocked, allowing the foot to be supple and pronate and accommodate to the floor. When the heel is inverted (varus), the transverse tarsal joint is divergent and locked, allowing for a stable hindfoot/midfoot complex for toe-off. CC, calcaneocuboid; TN, talonavicular.

3. During toe-off (hindfoot varus, forefoot adduction, and plantar flexion of the ankle), these joints become divergent and lock, providing stiffness to the foot for forward propulsion (Figure 6-6).
    - Failure of the posterior tibial tendon to lock the transverse tarsal joints is the biomechanical etiology for lack of a heel-rise in patients with posterior tibial tendon dysfunction.

H. The collective TMT joint complex is referred to as the Lisfranc joint.

I. The foot is also divided into three columns.

1. The medial column includes the first metatarsal, the medial cuneiform, and the navicular.
2. The middle column includes the second and third metatarsals, the middle cuneiform, and the lateral cuneiform.
3. The lateral column includes the fourth and fifth metatarsals and the cuboid.
4. The lateral column has the most sagittal mobility, and the middle column has the least.
5. The sagittal mobility of the lateral column imparts the flexibility necessary for walking on uneven ground.
6. The rigidity of the middle column allows for a rigid lever arm during push-off.

J. The foot has longitudinal and transverse arches. Stability of these arches is provided by a combination of the bony architecture, ligamentous attachments, and muscle forces.

1. The stability of the midfoot allows for push-off during gait or other activities.

K. Ligamentous stability to the midfoot is provided through longitudinal and transverse ligaments on the plantar and dorsal aspects of each joint.

1. The plantar ligaments are thicker and stronger than their dorsal counterparts.
2. The primary stabilizer of the longitudinal arch is the interosseous ligaments and not the plantar fascia. The plantar fascia is a secondary stabilizer.

L. The Lisfranc joint complex has a specialized bony and ligamentous structure, providing stability to this joint.

1. The middle cuneiform ends more proximally than the medial and lateral cuneiforms. The second metatarsal therefore extends more proximally than the surrounding metatarsals. This "keystone" effect imparts inherent bony stability.
2. Dorsal and plantar ligaments extend from the second metatarsal to each of the three cuneiforms.
3. The largest and strongest of these ligaments is the Lisfranc ligament, traveling from the medial cuneiform to the base of the second metatarsal.

M. The midfoot provides an important bridge between the hindfoot and forefoot. It provides both flexibility and stability necessary for normal gait and other activities.

II. FOREFOOT

A. The bony forefoot comprises the metatarsals and phalanges.

B. The first metatarsal is the widest and shortest and bears 50% of the weight during gait.

C. The second metatarsal is usually the longest and experiences more stress than the other lesser metatarsals.

1. The second metatarsal is more commonly involved in stress fractures.

D. The lesser toes are controlled by a balance among them.

1. Extrinsic muscles
   - Extensor digitorum longus (EDL)
   - Flexor digitorum longus (FDL)
2. Intrinsic muscles—metatarsophalangeal (MTP) flexion and proximal interphalangeal (PIP) extension
   - Interossei
   - Lumbricals
3. Passive restraints
   - Plantar plate—disrupted in a crossover toe
   - Extensor hood (primary distal insertion point of the long extensors), which functions to extend the MTP joint and NOT the PIP joint
   - Joint capsule
   - Collateral ligaments

E. The intrinsic tendons pass plantar (providing a flexion force) to the MTP joint axis proximally and pass dorsal to the axis distally (providing an extension force).

1. **Plantar migration of this axis after a Weil (oblique shortening) osteotomy of the metatarsal leads to a "cock-up" toe.** The tendons are now relatively dorsal to the MTP axis of rotation (Figure 6-7).
2. Loss of intrinsic function as seen in hereditary and motor sensory neuropathy or diabetic neuropathy predictably leads to claw toes.

III. FOOT POSITIONS VERSUS FOOT MOTIONS

A. Foot positions are defined in a manner different from that of foot motions.

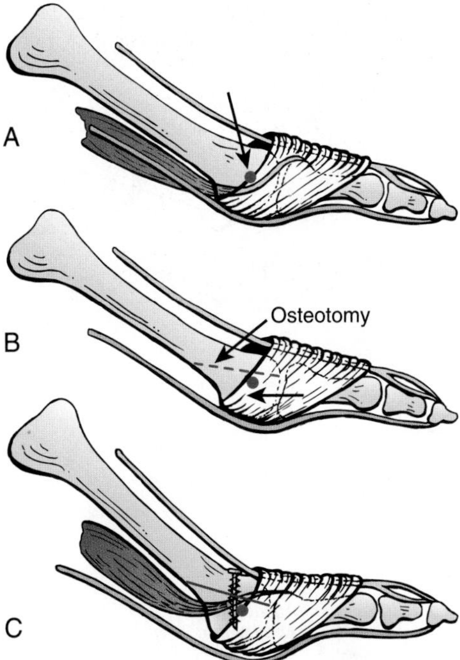

Figure 6-7 Axis of the metatarsophalangeal joint before and after Weil osteotomy. **A,** Lesser metatarsal before osteotomy; note intrinsics are plantar to the axis. **B,** Osteotomy is above the center of the metatarsal head. **C,** Following the osteotomy and proximal translation of the capital fragment, the intrinsics course dorsal to the axis of rotation. This can lead to metatarsophalangeal joint dorsiflexion. (From Coughlin M, et al: *Surgery of the foot and ankle,* ed 8, Philadelphia, 2006, Elsevier.)

B. The foot positions are

1. Varus/valgus (hindfoot)
2. Abduction/adduction (midfoot)
3. Equinus/calcaneus (ankle)

C. Foot motions in the three axes of rotation are illustrated in Figure 6-8 and summarized in Table 6-1.

1. The critical assessment is to determine the relationship of the forefoot to the hindfoot.

Table 6-1 Motions of the Foot and Ankle

Plane of Motion	Motion
Sagittal (X axis)	Dorsiflexion Plantar flexion
Frontal (coronal) (Z axis)	Inversion Eversion

Transverse (Y axis)	Forefoot/midfoot
	  Adduction
	  Abduction
	Ankle/hindfoot
	  Internal rotation
	  External rotation

Triplanar motion	Supination
	  Adduction
	  Inversion
	  Plantar flexion
	Pronation
	  Abduction
	  Eversion
	  Dorsiflexion

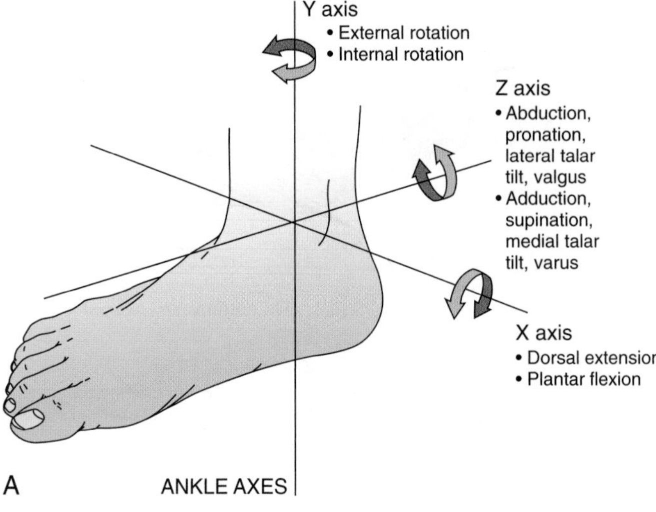

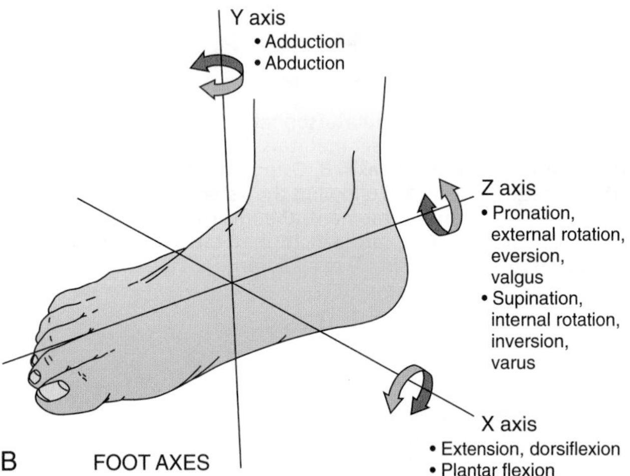

Figure 6-8 Axes of rotation of the ankle **(A)** and foot **(B).** (From Myerson MS: *Foot and ankle disorders,* Philadelphia, 2000, Elsevier.)

2. If the heel is in a neutral position (subtalar neutral), the forefoot should be parallel with the floor to meet the ground flush (plantigrade).
   - If the first ray is elevated, the forefoot is in varus position. If the first ray is flexed, the forefoot is in valgus position. This should not be confused with hindfoot varus or valgus.
   - For example, in a long-standing flatfoot deformity the heel is valgus and the forefoot has compensated by going into varus or supinating to keep the flat to the ground.
     - Once the heel has been corrected, the elevated first ray can be easily seen (Figure 6-9).

IV. THE GAIT CYCLE

A. One full gait cycle, from heel-strike to heel-strike, is termed a "stride."

1. Each stride is composed of a stance phase (heel-strike to toe-off, 62% of the cycle) and a swing phase (toe-off to heel-strike, 38% of the cycle) (Figure 6-10).
2. Walking is defined by a period of double-limb support in addition to always having one foot in contact with the ground throughout the gait cycle.
3. Ground reaction forces are approximately 1.5 times body weight during walking and 3 to 4 times body weight during running.
   - This difference is due to the increased load after the float phase of running, in which there is no foot in contact with the ground.
4. As the speed of gait increases, the stance phase decreases.

B. Soft tissue contributions to gait mechanics

1. Swing phase
   - Anterior tibialis—contracts concentrically
     - Loss of function results in a footdrop and steppage gait.

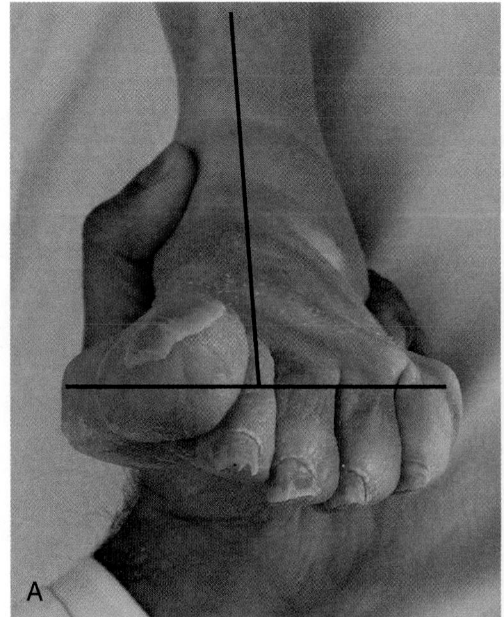

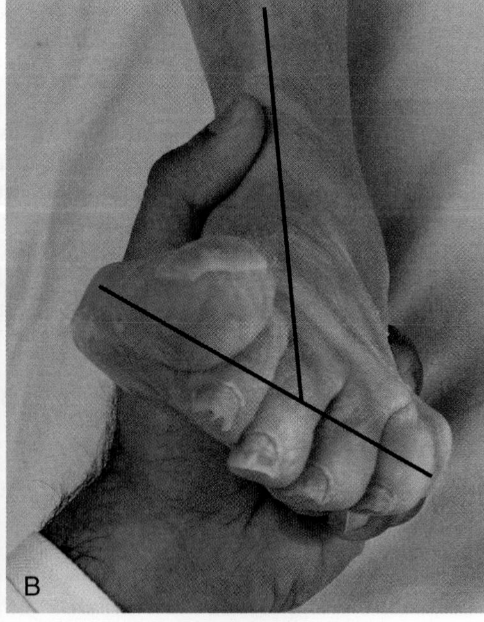

Figure 6-9 A patient with long-standing pes planovalgus deformity. With the hindfoot in valgus, the foot is plantigrade to the ground **(A).** With the hindfoot corrected to neutral, the forefoot supination becomes evident **(B)** with the elevated first ray. Failure to correct this deformity will cause any surgical correction to fail, because the hindfoot will go back into valgus as the first ray must contact the ground.

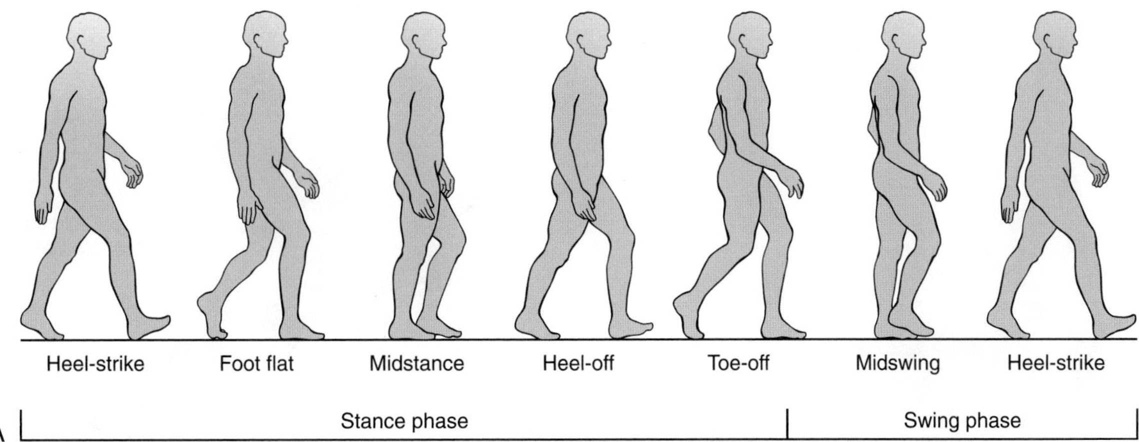

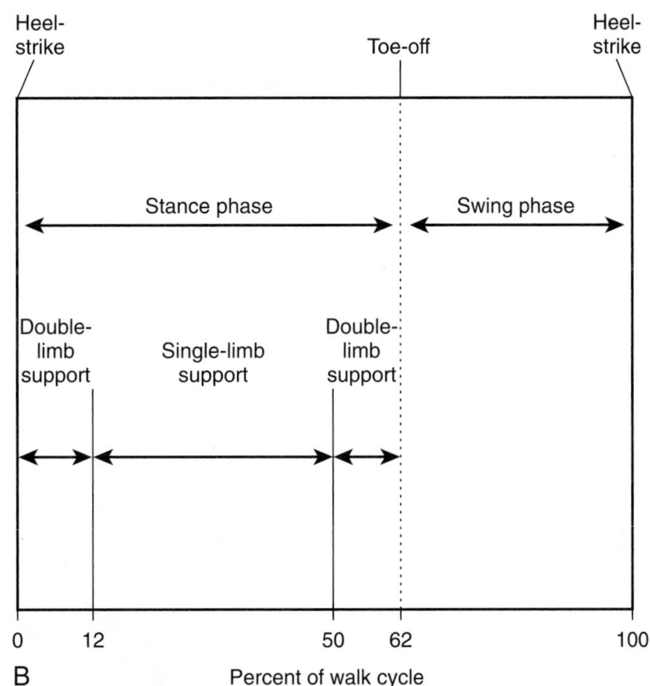

Figure 6-10 The gait cycle. **A,** The normal phases of gait. **B,** Time dimensions of normal gait cycle. (From Miller M: *Core knowledge in orthopaedics—sports medicine,* Philadelphia, 2006, Elsevier.)

2. Heel-strike
   - Anterior tibialis—contracts eccentrically
     - Controls the rate at which the foot strikes the ground. In patients with footdrop, the rapid strike of the foot can result in a loud "slap" during heel-strike.
   - Hindfoot—unlocked/everted for energy absorption
3. Foot flat
   - Gastrocnemius-soleus complex—eccentric contraction
     - Controls forward progression of the body over the foot
   - Hindfoot—unlocked/everted for ground accommodation
4. Toe-off
   - Gastrocnemius-soleus complex—concentric contraction

- In addition, as the foot progresses from heel-strike to toe-off, the following changes allow the foot to convert from a flexible shock absorber to a rigid propellant.
  - **The plantar fascia, which attaches to the plantar medial heel and runs the length of the arch to the bases of each proximal phalanx, is tightened as the MTP joints extend. The longitudinal arch is accentuated.**
    - **This is called the windlass mechanism** (Figure 6-11).
  - **The hindfoot supinates, with firing of the posterior tibial tendon.**
  - The transverse tarsal joint locks and provides a rigid lever arm for toe-off.

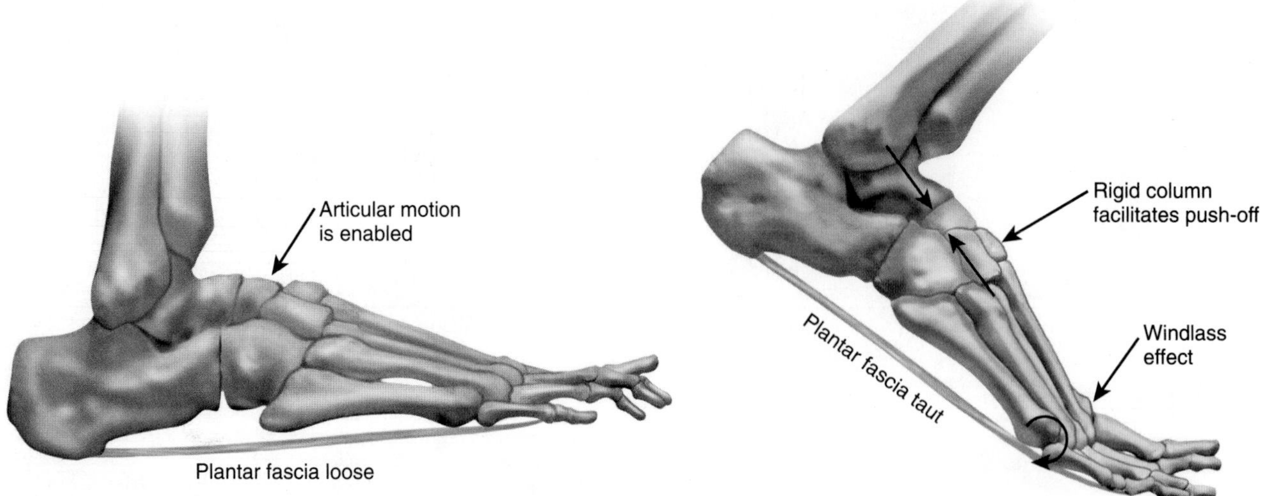

Figure 6-11 The windlass mechanism and function of the plantar fascia. When the foot is at rest, there is some mobility between the bones of the midfoot, allowing flexibility. During the push-off phase of gait, this flexibility would be detrimental. The plantar fascia, which inserts distal to the metatarsophalangeal (MTP) joints, tightens as the toes are dorsiflexed, which pulls the tarsal bones together and "locks" them into a rigid column. This effect has been likened to a windlass, which is a rope or chain extending over a drum used to raise and lower sails and anchors on a ship. (From Morrison W, Sanders T: *Problem solving in musculoskeletal imaging,* St. Louis, 2008, Mosby.)

SECTION 2 PHYSICAL EXAMINATION OF THE FOOT AND ANKLE

I. INSPECTION

A. The foot and ankle should be inspected for

1. Symmetry
2. Callouses—areas of abnormally increased pressure
3. Signs of peripheral vascular disease—lack of hair, increased skin pigmentation (hemosiderin deposition)
4. Swelling—symmetric (likely systemic etiology) versus asymmetric (trauma, venous thrombosis, cellulitis, osteomyelitis, focal musculoskeletal etiology) (Figure 6-12)
5. Ecchymosis—plantar ecchymosis associated with tarsometatarsal injury (Lisfranc injury) (Figure 6-13)
6. Alignment
   - Neutral
   - **Cavovarus—elevated longitudinal arch with hindfoot varus and plantar-flexed first ray** (Figure 6-14)
   - **Pes planus—flat longitudinal arch with hindfoot valgus** (Figure 6-15)
     - Must differentiate hindfoot-driven versus midfoot-driven etiology
       - Midfoot-driven secondary degenerative joint disease or chronic Lisfranc injury
         - Treatment—midfoot fusion with realignment
       - Hindfoot-driven (adult) secondary posterior tibial tendon dysfunction (most common)

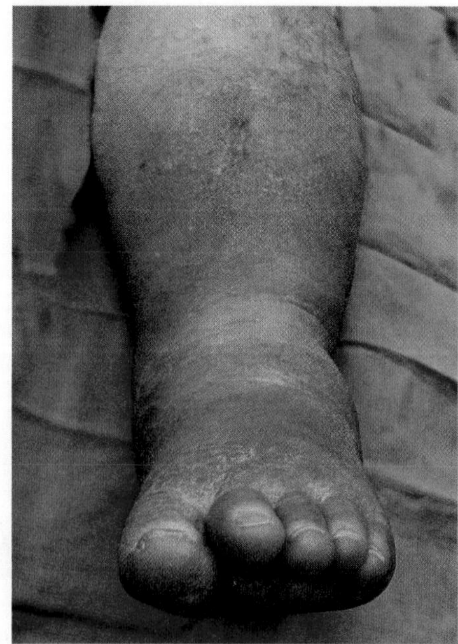

Figure 6-12 This patient presented with chronic osteomyelitis of the leg with a past medical history significant for diabetes mellitus and peripheral vascular disease. Note no hair growth in distal half of leg along with significant swelling of the limb.

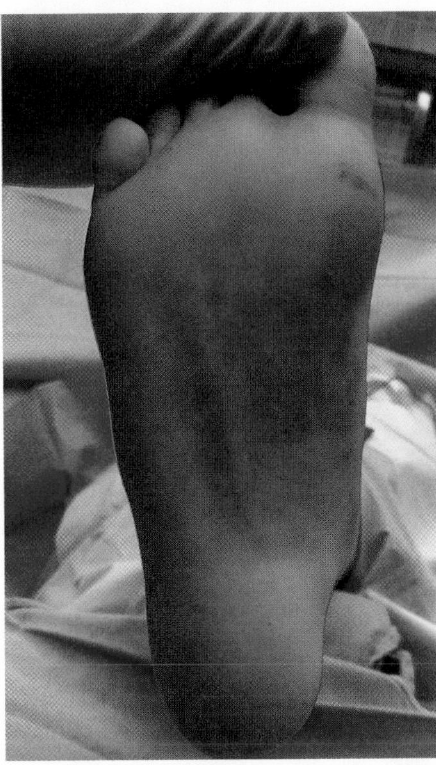

Figure 6-13 Plantar ecchymosis is noted in a patient with a Lisfranc (tarsometatarsal) injury.

- Treatment—FDL tendon transfer with medial slide calcaneal osteotomy
- Hindfoot-driven (pediatric) secondary to development
    - Treatment—lateral column lengthening

B. The patient's gait should be evaluated.

1. Steppage gait—increased knee and hip flexion during swing phase to ensure that the toes clear the floor (Figure 6-16)
    - Secondary to footdrop (peroneal nerve palsy or neuropathy)

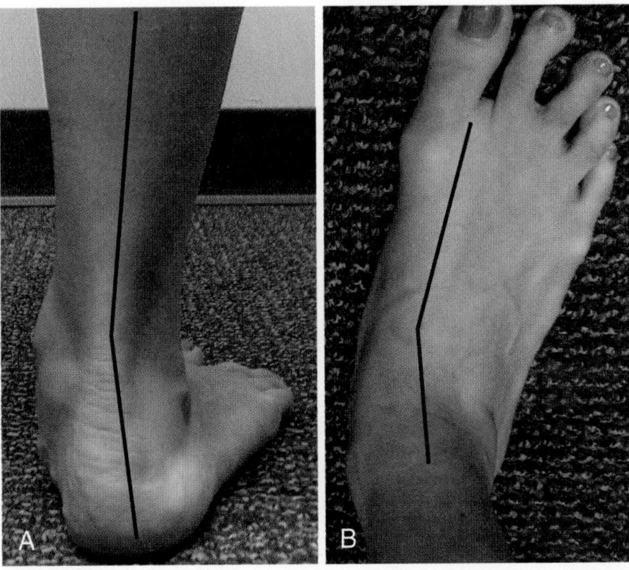

Figure 6-15 Valgus position of the hindfoot **(A)** with forefoot abduction **(B)** in a patient with a pes planovalgus deformity.

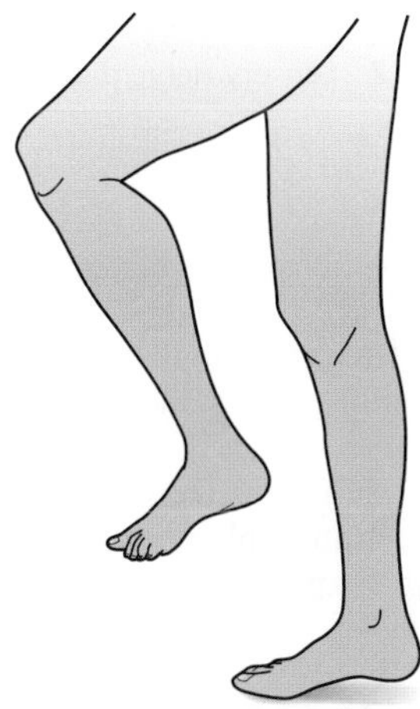

Figure 6-16 The steppage gait consists of each knee being excessively raised when walking. This maneuver compensates for a loss of position sense by elevating the feet to ensure that they will clear the ground, stairs, and other obstacles. It is a classical sign of posterior column spinal cord damage from tabes dorsalis. However, peripheral neuropathies more commonly impair position sense and lead to this gait abnormality. (From Kaufman D: *Clinical neurology for psychiatrists,* ed 6, Philadelphia, 2006, Elsevier.)

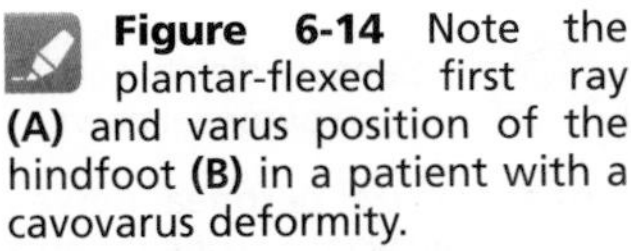

Figure 6-14 Note the plantar-flexed first ray **(A)** and varus position of the hindfoot **(B)** in a patient with a cavovarus deformity.

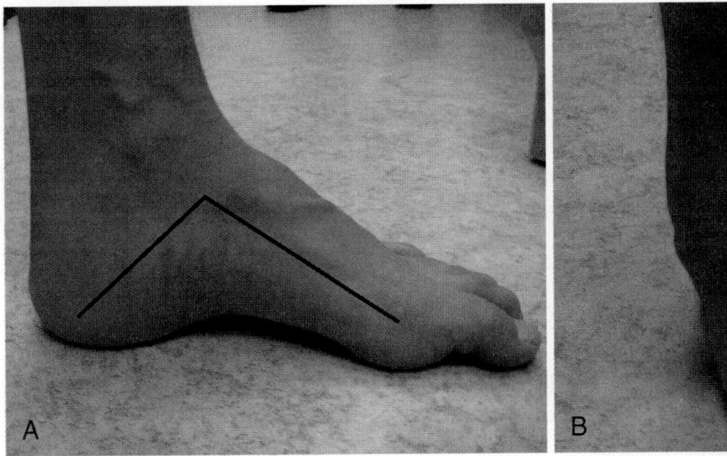

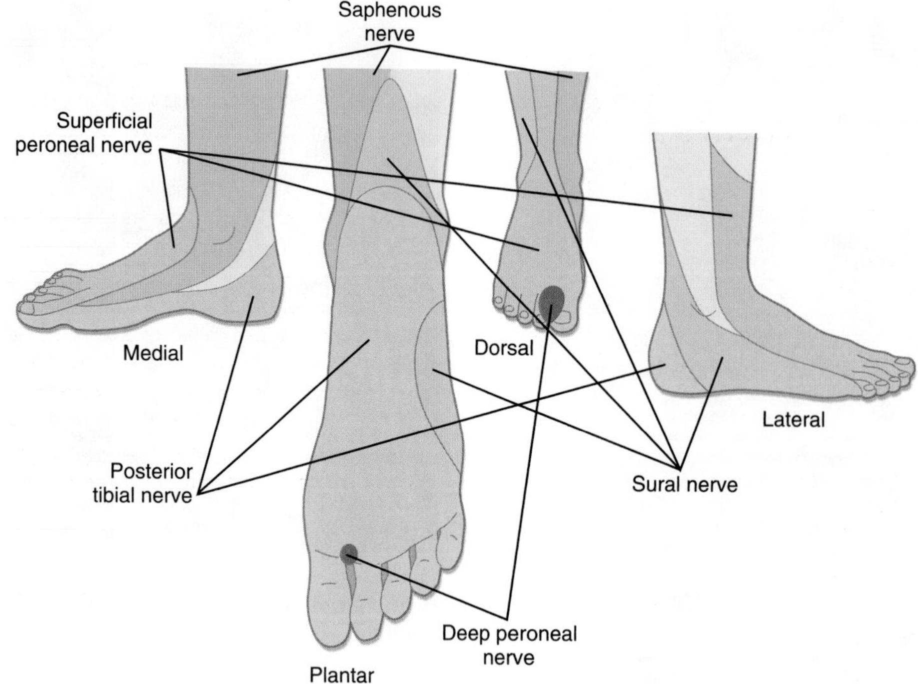

Figure 6-17 Sensory nerve distribution of the ankle. (From Adams J, et al: *Emergency medicine,* Philadelphia, 2008, Elsevier.)

2. Calcaneus gait—increased ankle dorsiflexion during heel-strike
   - Secondary to triceps surae weakness
3. Antalgic gait—shortened stance phase on the affected side
   - Secondary to pain, most commonly degenerative joint disease. Short stance phase minimizes the amount of time pressure is placed to affected limb, decreasing pain.

II. VASCULAR EXAMINATION

A. Palpate the dorsalis pedis and posterior tibial pulses. If they are not present, consider noninvasive studies.

1. Predictive for healing
   - Doppler ultrasonography
     - Triphasic waveforms are normal.
   - Ankle-brachial index
     - Greater than 0.5, with normal ranging from 0.9 to 1.3
     - Greater than 1.3 indicates inelastic vessel (calcified—common in diabetics); NOT indicative of good flow
   - **Toe pressure**
     - **Greater than 40 mm Hg**
   - **Transcutaneous oxygen pressure (TcPo$_2$)**
     - **Greater than 30 mm Hg**

III. NEUROLOGIC EXAMINATION

A. The sensory examination should assess the following five cutaneous nerves that supply the feet (Figure 6-17).

1. Saphenous—medial ankle and hindfoot
2. Superficial peroneal (Figure 6-18)

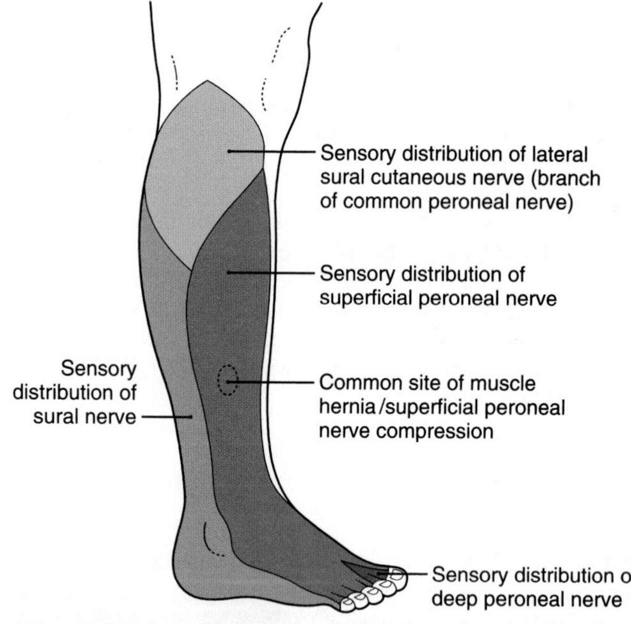

Figure 6-18 Sensory distribution of superficial peroneal nerve . Note typical location of muscle hernia/ superficial peroneal nerve compression. (From Frontera W, et al: *Clinical sports medicine: medical management and rehabilitation,* Philadelphia, 2006, Elsevier.)

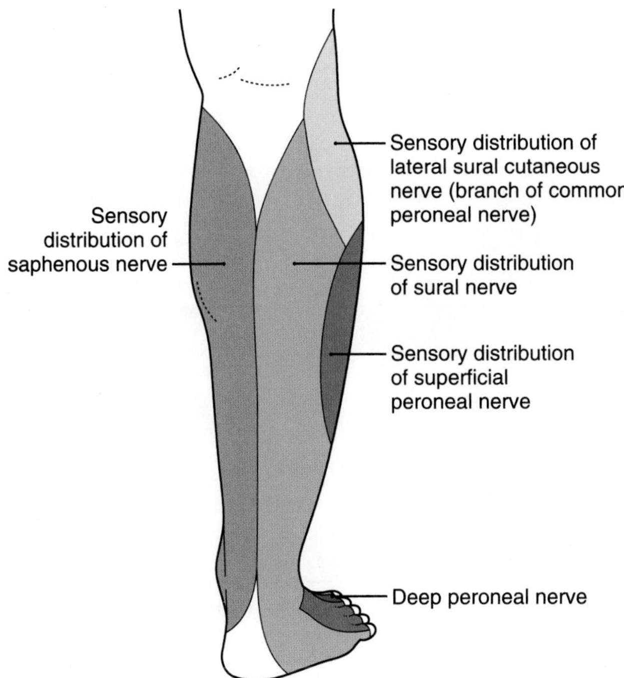

Figure 6-19 Sensory distribution of sural nerve. (From Frontera W, et al: *Clinical sports medicine: medical management and rehabilitation*, Philadelphia, 2006, Elsevier.)

- Medial dorsal cutaneous—dorsomedial foot
- Intermediate dorsal cutaneous—dorsolateral foot

3. Deep peroneal—first dorsal web space
4. Sural—posterolateral border of the leg and the lateral border of the foot (Figure 6-19)
5. Tibial—plantar foot (Figure 6-20)
   - Medial calcaneal
   - Medial plantar
   - Lateral plantar

B. Inability to sense a Semmes-Weinstein 5.07 monofilament is consistent with neuropathy.

1. **Most predictive sign for the development of a foot ulceration**

IV. MOTOR EXAMINATION

A. When assessing strength, keep in mind the relation the tendon has to the axis of the ankle. For example, if it passes medially and posteriorly, the function of that structure will be to provide plantar flexion and inversion (tibialis posterior).

B. When assessing motor function of the foot and ankle, the following muscles should be tested.

1. Tibialis anterior—ankle dorsiflexion, L3-4
2. Extensor hallucis longus—great-toe extension, L4-5
3. Peroneus longus and brevis—hindfoot eversion, L5-S1
4. Posterior tibialis—hindfoot inversion, L4-5
5. Gastrocnemius complex—ankle plantar flexion, S1

C. It is important to remember that neurologic deficits can be secondary to more proximal pathology (e.g., central nervous system, spinal cord, nerve root).

V. PALPATION AND STABILITY

A. Palpation of the tendinous and bony anatomy of the foot and ankle is facilitated by its subcutaneous nature. A detailed examination can typically reproduce the patient's source of pain, allowing the examiner to identify the cause without the need for supplementary studies.

B. The courses of all tendons are checked both at rest and during contraction for swelling, nodules, and subluxation.

C. A Tinel sign should be sought for

1. Tibial nerve at the tarsal tunnel
2. Superficial peroneal nerve as it exits the fascia of the lateral compartment (anterolateral leg)
3. Deep peroneal nerve (anterior tarsal tunnel syndrome) at the anterior ankle and hindfoot; may be compressed at the inferior extensor retinaculum

D. The web space can be palpated for evidence of interdigital neuromas with an associated Mulder sign.

1. With dorsal pressure applied to the web space, the metatarsal heads are compressed with the contralateral hand. An audible click, along with radiating pain into the affected toes, is a positive sign.

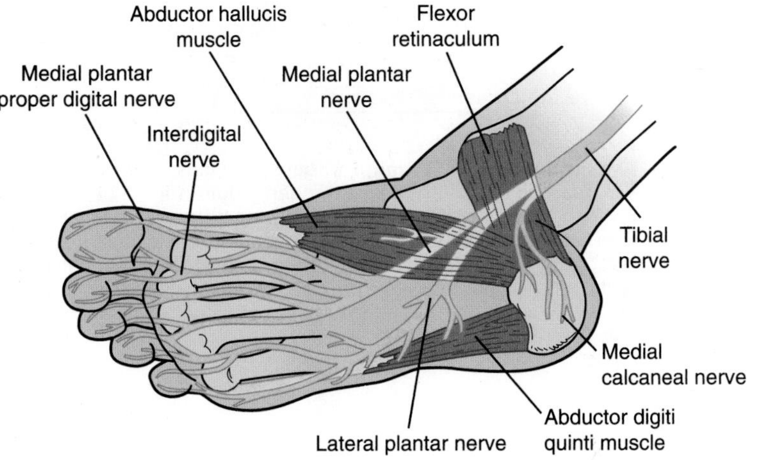

Figure 6-20 The tarsal tunnel and its neural contents—the terminal portion of the tibial nerve, the medial plantar nerve, the lateral plantar nerve, and the medial calcaneal nerve—are illustrated, as are the digital nerves. (From Dyck P, Thomas PK: *Peripheral neuropathy,* ed 4, Philadelphia, 2005, Elsevier.)

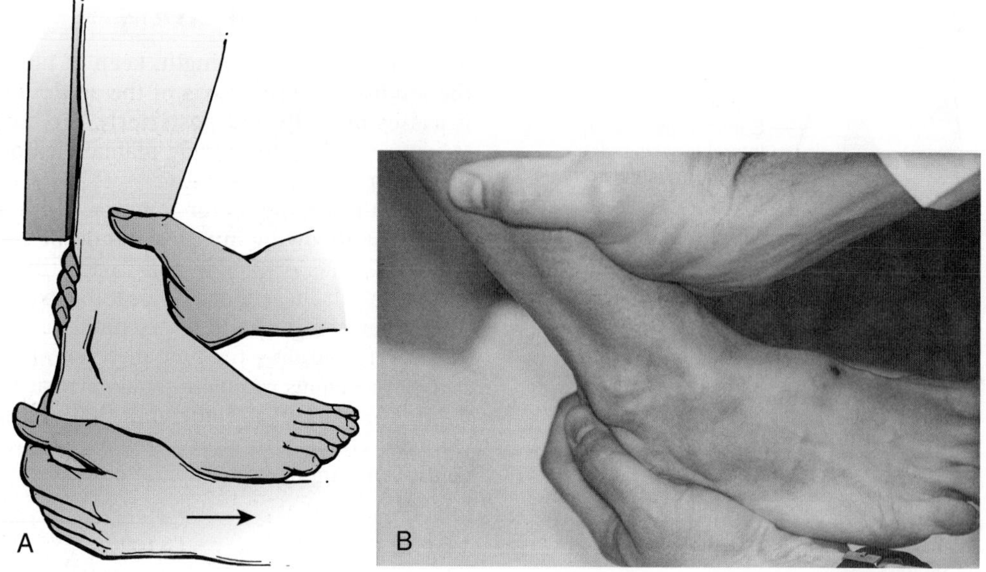

Figure 6-21 **A** and **B,** Anterior drawer test. (From Miller M: *Core knowledge in orthopaedics—sports medicine,* Philadelphia, 2006, Elsevier.)

E. Stability of the lateral ankle ligaments can be assessed with the anterior drawer and varus talar tilt tests (Figure 6-21).

1. Anterior drawer test
   - Anterior pressure on the hindfoot with the ankle in plantar flexion evaluates the anterior talofibular ligament.
2. **Varus stress test**
   - **Inversion of the ankle in dorsiflexion evaluates the calcaneofibular ligament.**

VI. RANGE OF MOTION

A. Both passive and active range of motion (ROM) should be compared with the contralateral side.

B. There is a high rate of variability of normal motion of the joints of the foot and ankle, with no defined absolute normal.

C. Range of motion that is limited to the contralateral side or is painful is abnormal.

D. Increased ROM, specifically ankle dorsiflexion, is critical to identify because that can be associated with an Achilles tendon rupture.

E. Silfverskiöld test (difference in ankle dorsiflexion with knee flexed versus extended) can help differentiate between gastrocnemius and Achilles contracture (Figure 6-22).

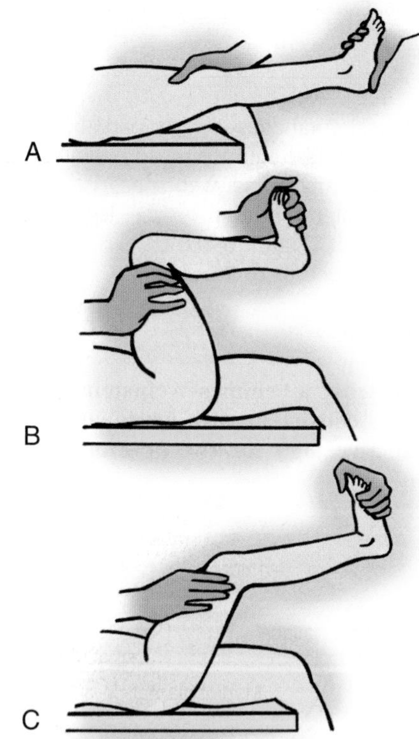

Figure 6-22 Testing for gastrocnemius contracture and spasticity. **A,** With knee extended, equinus in ankle is noted. **B,** With knee flexed, ankle is easily dorsiflexed, indicating no soleus contracture. **C,** As knee is extended, ankle dorsiflexion is resisted by tight or spastic gastrocnemius muscles. (From Canale ST, Beaty J: *Campbell's operative orthopedics,* ed 11, Philadelphia, 2007, Elsevier. Redrawn from Evans EB: Knee flexion deformity in cerebral palsy, *Instr Course Lect* 20:42, 1971.)

SECTION 3 RADIOGRAPHIC EVALUATION OF THE FOOT AND ANKLE

I. WEIGHT-BEARING VIEWS—should be obtained when possible

A. The standard views of the ankle are

1. Anteroposterior
2. Lateral
3. Mortise (a view of 15 degrees of internal rotation along the transmalleolar axis)
4. Gravity or manual external rotation stress is critical in the evaluation of suspected deltoid ligament (supination–external rotation stage IV [SER IV]) and syndesmotic injuries (Figure 6-23).
5. Anterior drawer and talar tilt views are helpful in cases of suspected ankle instability (Figures 6-24 and 6-25).
6. The standard views of the foot should include
   - Anteroposterior—medial and middle column visualized
   - Lateral
     - Sagittal alignment of the foot visualized (pes planus, cavus)
     - Dorsal osteophytes are easily identified at the hindfoot/midfoot that signify early degenerative joint disease.
   - Oblique—middle and lateral column visualized

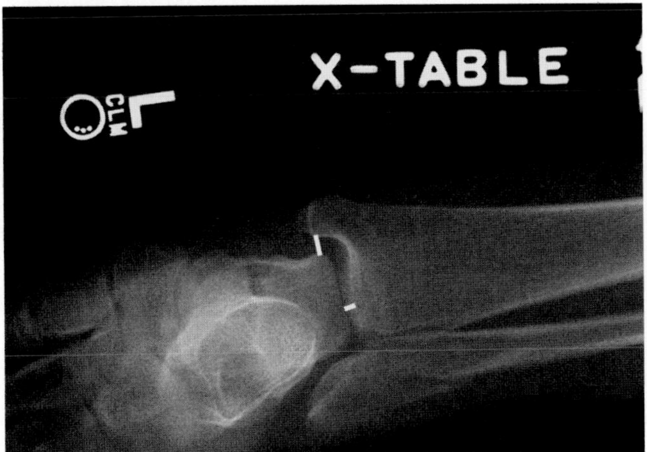

Figure 6-23 Gravity stress ankle radiograph demonstrating increased medial clear space (>4 mm) and greater than the superior clear space with associated fibular fracture displacement.

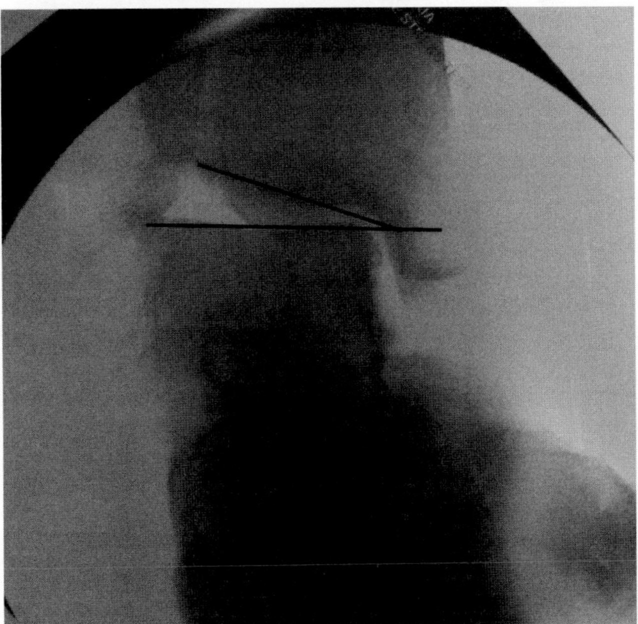

Figure 6-24 Varus stress radiograph of a patient with significant talar tilt of more than 15 degrees. (From Miller M, Sanders T: *Presentation, imaging and treatment of common musculoskeletal conditions,* Philadelphia, 2011, Elsevier.)

B. Special views are provided when the clinical presentation warrants it (Table 6-2).

C. Comparison views of the contralateral foot or ankle are not routinely ordered but can be helpful.

1. Primarily in the setting of a suspected ligamentous injury (syndesmotic, Lisfranc, or plantar plate of the first MTP)

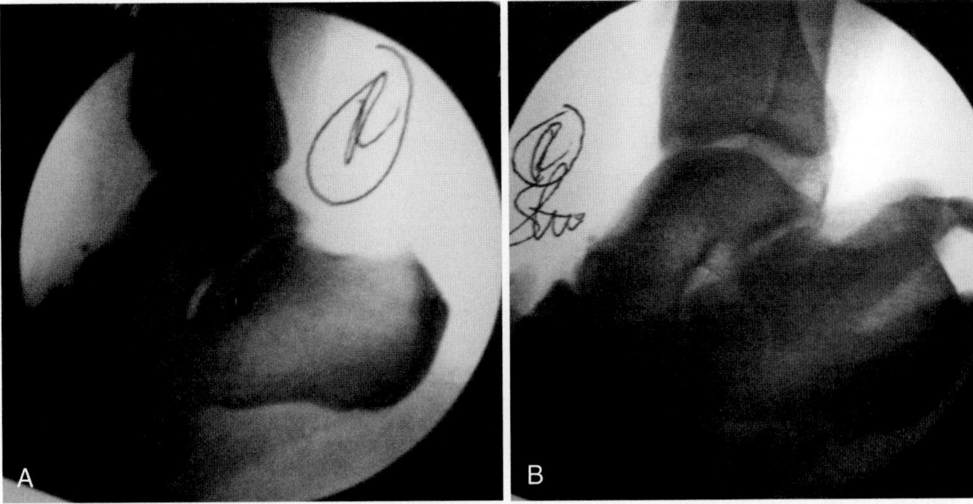

Figure 6-25 Anterior drawer stress radiograph demonstrating the anterior translation of the talus **(B)** relative to the normal position of the talus in the unstressed radiograph **(A).** (From Miller M, Sanders T: *Presentation, imaging and treatment of common musculoskeletal conditions,* Philadelphia, 2011, Elsevier.)

Table 6-2 Special Radiographic Views of the Foot and Ankle

View	Specific Purpose
Canale view—15-degree internal rotation for foot	Talar neck view for fracture
Harris view—axial heel view	Calcaneus fractures
Sesamoid view—axial sesamoid view	Sesamoid fracture or arthritis
Broden view—tibiocalcaneal (subtalar) medial oblique views at 10-degree variations	Posterior, medial, and anterior facets of subtalar joint for fracture or arthritis

II. IMAGING PROCEDURES

A. Computed tomography (CT) of the foot and ankle is especially useful for complex fractures (pilon, calcaneus, talus, midfoot, Lisfranc) and tarsal coalition.
B. Magnetic resonance imaging (MRI) aids the evaluation of osteochondral defects, osteonecrosis, neoplasm, and other soft tissue pathologies.
C. Bone scans are sensitive for the identification of stress fractures.
D. Indium-tagged white blood cell (WBC) scans are both sensitive and specific in the detection of osteomyelitis.

SECTION 4 ADULT HALLUX VALGUS

I. OVERVIEW

A. Hallux valgus is defined as a lateral deviation of great toe with medial deviation of first metatarsal.
B. The pathophysiology of hallux valgus is likely multifactorial.

1. Intrinsic factors such as genetic predisposition, ligamentous laxity, and predisposing anatomy (convex metatarsal head, pes planus) are contributory.
2. Extrinsic factors such as certain types of shoe wear (narrow toe box, high heels) also play a role.

II. PATHOANATOMY (FIGURE 6-26)

A. Medial capsular attenuation
B. Proximal phalanx drifts laterally, leading to the following conditions:

1. **Plantar-lateral migration of abductor hallucis; change in position causes the muscle to plantarflex and pronate the phalanx.**
2. Stretching of the extensor hood of the extensor hallucis longus
3. Lateral deviation of the extensor hallucis longus and flexor hallucis longus (FHL), causing a muscular imbalance and deforming force for valgus progression and pronation of the great toe (Figure 6-27)

C. First metatarsal head moves medially off the sesamoids, increasing the intermetatarsal angle (IMA).
D. Secondary contracture of the lateral capsule, adductor hallucis, lateral metatarsal-sesamoid ligament, and intermetatarsal ligament
E. Radiographs

1. Multiple measurements can be obtained from standard radiographs that guide treatment options.
   - Hallux valgus angle (HVA)—angle formed by line along first metatarsal shaft and line along shaft of proximal phalanx (Figure 6-28)
     - Normal less than 15 degrees

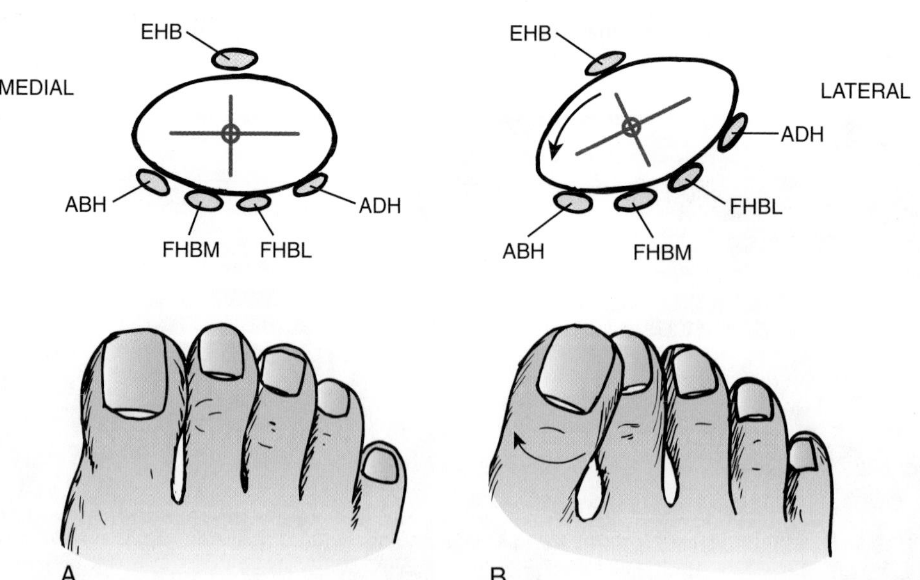

Figure 6-26 Schematic representation of tendons around the first metatarsal head. **A,** Normal articulation in a balanced state. **B,** Relationship of the tendons in hallux valgus deformity. ABH, abductor hallucis; ADH, adductor hallucis; EHB, extensor hallucis brevis; FHBL, flexor hallucis brevis lateral head; FHBM, flexor hallucis brevis medial head. (From Coughlin M, et al: *Surgery of the foot and ankle,* ed 8, Philadelphia, 2006, Elsevier.)

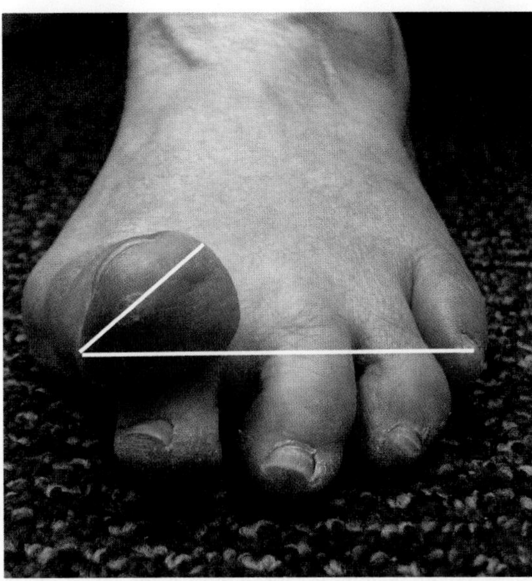

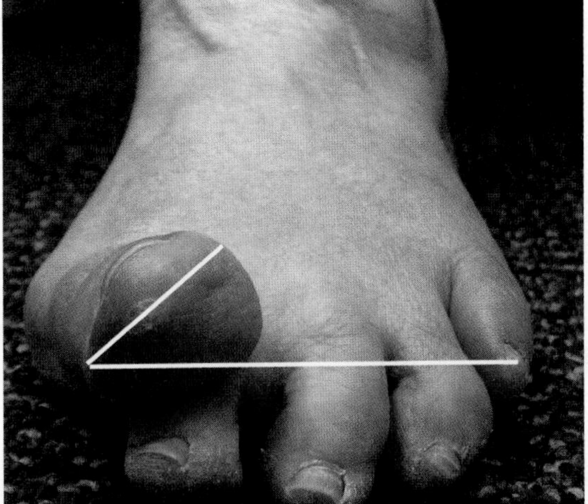

Figure 6-27 The pronation of the great toe is easily noted by comparing the angulation of the nail of the great toe relative to the floor. (From Miller M, Sanders T: *Presentation, imaging and treatment of common musculoskeletal conditions,* Philadelphia, 2011, Elsevier.)

- First-second IMA—angle formed by line along first metatarsal shaft and line along second metatarsal shaft (Figure 6-29)
  - Normal less than 9 degrees
- Hallux valgus interphalangeus (HVI) angle—angle formed by line along shaft of proximal phalanx and line along shaft of distal phalanx (Figure 6-30)
  - Normal—less than 10 degrees
  - Associated with a congruent deformity
- Distal metatarsal articular angle (DMAA)—angle formed by line along the articular surface of the first metatarsal and line perpendicular to axis of the first metatarsal (Figure 6-31)
  - Normal—less than 10 degrees
  - Associated with a congruent deformity

2. The congruency of the first MTP joint should be determined (Figure 6-32).
   - **Congruency is determined by comparing the line connecting the medial and lateral edge of the first metatarsal head articular surface with the similar line for the proximal phalanx.**
     - **When these lines are parallel, the joint is congruent.**

Hallux valgus (<15°) angle

A

B

C

D

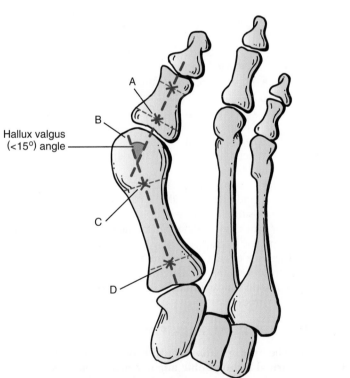

Figure 6-28 Hallux valgus angle. Marks are placed in the mid-diaphyseal region of the proximal phalanx and the first metatarsal at an equal distance from the medial and lateral cortices. The longitudinal axis of the proximal phalanx is determined by an axis drawn though points *A* and *B,* and the longitudinal axis of the first metatarsal is determined by a line drawn through points *C* and *D.* The hallux valgus angle is formed by the intersection of the diaphyseal axes of the first metatarsal (line CD) and the proximal phalanx (line AB). (From Coughlin M, et al: *Surgery of the foot and ankle,* ed 8, Philadelphia, 2006, Elsevier.)

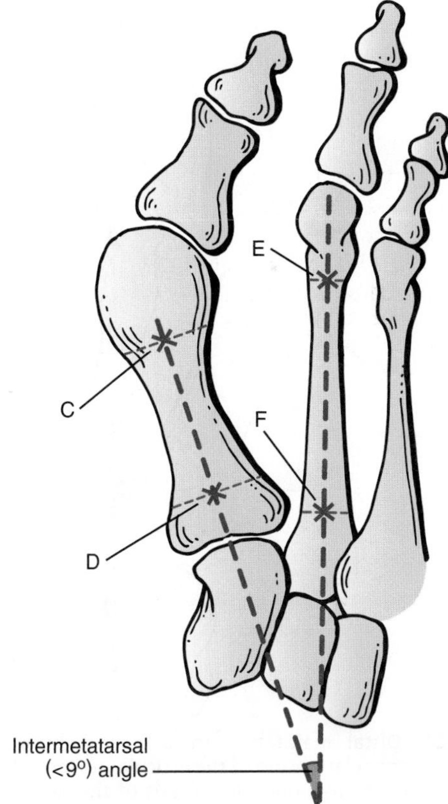

Figure 6-29 First-second intermetatarsal angle. Mid-diaphyseal reference points are placed equidistant from the medial and lateral cortices of the first and second metatarsals in both the proximal and distal mid-diaphyseal region. The longitudinal axis is drawn for both the first metatarsal *(line CD)* and the second metatarsal *(line EF).* The first-second intermetatarsal angle is formed by the intersection of these two axes (*line CD* and *line EF*). (From Coughlin M, et al: *Surgery of the foot and ankle,* ed 8, Philadelphia, 2006, Elsevier.)

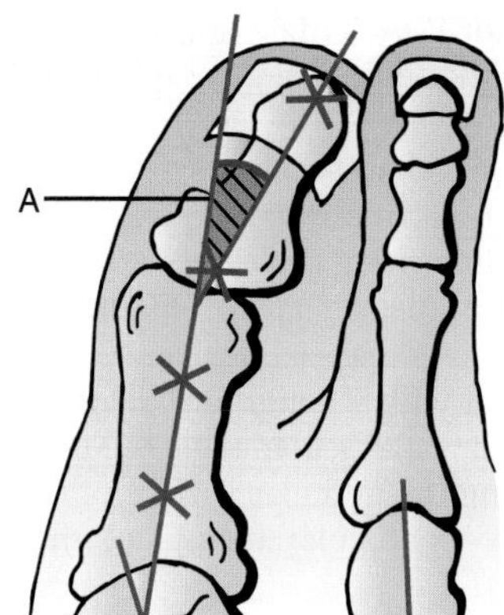

Figure 6-30 Hallux valgus interphalangeal angle. Mid-diaphyseal reference points are drawn on the proximal phalanx, and on the distal phalanx a reference point is placed at the distal tip of the phalanx and at the midpoint of the articular surface of the distal phalanx. A line is drawn to connect the reference points for the axes of each phalanx. Point *A* shows the proximal phalanx axis. The intersection of the axis of the distal phalanx with the longitudinal axis of the proximal phalanx forms the hallux valgus interphalangeal axis. (From Coughlin M, et al: *Surgery of the foot and ankle,* ed 8, Philadelphia, 2006, Elsevier.)

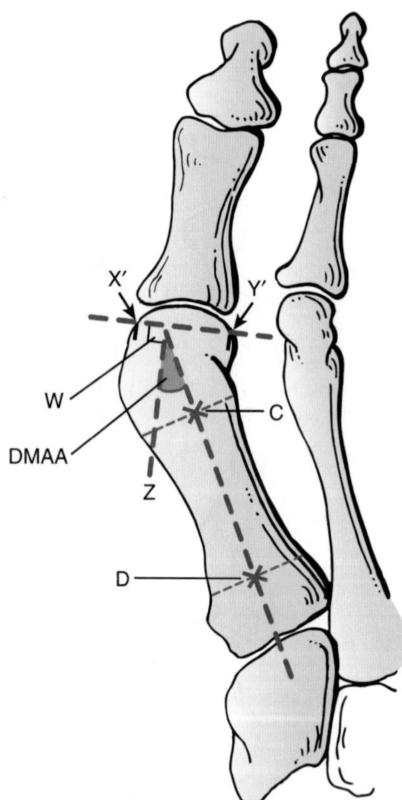

Figure 6-31 Distal metatarsal articular angle (DMAA). The DMAA defines the relationship of the articular surface of the distal first metatarsal with the longitudinal axis of the first metatarsal. Points are placed on the most medial and lateral extent of the distal metatarsal articular surface *(X′, Y′)*. A line drawn to connect these two points defines the "slope laterally of the articular surface." Another line through points *W* and *Z* is drawn perpendicular to the first line *X′Y′*. A third line through points *C* and *D* defines the longitudinal axis of the first metatarsal. The angle subtended by the perpendicular line *(W, Z)* and the longitudinal axis of the first metatarsal *(C, D)* defines the DMAA. (From Coughlin M, et al: *Surgery of the foot and ankle,* ed 8, Philadelphia, 2006, Elsevier.)

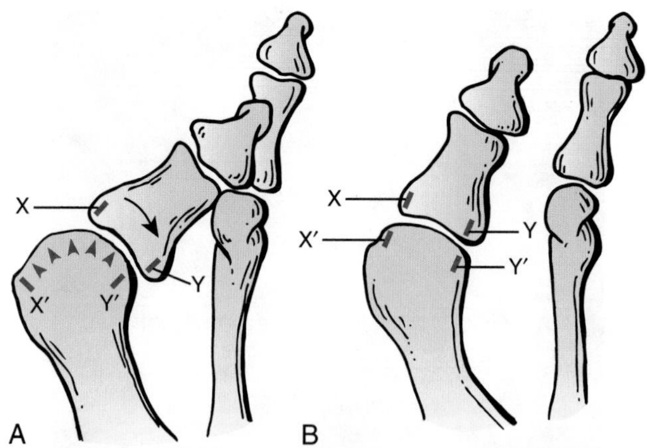

Figure 6-32 Congruency versus subluxation. **A,** Hallux valgus deformity with subluxation (noncongruent joint) is characterized by lateral deviation of the articular surface of the proximal phalanx in relation to the articular surface of the distal first metatarsal. **B,** Hallux valgus deformity with a nonsubluxated (congruent) metatarsophalangeal joint is caused most often by lateral inclination of the distal metatarsal articular surface. Points *X* and *Y* determine the medial and lateral extent of the articular surface of the proximal phalanx; points *X′* and *Y′* determine the medial and lateral extent of the metatarsal articular surface. Note the lateral slope of the distal metatarsal articular surface. (From Coughlin M, et al: *Surgery of the foot and ankle,* ed 8, Philadelphia, 2006, Elsevier.)

- Increased DMAA
  - Distal redirectional osteotomy of the metatarsal head (medial closed wedge)
- Increased HVI
  - Akin osteotomy to correct
    - Medial closed-wedge osteotomy of the phalanx
- Both of these operations may be required in addition to an osteotomy of the metatarsal to correct the increased IMA. Performing these osteotomies does NOT exclude additional distal or proximal metatarsal correction.

- When these lines are divergent, the joint is incongruent.
  - Patients may present with both an incongruent joint and increased DMAA or HVI in severe deformities.

3. The position of the sesamoids should be noted. In more severe or chronic deformities, the sesamoids are frequently displaced laterally.
4. Presence of first MTP joint and first metatarso-cuneiform joint degenerative changes should be noted.
   - A stiff or arthritic MTP joint requires a first MTP arthrodesis.

III. SURGICAL PROCEDURES (FIGURE 6-33)

A. The appropriate surgical procedure is dictated by the abnormal radiographic angular measurements in concordance with underlying clinical abnormalities.

1. The patient's physical examination and associated pathology dictates the appropriate surgical procedure regardless of the angular measurements.
   - **MTP fusion required**—The IMA will correct with realignment of the first MTP; concomitant metatarsal osteotomy is NOT required (Figure 6-34).
     - Rheumatoid arthritis
     - Osteoarthritis

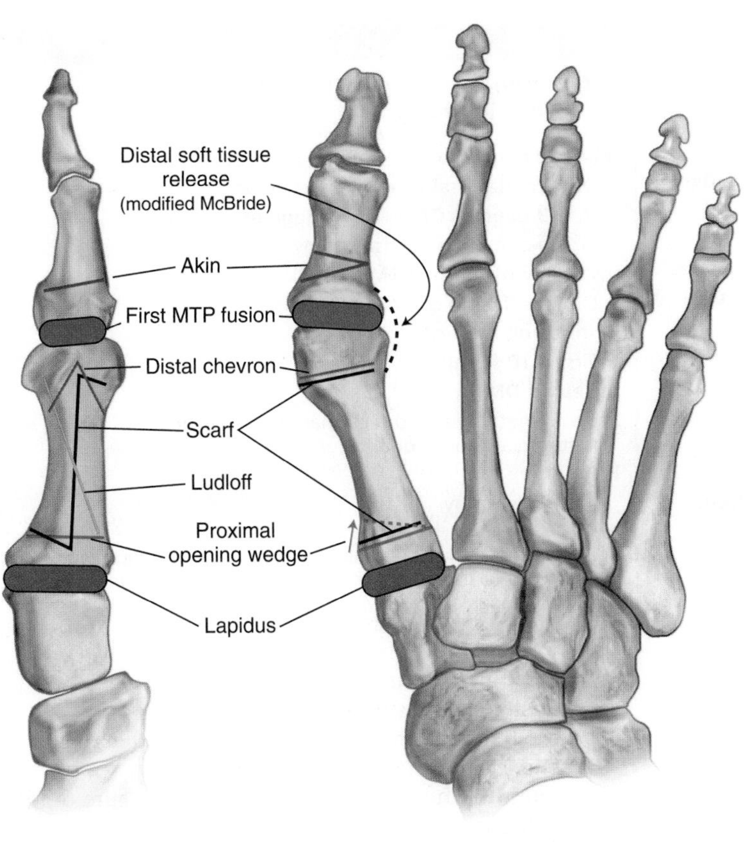

Figure 6-33 Lateral and AP figure depicting various surgical options for the correction of hallux valgus. Note that a distal soft tissue release is almost universally performed except in the case of a first MTP fusion. AP, anteroposterior; MTP, metatarsophalangeal.

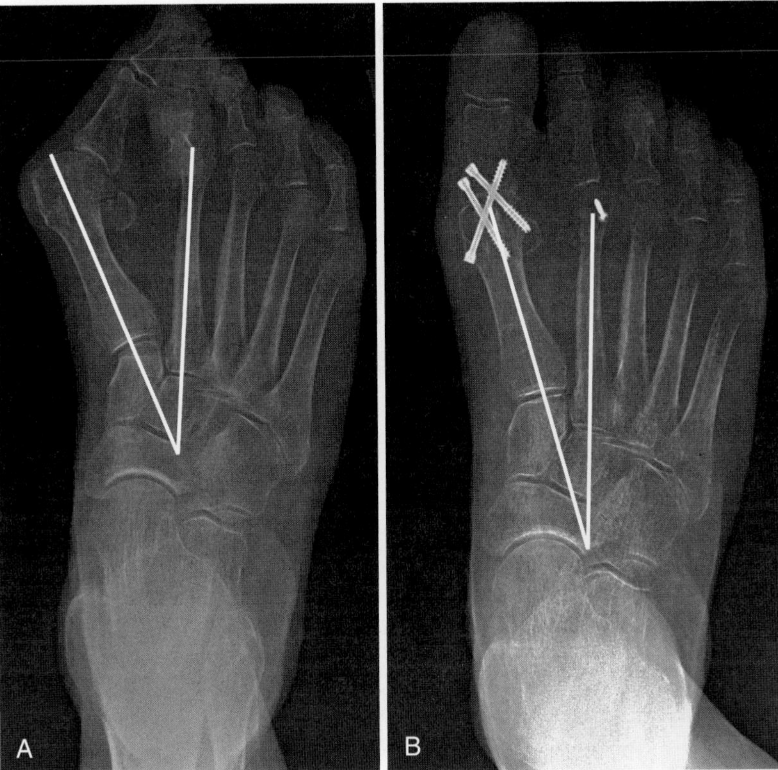

Figure 6-34 **A,** Preoperative anteroposterior radiograph of a patient with a hallux valgus deformity with associated stiffness and pain within the joint. **B,** Postoperative radiograph demonstrates correction of both the hallux valgus deformity and the intermetatarsal angle without the need for an additional metatarsal osteotomy.

- Painful or stiff first MTP
  - Deformity cannot be passively corrected.
- **Spasticity**
  - Stroke
  - **Cerebral palsy**

- **Lapidus (first tarsometatarsal realignment arthrodesis) required**
  - **Ligamentous laxity**
  - **First TMT degenerative joint disease**

2. **Procedures never appropriate in isolation (high recurrence rate)**
   - **Distal soft tissue release (modified McBride)**
     - Modification—retention of the lateral (fibular) sesamoid
   - Medial eminence resection
   - Medial capsular imbrication
   - Isolated osteotomy without associated soft tissue correction
3. Algorithmic approach to identifying the appropriate surgical intervention (Box 6-1)
   - **All patients should undergo a soft tissue release with all associated osteotomies and first TMT arthrodesis (Lapidus).**
   - **IMA is 13 degrees or less, AND HVA is 40 degrees or less.**
     - **Distal metatarsal osteotomy (chevron)**
     - **Distal soft tissue release**
     - **Medial eminence resection and capsular repair**
   - **IMA is greater than 13 degrees, OR HVA is greater than 40 degrees.**
     - **Proximal metatarsal osteotomy**
     - **Distal soft tissue release**
     - **Medial eminence resection and capsular repair**
   - **Instability of the first TMT/joint laxity**
     - **Lapidus (fusion of first TMT joint)** (Figure 6-35)
     - Soft tissue release
     - Medial eminence resection and capsular repair
   - Increased DMAA (>10 degrees)

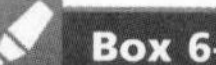

Box 6-1

Algorithm for Surgical Correction of Hallux Valgus

IMA ≤13 degrees AND HVA ≤40 degrees
Distal metatarsal osteotomy (chevron)
IMA >13 degrees OR HVA >40 degrees
Proximal metatarsal osteotomy
Instability of the first TMT/joint laxity
Lapidus (fusion of first TMT joint)
Arthritis or spasticity
First MTP fusion
Increased DMAA
Distal metatarsal redirectional osteotomy in addition to metatarsaltranslational osteotomy
HVI
Akin osteotomy

DMAA, distal metatarsal articular angle; HVA, hallux valgus angle; HVI, hallux valgus interphalangeus; IMA, intermetatarsal angle; MTP, metatarsophalangeal; TMT, tarsometatarsal.

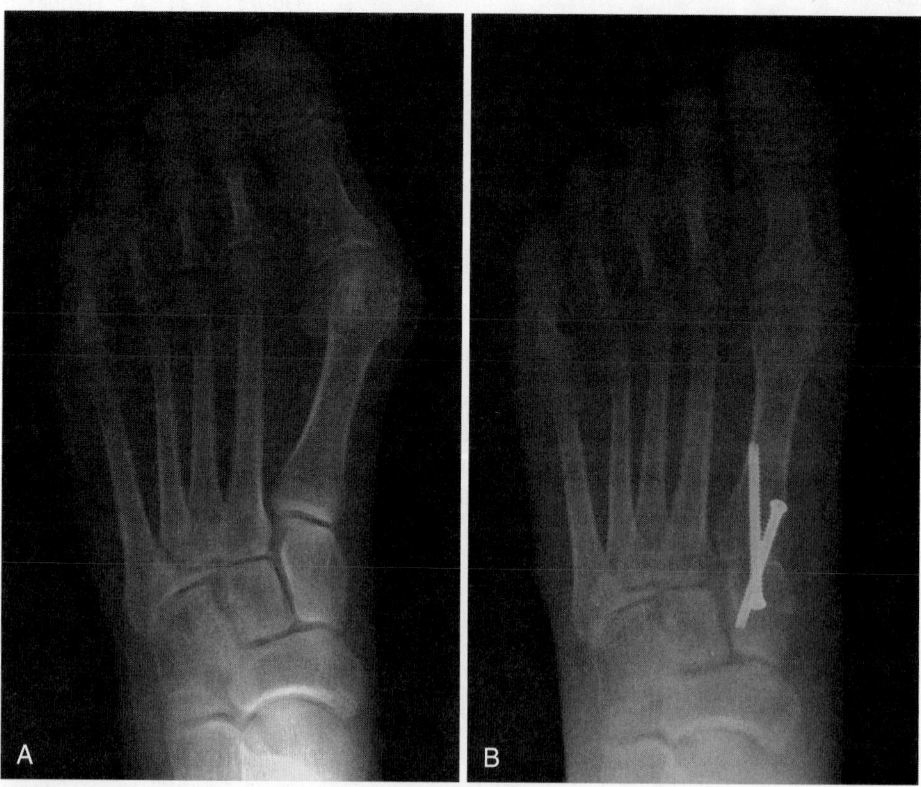

Figure 6-35 **A,** Preoperative radiograph of a patient with hallux valgus and first tarsometatarsal instability. **B,** Correction was successfully achieved with a Lapidus procedure using two crossed screws for fixation. (From Miller M, Sanders T: *Presentation, imaging and treatment of common musculoskeletal conditions,* Philadelphia, 2011, Elsevier.)

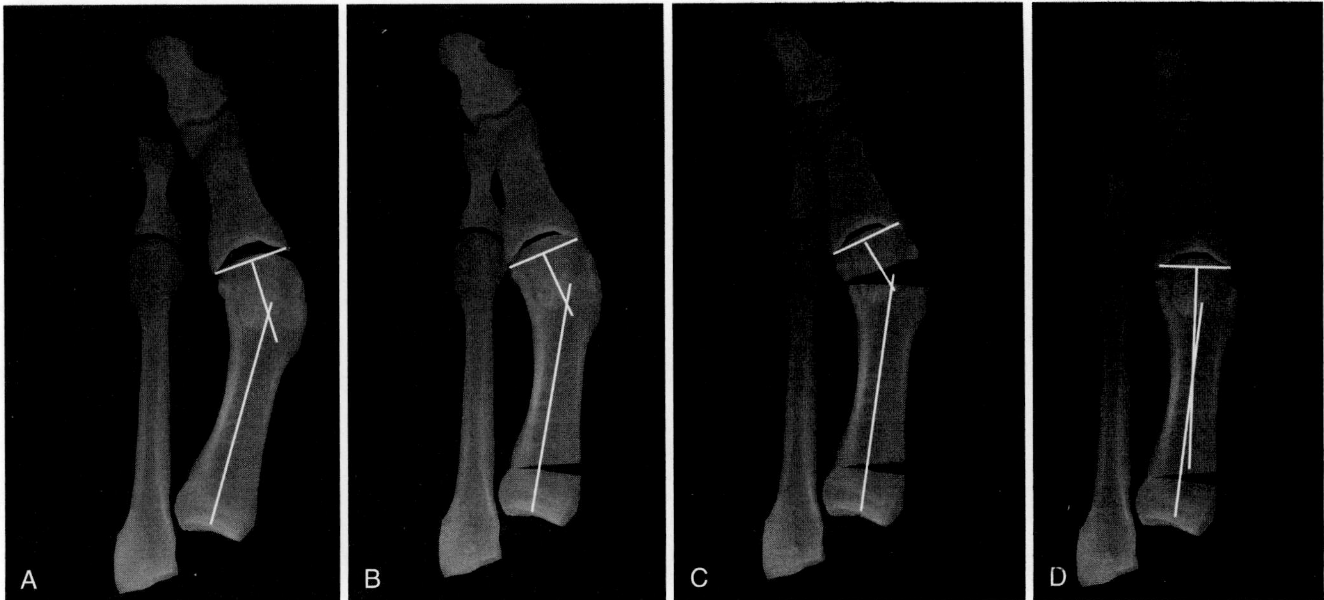

Figure 6-36 **A,** Hallux valgus deformity secondary to an increased intermetatarsal angle (IMA) and distal metatarsal articular angle (DMAA). **B,** Correction of the IMA with a proximal osteotomy causes the proximal phalanx to override the second toe secondary to the DMAA. **C,** A distal closed-wedge osteotomy is performed. **D,** With closure of the osteotomy, the phalanx is now directed parallel to the metatarsal shaft, correcting the overall deformity.

- Distal medial closed-wedge metatarsal osteotomy in addition to what is required based on the angular measurements (Figure 6-36)
  - IMA is 13 degrees or less, **AND** HVA is 40 degrees or less.
    - Distal biplanar closed-wedge metatarsal osteotomy
      - Translate and redirect the metatarsal head simultaneously.
  - IMA is greater than 13 degrees, **OR** HVA is greater than 40 degrees.
    - Proximal metatarsal osteotomy AND distal medial closed-wedge metatarsal osteotomy
- Instability of the first TMT/joint laxity
  - Lapidus AND distal medial closed-wedge metatarsal osteotomy
- Hallux valgus interphalangeus
  - Akin osteotomy—can be done in isolation if no other deformity present
    - Commonly performed in addition to procedures required to correct the HVA and IMA (Figure 6-37)

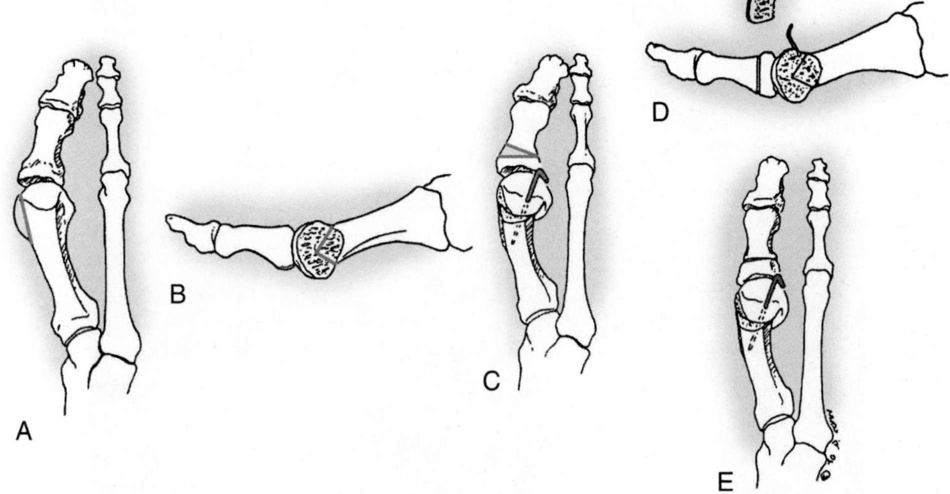

Figure 6-37 **A,** Resection of medial eminence parallel to medial border of foot. **B,** Chevron osteotomy cut is made, and metatarsal head is shifted laterally 2.5 to 3 mm. **C,** Osteotomy is fixed with 0.045-inch smooth pin, and protruding medial border of metatarsal is osteotomized flush with metatarsal head. **D,** Akin cut parallels concavity at base of proximal phalanx, and 1-mm wedge of bone is removed. **E,** Suture closure of Akin osteotomy corrects residual valgus of hallux. (From Canale ST, Beaty J: *Campbell's operative orthopedics,* ed 11, Philadelphia, 2007, Elsevier.)

IV. SURGICAL COMPLICATIONS

A. Avascular necrosis

1. Distal metatarsal osteotomy and lateral soft tissue release may be performed simultaneously without increased risk for avascular necrosis.
   - Intraoperative laser Doppler studies demonstrated medial capsulotomy primary insult to metatarsal head blood flow (45%).

B. Recurrence

1. **Can occur with any procedure; highly associated with**
   - **Undercorrection of the IMA**
   - **Isolated soft tissue reconstruction (modified McBride)**
   - **Isolated resection of the medial eminence**

C. Dorsal malunion

1. **Results in transfer metatarsalgia; highly associated with**
   - **Lapidus (first TMT fusion)**
   - **Proximal crescentic osteotomy**

D. Hallux varus

1. Resection of the fibular sesamoid (original McBride)
2. **Overresection of the medial eminence**
3. Excessive lateral release
4. Overcorrection of the IMA

E. Nonunion

1. Highest risk associated with a Lapidus

SECTION 5 JUVENILE AND ADOLESCENT HALLUX VALGUS

I. FACTORS

A. Several critical factors separate these patients from adult patients with hallux valgus deformity.

B. Recurrence of the deformity after surgical correction is the most common complication (Figure 6-38).

C. Proximal osteotomy is performed through the medial cuneiform in patients with an open first metatarsal physis.

1. If arthrodesis of the first TMT is required for laxity, surgical intervention is delayed until physeal closure.

D. The deformity is secondary to underlying bony and ligamentous anatomy that must be addressed to prevent recurrence.

1. Varus of the first metatarsal with a large IMA is commonly present.
2. DMAA is typically increased.

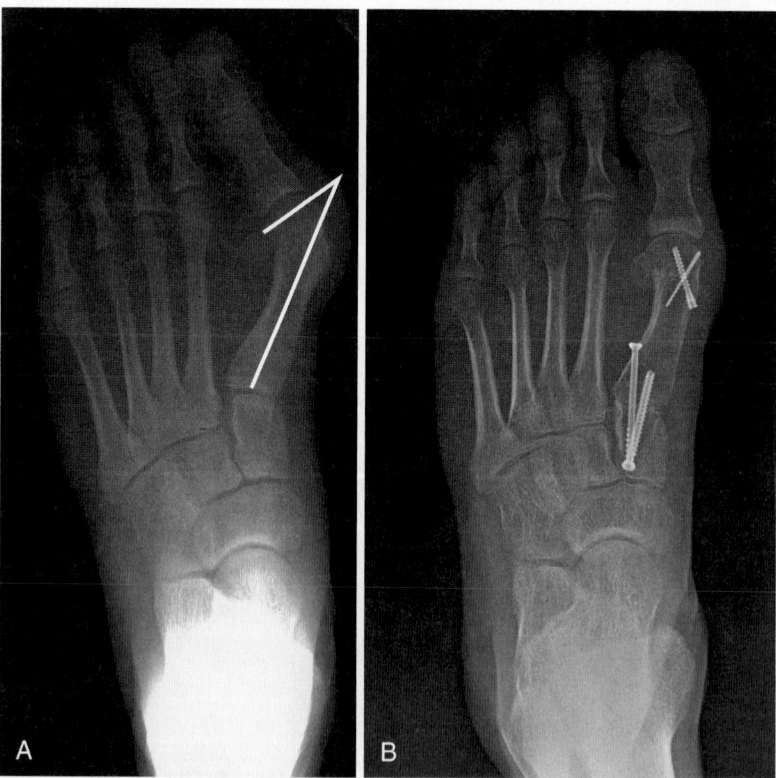

Figure 6-38 **A,** Juvenile hallux valgus recurrence in a patient that underwent a prior isolated proximal osteotomy. The deformity is associated with a large intermetatarsal angle and increased distal metatarsal articular angle. In addition, on examination the patient was noted to have hyperlaxity. **B,** A Lapidus procedure with a medial closed-wedge osteotomy of the distal metatarsal is required to achieve a long-lasting correction.

3. HVI may be present.
4. Ligamentous laxity may be present, and a history of Ehlers-Danlos or Marfan syndrome should be elicited.
   - Examine for generalized laxity to determine if a first TMT arthrodesis is required.
5. The family history is frequently positive for hallux valgus.

E. **Surgical correction**

1. Single, double, or triple osteotomies are required to correct the deformity, applying the same principles as described for the evaluation of adult hallux valgus.
2. In cases of ligamentous laxity—A first TMT arthrodesis substitutes for a proximal osteotomy to correct the IMA. The first metatarsal physeal plate must be closed.
   - Single osteotomy
     - HVI
       - Akin osteotomy
     - Increased DMAA, IMA 13 degrees or less
       - Biplanar distal chevron osteotomy for DMAA and IMA
   - Double osteotomy
     - HVI with increased DMAA, IMA 13 degrees or less
       - Akin osteotomy for HVI
       - Biplanar distal chevron osteotomy for DMAA and IMA
     - IMA greater than 13 degrees with increased DMAA
       - Biplanar distal chevron osteotomy for DMAA
       - Open-wedge medial cuneiform osteotomy
   - Triple osteotomy
     - HVI with increased DMAA, IMA greater than 13 degrees
       - Akin osteotomy for HVI
       - Biplanar distal chevron osteotomy for DMAA
       - Open-wedge medial cuneiform osteotomy

SECTION 6 HALLUX VARUS

I. CAUSE

A. Medial deviation of the great toe is most often an iatrogenic deformity secondary to overcorrection of hallux valgus.

B. Overresection of the medial eminence

C. Excessive lateral release

D. 0-degree or negative IMA (Figure 6-39)

II. NONOPERATIVE TREATMENT

A. Limited to accommodation of the deformity with shoe modifications and shoe stretching

III. OPERATIVE TREATMENT

A. Dependent upon if the deformity is flexible (reducible) or rigid (irreducible)

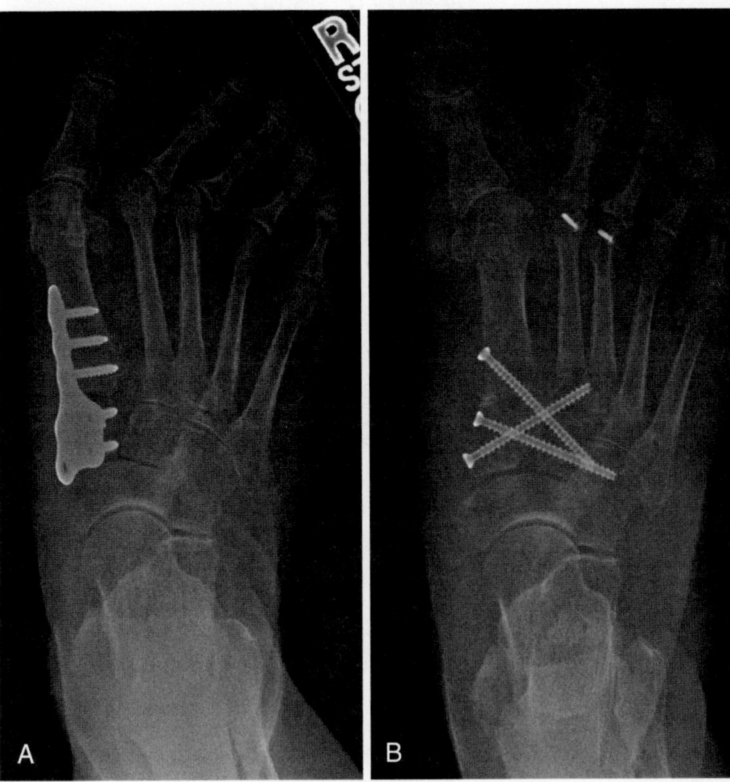

Figure 6-39 **A,** Recurrence of a hallux valgus deformity in a patient who underwent a prior Lapidus procedure. The increased intermetatarsal angle (IMA) occurred secondary to disruption of the intercuneiform. **B,** A revision procedure with arthrodesis of the intercuneiform joint resulted in an overcorrection of the IMA, resulting in hallux varus. The patient had a flexible deformity and was able to wear shoes without pain.

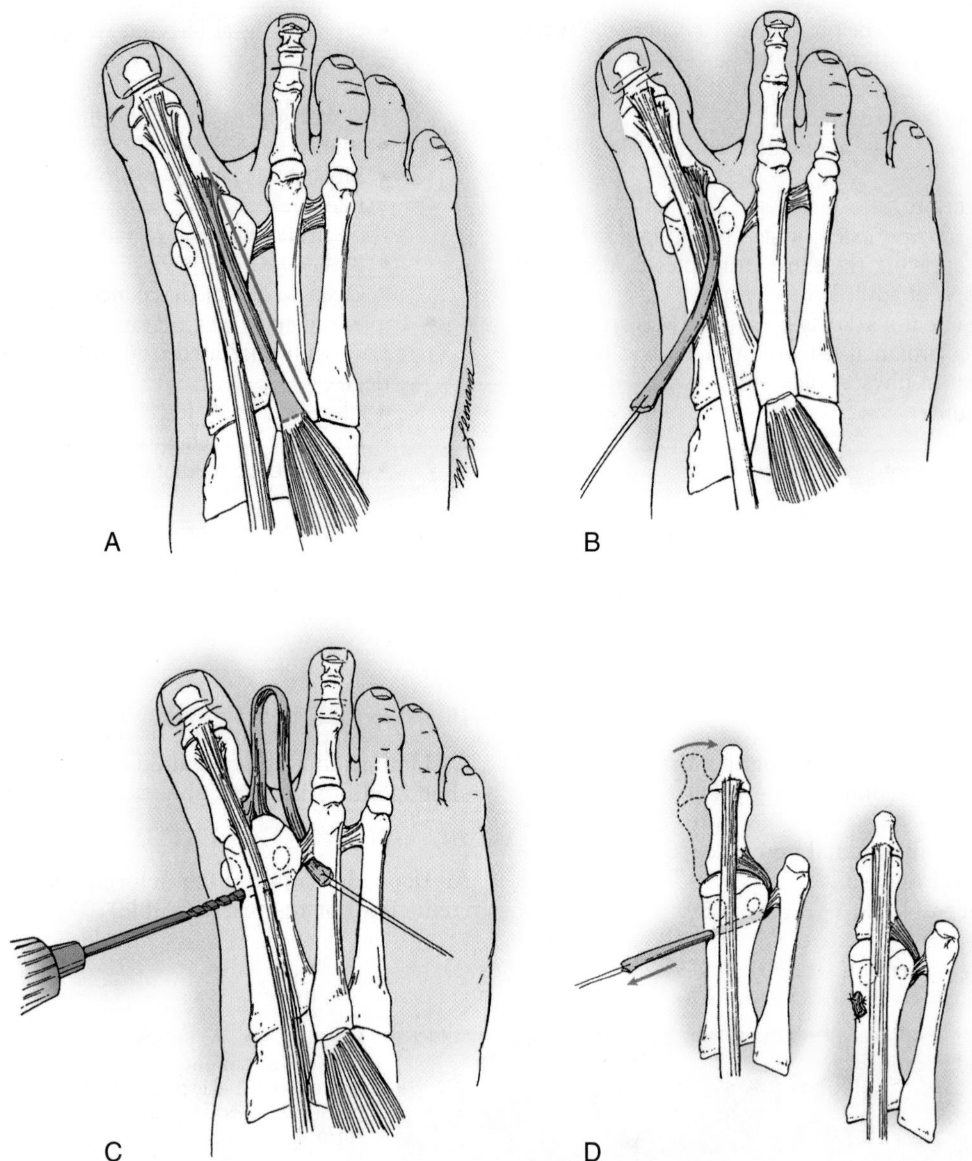

Figure 6-40 Hallux varus correction using extensor hallucis brevis tenodesis. **A,** Dorsal incision and transection of extensor hallucis brevis tendon. **B,** Transected tendon is passed deep to transverse metatarsal ligament from distal to proximal. **C,** Hole is drilled in dorsomedial first metatarsal. **D,** Extensor hallucis brevis tendon is pulled through drill hole and secured with sutures to periosteum or bone. (From Canale ST, Beaty J: *Campbell's operative orthopedics,* ed 11, Philadelphia, 2007, Elsevier. Redrawn from Juliano PJ, et al: Biomechanical assessment of a new tenodesis for correction of hallux varus, *Foot Ankle Int* 17:17, 1996.)

B. Flexible deformity can be corrected with a soft tissue procedure.

1. Release of the abductor hallucis muscle and fascia
2. Transfer of a portion of the extensor hallucis longus (EHL) or brevis tendon under the transverse intermetatarsal ligament to the distal metatarsal neck (taken from lateral to medial) (Figure 6-40)
   - The distal portion of the tendon is left intact, creating a static stabilizer to correct the deformity.

C. Fixed deformity or a deformity with limited first MTP motion is treated with a first MTP arthrodesis.

SECTION 7 LESSER-TOE DEFORMITIES

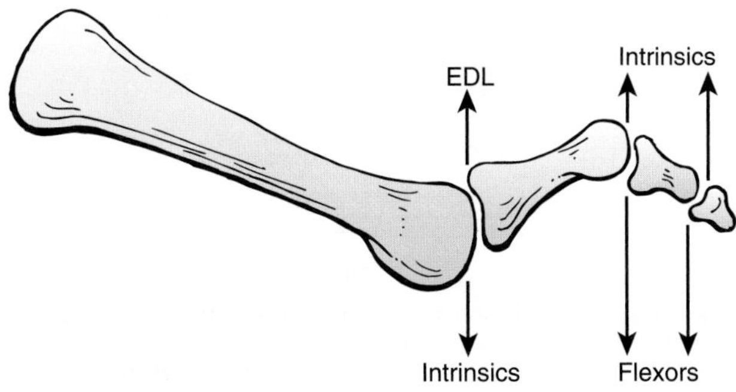

Figure 6-41 Diagram demonstrates the relationship of the intrinsic and extrinsic muscles about a lesser toe. The smaller intrinsic muscles are overpowered by the extrinsic muscles, leading to a hammer-toe deformity. EDL, extensor digitorum longus. (From Coughlin M, et al: *Surgery of the foot and ankle,* ed 8, Philadelphia, 2006, Elsevier.)

I. ANATOMY AND FUNCTION

A. Static stability of the lesser toes is provided by the congruency of the MTP and interphalangeal joints.

1. The plantar plate, which comprises the plantar aponeurosis and capsule, provides a soft tissue block to metatarsal head depression and prevents hyperextension of the MTP joint.
2. Persistent hyperextension at the MTP joint may lead to attenuation and weakening of the plantar structures.

B. Dynamic stability is provided by the various tendons that insert on the lesser toes (Figure 6-41).

1. The EDL is the primary extensor of the MTP joint.
   - The tendon runs through a sling over the dorsal surface of the MTP joint before splitting into a central slip that inserts on the middle phalanx and two dorsolateral slips that reconverge to insert at the base of the distal phalanx.
   - The distal extensor effect of the EDL is neutralized when the proximal phalanx is dorsiflexed, as in hammer-toe or claw-toe deformities.
2. The extensor digitorum brevis extends the PIP joints and inserts on the lateral aspect of the EDL tendon on all but the fifth toe.
3. The FDL is the primary plantar flexor of the distal interphalangeal (DIP) joints because it inserts on the plantar aspect of the distal phalanges. It also weakly plantar flexes the MTP joints.
4. The flexor digitorum brevis splits at the level of the MTP joint and inserts on the plantar lateral aspects of the middle phalanges. The flexor digitorum brevis is the primary plantar flexor of the PIP joints.
5. The intrinsic muscles of the foot include the lumbricals, which originate from the FDL tendon and insert on the extensor sheath over the MTP joints, and four dorsal and three plantar interossei muscles, which insert on the medial aspect of the proximal phalanges.
   - These muscles act similarly to the intrinsic muscles of the hand, flexing the MTP joints and extending the PIP and DIP joints.
   - The pull of the intrinsics is plantar to the rotational axis of the MTP joints.
     - Plantar translation of the metatarsal head after a distal osteotomy of the metatarsal places the intrinsics dorsal to the axis of rotation of the MTP joint, creating the "floating toe."

C. The extrinsic muscles (EDL and FDL) overpower the intrinsic muscles in positioning the lesser toes in hammer- and claw-toe deformities, with the EDL driving MTP joint extension and the FDL driving PIP and DIP joint flexion.

D. The EDL also is a weak antagonist to flexion at the interphalangeal joints, and likewise the FDL is a weak antagonist to extension at the MTP joint.

E. Dorsiflexion of the proximal phalanx at the MTP joint neutralizes these weak antagonist effects and accentuates the developing deformity.

F. Lesser-toe deformities occur much more commonly in women (up to 5:1 ratio), thought to be secondary to wearing high-fashion shoes that constrict the forefoot and maintain the MTP joints in hyperextension.

1. A hammer deformity most commonly involves the second toe because of its relative length compared to the remainder of the lesser toes. A short toe box will cause the second toe to buckle and extend at the MTP joint.
2. Chronic positioning of the MTP joint in hyperextension will attenuate the static plantar structures, allowing depression of the metatarsal head, migration of the fat pad distally, and imbalance of the dynamic forces on the toe as described above.

II. HAMMER-TOE DEFORMITY

A. The characteristic *hammer-toe* deformity is flexion of the PIP joint. With weight bearing, the MTP joint will appear dorsiflexed; however, this should correct with elevation of the foot off the ground (Figure 6-42).

B. The term "complex" hammer toe refers to concomitant dorsiflexion of the MTP joint that does not correct and is more appropriately termed and treated as a claw toe.

C. Treatment is dependent upon the flexibility of the deformity (Table 6-3).

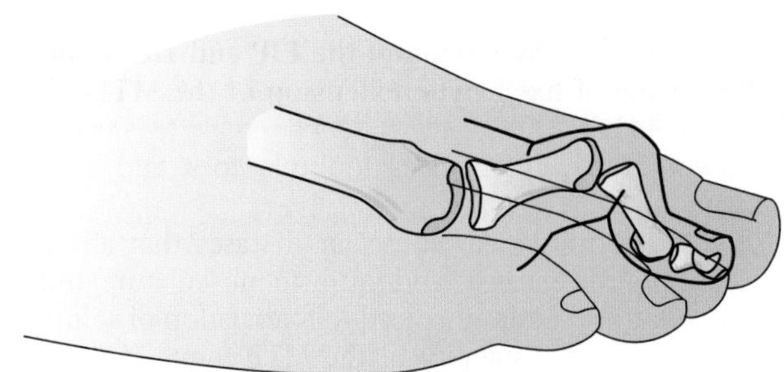

Figure 6-42 Hammer-toe deformity. (From DiGiovanni C: *Core knowledge in orthopaedics—foot and ankle,* Philadelphia, 2007, Elsevier.)

Table 6-3 Surgical Treatment of Lesser-Toe Deformities

Deformity	Surgical Options	Comments
Hammer toe		
Flexible	Girdlestone-Taylor FDL flexor-to-extensor tendon transfer	Add EDL lengthening or tenotomy if active flexion <10-15 degrees.
Fixed	PIP arthroplasty or arthrodesis	
Mallet toe		
Flexible	FDL tenotomy	
Fixed	Excisional arthroplasty or arthrodesis of the DIP joint	
Claw toe		
Flexible	FDL flexor-to-extensor tendon transfer with EDB tenotomy and EDL lengthening	Look for underlying neuromuscular etiology when more than two toes are involved.
Fixed	Weil osteotomy (oblique shortening osteotomy of the metatarsal) with MTP capsulotomy Extensor lengthening PIP arthroplasty or arthrodesis	
Crossover second toe	EDB tendon transfer with medial capsular release Flexor-to-extensor tendon transfer	Weil osteotomy should be performed if the MTP is dislocated.

DIP, distal interphalangeal; EDB, extensor digitorum brevis; EDL, extensor digitorum longus; FDL, flexor digitorum longus; MTP, metatarsophalangeal; PIP, proximal interphalangeal.

1. Flexible deformity
   - Nonoperative—Protective padding, shoes with tall toe boxes, and corrective hammer-toe splints are effective.
   - Operative—flexor tenotomy or flexor-to-extensor tendon transfer
2. Fixed deformity
   - Nonoperative—Accommodative shoes and protective padding can minimize callus formation. Corrective splint should NOT be used.
   - **Operative—PIP arthroplasty (resection of the distal neck and head of the proximal phalanx) or PIP arthrodesis (Figure 6-43)**

III. CLAW-TOE DEFORMITY (INTRINSIC MINUS TOE)

A. Characterized by flexion of the PIP and DIP joints in the setting of fixed hyperextension of the MTP joint (Figure 6-44)

1. Clawing typically involves multiple toes and is often bilateral.
2. Cavus deformity, neuromuscular diseases that affect the balance of the extrinsic and intrinsic musculature, inflammatory arthropathies that lead to attenuation of soft tissue structures and instability of the MTP joint, and trauma have all been implicated in the etiology of claw toes.
3. Claw toes are a noted complication of compartment syndrome involving the deep compartments of the foot.

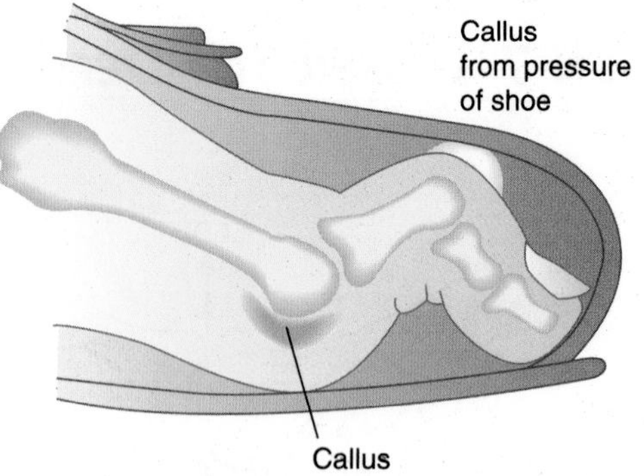

Figure 6-43 Dorsal aspect of the proximal interphalangeal joint strikes the toe box, leading to callus formation. An intractable plantar keratosis may develop beneath the metatarsal head. (From DeLee J: *DeLee and Drez's orthopedic sports medicine,* ed 3, Philadelphia, 2011, Elsevier.)

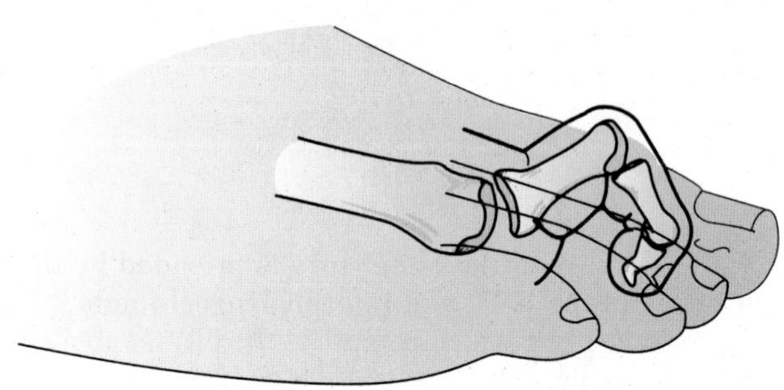

Figure 6-44 Claw toe deformity with fixed hyperextension of the MTP joint with PIP and DIP flexion. (From DiGiovanni C: *Core knowledge in orthopaedics—foot and ankle,* Philadelphia, 2007, Elsevier.)

B. Treatment is dependent upon the flexibility of the deformity (see Table 6-3).

1. Flexible deformity
   - Nonoperative—shoe modification, padding over any prominent or painful callosities, and use of orthotics to off-load and support a potentially painful, plantarly subluxed metatarsal head
   - **Operative—Flexor-to-extensor tendon transfer of the FDL alters the function of the FDL to function as an intrinsic and maintain correction (Figure 6-45).** Lengthening of the EDL and extensor digitorum brevis is typically required.
2. Fixed deformity
   - Nonoperative—shoe modification, padding over any prominent or painful callosities, and use of orthotics to off-load and support a potentially painful, plantarly subluxed metatarsal head
   - **Operative—PIP arthroplasty or arthrodesis along with MTP joint capsulotomy and extensor lengthening**
     - **Dislocated MTP joint**
       - **Requires the use of a Weil osteotomy (distal metatarsal osteotomy) to reduce the MTP joint (Figure 6-46).**

IV. MALLET-TOE DEFORMITY

A. A *mallet toe* consists of an isolated flexion deformity at the DIP joint (Figure 6-47).

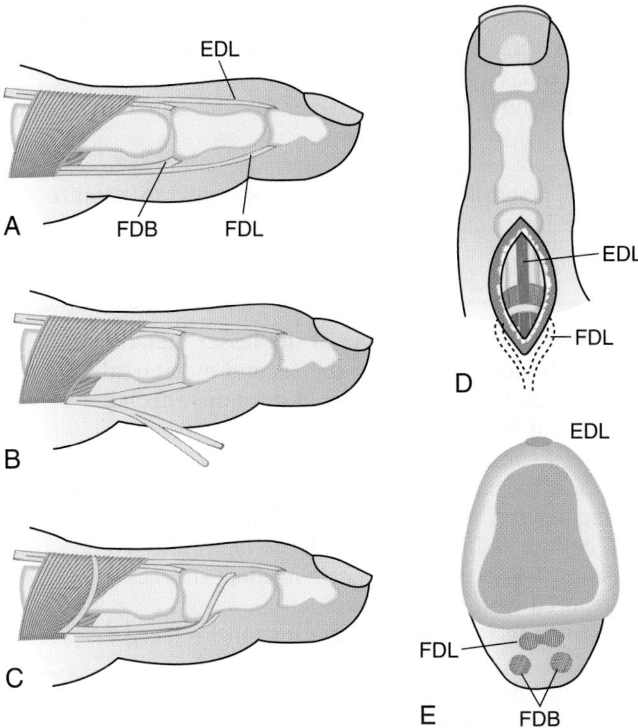

Figure 6-45 Technique of flexor tendon transfer. **A,** Lateral view shows flexor digitorum longus (FDL), flexor digitorum brevis (FDB), and extensor digitorum longus (EDL). **B,** The flexor digitorum longus is detached through a distal puncture wound and is delivered through a transverse incision at the plantar metatarsophalangeal joint flexion crease. **C,** The tendon is split longitudinally, and each half is delivered on either side of the proximal phalanx and is sutured into either the extensor expansion or the corresponding limb of the flexor tendon. **D,** Dorsal view shows transferred flexor digitorum longus tendon. **E,** Cross-sectional view shows the characteristic position of the flexor digitorum longus tendon. It is deep to the flexor digitorum brevis and is characterized by a midline raphe. (From DeLee J: *DeLee and Drez's orthopedic sports medicine,* ed 3, Philadelphia, 2011, Elsevier.)

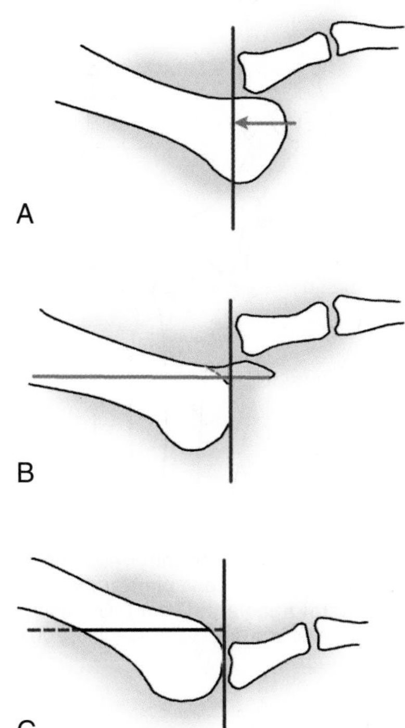

Figure 6-46 Weil osteotomy. **A,** Before surgery. **B,** After proximal displacement of metatarsal head. **C,** After resection of distal tip of dorsal fragment. (From Canale ST, Beaty J: *Campbell's operative orthopedics,* ed 11, Philadelphia, 2007, Elsevier. Redrawn from Vandeputte G, et al: The Weil osteotomy of the lesser metatarsals: a clinical and pedobarographic follow-up study, *Foot Ankle* 21:370, 2000.)

B. **Treatment (see Table 6-3)**
1. Nonoperative—These are similar to those used in treating patients with hammer-toe and claw-toe deformities.
2. Operative
   - Flexible
     - Flexor tenotomy
   - Fixed
     - DIP arthroplasty (excision of the distal neck and head of the middle phalanx) or DIP fusion
     - Extensor repair can be performed to minimize recurrence.

V. CROSSOVER-TOE DEFORMITY (SEE TABLE 6-3)

A. Multiplanar instability of the second toe may cause the toe to lie dorsomedially relative to the hallux (Figure 6-48).

B. Commonly referred to as a *crossover second toe,* this deformity

1. **Requires disruption of the plantar plate—KEY component**
2. Requires attenuation of the lateral collateral ligament
3. **May be iatrogenic—caused by steroid injection within the MTP joint—results in plantar plate attenuation**

C. **Nonoperative treatment**
1. Toe taping and corrective splints can minimize the discomfort but will not permanently correct the deformity.

D. **Operative treatment**
1. Flexor-to-extensor tendon transfer with release of the medial collateral ligament
2. Extensor digitorum brevis tendon transfer with rerouting plantar to the intermetatarsal ligament
3. Severe subluxation or dislocation of the MTP joint
   - Distal metatarsal osteotomy (Weil)

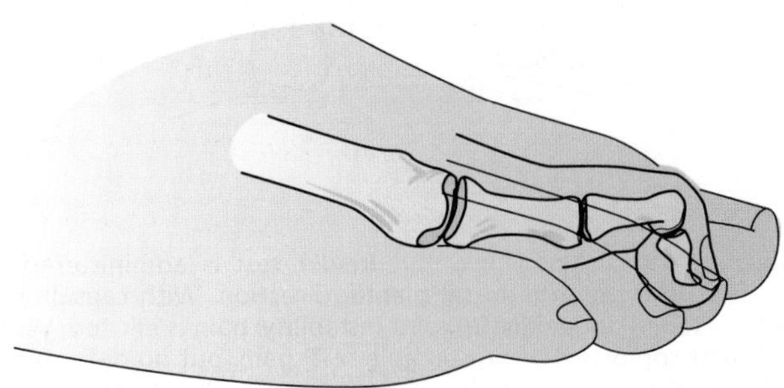

Figure 6-47 Mallet-toe deformity. (From DiGiovanni C: *Core knowledge in orthopaedics—foot and ankle,* Philadelphia, 2007, Elsevier.)

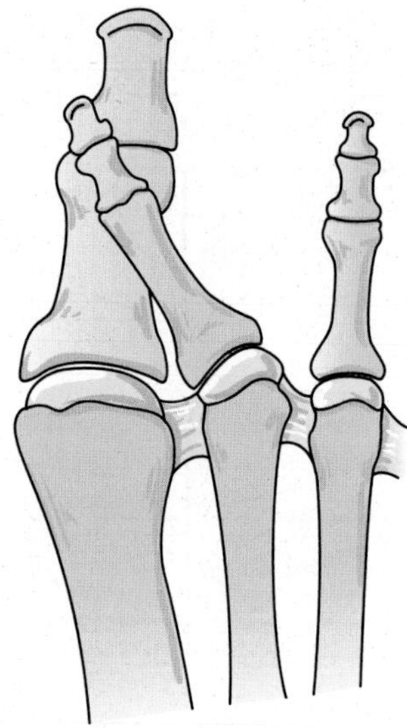

Figure 6-48 A crossover-toe deformity resulting from a rupture of the lateral collateral ligament and plantar plate and contracture of the medial collateral ligament. (From DiGiovanni C: *Core knowledge in orthopaedics—foot and ankle,* Philadelphia, 2007, Elsevier.)

VI. METATARSOPHALANGEAL INSTABILITY

A. Mild subluxation of the MTP joint that presents with pain and swelling without any deformity. Drawer test results in pain within the joint (Figure 6-49).

B. More commonly seen in athletes (runners, tennis players)

C. Nonoperative treatment

1. Toe taping and stabilizing lesser-toe orthotics

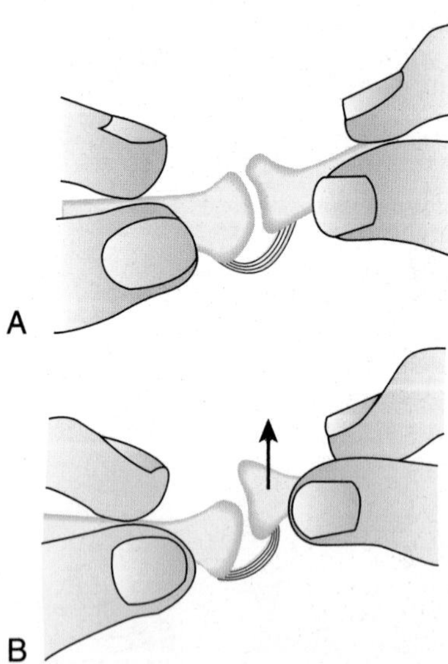

Figure 6-49 A dorsal plantar drawer test is administered by thrusting the toe in a dorsal plantar direction. With capsulitis or metatarsophalangeal (MTP) joint instability, pain is elicited. When a patient complains of presumable MTP pain, but no deformity is present, eliciting pain with a drawer test assists in making the correct diagnosis. (From DeLee J: *DeLee and Drez's orthopedic sports medicine,* ed 3, Philadelphia, 2011, Elsevier.)

2. Steroid injection is contraindicated and may result in the iatrogenic creation of a crossover-toe deformity.

D. Operative treatment

1. MTP synovectomy with reconstruction of the MTP joint capsule for isolated synovitis
2. If severe instability or deformity, a flexor-to-extensor tendon transfer is additionally performed to stabilize the MTP joint.

VII. FREIBERG DISEASE

A. Osteochondrosis of one of the lesser metatarsals, most commonly involving the second metatarsal

B. Patients have pain localized over the affected metatarsal head.

1. The second metatarsal is affected in over two thirds of cases. The third metatarsal accounts for most of the remaining cases. The fourth is affected in less than 5% of cases. The first and fifth metatarsals are rarely affected.
2. The pain is worse with ambulation and activities. It is relieved with sitting.

C. Common radiographic findings in Freiberg disease include

1. Resorption of the central metatarsal bone adjacent to the articular surface with flattening of the metatarsal head (Figure 6-50)

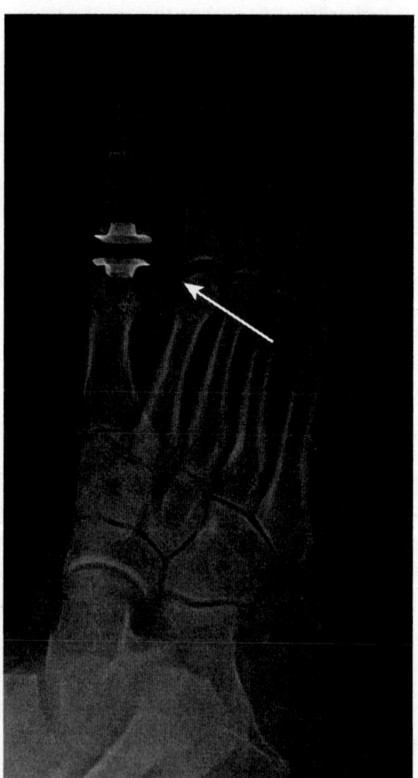

Figure 6-50 Note the flattening of the metatarsal head that is commonly seen with Freiberg disease *(arrow)*. This patient had a prior silicone arthroplasty of the great toe and developed Freiberg disease secondary to overload. (From Miller M, Sanders T: *Presentation, imaging and treatment of common musculoskeletal conditions,* Philadelphia, 2011, Elsevier.)

2. Osteochondral loose bodies
3. Joint space narrowing in late-stage disease with associated osteophyte formation along with collapse of the articular surface (Figure 6-51)

D. Nonoperative treatment

1. Common strategies consist of activity modification, shoewear modification (hard sole), orthotics (metatarsal bar), and a period of protected weight bearing.

E. Operative treatment

1. **For early-stage disease, joint débridement should be considered.**
   - **All synovitis, osteophytes, and loose bodies are débrided through a dorsal incision.**
   - This should be considered for patients with relatively good articular surface congruity and minimal metatarsal deformity.
2. Many studies have reported good results with dorsal closed-wedge metaphyseal osteotomy of the affected metatarsal (Figure 6-52).
   - This is done in conjunction with a thorough débridement of synovitis, abnormal cartilage, osteophytes, and necrotic bone.
   - This osteotomy serves to rotate the plantar aspect of the articular surface, which is typically well preserved, to a more superior position, where it then articulates with the phalanx.

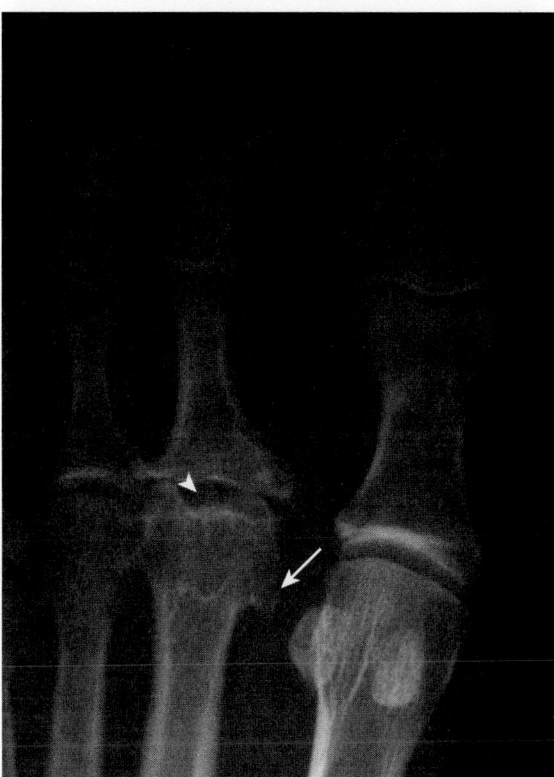

Figure 6-51 Coned-down anteroposterior view of the forefoot demonstrating the natural history and long-term sequela of untreated Freiberg disease. Note the significant subchondral cysts *(arrowhead)* and osteophyte formation *(arrow)* indicating osteoarthritis. (From Miller M, Sanders T: *Presentation, imaging and treatment of common musculoskeletal conditions,* Philadelphia, 2011, Elsevier.)

VIII. FIFTH-TOE DEFORMITIES

A. Several types of deformity exist, including underlapping, overlapping, rotatory, and cock-up fifth toe.

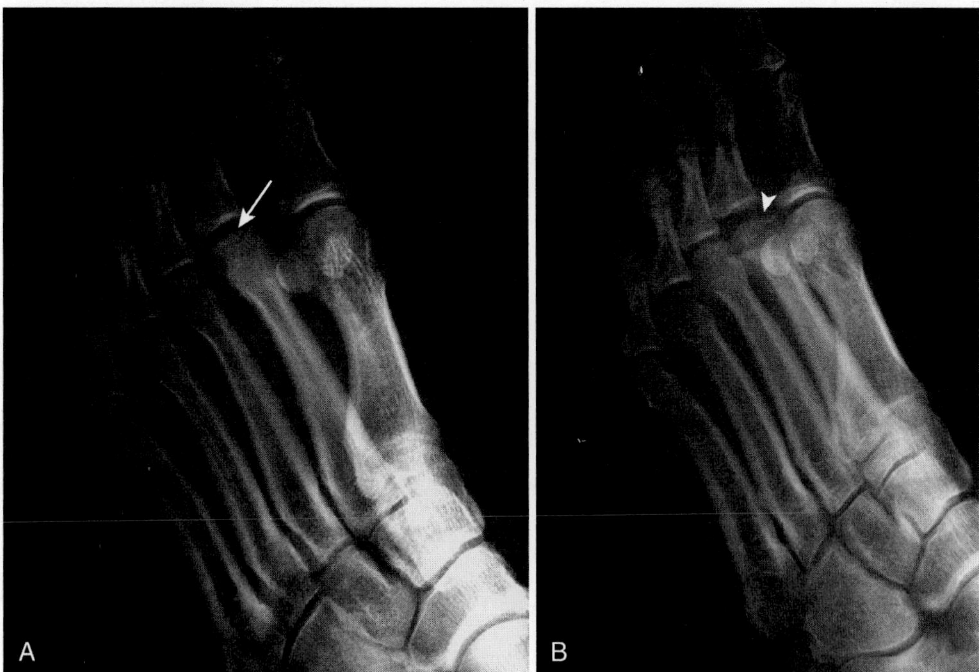

Figure 6-52 Oblique radiograph of a patient with Freiberg disease **(A)** with the characteristic flattening of the metatarsal head *(arrow)* treated with a dorsal closed-wedge osteotomy **(B)**. Note how the contour of the metatarsal head has been recreated ***(arrowhead).*** (From Miller M, Sanders T: *Presentation, imaging and treatment of common musculoskeletal conditions,* Philadelphia, 2011, Elsevier.)

B. Subluxation at the fifth MTP results in weakened push-off during ambulation, a loss of coverage of the fifth metatarsal head, and subsequent callus formation under the dorsolateral aspect of the fifth toe.

C. Nonoperative treatment

1. Stretching or taping may be helpful with an overlapping fifth toe, along with wide–toe box shoes.

D. Operative treatment

1. Cock-up fifth toe
   - EDL transfer into the abductor digiti minimi with rerouting inferior to the phalanx
   - Release of the dorsomedial capsule and Z-plasty of the skin may be required.
2. **Congenital curly toe (underlapping)**
   - **Tenotomy of FDL and flexor digitorum brevis has been recommended in children with flexible deformities.**
3. Syndactylization is reserved for salvage after failed operative intervention.

SECTION 8 HYPERKERATOTIC PATHOLOGIES

I. HARD CORNS (HELOMATA DURUM)

A. Diagnosis

1. Commonly occur over the metaphyseal aspect of the phalanges at the metatarsophalangeal or interphalangeal joints, especially of the fifth toe
   - Secondary to extrinsic pressure (on the border of the foot)
2. Secondary to frictional irritation or from pressure over bony prominences (Figure 6-53)

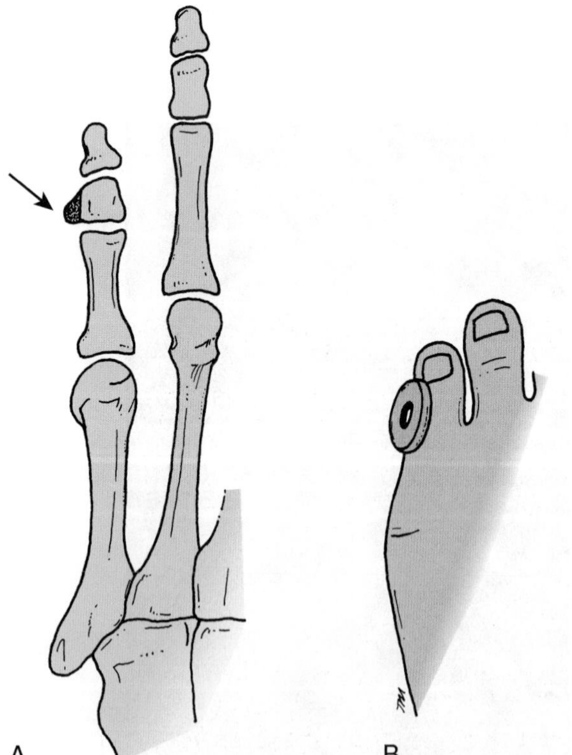

Figure 6-53 **A,** An underlying exostosis *(arrow)* combined with restrictive footwear leads to a hard corn. **B,** A pad may be used to relieve pressure. (From Porter D, Schon L: *Baxter's the foot and ankle in sport,* ed 2, Philadelphia, 2007, Elsevier.)

3. Examination reveals epidermal hyperplasia with a conical central area.

B. Treatment

1. Conservative management
   - Shaving or paring the corn with a pumice stone, followed by removal of the central inverted "seed" of the corn.
   - Modification of shoe wear and protective padding reduces extrinsic pressure.
2. Surgical treatment
   - Reserved for refractory cases that fail conservative management
   - Excision of bony prominences at the interphalangeal joint
   - Partial cheilectomy of the metatarsal head and hemiphalangectomy of the proximal phalanx can also be effective.

II. SOFT CORNS (HELOMATA MOLLE)

A. Diagnosis

1. Hyperkeratoses that develop as the result of moisture in web space and pressure from neighboring phalangeal condyles (Figure 6-54)
2. Two main types
   - Prominent medial condyle of the fifth proximal phalanx contacts the lateral base of the fourth proximal phalanx or metatarsal head.
   - Distal phalangeal exostosis abuts its neighboring toe at various locations.

B. Physical examination

1. Macerated and friable skin with thickened callus usually deep in the web space
2. Mediolateral squeezing of toes causes significant pain.

C. Treatment

1. Conservative treatment
   - Absorptive padding in web space and accommodative shoe wear
     - Decreases contact pressure between toes and wicks excess moisture
2. Surgical treatment
   - Excision of offending bony prominences and adjacent skin lesions

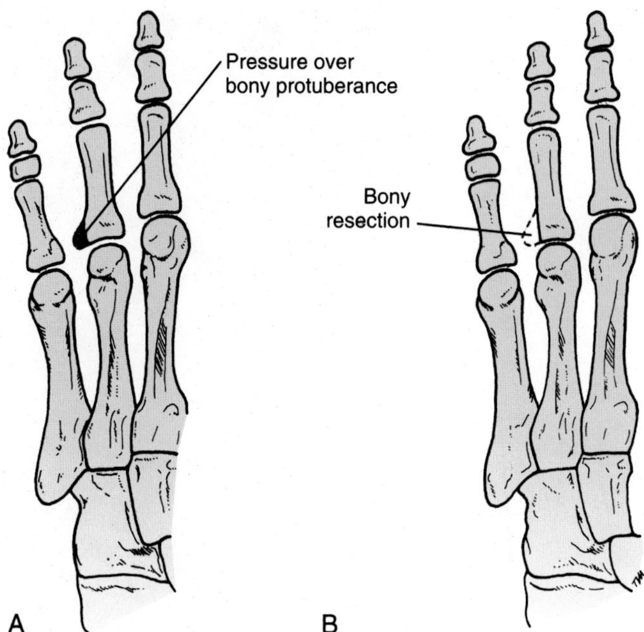

Figure 6-54 **A,** A soft corn may develop over the base of the proximal phalanx. **B,** Resection of the bony prominence. (From Porter D, Schon L: *Baxter's the foot and ankle in sport,* ed 2, Philadelphia, 2007, Elsevier.)

- Avoid web-space incisions to minimize the risk for infection.
- Proximal lesions
- Basilar hemiphalangectomy with lateral condyle excision of the metatarsal head
- Web-space syndactylization also effective

III. INTRACTABLE PLANTAR KERATOSIS

A. Plantar callus secondary to excess pressure from metatarsal head

B. Predisposing factors—fat pad atrophy, plantar-flexed first ray, equinus contracture, intrinsic minus toe contracture, and hypertrophy of the sesamoid

C. Two main types (Figure 6-55)

1. Discrete form
   - Localized callus with a hyperkeratotic core, usually caused by prominence of fibular condyle
   - Commonly associated with a prominent tibial sesamoid
   - Conservative treatment
     - Callus trimming and soft metatarsal pads
     - Consider total-contact orthosis or extended steel shank for patients with significant fat pad atrophy.
   - Surgical treatment
     - Tibial sesamoid shaving of the plantar surface or fibular metatarsal condylectomy
     - Consider complete excision of the tibial sesamoid in more advanced cases.
     - Consider dorsiflexion osteotomy in patients with a plantar-flexed first ray.
2. Diffuse form
   - Secondary to pressure phenomenon from the entire metatarsal head
   - Commonly associated with an elongated metatarsal, an excessively plantar-flexed metatarsal, or transfer lesion
   - Conservative management—similar to the discrete form of IPK
   - Surgical treatment
     - Shortening or dorsiflexion metatarsal osteotomy is the surgical treatment of choice.
     - Complete plantar condylectomy is also effective and favored over the original Duvries arthroplasty (which included resection of the metatarsal head that occasionally lead to transfer metatarsalgia).

IV. BUNIONETTE DEFORMITY (TAILOR'S BUNION)

A. Diagnosis

1. Prominence over the distal aspect of the fifth metatarsal head

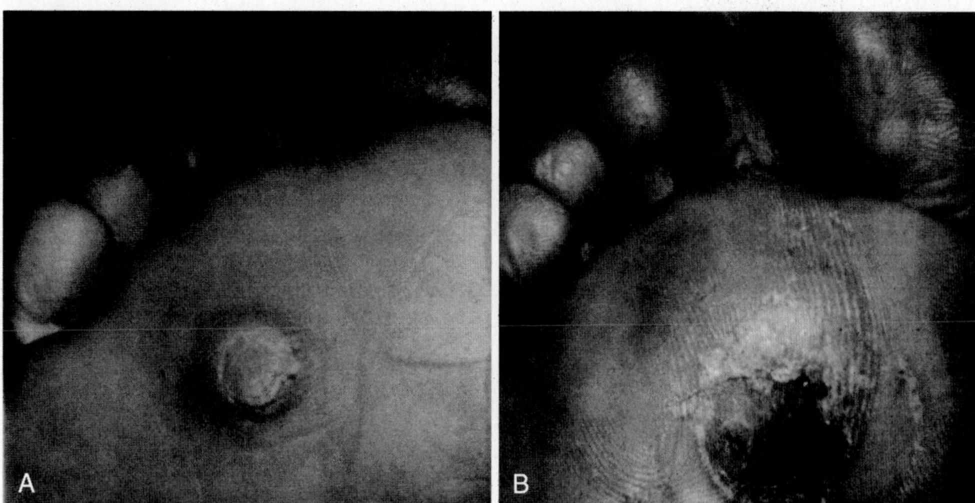

Figure 6-55 **A,** Discrete callus in a tennis player with an enlarged fibular condyle. **B,** Diffuse callus in a runner. (From Porter D, Schon L: *Baxter's the foot and ankle in sport,* ed 2, Philadelphia, 2007, Elsevier.)

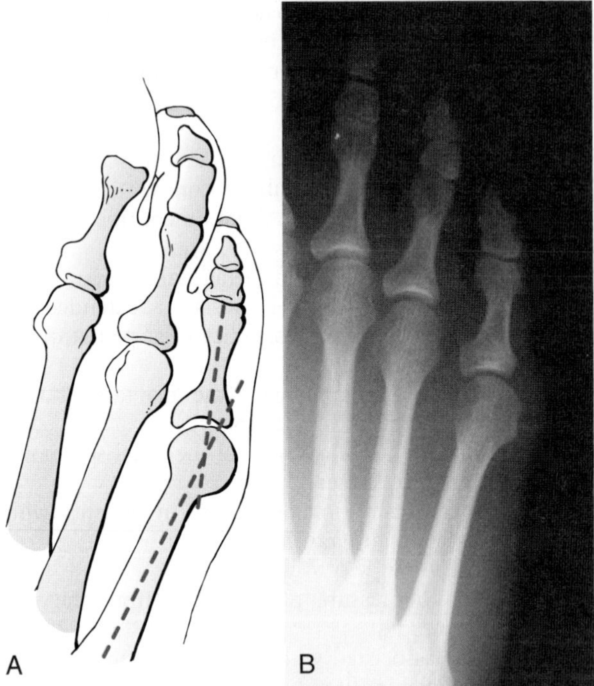

Figure 6-56 **A and B, Type I bunionette deformity is characterized by an enlarged fifth metatarsal head.** (From Coughlin M, et al: *Surgery of the foot and ankle,* ed 8, Philadelphia, 2006, Elsevier.)

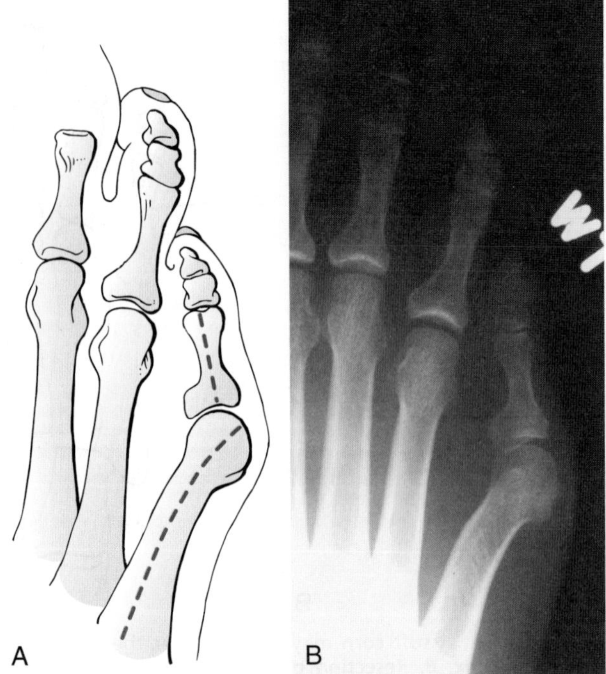

Figure 6-57 **A and B, Type II bunionette deformity is characterized by lateral bowing of the fifth metatarsal head.** (From Coughlin M, et al: *Surgery of the foot and ankle,* ed 8, Philadelphia, 2006, Elsevier.)

2. Causes pain over the lateral or plantar aspect of the MTP joint, particularly with compressive shoe wear
3. Bunionette deformity in conjunction with ipsilateral hallux valgus and metatarsus primus varus is termed "splayfoot."
4. Three distinct types have been described based on the anatomic location of the deformity along the fifth metatarsal.
   - Type I deformity—distinguished by the presence of an enlarged fifth metatarsal head (Figure 6-56)
     - Lateral metatarsal head condylectomy
   - **Type II deformity—demonstrates lateral bowing of the fifth metatarsal diaphysis (Figure 6-57)**
     - Distal fifth metatarsal osteotomy
   - Type III deformity—demonstrates an abnormally widened fourth-fifth metatarsal angle (intermetatarsal angle >8 degrees) (Figure 6-58)
     - Oblique diaphyseal osteotomy

B. Conservative treatment

1. Shoe-wear modification, strategic padding, and shaving the symptomatic callus is usually effective.
2. With plantar callus or associated pes planus, consider a metatarsal pad or custom orthotic device.

C. Surgical treatment

1. **Lateral metatarsal head condylectomy (type I)**
2. **Distal fifth metatarsal osteotomy (i.e., chevron) (type II)**
3. **Oblique diaphyseal osteotomy (type III)**
4. Consider metatarsal head resection for salvage.
5. Proximal osteotomy should be avoided owing to the tenuous blood supply at the proximal metadiaphyseal junction of the fifth metatarsal.

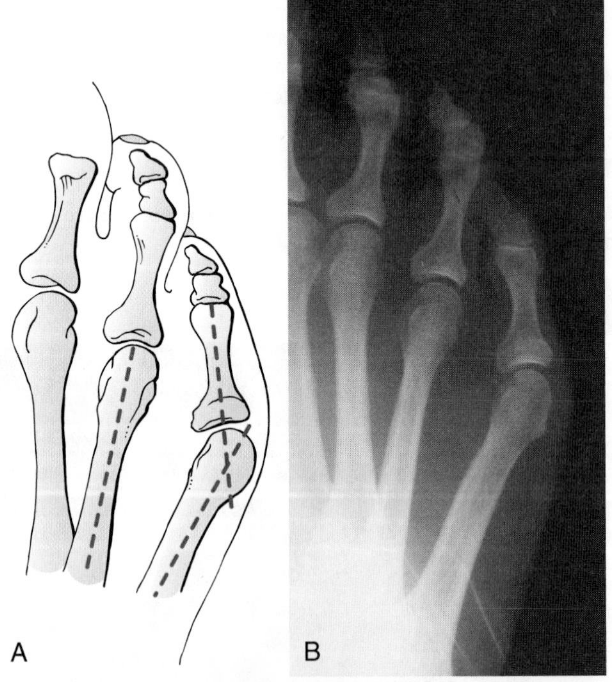

Figure 6-58 **A and B, Type III bunionette deformity is characterized by an abnormally wide fourth-fifth intermetatarsal angle.** (From Coughlin M, et al: *Surgery of the foot and ankle,* ed 8, Philadelphia, 2006, Elsevier.)

SECTION 9 SESAMOIDS

I. ANATOMY

A. The medial (tibial) and lateral (fibular) hallucal sesamoids are part of a strong sesamoid capsuloligamentous complex.

1. Enveloped within the two heads of the flexor hallucis brevis tendon, separated by an intersesamoid ridge called the crista
2. Attached to proximal phalanx via the plantar plate
3. Suspended by the collateral ligaments of MTP joint, metatarsosesamoid ligaments, intersesamoid ligament, abductor hallucis tendon, and adductor hallucis tendon

B. Analogous to the patella, as a mechanism to increase the mechanical advantage of the pulley function of the intrinsics (flexor hallucis brevis)

C. Protects the FHL and disperses the forces beneath the first metatarsal head

II. DEFORMITIES

A. Sesamoid disorders can include acute injury (fracture, dislocation, sprain/"turf toe"), sesamoiditis, stress fracture, arthrosis, avascular necrosis, and intractable plantar keratosis.

B. Diagnosis

1. Chief complaint is pain under the first metatarsal head, especially with toe-off.
2. Physical examination—tenderness with direct palpation of the involved sesamoid, pain with first MTP ROM
3. Radiographs—in addition to anteroposterior and lateral views, lateral oblique (fibular sesamoid) and medial oblique (tibial sesamoid) views isolate each bone, and the axial view shows the articulation with the metatarsal head (Figure 6-59).
4. Mechanism of injury—forced dorsiflexion of the first MTP joint, repetitive loading
   - **Turf toe**
     - **Forced dorsiflexion can result in avulsion of the plantar plate off the base of the phalanx and subsequent proximal migration of the sesamoids.**
   - The tibial sesamoid is more frequently involved in trauma but also more likely to be bipartite or multipartite.

C. Conservative treatment

1. Turf toe
   - Grade 1—capsular strain
     - Signs—normal ROM, weight bearing without difficulty, normal radiographs
     - Treatment—stiff insole, taping, with immediate return to play
   - Grade 2—partial capsular tear
     - Signs—painful ROM, limited weight bearing, normal radiographs
     - Treatment—no athletic activity for 2 weeks, stiff insole, return to play if painless 60-degree dorsiflexion present.
   - Grade 3—Complete tear of the plantar plate
     - Signs—severe pain with palpation, limited and painful ROM, abnormal radiographs (fracture, proximal sesamoid migration)
     - Treatment—superior results demonstrated with operative repair of the plantar plate over conservative care
2. Sesamoid fracture
   - Initial treatment with a fracture boot to limit the stress across the sesamoid
   - Transition to sesamoid relief pad (dancer's pad) with gradual resumption of activity
3. Sesamoiditis can be treated with anti-inflammatory medications, rest, ice, and activity and shoe-wear modification.

D. Surgical treatment

1. Symptomatic nonunions or cases that prove refractory to conservative care can be treated surgically with bone grafting or with partial or complete sesamoidectomy.
2. The results of sesamoidectomy are the most predictable.
   - Excision of the proximal or distal pole achieves the best results and should be performed if the fracture pattern allows.
3. **Complications of medial and lateral sesamoidectomy are hallux valgus and varus, respectively.**
   - Repairing the defect with capsule (or a slip of abductor hallucis for the tibial sesamoid) should help prevent this complication.
   - **Cock-up deformity (or claw toe) will occur if both sesamoids are excised (Figure 6-60).**
   - Care should be taken to avoid injury to the FHL and loss of flexor function, especially in the high-performance athlete.

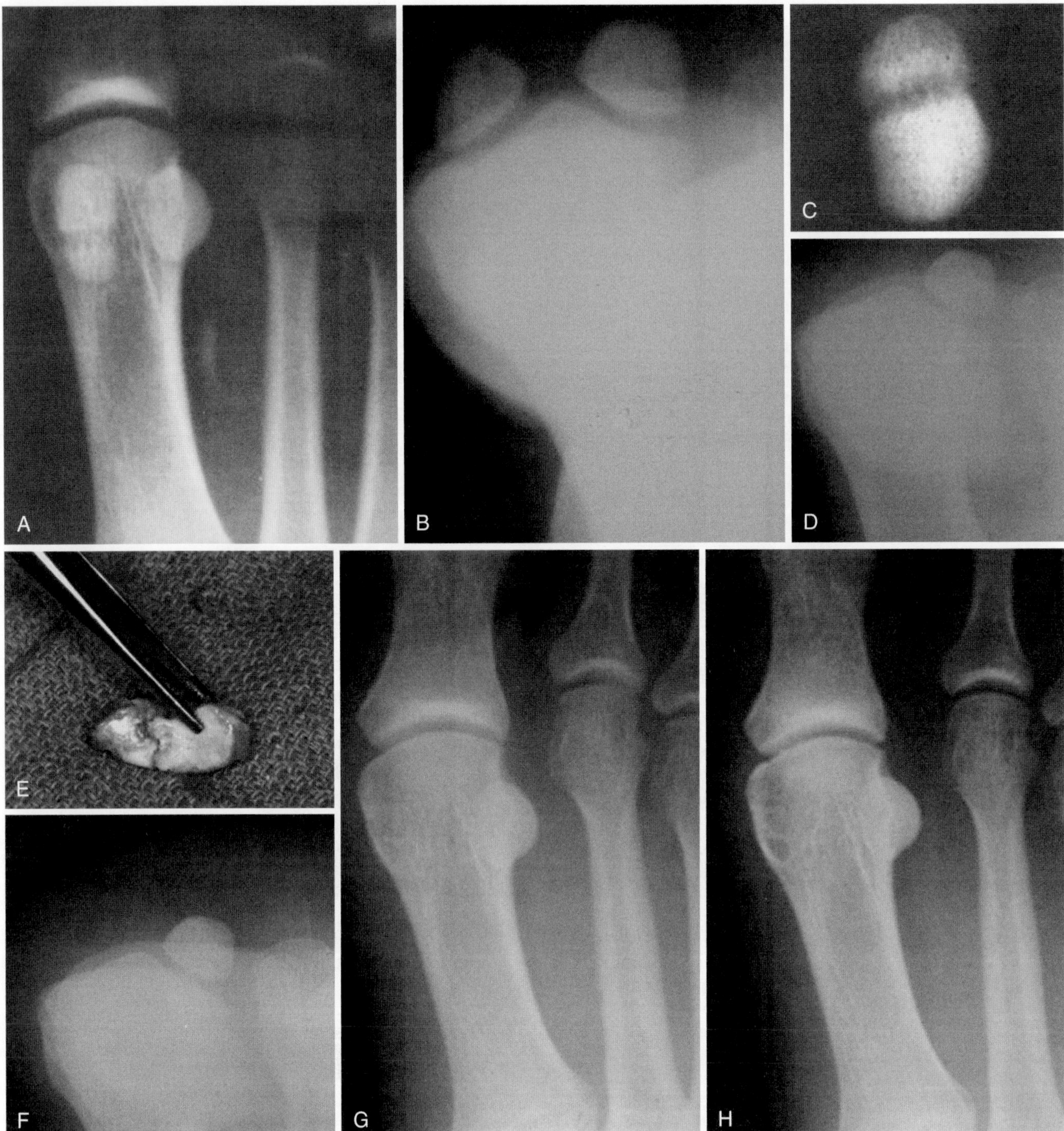

Figure 6-59 **A,** An anteroposterior radiograph demonstrates a painful bipartite sesamoid. **B,** An axial radiograph does not show evidence of a fracture or bipartite sesamoid. **C,** Radiograph of a pathology specimen showing rounded edges pathognomonic of a bipartite sesamoid. **D,** Axial view following excision of medial sesamoid. **E,** Gross pathology of a specimen. **F** and **G,** Immediately following surgery. **H,** At 19-year follow-up after medial sesamoid excision. Alignment of the first metatarsophalangeal joint is well maintained. (From Coughlin M, et al: *Surgery of the foot and ankle,* ed 8, Philadelphia, 2006, Elsevier.)

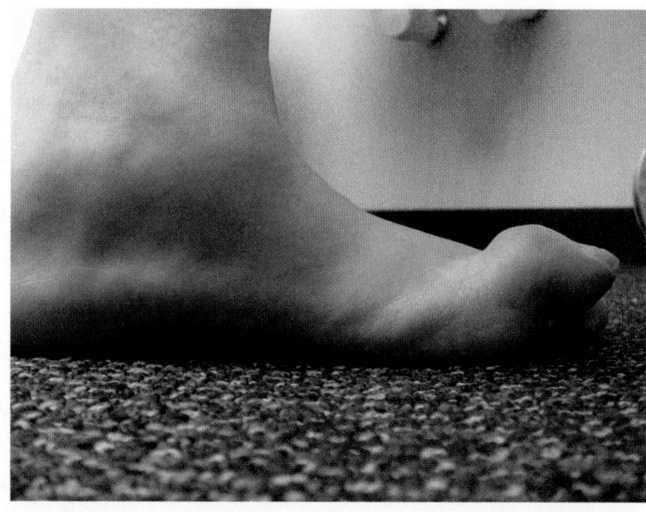

Figure 6-60 Cock-up toe in a patient who had undergone tibial and fibular sesamoidectomies. Both sesamoids should never be resected to prevent this complication. A first metatarsophalangeal joint fusion can be done concomitantly to prevent this from occurring.

SECTION 10 ACCESSORY BONES (FIGURE 6-61)

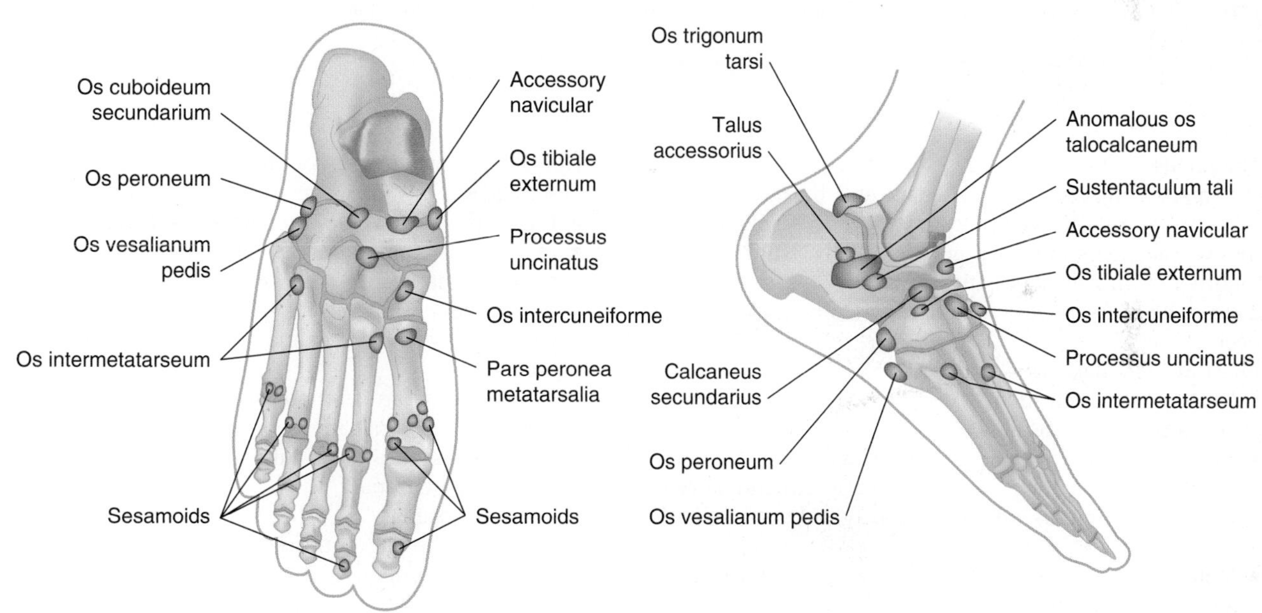

Figure 6-61 Accessory ossicles of the foot. (From Berquist TH, editor: *Radiology of the foot and ankle,* New York, 1989, Raven Press. In Mark J, et al: *Rosen's emergency medicine,* ed 7, Philadelphia, 2009, Elsevier.)

SECTION 11 NEUROLOGIC DISORDERS

I. INTERDIGITAL NEURITIS (MORTON NEUROMA)

A. Definition

1. **Compressive neuropathy of the interdigital nerve, usually between the third and fourth metatarsals (Figure 6-62)**
2. The pathophysiology of this condition is still poorly understood.
   - Theories include compression/tension around the intermetatarsal ligament, repetitive microtrauma, vascular changes, excessive bursal tissue, endoneural edema, and eventual neural fibrosis.

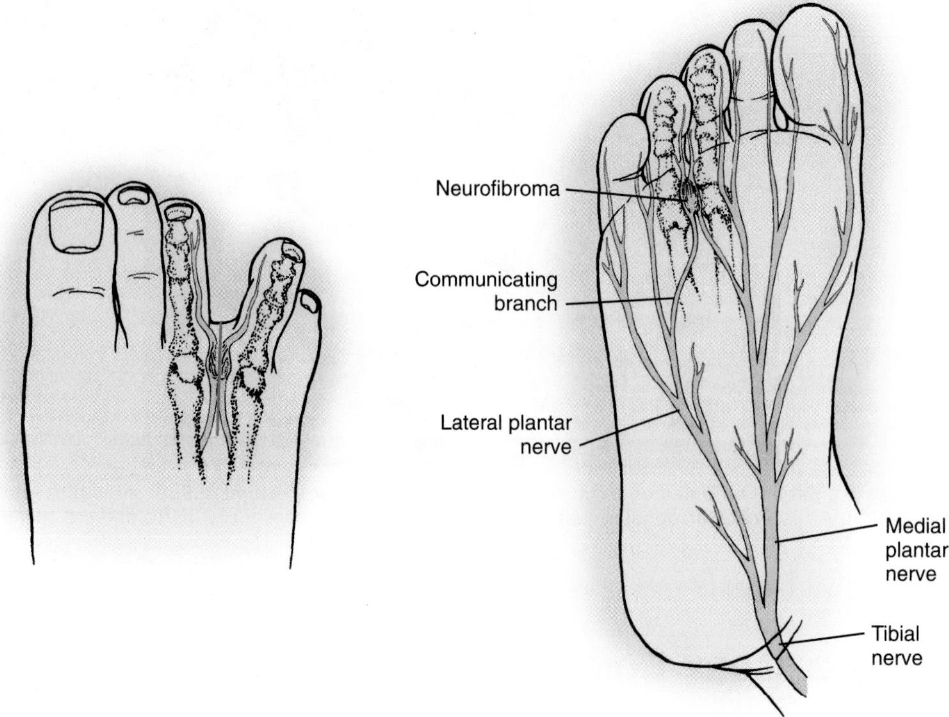

Figure 6-62 **Most common anatomic location of interdigital neuroma; plantar and dorsal views.** (From Canale ST, Beaty J: *Campbell's operative orthopedics,* ed 11, Philadelphia, 2007, Elsevier. Modified from McElvenny RT: The etiology and surgical treatment of intractable pain about the fourth metatarsophalangeal joint (Morton's toe), *J Bone Joint Surg* 25:675, 1943.)

B. Diagnosis

1. Patients will frequently report pain and burning on the plantar aspect of the web space, with over 60% of patients noting pain radiating into the toe distally. Numbness is reported in only 40% of patients.
2. Exacerbated by footwear with narrow toe boxes and high heels
3. Physical examination
   - Palpation between and just distal to the metatarsal heads elicits plantar tenderness.
   - Compressing the medial and lateral aspect of the forefoot while palpating the web space structures can provoke symptoms and occasionally a bursal "click" (Mulder click).
   - Metatarsalgia and MTP synovitis often present similarly and should be ruled out.
4. Radiography
   - Plain films should be performed to rule out bony masses or deformity.
   - MRI can be used to identify other pathologies but is not required for diagnosis.

C. Conservative treatment

1. Shoe-wear modification (avoiding high heels and narrow toe boxes) is the most important and effective intervention.
2. Metatarsal pads placed proximal to the focus of pain can prevent direct pressure and widen the intermetatarsal space during weight bearing, thereby indirectly decompressing the nerve.
3. Corticosteroid injections can have moderate effectiveness.

D. Surgical treatment—excision of neuroma

1. Dorsal approach most common (plantar approach also described)
   - **Incise the transverse intermetatarsal ligament.**
   - Identify the common digital nerve and its branches, and resect the nerve 2 to 3 cm proximal to the intermetatarsal ligament (proximal to the small plantar branches), which allows the proximal stump to retract (Figure 6-63).
     - Minimizes formation of stump neuroma, the most common complication
   - Difficult visualization results in a 4% rate of failure to excise the neuroma.
2. Plantar approach
   - Decreases the rate of missed neuroma excision
   - Does not require incision of the transverse intermetatarsal ligament
   - Increased risk (5%) of painful plantar scar

II. RECURRENT NEUROMA

A. Bulbous enlargement of the neural stump (or secondary glioma)

1. Usually caused by inadequate proximal resection or failure of the nerve to retract
2. Neural stump adheres to adjacent bone and soft tissue, causing a traction neuritis.

B. Diagnosis

1. Localized pain and tenderness to palpation (Tinel sign) in web space of previous neuroma resection, at or proximal to metatarsal heads
2. Must rule out "irritable" tibial nerve

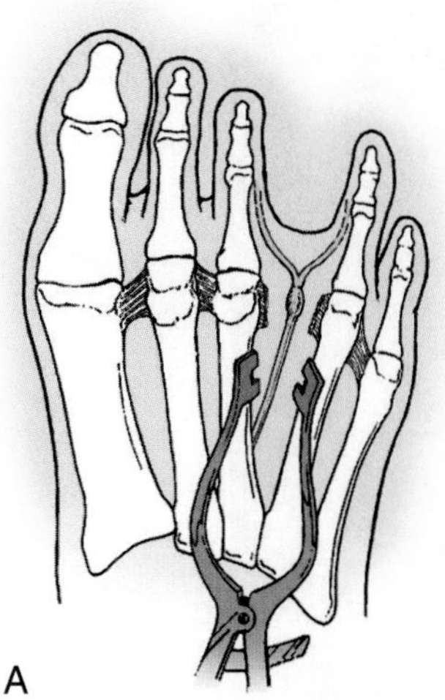

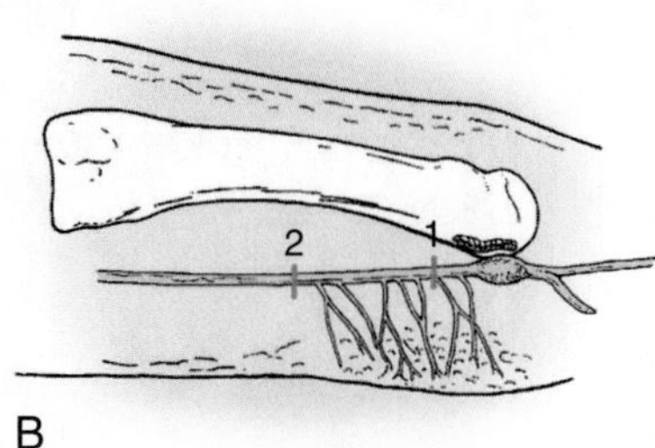

Figure 6-63 A, Lamina spreader used to expose neuroma. **B,** Lateral view of plantar branches of digital nerve. *1,* Previously recommended level of neurectomy; *2,* currently recommended level of neurectomy (3 cm proximal to ligament) to avoid plantarly directed nerve branches. (From Canale ST, Beaty J: *Campbell's operative orthopedics,* ed 11, Philadelphia, 2007, Elsevier. Modified from Weinfeld SB, Myerson MS: Interdigital neuritis: diagnosis and treatment, *J Am Acad Orthop Surg* 4:328, 1996.)

- Palpate along tibial nerve and branches distal to flexor retinaculum.

3. Recurrent neuroma is likely if symptoms are localized and reproducible.

C. Treatment

1. Conservative
   - Similar to primary neuroma—see the guidelines outlined previously
2. Surgical
   - Excision of the stump neuroma can be performed through another dorsal incision or through a plantar incision.
   - Plantar incision allows access to a very proximal location in which to place the resected neuroma stump.
     - Preferred approach for revision neuroma excision
   - The new stump should be transposed into muscle tissue, if possible.
   - The success rate after excision of a recurrent or stump neuroma is 65% to 75%, compared with the 80% to 85% success rate after initial excision.

III. TARSAL TUNNEL SYNDROME

A. Compressive neuropathy of the tibial nerve within the fibroosseous tunnel posterior and inferior to the medial malleolus

B. Anatomy

1. Bounded by the flexor retinaculum (laciniate ligament) superficially; the medial talus, medial calcaneus, and sustentaculum tali deep; and the abductor hallucis inferiorly
2. The tarsal tunnel also contains the tibialis posterior, FHL, and FDL tendons; the posterior tibial artery; the venae comitantes; and the numerous septa that subdivide the tunnel.

C. Reported causes of tarsal tunnel syndrome include tenosynovitis, engorged or varicose vessels, synovial or ganglion cysts, pigmented villonodular synovitis, nerve sheath tumors, lipomas, fracture of the sustentaculum tali or medial tubercle of the posterior process of the talus, middle facet tarsal coalition, and accessory muscles.

D. Systemic diseases such as diabetes mellitus, rheumatoid arthritis, and ankylosing spondylitis may have an indirect effect by causing inflammatory edema.

E. Clinical diagnosis

1. Symptoms of tarsal tunnel syndrome may be vague and misleading.
   - Include a burning sensation on the plantar surface of the foot and medial ankle and occasional sharp pains or paresthesias
   - Prolonged standing, walking, or running can exacerbate the symptoms.
2. Physical examination
   - Percussion of the entire course of the distal tibial nerve and its branches should be performed.
     - Tinel sign, radiating pain or discomfort with continuous deep compression over the nerve, or diminished two-point discrimination may be elicited.
   - Sensory examination is usually unpredictable.
   - Assess hindfoot alignment because pes planus may cause increased tension on the nerve.
   - Wasting of the abductor hallucis or abductor digiti quinti may be seen with involvement of the medial or lateral plantar nerve, respectively.

F. Diagnostic tests

1. Electrodiagnostic studies should be performed to help make the diagnosis, or determine a different level of compression.
   - Sensory nerve conduction studies are more commonly abnormal than motor nerve conduction studies.
   - Electromyogram abnormalities are less sensitive.
2. MRI can identify the presence of a mass-occupying lesion, which, if present, must be excised (Figure 6-64).
   - Surgical decompression with mass excision results in more predictable symptomatic improvement compared to patients who do not have a mass-occupying lesion.

G. Correlation with history and physical examination findings is essential.

H. Conservative treatment

1. Management should begin with conservative measures unless there is a suspicious mass or suspected malignancy.
2. Medications such as nonsteroidal anti-inflammatory drugs (NSAIDs), vitamin B_6, and tricyclic antidepressants are most commonly prescribed.
   - Selective serotonin reuptake inhibitors and antiseizure medications are also used.

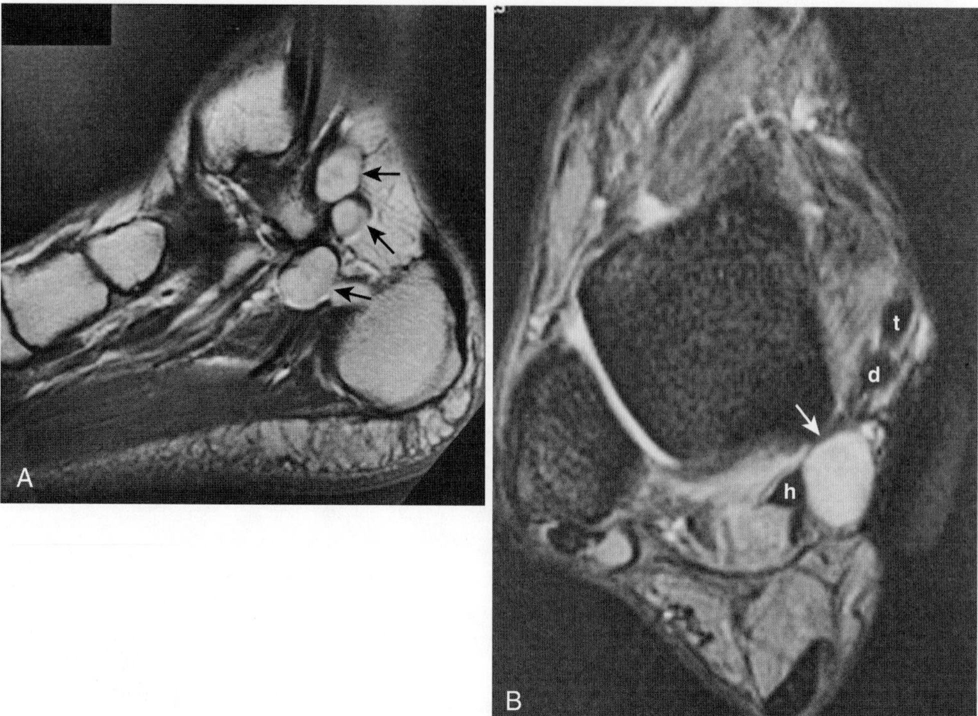

Figure 6-64 Tarsal tunnel syndrome from schwannomas. **A,** T1-weighted contrast-enhanced sagittal image of the hindfoot. Three round masses *(arrows)* that show enhancement are running through the tarsal tunnel. **B,** T2-weighted axial image of the hindfoot. One of the schwannomas is shown as a high-signal mass *(arrow)* in the space normally occupied by the posterior tibial nerve, artery, and vein. d, flexor digitorum tendon; h, flexor hallucis tendon; t, tibialis posterior tendon. (From Helms C, et al: *Musculoskeletal MRI,* ed 2, Philadelphia, 2009, Saunders.)

3. Physical therapy may include stretching, massage, desensitization, and iontophoresis.
4. Orthoses to correct hindfoot valgus (medial sole and heel wedge) play an important role as well.
5. In cases of acute inflammation or severe limitation because of pain, a brief course in short-leg casting can be helpful.

I. Surgical treatment

1. Space-occupying lesion should be excised with concomitant nerve release.
2. Appropriate conservative management for 3 to 6 months that is unsuccessful warrants surgical intervention.
3. Longitudinal incision is made over the course of the tibial nerve that curves distally behind the medial malleolus to the abductor musculature (Figure 6-65).
4. The nerve is identified proximally, and the proximal investing fascia and flexor retinaculum are released.
   - Care must be taken to release the superficial and deep fascia of the abductor hallucis muscle.
5. Endoscopic tarsal tunnel release is not recommended.
6. Recurrence of tarsal tunnel syndrome is a challenging problem.
   - Incomplete release is the most common etiology, though intrinsic nerve damage may play a role in recurrent symptoms.
   - Revision release may be of benefit if incomplete release is suspected, though results are often poor.

J. Lateral plantar nerve

1. Provides sensation to the plantar lateral aspect of the foot
2. **May be injured during surgical approaches that require a plantar incision, such as a tibiotalocalcaneal arthrodesis with an intramedullary nail**
3. First branch of the lateral plantar nerve (Baxter nerve) may a source of chronic plantar medial heel pain.

IV. ANTERIOR TARSAL TUNNEL SYNDROME

A. Compressive neuropathy of the deep peroneal nerve in the fibroosseous tunnel formed by the Y-shaped inferior extensor retinaculum (Figure 6-66)

B. The nerve divides into the lateral motor and the medial sensory branches within the tunnel and is accompanied by the dorsalis pedis artery.

C. The common causes of compression include tightly laced shoes; anterior osteophytes at the tibiotalar and TN articulations; a bony prominence associated with pes cavus deformity or fracture; ganglion cysts; and tendinitis of the EDL, EHL, and tibialis anterior (Figure 6-67).

D. Diagnosis

1. Patients present with burning pain and paresthesias along the medial second toe, lateral hallux, and first web space or even vague dorsal foot pain.
2. Symptoms are often worse at night as the ankle assumes a plantar-flexed posture and with shallow, laced shoes.
3. Physical examination
   - Decreased two-point discrimination, positive Tinel sign along course of deep peroneal nerve; may be worse with plantar flexion of ankle

E. Treatment

1. Night splints, NSAIDs, diagnostic/therapeutic injections, shoe tongue padding, and footwear with loose lacing or alternative lacing techniques are the conservative approaches.

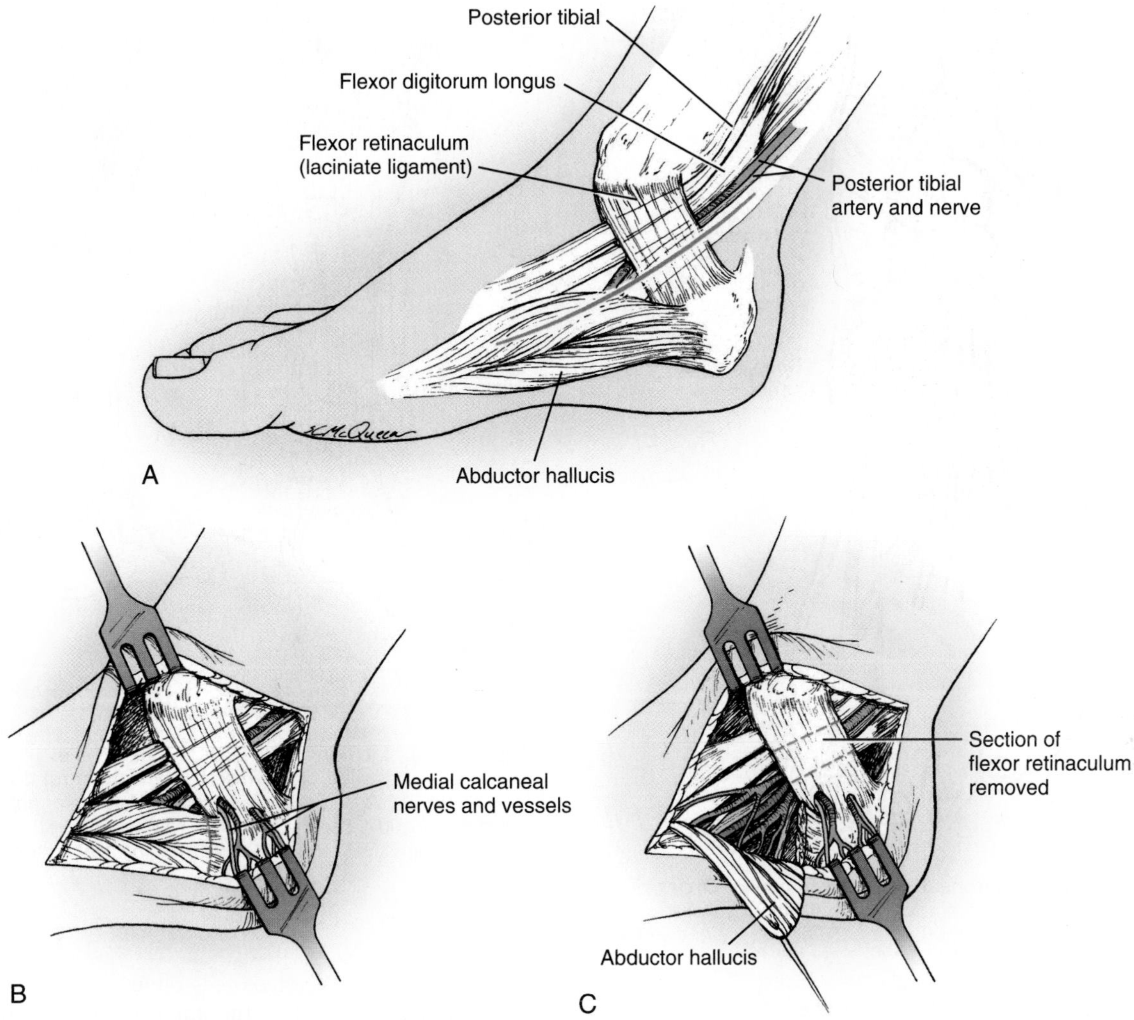

Figure 6-65 Tarsal tunnel release. **A,** Skin incision. **B,** Note branches of medial calcaneal nerve and artery penetrating retinaculum. *Broken line* indicates incision for reflecting abductor hallucis muscle. **C,** Abductor hallucis is reflected plantarward, and section of flexor retinaculum to be removed is outlined. (From Canale ST, Beaty J: *Campbell's operative orthopedics,* ed 11, Philadelphia, 2007, Elsevier.)

2. Surgical release involves incising the inferior extensor retinaculum, releasing both branches of the nerve, excising bone spurs, and carefully repairing the bony capsule to avoid exposing the nerve to bleeding bone while protecting the dorsalis pedis artery.
3. Patients should understand that relief of the paresthesias and dysesthesias may take weeks or months.

V. SEQUELAE OF UPPER MOTOR NEURON DISORDERS

A. Most commonly secondary to traumatic brain injury, stroke, and spinal cord injury

B. Pathology

1. Disruption of the upper motor neuron pathways can lead to paralysis, muscular imbalance, and acquired spasticity, which ultimately may cause deformity of the foot and ankle.
2. Secondary problems include fixed contractures, calluses, pressure sores, hygiene issues, joint subluxation, shoe-wear difficulties, and dissatisfaction with physical appearance.
3. **The most common deformity of the foot and ankle is equinovarus.**
   - **The equinus component is caused by overactivity of the gastrocnemius-soleus complex.**
   - **The varus is due to relative overactivity of the tibialis anterior, with lesser contributions from the FHL, FDL, and tibialis posterior.**

C. Treatment

1. Nonoperative care
   - Early intervention with physical therapy, stretching and strengthening, and maintenance of joint ROM
   - Other modalities include splinting, serial casting, oral muscle relaxants, phenol and lidocaine nerve blocks, and botulinum type A toxin injections.
   - Phenol blocks have a proven history, will often have longer-lasting effects, and are less expensive than botulinum toxin.
   - The advantage of botulinum is the ease of delivery; it needs only an injection into the muscle belly, rather than a precise injection around the motor nerve.
2. Surgical treatment
   - Surgery for acquired spasticity should be delayed at least 6 months after onset to allow for maximum recovery.

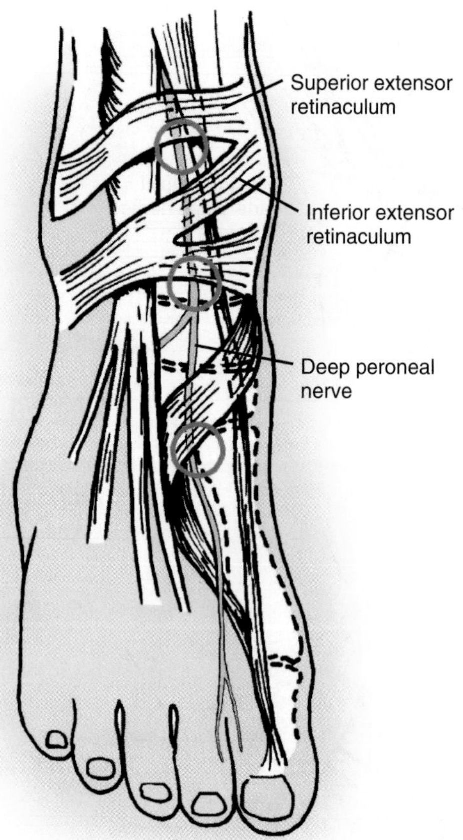

Figure 6-66 Deep peroneal nerve entrapment. *Circles* denote areas of impingement. (From Mann RA, Baxter DE: Diseases of the nerves. In Mann RA, Coughlin MJ, editors: *Surgery of the foot and ankle,* ed 6, St Louis, 1993, Mosby.)

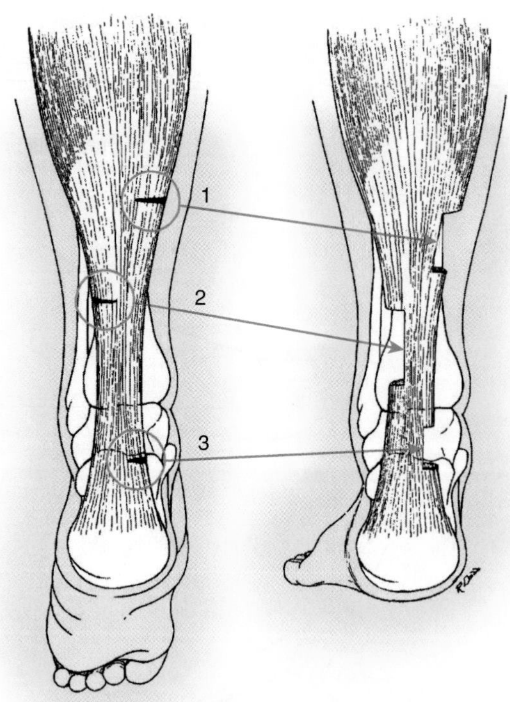

Figure 6-68 Incisions for percutaneous Achilles tendon lengthening. Cut ends slide on themselves with forceful dorsiflexion of foot. (From Canale ST, Beaty J: *Campbell's operative orthopedics,* ed 11, Philadelphia, 2007, Elsevier. Modified from Hsu JD, Hsu CL: Motor unit disease. In Jahss MH, editor: *Disorders of the foot,* Philadelphia, Saunders, 1982.)

- Equinus deformity is addressed with either an open Z-lengthening of the Achilles tendon, or a percutaneous triple-hemisection technique (Figure 6-68).
- **Varus deformity is addressed with a split anterior tibialis tendon transfer (SPLATT) to the lateral cuneiform or cuboid or total anterior tibial tendon transfer to the lateral cuneiform.**
  - If the varus deformity is fixed, lateral closed-wedge calcaneal osteotomy or subtalar fusion may be necessary.
- Release of the toe flexors is often required secondary to a tenodesis effect as the ankle is brought into a more plantigrade position.

VI. CHARCOT-MARIE-TOOTH DISEASE

A. Charcot-Marie-Tooth disease (CMT) is the most common inherited progressive peripheral neuropathy, affecting approximately 1 in every 2500 people.

1. There are many genetic variants of CMT, and as a group they are referred to as hereditary motor-sensory neuropathies.
2. **Type I hereditary motor-sensory neuropathy is the most common presentation of CMT.**

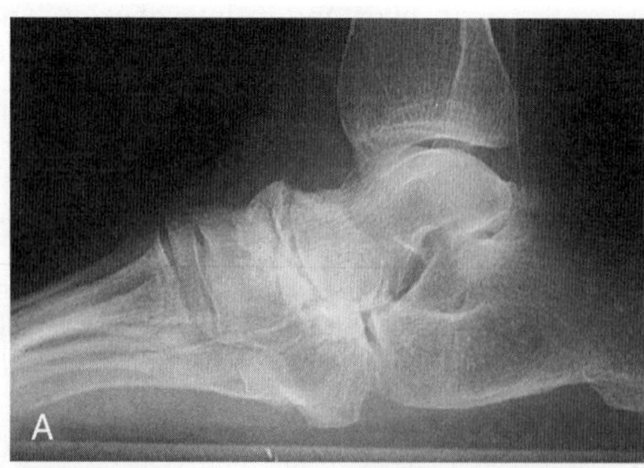

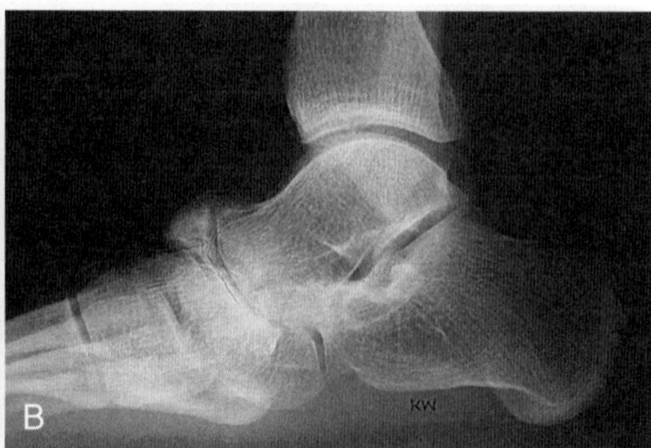

Figure 6-67 Arthritis of the talonavicular joint **(A)** or nonunion of a navicular fracture **(B)** can compress the deep peroneal nerve. (From Myerson MS: *Foot and ankle disorders,* Philadelphia, 2000, Elsevier.)

- **Usually autosomal dominant with a duplication of chromosome 17**

3. An abnormal myelin sheath protein is the basis of CMT degenerative neuropathy.
4. The earlier the onset, the more severe the neurologic findings

B. **Diagnosis**

1. Deformity and awkward gait are common initial complaints, with weakness, lateral ankle instability, and lateral foot pain presenting later.
2. Physical examination
   - Bilateral, symmetric pes cavovarus deformity is caused by motor imbalance.
     - Tibialis anterior and peroneus brevis weakness seen early
     - **First ray is plantar flexed due to relative unopposed pull of the peroneus longus (peroneus longus > tibialis anterior)** (Figure 6-69).
       - **This creates forefoot cavus and compensatory hindfoot varus (tripod effect).**
     - Hindfoot pulled further into varus because of relative unopposed pull of the posterior tibial muscle (posterior tibial > peroneus brevis).
       - Plantar-flexed first ray and hindfoot varus leads to external rotation of distal tibia and fibula.
   - **Intrinsic (extensor digitorum brevis, extensor hallucis brevis, interossei) wasting leads to overpull of extrinsics (EHL, EDL, FHL, FDL), which causes claw-toe deformity.**
     - Weak tibialis anterior leads to recruitment of EHL and EDL during swing phase of gait, worsening the claw-toe deformity.
     - Prominent and tender calluses may be present beneath the metatarsal heads.
   - The Coleman block test (Figure 6-70) should be used to determine if a hindfoot varus deformity is secondary to the plantar-flexed first ray or an independent component.
     - Deformity corrects with Coleman block—forefoot-driven hindfoot varus
       - Surgical correction involves dorsiflexion osteotomy of the first metatarsal.
     - Deformity does not correct with Coleman block—hindfoot varus independent of the forefoot
       - Surgical correction involves both
         - Dorsiflexion osteotomy of the first metatarsal (forefoot)
         - Lateral closing calcaneal osteotomy (hindfoot)
   - Sensory deficit is variable.
     - Proprioception, vibration, and two-point discrimination affected first
     - Severe sensory loss may lead to recurrent ulceration, deep infection, and even neuropathic arthropathy.

C. **Treatment**

1. Flexible deformity (hindfoot can be passively manipulated)
   - Surgical rather than brace management is currently recommended in an adolescent with closed physes and a supple deformity because of the progressive pattern of this disease.

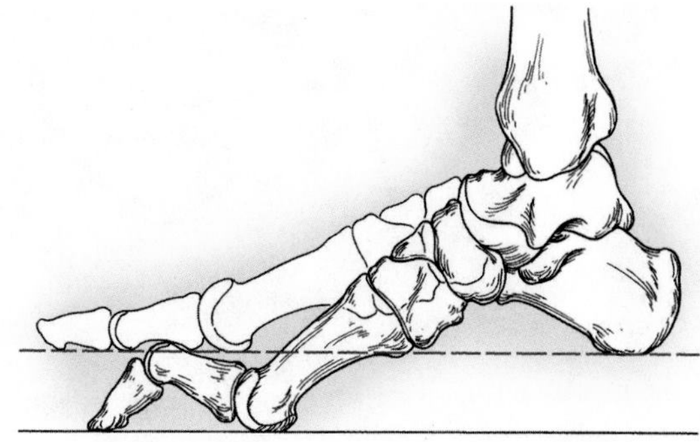

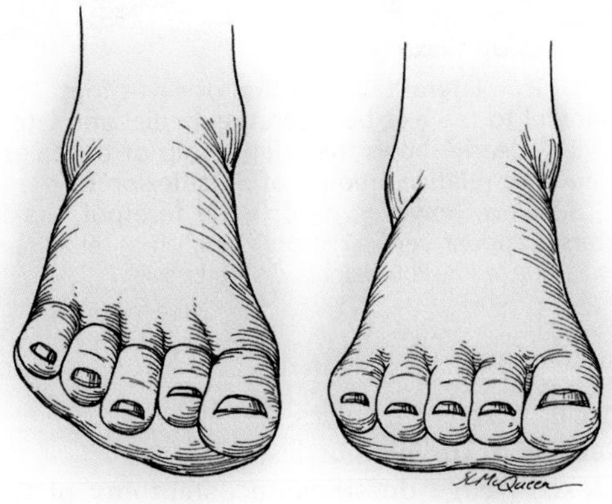

Figure 6-69 Lateral and frontal view of plantar-flexed first ray as seen in Charcot-Marie-Tooth disease. (From Canale ST, Beaty J: *Campbell's operative orthopedics,* ed 11, Philadelphia, 2007, Elsevier.)

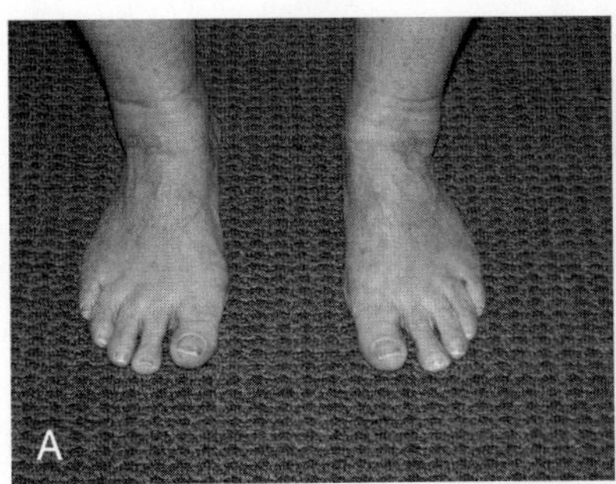

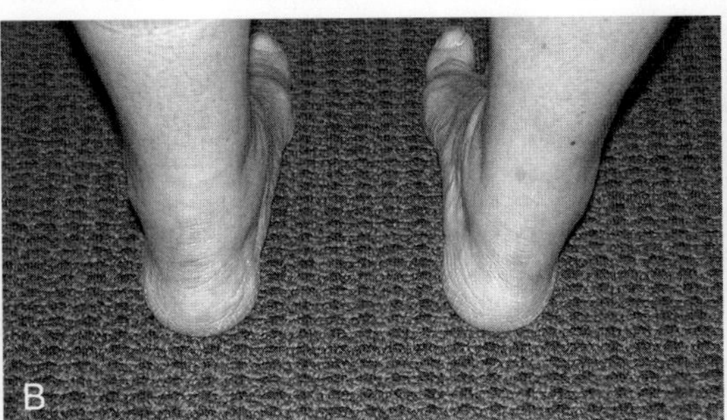

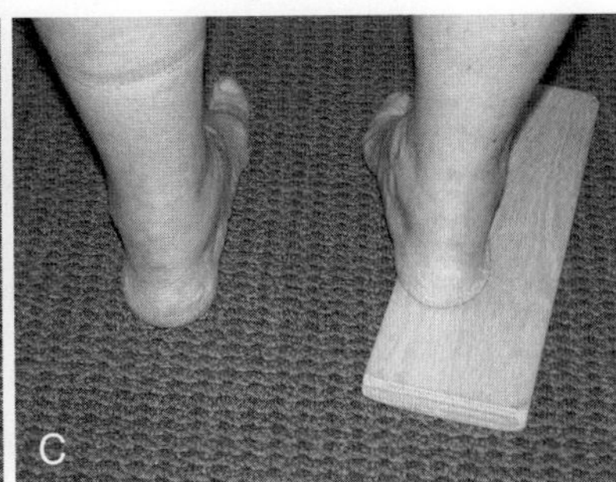

Figure 6-70 **A,** Unilateral cavus foot on left (patient's right foot). Note the appearance of the medial heel on the left, while on the opposite side the medial heel is not visible. **B,** Right varus heel alignment on the same patient, viewed from behind. Note the normal heel alignment of the left foot. **C,** Correction of heel alignment on Coleman block testing on the same patient. Note the same alignment of both feet while right foot is on the block, implying forefoot-driven cavus. (From DiGiovanni C: *Core knowledge in orthopaedics—foot and ankle,* Philadelphia, 2007, Elsevier.)

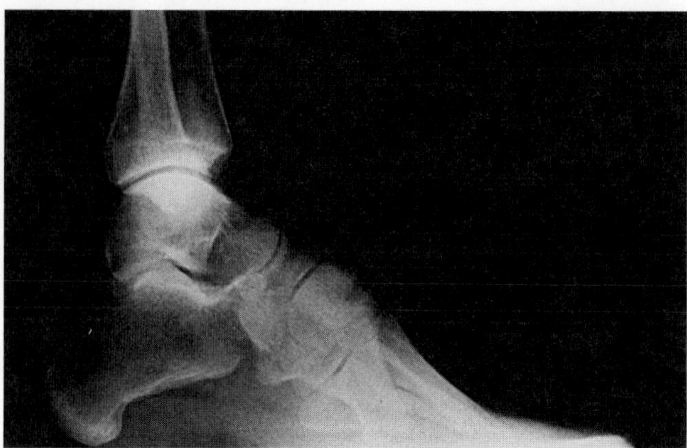

Figure 6-71 True lateral talar position of cavus foot. The radiograph is parallel to the axis between the medial and lateral malleoli. This view clearly shows the relationship of the talus to the calcaneus and the relative amount of dorsiflexion of the talus to the tibia. This view, however, distorts the forefoot, making the first metatarsal appear vertical. (From Coughlin M, et al: *Surgery of the foot and ankle,* ed 8, Philadelphia, 2006, Elsevier.)

- Surgical treatment involves
  - **Release of the plantar fascia**
  - **Closed-wedge dorsiflexion osteotomy of the first metatarsal**
    - **Always required. If the deformity corrects with a Coleman block test, no other bony correction is required.**
  - Lateral calcaneal slide and/or closed-wedge osteotomy
    - If deformity does NOT correct with the Coleman block (Figure 6-71)
  - **Transfer of the peroneus longus into the peroneus brevis at the level of the distal fibula**
  - Frequently an Achilles tendon lengthening is required.
  - Forefoot correction is performed according to the guidelines outlined previously.
  - The clawed hallux can be surgically treated with a Jones procedure (arthrodesis of the interphalangeal joint and transfer of the EHL to the first metatarsal).

2. Fixed deformity (hindfoot cannot be passively manipulated)
   - **Conservative management can be attempted with a brace.**
     - **Locked-ankle, short-leg ankle-foot orthosis (AFO) with an outside (varus-correcting or lateral) T-strap is recommended.**
     - **Rocker sole can improve gait and decrease energy expenditure.**
   - Surgical management
     - Triple arthrodesis usually required for hindfoot correction
     - Posterior tibial tendon transfer through the interosseous membrane and Achilles tendon lengthening can correct equinus contracture and dorsiflexion weakness.
     - Plantar fascia release and dorsiflexion osteotomy of the first metatarsal
     - Forefoot correction is performed according to the guidelines outlined previously.

VII. PERIPHERAL NERVE INJURY AND TENDON TRANSFERS

A. Traumatic injuries to the lower extremity can result in injury to the nerves and/or musculature resulting in a paralytic deformity.

B. Use of an AFO can be a successful nonsurgical management; however, many patients desire to become brace-free.

C. Principles of tendon transfers

1. Deformity must be flexible (passive ROM must be present). A rigid deformity requires an arthrodesis.
2. Preoperative physical examination is critical to determine which tendons should be transferred.
   - Assess which muscles are still active—must have at least four-fifths strength to transfer
   - Redirect a deforming force to create a restoring force.

D. Peroneal nerve palsy

1. **Loss of the anterior and lateral compartment—loss of active dorsiflexion and eversion**
2. **Deformity—equinovarus**
3. **Transfer posterior tibial tendon (PTT) (deforming force) through the interosseous membrane anteriorly to the dorsal midfoot (restores dorsiflexion) with an Achilles tendon lengthening.**

E. Compartment syndrome example—loss of the anterior and deep posterior compartments

1. Deformity—cavovarus (PL) with equinus (Achilles)
2. Treatment—Achilles tendon lengthening with transfer of the PL (deforming force) to the dorsolateral midfoot (restores dorsiflexion)

F. Unique cases such as compartment syndrome or traumatic injury can create variable patterns of motor loss. Correction of the deformity is unique to each case dependent upon the remnant motor function.

SECTION 12 ARTHRITIC DISEASE

I. CRYSTALLINE DISEASE

A. Gout

1. Pathology
   - Abnormal purine metabolism results in precipitation and deposition of monosodium urate crystals into synovium-lined joints.
   - Induces a severe inflammatory response
   - Induced by certain medications that increase serum uric acid, localized trauma, alcohol, or purine-rich foods as well as by the postsurgical state
   - Men are more commonly affected than women.
2. Diagnosis

- Patients complain of sudden joint pain, with a characteristic history ("Not even a sheet could touch it").
- Physical examination—intense signs of inflammation (redness, swelling, warmth, tenderness) and pain with ROM
- The great toe MTP joint is most often involved (50% to 75% of initial attacks).
  - 90% of patients with chronic gouty attacks will have one or more episodes involving the hallux MTP joint (podagra).
- Characteristic radiographic signs
  - Inordinate soft tissue enlargement about the MTP joint
  - Bony erosions both at a distance from and within the joint articular surface
    - Extensive articular and periarticular destruction can occur in chronic conditions (Figure 6-72).
    - Secondary to large deposits of gouty residue (tophi)

3. Definitive diagnosis—Needle aspiration of the joint. Indicated in the presence of an acute swollen painful joint. Fluid is sent for crystals and Gram stain with culture.
   - Pathognomonic signs are needle-shaped monosodium urate crystals, which under polarized light are strongly negatively birefringent.
   - Critical to rule out an acute septic joint, which will be determined from the aspiration
   - The serum uric acid may or may not be elevated and should be not used to confirm or refute the diagnosis.
4. Treatment
   - Acute attacks treated with indomethacin or colchicine
   - Chronic attacks treated with allopurinol
   - Joint destruction or deposition of large quantities of tophi may require arthrodesis and/or débridement of tophaceous debris.

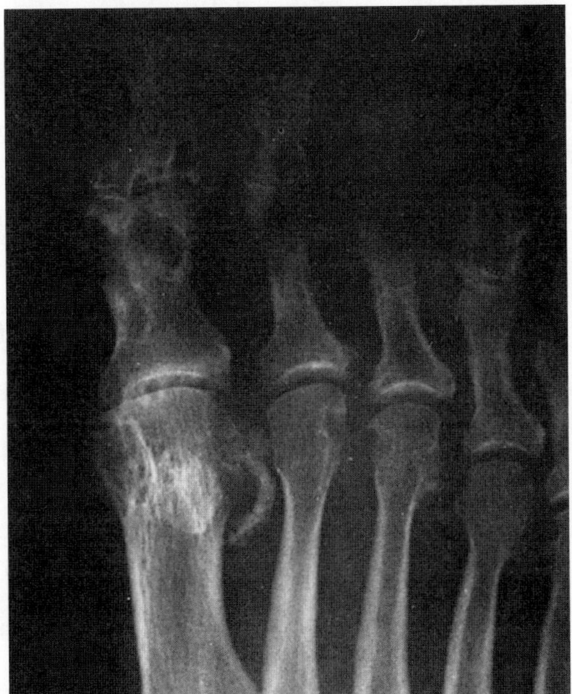

Figure 6-72 Gouty arthritis. Multiple punched-out lesions are present. (From Mercier L: *Practical orthopaedics,* ed 6, Philadelphia, 2008, Elsevier.)

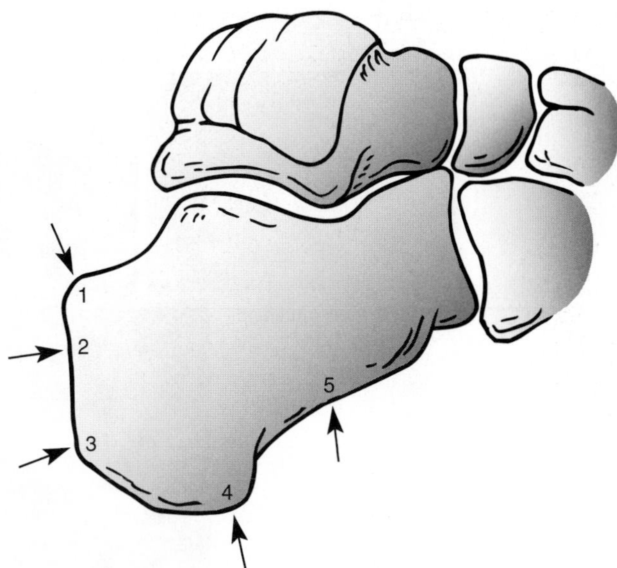

Figure 6-73 Common areas of enthesopathy associated with inflammatory arthritis. *1,* Superior aspect of calcaneus. *2* and *3,* Achilles tendon insertion. *4,* Plantar fascia insertion. *5,* Plantar aspect of calcaneus. (From Coughlin MJ, et al: *Coughlin surgery of the foot and ankle,* ed 8, St. Louis, 2007, Mosby.)

B. Pseudogout (chondrocalcinosis)

1. Commonly affects the knee but may present in an articulation of the foot or ankle
2. Pathology
   - Deposition of calcium pyrophosphate dihydrate (CPPD) crystals in or about a joint may lead to severe initial inflammatory response.
   - Usually articular, with less periarticular soft tissue involvement than gout
3. Diagnosis
   - Joint aspiration reveals weakly positive birefringent crystals under polarized light microscopy with varied shapes.
   - Lesser MTP, TN, and subtalar joints can be affected.
   - Uncommonly involved in gout
   - Radiographs
     - Intraarticular calcifications commonly seen (unlike gout)
     - Joint destruction can occur with recurrent attacks over a long period, but this is rare.
4. Treatment—rest, oral NSAIDs for acute synovitis, protected weight bearing, and corticosteroid injections

II. SERONEGATIVE SPONDYLOARTHROPATHY

A. Diagnosis

1. Inflammatory arthritides that are negative for rheumatoid factor
2. Distinguished from rheumatoid arthritis clinically by a higher incidence of involvement of entheses (i.e., the interface between collagen and bone where ligament, tendon, and capsular tissue insert into bone) (Figure 6-73)
3. Involvement of this transitional tissue is found in psoriatic arthritis, ankylosing spondylitis, Reiter syndrome, and inflammatory bowel disease.
4. May destroy articular cartilage but characteristically is more destructive toward collagen and fibrocartilage

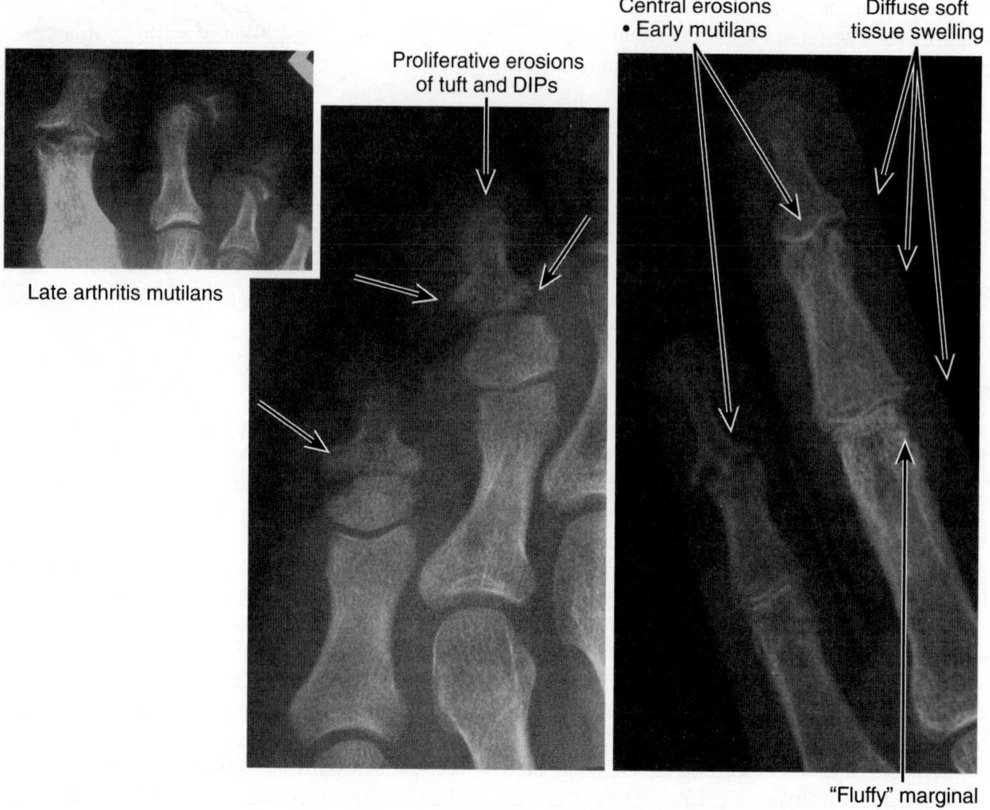

Figure 6-74 Psoriatic arthritis. Erosions classically have a proliferative appearance, with a fluffy or whiskered quality. Central erosions can lead to joint destruction with a "pencil-in-cup" pattern. DIPs, distal interphalangeal joints. (From Morrison W, Sanders T: *Problem solving in musculoskeletal imaging,* Philadelphia, 2008, Elsevier.)

- Often presents in the foot as plantar fasciitis, Achilles tendinitis, or posterior tibial tendinopathy

5. Psoriatic arthritis can present with swollen and inflamed distal joints or, more classically, as dactylitis, or "sausage digit."
   - Periarticular bony erosion may occur, causing a classical "pencil-in-cup" sign typical of psoriatic arthritis (Figure 6-74).
6. Additional findings may include nail pitting, onycholysis, and keratosis.

B. **Treatment**

1. Pharmacologic agents such as NSAIDs, or occasionally salicylates or cytotoxic drugs under the direction and observation of a rheumatologist, are the mainstay of treatment.
2. Intraarticular corticosteroid injections may improve symptoms.
3. Surgical intervention is sometimes required for small joint erosions, recalcitrant Achilles tendinopathy, and plantar fasciitis.

III. RHEUMATOID ARTHRITIS

A. Chronic, symmetric polyarthropathy that most commonly presents in the third and fourth decades and is more prevalent in women

B. Synovitis causes ligament and capsular laxity and cartilage and bony erosion.

C. Vasculitis and soft tissue fragility is common, requiring diligent care of the soft tissues during nonoperative and operative management.

D. The use of immune-mediating pharmacologic therapies in the perioperative period should be discussed with a rheumatologist because complications can result.

1. Although most can be continued (prednisone, methotrexate, plaquenil), the newer biologic agents (such as tumor necrosis factor antagonists) should be discontinued.

E. **Diagnosis**

1. **Foot involvement very common in rheumatoid patients**
   - **Forefoot more commonly involved than the midfoot or hindfoot.**
2. Patients complain of forefoot swelling, poorly defined pain, and eventually deformity.
3. MTP joint pathophysiology
   - Chronic synovitis leads to incompetence of the joint capsules and collateral ligaments.
   - **The toes sublux or dislocate dorsally, deviate laterally into valgus, and develop hammering (Figure 6-75).**
   - The intrinsic muscles worsen the claw-toe deformity.
   - The plantar fat pad migrates distally and atrophies, causing metatarsalgia and forming keratoses.
   - As the lesser toes deviate laterally, hallux valgus occurs and transfer metatarsalgia worsens.
4. The midfoot and hindfoot are less commonly and less severely involved in rheumatoid arthritis.

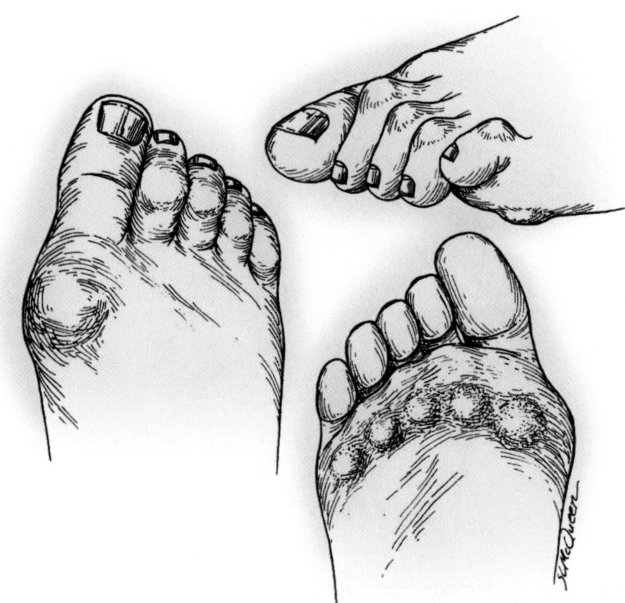

Figure 6-75 Rheumatoid foot. Note multiple deformities of rheumatoid arthritis of forefoot with hallux valgus, subluxed and dislocated metatarsophalangeal joints, claw toes, hammer toes, and bursal formation. (From Canale ST, Beaty J: *Campbell's operative orthopedics,* ed 11, Philadelphia, 2007, Elsevier.)

- Significant midfoot/hindfoot arthrosis (TN joint characteristic)
- Often results in a pes planovalgus deformity
  - The underlying cause of the flatfoot deformity must be carefully assessed to determine whether it is midfoot driven or hindfoot driven.
  - Midfoot etiology—The tarsometatarsal joints are subluxated with a congruent hindfoot (Figure 6-76).
    - Treatment—realignment midfoot arthrodesis
  - Hindfoot etiology—The transverse tarsal and subtalar joint is subluxated with a normal midfoot.
    - Treatment—triple arthrodesis

5. The tibiotalar joint is also commonly involved. Easily differentiated from osteoarthritis with lack of osteophyte formation, osteopenia, and symmetric joint space narrowing (Figure 6-77)
   - Ankle arthrodesis is currently the treatment of choice, with ankle replacement emerging as a more reliable technique.
     - A tibiotalar and subtalar (tibiotalocalcaneal) arthrodesis performed with an intramedullary nail risks a tibial stress fracture in these patients.
       - This complication is best treated conservatively with a cast.
   - Risks for wound complications have been shown to higher in patients with rheumatoid arthritis when performing an ankle replacement.

F. **Treatment**

1. Conservative—Rest, NSAIDs, immune-modulating drugs under the direction of rheumatologists, toe taping, orthoses, and careful use of corticosteroid injections may help symptoms related to synovitis.
2. Surgical
   - Late (in presence of deformity)—"rheumatoid forefoot reconstruction" (Figure 6-78)
     - **First MTP arthrodesis, lesser metatarsal head resection with pinning of the lesser MTP joints, and closed osteoclasis of the interphalangeal joints versus PIP arthroplasty**
       - Silicone arthroplasty not recommended due to cock-up deformity, silicone synovitis, and osteolysis
     - Accomplished through three well-placed longitudinal dorsal incisions (Figure 6-79)
     - Extensor brevis tenotomy and Z-lengthening of the extensor longus tendons may be necessary.

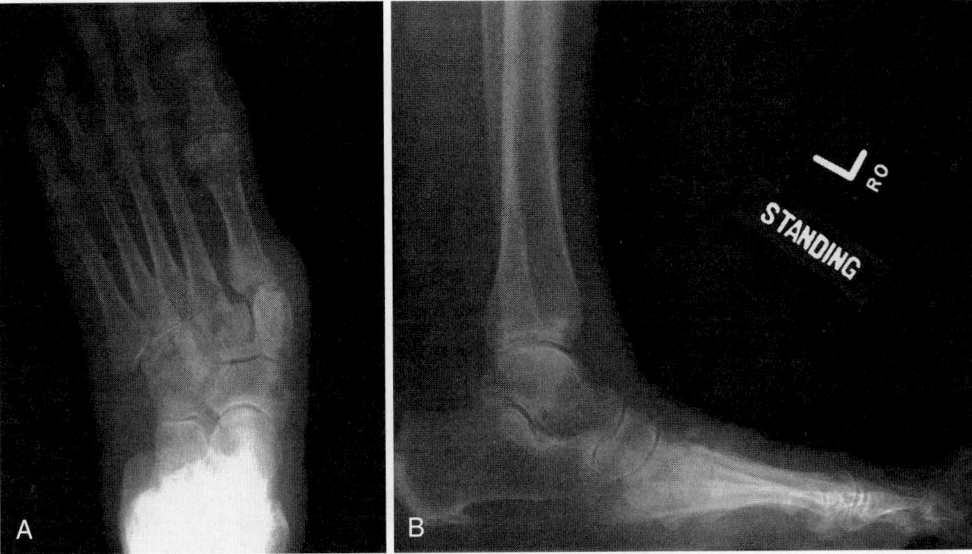

Figure 6-76 **A,** Anteroposterior radiograph of a patient with rheumatoid arthritis with a flatfoot deformity that is secondary to midfoot arthritis. Note how the first and second metatarsals are subluxated laterally relative to the cuneiforms. **B,** The lateral radiograph demonstrates loss of the longitudinal arch centered at the tarsometatarsal joints with obvious degenerative changes. The surgical treatment is a realignment midfoot arthrodesis. Care must be taken in differentiating this from a hindfoot-driven flatfoot, where the deformity is centered at the talonavicular joint.

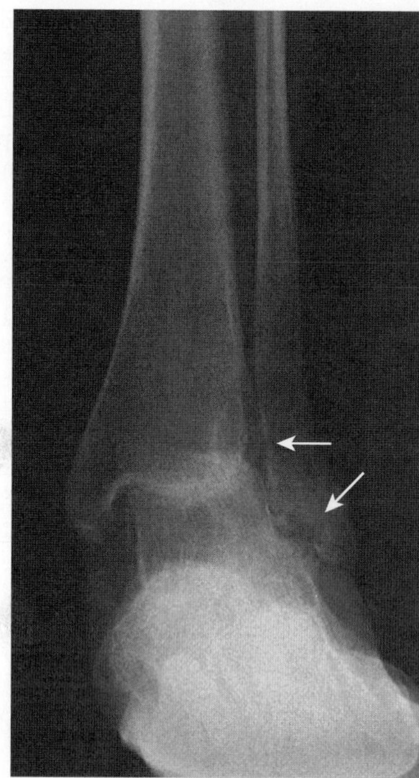

Figure 6-77 Rheumatoid arthritis of the ankle. There is diffuse loss of cartilage space with erosions of the fibula *(arrows)*. The scalloping along the medial border of the distal fibula is designated the fibular notch sign and is a characteristic finding in rheumatoid arthritis. The hindfoot is in valgus alignment. (From Firestein G, et al: *Kelley's textbook of rheumatology,* ed 8, Philadelphia, 2008, Elsevier.)

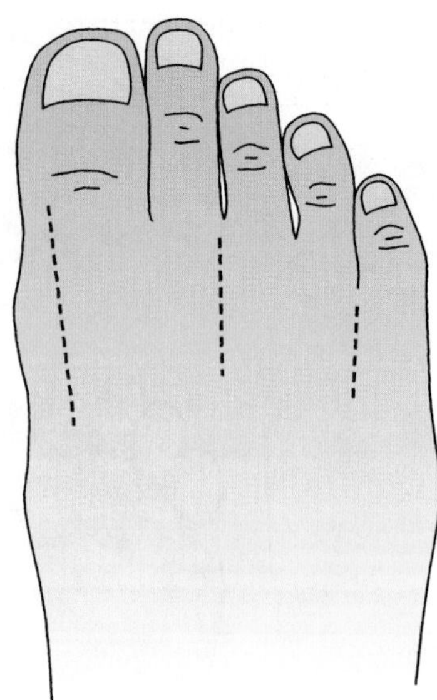

Figure 6-79 Incisions for first metatarsophalangeal (MTP) joint arthrodesis and lesser MTP joint resection arthroplasty for rheumatoid arthritis.

- Most common complication of forefoot arthroplasty is intractable plantar keratoses.

IV. OSTEOARTHRITIS

A. Osteoarthritis and post-traumatic arthritis share similarities in the mechanical nature of the problem, clinical presentation, and treatment algorithm.

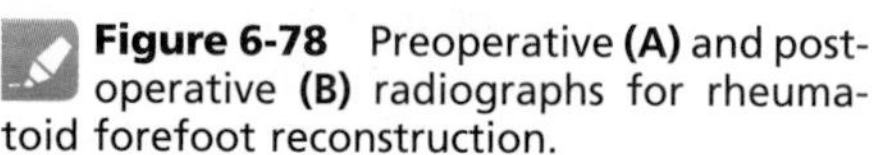

Figure 6-78 Preoperative **(A)** and postoperative **(B)** radiographs for rheumatoid forefoot reconstruction.

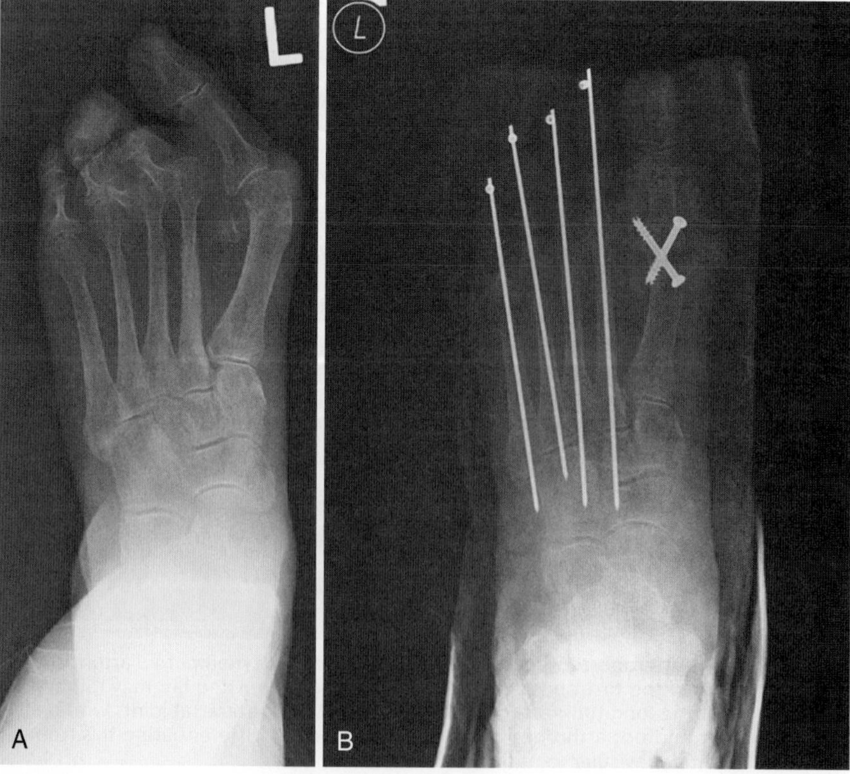

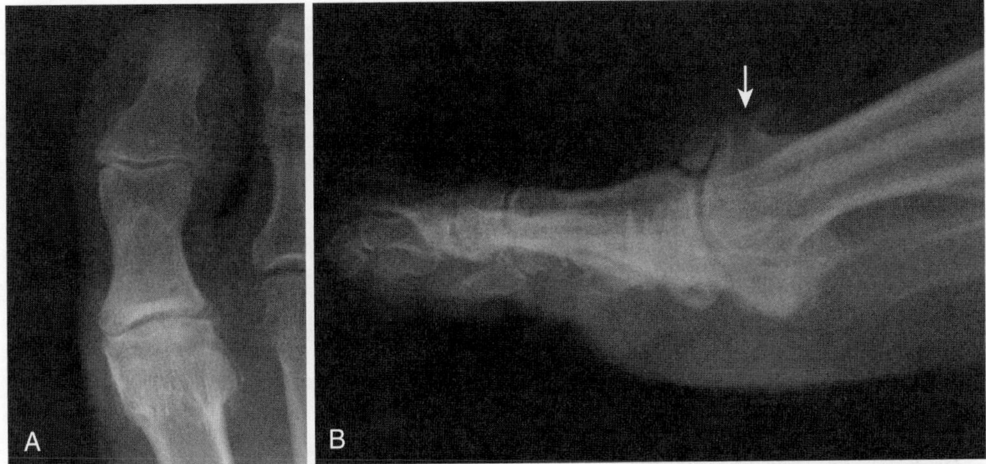

Figure 6-80 Hallux rigidus. **A,** Posteroanterior radiograph of the great toe shows cartilage space narrowing and hypertrophic lipping. **B,** The lateral radiograph shows a prominent dorsal osteophyte *(arrow).* (From Weissman B: *Imaging of arthritis and metabolic bone disease,* Philadelphia, 2009, Elsevier.)

B. Post-traumatic arthritis is most common in the hindfoot and tibiotalar articulations.

C. Osteoarthritis commonly affects the first MTP joint and the midfoot joints (tarsometatarsal, intercuneiform, navicular-cuneiform, and TN joints).

D. Lateral ankle instability, posterior tibial tendon insufficiency, and neuromuscular deformities also commonly contribute to degenerative arthritis.

E. Diagnosis

1. Patients complain of dull, achy pain at the involved joint, usually worse with activity.
2. Physical examination—tenderness to palpation at the joint surface, with loss of ROM, and pain with passive ROM
3. Radiographs—loss of joint space, subchondral sclerosis and cysts, osteophyte formation (Figure 6-80)
4. **First MTP joint**
   - **Tenderness over the dorsum of the joint, limited dorsiflexion secondary to large dorsal osteophyte, and pain with grind test;** graded clinically and radiographically
     - Grade 0—normal radiograph, stiff on examination
     - Grade I—mild dorsal osteophyte, joint space preservation, mild pain at extremes of ROM
     - Grade II—moderate osteophyte formation, joint space narrowing (<50%), moderate pain with ROM that may be more constant
     - **Grade III—severe osteophyte formation, substantial joint space narrowing (>50%), significant stiffness with pain at extreme ROM but not at midrange**
     - Grade IV—same as III but with pain at midrange of passive motion
5. Subtalar, TN, CC joints
   - Tenderness at the sinus tarsi (subtalar joint), dorsal TN joint, and/or lateral column
   - Pain with passive hindfoot inversion/eversion (subtalar), midfoot ROM (TN, CC)
   - Radiographs show varying severity of joint space narrowing and osteophyte formation.
   - Rigid flatfoot without arthritis is also a common presentation, is not amenable to joint preservation surgery, and should be treated with a triple arthrodesis.
6. Tibiotalar joint
   - Tenderness in anterior ankle joint line
   - Limited ROM with pain, especially in extreme dorsiflexion
   - May have associated varus or valgus deformity, either at ankle or more proximal
   - Radiographs show joint space narrowing, sclerosis and cysts, osteophytes, and possibly varus or valgus deformity
     - Standing radiographs essential; may need long-leg alignment view with history of leg trauma
   - May be associated with cavovarus deformity, rigid flatfoot (valgus), or chronic lateral ankle instability (varus)

F. Treatment

1. Conservative—Initial treatment should include anti-inflammatory medications, activity modification, orthotic support or bracing, and corticosteroid injections.
   - **Hallux rigidus—stiff foot plate with an extension under the great toe (Morton extension)**
   - **Midfoot (tarsometatarsal) arthritis—stiff-soled or steel shank–modified shoe with a rocker bottom in addition to a cushioned heel. Use of a full-length rigid foot orthotic can also be beneficial.**
   - Hindfoot (subtalar, TN, CC) arthritis—AFO or rigid lace-up leather brace (Arizona type)
   - Tibiotalar arthritis—AFO with a rocker bottom or rigid lace-up leather brace (Arizona type)
2. Surgical management
   - **Hallux rigidus**
     - **Grades I and II (pain at extreme ROM only)—usually treated with dorsal cheilectomy (removal of all osteophytes, including portion of dorsal metatarsal head with loss of cartilage) (Figure 6-81)**
     - **Grades III and IV (pain throughout the ROM with positive grind)—best treated with arthrodesis (Figure 6-82)**
       - **Position—neutral rotation, 10 to 15 degrees of dorsiflexion, and slight valgus**
     - Interposition arthroplasty with varying results
     - Implant arthroplasty not recommended due to poor results

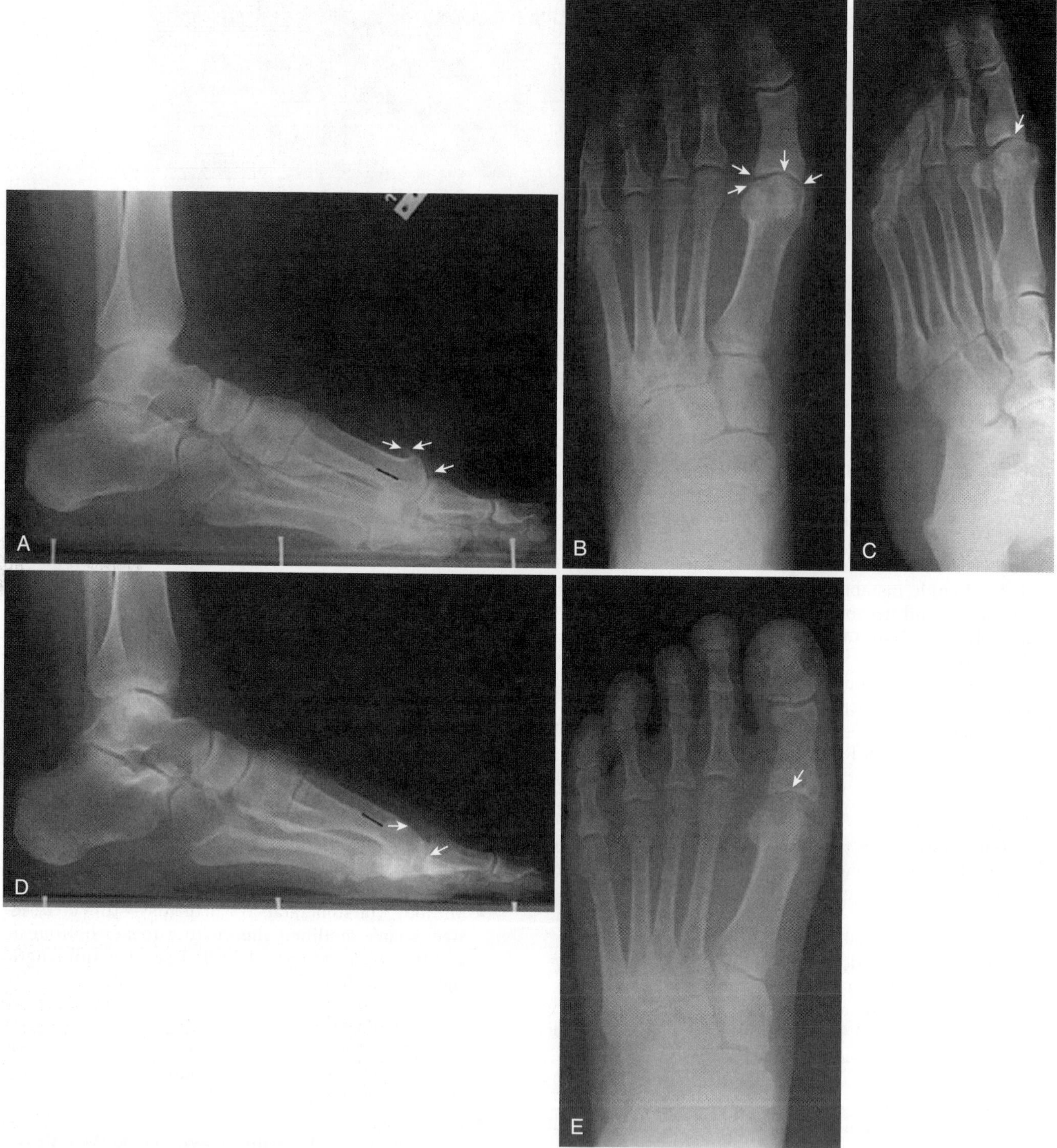

Figure 6-81 Hallux rigidus of left foot treated with cheilectomy. **A** to **C,** After surgery. **D** and **E,** One year after surgery. Radiographic hallmarks of hallux rigidus denoted by *white arrows* (dorsal osteophyte, **A** and joint space narrowing, **B** and **C**). Postoperative radiograph after cheilectomy (*white arrow*; **D**) with diminished but preserved joint space (*white arrow*; **E**). (From Canale ST, Beaty J: *Campbell's operative orthopedics,* ed 11, Philadelphia, 2007, Elsevier.)

- Silicone arthroplasty can result in a heavy synovitis with destruction of the joint.
  - Isolated pain within the great toe
    - Removal of implant with synovectomy only is successful in providing pain relief.
  - Great toe pain with lesser metatarsalgia
    - Implant removal with bone grafting and arthrodesis to restore the function of the great toe
- Midfoot joints
  - Midfoot arthrodesis is the treatment of choice.
    - In the setting of deformity (flatfoot) the joints must be reduced back into an anatomic position to achieve a satisfactory result (realignment arthrodesis) (Figure 6-83).
    - Medial column arthrodesis refers to fusion of both the naviculo-cuneiform and first TMT joints, occasionally required for a flatfoot deformity to stabilize

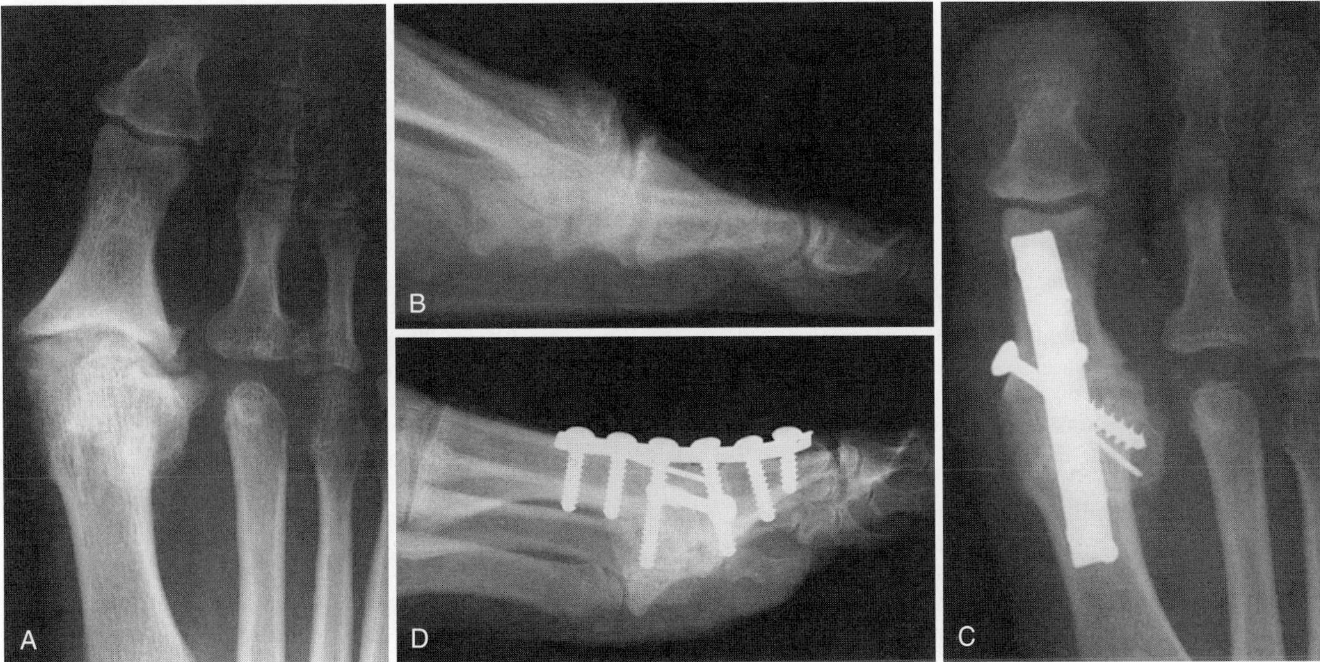

Figure 6-82 Fusion for severe hallux rigidus. **A** and **B,** Preoperative radiographs. **C** and **D,** Postoperative radiographs. (From Coughlin M, et al: *Surgery of the foot and ankle,* ed 8, Philadelphia, 2006, Elsevier.)

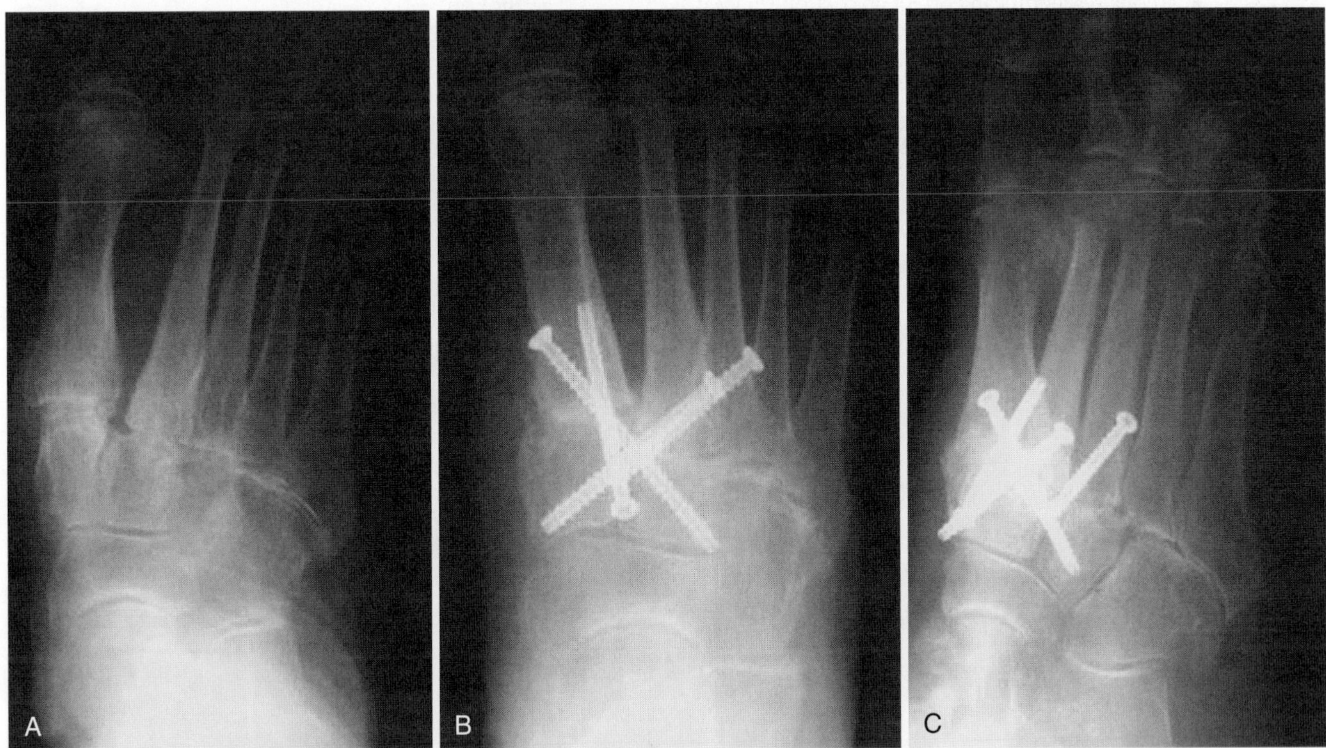

Figure 6-83 **A,** This post-traumatic deformity involved the entire midfoot, with all three columns seemingly affected. Despite the severity of the deformity, only the medial and middle columns were clinically symptomatic. **B** and **C,** Arthrodesis was performed with realignment and screw fixation. (From Myerson M: *Reconstructive foot and ankle surgery: management of complications,* ed 2, Philadelphia, 2010, Elsevier.)

the collapsed midfoot and restore the lateral talo–first metatarsal angle.
- In situ fusion in the setting of a deformity will predictably lead to a poor result.

- Hindfoot (subtalar, TN, CC) joints
  - Arthrodesis of single joints leads to significant limitation in hindfoot inversion/eversion (TN > subtalar > CC).
    - Isolated TN fusion has a high rate of nonunion and given the significant restriction of hindfoot motion from a TN fusion, a subtalar fusion is commonly performed in addition to ensure a union without causing any incremental functional deficit. A triple arthrodesis is also an appropriate option. If the CC joint is unaffected, it is becoming more common to not include the CC joint in the arthrodesis.
  - **Triple arthrodesis usually performed to correct arthritis secondary to deformity** (Figure 6-84)
    - Position—0 to 5 degree of hindfoot valgus, neutral abduction/adduction, plantigrade (both the first and fifth metatarsal evenly strike the ground)
    - **Revision of a malunited triple arthrodesis requires**
      - **Calcaneal osteotomy (corrects varus or valgus)**
      - **Transverse tarsal osteotomy (allows rotation of the foot into a plantigrade position)**
        - Wedge resection can correct abduction (medial wedge) or adduction (lateral wedge).
  - Subtalar arthrodesis
    - Indications
      - Subtalar degenerative joint disease
      - Calcaneus fracture (Sanders IV) or late sequelae
      - Post-traumatic degenerative joint disease secondary talus fracture (no deformity) (Figure 6-85)
      - Talocalcaneal coalition
      - Subtalar degenerative joint disease
    - **Increased nonunion rate with history of**
      - Ankle arthrodesis or smoking; nonunion rate higher with ankle arthrodesis than with smoking
    - Subtalar bone-block arthrodesis (Figure 6-86)
      - **Prior calcaneal fracture with loss of height**
        - **Results in anterior impingement, complaints of anterior ankle pain with ambulation in addition to hindfoot pain**
      - Autograft or allograft bone-block arthrodesis restores the height of the calcaneus.
        - Less successful at correcting residual hindfoot varus
- Tibiotalar joint
  - **Arthrodesis provides excellent pain relief with some restricted function (Figure 6-87).**
    - **Position—neutral dorsiflexion (90 degrees), 0 to 5 degrees hindfoot valgus, 5 to 10 degrees external rotation**
      - Valgus and external rotation keep the hindfoot unlocked to allow for accommodative hindfoot motion.
    - **Leads to eventual arthritis in surrounding foot joints**

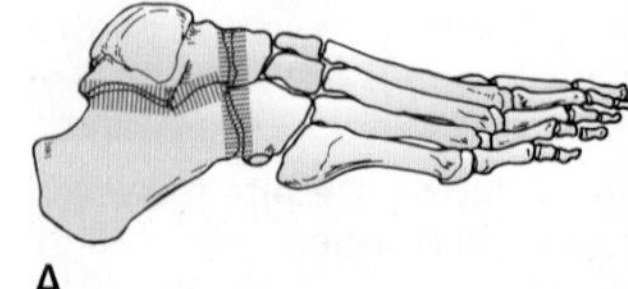

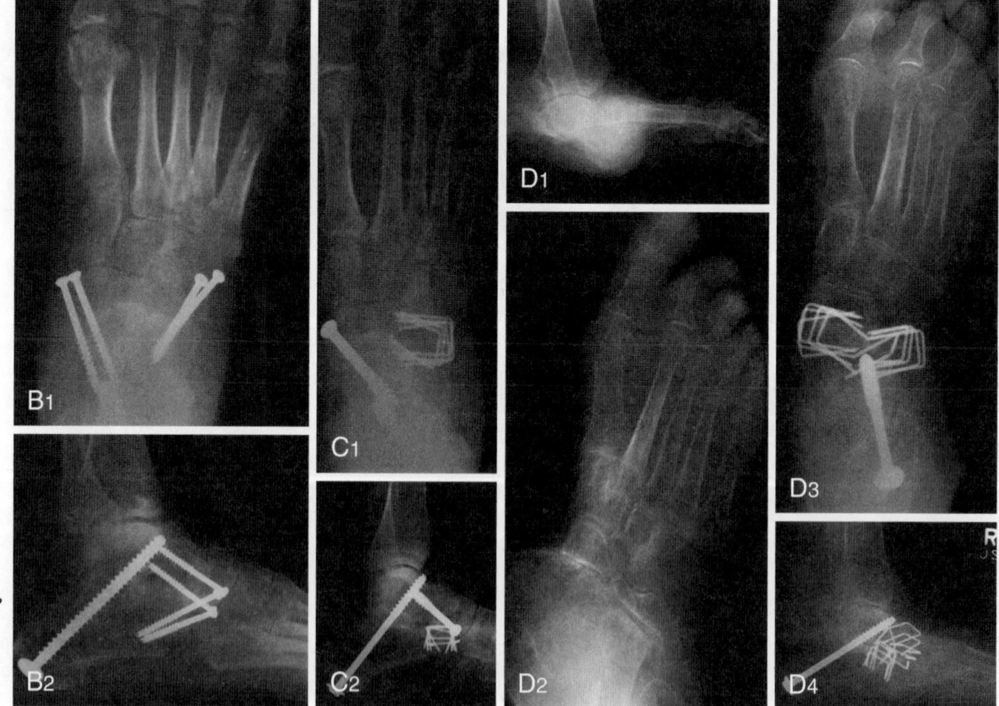

Figure 6-84 Triple arthrodesis, methods of internal fixation. **A,** Diagram of triple arthrodesis. **B,** Postoperative radiograph demonstrating triple arthrodesis with anatomic restoration of foot posture. **C,** Triple arthrodesis using 7.0-mm cannulated screws for the subtalar and talonavicular joints and multiple power staples for the calcaneocuboid joint. **D,** Correction of severe hindfoot deformity secondary to long-standing posterior tibial tendon dysfunction with restoration of the longitudinal arch using a 7.0-mm cannulated screw for the subtalar joint and power staples for the talonavicular and calcaneocuboid joints. Note that the height of the longitudinal arch has been restored and severe abduction of the foot is corrected. (From Coughlin M, et al: *Surgery of the foot and ankle,* ed 8, Philadelphia, 2006, Elsevier.)

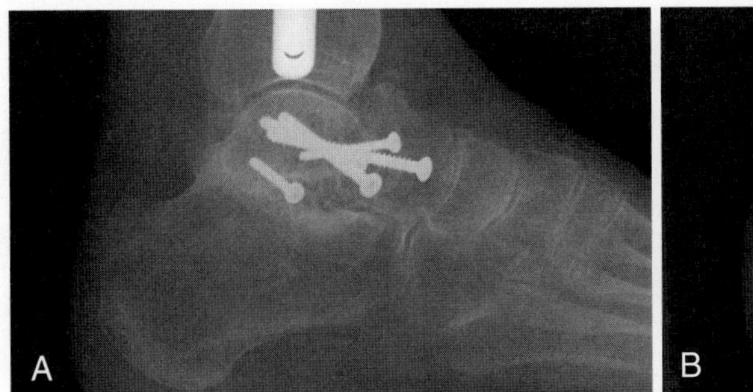

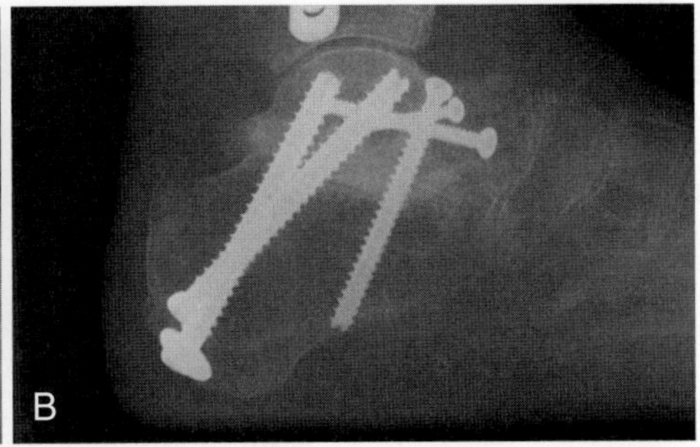

Figure 6-85 **A,** Preoperative radiograph of a patient with subtalar arthritis, the most common complication following a talus fracture. Importantly, the patient did not have a varus deformity with shortening of the medial column. **B,** Postoperative radiograph demonstrates a subtalar fusion that eliminated the patient's pain. If the patient had had a varus deformity, a triple arthrodesis would have been required.

    - **Subtalar joint is the most common location of adjacent joint arthritis.**
    - No evidence to show causation or progress of knee or hip arthritis
- Total ankle arthroplasty outcomes are improving and are no longer considered experimental.
    - Pain relief equivalent to arthrodesis, function may be slightly improved, higher risk of revision surgery
    - **Ankle replacement has shown the best outcome in patients with osteoarthritis.**
        - This is superior to that shown in patients with rheumatoid or post-traumatic etiology.
        - **Syndesmotic fusion associated with decreased rate of failure with the Agility ankle replacement**
- Distraction arthroplasty using thin-wire external fixation—limited role, may be option in younger patients
- Bipolar osteochondral allograft transplantation—not recommended

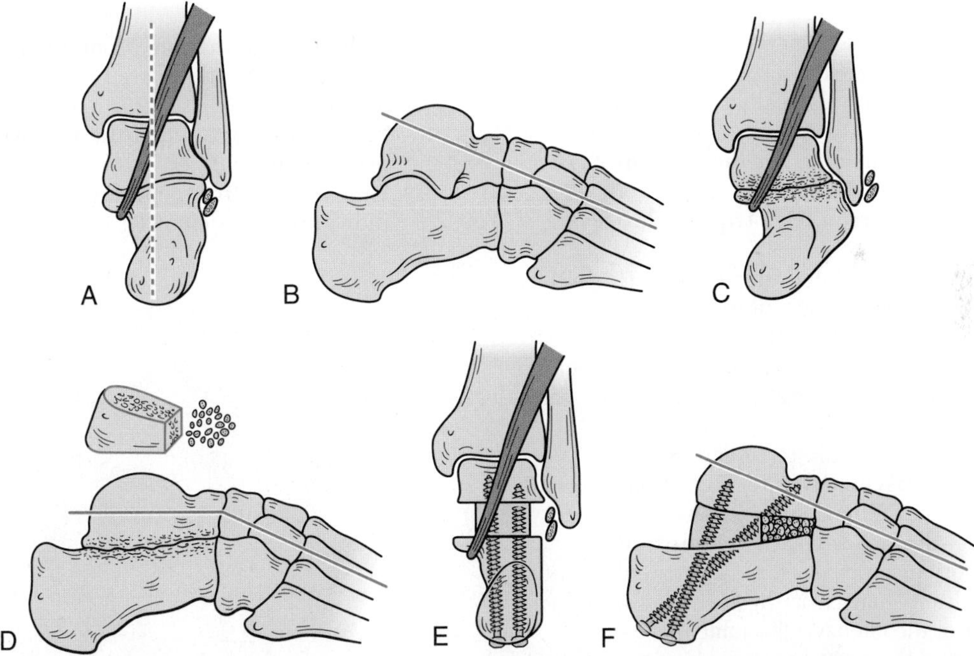

Figure 6-86 Subtalar fusion with distraction. **A,** The *dashed line* shows the alignment of the tibia through the tuber, the area where the flexor hallucis longus crosses at the back of the joint, and the location of the peroneal tendons under the fibular tip. **B,** Normal alignment of the subtalar joint and inclination of the talus are depicted. Notice that the all-important midaxial line of the talus continues directly through the midfoot and the apex of the first metatarsal in the medial column. **C,** After a typical high-energy calcaneal crush injury, the tuber is angled into varus while the lateral wall is angled and has exploded laterally toward valgus and impinges on the distal fibula, pushing the peroneal tendons out of their normal position. The subtalar joint is crushed, and the hindfoot has lost height. **D,** The inclination of the talus is out of line with the medial column and markedly limits the range of dorsiflexion in the anterior dome of the talus. A wedge of posterior iliac crest tricortical bone will be used to open the talocalcaneal joint and restore height. **E,** Two large 6.5-mm bolts or fully threaded screws are positioned much as they would be for subtalar arthrodesis in situ. In this case, however, they serve as positioning screws rather than lag screws and maintain distraction of the talus from the calcaneus instead of compressing the graft. The exploded lateral wall is excised and the tuber repositioned with less varus tilt and in slight valgus alignment to the weight-bearing line of the tibia. **F,** Reconstruction restores ideal talar inclination and talar–naviculo-cuneiform–first metatarsal axial alignment. An anteroposterior radiographic view of the foot should be taken intraoperatively to ensure that the talocalcaneal alignment is correct in the transverse plane and that the foot is not significantly pronated or supinated. (From Browner B et al: *Skeletal trauma,* ed 4, Philadelphia, 2008, Elsevier. Adapted and redrawn from Hansen ST Jr: *Functional reconstruction of the foot and ankle,* Philadelphia, 2000, Lippincott Williams & Wilkins.)

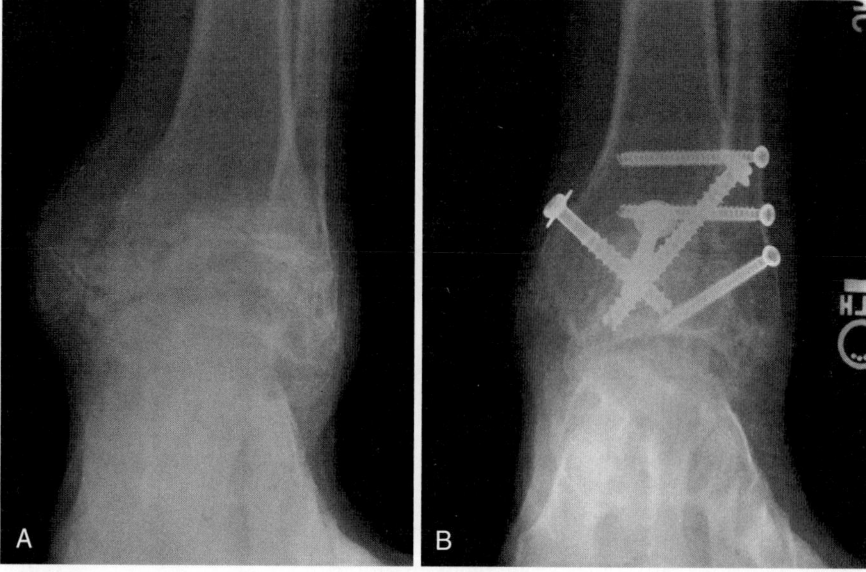

Figure 6-87 **A,** Preoperative anteroposterior radiograph of end-stage ankle arthritis with varus deformity. **B,** Cross screws were used to perform the ankle arthrodesis with realignment of the ankle into a neutral position. Additional syndesmotic fusion was performed in this case. (From Miller M, Sanders T: *Presentation, imaging and treatment of common musculoskeletal conditions,* Philadelphia, 2011, Elsevier.)

SECTION 13 Postural Disorders

I. PES PLANUS (FLATFOOT) DEFORMITY

A. May be congenital (see Chapter 3, Pediatric Orthopaedics) or acquired (also called adult-acquired flatfoot deformity)

B. Important to determine whether the deformity is flexible or fixed

Fixed or rigid deformity requires a triple arthrodesis.

C. Pathology

1. Most common cause of adult-acquired flatfoot deformity is posterior tibial tendon dysfunction (PTTD)
   - PTT is the primary dynamic support for the arch.
   - PTT fires after the foot is flat to generate heel-rise and locking of the transverse tarsal joint for a rigid, stable foot during push-off.
   - Etiology of PTTD is multifactorial and includes
     - **Zone of hypovascularity 2 to 6 cm from the PTT attachment on the navicular**
     - Overload of the arch from activity or obesity
     - Inflammatory disorders such as rheumatoid arthritis
2. The spring (calcaneo-navicular) ligament is the primary static stabilizer of the talonavicular joint.
   - Incompetence of the spring ligament is associated with increasing flatfoot deformity.
   - Isolated acute rupture of the spring ligament has been reported to cause an acute deformity without disease of the PTT.
   - Reconstruction of the spring ligament with allograft or autograft as an adjunct to standard flatfoot reconstruction has shown success in early series.

D. Diagnosis

1. Patients complain of medial ankle/foot pain early, progressive loss of arch, and lateral ankle pain late (subfibular impingement).
2. Physical examination
   - **Standing examination demonstrates asymmetric hindfoot valgus, depressed arch, and an abducted forefoot.**
     - **"Too many toes" when the foot is viewed posteriorly (Figure 6-88)**
     - **Pain or inability to perform single-limb heel-rise indicates insufficient PTT.**

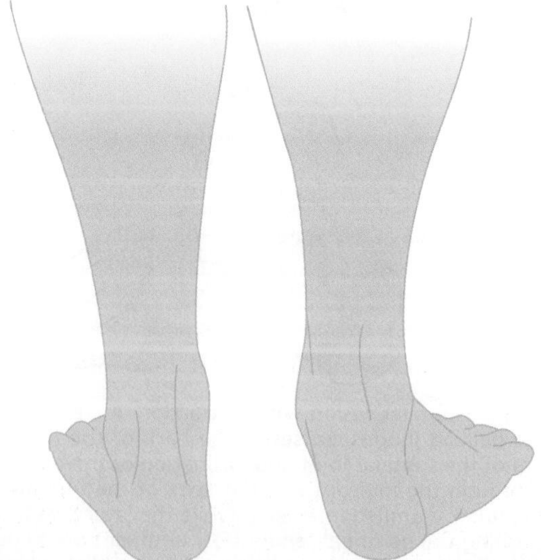

Figure 6-88 Patients with tendon ruptures have either a unilateral flatfoot or, in those who had previous flat feet, a relatively flatter foot on the involved side. Excessive forefoot abduction also can be suspected from posterior observation when more toes are visible lateral to the patient's heel on the involved side. This finding is called the *too-many-toes sign.* (From DeLee J: *DeLee and Drez's orthopedic sports medicine,* ed 3, Philadelphia, 2011, Elsevier.)

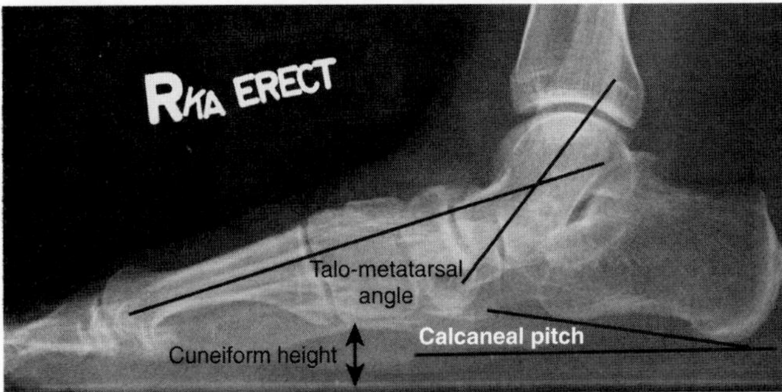

Figure 6-89 The lateral foot radiograph images the loss of alignment between the first metatarsal and midfoot. A talo–first metatarsal angle greater than 4 degrees signifies pes planus; as shown, 32 degrees. The calcaneal pitch angle is also determined on the lateral radiograph; a normal angle is between 17 and 32 degrees (12 degrees in this patient). Arch height loss is documented by a decrease in this angle. A loss of medial cuneiform-floor height is also indicative of loss of arch height. This is shown by the *black arrow.* (From DiGiovanni C: *Core knowledge in orthopaedics—foot and ankle,* Philadelphia, 2007, Elsevier.)

- **Determine whether deformity is flexible (passively correctable to a plantigrade foot) or fixed (rigid deformity that is not passively correctable).**

3. Radiographs (Figure 6-89)
   - **Pes planus indicated by negative lateral talo–first metatarsal angle** (Meary angle)
   - **Forefoot abduction indicated by TN uncoverage**

E. **Treatment—based upon the stage of the deformity**

1. Stage I—Synovitis without deformity
   - Conservative
     - Immobilization (cast or boot)
     - Orthotic after acute swelling and pain subsided
       - Arch support with medial heel wedge
   - Surgical
     - Synovectomy
2. **Stage II—Flexible deformity is the critical feature. The PTT is degenerated and functionally incompetent.**
   - Conservative
     - **AFO in conjunction with physical therapy has demonstrated the highest success rate.**
     - **A full-length orthotic with an arch support, medial heel wedge, and medial forefoot support (if supination/forefoot varus present) is used after the acute pain has resolved.**
     - A lace-up ankle brace may also be used.
   - Surgical
     - **Correction of all stage II deformities includes a tendon transfer (FDL or FHL) into the navicular to reconstruct the PTT.**

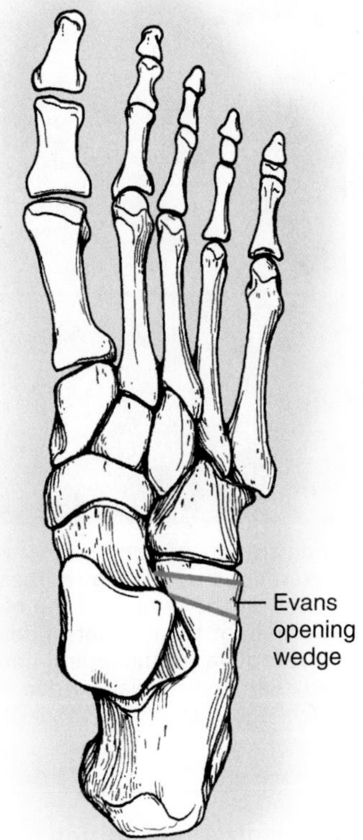

Figure 6-91 Evans anterior calcaneal osteotomy helps restore and stabilize longitudinal arch by elongating lateral column of foot. (From Coughlin M, et al: *Surgery of the foot and ankle,* ed 8, Philadelphia, 2006, Elsevier. Modified from Pedowitz WJ, Kovatis P: Flatfoot in the adult, *J Am Acad Orthop Surg* 3:293, 1995.)

     - **The presence of a gastrocnemius contracture should be assessed for and corrected with a gastrocnemius recession if present.**
     - Further subdivided into three categories that guide bony operative treatment
     - Stage IIA—defined by hindfoot valgus without significant forefoot abduction (<40% uncovering of the talus)
       - Medial slide calcaneal osteotomy (Figure 6-90)
     - Stage IIB—defined by forefoot abduction (>40% talar uncovering) in addition to hindfoot valgus
       - Lateral column lengthening (Figure 6-91)
       - Additional medial slide calcaneal osteotomy may be required.
     - **Stage IIC—defined by fixed forefoot supination/varus (first ray is elevated after correction of the**

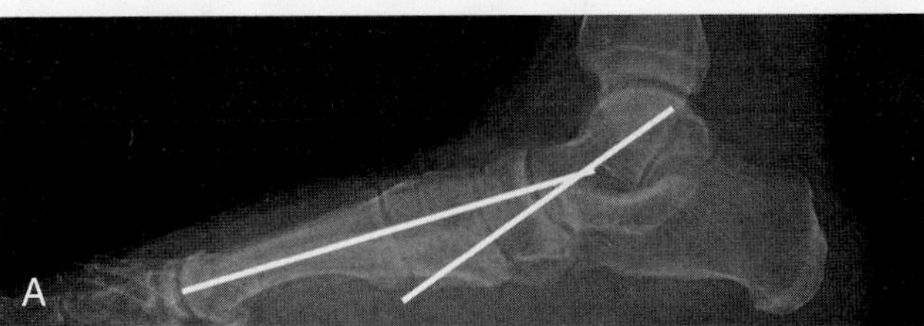

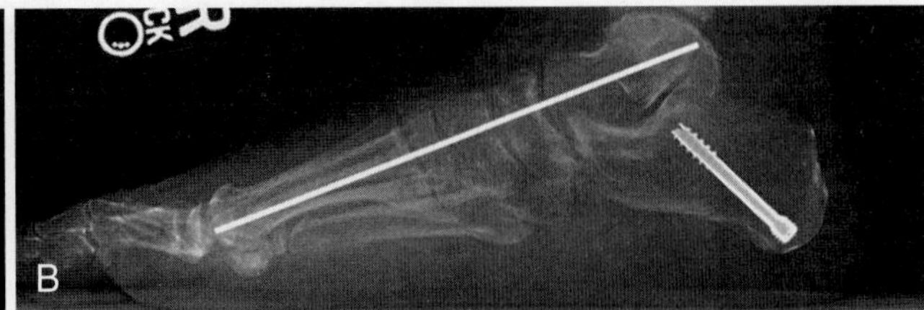

Figure 6-90 **A,** Preoperative radiograph of a patient with stage II posterior tibial tendon dysfunction. Note the break in the lateral talo–first metatarsal angle centered at the talonavicular joint. **B,** Excellent correction is noted on the postoperative radiograph, with restoration of the lateral talo–first metatarsal angle with colinearity of the first metatarsal and the talus.

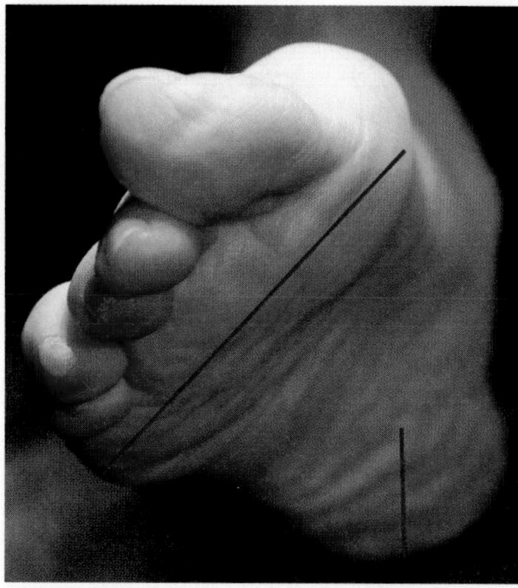

Figure 6-92 Demonstration of forefoot varus. The degree of forefoot varus is determined by placing the heel in neutral position, covering the head of the talus with the navicular, and then observing the relationship of the metatarsal heads to the neutral hindfoot. In fixed forefoot varus, the lateral border of the foot is more plantar flexed than the medial border. (From Coughlin M, et al: *Surgery of the foot and ankle,* ed 8, Philadelphia, 2006, Elsevier.)

hindfoot to neutral) in addition to hindfoot valgus (Figure 6-92). Forefoot abduction may also be present.

- **Stable medial column—Navicular is colinear with the first metatarsal.**
  - **Cotton osteotomy (dorsal open-wedge osteotomy of the cuneiform) to plantar flex the first ray**
- Unstable medial column—plantar sag at naviculocuneiform or first TMT joint
  - Medial column fusion (based upon point of collapse)
    - Isolated first TMT fusion
    - Isolated navicular fusion
    - Combined navicular and TMT fusion (both joints are involved radiographically)
    - **Hindfoot treated based upon talar uncovering**
      - **Less than 40%—medial slide calcaneal osteotomy**
      - Greater than 40%—lateral column lengthening and possible medial slide calcaneal osteotomy if residual hindfoot valgus
- **Stage II surgical summary**
  - **FDL or FHL tendon transfer for ALL patients**
  - **Gastrocnemius recession if contracture present**
  - **Hindfoot valgus—medial slide calcaneal osteotomy**
  - **Forefoot abduction—lateral column lengthening**
  - **Forefoot supination**
    - **Stable medial column—cotton osteotomy**
    - **Unstable medial column—first TMT arthrodesis**

3. **Stage III—defined by a fixed/rigid pes planovalgus deformity**
   - Conservative
     - Rigid AFO or Arizona brace. Do not attempt to correct the deformity.
   - Surgical
     - **Triple arthrodesis**
     - Additional medial column stabilization is occasionally required for severe deformities (Figure 6-93).
     - Achilles lengthening if equinus contracture present
4. Stage IV—Defined by incompetence of the deltoid ligament. Standing anteroposterior ankle radiograph demonstrates lateral talar tilt (valgus) or ankle arthritis.
   - If the ankle valgus is passively correctable, an attempt can be made at deltoid ligament reconstruction with hindfoot reconstruction.
   - Rigid deformity requires tibiotalocalcaneal arthrodesis (Figure 6-94).
     - The most reliable operation for a stage IV deformity is a tibiotalocalcaneal fusion (Figure 6-95).

II. PES CAVUS DEFORMITY

A. Defined by a highly arched foot, often with associated heel varus (cavovarus)

B. Etiology

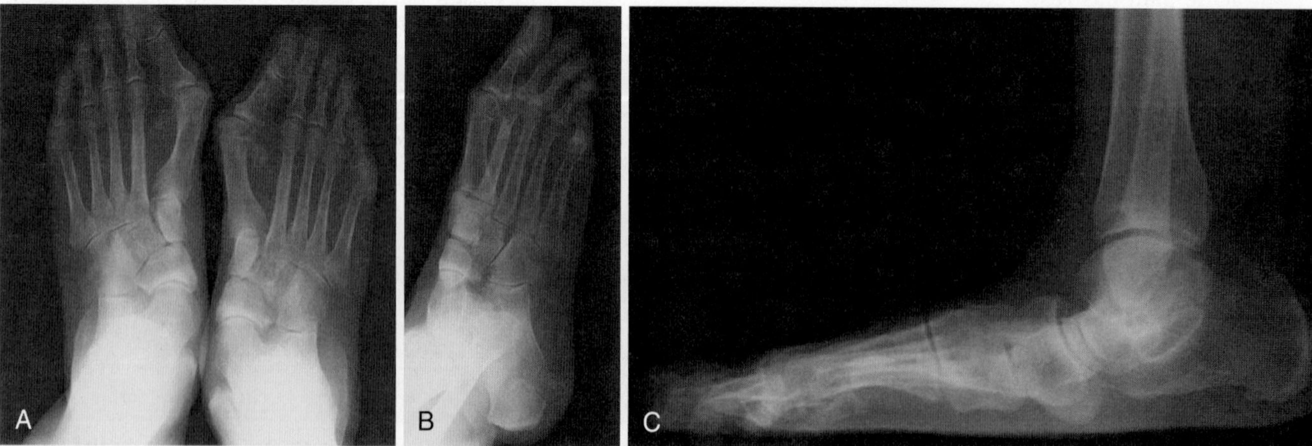

Figure 6-93 **A to C, Rigid flatfoot deformity before treatment with a triple arthrodesis.** (From Myerson M: *Reconstructive foot and ankle surgery: management of complications,* ed 2, Philadelphia, 2010, Elsevier. [Photos courtesy of John Campbell, MD, Baltimore, Md.])

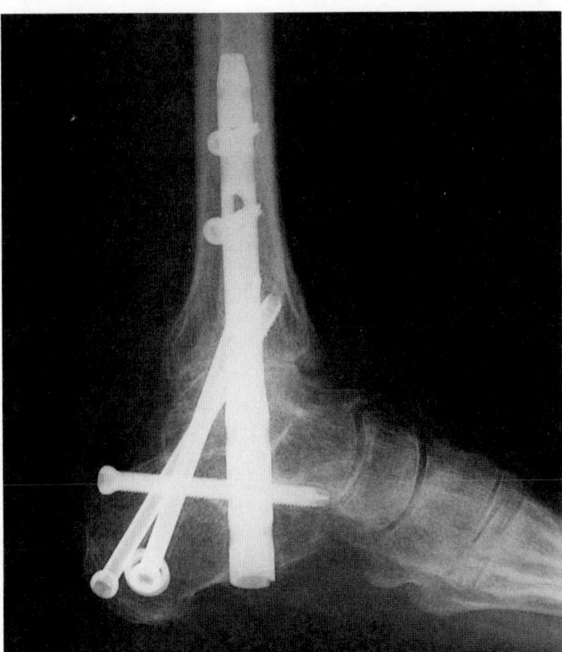

Figure 6-94 Radiograph showing tibiotalocalcaneal arthrodesis for involvement of the ankle and subtalar joints performed with an intramedullary device and augmented with screw fixation. (From DiGiovanni C: *Core knowledge in orthopaedics—foot and ankle,* Philadelphia, 2007, Elsevier.)

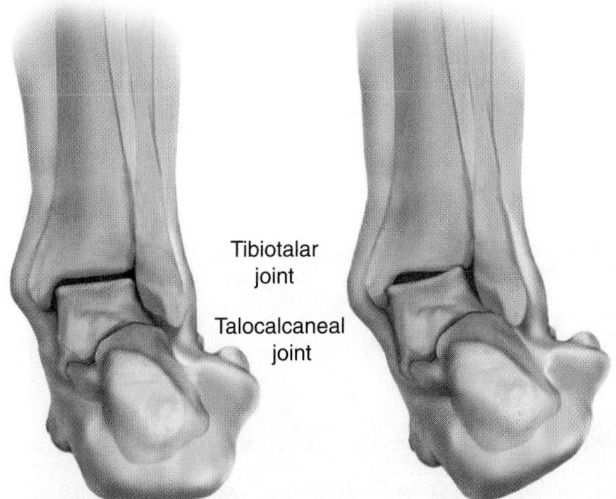

Figure 6-95 Stages I, II, and III PTTD have neutral alignment of the ankle **(A)**. Stage IV **(B)** posterior tibial tendon dysfunction is defined by a structural abnormality within the ankle. This can be either ankle valgus or ankle arthritis or a combination of both. The most common method of treatment is a tibiotalocalcaneal arthrodesis to correct both the hindfoot and ankle. However, newer emerging techniques involve hindfoot reconstruction with an associated ankle replacement (arthritis) or deltoid reconstruction (ankle valgus without arthritis).

1. Neuromuscular
   - Unilateral—Rule out tethering of the spinal cord or spinal cord tumors.
   - Bilateral—most commonly CMT (see the section Neurologic Disorders)
2. Idiopathic—usually subtle, bilateral
3. Traumatic—secondary to talus fracture malunion, compartment syndrome, crush injury

C. **Diagnosis**

1. Patients complain of painful calluses under the first metatarsal, fifth metatarsal, and medial heel.
   - Secondary to the plantar-flexed first ray and varus hindfoot
2. Often associated with lateral ankle ligament instability, peroneal tendon pathology
3. The Coleman block test is used to assess the flexibility of the hindfoot (out of varus) when the first metatarsal plantar flexion (forefoot valgus) is eliminated.
   - Wooden block placed just lateral to the first ray; first metatarsal head then lies off the block with the remainder of the block on the weight-bearing foot.
     - **If the hindfoot passively corrects into valgus, the deformity is forefoot driven (due to plantar-flexed first ray).**

D. **Treatment**

1. **Conservative—Orthotics with lateral heel wedge, decreased arch, and depressed first ray may be effective (Figure 6-96).**
2. Surgical
   - In forefoot driven deformity—First metatarsal dorsiflexion osteotomy is indicated.
   - With no or incomplete correction of the hindfoot with the Coleman block test, a lateral calcaneal closed-wedge osteotomy (Figure 6-97) is indicated in addition to a dorsiflexion osteotomy of the first metatarsal (Figure 6-98).
     - Subtalar fusion may be needed if arthritic symptoms are present.

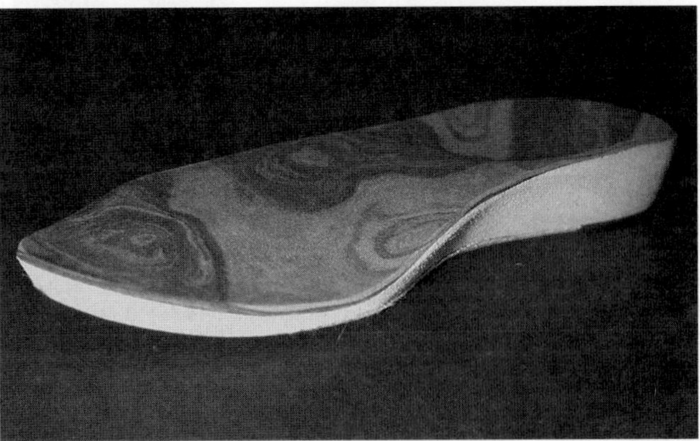

Figure 6-96 Cavus foot orthotic. Note the hollowed-out recess under the first metatarsal head and the laterally based forefoot wedge and lowered medial arch. (From DiGiovanni C: *Core knowledge in orthopaedics—foot and ankle,* Philadelphia, 2007, Elsevier.)

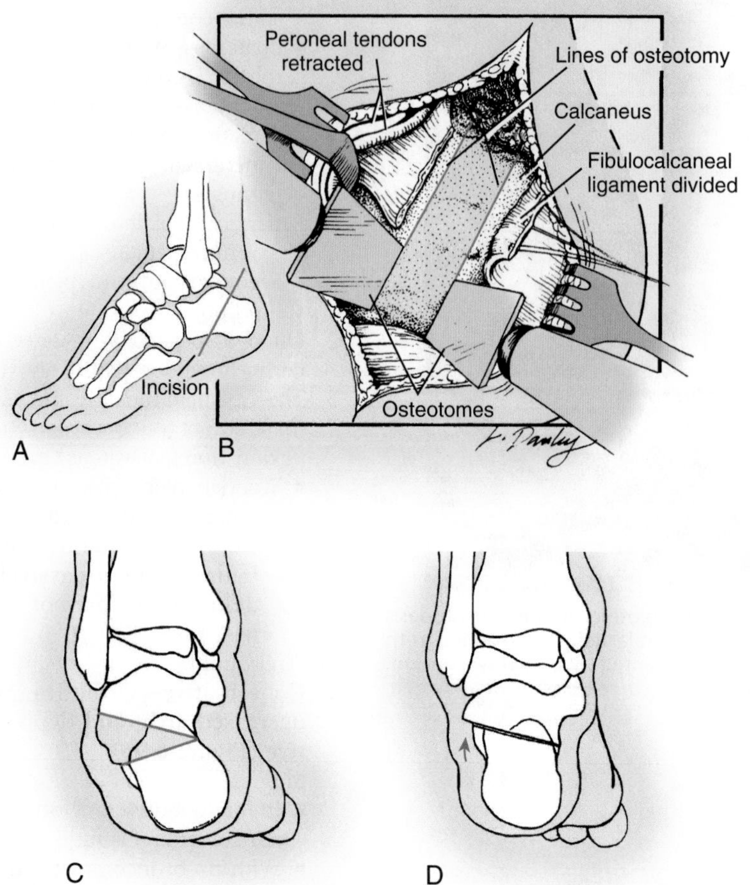

Figure 6-97 Dwyer closed-wedge osteotomy of calcaneus for varus heel. **A,** Lateral skin incision is made inferior and parallel to peroneal tendons. **B,** Wedge of bone is resected with its base laterally. **C,** Wedge of bone is tapered medially. **D,** Calcaneus is closed after bone has been removed, and varus deformity is corrected to slight valgus. (From Canale ST, Beaty J: *Campbell's operative orthopedics,* ed 11, Philadelphia, 2007, Elsevier.)

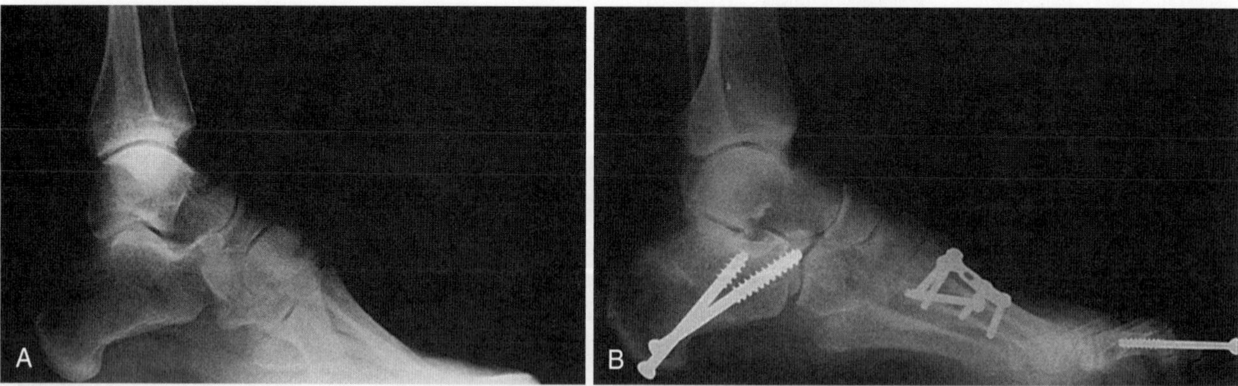

Figure 6-98 **A,** True lateral talar position of cavus foot. The radiograph is parallel to the axis between the medial and lateral malleoli. This view clearly shows the relationship of the talus to the calcaneus and the relative amount of dorsiflexion of the talus to the tibia. This view, however, distorts the forefoot, making the first metatarsal appear vertical. **B,** Postoperative radiograph demonstrates corrections of the foot. Hindfoot was repaired with a calcaneal slide transfixed with two screws. Note the slight cephalad positioning of the posterior fragment of the calcaneus. A majority of the correction was achieved by sliding this fragment laterally (out of varus). Midfoot was corrected with internal fixation with a dorsal closed-wedge osteotomy of the first metatarsal. In the forefoot correction, a single screw transfixes the interphalangeal joint of the hallux. The lesser toes were not corrected in this case. (From Coughlin M, et al: *Surgery of the foot and ankle,* ed 8, Philadelphia, 2006, Elsevier.)

SECTION 14 TENDON DISORDERS

I. ACHILLES TENDON

The achilles tendon is addressed in the section, Heel Pain.

II. PERONEAL TENDONS

A. Most common disorders include tendinitis/ tenosynovitis and tendon subluxation/dislocation, which often causes peroneus brevis degenerative tears.

B. Diagnosis

1. Acute or chronic localized swelling and tenderness over peroneal tendons
2. Common cause for chronic pain following an ankle sprain or chronic instability
3. Associated with cavovarus foot deformity
4. Peroneal subluxation or dislocation
   - **Caused by forced eversion and dorsiflexion, leading to disruption of superior peroneal retinaculum**
   - Pain and/or sensation of snapping in the retrofibular groove
   - Often causes peroneus brevis degenerative tears
5. Acute rupture of the peroneus longus tendon at or through a fracture of the os peroneum can occur.
   - Radiographs show a retraction or fracture of the os peroneum.

C. Treatment

1. Nonoperative treatment
   - Chronic peroneal tendinosis or tenosynovitis is initially treated with activity modification, NSAIDs, lace-up ankle brace, and physical therapy.
   - Ultrasound or MRI can be used to aid diagnosis (Figure 6-99).

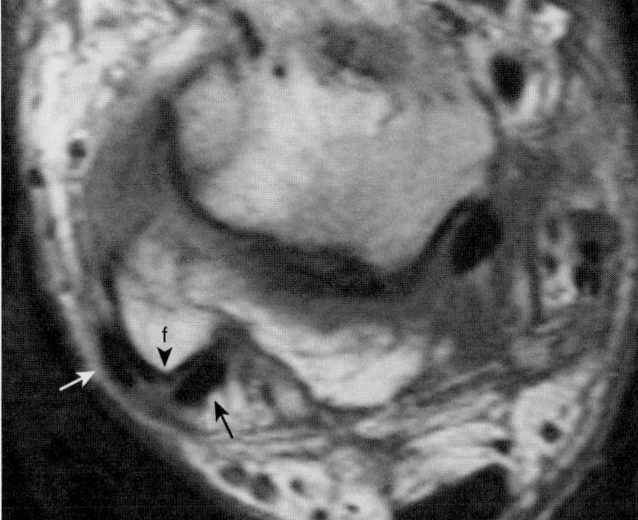

Figure 6-99 Peroneal tendon subluxation. Axial proton density magnetic resonance image shows longitudinally torn peroneus brevis *(white arrow)* subluxed laterally and anteriorly from its normal position adjacent to the peroneus longus *(black arrow)*. Note that the distal fibula has a rounded contour *(small black arrowhead)*, a finding that can be associated with peroneal subluxation. f, fibula. (From Manaster BJ, et al: *Musculoskeletal imaging—the requisites,* ed 3, Philadelphia, 2006, Elsevier.)

     - Ultrasound useful as dynamic tool to evaluate subluxation/dislocation
     - False-positive results showing longitudinal tears common with MRI
2. Surgical treatment—based on the pathology
   - Tenosynovectomy, débridement, and repair of degenerative tears (usually the peroneus brevis)
     - Synovitis or less than 50% diseased tendon
     - Groove deepening if shallow fibular groove
   - Excision and tenodesis
     - Required when there is a complete rupture or severely degenerative tendon (>50%) that prohibits repair
   - Hindfoot varus
     - Dwyer osteotomy (lateral closed-wedge osteotomy of the calcaneus)
   - **Peroneal subluxation or dislocation**
     - **Requires repair/reconstruction of the superior peroneal retinaculum and fibular groove deepening**
   - FHL transfer to the fifth metatarsal
     - Greater than 50% degeneration of both the peroneus longus and brevis that requires excision of both tendons

III. POSTERIOR TIBIAL TENDON

The posterior tibial tendon is addressed in the section, Pes Planus (Flatfoot) Deformity.

IV. ANTERIOR TIBIAL TENDON

A. Tenosynovitis uncommon but can be observed in patients with inflammatory arthritis

1. NSAIDs and walking cast or boot is recommended.
2. Corticosteroid injections can provide relief but increase the risk of tendon rupture.

B. Complete ruptures rare; mainly occur in older patients

1. Present as painless anterior ankle mass
2. Surgical repair in the older population has recently demonstrated successful results. Primary repair is appropriate for an acute rupture; however, an interpositional graft may be required in delayed cases.

V. FHL—STENOSING FHL TENOSYNOVITIS

A. Usually seen in dancers on pointe

B. Posterior or postero-medial ankle pain, triggering of the hallux interphalangeal, and pain with resisted hallux plantar flexion

C. Stenosis occurs along course of FHL between the posterolateral and posteromedial tubercles of the talus.

D. MRI is the diagnostic modality of choice.

1. **Fluid (high signal intensity) will be noted surrounding the FHL at the level of the ankle joint** (Figure 6-100).

E. Nonoperative treatment—activity modification

F. Operative treatment—open (posteromedial approach) or arthroscopic FHL tenosynovectomy and release of the fascia

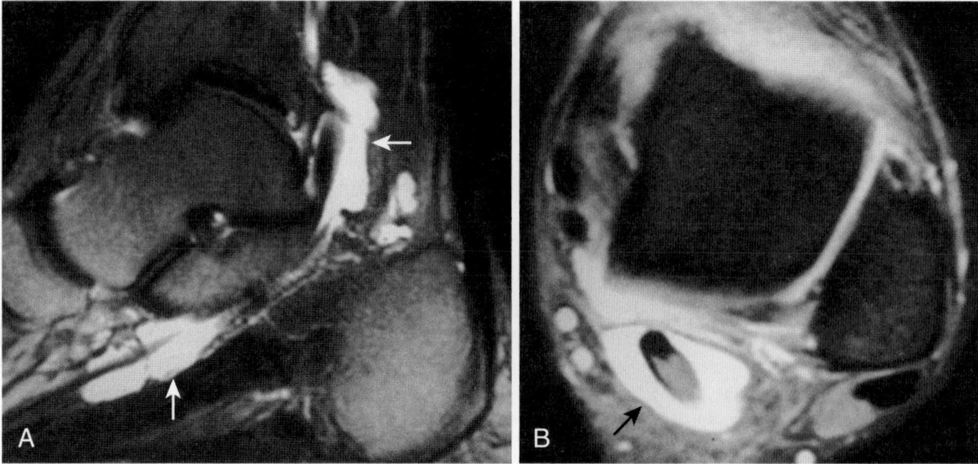

Figure 6-100 Abnormalities of the flexor hallucis longus tendon: tenosynovitis. Sagittal (TR/TE, 3400/98) **(A)** and transverse (TR/TE, 4000/14) **(B)** fast spin-echo magnetic resonance images reveal considerable fluid within the sheath *(arrows)* about the flexor hallucis longus tendon. The amount of fluid is out of proportion to that present in the ankle joint. (From Resnick D: *Internal derangements of joints,* ed 2, Philadelphia, 2006, Elsevier.)

SECTION 15 HEEL PAIN

I. PLANTAR HEEL PAIN

A. Plantar fasciitis

1. Painful heel condition that can affect both sedentary and active individuals and is most often seen in the adult population.
   - **Associated with a contracture of the gastrocnemius-soleus complex (Achilles tendon)**
2. Presentation
   - **Exquisite pain and tenderness over the plantar medial tuberosity of the calcaneus at the proximal insertion of the plantar fascia**
   - **Classic symptoms include pain with the first step in the morning and after prolonged sitting.**
   - Bilateral symptoms are common.
   - Small subset of patients may experience pain and tenderness at the origin of the abductor hallucis, which may indicate entrapment or inflammation of the first branch of the lateral plantar nerve.
3. Pathology—likely involves microtears at the origin of the plantar fascia, which initiates inflammation and an injury-repair process that leads to a traction osteophyte
   - Approximately 10% of patients will develop persistent, disabling symptoms.
4. Treatment
   - Nonoperative
     - **Plantar fascia–specific stretching protocols and Achilles tendon (heel cord) stretching are the key to effective nonoperative management.**
     - **Also includes cushioned heel inserts, night splints, physical therapy, walking casts, cortisone injections, and anti-inflammatory medications**
   - Operative
     - Limited (medial one-half) release of the plantar fascia may be necessary in refractory cases.
       - **Complete release can place the longitudinal arch of the foot at risk, overload the lateral column, and lead to dorsolateral foot pain.**
       - Concomitant release of the deep fascia of the abductor hallucis may relieve entrapment of the lateral plantar nerve and improve the surgical result (Figure 6-101).
     - **Other invasive options with evolving evidence include gastrocnemius recession and high-energy extracorporeal shock wave therapy.**

B. Baxter neuritis (compression of the first branch of the lateral plantar nerve)

1. **Baxter neuritis presents as plantar medial heel pain that can be difficult to differentiate from plantar fasciitis.**
   - Associated with athletes involved in running sports
   - Pain is located more medial over the abductor hallucis as compared to the more plantar pain seen with plantar fasciitis.
   - Compression over Baxter nerve will reproduce the pain and may cause radiation into the plantar lateral foot.
2. Diagnostic tests
   - Electromyogram/nerve conduction velocity may demonstrate increased motor latency within the abductor digiti quinti.
   - MRI may demonstrate fatty infiltration of the abductor digiti quinti, best seen on the coronal views.
3. Treatment
   - Standard conservative management uses heel cord stretching and cushioned heel inserts.

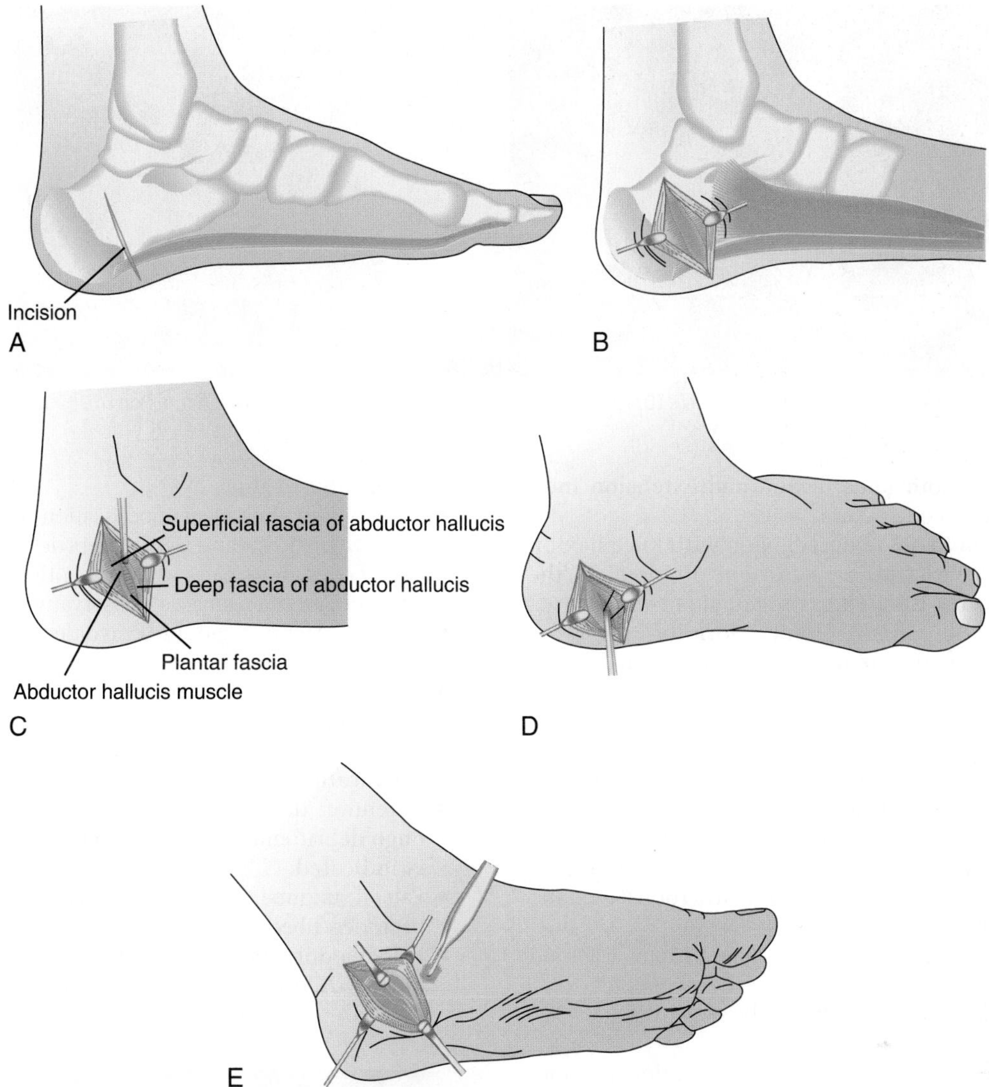

Figure 6-101 Plantar fascia and nerve release. **A,** Incision. **B,** Release of the abductor hallucis muscle. **C,** Abductor hallucis muscle is reflected proximally. **D,** Abductor hallucis is retracted distally. **E,** Resection of small medial portion of the plantar fascia. (From DeLee J: *DeLee and Drez's orthopedic sports medicine,* ed 3, Philadelphia, 2011, Elsevier.)

- Surgical treatment
  - Open release of Baxter nerve must include release of the deep fascia of the abductor hallucis.

C. Bony causes

1. Calcaneal stress fractures
   - Most commonly in the active individual or military recruit
   - Bone scintigraphy or MRI (more sensitive and specific) used to aid diagnosis
   - Treat with rest, protected weight bearing.
2. Periostitis
   - Pain and tenderness in the central portion of the heel pad
   - Represents traumatic periosteal or bursal inflammation secondary to a known injury or atrophic heel pad
   - Treat with cushioned shoe inserts or a short course in a well-padded cast.
   - The examiner should be vigilant for other signs or symptoms suggesting inflammatory arthritis.

II. POSTERIOR HEEL PAIN

A. Anatomy

1. The Achilles tendon (comprising the gastrocnemius and soleus tendons) rotates 90 degrees laterally to insert on the posterior aspect of the calcaneal tuberosity.
2. The retrocalcaneal bursa lies between the anterior surface of the Achilles tendon and the posterosuperior aspect of the calcaneus.
3. Haglund deformity refers to an enlarged prominence of the posterosuperior calcaneal tuberosity.
4. The Achilles accepts 2000 to 7000 N of stress, depending on the applied load, and transfers forces of 6 to 10 times body weight during a running stride.

B. Physical examination

1. Bony prominence, tendon thickening, and area of tenderness should be evaluated.
2. **The Silfverskiöld test evaluates for contracture.**
   - **Test ankle dorsiflexion with the knee extended and flexed.**

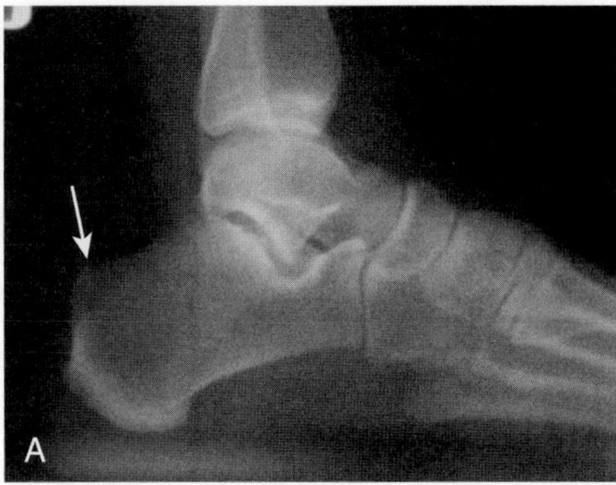

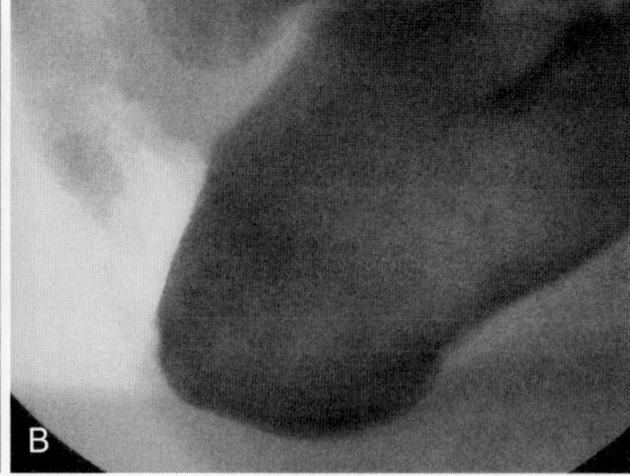

Figure 6-102 Preoperative **(A)** and intraoperative **(B)** radiographs of Haglund deformity ***(arrow).*** (From Porter D, Schon L: *Baxter's the foot and ankle in sport,* ed 2, Philadelphia, 2007, Elsevier.)

- **Tightness in both knee flexion and extension indicates Achilles contracture.**
- **Improvement in ankle dorsiflexion with knee flexion (relaxing the gastrocnemius origin proximal to the knee) indicates isolated gastrocnemius contracture.**

C. **Retrocalcaneal bursitis/Haglund deformity**

1. Inflammation of the retrocalcaneal bursa that often occurs along with insertional tendinopathy and Haglund deformity
2. Diagnosis
   - Patients present with deep posterior heel pain, fullness and tenderness with palpation medial and lateral to the tendon, and increased pain with ankle dorsiflexion.
   - Symptoms often seen in conjunction with insertional Achilles tendinopathy (see section, Insertional Achilles Tendinopathy)
   - Lateral foot radiographs will demonstrate Haglund deformity.
   - MRI is rarely necessary to make the diagnosis.
3. Treatment
   - Nonoperative management of this condition includes NSAIDs, external padding, ice, and shoe-wear modification.
   - Steroid injection should be avoided due to inherent risk of Achilles rupture.
   - Operative treatment includes débridement of the inflamed retrocalcaneal bursa along with excision of the Haglund deformity when present (Figure 6-102).

D. **Insertional Achilles tendinopathy**

1. Diagnosis
   - Patients complain of pain, swelling, burning, and stiffness in the posterior heel.
   - Progressive enlargement of the bony prominence of the heel along with pain caused by direct pressure from shoe wear is common.
   - Tenderness localized to the Achilles tendon insertion on the posterior calcaneus, most often midline
   - Imaging
     - Bone spur and intratendinous calcification seen on lateral foot radiograph (Figure 6-103)
     - MRI and ultrasonography can be helpful to determine extent of Achilles tendon degeneration.
   - Histopathology—degenerative process showing disorganized collagen and mucoid degeneration with minimal inflammatory cells
     - Tendinopathy is preferred description.
2. Nonoperative treatment
   - Activity and shoe-wear modification, heel lifts, stretching, physical therapy with eccentric training, and silicone heel sleeves/pads to decrease the pain from direct pressure are mainstays of conservative treatment.
   - Steroid injections should be avoided.
3. Operative treatment
   - **Includes excision of retrocalcaneal bursa, resection of prominent superior calcaneal tuberosity, and débridement of degenerative tendon including calcification**
   - **If tendon detachment (>50%) is required for thorough débridement, reattachment with suture anchors is indicated.**
   - Lateral, midline, and medial J-shaped incisions have all been described.
   - **FHL tendon transfer is indicated if more than 50% of the Achilles tendon requires excision (Figure 6-104).**

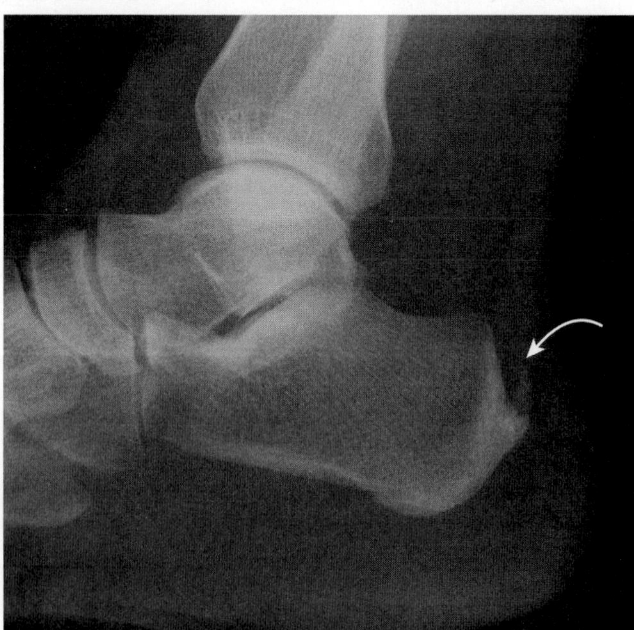

Figure 6-103 Radiography of the Achilles tendon. Insertional tendinosis. The distal tendon is thickened at its site of insertion onto the calcaneus, and an insertional enthesophyte has formed ***(curved arrow).*** (From Weissman B: *Imaging of arthritis and metabolic bone disease,* Philadelphia, 2009, Elsevier.)

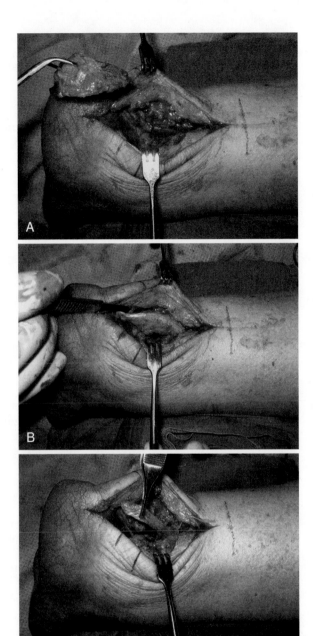

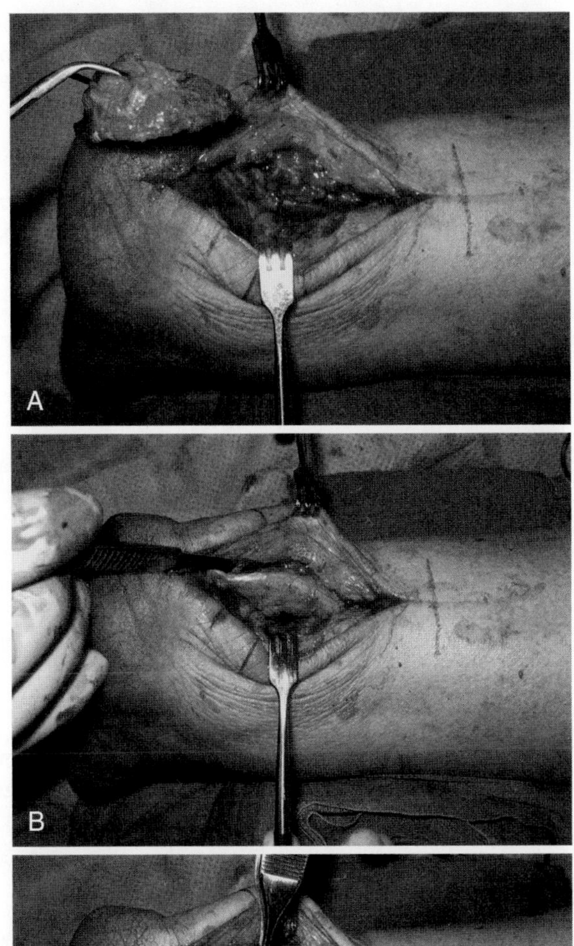

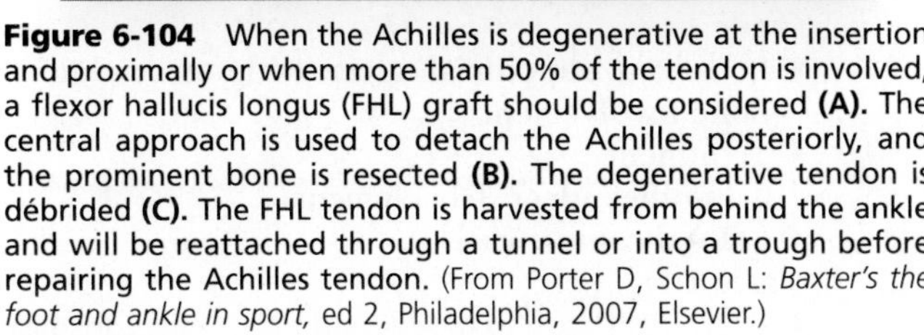

Figure 6-104 When the Achilles is degenerative at the insertion and proximally or when more than 50% of the tendon is involved, a flexor hallucis longus (FHL) graft should be considered **(A).** The central approach is used to detach the Achilles posteriorly, and the prominent bone is resected **(B).** The degenerative tendon is débrided **(C).** The FHL tendon is harvested from behind the ankle and will be reattached through a tunnel or into a trough before repairing the Achilles tendon. (From Porter D, Schon L: *Baxter's the foot and ankle in sport,* ed 2, Philadelphia, 2007, Elsevier.)

E. Noninsertional Achilles tendinopathy

1. Includes inflammation of the paratenon alone, peritendinitis with a component of tendon thickening (commonly referred to as tendinosis), or tendinosis alone
2. Multifactorial etiology includes overuse, mechanical imbalance, poor tissue vascularity and genetic predisposition, and fluoroquinolone antibiotics.
3. Pathophysiology—thought to involve the response to microscopic tearing of the tendon
   - Abnormal vascularization of the ventral mesotenal vessels 2 to 6 cm proximal to the insertion thought to contribute
4. Diagnosis
   - Patients often present with pain, swelling, and impaired performance, especially with running.
   - Tender area of fusiform thickening localized approximately 2 to 6 cm proximal to the insertion of the tendon
   - MRI will demonstrate thickening of the tendon with intrasubstance intermediate signal intensity consistent with the disorganized tissue. In the setting of a chronic rupture a large gap will be present between the hypoechoic (dark) tendon ends (Figure 6-105).
5. Nonoperative treatment
   - Eccentric strengthening has demonstrated the highest success rate; includes rest, activity modification, heel lifts, physical therapy with emphasis on modalities and eccentric strengthening exercises and shock-wave therapy
   - Other treatments with evolving evidence include glyceryl trinitrate patches, prolotherapy, and aprotinin injections.
6. Operative treatment
   - Less invasive options include percutaneous longitudinal tenotomies in the area of degeneration, as well as

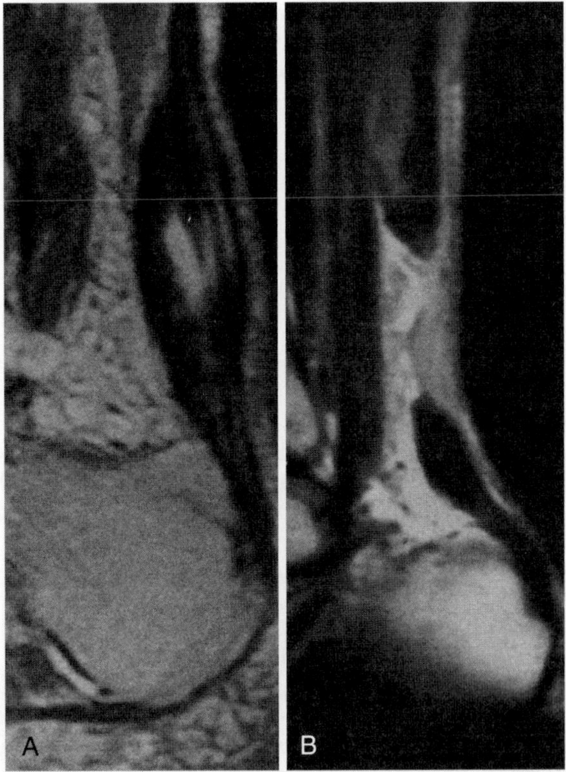

Figure 6-105 Chronic Achilles tendinosis with a partial or complete tear. **A,** Partial tear. Sagittal T2-weighted (TR/TE, 2000/70) spin-echo magnetic resonance (MR) image shows an enlarged Achilles tendon containing irregular regions of high signal intensity. **B,** Complete tear. Sagittal intermediate-weighted (TR/TE, 3000/30) spin-echo MR image shows complete disruption of the Achilles tendon and a proximal segment that is inhomogeneous in signal intensity. Note the edema and hemorrhage of high signal intensity about the acutely torn tendon. (From Resnick D, Kransdorf M: *Bone and joint imaging,* ed 3, Philadelphia, 2004, Elsevier.)

stripping the anterior aspect of the tendon with large suture to free adhesions.
- For moderate to severe disease, open excision of the degenerated tendon tissue with tubularization has shown good results.
- **For more than 50% degenerative involvement of the Achilles, a tendon transfer with FHL is recommended.**
  - **MRI evidence of significant involvement (diffuse thickening of the tendon without a focal area of disease) indicates the need for an FHL transfer.**

F. **Chronic Achilles tendon rupture**
1. Nonoperative—AFO
2. **Operative treatment—In the setting of a chronic rupture an FHL transfer is the treatment of choice.**

SECTION 16 THE DIABETIC FOOT

I. PATHOPHYSIOLOGY

A. **Diabetic neuropathy**
1. The diagnosis of foot ulcerations results in the greatest rate of hospital admissions in diabetic patients, as well as lower extremity amputations.
2. The combination of neuropathy and excess pressure on the plantar foot leads to ulceration.
3. Sensation
   - Polyneuropathic loss of sensation begins in a stocking distribution of the feet and progresses proximally.
   - Diagnosed by the inability to perceive the 5.07 Semmes-Weinstein monofilament
   - **90% of patients who cannot feel the 5.07 monofilament have lost protective sensation to their feet and are at risk for ulceration.**
   - With the Therapeutic Shoe Bill, money is allocated for neuropathic patients to purchase extradepth shoes and total contact inserts (three per year) for ulcer prevention.
4. Autonomic neuropathy
   - An abnormal sweating mechanism leads to a dry foot.
   - Vulnerable to fissuring cracks, which then become portals for infection.
5. Motor neuropathy
   - Most commonly involves the common peroneal nerve
   - Resultant loss of tibialis anterior motor function and a footdrop
   - **Small intrinsic musculature of the foot also commonly affected, resulting in claw toes and subsequent toe-tip ulcerations due to excessive pressure**

B. **Hypomobility syndrome**
1. Result of excessive glycosylation of the soft tissues of the extremities
2. Leads to decreased joint ROM

C. **Peripheral vascular disease**
1. Occurs in 60% to 70% of patients who have had diabetes for over 10 years, involving both large and small vessels
2. **Noninvasive vascular examination should be performed when pulses are not palpable.**
   - Waveforms (normal is triphasic)
   - Ankle-brachial indices (minimum for healing, 0.45; normal, 1.0)
     - Calcifications in the artery can falsely elevate the ankle-brachial index. Greater than 1.3 is nonphysiologic and consistent with calcification of the vessels.
   - **Absolute toe pressures (minimum for healing, 40 mm Hg; normal, 100 mm Hg)**
3. **Transcutaneous oxygen pressure of the toes greater than 40 mm Hg have been found to be predictive of healing.**

D. **Immune system impairment**
1. Poor cellular defenses such as abnormal phagocytosis, altered chemotaxis of the WBCs, and a poor cytotoxic environment (due to hyperglycemia) to fight off bacteria lead to difficulty in fighting off infection once it has developed.

E. **Metabolic deficiency**
1. **Reduced total protein less than 6.0 g/dL, WBC count less than 1500, and albumin levels less than 2.5 g/dL result in poor healing potential.**

II. CLINICAL PROBLEMS

A. **Ulcers**
1. Classification and treatment
   - **Ulcer location (forefoot, midfoot, and heel) and the presence or absence of arterial disease influence healing rates.**
   - Depth-ischemia classification (modification of Wagner-Meggitt classification)
   - Depth
     - Grade 0
       - Skin intact with bony deformity—at risk
       - Treatment
         - Extradepth shoe and pressure-relief insoles
     - Grade 1
       - **Localized superficial ulcer without tendon or bone involvement**
       - **Treatment**
         - **In-office ulcer débridement**
         - **Total-contact cast**
     - Grade 2
       - Deep ulcer with exposed tendon or joint capsule
       - Treatment
         - Formal operative débridement of all exposed tendon and nonviable tissue
         - Followed by dressing changes and total-contact casting once wound bed is healthy
     - **Grade 3**
       - **Extensive ulcer with exposed bone/osteomyelitis or abscess**
       - **Treatment**
         - **Surgical débridement of exposed bone/osteomyelitis and nonviable tissue**

- **Followed by dressing changes and total-contact casting once wound bed is healthy**
- Ischemia
  - Grade A—normal vascularity
  - **Grade B—ischemia without gangrene**
    - **Noninvasive vascular studies and surgical revascularization if indicated**
  - Grade C—partial (forefoot) gangrene
    - Noninvasive vascular studies and surgical revascularization if indicated
    - Metabolic assessment
      - Delay surgery if albumin is less than 2.5 g/dL or total protein is less than 6 g/dL, and improve nutritional status of the patient.
    - Operative intervention—partial foot amputation
  - Grade D—complete foot gangrene
    - Same as with grade C
    - Operative intervention—below-the-knee or above-the-knee amputation

2. Additional treatment
   - Midfoot collapse may require ostectomy of bony prominence or midfoot fusion if instability of the midfoot is present.
   - **Equinus contracture is very common, and tendo-Achilles lengthening will offload the midfoot/forefoot.**
     - **Achilles lengthening required**
       - **Recurrent forefoot/midfoot ulceration**
       - **Ulceration with equinus deformity**
   - Toe deformities often require joint resection or amputation.
3. The ultimate goal is an ulcer-free, functional, plantigrade foot that can fit within a brace or shoe.

B. **Charcot arthropathy**

1. **Chronic, progressive, destructive process affecting bone architecture and joint alignment in people lacking protective sensation**
2. Two theories regarding pathophysiology are neurotraumatic and neurovascular destruction.
3. Classification—Eichenholtz stages of Charcot arthropathy (Table 6-4)
   - Related to the degree of warmth, swelling, and erythema
   - Continuum from bone resorption and fragmentation to bone formation and consolidation that takes 6 to 18 months
   - **Also classified by location—type 1 midfoot (most common);** type 2 hindfoot (subtalar, TN, CC joints); type 3 tibiotalar joint
4. **Patients complain of swelling, warmth, redness, and deformity that is usually painless.**
   - **Swelling and redness is typically resolved in morning.**
   - **Often confused with osteomyelitis clinically**
5. Treatment
   - Goal is to achieve stage 3 (resolution) while maintaining alignment, ambulatory status, and minimizing soft tissue breakdown.
   - **Initial treatment is immobilization and non–weight bearing.**
     - **Best with total-contact cast**
     - **Can transition to custom brace (AFO, or Charcot restraint orthosis walker boot) once swelling and warmth subsides**
   - Surgical treatment
     - Stable deformity with recurrent ulcers secondary to prominence—exostectomy
     - Unstable/unbraceable deformity—arthrodesis
       - Ankle and hindfoot Charcot best treated with arthrodesis given the high likelihood of failure of nonoperative management
     - Tendo-Achilles lengthening almost universally required
     - Amputation as salvage

C. **Diabetic foot infections**

1. Occur contiguous to an open skin wound (ulceration, skin fissure, or cut)
   - Hematogenous spread of infection into the foot or ankle is rare.
2. Infections in the diabetic foot or ankle are either isolated soft tissue infections (cellulitis or abscess) or osteomyelitis.
   - If abscess is suspected, perform needle aspiration or MRI.
     - MRI has high false-positive rate in the diagnosis of osteomyelitis, particularly with concurrent Charcot arthropathy.
   - WBC-labeled scan or dual-image Tc/In scan is more sensitive and specific for osteomyelitis than isolated technetium scan.
   - 67% of the foot ulcerations that probe to bone have contiguous osteomyelitis.
3. Diabetic foot infections are polymicrobial.
   - Superficial wound culture does not identify the organism responsible for the infection and should not be performed.
   - **Deep surgical cultures (or bone biopsy if exposed bone) provide most accurate result.**

Table 6-4 Stages of Charcot Arthropathy (Eichenholtz)*

Stage	Signs and Symptoms	Radiographs
0: Clinical (prefragmentation)	Acute inflammation; confused with infection	Regional bone demineralization
1: Dissolution (fragmentation)	Acute inflammation, swelling, erythema, warmth; confused with infection	Regional bone demineralization, periarticular fragmentation, joint dislocation
2: Coalescence	Less inflammation, less swelling, less erythema	Absorption of bone debris; early bone healing and periosteal new bone formation
3: Resolution	Resolved erythema, swelling, and warmth; consolidation of healing	Smoothed bone edges, bony/fibrous ankylosis

*Based on the signs, symptoms, and radiographic changes that occur with the neuropathic joint/fracture over time.

4. **Treat with initial broad-spectrum antibiotic coverage once surgical cultures are obtained, and adjust once sensitivity results return.**
5. Abscesses require surgical drainage and antibiotics.
6. Osteomyelitis is treated with antibiotics and usually surgical débridement.
   - Culture-specific antibiotics from a bone biopsy have proven to be an effective tool in treating osteomyelitis without the need for bone resection. Resection of all nonviable or infected soft tissue should also be performed.
   - If culture-specific antibiotic therapy fails, then surgical resection of infected bone and débridement of surrounding tissue is required in addition to antibiotic therapy.
   - **Often results in more extensive débridement, including ray resection, partial calcanectomy (calcaneal involvement), and partial or complete foot amputation**

D. Amputation level

1. Transmetatarsal
   - Lowest energy expenditure
   - No tendon transfer needed
2. **Lisfranc**
   - **Must transfer peroneal tendons to the cuboid to prevent varus**
   - **Achilles lengthening to prevent equinus**
3. **Chopart**
   - **Transfer anterior tibialis to talus to prevent equinus.**
   - **Achilles lengthening to prevent equinus**
4. Syme
   - Amputation level with the next lowest energy expenditure after a transmetatarsal amputation. Superior to both a Lisfranc and Chopart amputation with regard to the amount of energy required to ambulate
5. Transtibial
   - Superior results with postoperative casting for 3 to 5 days with conversion to rigid removal dressing

E. Total-contact casting

1. **Proximal transfer of plantar weight-bearing forces to calf and leg**
2. Edema control and bony protection in Charcot arthropathy
3. Indicated for ulcers that are plantar and with a healthy wound bed

SECTION 17 TRAUMA

I. PHALANGEAL FRACTURES

A. Diagnosis

1. Most common injuries to the forefoot
2. Usually caused by stubbing mechanism (axial loading with varus or valgus force) or by crush mechanism (heavy load dropped on the foot)
3. Present with pain, ecchymosis, and swelling

B. Treatment

1. Nondisplaced fractures with or without articular involvement
   - Stiff-soled shoes and protected weight bearing, "buddy taping"
2. Displaced fractures
   - Closed reduction can be attempted with gravity traction, followed by stiff-soled shoe and "buddy taping."
3. Hallux fractures carry greater functional significance than those of the lesser toes.
   - Distal phalanx fractures often the result of a crush mechanism
     - If concomitant nail bed injury is present, considered an open fracture.
     - Should be irrigated and treated with antibiotics
   - Operative treatment—indicated for gross instability or intraarticular discontinuity
     - Fixation achieved with crossed Kirschner wires (K-wires) or minifragment screws
     - Most common complication—stiffness

II. METATARSAL FRACTURES

A. Anatomy

1. Stability achieved by the bony architecture of the midfoot and the ligamentous attachments at the metatarsal bases and necks (intermetatarsal ligaments)
2. Severe displacement of shaft fractures is uncommon unless multiple metatarsals are fractured.
3. First and fifth metatarsals are more mobile and susceptible to injury.

B. Mechanisms of injury—crush-type injury (which can result in severe soft tissue trauma), twisting forces

1. When multiple metatarsals are fractured, a Lisfranc injury must be ruled out.

C. Radiographs—Anteroposterior, lateral, and oblique radiographs are usually suitable to detect fractures.

D. First metatarsal fracture

1. Bears approximately one third of the body weight
   - Maintenance of alignment is very important.
2. Nondisplaced fracture—boot or hard-soled shoe, weight bearing as tolerated
3. Displaced fracture—Surgical fixation; open reduction with internal fixation (ORIF) with lag screws or plate fixation

E. Second, third, and fourth metatarsal fractures

1. Majority are minimally displaced.
   - Treat with a low-tide walking boot or hard-soled shoe with arch support.
   - Isolated fractures are stable secondary to the intermetatarsal ligaments that are present both at the base and neck that help to prevent displacement.
2. Surgical fixation indicated in fractures with significant sagittal plane deformity (more than 10 degrees) or if the three central metatarsals are fractured. With multiple fractures, the intermetatarsal ligaments cannot provide stability, and therefore these are inherently unstable.
   - ORIF with intramedullary antegrade-retrograde pinning technique
   - Care should be taken to maintain proper metatarsal length in order to minimize the risk of transfer metatarsalgia or plantar keratosis.

3. Metatarsal neck fractures
   - Most treated conservatively in boot or shoe
   - With multiple (central three) and/or complete displacement—Treat with open reduction and antegrade-retrograde pinning.
4. Metatarsal base fractures
   - Primarily through metaphyseal bone, heal rapidly
   - High suspicion for a Lisfranc injury should be present when this fracture is seen.
5. Metatarsal stress fractures
   - Common, often secondary to repetitive stress, cavovarus foot posture
   - MRI or bone scans will aid in the diagnosis.
   - **Second metatarsal stress fracture is the most common and is classically described in amenorrheal dancers.**
   - **Treat in weight-bearing boot or hard-soled shoe.**
   - **Evaluate for metabolic bone disease in these patients, especially if insidious onset or if there is no distinct causal event (increase in training, initiation of new activity).**
   - Recurrent stress fracture in the presence of a cavovarus foot—may require reconstruction of the alignment to prevent recurrence

F. **Fifth metatarsal fracture**

1. These fractures represent a unique subset of forefoot injuries.
2. Best classification involves anatomic description of the fracture (Figure 6-106).
   - Zone 1—avulsion fracture of the proximal fifth metatarsal tuberosity
     - Occurs secondary to an inversion mechanism and subsequent pull of the lateral band of the plantar fascia and/or peroneus brevis tendon
     - Sometimes extends into the cubometatarsal joint
     - **Most treated with protected weight bearing in shoe or boot**
     - Open reduction required if the fifth metatarso-cuboid articular is displaced or if the fracture is rotated—with the fractured surface of the proximal fragment no longer facing the distal fragment
     - Tenting of the skin is also an indication for fixation.
     - A lag screw placed obliquely from the base of the fifth metatarsal into the medial cortex of the fifth metatarsal is the surgical treatment of choice.
   - Zone 2—fractures of the metaphyseal-diaphyseal junction that extend into the fourth-fifth intermetatarsal articulation
     - Also known as Jones fractures (Figure 6-107)
     - **Acute Zone 2 fractures can be treated with non–weight-bearing immobilization for 6 to 8 weeks.**
       - **Recurrent fracture after nonoperative intervention should be treated with intramedullary screw fixation.**
     - **Elite athletes should be treated with intramedullary screw fixation.**
   - Zone 3—fractures of the proximal diaphysis usually secondary to stress
     - Mostly in athletes secondary to repetitive microtrauma
     - Occur in the vascular watershed region of the proximal fifth metatarsal
       - Slow healing time and greater risk of nonunion
     - High risk of refracture with nonoperative treatment when fracture is stress related (33%)
     - Intramedullary screw fixation is surgical treatment of choice.
       - Bone grafting may be required in case of nonunion, significant resorption.
     - The presence of a varus foot deformity is not uncommon in these patients, and concomitant lateral

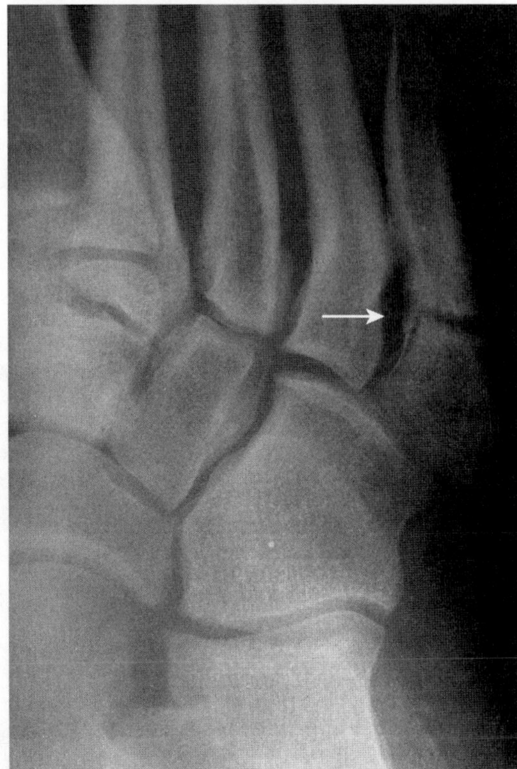

Figure 6-107 Jones fracture of the fifth metatarsal *(arrow).* (From Coughlin M, et al: *Surgery of the foot and ankle,* ed 8, Philadelphia, 2006, Elsevier.)

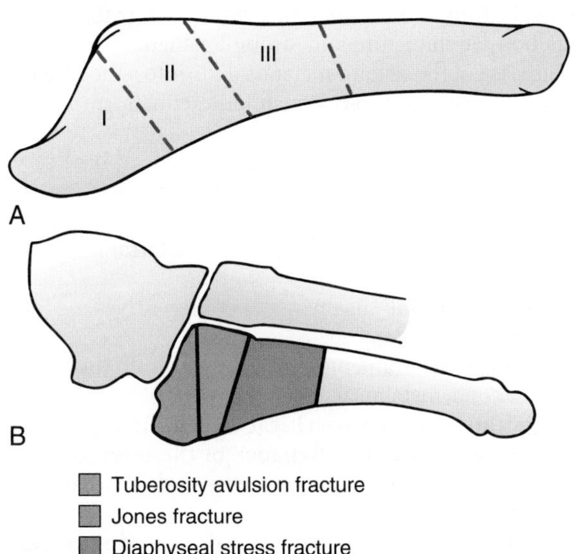

Figure 6-106 A and B, Three-part classification scheme as described by Botte. (From Coughlin M, et al: *Surgery of the foot and ankle,* ed 8, Philadelphia, 2006, Elsevier. [Courtesy of M. Botte.])

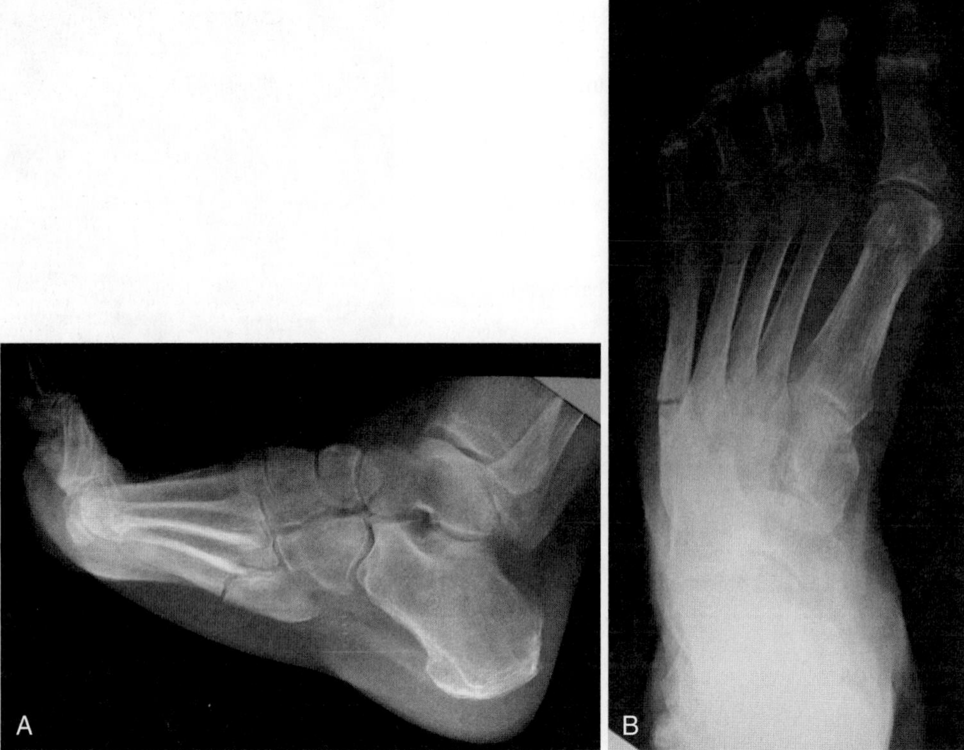

Figure 6-108 **Watch for the Jones fracture in the varus foot. A, This patient had a cavovarus foot deformity secondary to a stroke. Chronic lateral foot overload resulted in a fifth metatarsal fracture and subsequent nonunion. B, The fracture appears incompletely healed after 6 months of symptoms. The patient underwent surgery, including intramedullary screw placement and hindfoot osteotomy with muscle transfers, to balance the deformity.** (From DiGiovanni C: *Core knowledge in orthopaedics—foot and ankle,* Philadelphia, 2007, Elsevier.)

closed-wedge calcaneal osteotomy should be considered to prevent recurrence (Figure 6-108).

- If joint is unstable after reduction, pinning the joint for 3 to 4 weeks is indicated.

III. FIRST METATARSOPHALANGEAL JOINT INJURIES

A. Hallux MTP sprain (turf toe)—see the section, Sesamoids

B. Hallux MTP dislocation

1. Usually a dorsal dislocation secondary to hyperextension
2. Results in volar plate rupture at its insertion on the metatarsal neck
3. The classification indicates which structures are injured as well as likelihood of achieving closed reduction.
   - Type I—intersesamoid ligament is intact, likely plantar incarceration of the metatarsal head. Sesamoids may be intraarticular. No fracture present
     - Irreducible by closed methods
   - Type IIA—intersesamoid ligament ruptured
   - Type IIB—associated sesamoid fracture (usually tibial sesamoid) (Figure 6-109)
     - High possibility of closed reduction
   - Type IIC—combination of type IIA and IIB
4. Treatment
   - Type I injuries require open reduction with dorsal longitudinal approach.
   - Type II injuries are possible to close reduce.
     - They may have associated intraarticular fracture fragments that require excision.

IV. TARSOMETATARSAL FRACTURES AND DISLOCATIONS (LISFRANC INJURY)

A. Anatomy

1. The Lisfranc articulation is a stable construct because of its bony architecture and strong ligaments.
2. The base of the second metatarsal fits into a mortise formed by the proximally recessed middle cuneiform ("keystone configuration").
3. In the coronal plane, the second metatarsal base serves as the cornerstone in a "Roman arch" configuration (Figure 6-110).
4. Ligamentous anatomy of the tarsometatarsal joints (Figure 6-111)
   - Intermetatarsal ligaments between the second-fifth metatarsal bases.
     - No direct ligamentous attachment from the first to the second metatarsal
   - **Lisfranc ligament—critical to stabilizing the second metatarsal and maintenance of the midfoot arch**
     - **Between medial cuneiform and base of second metatarsal**
     - **Interosseous ligament is stiffest and strongest.**
     - **Plantar ligament inserts on base of second and third metatarsal.**

B. Diagnosis

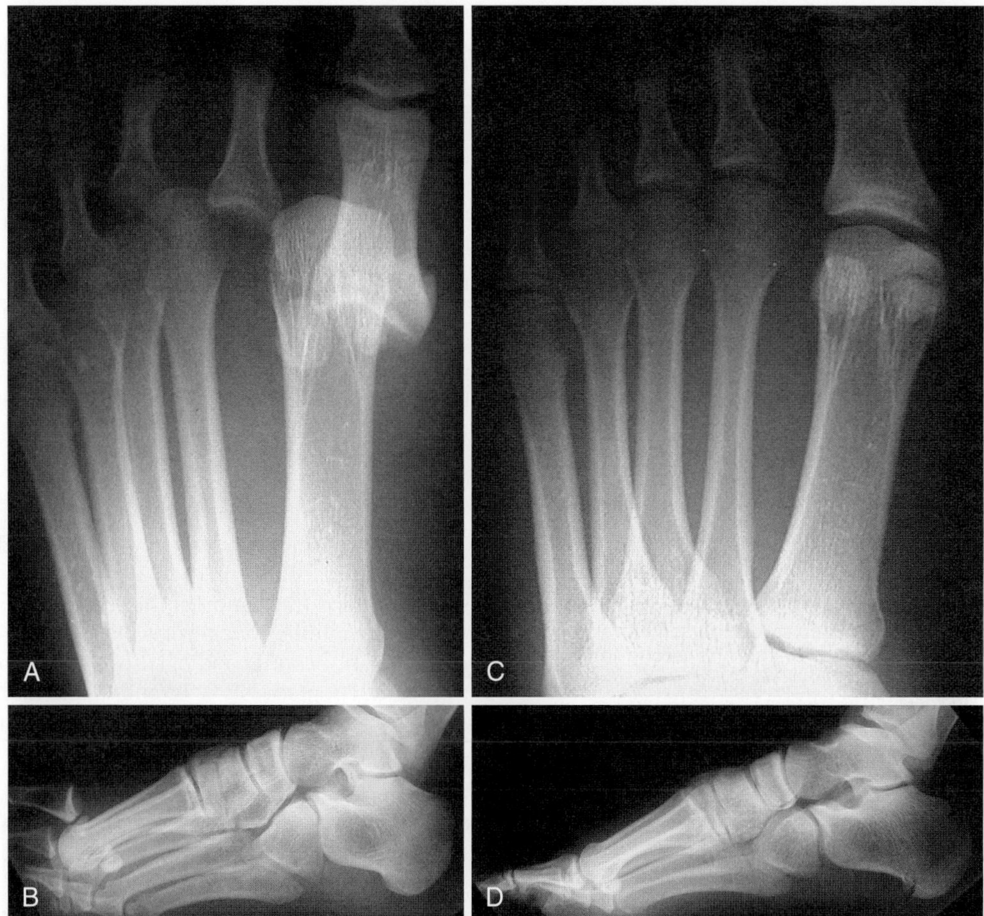

Figure 6-109 Type IIB dorsal dislocation of the first metatarsophalangeal joint, as seen on anteroposterior **(A)** and lateral **(B)** radiographs. Fracture through the medial sesamoid is best seen on the lateral view. Closed reduction was performed, also reducing the sesamoid fracture **(C and D)**. (From Coughlin M, et al: *Surgery of the foot and ankle,* ed 8, Philadelphia, 2006, Elsevier.)

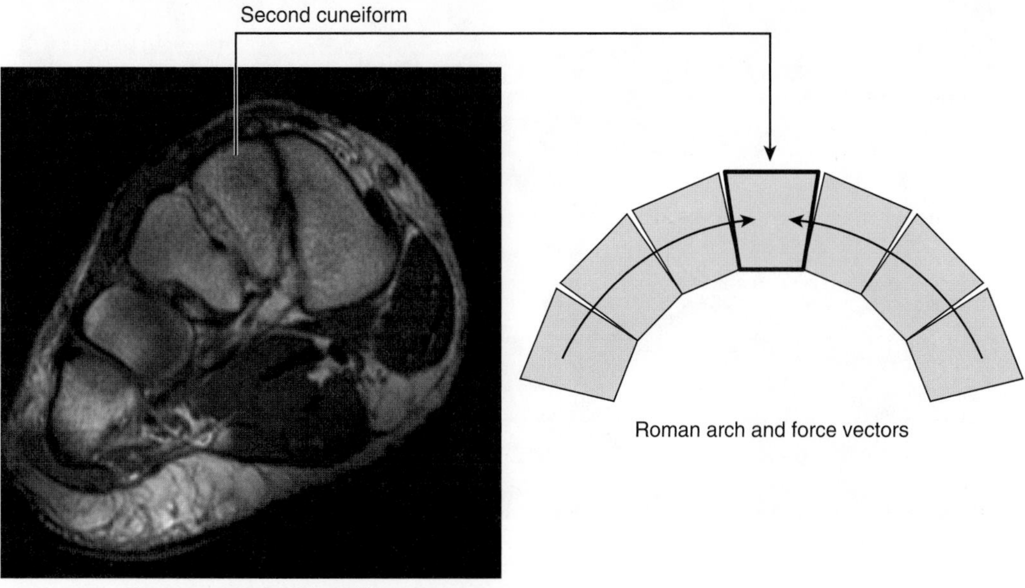

Figure 6-110 The second cuneiform and second metatarsal base are shaped like a keystone in the coronal plane. The Lisfranc joint is shaped like a Roman arch. This anatomy, and stabilization by the Lisfranc ligament, is important for support of the arch of the foot. (From Morrison W, Sanders T: *Problem solving in musculoskeletal imaging,* Philadelphia, 2008, Elsevier.)

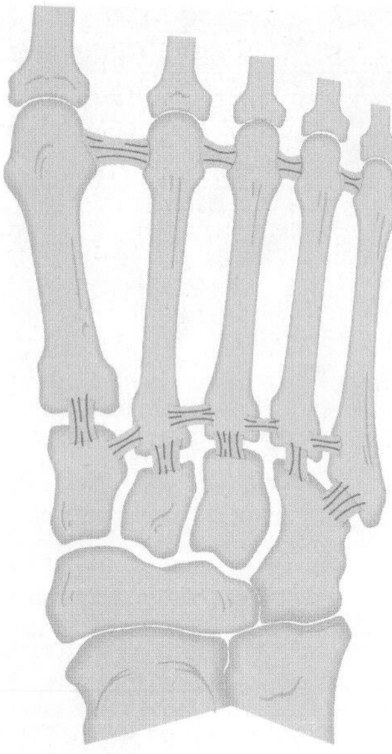

Figure 6-111 The Lisfranc articulation with its ligamentous attachments. Note the recessed second tarsometatarsal joint and the Lisfranc ligament in place of the first-second intermetatarsal ligament. (From DeLee J: *DeLee and Drez's orthopedic sports medicine,* ed 3, Philadelphia, 2011, Elsevier.)

1. Injuries range from nondisplaced, purely ligamentous disruptions to severe fracture-dislocations (Figure 6-112).
2. More common in men
3. Mechanism of injury
   - Indirect
     - Axial loading of a plantar-flexed foot
     - Athletic injury (most common), fall from height
     - Subtle and have a higher likelihood of being misdiagnosed
   - Direct
     - Motor vehicle accidents, crush injuries
     - Significant soft tissue injury, often open
4. Presentation
   - Severe pain, an inability to bear weight, marked swelling, and tenderness
   - Plantar ecchymosis should raise suspicion for a TMT injury.
5. Imaging
   - Anteroposterior, lateral, and oblique radiographs should be obtained (Figure 6-113).
     - Lateral translation of the second metatarsal relative to the middle cuneiform is diagnostic of a Lisfranc injury.
   - Weight-bearing radiographs with comparison view, abduction stress views, and single-limb weight-bearing views may be necessary to confirm diagnosis when clinical suspicion is high (Figure 6-114).

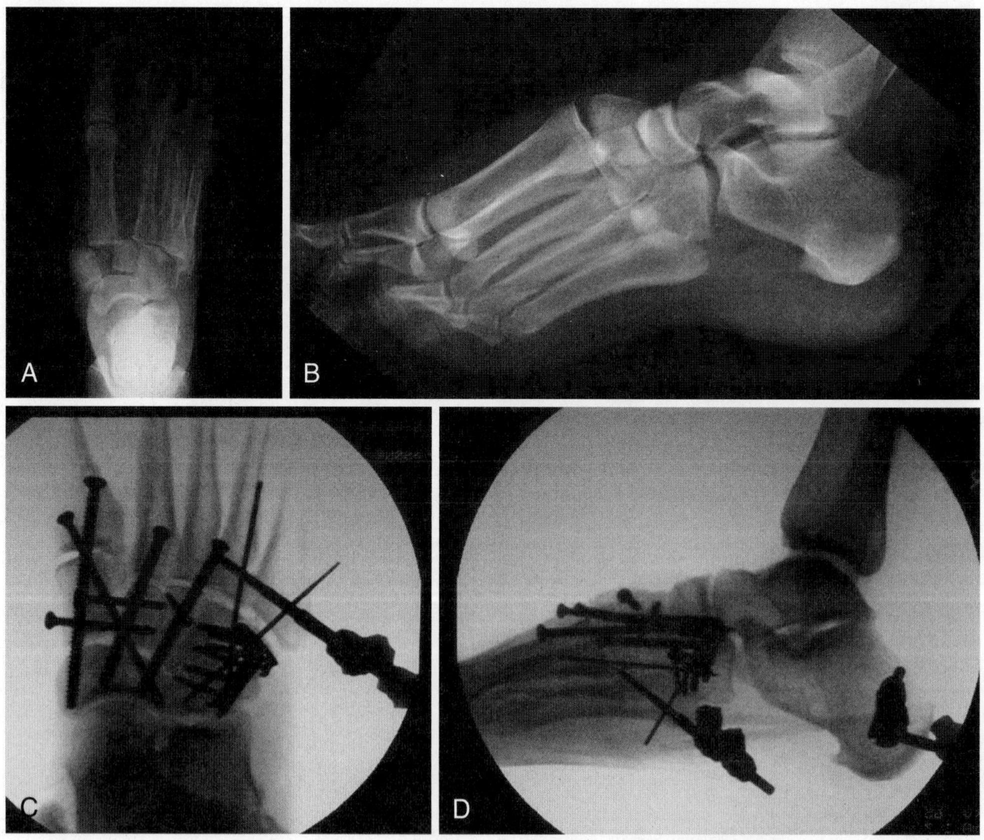

Figure 6-112 Commonly, intertarsal instability accompanies a Lisfranc (tarsometatarsal) injury. Sometimes it is occult, so a high index of suspicion should always be maintained intraoperatively and both clinical and radiographic stress examinations performed. Usually, however, it is overt (as in this case—**A, B**), and treatment is the same and demands rigid anatomic open reduction with internal fixation (ORIF) **(C, D).** The intertarsal instability can often be initially aligned with a medial or lateral column external fixator, as was used for this patient, after which fixation is made easier for the surgeon and should begin proximally and proceed distally so that abnormal anatomy can be realigned to normal anatomy in a sequential manner. Note that this technique helped with disimpaction of the lateral cuboid nutcracker injury, which also required ORIF with bone grafting to restore integrity to the lateral column. (From Browner B, et al: *Skeletal trauma,* ed 4, Philadelphia, 2008, Elsevier.

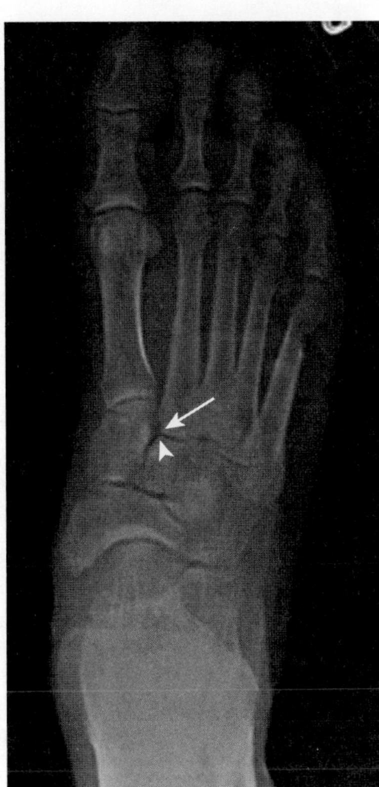

Figure 6-113 Normal anteroposterior weight-bearing radiograph demonstrating the alignment relationship between the base of the second metatarsal *(arrow)* and middle cuneiform *(arrowhead)*. Any lateral deviation of the second metatarsal relative to the middle cuneiform is consistent with a Lisfranc disruption and must be operatively treated. (From Miller M, Sanders T: *Presentation, imaging and treatment of common musculoskeletal conditions,* Philadelphia, 2011, Elsevier.)

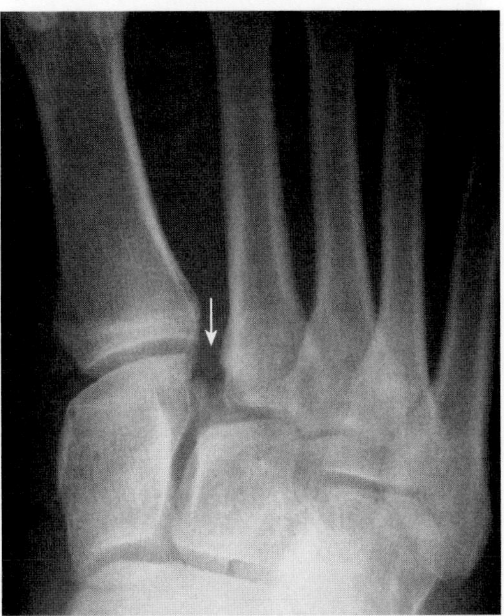

Figure 6-115 Lisfranc injury showing the fleck sign *(arrow)*. (From Mercier L: *Practical orthopaedics,* ed 6, Philadelphia, 2008, Elsevier.)

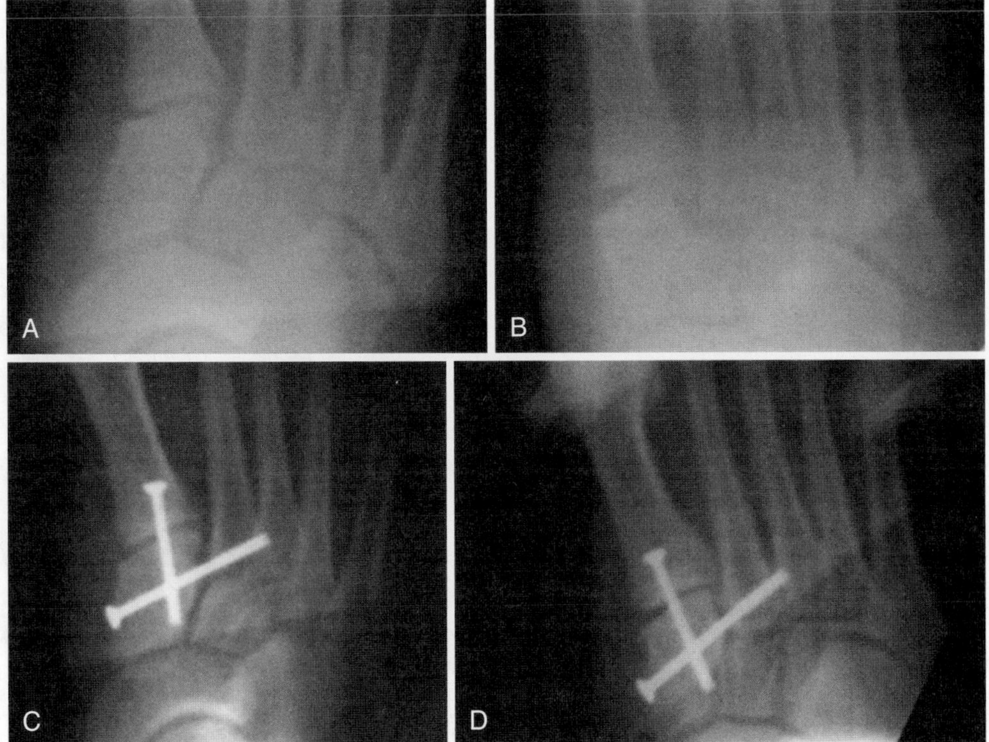

Figure 6-114 Anteroposterior and stress radiographs of foot with subtle Lisfranc dislocation. **A,** Radiograph appears normal. **B,** With stress into everted position, metatarsals sublux laterally. **C,** Postreduction radiograph reveals satisfactory reduction and internal fixation. **D,** Reduction maintained on eversion stress radiograph. (From Canale ST, Beaty J: *Campbell's operative orthopedics,* ed 11, Philadelphia, 2007, Elsevier.)

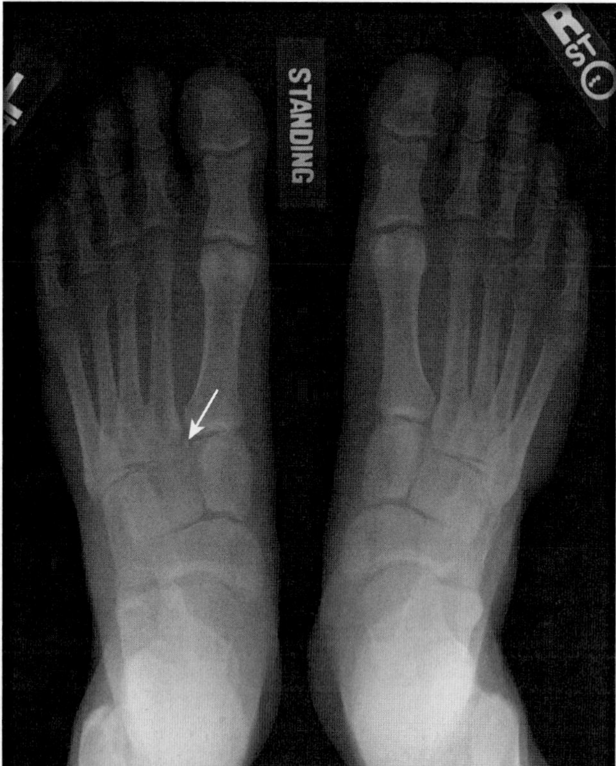

Figure 6-116 Patient with a Lisfranc injury identified by the fleck sign *(arrow)*. In this case, the ligament itself remained intact and the injury occurs by avulsion of the ligament from the base of the second metatarsal. The function of the ligament is compromised, and operative intervention is indicated. (From Miller M, Sanders T: *Presentation, imaging and treatment of common musculoskeletal conditions,* Philadelphia, 2011, Elsevier.)

- "Fleck sign" (Figure 6-115)
  - Small, bony avulsion from the base of the second metatarsal seen in the first intermetatarsal space
  - Diagnostic of a Lisfranc injury
- Proximal variant—forces transmit through the intercuneiform joint, may be subtle (Figure 6-116)

6. Classification
   - Differentiating between purely ligamentous injuries and fracture-dislocations may have treatment implications.
     - **Primary arthrodesis of the tarsometatarsal joints is an alternative to ORIF in a purely ligamentous injury.**
   - Multiple described classification schemes are not useful for determining treatment and prognosis.
7. Treatment
   - Anatomic reduction is most predictive of good clinical results.
   - Nonsurgical management is indicated only in cases with no displacement on weight-bearing and stress radiographs and no evidence of bony injury on CT (usually dorsal sprains).
     - Operative treatment—Any displacement on radiographs or evidence of a bony injury is treated with ORIF.
     - Should be delayed until the soft tissue swelling has resolved
     - Anatomic reduction is mandatory; therefore open reduction is preferred to closed reduction with percutaneous fixation.
     - Fixation should proceed from proximal to distal and medial to lateral.
     - Medial and middle column (first, second, and third TMT joints, intercuneiform joint)
       - Typically stabilized with screw fixation across the involved joints (Figure 6-117)
       - Dorsal plating is gaining in popularity because of less iatrogenic articular damage.
       - Fixation is commonly removed after 4 months to minimize the risk of hardware failure and restore the normal joint mechanics.
     - Lateral column (fourth, fifth TMT joint)
       - Temporary fixation with K-wires due to mobile segment
       - Removed at 6 weeks
     - **Primary arthrodesis is an alternative treatment option, with some benefit seen in patients with purely ligamentous injury or significant intraarticular comminution (Figure 6-118).**
   - Complications
     - **Missed diagnosis or improper treatment may lead to traumatic planovalgus deformity or posttraumatic arthritis.**
     - **Midfoot realignment and arthrodesis is the appropriate salvage procedure (Figure 6-119).**

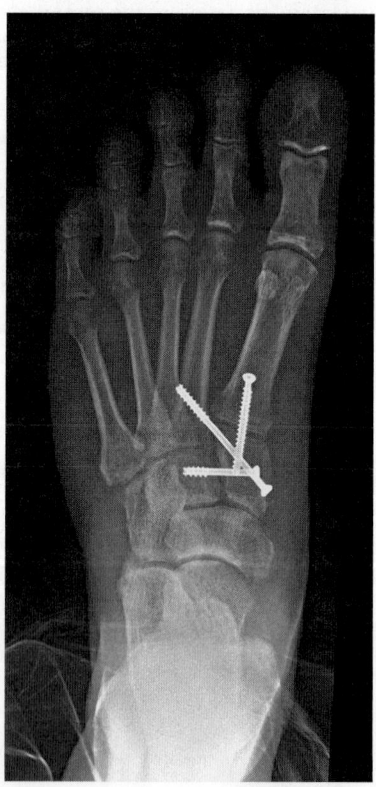

Figure 6-117 Postoperative radiograph of patient that was treated with screw fixation. In addition to a screw transfixing the first tarsometatarsal joint, the "Lisfranc" screw was used to hold the second metatarsal reduced. In this case instability of the intercuneiform joint was noted and required fixation. (From Miller M, Sanders T: *Presentation, imaging and treatment of common musculoskeletal conditions,* Philadelphia, 2011, Elsevier.)

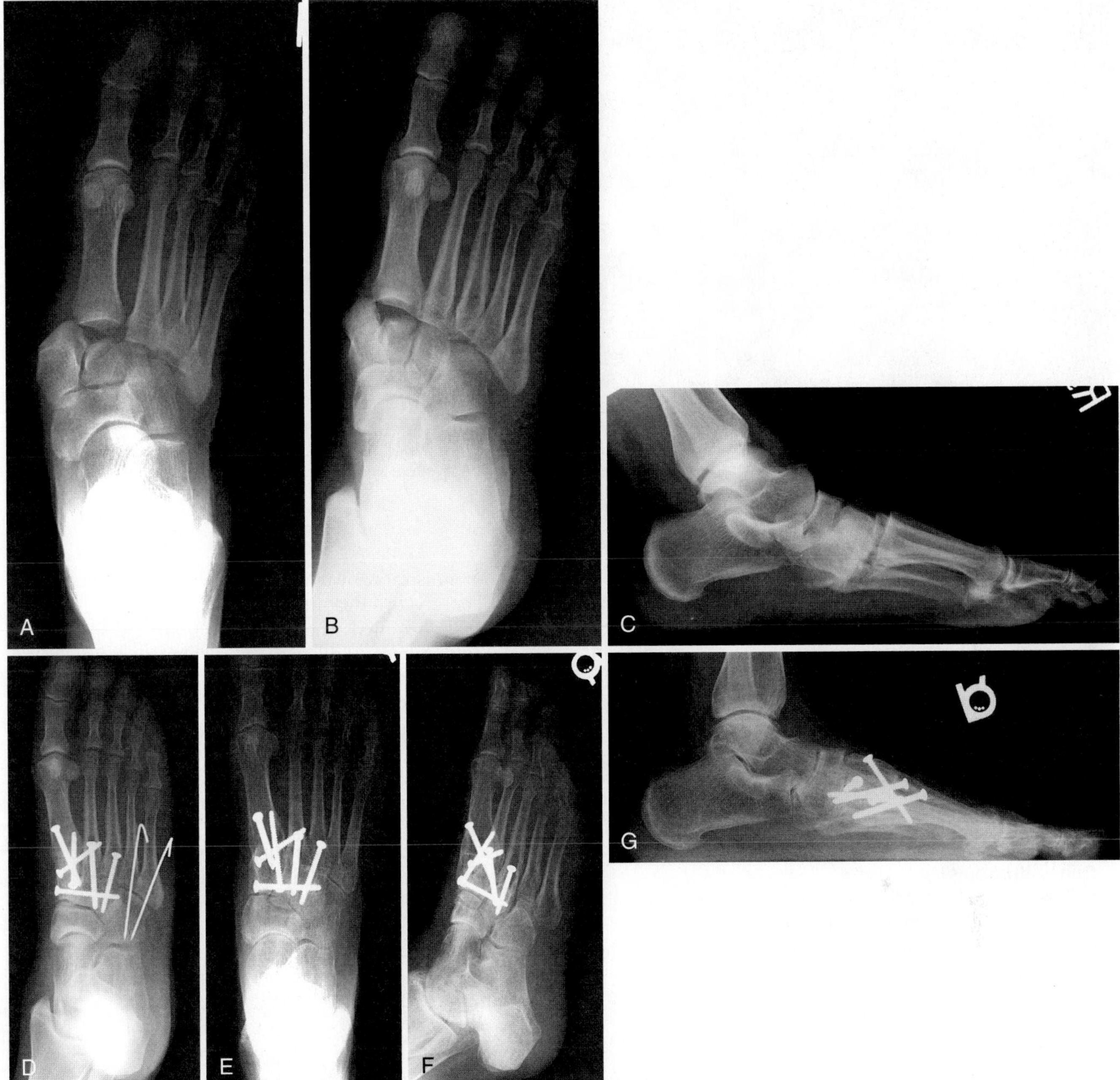

Figure 6-118 Lisfranc and midtarsal injury treated with primary arthrodesis of the first through third tarsometatarsal (TMT) joints. Anteroposterior **(A)**, oblique **(B)**, and lateral **(C)** radiographs of a Lisfranc injury with dorsolateral dislocation of all metatarsal bases without associated fracture. The lateral radiographs also show associated injury to the midtarsal joint with plantar fracture-dislocation of the navicular, which required open reduction internal fixation to stabilize this articulation. Primary arthrodesis may be indicated in true TMT dislocations because the long-term stability of these joints depends on ligamentous healing, which is less reliable than bony healing. **D,** Oblique postoperative radiograph showing arthrodesis of the medial three TMT joints and provisional Kirschner-wire fixation of the fourth and fifth TMT joints. Weight-bearing anteroposterior **(E)**, oblique **(F)**, and lateral **(G)** radiographs 1 year postoperatively. (From Coughlin M, et al: *Surgery of the foot and ankle,* ed 8, Philadelphia, 2006, Elsevier.)

V. MIDFOOT INJURIES (EXCLUDING LISFRANC INJURIES)

A. Anatomy

1. Midfoot consists of the navicular, the three cuneiforms, the cuboid, and their corresponding articulations.
2. Acts as a stout connection between the forefoot and hindfoot
   - Relatively immobile, with strong plantar ligaments
   - Serves an important shock-absorbing function
   - Chopart and Lisfranc joints are therefore of greater functional importance than the articulations among the midfoot bones.
   - Cuboid is critical to the integrity of the lateral column.

B. Cuboid injuries

1. Often associated with other midfoot or Lisfranc fractures/ dislocations

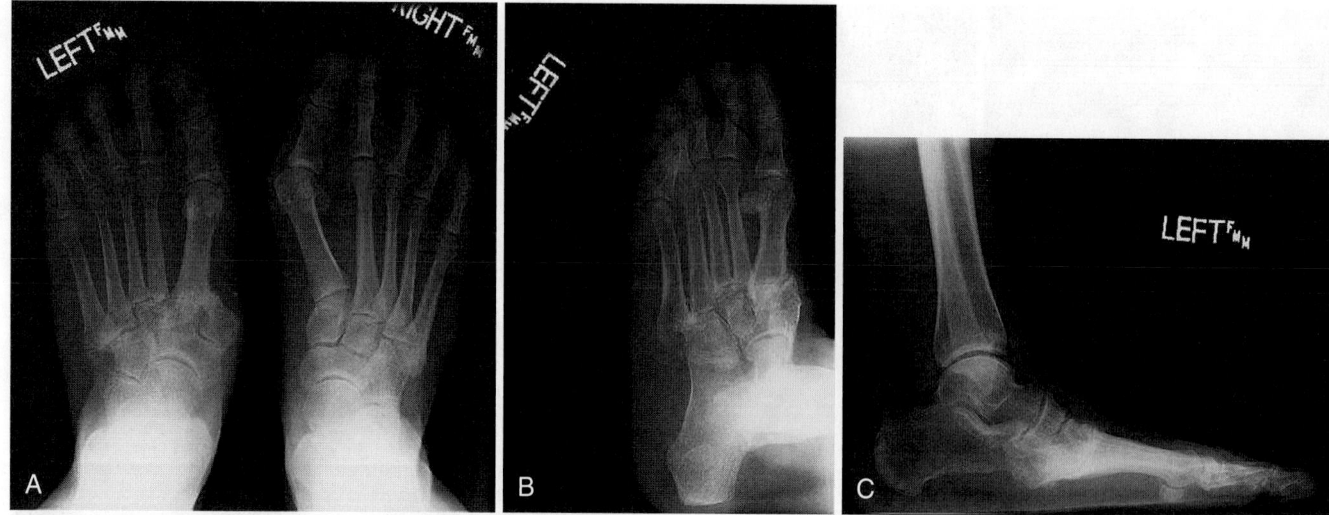

Figure 6-119 A to C, This severe post-traumatic deformity was symptomatic in each of the three midfoot columns. Note the severe abduction of the entire tarsometatarsal joint complex. (From Myerson M: *Reconstructive foot and ankle surgery: management of complications,* ed 2, Philadelphia, 2010, Elsevier.)

2. Radiographic evaluation
   - Anteroposterior, lateral, and oblique (30-degree medial oblique is ideal) views
   - Weight-bearing/stress views can help ascertain midfoot stability if there is clinical concern.
   - CT may be required to define fracture fragments and articular congruity.
3. Cuboid avulsion from the CC articulation
   - Most common, due to an inversion force (lateral ankle sprain)
   - Treat conservatively, with weight bearing as tolerated in boot or brace.
4. Cuboid fractures
   - Results from forced plantar flexion and abduction of the forefoot resulting in an axial load
   - Often causes comminuted, impacted fracture, or "nutcracker" fracture (Figure 6-120)
   - Treatment
     - Nondisplaced, minimal articular involvement—conservative treatment in boot
     - ORIF required when comminution or displacement compromises the length and alignment of the lateral column.
     - Lateral column external fixation can be used as an aid to obtain length or for definitive fixation in severely comminuted cases (Figure 6-121).
5. Cuboid syndrome
   - Painful subluxation seen in athletes, especially ballet dancers
   - The patient may have pain or a palpable "click" as the foot is brought from plantar flexion and inversion to dorsiflexion and eversion.
6. Complete dislocation of the cuboid
   - Extremely rare, often due to higher-energy mechanisms
   - Usually displaced in a plantar and medial direction

C. **Cuneiform injuries**

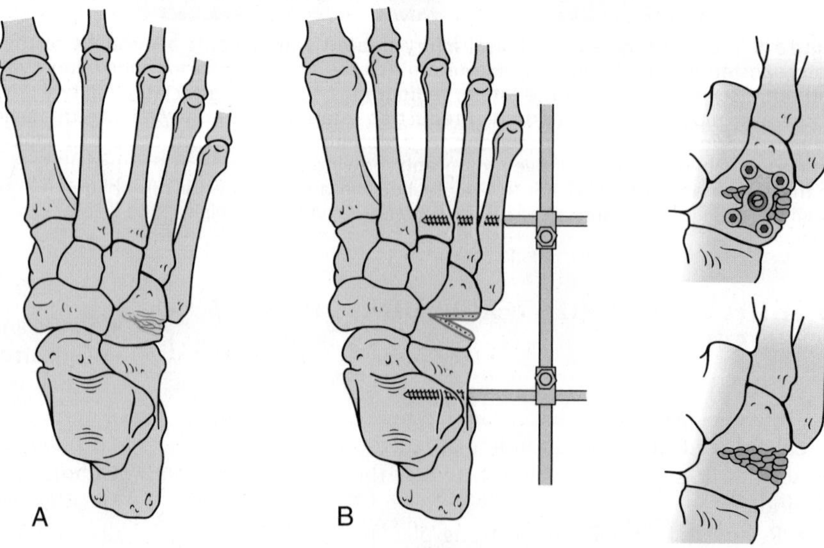

Figure 6-120 A, A so-called "nutcracker impaction" injury of the cuboid shortens the lateral column of the foot, thereby causing a pes planus deformity because of a relative mismatch with the medial column. **B,** External fixation to distract the fracture corrects the deformity but leaves a void. Stable healing requires bone grafting, often augmented with a small buttress plate. (From Browner B, et al: *Skeletal trauma,* ed 4, Philadelphia, 2008, Elsevier.)

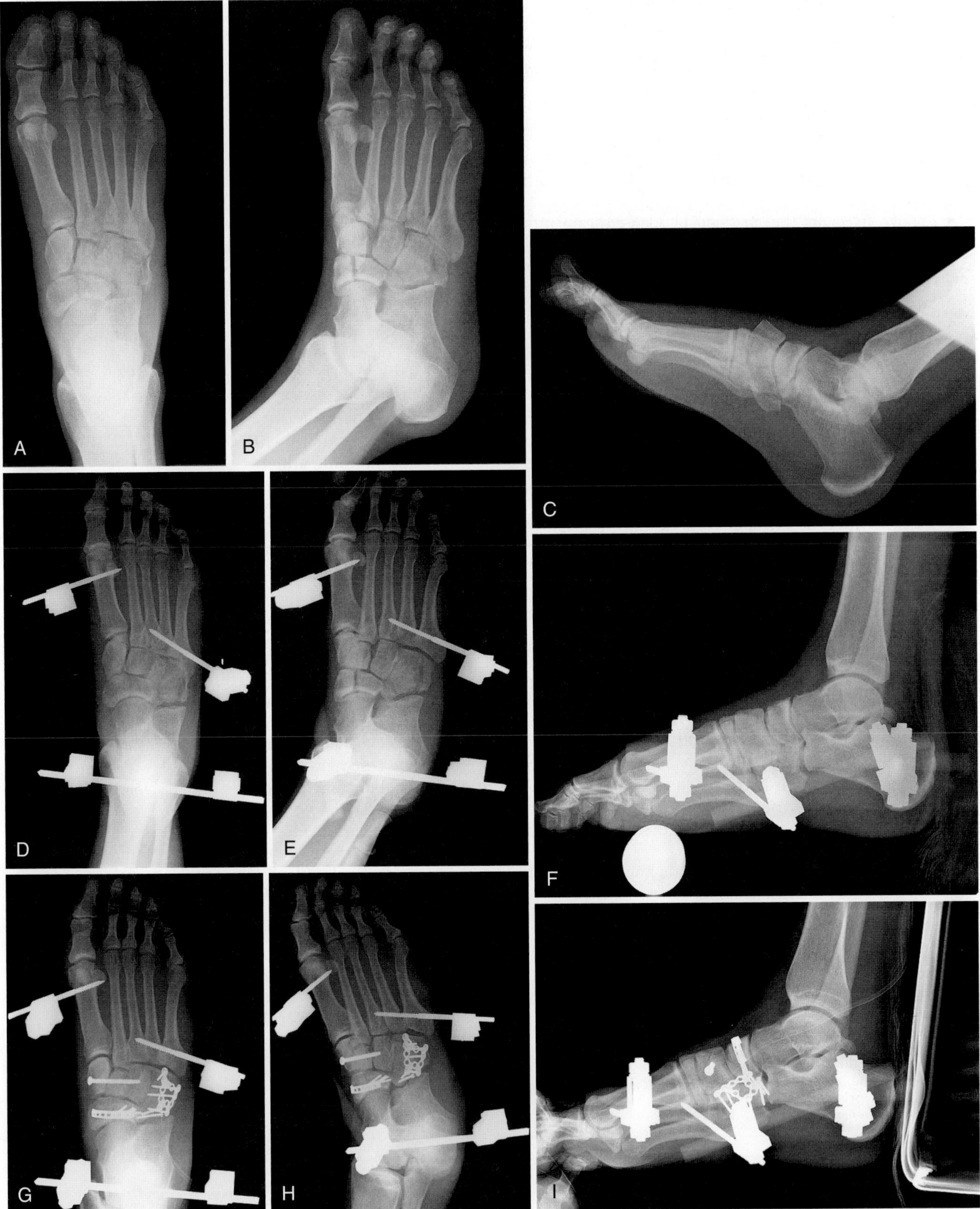

Figure 6-121 Navicular and cuboid fractures with middle (second) cuneiform dislocation. This patient sustained these injuries in a motor vehicle crash. **A** and **B,** Anteroposterior and oblique injury radiographs. **C,** Lateral injury radiograph. **D** to **F,** Definitive open reduction with internal fixation (ORIF) of this patient's injuries could not be accomplished acutely due to profuse edema. Closed reduction of middle (second) cuneiform dislocation and of foot alignment was accomplished and held using a through-and-through calcaneal tuberosity pin, attached via carbon fiber rods to a distal first metatarsal pin medially and a proximal fourth and fifth metatarsal pin laterally. **G** to **I,** Definitive ORIF was accomplished after foot edema was controlled. A single intercuneiform screw holds the middle (second) cuneiform reduced. Plate fixation is noted on the navicular and cuboid, maintaining anatomic reduction. The medial and lateral external fixator was left in place for 6 weeks to supplement fixation support. (From DiGiovanni C: *Core knowledge in orthopaedics—foot and ankle,* Philadelphia, 2007, Elsevier.)

1. Most occur in association with other midfoot injuries, in particular Lisfranc injuries
2. The medial cuneiform is the most commonly injured.
   - Displaced or unstable medial cuneiform injuries require anatomic reduction and stable fixation.

D. Navicular fractures

1. Anatomy
   - The navicular articulates with the talar head on its concave proximal surface and with the three cuneiforms distally.
   - Rigidly fixed in the midfoot by dense ligamentous attachments
   - Blood supply—Dorsalis pedis supplies the dorsum, medial plantar branch of the posterior tibial artery supplies the plantar surface, and branches of these arteries create a plexus to supply the tuberosity.
     - The central portion of the bone is relatively less vascular and therefore at risk for stress injuries and nonunions.
2. Classification
   - Navicular fractures classified as avulsion, tuberosity, body, and stress injuries
   - Avulsion fractures
     - Ligamentous attachments (usually from dorsal TN joint) avulse a fragment of bone during inversion, twisting, and hyper–plantar flexion injuries.
     - Most common, treated symptomatically
   - Navicular tuberosity fractures
     - Secondary to acute eversion of the foot with simultaneous contraction of the tibialis posterior
     - Displacement usually minimal due to broad attachment of the posterior tibial tendon
     - Concomitant lateral injury is common (anterior process of the calcaneus, cuboid fracture).
     - Treatment
       - Nondisplaced or minimally displaced fractures treated in cast or boot
       - Fractures displaced more than 5 mm have high chance of nonunion; surgical fixation recommended
       - Small avulsions or symptomatic nonunions can be treated with excision.
   - Navicular body fractures
     - Mechanism of injury—axial load to a plantar-flexed foot with either abduction or adduction through the midtarsal joints
     - Type I fracture—transverse in the coronal plane, dorsal fragment less than 50% of body
     - Type II fracture—dorsal-lateral to plantar-medial with resultant medialization (adduction) of the fragment and forefoot
     - Type III fracture—central or lateral comminution with possible lateral displacement of the foot
     - Treatment—ORIF of even minimally displaced fractures is recommended.
       - Goal is to preserve TN and therefore hindfoot motion.
       - May require external fixation to preserve medial column length or as aid in fracture reduction
       - Primary or delayed arthrodesis of involved joints may be required with extensive comminution.
   - Navicular stress fractures
     - **Secondary to repetitive trauma, especially running and jumping athletes**
     - Cavus feet a predisposing factor
     - **Typically occur in the central one third of the navicular**
     - **Patients complain of vague dorsal midfoot or ankle pain.**
     - Physical examination reveals tenderness at dorsal central navicular.
     - Imaging
       - Anteroposterior, lateral, and oblique foot views may or may not show fracture.
       - MRI and bone scan can aid in the diagnosis.
       - **CT gold standard, defines complete and incomplete fractures, displaced versus nondisplaced**
         - Best viewed on coronal images (Figure 6-122)
         - Fracture line extends from dorsolateral to plantar medial.
     - Treatment
       - **Conservative treatment recommended for nondisplaced fractures—Non–weight bearing (usually in cast for 6 to 8 weeks) is critical.**

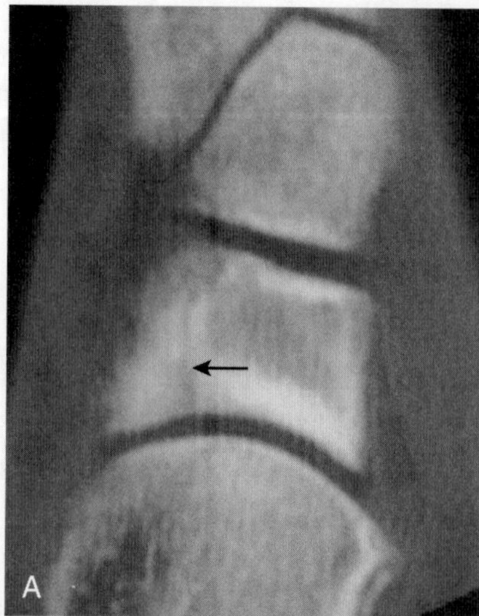

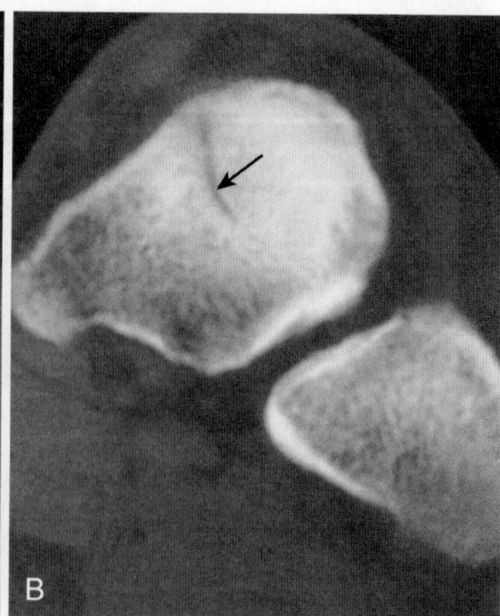

Figure 6-122 Stress fractures: computed tomographic (CT) scanning. Tarsal navicular bone. Transverse **(A)** and coronal **(B)** CT scans show a typical fatigue fracture *(arrows)* of the tarsal navicular bone. These fractures are usually located in the proximal and dorsal aspect of the bone, and they have a vertical or vertical-oblique orientation. (From Resnick D: *Internal derangements of joints,* ed 2, Philadelphia, 2006, Elsevier.)

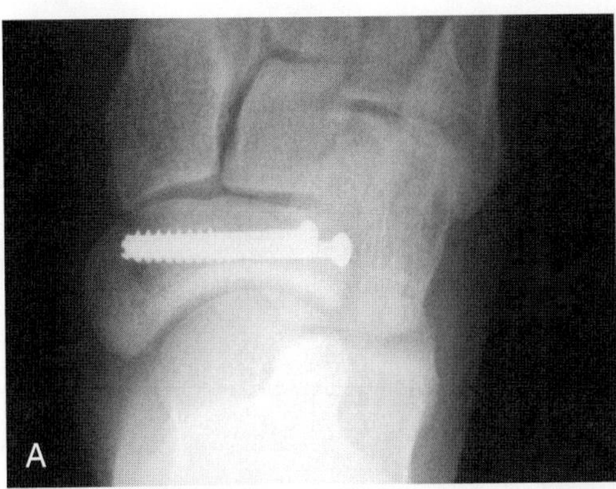

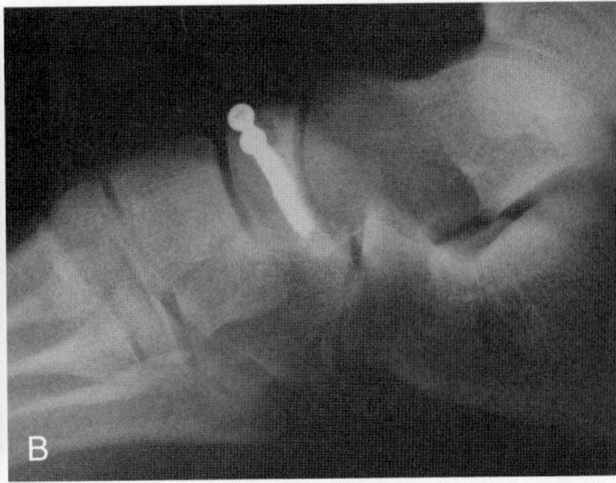

Figure 6-123 Anteroposterior **(A)** and lateral **(B)** radiographs of completed screw fixation. (From Coughlin M, et al: *Surgery of the foot and ankle,* ed 8, Philadelphia, 2006, Elsevier.)

- Surgical treatment with transverse screw placement recommended for displaced fractures or fractures with evidence of nonunion
  - Screw should be placed from dorsolateral to plantar medial (Figure 6-123).
- Bone grafting may be necessary.
- Initial surgical treatment may be considered in elite athletes, though controversy remains.
- The two most common complications of navicular fractures are degenerative arthritis and avascular necrosis.

VI. ANKLE FRACTURES

(See Chapter 17, Trauma)

VII. TALUS FRACTURES

A. Constitute less than 1% of all fractures, but rank second (behind calcaneus fractures) among all tarsal bone injuries

B. Anatomy

1. More than half of the surface area of the talus is covered by articular cartilage.
2. The neck is angled in a medial and plantar direction relative to the axis of the body.
3. There are no muscular or ligamentous attachments.
4. **Blood supply—provided by three main vessels: the posterior tibial artery, the dorsalis pedis artery, and the perforating peroneal artery**
   - The arteries of the tarsal sinus, the tarsal canal, and the deltoid are important branches of the main vessels.
   - **The artery of the tarsal canal carries the main supply to the talar body.**
   - The head and neck are vascularized by the artery of the tarsal sinus and the dorsalis pedis.
5. A thorough understanding of the relationship between fracture displacement and those vessels that are disrupted is extremely important when operative approaches and fixation are planned.

C. Classification

1. Talar neck fractures—Hawkins classification (Figure 6-124)
   - Type I fracture—only one of three main sources of blood supply disrupted
     - Truly nondisplaced talar neck fractures are rare—Any amount of displacement should be treated as a type II injury.
   - Type II fracture—two of three main sources of blood supply disrupted (artery of the tarsal canal and tarsal sinus)
     - The deltoid branch of the posterior tibial artery is the only remaining blood supply, emphasizing the critical requirement to preserve the deltoid ligament during all surgical approaches.
   - Type III fracture—The blood supply has theoretically been completely compromised. However, in minimally displaced fracture, the deltoid branch of the posterior tibial artery may remain intact.
   - Type IV fracture—may also have disrupted vascularity to the talar head and neck
2. Talar body fractures
   - Lateral process acts as dividing line.
     - Inferior fracture lines that exit anterior to the lateral process are identified as talar neck fractures.
     - Fractures posterior to the lateral process are classified as body fractures.
   - Talar body fractures affect both the subtalar and tibiotalar articulations.

D. Mechanism of injury

1. Most common mechanism is a fall from a significant height or a motor vehicle collision.
2. Forceful dorsiflexion of the foot leads to impaction of the more narrow talar neck on the anterior tibia.
   - The energy propagates through the ligaments that stabilize the subtalar joint, leading to subluxation or dislocation of the body.
   - If the hindfoot deviates into supination, the talar neck can fracture the medial malleolus, become impacted and comminuted, and result in talar head rotation and displacement.

E. Diagnosis

1. Marked swelling, gross deformity, and soft tissue compromise common
2. Decreased plantar sensation may be present with posteromedial extrusion of talar body in type III injuries.
3. Imaging
   - Anteroposterior, lateral, and Canale oblique radiographs should be routine.
   - CT scanning is very useful for evaluating the fracture pattern, comminution, and angulation during preoperative planning.

F. Treatment

1. Goal is to obtain anatomic reduction (length, rotation, angulation) and rigid stabilization.

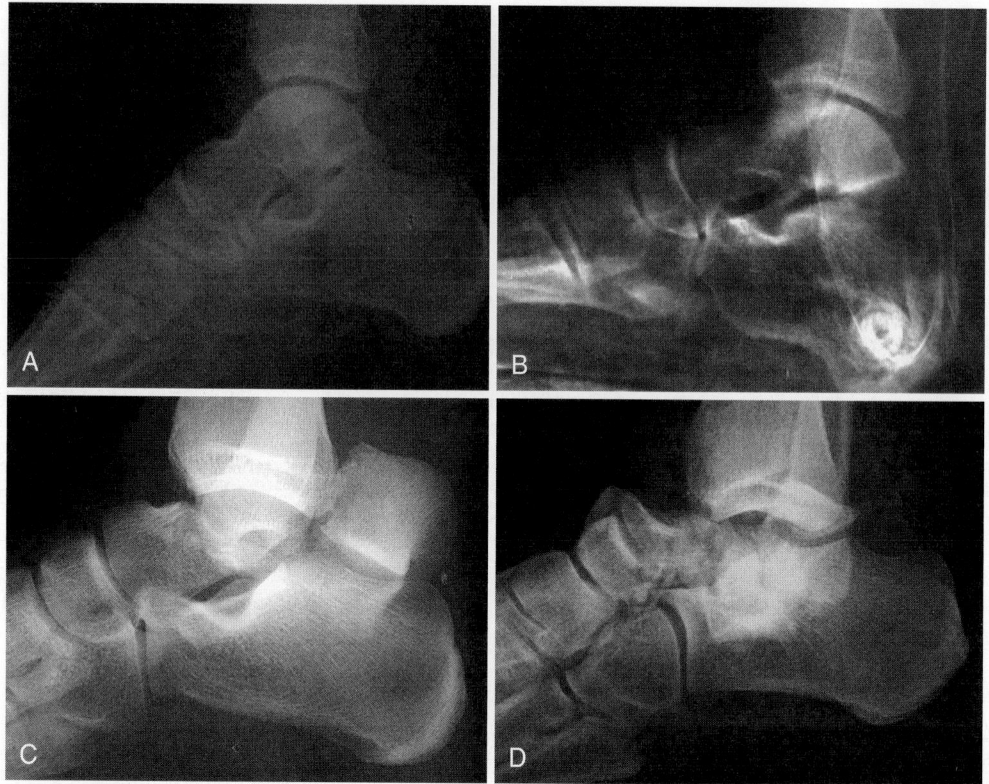

Figure 6-124 **The Hawkins classification of talar neck fractures remains useful because it is relatively simple, guides treatment, and has prognostic value. A, Type I fracture (minimally displaced). B, Type II fracture with displacement of the subtalar joint. C, Type III fracture with displacement of the subtalar and tibiotalar joints. D, The type IV fracture as described by Canale includes a talar neck fracture with displacement of the subtalar, tibiotalar, and talonavicular joint.** (From Browner B, et al: *Skeletal trauma,* ed 4, Philadelphia, 2008, Elsevier.)

- Even slight displacement can significantly alter the contact characteristics of the subtalar joint.

2. Controversy exists regarding the timing of surgical fixation of displaced talar neck fractures.
   - Most recent studies show no correlation between time to fixation and development of osteonecrosis.
   - Dislocations should be urgently reduced.
3. Talonavicular incongruity or instability warrants operative fixation to minimize post-traumatic arthrosis.
   - The TN joint is critical to overall hindfoot motion.
   - Talonavicular fusion for talar head fractures should be a salvage procedure.
4. Talar neck fractures
   - Medial malleolar osteotomy NOT required for open reduction
   - Type I—immobilization in a non–weight-bearing cast for 6 to 8 weeks
     - Frequent radiographs required to evaluate for fracture displacement
     - CT required to ensure that the fracture is non-displaced
   - Type II
     - Significant displacement may lead to skin compromise.
       - Closed reduction should be performed with plantar flexion and heel manipulation.
     - **Medial neck comminution is common, leading to varus deformity.**
     - ORIF required
       - Dual medial and lateral incisions is best approach to appropriately gauge talar length and angulation.
       - **Be careful to preserve medial blood supply from the deltoid artery.**
       - Fixation achieved with combination of screws and/or minifragment plates
         - A minimally displaced fracture without comminution is ideal for percutaneous screw fixation (Figure 6-125).
         - Medial compression screw may worsen varus deformity if comminution is present. A fully threaded screw or plate should be used medially to avoid this complication.
         - Be careful not to underestimate the degree of varus angulation and medial impaction.
   - Type III
     - Requires immediate closed or, if necessary, open reduction
     - Similar approach to type II injuries. Comminution is more common, and fixation with minifragment plate is commonly required (Figure 6-126).
     - Associated medial malleolus fracture is common.
     - These are at significant risk for avascular necrosis, subtalar and ankle post-traumatic arthritis, malunion, and nonunion.
   - Type IV
     - Similar treatment and approach to type II and III injuries

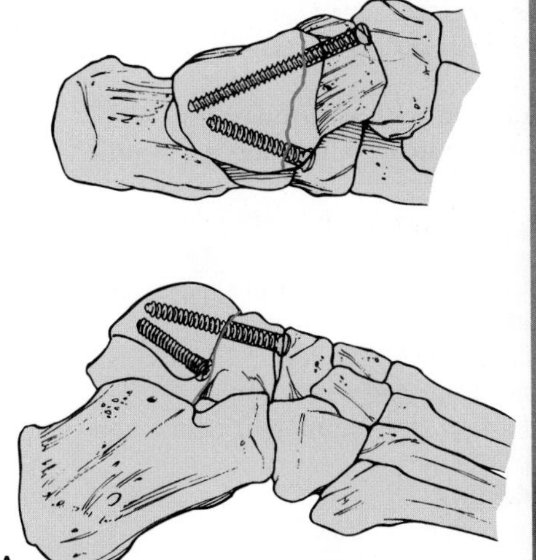

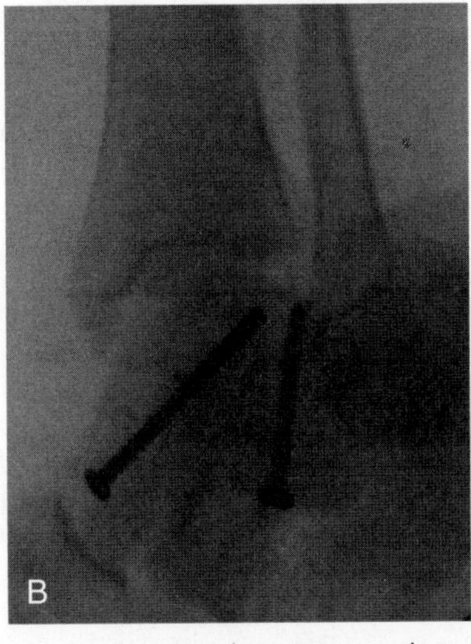

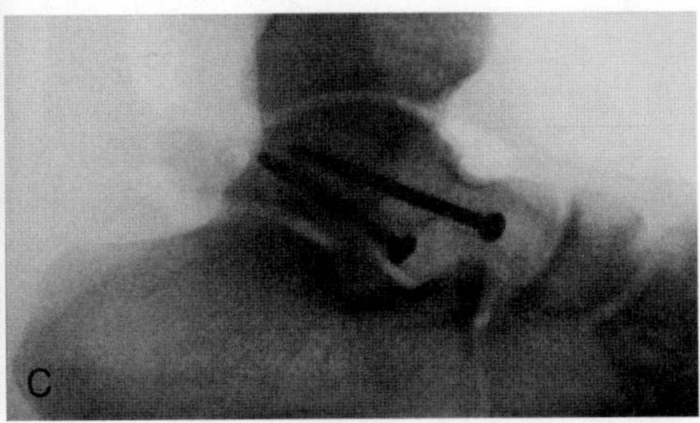

Figure 6-125 Screws placed anterior to posterior can be placed percutaneously to stabilize a minimally displaced talar neck fracture. Two 3.5-mm cortical screws are placed across a fracture located at the base of the neck of the talus. The first screw, which is placed medially, is countersunk into the articular surface. The second screw is placed through a 3.5-mm gliding hole in the sinus tarsi and a 2.5-mm thread hole in the body. **A,** In this case, both screws are inserted approximately perpendicular to the fracture line and along the midaxial line of the talar neck to avoid creating dorsal or plantar gapping along the fracture line during compression. **B,** Intraoperative Canale view demonstrating screw placement. **C,** Intraoperative lateral view showing screw location. (From Browner B, et al: *Skeletal trauma,* ed 4, Philadelphia, 2008, Elsevier.)

- May require stabilization of the TN joint
- Increased risk of avascular necrosis of the talar head and body
- Type IV injuries offer the worst prognosis.

- Complications
  - Subtalar arthritis is the most common complication.
  - **Varus malunion**
    - **Highly associated with use of medial compression screws**
    - **Results in a cavovarus deformity, limiting hindfoot eversion that results in lateral border foot pain**
    - If arthritis present—triple arthrodesis
      - Isolated subtalar fusion cannot correct the deformity because the site of the deformity is distal to the subtalar joint in the talar neck (Figure 6-127).
    - No arthritis present
      - Open-wedge osteotomy of medial talar neck
  - Avascular necrosis (Table 6-5)
    - Increases with severity of the injury—approaches 100% with a type IV injury
    - **Hawkins sign—subchondral linear lucency of the talar dome that is indicative of talar revascularization (Figure 6-128). Sclerosis of the talar dome (increased density) does not guarantee that avascular necrosis has occurred, although it is suggestive.**

5. Talar body fractures
   - Nondisplaced fractures treated with immobilization for 6 to 8 weeks
   - Any displacement requires anatomic reduction and stable internal fixation.
     - Usually achieved with small-fragment or minifragment lag screws
   - Medial or lateral malleolar osteotomy may be required for adequate visualization.

Table 6-5 Hawkins Classification of Talar Neck Fractures

Type	Description	Treatment	Complications
I	Nondisplaced talar neck fracture	Non–weight-bearing cast until union (usually 6-8 wk)	AVN, 13% (fractures that develop AVN may have reduced spontaneously)
II	Displaced talar neck fracture with subluxation or dislocation of subtalar joint but intact ankle mortise	Occasionally closed reduction and internal fixation in sagittal plane with fluoroscopy (usually ORIF)	AVN, 30%-45% Post-traumatic arthritis of the subtalar joint, 40%-90%
III	Displaced talar neck fracture with dislocation of talar body from ankle mortise	ORIF	AVN, 90%-100% Post-traumatic arthritis of the subtalar and tibiotalar joints, 40%-90% Nonunion, 13% Malunion, 27%
IV	Displaced talar neck fracture with dislocation of talar body from ankle mortise and subluxation or dislocation of talonavicular joint	ORIF	AVN, 90%-100% Post-traumatic arthritis of the subtalar and tibiotalar joints, 40%-90% Nonunion, 13% Malunion, 27%

AVN, avascular necrosis; ORIF, open reduction with internal fixation.

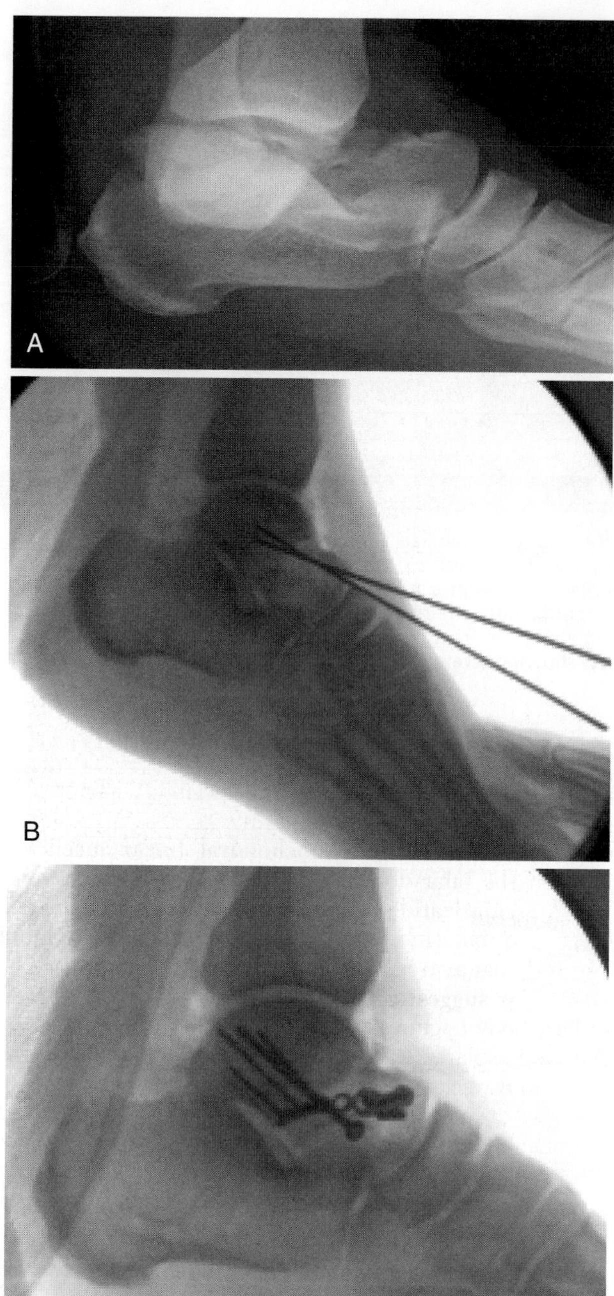

Figure 6-126 In Hawkins type III injuries, the talar body is often extruded posteromedially from the ankle and subtalar joint **(A)**. The fracture is then reduced through standard medial and lateral approaches, and provisional fixation is achieved with K wires **(B)**. Stable fixation is achieved with a 2.0-mm blade plate on the lateral side and a compression screw medially **(C)**.

6. Talar body extrusion
   - With minimal contamination and any remaining soft tissue attachment, talar body should be copiously irrigated, débrided, and reimplanted.
   - In the presence of gross contamination, may be appropriate to disregard the body and perform a delayed reconstruction
     - Rates of deep infection and overall failure are very high.
7. Lateral process talus fractures
   - Mechanism—dorsiflexion, inversion, and external rotation of the foot
   - **Highly associated with snowboarding**
   - **Source of continued pain after a "simple" ankle sprain**
     - Best seen on the anteroposterior ankle radiograph (Figure 6-129)
     - CT should be performed to evaluate the extent of comminution.
   - Treatment depends on the degree of articular involvement, displacement, and comminution.
   - Nondisplaced fractures—immobilized in a non–weight-bearing cast or boot
   - Displaced fractures
     - ORIF if amenable to screw fixation
   - Excision if small or significantly comminuted

VIII. CALCANEUS FRACTURES

A. Extraarticular calcaneal fractures

1. Avulsion fractures of the tuberosity
   - Caused by forceful Achilles tendon contraction
   - Nondisplaced treated with immobilization
   - **May endanger posterior skin if significant displacement (Figure 6-130)**
   - **Urgent operative reduction and fixation required if skin is compromised**
   - Fixation achieved with lag screws from the posterior superior tuberosity directed inferior and distal
   - Percutaneous technique is most commonly used for this fracture.
2. Anterior process fractures
   - Avulsions at the bifurcate ligament caused by forced inversion and plantar flexion
   - Often misdiagnosed as ankle sprains
   - Most can be treated with immobilization in boot or brace
   - Significant displacement involving greater than 25% of the CC joint may benefit from ORIF.
   - Late symptoms secondary to nonunion may benefit from excision of the fragment.
3. Sustentaculum fractures
   - Rarely present without posterior facet involvement
   - CT scan aids diagnosis when medial hindfoot pain persists after an injury.
   - Displaced fractures treated with ORIF via lag screws through a medial approach

B. Intraarticular fractures

1. Approximately 75% of all fractures of the calcaneus are posterior facet fractures, and most of them have some degree of displacement.
2. Mechanism of injury—usually secondary to high-energy trauma such as fall from height or motor vehicle accident
   - Result in axial loading and shear forces to the calcaneus
   - One or more posterior facet fragments are impacted into the body of the calcaneus.
   - **The lateral wall is "blown out," causing subfibular impingement and peroneal tendon encroachment.**
   - Heel pad crush occurs.

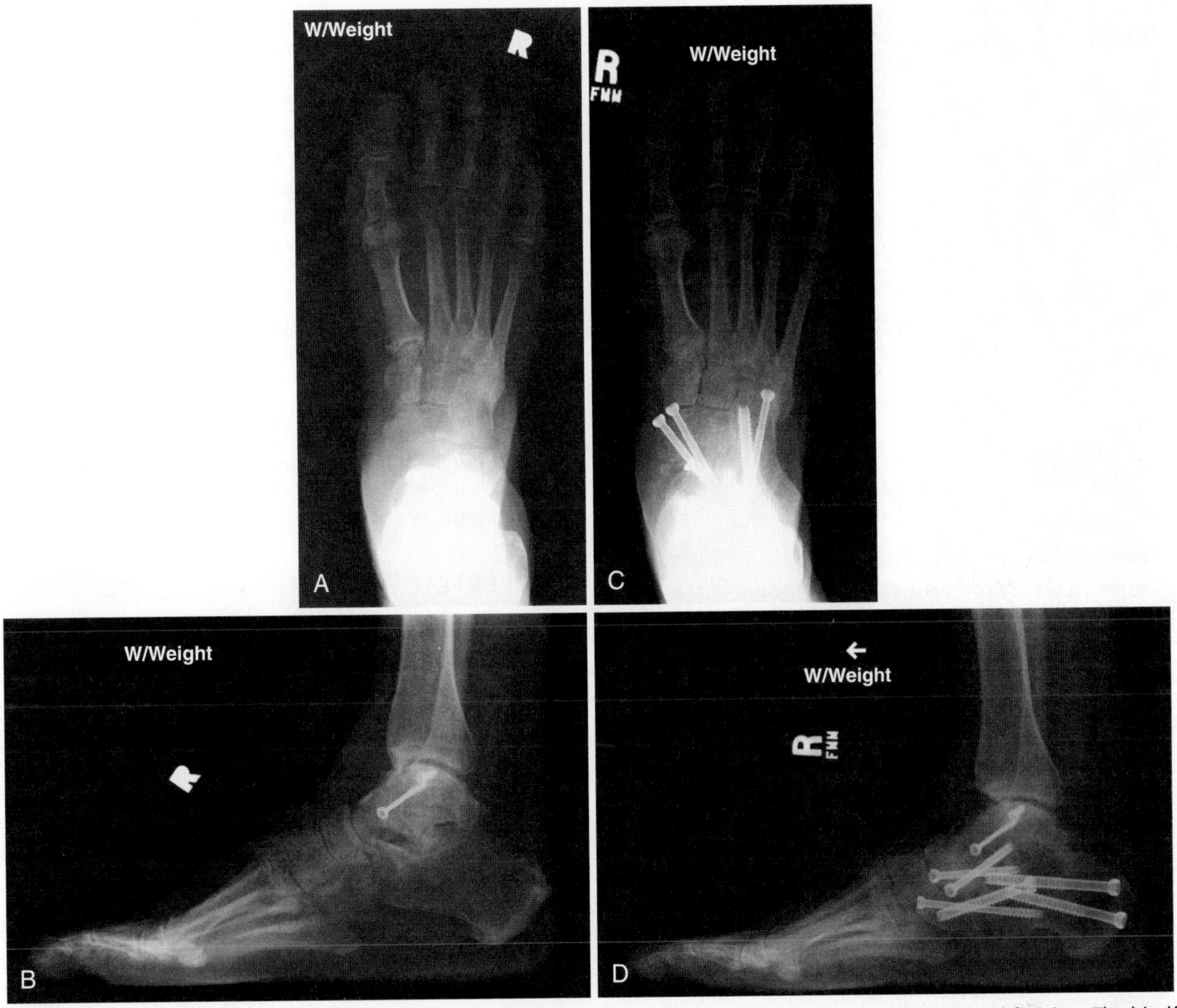

Figure 6-127 **A** and **B,** Malunion of a fracture of the neck of the talus treated with open reduction and internal fixation. The hindfoot was fixed in varus as a result of shortening of the medial column of the hindfoot. **C** and **D,** Correction was accomplished with a triple arthrodesis achieved by resecting a small wedge from the lateral aspect of the calcaneocuboid joint. (From Myerson M: *Reconstructive foot and ankle surgery: management of complications,* ed 2, Philadelphia, 2010, Elsevier.)

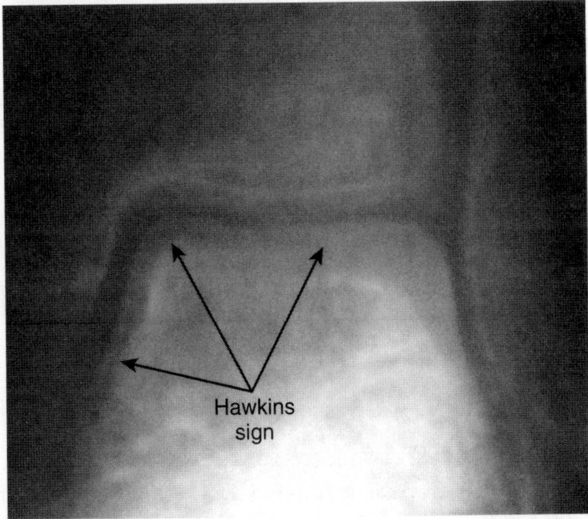

Figure 6-128 Hawkins sign. *Arrows* indicate revascularization. (From Coughlin M, et al: *Surgery of the foot and ankle,* ed 8, Philadelphia, 2006, Elsevier.)

- Results in shortened, widened, and flattened calcaneus
- Significant soft tissue disruption is common, with open fractures accounting for 17% of calcaneus fractures.
  - **Disruption of the medial soft tissue does not increase the complication rate for ORIF as opposed to lateral soft tissue trauma.**
- Must evaluate for concomitant injuries such as vertebral fractures

3. Imaging
   - Anteroposterior, lateral, oblique, and axial os calcis radiographs performed initially
   - Reduction in the Böhler angle, the angle of Gissane calcaneal shortening, and varus deformity to the tuberosity are common in joint depression fractures (Figure 6-131).
   - Broden oblique view of the ankle is helpful to evaluate posterior facet displacement.
   - CT scanning in the 30-degree semicoronal (posterior and middle facets displacement), axial (CC joint involvement), and sagittal (tuberosity displacement) planes is

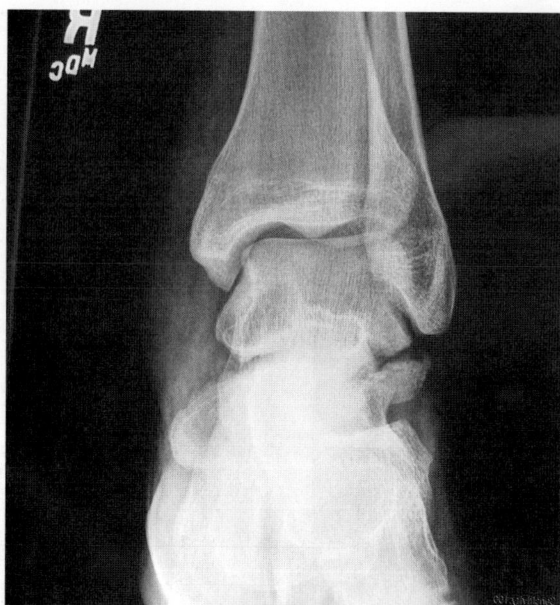

Figure 6-129 Snowboarder's ankle (fracture of the lateral process of the talus). (From Miller M: *Core knowledge in orthopaedics—sports medicine,* Philadelphia, 2006, Elsevier.)

helpful in evaluating this multiplanar injury as well as in preoperative planning.

4. Classification
   - Sanders classification system is most widely used (Figure 6-132).
     - Based on CT scan in coronal plane
     - Correlates with treatment and prognosis
   - Essex-Lopresti noted the difference between joint depression fractures and tongue-type fractures (articular surface attached to displaced tuberosity fragment).
5. Treatment
   - Sanders type I—immobilize 2 to 3 weeks, early motion, non–weight bearing 6 weeks.
   - Sanders type II and III
     - **Indications for ORIF—posterior facet fracture displacement more than 2 to 3 mm, flattening of Böhler angle, varus malalignment of tuberosity**
     - Extensile lateral exposure provides access to subtalar and CC joint, allows for lateral plate placement; however, has a high rate of wound complications
       - **Delayed wound healing can occur in 25% of patients from an extensile approach. Risk of a deep infection is much lower at 1% to 4%.**
       - Decreased rate of subtalar arthrosis compared to nonoperative intervention
       - **FHL at risk during placement of screws from lateral to medial—specifically at the level of the sustentaculum (constant fragment)**
     - Less-invasive techniques (sinus tarsi incision, percutaneous screws) gaining in popularity
   - Sanders type IV
     - Significant comminution and displacement leads to relatively poor prognosis.
     - ORIF with primary subtalar arthrodesis is treatment of choice (Figure 6-133).
   - Prognosis
     - **Worse outcomes correlate to higher fracture types.**
     - **Patients with significant intraarticular displacement, flatter Böhler angle, age less than 29 years, women, and those not involved in workers' compensation have improved clinical outcomes with surgical compared to nonoperative management.**
     - **Post-traumatic subtalar arthritis is common and may require arthrodesis. Patients complain of pain over the sinus tarsi with limited inversion/eversion.**
       - Superior outcomes demonstrated with arthrodesis after ORIF compared to patients who had prior nonoperative treatment.
         - Secondary to restoration of height and width of the hindfoot in operatively treated patients
     - **In cases with significant loss of calcaneal height, horizontal talus, and resultant anterior ankle pain, bone-block distraction arthrodesis of the subtalar joint is required.**

IX. PERITALAR (SUBTALAR) DISLOCATIONS

A. Medial dislocation (Figure 6-134)
1. **More common than lateral dislocations**
2. Results from forceful inversion of the hindfoot, resulting in medial displacement of the calcaneus
3. Reduction can usually be accomplished under sedation or general anesthesia.
4. **Most common obstacles to reduction are the extensor digitorum brevis, the extensor retinaculum, the peroneal tendons, and the TN capsule.**

B. Lateral dislocation (Figure 6-135)
1. Occurs with forceful eversion of the hindfoot, resulting in lateral displacement of the calcaneus
2. **Most common obstacles to reduction are an interposed posterior tibial tendon and FHL tendon.**

C. **CT scan strongly recommended in all cases to rule out small intraarticular fragments**

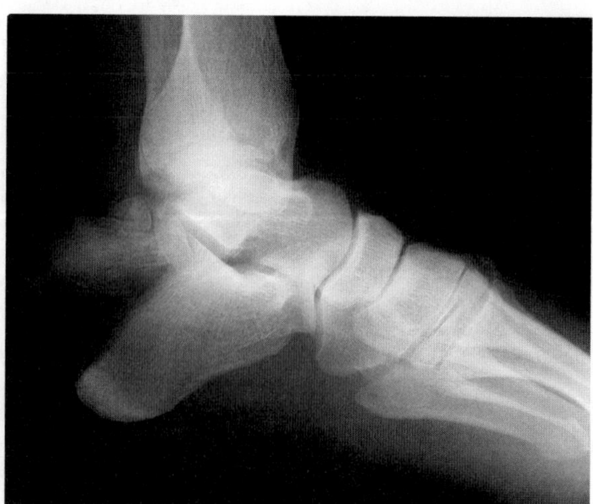

Figure 6-130 This patient suffered a displaced tuberosity fracture that was tenting the skin over the posterior heel. Urgent percutaneous reduction and fixation was performed to prevent skin necrosis. (From DiGiovanni C: *Core knowledge in orthopaedics—foot and ankle,* Philadelphia, 2007, Elsevier.)

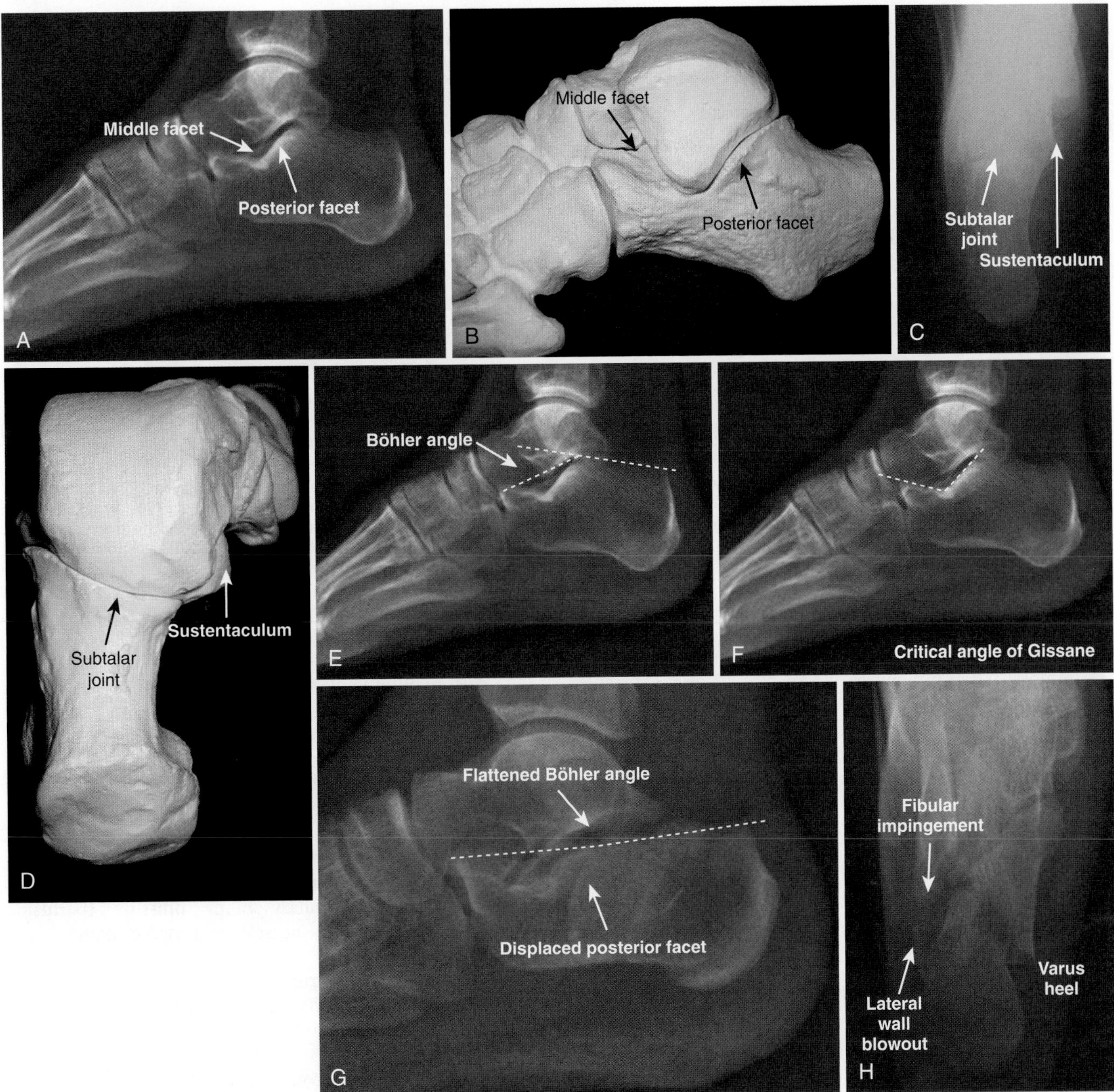

Figure 6-131 The normal **(A, C)** and pathologic **(G, H)** radiographic anatomy of the calcaneus. The lateral **(A, E, G)** and Harris axial **(C, H)** views of the calcaneus are useful in assessing the shape and alignment of the calcaneus. The lateral view **(A, E)** allows for the assessment of the posterior and middle facet positions as well as an assessment of calcaneal height (Böhler angle, ***E***). The Böhler angle is formed by drawing two lines. The first is drawn from the highest point on the anterior process to the highest point on the posterior facet. The second line is tangential to the superior edge of the tuberosity. The normal value of the Böhler angle is 25 to 40 degrees. In the injured calcaneus **(G)**,the Böhler angle diminishes, corresponding to the loss of height ("flattening"). The critical angle of Gissane **(F)** is the angle formed by the intersection of a line drawn along the dorsal aspect of the anterior process of the calcaneus and a line drawn along the dorsal slope of the posterior facet. The normal value of the Gissane angle is 120 to 145 degrees. The axial view **(C, H)** is useful for determining displacement of the tuberosity, varus angulation, fibular abutment, and displacement of the lateral wall. (From Browner B, et al: *Skeletal trauma,* ed 4, Philadelphia, 2008, Elsevier.)

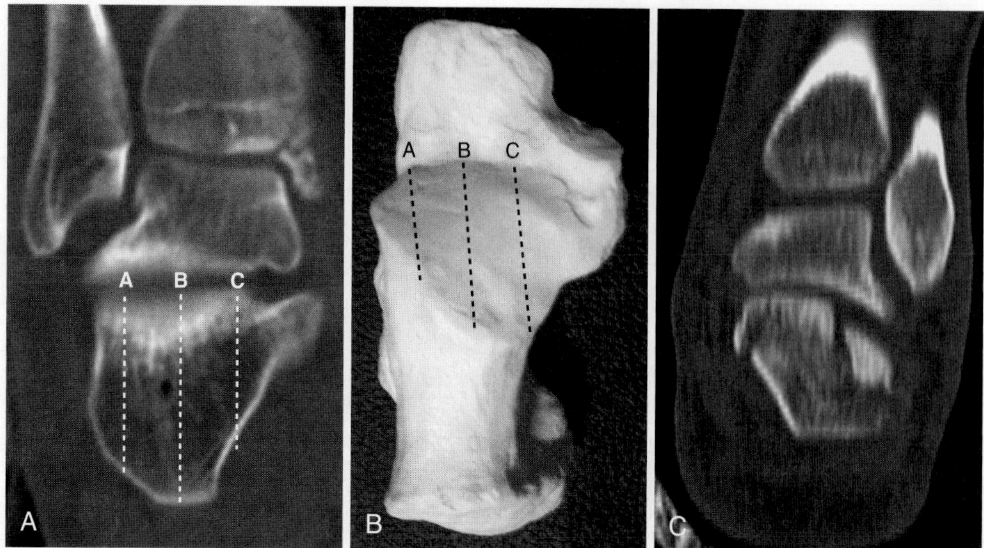

Figure 6-132 The Sanders classification is based on the fracture pattern through the posterior facet as seen on coronal computed tomography scan. Type 1 fractures are nondisplaced. Type 2 fractures are two-part fractures of the posterior facet. Type 3 fractures are three-part fractures of the posterior facet. Type 4 fractures are highly comminuted, with four or more fragments to the posterior facet. **A** and **B,** Type 2 and type 3 fractures are further classified based on the location of the fracture lines (*A, B,* and *C*), as shown. **C,** Based on this classification system, this fracture would be a Sanders type 3AC. The prognosis for calcaneus fractures worsens as the comminution of the posterior facet worsens. (From DiGiovanni C: *Core knowledge in orthopaedics—foot and ankle,* Philadelphia, 2007, Elsevier.)

D. **Treatment**
1. Immobilization in boot or cast for 6 to 12 weeks if stable reduction
2. Unstable reduction requires temporary stabilization with either K-wire fixation or external fixation.
3. Intraarticular fragments should be removed surgically.

X. COMPARTMENT SYNDROME

A. **Anatomy**
1. Medial compartment—abductor hallucis, flexor hallucis brevis

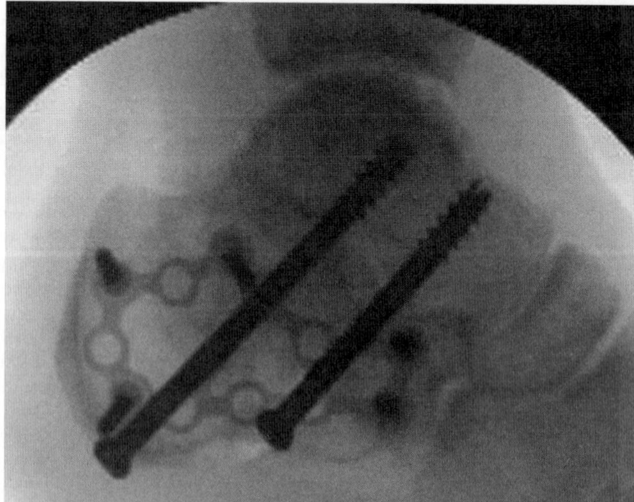

Figure 6-133 Primary subtalar fusion may be indicated in cases of severe comminution or destruction of the articular cartilage. Once reduction and fixation of the calcaneus is complete, the subtalar joint is denuded of cartilage. Compressive fixation is then applied across the subtalar joint. (From Browner B, et al: *Skeletal trauma,* ed 4, Philadelphia, 2008, Elsevier.)

2. Central compartment—flexor digitorum brevis, the lumbricals, quadratus plantae, adductor hallucis
3. Lateral compartment—flexors, abductors, and opponens to the fifth toe
4. Interosseous compartment—the seven interossei muscles
5. The dorsalis pedis artery forms an anastomosis with the plantar arch by passing between the first and second metatarsal bases.

B. **Mechanism of injury**
1. When the intracompartmental fluid pressure meets or exceeds the capillary filling pressure (perfusion pressure), irreversible muscle and nerve damage can occur.
2. In the foot, crush injuries are the most common cause.
3. Calcaneus fractures carry a 10% incidence of compartment syndrome.

C. **Diagnosis**
1. Diagnosis is made by constellation of clinical findings and high index of suspicion.
2. Clinical findings include massive swelling, pain out of proportion to the injury that is not relieved by immobilization or appropriate analgesics, severe pain with passive motion of the toes (stretching the intrinsic muscles), and paresthesias and/or loss of light-touch and two-point discrimination.
3. Presence of normal capillary refill and palpable and/or Doppler positive pulses does not rule out compartment syndrome.
4. Compartment pressures can be measured to aid in the diagnosis.
   - Values greater than 30 mm Hg or those within 20 mm Hg of the diastolic pressure should raise suspicion of a compartment syndrome.

D. **Treatment**
1. Fasciotomies can be performed through three incisions: one over the second metatarsal, one over the fourth

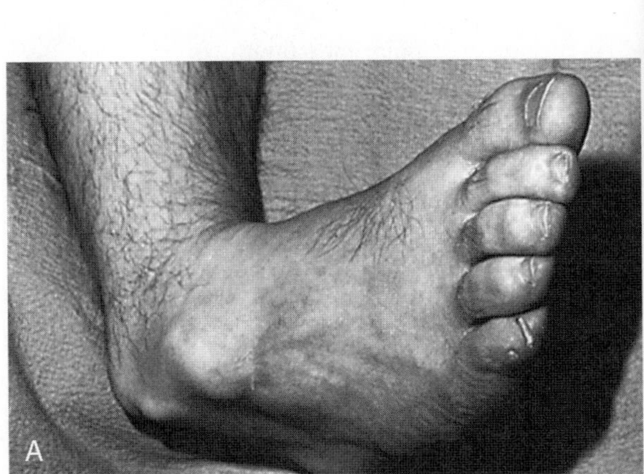

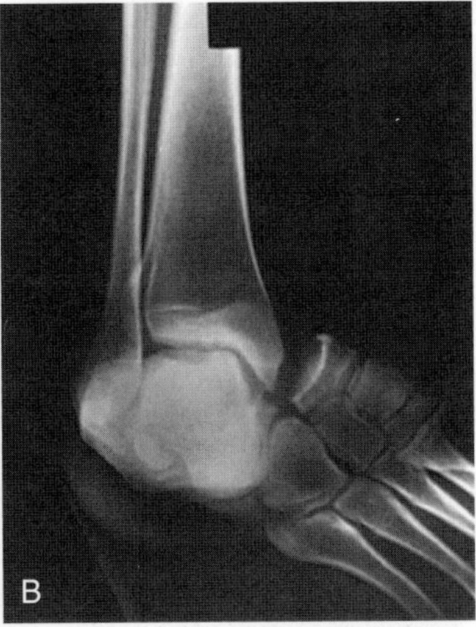

Figure 6-134 Medial subtalar dislocation. **A,** Posture of foot. Note prominence of head of talus. **B,** Radiographic appearance of dislocation. (From Canale ST, Beaty J: *Campbell's operative orthopedics,* ed 11, Philadelphia, 2007, Elsevier; and DeLee JC, Curtis R: Subtalar dislocation of the foot, *J Bone Joint Surg* 64A:433, 1982.)

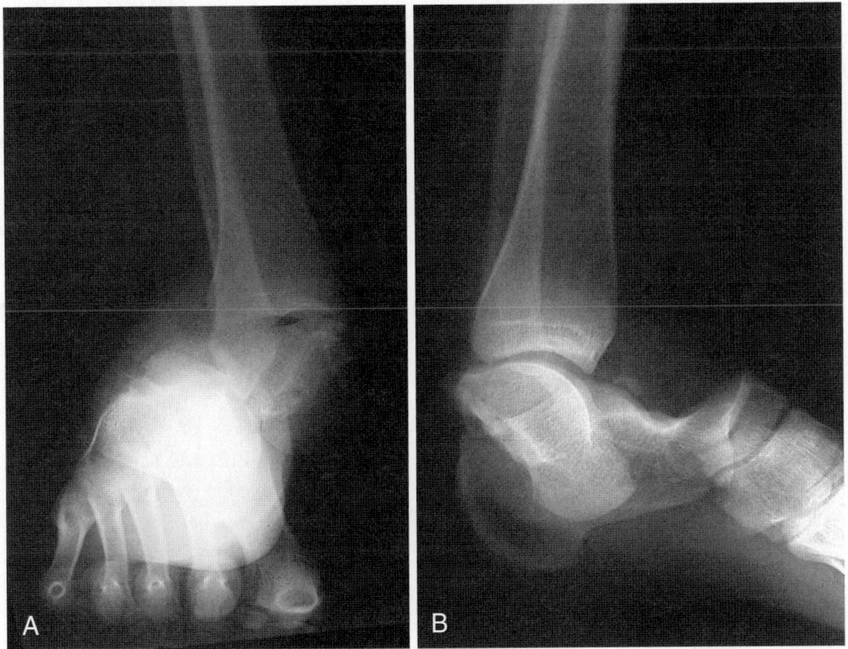

Figure 6-135 Anteroposterior **(A)** and lateral **(B)** radiographs of lateral subtalar dislocation. (From Coughlin M, et al: *Surgery of the foot and ankle,* ed 8, Philadelphia, 2006, Elsevier.)

metatarsal, and a medial approach along the inferior border of the first metatarsal.

2. The wounds should be left open for approximately 5 days and may require skin grafting.
3. Definitive treatment is compartment release.
   - **The result of unrecognized and untreated compartment syndrome is NOT isolated claw toes.**
   - Damage is not isolated to the musculature but also affects the peripheral nerves. This commonly results in chronic pain with hypersensitivity that can be difficult or impossible to treat.
   - Benign neglect of a foot compartment syndrome is not appropriate management.

TESTABLE CONCEPTS

SECTION 1 BIOMECHANICS OF THE FOOT AND ANKLE

- At the distal tibiofibular joint, the fibula externally rotates and proximally translates with ankle dorsiflexion.
- The foot has longitudinal and transverse arches. Stability is provided by a combination of bony architecture, ligamentous attachments, and muscle forces.
- In the toe-off phase of gait, the plantar fascia is tightened as the metatarsophalangeal (MTP) joints extend. The longitudinal arch is accentuated. This is termed the windlass mechanism. The hindfoot supinates, with firing of the posterior tibial tendon.

SECTION 2 PHYSICAL EXAMINATION OF THE FOOT AND ANKLE

- Cavovarus alignment is an elevated longitudinal arch with hindfoot varus and plantar-flexed first ray. Pes planus is a flat longitudinal arch with hindfoot valgus.
- Vascular examination findings that are predictive for healing include toe pressure greater than 40 mm Hg and transcutaneous oxygen pressure greater than 30 mm Hg.
- Neurologic examination should include use of a Semmes-Weinstein 5.07 monofilament. Inability to sense this is consistent with neuropathy and is the most predictive sign for the development of a foot ulceration.
- Stability of the lateral ankle ligaments can be assessed with the anterior drawer and varus talar tilt tests.
  - Anterior drawer test—Anterior pressure on the hindfoot with the ankle in plantar flexion evaluates the anterior talofibular ligament.
  - Varus stress test—Inversion of the ankle in dorsiflexion evaluates the calcaneofibular ligament.
- The Silfverskiöld test evaluates for contracture.
  - Test ankle dorsiflexion with the knee extended and flexed.
  - Tightness in both knee flexion and extension indicates Achilles contracture.
  - Improvement in ankle dorsiflexion with knee flexion (relaxing the gastrocnemius origin proximal to the knee) indicates isolated gastrocnemius contracture.

SECTIONS 4 AND 5 ADULT AND JUVENILE AND ADOLESCENT HALLUX VALGUS

- A key feature in the pathoanatomy of hallux valgus is lateral drift of the proximal phalanx, leading to plantar lateral migration of abductor hallucis, which results in plantar flexion and pronation.
- There are four key radiographic angular measurements in hallux valgus.
  - Hallux valgus angle (HVA), first-second intermetatarsal angle (IMA), hallux valgus interphalangeus (HVI) angle, and the distal metatarsal articular angle (DMAA)
- Congruency of the first MTP must also be determined by comparing the line connecting the medial and lateral edge of the first metatarsal head articular surface with the similar line for the proximal phalanx. When these lines are parallel, the joint is congruent.
- Appropriate surgical procedures are determined by two factors.
  - Angular measurements
  - Clinical scenario
- Regardless of angular measurements, the following clinical abnormalities dictate surgical procedure.
  - Spasticity (stroke or cerebral palsy)—first MTP fusion
  - Osteoarthritis or rheumatoid arthritis—first MTP fusion
  - Ligamentous laxity—Lapidus (first tarsometatarsal [TMT] realignment arthrodesis)
  - First TMT degenerative joint disease—Lapidus
- A distal soft tissue release (modified McBride) is never appropriate in isolation.
- In general, all patients should undergo a soft tissue release with all associated osteotomies and first TMT arthrodesis.
- Angular measurement guides for surgical procedure
  - IMA less than or equal to 13 degrees AND HVA less than or equal to 40 degrees—chevron
  - IMA greater than 13 degrees OR HVA greater than 40 degrees—proximal metatarsal osteotomy
- Complications
  - Recurrence—undercorrection of IMA or isolated soft tissue reconstruction. Recurrence of the deformity after surgical correction is the most common complication in juvenile and adolescent hallux valgus.
  - Dorsal malunion—Lapidus or proximal crescentic osteotomy; results in transfer metatarsalgia
  - Hallux varus—overresection of the medial eminence

SECTION 7 LESSER-TOE DEFORMITIES

- Hammer toe—proximal interphalangeal (PIP) flexion (MTP dorsiflexed, but should correct with elevation). Fixed deformity is treated with PIP arthroplasty (resection of distal neck and head of proximal phalanx) or PIP arthrodesis.
- Claw toe—PIP and distal interphalangeal (DIP) flexion with fixed MTP hyperextension
  - Flexible—flexor-to-extensor tendon transfer of flexor digitorum longus (FDL)
  - Fixed—PIP arthroplasty/arthrodesis with MTP capsulotomy and extensor lengthening. A dislocated MTP joint requires use of a Weil osteotomy (distal metatarsal osteotomy) to reduce MTP joint.
- Mallet toe—DIP flexion; flexible deformity treated with flexor tenotomy; fixed deformity with DIP arthroplasty or fusion/
- Crossover toe—sagittal and axial plane deformities. Key component is disruption of the plantar plate. May be iatrogenic from steroid injection within MTP joint
- Freiberg disease—osteochondrosis of metatarsal head. Early-stage disease is treated with joint débridement. A dorsal closed-wedge metaphyseal osteotomy may also be performed.
- Congenital curly toe—Perform tenotomy of FDL and flexor digitorum brevis in children with flexible deformities.

SECTION 8 HYPERKERATOTIC PATHOLOGIES

- Bunionette deformity is treated based on the anatomic location of deformity.
  - Enlarged fifth metatarsal head—lateral condylectomy
  - Lateral bowing of fifth metatarsal diaphysis—distal metatarsal osteotomy
  - Widened fourth-fifth metatarsal angle—oblique diaphyseal osteotomy

SECTION 9 SESAMOIDS

- Turf toe mechanism of injury is a forced dorsiflexion resulting in avulsion of the plantar plate off the base of the phalanx and subsequent proximal migration of the sesamoids.
  - Complete tears of the plantar plate treated with operative repair have demonstrated superior results compared to conservative care.
- Complications of medial and lateral sesamoidectomy are hallux valgus and varus, respectively.
- Cock-up deformity (or claw toe) will occur if both sesamoids are excised.

SECTION 11 NEUROLOGIC DISORDERS

- Interdigital neuritis (Morton neuroma) is a compressive neuropathy of the interdigital nerve, usually between the third and fourth metatarsals. Surgical treatment is via a dorsal approach, incision of the transverse intermetatarsal ligament, and resection of the nerve 2 to 3 cm proximal to the intermetatarsal ligament.
- The lateral plantar nerve may be injured during surgical approaches that require a plantar incision, such as a tibiotalocalcaneal arthrodesis with an intramedullary nail.
- Upper motor neuron disorders most commonly result in an equinovarus foot deformity.
  - Equinus—overactivity of gastrocnemius-soleus complex
    - Equinus deformity is addressed with either an open Z-lengthening of the Achilles tendon or a percutaneous triple-hemisection technique.
  - Varus—overactivity of tibialis anterior (lesser contributions from flexor hallucis longus [FHL], FDL, and tibialis posterior)
    - Varus deformity is addressed with a split anterior tibialis tendon transfer (SPLATT) to the lateral cuneiform or cuboid or total anterior tibial tendon transfer to the lateral cuneiform.
- Type I hereditary motor-sensory neuropathy is the most common presentation of Charcot-Marie-Tooth disease (CMT).
  - Usually autosomal dominant with a duplication of chromosome 17
  - Characterized by the following
- Treatment of a flexible deformity involves
  - Release of the plantar fascia
  - Transfer of the peroneus longus into the peroneus brevis at the level of the distal fibula
  - A closed-wedge dorsiflexion osteotomy of the first metatarsal is always required.
    - If the deformity does not correct with Coleman block, perform a lateral calcaneal slide and/or closed-wedge osteotomy.
- Nonoperative treatment of a fixed deformity
  - Locked-ankle, short-leg ankle-foot orthosis with an outside (varus-correcting or lateral) T-strap is recommended.
  - Rocker sole can improve gait and decrease energy expenditure.
- Peroneal nerve palsy results in loss of the anterior and lateral compartments with loss of active dorsiflexion and eversion. This results in equinovarus.
  - Transfer posterior tibial tendon (PTT) through the interosseous membrane anteriorly to the dorsal midfoot to restore dorsiflexion. Achilles tendon should be lengthened.

SECTION 12 ARTHRITIC DISEASE

- Foot involvement very common in rheumatoid patients with the forefoot more commonly involved than the midfoot or hindfoot
  - The toes sublux or dislocate dorsally, deviate laterally into valgus, and develop hammering.
  - "Rheumatoid forefoot reconstruction"—first MTP arthrodesis, lesser metatarsal head resection with

Foot Deformities in Charcot-Marie-Tooth Disease

Deformity	Weak Agonist Muscle(s)	Intact Antagonist Muscle(s)	Action
Equinus	Tibialis anterior	Gastrocnemius-soleus	Plantar flexion
Adduction and hindfoot varus	Peroneus brevis	Tibialis posterior	Adducts the foot, inverts the subtalar joint
Plantar flexion of the first ray*	Tibialis anterior	Peroneus longus	Plantar flexes the first ray, creates a secondary forefoot cavus*
Toe deformities	Foot intrinsics	Long toe flexors	Clawing occurs as the extrinsic forces are unmodified by the intrinsics; also depresses the metatarsal heads and accentuates cavus
Hallux claw toe	Foot intrinsics	EHL and FHL	Severe hallucal clawing occurs when a spared EHL is used to assist a weak tibialis anterior dorsiflex the foot

From Coughlin M, et al: *Surgery of the foot and ankle,* ed 8, Philadelphia, 2006, Elsevier.
*Plantar flexion of the first ray is the primary deformity in CMT.
EHL, extensor hallucis longus; FHL, flexor hallucis longus.

Continued

pinning of the lesser MTP joints, and closed osteoclasis of the interphalangeal joints versus PIP arthroplasty
- The most common complication of forefoot arthroplasty is intractable plantar keratoses.

- Osteoarthritis etiology is typically post-traumatic in the hindfoot and tibiotalar articulations, while idiopathic in the first MTP and midfoot joints.
  - First MTP (hallux rigidus)—tenderness over dorsum of joint, limited dorsiflexion due to large dorsal osteophyte and pain with grind test
    - Initial treatment is a stiff foot plate with extension under great toe (Morton extension).
    - Surgical treatment in those with pain at extremes of range of motion (ROM)—dorsal cheilectomy
    - Pain throughout ROM with positive grind—arthrodesis (neutral rotation, 10 to 15 degrees of dorsiflexion, and slight valgus)
  - Hindfoot arthritis—triple arthrodesis to correct arthritis secondary to deformity (0 to 5 degrees of hindfoot valgus, neutral abduction/adduction, plantigrade)
    - Revision of malunited triple arthrodesis requires calcaneal osteotomy and/or transverse tarsal osteotomy.
  - Subtalar arthritis—Subtalar fusion nonunion risk is increased with history of ankle arthrodesis and smoking.
    - Prior calcaneal fracture with loss of height results in anterior impingement, anterior ankle pain, and hindfoot pain and is treated with subtalar bone-block arthrodesis.
  - Tibiotalar arthritis—Arthrodesis provides excellent pain relief with some restricted function (neutral dorsiflexion, 0 to 5 degrees of hindfoot valgus, and 5 to 10 degrees of external rotation).
    - Leads to eventual arthritis in surrounding foot, most commonly the subtalar joint
    - Total ankle arthroplasty has shown the best outcome in patients with osteoarthritis. Syndesmotic fusion is associated with a decreased rate of failure for the Agility ankle replacement.

SECTION 13 POSTURAL DISORDERS

- Pes planus (flatfoot) deformity is most commonly caused by posterior tibial tendon dysfunction in the adult. There is a zone of hypovascularity 2 to 6 cm from the PTT attachment on the navicular.
  - Standing examination demonstrates asymmetric hindfoot valgus, depressed arch, and an abducted forefoot.
  - "Too many toes" when the foot is viewed posteriorly
  - Pain or an inability to perform a single-limb heel-rise indicates an insufficient PTT.
  - Radiographs demonstrate a negative lateral talo–first metatarsal angle (Meary angle) and talonavicular un-coverage
  - Treatment is based on whether the deformity is flexible or fixed.
  - Pes cavus etiology is neuromuscular, idiopathic, or traumatic (talus fracture malunion).
  - The Coleman block test is used to assess the flexibility of the hindfoot (out of varus) when the first metatarsal plantar flexion (forefoot valgus) is eliminated.
  - If the hindfoot passively corrects into valgus, the deformity is forefoot driven (due to plantar-flexed first ray).
  - Conservative treatment is orthotics with a lateral heel wedge, decreased arch, and depressed first ray.
  - Surgical treatment for forefoot-driven deformity—first metatarsal dorsiflexion osteotomy
  - Surgical treatment for rigid hindfoot—lateral calcaneal closed-wedge osteotomy and first metatarsal dorsiflexion osteotomy

SECTION 14 TENDON DISORDERS

- Peroneal tendon subluxation is caused by forced eversion and dorsiflexion, leading to disruption of superior peroneal retinaculum. This requires repair/reconstruction of the superior peroneal retinaculum and fibular groove deepening.
- FHL tenosynovitis is classically seen in dancers.

Stage	Features	Nonoperative	Operative
I	Synovitis without deformity	Immobilization; orthotic after swelling and pain subsided	Synovectomy
II	Flexible deformity; PTT functionally incompetent	AFO; orthotic after acute pain subsided; full length with arch support, medial heel wedge, and medial forefoot support	FDL or FHL transfer into navicular to reconstruct PTT Gastrocnemius recession if contracted
IIA	Hindfoot valgus without significant forefoot abduction (<40% uncovering of talus)		Add medial calcaneal osteotomy
IIB	Hindfoot valgus with forefoot abduction (>40% uncovering of talus)		Add lateral column lengthening (Medial calcaneal osteotomy may still be required)
IIC	Hindfoot valgus and fixed forefoot supination/varus		If stable medial column—add cotton osteotomy If unstable medial column—add first TMT arthrodesis
III	Rigid deformity	Rigid AFO or Arizona brace	Triple arthrodesis; Achilles lengthening if equinus contracture
IV	Incompetent deltoid ligament and either lateral talar tilt or ankle arthritis		Flexible—deltoid ligament reconstruction and hindfoot reconstruction Rigid—tibiotalocalcaneal arthrodesis

AFO, ankle-foot orthosis; FDL, flexor digitorum longus; FHL, flexor hallucis longus; PTT, posterior tibial tendon; TMT, tarsometatarsal.

- Posteromedial ankle pain, triggering of first interphalangeal joint, and pain with resisted hallux plantar flexion
- Magnetic resonance imaging (MRI) demonstrates fluid surrounding FHL at ankle joint.
- Operative treatment is FHL tenosynovectomy and release of the fascia.

SECTION 15 HEEL PAIN

- Plantar fasciitis classically presents with exquisite pain and tenderness over the plantar medial tuberosity of the calcaneus at the proximal insertion of the plantar fascia. There is pain with the first step in the morning and after prolonged sitting. It is frequently associated with an Achilles tendon contracture.
  - Nonoperative management includes both plantar fascia–specific stretching and Achilles stretching. Management also includes cushioned heel inserts, night splints, physical therapy, walking casts, cortisone injections, and anti-inflammatory medications.
  - Operative management includes limited (medial one-half) release of the plantar fascia. Complete release can place the longitudinal arch of the foot at risk, overload the lateral column, and lead to dorsolateral foot pain.
  - Other invasive options with evolving evidence include gastrocnemius recession and high-energy extracorporeal shock wave therapy.
- Baxter neuritis is compression of the first branch of the lateral plantar nerve. It presents as plantar medial heel pain and can be difficult to differentiate from plantar fasciitis.
- Insertional Achilles tendinopathy treatment includes excision of the retrocalcaneal bursa, resection of a prominent superior calcaneal tuberosity, and débridement of the degenerative tendon.
  - If more than 50% tendon detachment is required, reattachment with suture anchors is indicated. FHL tendon transfer is indicated if more than 50% of tendon requires excision.
- In noninsertional Achilles tendinopathy, MRI evidence of significant diffuse involvement without a focal area of disease, indicates need for an FHL transfer.
  - Chronic rupture of the Achilles tendon requires FHL transfer.

SECTION 16 THE DIABETIC FOOT

- 90% of patients who cannot feel the 5.07 monofilament have lost protective sensation to their feet and are at risk for ulceration.
- Motor neuropathy most commonly involves the common peroneal nerve and resultant loss of tibialis anterior motor function with a footdrop. The small intrinsic musculature is also commonly affected, resulting in claw toes and subsequent toe-tip ulcerations.
- Peripheral vascular disease occurs in 60% to 70% of diabetic patients, and noninvasive vascular examination should be performed when pulses are not palpable. Absolute toe pressures are normally 100 mm Hg, and the minimum for healing is 40 mm Hg.
  - Transcutaneous oxygen measurements ($TcPo_2$) of the toes greater than 40 mm Hg have been found to be predictive of healing.
- Metabolic deficiency also impairs wound healing with reduced total protein less than 6.0 g/dL, white blood cell (WBC) count less than 1500, and albumin levels less than 2.5 g/dL, all predictive of poor healing potential.

II. Clinical Problems

Diabetic Ulcers

- Diabetic ulcer management is based on the depth-ischemia classification
- Equinus contracture is very common, and tendo-Achilles lengthening will offload the midfoot/forefoot; required in recurrent forefoot/midfoot ulceration or ulceration with equinus deformity

Charcot Arthropathy

- Charcot arthropathy is a chronic, progressive, destructive process affecting bone architecture and joint alignment in people lacking protective sensation.
- Eichenholtz classification
  - I—Fragmentation: hyperemia, hot, swollen, erythematous

Grade	Clinical	Treatment
Depth		
0	At risk: Skin intact with bony deformity	Extradepth shoe and pressure-relief insoles
1	Localized superficial ulcer NO tendon or bone involvement	In-office ulcer débridement Total-contact cast
2	Deep ulcer Exposed tendon or joint	Formal operative débridement Dressing changes; total-contact cast only when wound bed healthy
3	Extensive ulcer Exposed bone/osteomyelitis OR abscess	Surgical débridement of bone/tissue Dressing changes; total-contact cast only when wound bed healthy
Ischemia		
A	Normal	
B	Ischemia without gangrene	Noninvasive vascular studies; vascular reconstruction as needed
C	Forefoot gangrene	Same as in grade B Partial foot amputation
D	Complete gangrene	Same as in grade B BKA vs. AKA

AKA, above-the-knee amputation; BKA, below-the-knee amputation.

Continued

- II—Coalescence: beginning of reparative process
- III—Resolution/Consolidation: smoothed bone edges with bony/fibrous ankylosis
- Midfoot most common location
- Swelling and redness is classically diminished with elevation. It is often confused with osteomyelitis clinically.
- Initial treatment is immobilization and non–weight bearing; best with a total-contact cast; transition to ankle-foot orthosis (AFO) or Charcot restraint orthosis walker boot once swelling/erythema subsides

Diabetic Foot Infections

- Diabetic foot infections are polymicrobial. Deep surgical cultures provides the most accurate result.
- Treatment with initial broad-spectrum antibiotic coverage once surgical cultures obtained. Adjust once sensitivity returns.
- Surgical resection of infected bone is indicated if culture specific antibiotic therapy fails. Ray resection, partial calcanectomy or partial/complete foot amputation may be required

Amputation Level

- Lisfranc—tarsometatarsal disarticulation; must transfer peroneal tendons to cuboid to prevent varus and perform Achilles lengthening to prevent equinus
- Chopart—talonavicular and calcaneocuboid joint combined disarticulation; nust transfer anterior tibialis to talus to prevent equinus and perform Achilles lengthening to prevent equinus
- Syme—ankle disarticulation; second lowest energy expenditure after a transmetatarsal amputation. Heel ulcers are absolute contraindication.

SECTION 17 TRAUMA

II. Metatarsal Fractures

- Second metatarsal stress fracture is the most common and is classically described in amenorrheal dancers.
  - Treat in weight-bearing boot or hard-soled shoe.
  - Evaluate for metabolic bone disease in these patients, especially if insidious onset or if there is no distinct causal event (increase in training, initiation of new activity).
- Fifth metatarsal fractures can be divided anatomically into avulsion fractures, fractures of the metaphyseal-diaphyseal junction, and fractures of the proximal diaphysis.
  - Avulsion fractures—protected weight bearing
  - Metaphyseal-diaphyseal fractures—non–weight bearing; elite athletes treated with intramedullary screw fixation
  - Proximal diaphysis—intramedullary fixation

IV. Tarsometatarsal Fractures and Dislocations (Lisfranc Injury)

- Lisfranc ligament is between the medial cuneiform and base of second metatarsal.
  - Nonsurgical management of Lisfranc injuries is indicated in nondisplaced injuries.
  - Anatomic reduction is mandatory, necessitating open reduction instead of closed reduction and percutaneous fixation.
  - Primary arthrodesis is an alternative treatment option, with some benefit seen in patients with purely ligamentous injury or significant intraarticular comminution.
  - Missed diagnosis or improper treatment may lead to traumatic planovalgus deformity or post-traumatic arthritis.
  - Midfoot realignment and arthrodesis is the appropriate salvage procedure.

V. Midfoot Injuries (Excluding Lisfranc Injuries)

Navicular Fractures

- Navicular stress fractures are secondary to repetitive trauma, especially running and jumping. They typically occur in the central one-third, and patients complain of vague dorsal midfoot or ankle pain.
  - Computed tomography (CT) is the gold standard for diagnosis.
  - Nondisplaced fractures should be treated with non–weight bearing.

VII. Talus Fractures

- The talus blood supply is provided by the posterior tibial artery, the dorsalis pedis artery, and the perforating peroneal artery. The artery of the tarsal canal carries the main supply to the talar body.
- Talar neck fractures are commonly associated with medial neck comminution, leading to a varus deformity.
  - Varus malunion is highly associated with use of medial compression screws. This leads to a cavovarus deformity, limiting hindfoot eversion that results in lateral border foot pain.
  - Avascular necrosis increases with the severity of the injury. Hawkins sign is a subchondral linear lucency of the talar dome that is indicative of talar revascularization. Sclerosis of the talar dome does not guarantee that avascular necrosis has occurred, but it is suggestive.
  - Lateral process talus fractures are highly associated with snowboarding. They are also a source of continued pain after an ankle sprain.

VIII. Calcaneus Fractures

- Extraarticular calcaneal fractures may endanger posterior skin if there is significant displacement. Urgent operative reduction and fixation is required.
- Intraarticular calcaneal fractures result in lateral wall blowout, resulting in subfibular impingement and peroneal tendon encroachment.
  - Indications for open reduction with internal fixation (ORIF)—posterior facet fracture displacement greater than 2 to 3 mm, flattening of Böhler angle, varus malalignment of tuberosity
  - Disruption of the medial soft tissue does not increase the complication rate for ORIF as opposed to lateral soft tissue trauma.

- Delayed wound healing can occur in 25% of patients from an extensile approach. Risk for a deep infection is much lower at 1% to 4%.
- FHL at risk during placement of screws from lateral to medial—specifically at the level of the sustentaculum (constant fragment)
- Worse outcomes correlate to higher fracture types.
- Patients with significant intraarticular displacement, flatter Böhler angle, age less than 29 years, women, and those not involved in workers' compensation have improved clinical outcomes with surgical compared to nonoperative management.
- Post-traumatic subtalar arthritis is common and may require arthrodesis. Patients complain of pain over the sinus tarsi with limited inversion/eversion.
    - In cases with significant loss of calcaneal height, horizontal talus, and resultant anterior ankle pain, bone-block distraction arthrodesis of the subtalar joint is required.

IX. Peritalar (Subtalar) Dislocations

- Subtalar dislocations are most commonly medial. The most common obstacles to reduction are the extensor digitorum brevis, the extensor retinaculum, and the peroneal tendons.
    - Most common obstacles to reduction of a lateral dislocation are an interposed posterior tibial tendon and FHL tendon.

SELECTED BIBLIOGRAPHY

The selected bibliography for this chapter can be found on www.expertconsult.com.

Chapter 7

HAND, UPPER EXTREMITY, AND MICROVASCULAR SURGERY

Lance M. Brunton and A. Bobby Chhabra

CONTENTS

I. ANATOMY*

A. Extensor anatomy

1. Extensor (dorsal) compartments of the wrist (Figure 7-1 and Table 7-1)
2. Extensor retinaculum—prevents tendon bowstringing at wrist
3. Juncturae tendinum—extensor tendon interconnections in hand that may mask proximal tendon lacerations
4. Sagittal bands—aid in metacarpophalangeal (MCP) joint extension, centralize the extensor mechanism, and attach to the volar plate (Figure 7-2)
5. Central slip—inserts on base of middle phalanx (P2), aids in proximal interphalangeal (PIP) joint extension (Figure 7-3)
6. Extensor mechanism receives contributions from the intrinsic muscles—interossei and lumbricals (see Figures 7-3 and 7-4)
7. Lateral bands—receive contributions from common extensor and intrinsics, converge to form terminal extensor tendon, which inserts on base of distal phalanx (P3) (see Figures 7-3 and 7-4)
8. Transverse retinacular ligament—prevents dorsal subluxation of lateral bands (see Figure 7-4)
9. Triangular ligament—prevents volar subluxation of lateral bands (see Figure 7-3)
10. Oblique retinacular ligament (ligament of Landsmeer)—helps to link PIP and distal interphalangeal (DIP) joint extension (see Figure 7-4)
11. Grayson/Cleland ligaments—volar and dorsal to digital neurovascular bundles, respectively (Grayson is ground; Cleland is ceiling)

B. Flexor anatomy

1. Flexor digitorum profundus (FDP)—flexes the DIP joint, aids in PIP and MCP flexion, typically shares common muscle belly in forearm
   - Index FDP often distinct muscle belly
2. Flexor digitorum superficialis (FDS)—flexes the PIP joint, aids in MCP flexion, individual muscle bellies in forearm
   - Small FDS—absent approximately 20% of the time
3. FDP tendon splits FDS at the Campers chiasm at level of proximal phalanx (P1) (Figure 7-5).
4. Flexor tendon sheath—encompasses tendons distal to MCP joint
5. **Vascular supply to flexor tendons is twofold.**
   - **Diffusion via synovial sheath**
     - **More important proximal to MCP**
   - Direct vascular supply
6. Each digit has five annular pulleys (A1 to A5) and three cruciate pulleys (C1 to C3).
   - A2 and A4 pulleys—prevent flexor tendon bowstringing (Figure 7-6)

Table 7-1 Extensor (Dorsal) Compartments of the Wrist

Compartment	Tendons	Associated Pathology	Other Points
1	APL/EPB	de Quervain tenosynovitis	APL may have multiple slips, and EPB may have a separate compartment
2	ECRL/ECRB	Intersection syndrome	Radial to Lister tubercle
3	EPL	Late rupture after closed treatment of distal radius fracture	Ulnar to Lister tubercle; test by placing palm flat on table and lifting thumb
4	EDC/EIP	Extensor tenosynovitis	EIP ulnar to index EDC Small EDC present in only 25%
5	EDM	Vaughn-Jackson syndrome (initial)	EDM ulnar to small EDC
6	ECU	ECU instability	ECU subsheath part of TFCC

APL, abductor pollicis longus; ECRB, extensor carpi radialis brevis; ECRL, extensor carpi radialis longus; ECU, extensor carpi ulnaris; EDC, extensor digitorum communis; EDM, extensor digiti minimi; EIP, extensor indicis proprius; EPB, extensor pollicis brevis; EPL, extensor pollicis longus; TFCC, triangular fibrocartilage complex.

7. Thumb has two annular pulleys and an oblique pulley in between that prevents bowstringing.
8. **Carpal tunnel contains median nerve and nine flexor tendons (one flexor pollicis longus [FPL], four FDS, and four FDP tendons).**
   - FPL tendon—most radial structure in carpal tunnel
   - Long and ring FDS tendons are volar to index and small FDS (Figure 7-7).
   - Transverse carpal ligament (TCL)—roof of carpal tunnel
9. The Guyon canal (ulnar tunnel)—contains the ulnar nerve and artery
   - Volar carpal ligament—roof of Guyon canal (TCL is floor)
10. Linburg sign—interconnections between FPL and index FDP in forearm; unilateral in 25% to 30%, bilateral in 5% to 15%
11. Palmaris longus (PL) tendon—present 80% to 85% of the time, common source of autograft for upper extremity reconstructive procedures
12. Flexor carpi radialis (FCR)/flexor carpi ulnaris (FCU)—primary wrist flexors, insert on base of second metacarpal and pisiform, respectively

C. **Intrinsic anatomy**

1. Four dorsal interosseous (digit abductors) and three palmar interosseous (digit adductor) muscles
   - Contribute to MCP flexion and interphalangeal extension—innervated by ulnar nerve (Figure 7-8)

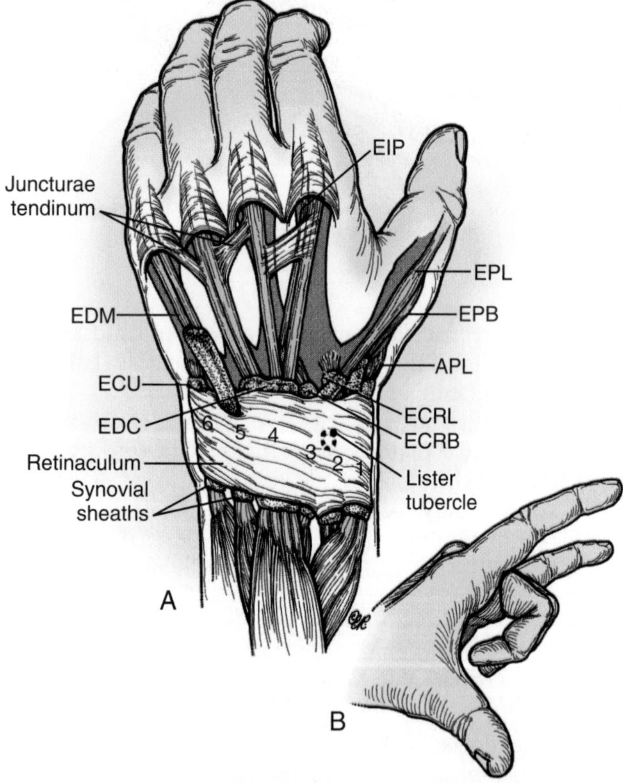

Figure 7-1 **A,** Extensor (dorsal) compartments of the wrist. The first compartment contains the abductor pollicis longus *(APL)* and extensor pollicis brevis *(EPB)*; the second contains the radial wrist extensors, extensor carpi radialis longus *(ECRL)*, and extensor carpi radialis brevis *(ECRB)*; the third contains the extensor pollicis longus *(EPL)*; the fourth contains the extensor digitorum communis *(EDC)* and extensor indicis proprius *(EIP)*; the fifth contains the extensor digiti minimi *(EDM)*; and the sixth contains the extensor carpi ulnaris *(ECU)*. **B,** Depiction of independant index and small digit extension from EIP and EDM. (From Doyle JR: Extensor tendons—acute injuries. In Green DP, et al, editors: *Green's operative hand surgery,* ed 5, New York, 2005, Churchill Livingstone, p 1881.)

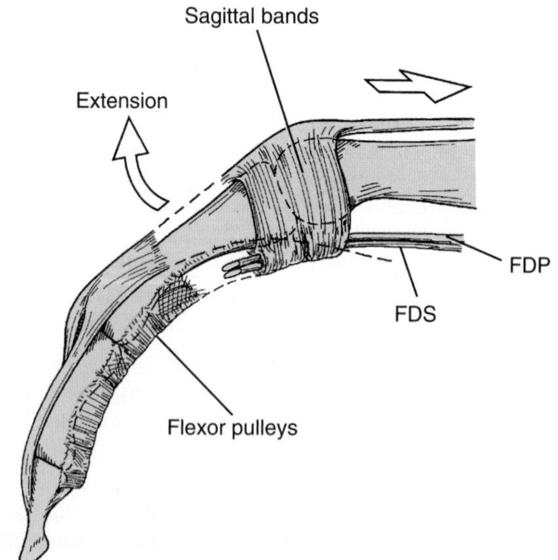

Figure 7-2 Sagittal bands of the extensor mechanism contribute to metacarpophalangeal joint extension. FDP, flexor digitorum profundus; FDS, flexor digitorum superficialis. (From Trumble TE, editor: *Principles of hand surgery and therapy,* Philadelphia, 2000, WB Saunders.)

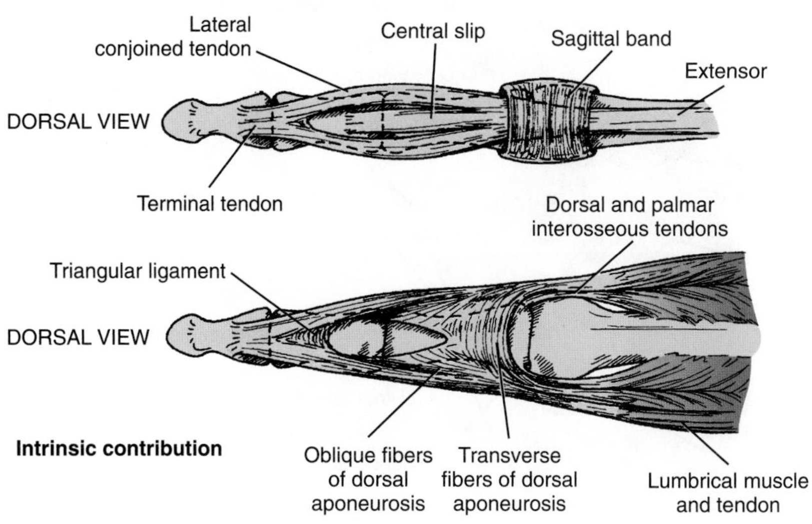

Figure 7-3 Dorsal view of the digital extensor mechanism. (From Trumble TE, editor: *Principles of hand surgery and therapy,* Philadelphia, 2000, WB Saunders.)

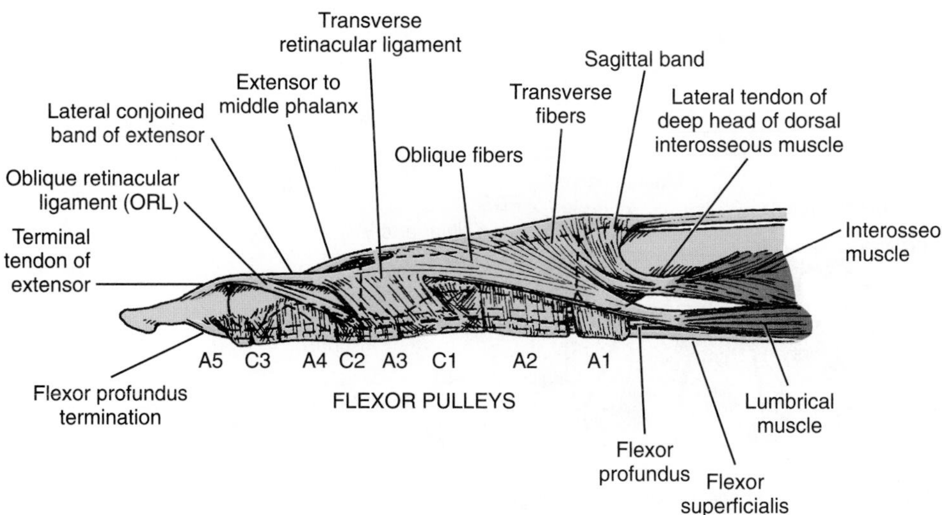

Figure 7-4 Lateral view of digital extensor mechanism. (From Trumble TE, editor: *Principles of hand surgery and therapy,* Philadelphia, 2000, WB Saunders.)

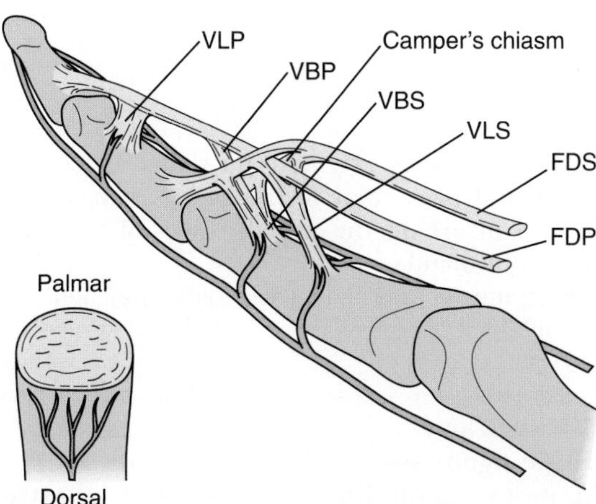

Figure 7-5 Decussation of the flexor digitorum superficialis (FDS) produces the Camper's chiasm. Both the FDS and flexor digitorum profundus (FDP) receive their blood supply via the vinculum longus and brevis. VBP, vinculum brevis profundus; VBS, vinculum brevis superficialis; VLP, vinculum longus profundus; VLS, vinculum longus superficialis. (From Trumble TE, et al, editors: *Core knowledge in orthopaedics: hand, elbow, and shoulder,* Philadelphia, 2006, Mosby, p 190.)

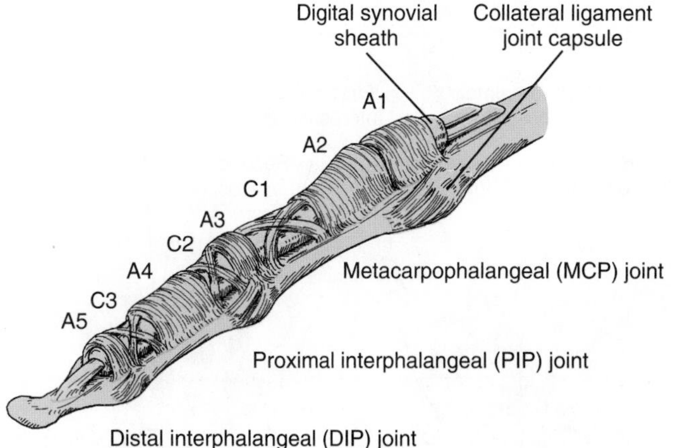

Figure 7-6 The flexor tendon sheath is composed of annular and cruciate pulleys. (From Trumble TE, editor: *Principles of hand surgery and therapy,* Philadelphia, 2000, WB Saunders.)

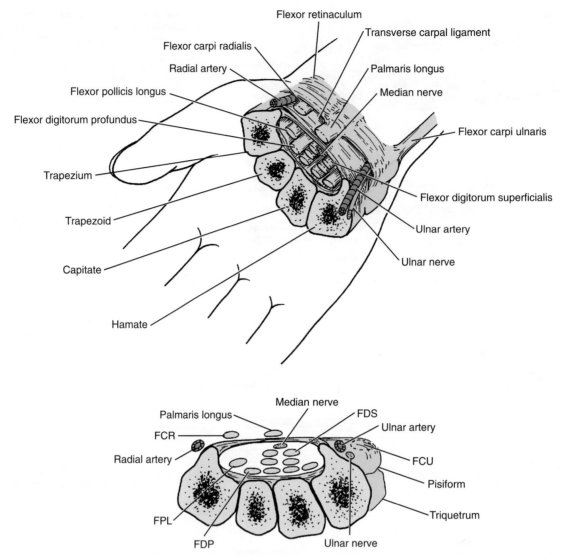

Figure 7-7 The median nerve, digital flexor tendons, and the flexor pollicis longus (FPL) pass through the carpal tunnel. FCR, flexor carpi radialis; FCU, flexor carpi ulnaris; FDP, flexor digitorum profundus; FDS, flexor digitorum superficialis. (From Trumble TE, editor: *Principles of hand surgery and therapy,* Philadelphia, 2000, WB Saunders.)

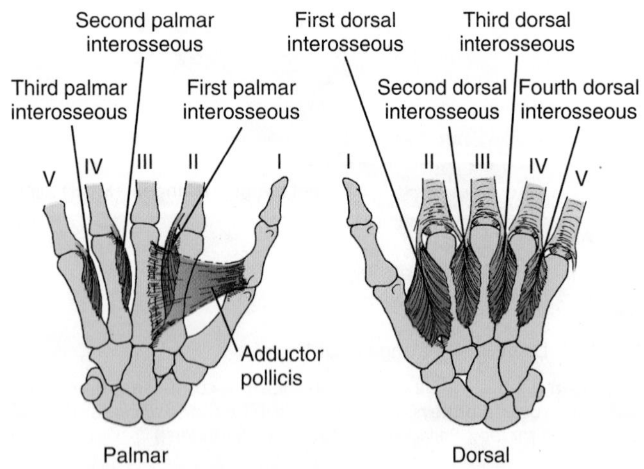

Figure 7-8 Four dorsal interossei provide abduction and three volar interossei provide adduction of the fingers. (From Trumble TE, editor: *Principles of hand surgery and therapy,* Philadelphia, 2000, WB Saunders.)

2. **Lumbrical muscles originate on radial aspect of FDP tendons and pass volar to transverse metacarpal ligaments to insert on the radial aspect of the extensor hood lateral bands.**
   - Contribute to interphalangeal joint extension through radial lateral bands, relax extrinsic flexor system (Figure 7-9)
   - Radial two lumbricals—innervated by median nerve
   - Ulnar two lumbricals—innervated by ulnar nerve
3. **Intrinsic tightness—PIP flexion less with MCP joints held in extension (intrinsics on stretch, extrinsics relaxed)**
4. Extrinsic tightness—PIP flexion less with MCP joints held in flexion (extrinsics on stretch, intrinsics relaxed)

D. Neurovascular anatomy

1. Entire hand supplied by branches of median, radial, and ulnar nerves
2. Sensory innervation of hand—Figure 7-10

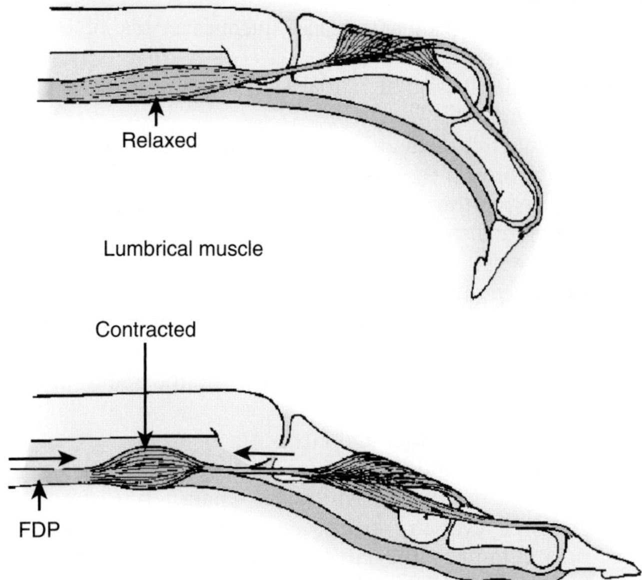

Figure 7-9 **The lumbrical muscles flex the metacarpophalangeal joint and extend the proximal interphalangeal joint. FDP, flexor digitorum profundus.** (From Trumble TE, editor: *Principles of hand surgery and therapy,* Philadelphia, 2000, WB Saunders.)

3. Median nerve—innervates pronator teres, FDS, FCR, PL, radial two lumbricals
   - Anterior interosseous branch of median nerve—innervates FPL, index and long FDP (50% of time), pronator quadratus
   - Palmar cutaneous branch of median nerve—usually lies between PL and FCR at distal wrist flexion crease
   - Recurrent motor branch of median nerve—innervates abductor pollicis brevis, opponens pollicis, and superficial head of flexor pollicis brevis
4. Ulnar nerve—innervates FCU, ring/small FDP (50% of time), ulnar two lumbricals
   - Deep motor branch of ulnar nerve—innervates hypothenar and interosseous muscles, adductor pollicis, and deep head of flexor pollicis brevis
5. Martin-Gruber anastomoses—crossover variations between median and ulnar nerves, approximately 15% of population
6. Radial nerve proper—innervates lateral portion of brachialis (also musculocutaneous), triceps, anconeus, brachioradialis, extensor carpi radialis longus (ECRL)
   - Divides into superficial sensory branch and posterior interosseous nerve (PIN), which innervates remaining extensor muscles
   - Extensor carpi radialis brevis (ECRB) has variable innervation.
   - Terminal branch of PIN—lies at floor of fourth extensor compartment
7. Proper digital nerves lie volar to proper digital arteries.
8. Vascular anatomy is covered in the section Vascular Disorders.

II. DISTAL RADIUS FRACTURES

A. Introduction

1. Most common fracture of the upper extremity (>300,000 per year in United States)
2. High-energy trauma in young
3. Low-energy falls in elderly persons with osteoporotic bone
4. Most prevalent group—white women over age 50 years

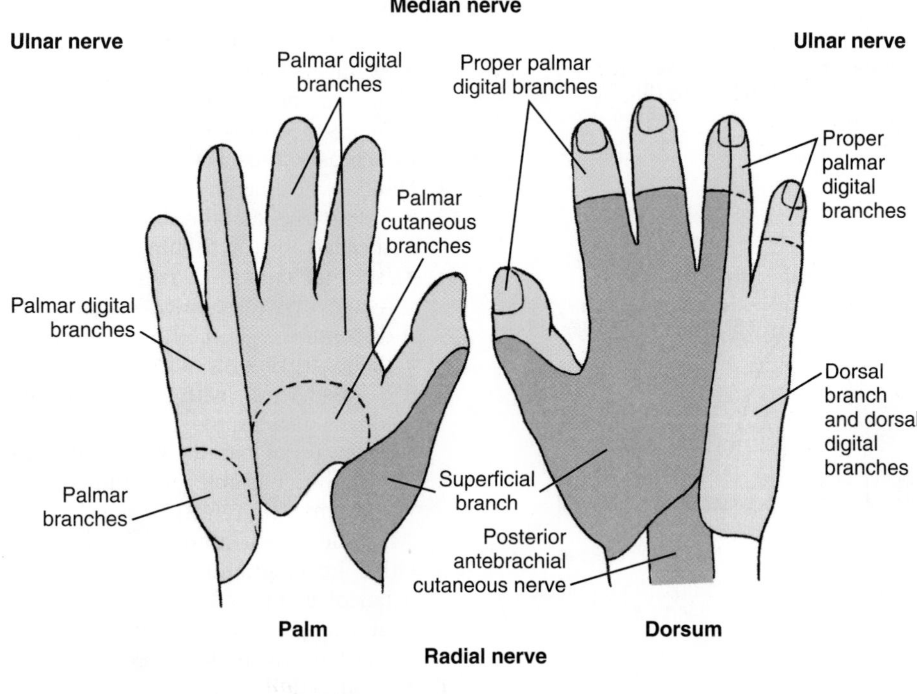

Figure 7-10 Sensory patterns of the median, ulnar, and radial nerves for the volar *(left)* and dorsal *(right)* aspects of the hand. (From Trumble TE, editor: *Principles of hand surgery and therapy,* Philadelphia, 2000, WB Saunders.)

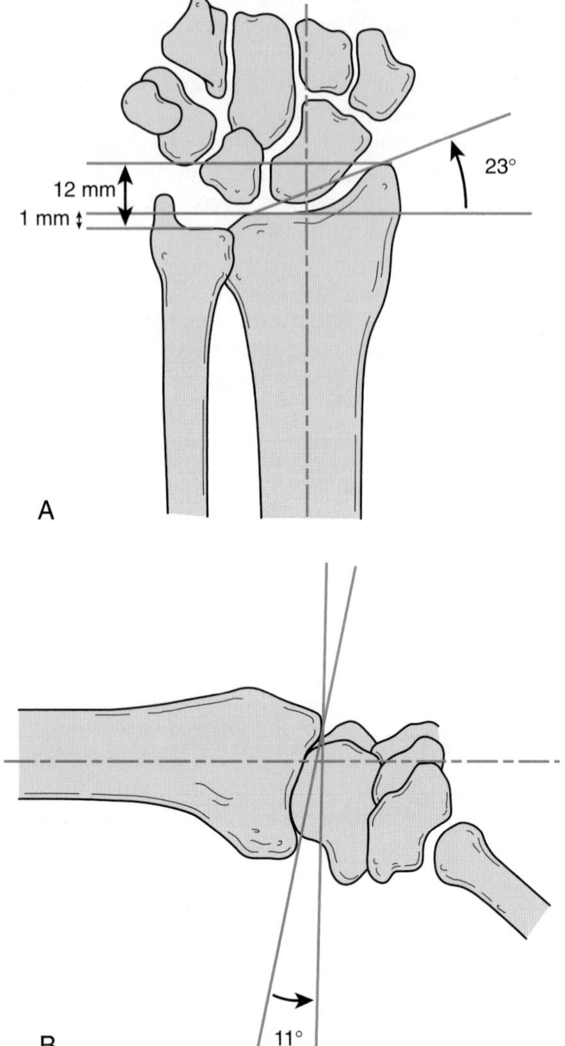

Figure 7-11 Schematic drawings of the average radial inclination **(A)** and volar tilt of the distal radius **(B).** (From Trumble TE, et al, editors: *Core knowledge in orthopaedics: hand, elbow, and shoulder,* Philadelphia, 2006, Mosby, p 89.)

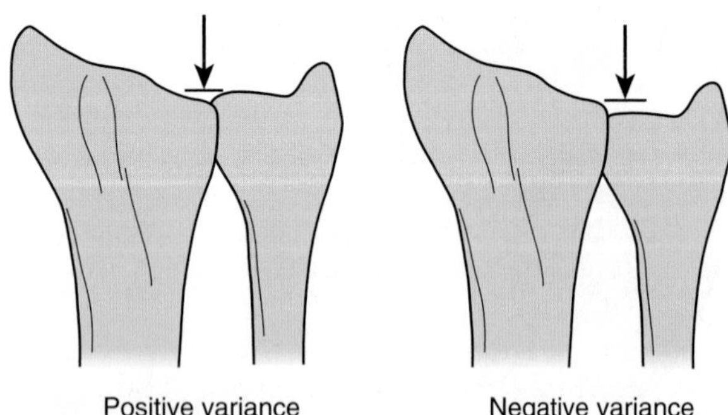

Figure 7-12 Ulnar variance of the distal radius. (From Trumble TE, et al, editors: *Core knowledge in orthopaedics: hand, elbow, and shoulder,* Philadelphia, 2006, Mosby, p 89.)

B. Anatomy
1. Distal radius articular surface—biconcave, scaphoid and lunate facets
2. Distal radioulnar joint (DRUJ)—articulation with ulna at sigmoid notch
3. Lister tubercle—small dorsal prominence, landmark for dorsal approach to wrist
4. Metaphysis—thin cortex, vulnerable to bending forces
5. Brachioradialis insertion—major deforming force
6. Normal wrist—Distal radius bears 80% of axial load.

C. Clinical evaluation
1. Pain, swelling, and deformity at the wrist after trauma
2. Open injuries more common in young patients
3. Examine for concurrent anatomic snuffbox and **ulnar-sided tenderness.**
4. Evaluate the shoulder and elbow.
5. Assess median and ulnar nerve function.
   - Acute carpal tunnel syndrome—characterized by progressive, evolving paresthesias and disproportionate pain; requires emergency median nerve decompression (carpal tunnel release)
   - Mild, vague, and nonprogressive sensory dysfunction is not indicative of acute carpal tunnel syndrome.
   - Ulnar nerve palsy after high-energy displaced distal radius fractures has also been described.

D. Radiographic evaluation (posteroanterior, lateral, and oblique views)
1. Intraarticular involvement
   - Evaluate pattern, gap, and step-off.
2. Distal fragment angulation
   - Apex dorsal—Smith
   - Apex volar—Colles
3. Radial height
   - Average 11 mm
4. Radial inclination
   - Average 22 degrees (Figure 7-11)
5. Volar tilt (lunate fossa inclination)
   - Average 11 degrees
6. Ulnar variance—neutral (normal), positive, or negative
   - Assessed with forearm in neutral rotation
   - Compare to contralateral side (Figure 7-12).
7. DRUJ involvement
   - Assess true lateral radiograph for DRUJ alignment.
8. Associated fractures—ulnar styloid, distal ulna, carpus
   - Isolated fracture of radial styloid (chauffeur's fracture) —may be associated with scapholunate ligament disruption
   - Radiocarpal dislocation may be purely ligamentous or associated with styloid fractures (radial and/or ulnar).
     - Beware of extremely distal fracture patterns.
     - Highly unstable and difficult to reduce by closed means
     - "Inferior arc" injury
9. Other imaging studies—computed tomography (CT) for detail of complex intraarticular patterns; magnetic resonance imaging (MRI) for occult fracture, bone contusion, associated soft tissue injury

E. Classification
1. Mostly descriptive
2. Common eponyms (Colles, Smith, Barton, Hutchinson) predate radiography.

3. Over 10 other schemes exist (e.g., AO, Frykman, Fernandez, Melone, Mayo) but largely fail to help predict treatment or prognosis.

F. **Treatment**

1. General goals—maintain reduction until union, restore function, prevent symptomatic post-traumatic radiocarpal osteoarthrosis
2. Factors considered—age, medical condition, activity demands, bone quality, fracture stability, associated injuries
3. Closed treatment
   - Definitive cast immobilization (favored over removable splints) sufficient in minimally displaced low-energy injuries, especially in functionally low-demand patients
     - Minimal initial displacement likely to remain stable
   - Closed reduction indicated in displaced fractures with abnormal radiographic parameters, especially in functionally high-demand patients
     - Dorsal hematoma block with local anesthetic
     - Finger traps, upper arm counterweight for ligamentotaxis
     - Recreate deformity, manipulate distal fragment.
     - Sugar tong plaster splint with three-point mold
     - Keep MCP and interphalangeal joints free for motion.
     - Radiographs obtained weekly for first 3 weeks
     - Loss of reduction correlates with increasing age.
     - **Postreduction benchmarks (American Academy of Orthopaedic Surgeons guideline)**
       - Radial shortening less than 3 mm
       - Dorsal articular tilt less than 10 degrees
       - Intraarticular step-off less than 2 mm
   - Immobilization for 6 to 8 weeks (no evidence to support any particular type)
   - Wrist and digit stiffness, muscle atrophy, and disuse osteopenia may result from prolonged immobilization.
     - Aggressive therapy for motion recovery and progressive strengthening
     - **Formal physical therapy compared to home exercise demonstrates no significant difference.**
4. Operative treatment
   - Closed reduction and percutaneous pinning (CRPP)
     - Kapandji intrafocal pinning used rarely
   - External fixation
     - Bridging and nonbridging techniques described
   - Open reduction with internal fixation (ORIF)
     - Dorsal plating
       - Approach between third and fourth extensor compartments
       - Articular reduction directly visualized
       - **Best for dorsally displaced fractures with dorsal bony defects**
       - Historical disadvantage—extensor tendon irritation/rupture from prominent hardware
     - Volar plating
       - Henry approach between FCR and radial artery or through floor of FCR tendon sheath
       - Articular reduction not directly visualized, relies on fluoroscopic guidance
       - Fixed-angle and variable-angle plates available
       - Best for Smith and Barton fracture patterns, increasingly used for dorsally displaced injuries
     - Fragment-specific
       - Low-profile constructs, technically challenging
     - Intramedullary nailing
       - May have role in stable, extraarticular patterns
       - Minimal long-term data to support use
     - Arthroscopic assistance
       - Aids in articular reduction
       - Ensures that screws do not penetrate joint
     - Injectable bone graft substitutes
       - Calcium phosphate
       - Coralline hydroxyapatite
   - Evidence does not support any advantage of early versus delayed motion recovery after surgical fixation of distal radius.
   - Concurrent treatment of ulnar styloid fracture not routinely necessary
     - No difference in multiple outcome measures when comparing patients undergoing ORIF of distal radius with and without ulnar styloid fracture
     - In small number of cases painful nonunion and DRUJ instability
5. Complications
   - Median nerve dysfunction is the most common complication following a distal radius fracture.
   - **Extensor pollicis longus (EPL) tendon rupture**
     - Most commonly occurs as a late complication following closed treatment because of attritional wear and/or vascular insufficiency near the Lister tubercle
     - Typically presents as a painless, acute loss of thumb extension
     - Treat with PL intercalary autograft or extensor indicis proprius (EIP)-to-EPL tendon transfer.
       - Primary repair often not possible
   - Nonunion uncommon
   - Asymptomatic malunion in a functionally low-demand patient does not require treatment.
   - Low-demand patients with pain from ulnocarpal impaction may benefit from a distal ulna resection (Darrach procedure).
   - A corrective radius osteotomy with ORIF and bone grafting may be indicated for high-demand patients.
   - Presence of radiocarpal osteoarthrosis following intraarticular distal radius fracture with residual step-off is prevalent but does not necessarily correlate with patient-reported symptoms.
   - Multiple case reports of flexor tendon ruptures after volar plating
     - FPL is the most common rupture after volar locking plating.
     - EPL is the most common extensor tendon injured, potentially due to drill-bit penetration or prominent screws.
   - Vitamin C in doses of at least 500 mg/day may decrease the incidence of complex regional pain syndrome (disproportionate pain).

III. CARPAL FRACTURES AND INSTABILITY

A. **Anatomy**

1. Eight carpal bones aligned in two rows
2. Proximal row—scaphoid, lunate, and triquetrum
   - Flexes with radial deviation, extends with ulnar deviation

Table 7-2 Incidence of Carpal Fractures

Bone	Number of Fractures*	% of Total
Scaphoid	5036	78.8
Triquetrum	880	13.8
Trapezium	144	2.3
Hamate	95	1.5
Lunate	92	1.4
Pisiform	67	1.0
Capitate	61	1.0
Trapezoid	15	0.2
Total	**6390**	

From Green DP, et al, editors: *Green's operative hand surgery,* ed 5, Philadelphia, 2005, Churchill Livingstone, p 711.

*The number of fractures represents a total of 6390 fractures compiled from three referenced studies to accumulate incidence of carpal bone fractures.

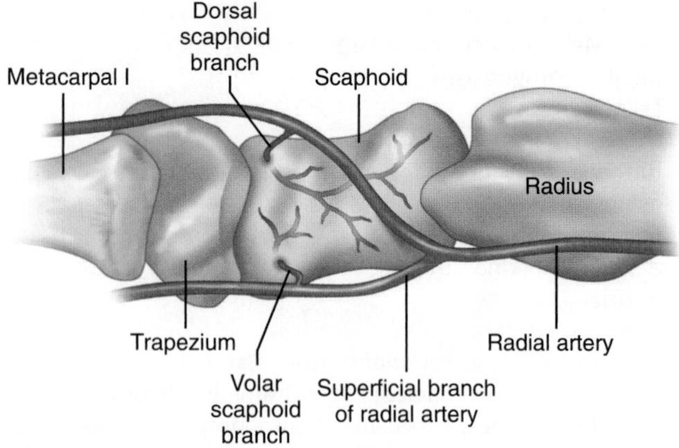

Figure 7-13 Dorsal and volar blood supply to the scaphoid from branches of the radial artery. (From Trumble TE, et al, editors: *Core knowledge in orthopaedics: hand, elbow, and shoulder,* Philadelphia, 2006, Mosby, p 117.)

3. Distal row—trapezium, trapezoid, capitate, and hamate
   May be considered as one unit
4. Pisiform is sesamoid within the FCU tendon.
5. Dart-thrower's motion is combined wrist extension–radial deviation to wrist flexion–ulnar deviation.
   - Occurs through midcarpal joint; proximal row remains relatively immobile
   - Functional arc for activities of daily living
6. Carpus has a rich vascular supply with multiple anastomoses.
7. Scaphoid, lunate, and capitate may each have large area supplied by a single interosseous vessel.
8. Some evidence suggests a proprioceptive role for the terminal branch of the posterior interosseous nerve, which may be compromised when this branch is sacrificed during dorsal approaches to the wrist.

B. Scaphoid fractures

1. Most common carpal fracture (Table 7-2), accounting for up to 15% of all acute wrist injuries
   - Anatomy
     - Approximately 75% covered by articular cartilage
     - Main blood supply comes from a dorsal branch of the radial artery, enters at dorsal ridge just distal to waist, and flows in retrograde fashion toward proximal pole.
     - Additional branches off superficial volar branch of radial artery enter at distal tubercle and perfuse distal one third.
     - Tenuous vascular anatomy renders waist and proximal pole fractures at risk for nonunion and post-traumatic osteonecrosis (Figure 7-13).
   - Diagnosis
     - Suspect when chief complaint is radial-sided wrist pain after injury or trauma
     - Most common mechanism is forced hyperextension and radial deviation of the wrist.
       - **This results in force transmission through the radioscaphoid articulation and concentration at the scaphoid.**
     - Swelling, anatomic snuffbox/volar tubercle tenderness, limited wrist motion
     - Posteroanterior, lateral, oblique, and scaphoid radiographic views
       - Scaphoid view—approximately 30 degrees of wrist extension and approximately 20 degrees of ulnar deviation
       - Radiographs initially nondiagnostic in more than 30% of cases
       - With negative radiographs and high clinical suspicion, thumb spica splint immobilization and repeat examination and radiographs in 2 weeks
     - Bone scan, ultrasonography, CT, and MRI have all been used for earlier diagnosis.
       - MRI has highest sensitivity, specificity, and accuracy (all >95%) with high positive and negative predictive values.
       - CT has lower predictive values.
       - Bone scan and ultrasonography lowest specificity and positive predictive value
       - All of these are better for ruling out rather than ruling in a scaphoid fracture.
     - Neglect of injury for 4 weeks increases nonunion rate from approximately 5% to 45%.
   - Classification
     - Location (Figure 7-14)
       - Tubercle, distal pole, waist (most common), proximal pole
     - Stability

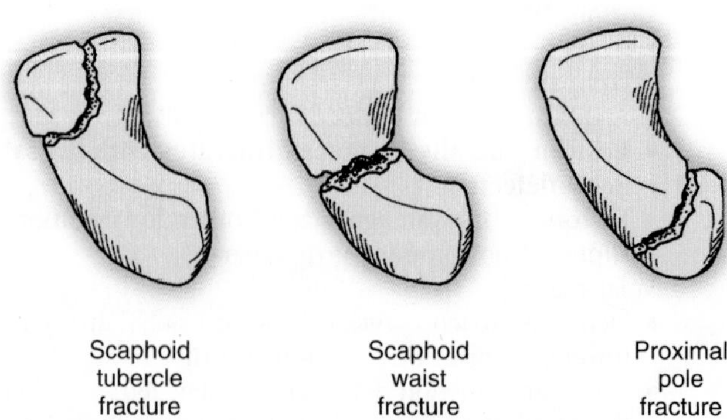

Figure 7-14 Scaphoid fractures can be simply described as involving the distal pole or tubercle, waist, or proximal pole. (From Trumble TE, editor: *Principles of hand surgery and therapy,* Philadelphia, 2000, WB Saunders.)

- Stable fractures characterized by transverse pattern, minimal comminution, and impaction
- Unstable fractures often demonstrate more vertical or oblique patterns, significant comminution, and wide displacement.
- CT probably best for characterizing displacement and stability

2. Treatment
   - Nonoperative
     - Cast immobilization for nondisplaced fractures
     - There is no evidence to suggest that the type of cast affects outcome (e.g., long-arm versus short-arm, standard versus additional thumb spica component).
     - Expected time to union increases and overall union rate decreases as the fracture becomes more proximal.
     - Consequently, length of cast immobilization should be greater for more proximal fractures.
   - Operative
     - **Indications include greater than 1 mm displacement, intrascaphoid angle greater than 35 degrees (humpback deformity), and trans-scaphoid perilunate dislocation.**
     - Proximal pole fracture is also a relative indication
     - **Minimally displaced fractures may be treated with percutaneous internal fixation.**
       - **Commonly performed via a dorsal approach**
       - **Direct visualization of the screw via a limited incision is recommended to ensure seating of the screw in subchondral bone.**
       - **Results in faster radiographic union and return to activity**
     - **Formal ORIF with headless compression screw for displaced injuries**
       - **Guide-pin placement should be along the central axis of both the proximal and distal fragments.**
     - Approach dictated by fracture location and surgeon preference
       - **Volar approach potentially avoids disruption to the blood supply of the scaphoid and is the most commonly employed approach.**
     - Union rates of over 90% to 95% expected
     - Aggressive physical therapy typically delayed until radiographic union achieved
     - CT may be necessary to confirm union (bridging trabeculae).
   - Complications
     - Include nonunion, malunion, osteonecrosis, and post-traumatic osteoarthrosis
     - **Symptomatic, early-stage scaphoid nonunion may be treated with ORIF and bone grafting.**
     - Inlay (Russe) technique best used in cases with minimal deformity and vascularized proximal pole
     - Scaphoid nonunion with accompanying humpback deformity requires open-wedge interposition (Fisk) graft to restore scaphoid length and angulation.
     - Grafts obtained from distal radius or iliac crest
     - Most surgeons typically use supplemental headless compression screw in nonunion cases.
     - Presence of intraoperative punctate bleeding is most reliable sign of vascular proximal pole.
     - Vascularized bone grafting has gained popularity in nonunions with avascular proximal pole.
       - Most commonly harvested from dorsal aspect of distal radius, based on 1,2 intercompartmental supraretinacular artery (1,2 ICSRA)
     - **Untreated, chronic scaphoid nonunion may lead to characteristic progression of post-traumatic osteoarthrosis called scaphoid nonunion advanced collapse (SNAC) wrist.**
       - Distal portion flexes, while proximal pole is tethered by intact scapholunate ligament and follows lunate into extension. This produces the humpback deformity.
       - **Staging**
         - **Stage I—radioscaphoid arthritis**
         - **Stage II—involvement of scaphocapitate joint**
         - **Stage III—lunocapitate joint**
       - Options for treatment of SNAC wrist include radial styloidectomy, proximal row carpectomy, scaphoid excision and four-corner (bone) fusion, and total wrist fusion, depending on stage of presentation and surgeon preference.

C. Other carpal bone fractures—small fraction of wrist injuries (see Table 7-2)

1. Lunate—rarely encountered in isolation
   - May be seen in setting of perilunate dislocation
   - Treat with ORIF for displaced fractures.
   - High rate of post-traumatic osteonecrosis
2. Capitate neck—may occur in combination with scaphoid fracture or perilunate dislocation, treated with ORIF or intercarpal fusion
3. Triquetrum—Majority of injuries are dorsal capsular avulsion fractures (wrist sprain) and require only brief period of immobilization.
4. **Hook of hamate—often from blunt trauma to palm, frequently associated with certain sports (e.g., golf, baseball, hockey, racquet sports)**
   - Imaging—**carpal tunnel view**, CT scan (Figure 7-15)
   - Symptomatic patients who fail trial of cast immobilization are treated with fracture fragment excision.
   - ORIF has been described for larger fracture fragments but has high complication rate and little clinical benefit.
   - Flexor tendon rupture may be seen with chronic nonunion.
   - Be aware of the bipartite hamate, which may be differentiated from a fracture by smooth cortical surfaces.

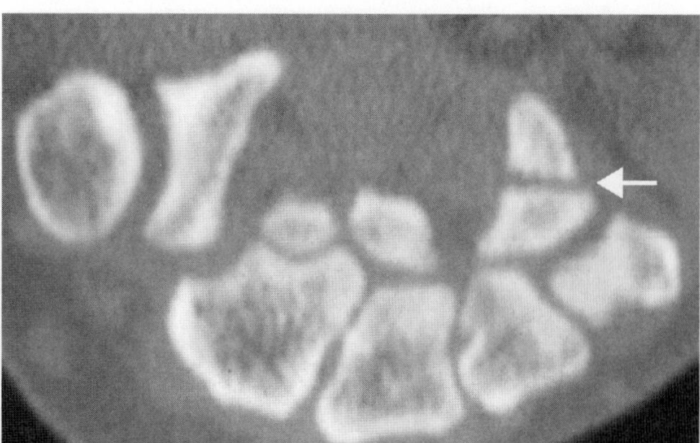

Figure 7-15 Sagittal computed tomographic scan of a hook-of-hamate fracture *(arrow)*. (From Trumble TE, editor: *Principles of hand surgery and therapy*, Philadelphia, 2000, WB Saunders.)

5. Fractures of trapezoid or pisiform—extremely rare
   - Pisiform fractures are treated with cast immobilization.
   - **If symptomatic nonunion occurs, pisiform excision can be performed.**

D. Carpal instability

1. Disruption of normal kinematics of wrist
2. Characterized by wrist pain, loss of motion, weakness
3. If untreated, may lead to degenerative arthritis and disability
4. Spectrum of injury from occult (predynamic) to dynamic to static
5. Static instability detected on standard radiographs, whereas dynamic instability requires either stress radiographs requires either stress radiographs, cineradiography, or live fluoroscopy
6. Carpal instability dissociative (CID) describes instability between individual carpal bones of single carpal row.
   - Examples include classical patterns of dorsal intercalated segmental instability (DISI) and volar intercalated segmental instability (VISI) (Figure 7-16).
7. Carpal instability nondissociative (CIND) describes instability between carpal rows, such as midcarpal or radiocarpal instability.
8. Carpal instability resulting from malunited distal radius fracture is an example of carpal instability adaptive.
9. Perilunate dislocations combine CID and CIND and are classified as carpal instability complex.
   - DISI—most common form of carpal instability
     - **Scapholunate ligament disruption**
     - **Dorsal fibers are stronger than volar fibers.**
     - Secondary injury to stabilizing dorsal and/or volar extrinsic ligaments, volar scaphoid-trapezo-trapezoid ligaments
     - Scaphoid hyperflexion and lunate hyperextension
     - May be traumatic or result from inflammatory or crystalline arthropathy
     - Physical examination findings
       - Dorsal wrist pain, often with loading
       - Diminished grip strength
       - Reproduction of pain/palpable clunk with scaphoid shift test (dorsally directed pressure over volar scaphoid tubercle while wrist brought from ulnar to radial deviation subluxates or dislocates scaphoid over dorsal ridge of distal radius that when released causes scaphoid to reduce with painful clunk) (Figure 7-17)
       - A bilateral nonpainful clunk is a negative test result.
     - Standard radiographs may reveal cortical ring sign (Figure 7-18), increased scapholunate angle (>70 degrees), or widened scapholunate interval (>3 mm) in static DISI.
     - Bilateral clenched-fist (anteroposterior grip) comparison views may reveal a dynamic DISI with relatively widened scapholunate interval on affected side (stress radiographs).
     - MRI best, but not perfect, for detection of scapholunate ligament injury (see Figure 7-18)
     - Gold standard is wrist arthroscopy.
       - Geissler classification (Table 7-3)
     - Treatment depends on stage of instability.
       - Partial injuries may improve with nonoperative treatment or arthroscopic débridement.
       - Acute scapholunate ligament rupture may be amenable to primary repair.
       - Delayed treatment may require open reduction of scapholunate interval and pinning with or without dorsal capsulodesis.
       - Limited clinical data on reduction-association of scaphoid and lunate (RASL) procedure
       - Tendon and bone-retinaculum-bone grafts have been attempted for scapholunate reconstruction.

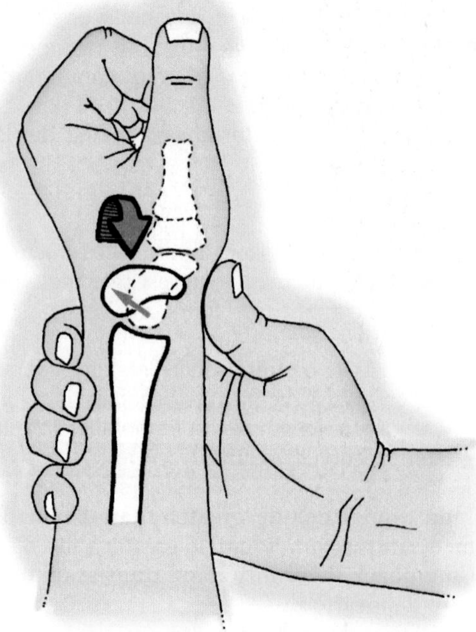

Figure 7-17 Watson scaphoid shift test. **Firm pressure is applied to the volar tubercle of the scaphoid while the wrist is moved from ulnar to radial deviation *(curved arrow)*. This may produce pain over the dorsal aspect of the scapholunate interval due to synovial irritation. The scaphoid is no longer constrained proximally and will dorsally subluxate from the scaphoid fossa *(straight arrow)*. When pressure on the scaphoid is removed, the scaphoid goes back into position, and a typical snapping or clunk occurs. Because this phenomenon may be present bilaterally in asymptomatic patients, the test is positive only when pain is elicited.** (From Green DP, et al, editors: *Green's operative hand surgery,* ed 5, Philadelphia, 2005, Churchill Livingstone, p 557.)

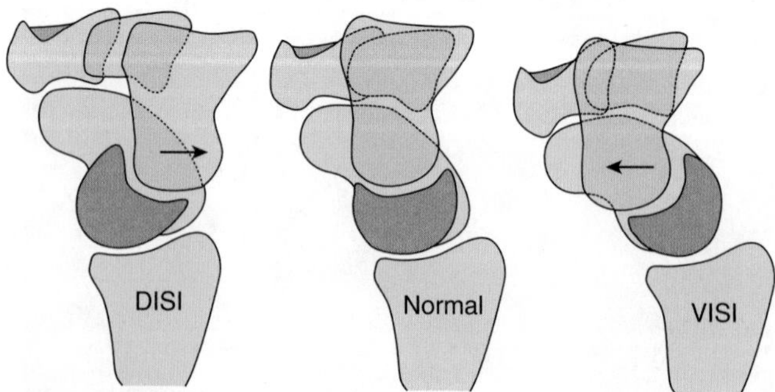

Figure 7-16 **The two major patterns of sagittal carpal malalignment are dorsal intercalated segment instability (DISI) and volar intercalated segment instability (VISI).** (From Green DP, et al, editors: *Green's operative hand surgery,* ed 5, Philadelphia, 2005, Churchill Livingstone, p 541.)

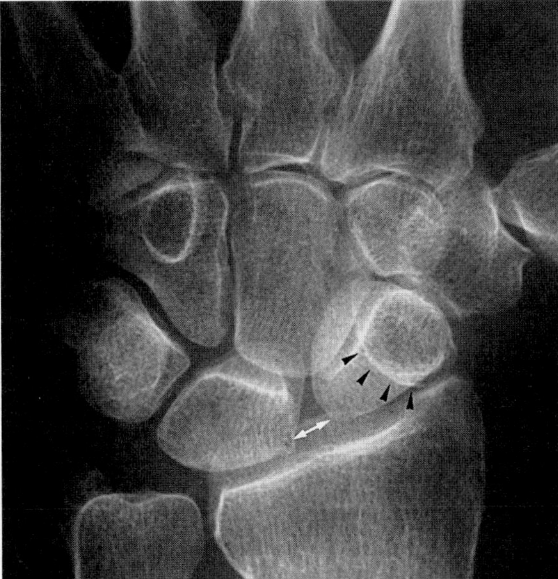

Figure 7-18 Posteroanterior view of the wrist of a 35-year-old man who sustained a hyperextension injury 4 months before seeking medical attention. Note the foreshortened scaphoid with a cortical ring sign *(arrowheads)*, representing the frontal projection of the volar tubercle, and the increased scapholunate joint space *(white arrow)*, indicating the presence of scapholunate dissociation with rotatory subluxation of the scaphoid. (From Green DP, et al, editors: *Green's operative hand surgery,* ed 5, Philadelphia, 2005, Churchill Livingstone, p 557.)

- Cases of chronic, static instability may result in scapholunate advanced collapse (SLAC wrist).
  - Three stages are described (Figure 7-19).
  - Radioscaphoid and capitolunate joints are affected, radiolunate joint is spared.
  - Treatment depends on condition of articular surfaces and competency of radioscaphocapitate ligament.
  - Options include radial styloidectomy, proximal row carpectomy, scaphoid excision and four-corner fusion, total wrist fusion.

Table 7-3 Geissler Classification of Arthroscopic Scapholunate Ligament Disruption

Grade	Description
I	Attenuation or hemorrhage of interosseous ligament as seen from radiocarpal space. No incongruity of carpal alignment in midcarpal space.
II	Attenuation or hemorrhage of interosseous ligament as seen from radiocarpal space. There may be a slight gap (less than width of probe) between carpal bones in midcarpal space.
III	Incongruity or step-off of carpal alignment as seen from both radiocarpal and midcarpal space. Probe may be passed through gap between carpal bones.
IV	Incongruity or step-off of carpal alignment as seen from both radiocarpal and midcarpal space. There is gross instability with manipulation. A 2.7-mm arthroscope may be passed through the gap between carpal bones ("drive-through sign").

- VISI—second most common form of carpal instability
  - Disruption of lunotriquetral interosseous ligament
  - Volar fibers are stronger than dorsal fibers.
  - Accompanying injury of the dorsal extrinsic ligaments may result in static instability.
    - Dorsal radiocarpal (DRC)
    - Dorsal intercarpal (DIC)
  - Both the scaphoid and lunate tilt volarly.
  - Ulnar-sided wrist pain
  - Physical examination
    - Positive lunotriquetral shear test
  - Radiographs may show break in Gilula arc on posteroanterior view and decreased scapholunate angle on lateral view.
  - MRI may show pathology of lunotriquetral ligament.
  - Arthroscopy is gold standard for diagnosis.
  - Treatment
    - Direct volar lunotriquetral repair
    - FCU tendon augmentation

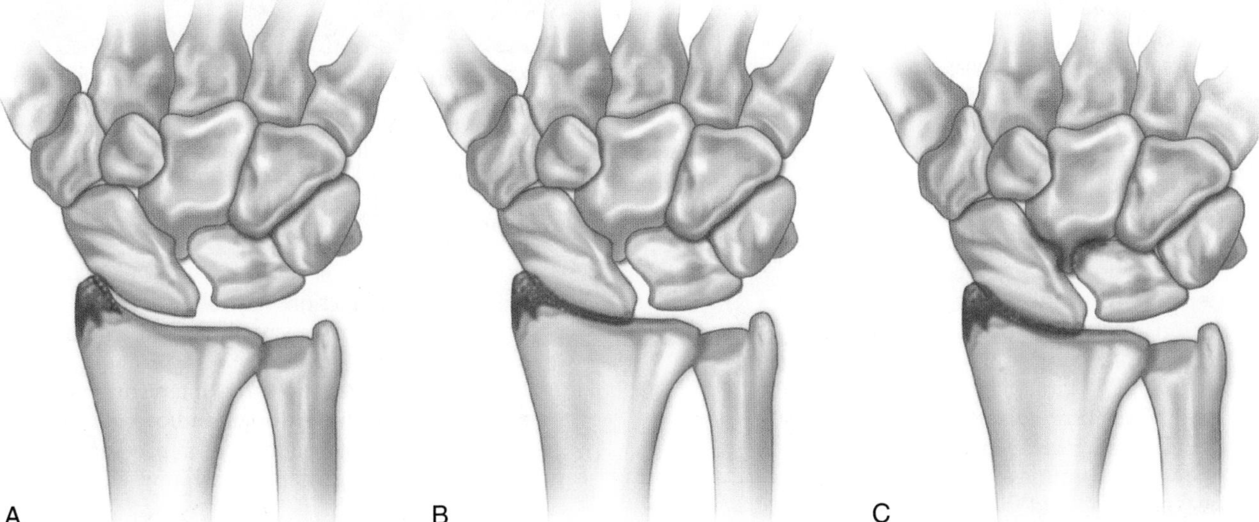

Figure 7-19 Progression of scapholunate advanced collapse. **A** and **B** depict progressive degenerative changes at the radioscapnoid joint. With advancing carpal collapse, the capitate may migrate proximally, resulting in midcarpal arthritis **(C)** and disruption of the Gilula lines radiographically. (© Mayo Clinic. Reproduced with permission of the Mayo Foundation.)

    - Lunotriquetral arthrodesis
    - Ulnar-shortening osteotomy for patients with concurrent ulnocarpal impaction syndrome
- Midcarpal CIND
  - Clunking wrist that may or may not be painful
  - Many patient have generalized ligamentous laxity.
  - History of trauma often absent
  - Sudden shift of proximal carpal row with active radial or ulnar deviation (cineradiographic studies)
  - Maximize nonoperative management.
  - Midcarpal fusion preferred over ligamentous reconstruction
- Radiocarpal dislocation (CIND)
  - Rare, high-energy injuries
  - "Inferior arc" injury
  - May be associated with intracarpal injury, acute carpal tunnel syndrome, possible compartment syndrome, other major musculoskeletal and/or organ injuries
  - Volar more severe than dorsal dislocation
  - May be purely ligamentous or include radial and/or ulnar styloid fractures
  - Ulnar translocation of the carpus signifies global ligamentous disruption.
    - Volar extrinsic ligaments
      - Radioscaphocapitate
      - Long radiolunate
      - Short radiolunate
      - Radioscapholunate, also termed ligament of Testut—neurovascular contents
  - Moneim proposed two types based on accompanying intracarpal fracture or interosseous ligament injury
  - Dumontier and Graham stressed the distinction between injuries with small versus large radial styloid fractures.
  - ORIF of styloid fractures may be enough to restore stability.
  - May also require direct ligamentous repair and/or external fixation to neutralize forces
  - Associated intracarpal injuries treated simultaneously
- Carpal instability adaptive from distal radius malunion
  - Correct distal radius alignment with osteotomy
- Perilunate dislocations (carpal instability complex)
  - Potentially devastating injuries resulting from forced dorsiflexion, ulnar deviation, and supination of wrist
  - **Approximately 25% of cases may be missed in the emergency department**
  - Mayfield described four stages of perilunar disruption of ligamentous constraints, proceeding in counterclockwise direction
    - Stage I—scapholunate disruption
    - Stage II—scaphocapitate disruption
    - Stage III—lunotriquetral disruption
      - Dorsal midcarpal dislocation
      - Capitate dorsal to lunate on lateral view
    - Stage IV—circumferential disruption
      - Volar lunate dislocation (Figure 7-20)
  - Lesser-arc injuries—purely ligamentous
  - Greater-arc injuries—carpal fracture
    - Trans-scaphoid
  - **Prompt treatment recommended**
  - **May attempt immediate closed reduction, especially in setting of acute carpal tunnel syndrome**

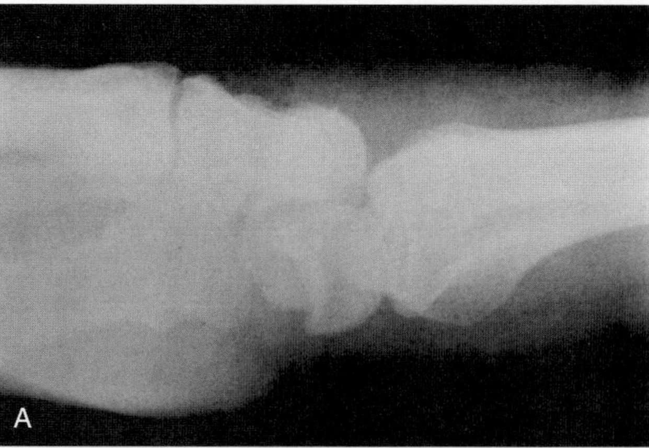

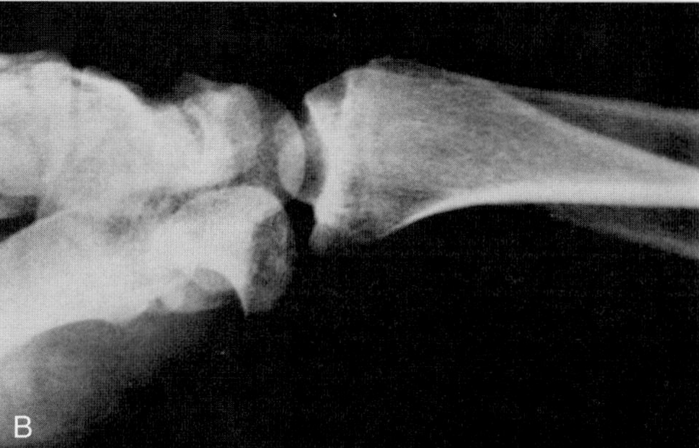

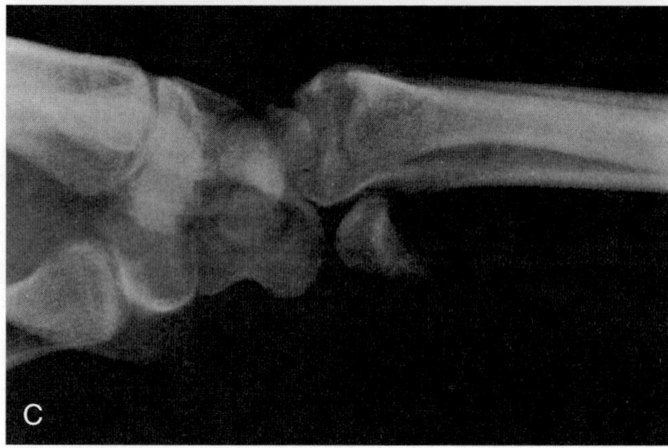

Figure 7-20 Carpal dislocations constitute a spectrum of injury, and the initial lateral radiograph in a patient with a carpal dislocation may depict a configuration at any point on that spectrum. **A,** A "pure" dorsal perilunate dislocation. **B,** An intermediate stage. **C,** A "pure" volar lunate dislocation. (From Green DP, et al, editors: *Green's operative hand surgery,* ed 5, Philadelphia, 2005, Churchill Livingstone, p 592.)

  - Stable closed reduction may allow for delayed definitive surgical management, but there is no role for closed treatment alone.
  - If irreducible, urgent operative intervention warranted
    - **ORIF, may require dorsal and/or volar approach**
    - Combination of ligamentous repair, dorsal capsulodesis, pinning of proximal row and midcarpal joint
    - Carpal tunnel release for associated acute carpal tunnel syndrome
    - Cast immobilization for 2 to 3 months

- Late diagnosis leads to consistently poor outcomes.
  - Methods of treating delayed and chronic perilunate dislocations are controversial.

IV. METACARPAL AND PHALANGEAL INJURIES

A. Introduction

1. Most frequently encountered injuries of skeletal system
2. Vast majority treated nonoperatively
   - Many initially splinted with hand in intrinsic-plus or "safe" position
     - Wrist in 15 to 30 degrees of extension
     - MCP joints in 70 to 90 degrees of flexion
     - Interphalangeal joints in neutral
   - Immobilization for 3 to 4 weeks at most
3. Surgical intervention may be indicated in open injuries, intraarticular fractures, irreducible fractures, digit malrotation, and multiple fractures.
4. Digit rotation assessed statically with wrist tenodesis and dynamically as patient initiates making a fist
   - All digits should point toward volar scaphoid tubercle.
5. Goals of treatment are stable reduction, edema control, and early range of motion.

B. Fractures and dislocations

1. Metacarpal head
   - Rare intraarticular injury
   - Most commonly occurs in index or middle finger
   - Greater than 1 mm of articular step-off may warrant ORIF.
   - Severe open or comminuted fractures (e.g., gunshot wounds) may be treated with spanning external fixation.
   - Associated open "fight bites" require surgical débridement.
2. Metacarpal neck
   - Weakest portion of metacarpal
   - Most frequently involves the ring and small finger
   - "Boxer's fracture"—metacarpal neck fracture of the small finger
   - Intrinsic muscles are major deforming force leading to apex dorsal angulation.
   - Check rotation, MCP joint extensor lag.
   - Many treated with closed reduction (Jahss maneuver) and 3 to 4 weeks of immobilization (Figure 7-21)
   - Suggested acceptable angulation of each metacarpal neck
     - Index and long fingers less than 20 degrees
     - Ring finger less than 40 degrees
   - Small finger less than 70 degrees (controversial)
   - Greater compensation from more mobile fourth and fifth carpometacarpal (CMC) joint
   - CRPP for irreducible fractures
3. Metacarpal shaft
   - May be transverse, oblique, or spiral
   - May be associated with higher risk of malrotation
     - Just 5 degrees of malrotation results in 1.5 cm of digital overlap.
   - Suggested acceptable angulation of each metacarpal shaft
     - Index and long fingers less than 10 degrees
     - Ring and small fingers less than 30 degrees

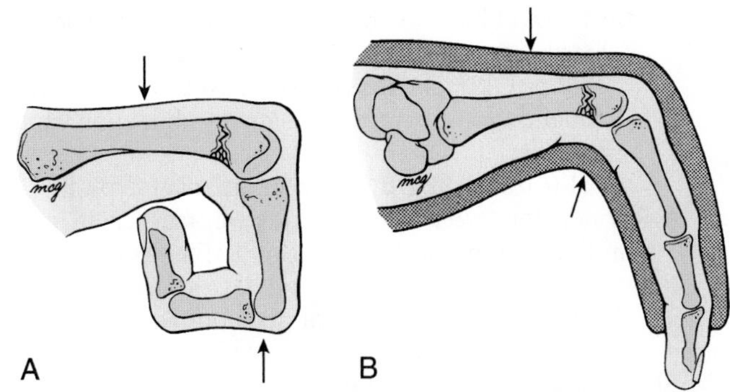

Figure 7-21 **A,** The Jahss maneuver for reduction of a metacarpal neck fracture. *Arrows* indicate the direction of pressure application for fracture reduction. **B,** After reduction, the fingers are held in an intrinsic-plus (safe) position with an ulnar gutter splint molded as indicated by arrows. (From Green DP, et al, editors: *Green's operative hand surgery,* ed 5, Philadelphia, 2005, Churchill Livingstone, p 283.)

   - Every 2 mm of metacarpal shortening leads to 7 degrees of extensor lag.
   - Up to 5 mm is acceptable without significant functional deficit.
   - Irreducible fractures are treated with CRPP or ORIF.
     - Prominent dorsal plates may interfere with extensor tendon function and necessitate later removal after union.
   - Multiple metacarpal shaft fractures are unstable injuries that often necessitate surgical intervention regardless of deformity.
4. Metacarpal base fracture and CMC joint dislocation
   - Stable, minimally displaced fractures of metacarpal base are typically treated nonoperatively.
   - Ring and small CMC joint fracture-dislocations often result from higher-energy mechanisms.
     - Pronated 30-degree oblique radiograph provides best view.
     - CT scan for better detail of complex injuries
   - Small-finger CMC joint fracture-dislocation is termed a "reverse" or "baby" Bennett fracture.
     - Extensor carpi ulnaris (ECU) tendon is major deforming force.
   - Accompanying distal row carpal fractures may be seen.
   - Attempt at closed reduction is warranted, but these unstable injuries often require surgical stabilization.
     - CRPP or ORIF
   - Delayed treatment, painful malunion, or post-traumatic osteoarthrosis may require arthrodesis.
5. Thumb metacarpal
   - Most common pattern is extraarticular epibasal fracture.
     - Up to 30 degrees of angulation acceptable secondary to compensatory CMC joint motion
     - Excessive angulation may lead to MCP joint hyperextension and requires CRPP.
   - Bennett fracture is an intraarticular fracture-dislocation.
     - **Abductor pollicis longus (APL) and thumb extensors cause proximal, dorsal, and radial displacement of the metacarpal shaft.**
     - Adductor pollicis causes supination and adduction of the metacarpal shaft.

- Anterior oblique or "beak" ligament keeps the volar-ulnar base fragment reduced to trapezium.
- CRPP or ORIF is chosen based on size of fragment.
- Reduction with traction, palmar abduction and pronation
- Goal is less than 1 to 2 mm of articular step-off.

- Rolando fracture is a comminuted intraarticular fracture that may be in shape of Y or T (Figure 7-22).
  - Degree of comminution guides treatment because CRPP, ORIF, and external fixation are all viable options.

6. Skier's or gamekeeper's thumb
   - **Acute (skier's) or chronic (gamekeeper's) injury to the thumb MCP joint ulnar collateral ligament (UCL)**
   - Competent UCL is critical for strong, effective pinch.
   - Mechanism of injury is usually forceful thumb hyperextension and/or hyperabduction.
   - Spectrum of injury potentially involving proper UCL, accessory UCL, and volar plate
   - Radiographs should be obtained before stress examination to rule out bony avulsion injury.
   - **Stress joint with radial deviation both at neutral and 30 degrees of flexion.**
     - **Instability in 30 degrees of flexion indicates injury to proper UCL.**
     - Additional instability in neutral indicates additional injury to accessory UCL and/or volar plate.
     - Threshold is greater than 35 degrees of opening or greater than 20 degrees difference compared to uninjured thumb.
   - Differentiation between complete and partial tears is difficult to determine by physical examination alone.
     - Stress radiographs and/or MRI may aid in the diagnosis.
   - Partial injuries may be initially treated with thumb spica cast immobilization for 4 to 6 weeks.
   - **In over 85% of cases, a complete injury is accompanied by a Stener lesion, in which the adductor pollicis aponeurosis is interposed between the avulsed UCL and its insertion site on the base of the proximal phalanx** (Figure 7-23).
     - Presence of a Stener lesion may be palpable on examination, prevents proper healing, and requires surgical intervention to reattach the ligament through drill holes or suture anchor.
   - A displaced avulsion fracture of the base of the proximal phalanx may occasionally require ORIF if large enough fragment.

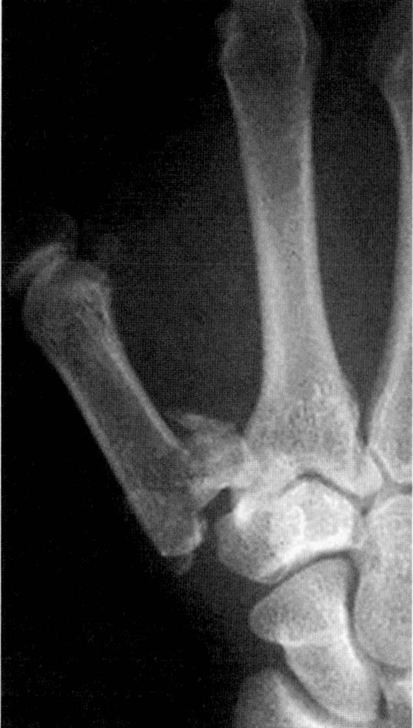

Figure 7-22 Comminuted metacarpal base fracture. (From Trumble TE, et al, editors: *Core knowledge in orthopaedics: hand, elbow, and shoulder,* Philadelphia, 2006, Mosby, p 66.)

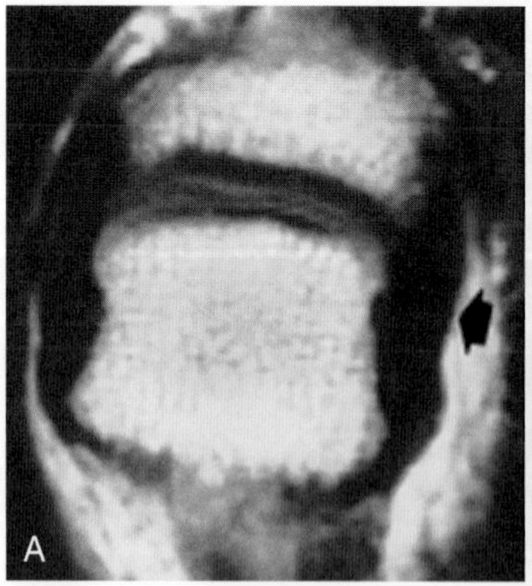

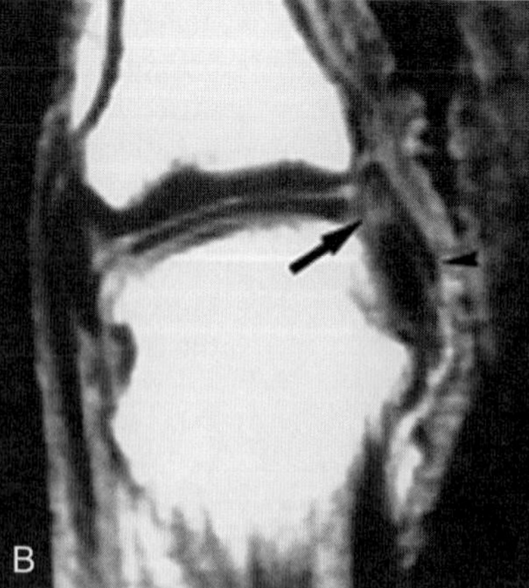

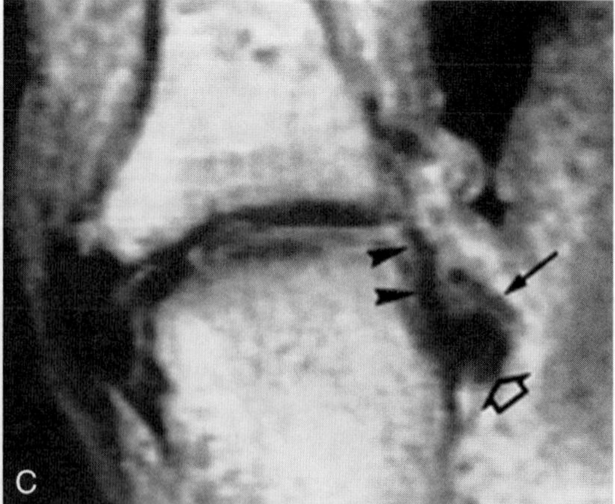

Figure 7-23 MRI of the thumb MCP joint and ulnar collateral ligament [UCL]. **A,** Normal UCL *(thick arrow)*. **B,** Partially torn UCL from its distal insertion without significant retraction *(thin arrow)*. Arrowhead indicates intact adductor aponeurosis. **C,** Completely torn UCL from its distal insertion with Stener lesion *(thick open arrow)*. Arrowheads indicate intact accessory fibers. *Thin arrow* shows leading edge of adductor aponeurosis. A Stener lesion occurs when the torn proper ulnar collateral ligament of the thumb metacarpophalangeal joint lies superficial to the leading edge of the adductor aponeurosis, preventing proper healing. (From Trumble TE, et al, editors: *Core knowledge in orthopaedics: hand, elbow, and shoulder,* Philadelphia, 2006, Mosby, p 61.)

- Chronic UCL injuries require ligament reconstruction with either adjacent joint capsule or tendon graft with or without pinning of joint
  - Associated post-traumatic osteoarthrosis best treated by MCP fusion

7. MCP joint dislocation
   - Classified as simple or complex
   - Dorsal dislocations are most common.
     - Skin dimpling in distal palm pathognomonic
   - Index, small fingers most frequently involved
   - In simple dislocation, P1 is perched on metacarpal and closed reduction usually possible
     - Longitudinal traction and MCP hyperextension avoided
     - Direct pressure over P1 with wrist in flexion to relax extrinsic flexors
   - In complex dislocation, P1 and metacarpal are in bayonet position and interposition of volar plate and/or sesamoids likely
     - Usually irreducible by closed means
     - Open reduction through dorsal or volar approach
     - Volar approach risks iatrogenic neurovascular injury.
       - A1 pulley divided to loosen noose around metacarpal head and volar plate removed
8. Boxer's knuckle
   - Most common hand injury in both amateur and professional fighters
   - The extensor hood of the MCP joint is ruptured, leading to increased risk of chondral injury and osteoarthrosis of the joint.
   - Presents with swelling, reduced range of motion, and occasional extensor lag
   - **Treatment is via direct repair of the extensor hood.**
9. P1 and P2 phalanges
   - Fractures of P1 deform with apex volar angulation.
     - Proximal fragment flexion (interossei)
     - Distal fragment extension (central slip)
   - Fractures of P2 deform with apex dorsal or volar angulation.
     - Apex dorsal if fracture proximal to FDS insertion
     - Apex volar if fracture distal to FDS insertion
   - **Majority treated nonoperatively if less than 10 degrees of angulation and no rotational deformity**
   - Three weeks of immobilization followed by aggressive motion recovery
   - Radiographic union lags behind clinical union by several weeks.
   - **Irreducible or unstable fracture patterns may require surgery.**
   - Operative techniques
     - Crossed Kirschner wires
     - Eaton-Belsky pinning through metacarpal head
     - Minifragment fixation
       - Lag screws
       - Plate and screw construct
     - External fixation reserved for highly comminuted intraarticular fractures or those associated with gross contamination and segmental bone loss
10. PIP joint dislocation
    - Dorsal dislocation—most common
      - **Injury to volar plate** and at least one collateral ligament
      - "Simple" dislocation—middle phalanx in contact with condyles of proximal phalanx
        - Easily reduced with longitudinal traction
      - "Complex" dislocation—base of middle phalanx no longer in contact with condyle of proximal phalanx, giving a bayonet appearance
        - Volar plate acts as block to reduction if longitudinal traction applied.
        - Reduction via hyperextension of middle phalanx followed by a palmar force
      - Short-term buddy taping is sufficient aftercare.
      - Persistent instability is rare but may be treated by dorsal block splinting.
      - Persistent swelling and soreness for months is common.
      - Irreducible complex dislocations require open reduction via a dorsal approach and incision between the central slip and lateral band.
    - Volar dislocation
      - **Injury to central slip** and at least one collateral ligament
      - Splinted in full extension for 6 weeks after reduction
      - **Inadequate treatment will lead to boutonniere deformity.**
    - **Rotatory dislocation**
      - **One of the phalangeal condyles is buttonholed between central slip and lateral band.**
      - Often requires open reduction
11. PIP joint fracture-dislocation
    - Inappropriate recognition and treatment of these injuries may result in significant functional deficits.
    - Dorsal dislocation accompanied by fracture at P2 base (Figure 7-24)
    - Hastings classification based on amount of P2 articular surface involvement (Table 7-4)
    - Treatment options include dorsal block splinting, ORIF, and volar plate arthroplasty.
      - **Regardless of treatment, maintenance of adequate joint reduction is the most important factor for favorable long-term outcome.**
    - Highly comminuted "pilon" fractures may be treated with the dynamic distraction external fixation method for ligamentotaxis and early range of motion.
    - Chronic PIP fracture-dislocations are best treated with volar plate arthroplasty or arthrodesis.

Table 7-4 Classification of PIP Joint Fracture-Dislocations (Hastings)

Type	Amount of P2 Articular Surface Involved	Treatment
I—Stable	<30%	Dorsally based extension block splint
II—Tenuous	30%-50%	If reducible in flexion, dorsally based extension block splint
III—Unstable	>50%	ORIF, hamate autograft, or volar plate arthroplasty

ORIF, open reduction with internal fixation; PIP, proximal interphalangeal; P2, middle phalanx.

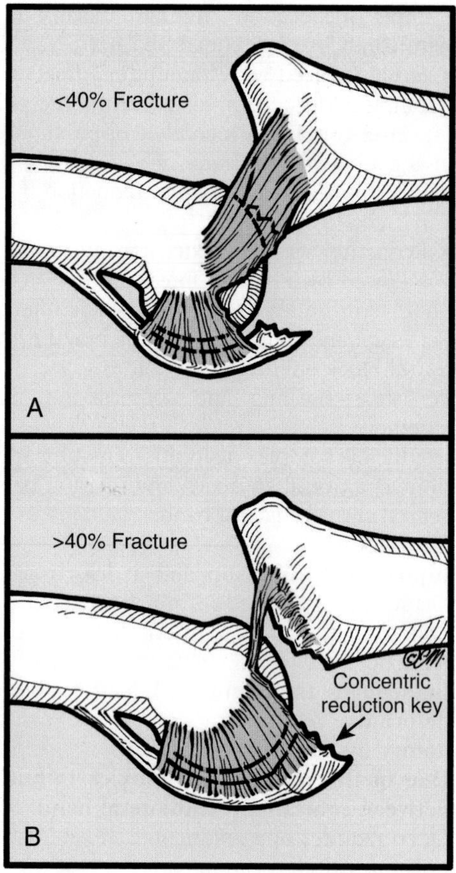

Figure 7-24 Fracture-dislocations of the proximal interphalangeal (PIP) joint. **A,** Fracture-dislocations with 40% or less of the articular surface involved may be successfully treated with dorsal extension block splinting. The patient is allowed to actively flex the PIP joint, while extension is slowly progressed over the course of approximately 4 weeks. **B,** Fracture-dislocations with more than 40% of the articular surface involved are highly unstable and may require open reduction and internal fixation. The key to all treatment is concentric reduction of the PIP joint. (From Green DP, et al, editors: *Green's operative hand surgery,* ed 5, Philadelphia, 2005, Churchill Livingstone, p 349.)

12. DIP dislocation and distal phalanx fractures
    - DIP dislocation is treated with closed reduction followed by immobilization in slight flexion with a dorsal splint for 2 weeks.
    - **Irreducible DIP dislocations are typically due to interposition of the volar plate; treatment is via open reduction and extraction of the volar plate.**
    - May accompany extensive soft tissue and/or nail bed disruption in severe fingertip injuries
    - Open injuries initially treated with irrigation and débridement, reduction, nail bed repair (if necessary), antibiotics, tetanus prophylaxis, and splinting
    - Unstable, displaced fractures of the distal phalanx may require percutaneous pinning to support the nail bed repair.
    - A stable tuft fracture is more common with these injuries and requires no specific treatment apart from temporary splinting.
    - Soft tissue loss treated accordingly
    - Highly comminuted injuries with significant soft tissue loss may be more amenable to revision amputation (shortening and closure).
    - For further details see the section "Nail and Fingertip Injuries"

V. TENDON INJURIES AND OVERUSE SYNDROMES

A. Extensor tendon injury

1. Description and treatment are based on zones of injury (Figure 7-25).
2. Most commonly injured digit is long finger.
3. Partial lacerations less than 50% of tendon width do not require direct repair if patient can extend finger against resistance.
    - Early protected motion to prevent adhesions
4. After direct suture repair of complete lacerations or those constituting more than 50% of tendon width, rehabilitation is based on zone of injury.
    - Zone I injury (mallet finger)
        - Disruption of terminal extensor tendon at or distal to the DIP joint
        - Sudden forced flexion of the extended fingertip
        - Patient cannot actively extend at DIP joint, and finger remains in flexed posture.
        - May be accompanied by bony avulsion injury from dorsal base of P3 (bony mallet)
        - If detected within 12 weeks of injury, closed management with full-time DIP joint extension splinting for at least 6 weeks, followed by part-time splinting for an additional 4 to 6 weeks
        - No consensus on best type of splint to use

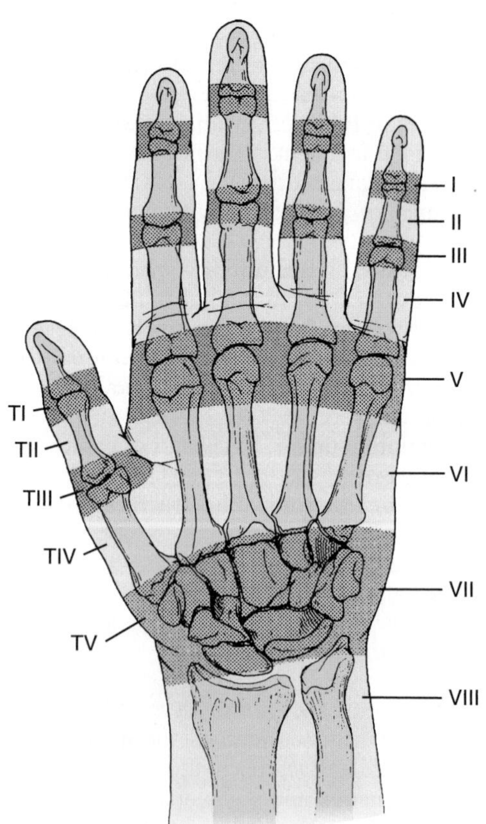

Figure 7-25 Zones of the extensor tendon system. (From Trumble TE, et al, editors: *Core knowledge in orthopaedics: hand, elbow, and shoulder,* Philadelphia, 2006, Mosby, p 203.)

- Hyperextension should be avoided; skin necrosis can occur.
- Noncompliance is common.
- Maintenance of PIP joint motion often overlooked
- A nondisplaced, bony mallet finger may also be treated with extension splinting until fracture union.
- **A relative surgical indication is a displaced bony mallet injury with significant volar subluxation of P3.**
  - CRPP through DIP joint
  - Extension block pinning
  - ORIF if large fragment (>50% articular surface)
- Chronic mallet finger detected more than 12 weeks after injury
  - Closed treatment only if joint supple, congruent, and without arthritic changes
  - Dynamic splinting, serial casting for contracted joint
  - Operative—tenodermodesis
- Prolonged DIP flexion may lead to swan neck deformity (Figure 7-26), caused by dorsal subluxation of lateral bands and corresponding PIP joint hyperextension.
  - Fowler central slip tenotomy
  - Spiral oblique retinacular ligament reconstruction
- A painful, stiff, arthritic DIP joint is treated with arthrodesis.

- Zone II injury
  - Occurs over middle phalanx of digit or over proximal phalanx of thumb
  - Mechanism of injury usually involves a dorsal laceration or crush component.
  - Partial disruptions (<50%) are treated nonoperatively with local wound care and early mobilization.
  - Direct repair may be attempted for greater than 50% lacerations.
  - Some surgeons will temporarily pin across terminal joint after direct repair.
- Zone III injury (boutonniere)
  - **Occurs over PIP joint of digit (central slip) or MCP joint of thumb**
  - Open injuries are directly repaired if possible.
    - Loss of tendon substance may require a free-tendon graft or extensor mechanism turndown flap.
  - For closed injuries, the Elson test is performed by flexing the patient's PIP joint 90 degrees over the edge of a table and asking patient to extend the PIP joint against resistance (Figure 7-27).
    - If the central slip is intact, the DIP joint will remain supple.
    - If the central slip is ruptured, the DIP joint will be rigid.
  - **An acute boutonniere deformity results from central slip disruption and volar subluxation of the lateral bands, resulting in DIP hyperextension** (Figure 7-28).
  - Closed injuries are treated with full-time PIP extension splinting for at least 6 weeks, followed by part-time splinting for an additional 4 to 6 weeks.
    - DIP flexion maintained to balance extensor mechanism
  - **Chronic (untreated) boutonniere deformity**
    - May require dynamic splinting or serial casting to achieve maximal passive motion first
    - Terminal extensor tenotomy, PIP volar plate release
    - **Central slip reconstruction techniques**
      - Tendon graft
      - Extensor turndown
      - Lateral band mobilization
      - Transverse retinacular ligament
      - FDS slip
  - A painful, stiff, arthritic PIP joint is treated with arthrodesis.
- Zone IV injury
  - Occurs over proximal phalanx of digit or over the metacarpal of thumb
  - Treatment is similar to that for injuries in zone II.
  - A common complication in this zone is adhesion formation, with resulting loss of digital flexion.
    - Adhesion formation may be reduced with early protected range of motion and dynamic splinting.
    - Failure of nonoperative management may require extensor tenolysis.
- Zone V injury
  - Occurs over MCP joint of digit or over CMC joint of thumb
  - Lacerations involving more than 50% of the tendon substance should be repaired.

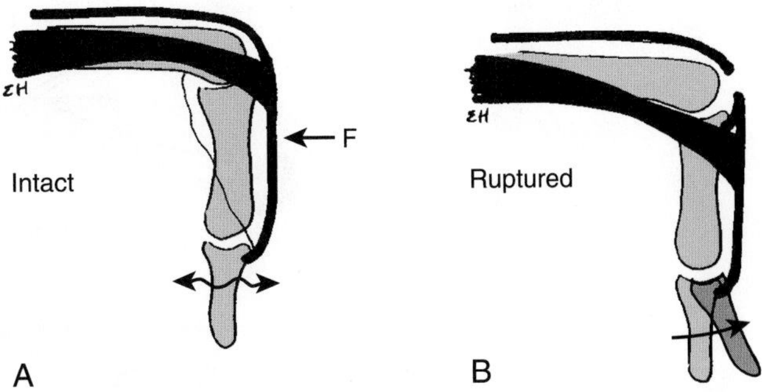

Figure 7-27 Elson test for acute rupture of the central slip. **A,** Intact central slip renders the DIP joint supple or floppy with forced extension against resistance at the PIP joint. The lateral bands are relatively relaxed. **B,** Ruptured central slip renders the DIP joint rigid because of lateral band activation to extend digit. F, static force. (From Trumble TE, et al, editors: *Core knowledge in orthopaedics: hand, elbow, and shoulder,* Philadelphia, 2006, Mosby, p 206.)

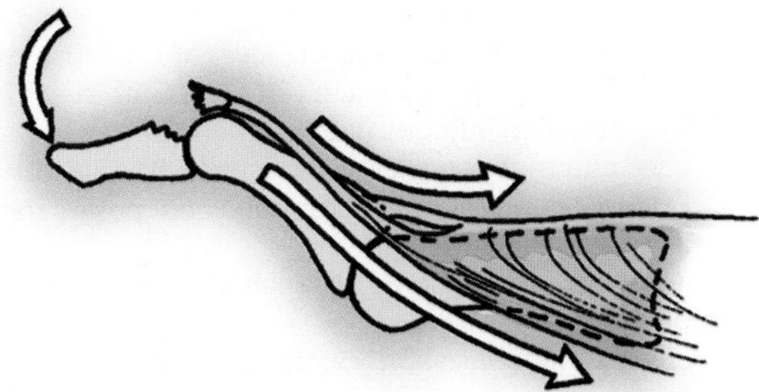

Figure 7-26 Swan neck deformity resulting from disruption of the terminal extensor tendon, dorsal subluxation of the lateral bands, and subsequent hyperextension of the proximal interphalangeal joint. (From Trumble TE, editor: *Principles of hand surgery and therapy,* Philadelphia, 2000, WB Saunders.)

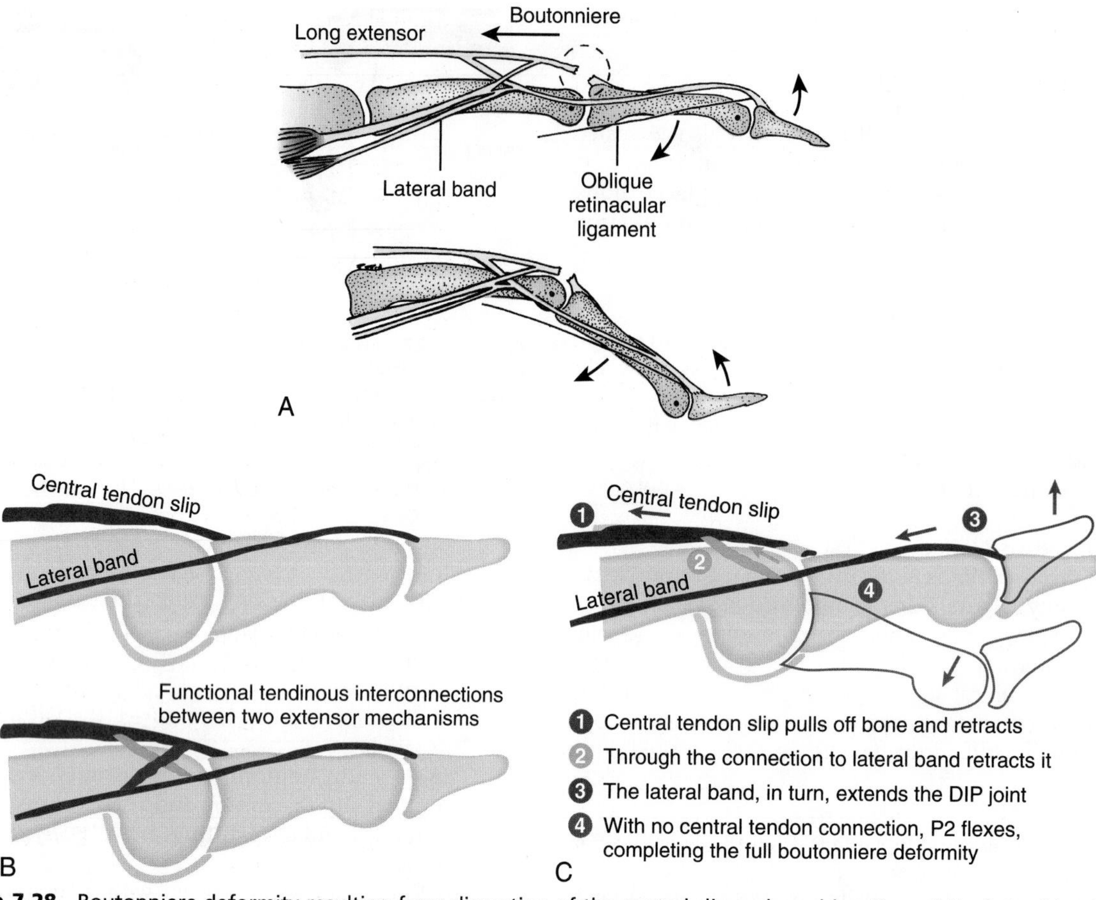

Figure 7-28 Boutonniere deformity resulting from disruption of the central slip, volar subluxation of the lateral bands, and subsequent hyperextension of the distal interphalangeal joint. **A,** Schematic depicting changes to extensor mechanism resulting from central slip disruption. Contribution of oblique retinacular ligaments is controversial. **B,** Typical interconnections are present between central slip and lateral bands. **C,** Progression of changes following central slip rupture resulting in boutonniere deformity. (From Trumble TE, et al, editors: *Core knowledge in orthopaedics: hand, elbow, and shoulder,* Philadelphia, 2006, Mosby, p 206.)

- Early mobilization and dynamic splinting is advocated.
- A fight bite requires surgical débridement of the MCP joint with loose or delayed wound closure.
  - Treat with culture-specific antibiotics. Eikenella corrodens is a common mouth organism.
  - Extensor lag and loss of flexion are common.
- A sagittal band rupture ("flea-flicker" injury) may result from forced extension of flexed digit.
  - Long finger most common
  - Rupture of the stronger radial fibers may lead to extensor tendon subluxation/dislocation
  - Finger will be held in flexed position at MCP joint with no active extension
  - Passive extension of the MCP joint is possible, and the patient can then usually maintain the finger in an extended position
  - Acute injuries may be treated with 4-6 weeks of extension splinting of the MCP joint (one of the only exceptions to splinting the MCP joints in flexion)
  - Failure of nonoperative management or missed injuries with delayed diagnosis may require repair or reconstruction of the sagittal band
- Zone VI injury
  - Occurs over metacarpal and represents most frequently injured zone
  - Associated lacerations of superficial veins and nerves are likely.
  - Direct repair is indicated when the disruption constitutes more than 50% of the tendon substance.
  - Early protected motion advocated postoperatively
    - Dynamic splinting may offer better short-term range of motion and strength without increased complications over static splinting.
    - No long-term difference
  - The prognosis is good in the absence of concurrent skeletal injury.
- Zones VII and VIII injury
  - Zone VII injury occurs at the level of the wrist joint, and zone VIII injury occurs in the distal forearm at the musculotendinous junction.
  - Lacerations at wrist level are usually associated with extensor retinaculum disruption, and postoperative adhesions are common.
  - The retinaculum should be repaired to prevent tendon bowstringing.
  - Static immobilization with the wrist held in extension and the MCP joints partially flexed is advised for the first 3 weeks, followed by protected motion.
  - The results of surgical repair in these zones are not as good as those in zones IV, V, and VI.

B. Flexor tendon injury

1. Overview
- This injury usually results from volar lacerations, and concomitant neurovascular injury is common.
- Rather than attempting to probe wounds acutely, note the resting posture of the hand and check the tenodesis effect with passive wrist flexion and extension.
- Each digit is then tested in isolation for active DIP and PIP flexion, especially in setting of multiple digit trauma.
  - The profundus tendons (middle through small) typically share a common muscle belly so that DIP flexion of each digit must be tested while blocking the other digits in extension.
  - The superficialis tendons have independent muscle bellies and may be tested without blocking other digits.
  - FDS to small absent in approximately 25% of population
- Patial lacerations may be associated with gap formation or triggering with nonoperative treatment.
- Triggering may be alleviated by trimming tendon ends under flexor tendon sheath.
- Standard of care for lacerations greater than 60% of tendon width is simultaneous core and epitendinous repair within 3 weeks, but preferrably within 7 to 10 days of injury.
- **Basic surgical techniques of flexor tendon repair**
  - **Strength of repair proportional to number of suture strands that cross repair site**
    - Six to eight strands have superior strength and stiffness.
  - **High-caliber (e.g., 5-0 instead of 6-0) suture material decreases gap formation and increases strength and stiffness.**
  - **A locking-loop configuration decreases gap formation.**
  - **Epitendinous repair decreases gap size and increases overall strength by 10% to 50%.**
  - Purchase, defined as the longitudinal distance from cut tendon end to transverse component of the core suture, should be 0.7 to 1.2 cm.
  - Dorsally placed core sutures are stronger.
  - **Repair of the flexor tendon sheath has no effect on flexor tendon repair.**
- An atraumatic minimal-touch technique minimizes adhesions.
- To prevent tendon bowstringing, A2 and A4 pulleys should be preserved in digits and oblique pulley preserved in thumb.
- Risk of tendon rupture greatest 3 weeks after repair, and failure typically occurs at suture knots.
- **In general, early protected range of motion is advocated to increase tendon excursion, decrease adhesion formation, and increase repair strength.**
  - **Use of an active flexion protocol postoperatively requires a minimum four-strand repair with epitendinous suture.**
  - **Young children cannot comply with protected motion protocols and require cast immobilization for 4 weeks.**
- Tendon healing factors
  - Abundant research continues to be focused on flexor tendon injuries.
  - No repair tissue matches the strength and stiffness of a normal uninjured tendon.
  - Intrinsic healing is directed by tendon fibroblasts (tenocytes).
  - Extrinsic healing potential is limited.
    - Only small contribution from repair cells within tendon sheath or from vascular invasion
  - Tendon healing is strongly influenced by biomechanical stimuli, and early mobilization has been shown to decrease adhesion formation and increase the strength of repair tissue.
  - Many recent studies have investigated the use of growth factor augmentation of flexor tendon repair, but no definitive conclusions can be made at this point.
- Treatment according to Verdan zones (Figure 7-29)
  - Zone I injury ("rugger jersey" finger)
    - **Closed FDP avulsion occurring distal to the FDS insertion**
    - **Mechanism of injury is forced extension of the DIP joint during grasping.**
    - The ring finger is involved in 75% of cases.
    - Leddy and Packer classification (Figure 7-30)
      - Type I injuries, in which the FDP is retracted to the palm, require direct repair within 7 to 10 days.
      - Type II injuries may be directly repaired up to 6 weeks later, because the intact vincula prevent FDP retraction proximal to the PIP joint.

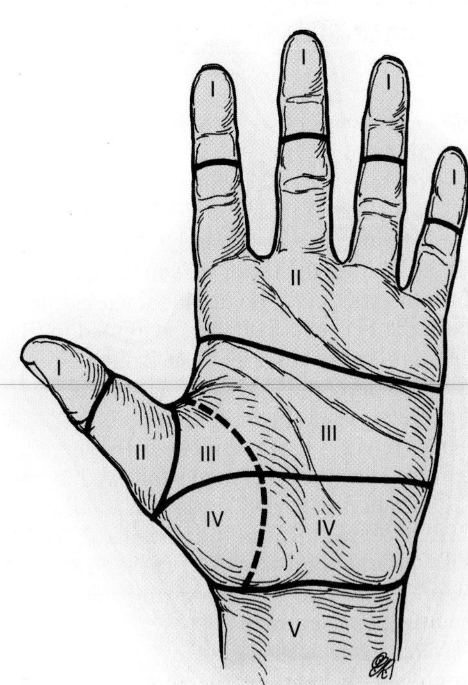

Figure 7-29 The flexor tendon system has been divided into five zones for the purposes of discussion and treatment. Zone II, which lies within the fibroosseous sheath, has been called "no man's land" because it was once believed that primary repair should not be done in this zone. (From Green DP, et al, editors: *Green's operative hand surgery,* ed 5, Philadelphia, 2005, Churchill Livingstone, p 221.)

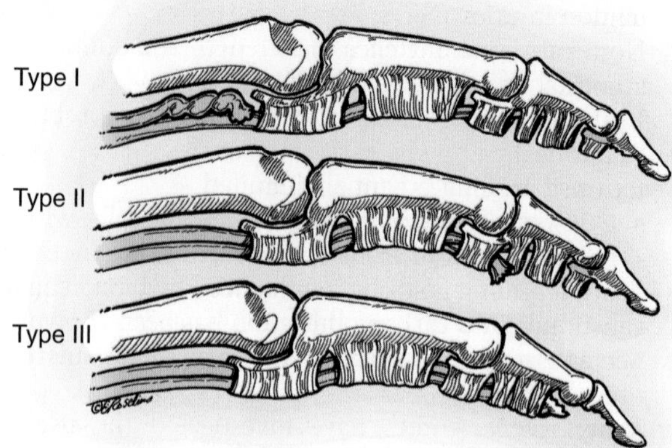

Figure 7-30 Profundus avulsion classification of Leddy and Packer. In *type I,* the flexor digitorum profundus tendon is avulsed from its insertion and retracts into the palm. In *type II,* the tendon stump remains within the digital sheath, implying that the supporting vincula are still intact. In *type III,* a bony fragment is attached to the tendon stump, which remains within the flexor sheath. Further proximal retraction is prevented at the distal end of the A4 pulley. (From Green DP, et al, editors: *Green's operative hand surgery,* ed 5, Philadelphia, 2005, Churchill Livingstone, p 226.)

- Type III injuries associated with small bony avulsion fragment with little retraction and may be successfully repaired up to 6 weeks after injury
- **Profundus advancement of 1 cm or more carries a risk of DIP joint flexion contracture or quadrigia.**
  - **The latter phenomenon occurs because the FDP tendons (middle ring, small) share a common muscle belly, and distal advancement of one tendon will compromise flexion of the adjacent digits, resulting in forearm pain.**
- If full PIP flexion is present, chronic injuries may be treated with observation or DIP arthrodesis in a functional position.
  - Two-stage flexor tendon reconstraction may be considered in young motivated patients.
- Zone II injury ("no man's land")
  - Occurs within the flexor tendon sheath between the FDS insertion and the distal palmar crease
  - Both the FDS and FDP may be injured in this zone.
  - Tendon lacerations may be at a different level than the skin laceration, depending on the position of the finger when the laceration occurred.
  - Direct repair of both tendons with a core and epitendinous suture technique followed by an early mobilization protocol is typically advocated.
  - Results of treatment in this zone have been historically poor and attributed to the high rate of adhesion formation at the pulleys and associated digital neurovascular injuries.
  - Advances in postoperative rehabilitation have improved the clinical outcomes, although up to 50% of patients require subsequent tenolysis to enhance active motion at least 3 months after repair.
- Zone III injury
  - Occurs between the distal palmar crease and the distal end of the carpal tunnel
  - Compared with zone II injuries, the results of direct repair are much better.
  - Lumbrical muscles originate from the radial aspect of FDP tendons in zone III.
- Zone IV injury
  - Occurs within the carpal tunnel
  - Transverse carpal ligament should be repaired in a lengthened fashion to prevent bowstringing and allow for immobilization of wrist in flexion.
- Zone V injury
  - Occurs between proximal end of carpal tunnel and musculotendinous junction
  - Direct repair in this zone has a favorable prognosis.
  - Results may be compromised by coexisting nerve injury V
- FPL injury
  - Zone I injuries—occur distal to interphalangeal joint
  - Zone II injuries—occur between interphalangeal and MCP joints
  - Zone III injuries—occur deep to thenar muscles
- Postoperative rehabilitation
  - Two most common postoperative rehabilitation protocols are those of Kleinert and Duran.
  - Kleinert protocol employs dynamic splinting, which allows for active digit extension and passive digit flexion.
  - Duran protocol requires strict patient compliance because other hand is used to perform passive digital flexion exercises.
  - Both programs restrict active flexion for approximately 6 weeks.
  - Newer protocols add components of early active digital flexion with the hope of further reducing adhesion formation and increasing tendon excursion.
  - These protocols require stronger repair methods, such as the use of more than four core strands.
- Flexor tendon reconstruction
  - Indicated for failed primary repair or chronic, untreated injuries
  - Requirements include supple skin, a sensate digit, adequate vascularity, and full passive range of motion of adjacent joints.
  - The majority of cases require two-stage reconstruction.
    - In stage I, a temporary silicone (Hunter) rod is implanted, secured distally, and allowed to glide proximally.
      - A2 and A4 pulleys are either preserved or reconstructed.
    - Stage II is performed at least 3 months later, after full passive range of motion has been attained and a sheath has formed around the silicone rod.
      - The rod is removed, and a tendon autograft is passed through the sheath.
      - Extrasynovial graft choices such as palmaris longus or plantaris act as scaffold and heal by tenocyte repopulation.
      - Intrasynovial grafts such as FDS retain their gliding surface and heal intrinsically.
  - Postoperative rehabilitation is intensive, and subsequent tenolysis is needed more than 50% of the time.

C. **Stenosing tenosynovitis (trigger finger)**

1. Most common in women over 50 years of age
2. Common in diabetic patients and patients with inflammatory arthropathy

Table 7-5 Classification of Trigger Digit (Green)

Grade	Description
I	Pain and tenderness at the A1 pulley
II	Catching of digit
III	Locking of digit; passively correctable
IV	Fixed, locked digit

3. May simply result from repetitive grasping activities (idiopathic form)
4. Inflammation of the flexor tendon sheath, which inhibits the smooth gliding motion of flexor tendons in the digits or thumb
5. Initially characterized by pain and tenderness at the distal palm near the A1 pulley
6. If left untreated, stenosing tenosynovitis may lead to catching and locking of the digit as the space available for the flexor tendon narrows.
7. Green classification (Table 7-5)
8. Ring finger most common in adults
9. Many respond to corticosteroid injection into flexor tendon sheath.
   - Review of best evidence indicates that injection effective in approximately 60%
   - Diabetic patients generally less responsive to injection
10. Failure of nonoperative management treated surgically with release of A1 pulley
11. Pediatric trigger digits
   - Thumb most common (pediatric trigger thumb)
     - **Presents with fixed flexion deformity of interphalangeal joint**
     - In contrast to adults, pathology is in tendon, with a nodular thickening referred to as a Notta node.
     - **May initially be treated nonoperatively, but generally annular pulley release is required**
   - Trigger finger
     - Etiology unknown
     - **Treatment on a case-by-case basis, depending on intraoperative findings**
     - A1 pulley release may not resolve triggering; A3 release or resection of a FDS slip may be required.

D. de Quervain tenosynovitis

1. Attritional and degenerative condition affecting the first extensor compartment (APL/EPB)
2. Commonly affects middle-age women
3. Other high-risk groups—**new mothers**, golfers, and racquet-sport athletes
4. Dorsoradial wrist tenderness, swelling, crepitus
5. Finkelstein test and/or Eichoff maneuver places first extensor compartment tendons under maximum tension and exacerbates symptoms.
6. **Nonoperative management includes rest, activity modification, thumb spica splinting/bracing, nonsteroidal anti-inflammatory drugs (NSAIDs), and corticosteroid injections into the first dorsal extensor compartment.**
   - **Corticosteroid injections successful in more than 80% of patients**
7. When these measures fail, surgical release of the first extensor compartment may be performed.
   - Dorsal retinaculum is released to prevent volar tendon subluxation.
   - Anatomic variation within the first extensor compartment is frequently encountered in recalcitrant cases.
     - APL may have multiple slips (two to four), and EPB may have its own separate compartment.
     - Outcomes generally excellent
   - Complications of operative treatment include iatrogenic injury to the superficial sensory radial nerve, tendon subluxation, complex regional pain syndrome, and recurrence from incomplete release.

E. Intersection syndrome

1. Tenosynovitis and/or bursitis occurring at the junction between the first and second extensor compartments, where APL and EPB tendons cross ECRL and ECRB
2. Affects **rowers**, weight lifters, football lineman, martial artists, and golfers
3. Tenderness, swelling, and crepitus are localized to an area approximately 4 to 5 cm proximal to the radiocarpal joint.
4. **Initially treated with ice, splinting, NSAIDs, corticosteroid injection into the second extensor compartment**
5. When nonoperative measures fail, surgical release of the second extensor compartment and débridement of inflamed bursae may be effective.

F. Acute calcific tendonitis

1. Overuse syndrome from repetitive resisted wrist flexion
2. Most frequently described for FCU but may also involve FCR
3. Acute onset of wrist pain, swelling, and discoloration that mimics infection or crystalline arthropathy in severity
4. Fluffy calcium deposits may be detected on plain radiographs
5. Usually responds to short course of oral steroids or high-dose NSAIDs, ice, and immobilization

G. ECU tendonitis and subluxation

1. ECU tendon held tightly within a groove in the distal ulna, tethered by a fibroosseous sheath
2. Overuse tendonitis often affects racquet-sport athletes.
3. MRI may reveal thickening (hypertrophy), partial longitudinal tears, or generalized increased signal intensity within tendon.
4. Nonoperative management with rest, activity modification, splinting, NSAIDs, and corticosteroid injections recommended
5. Traumatic subluxation of ECU tendon may result from forceful hypersupination and ulnar deviation of wrist.
   - A painful audible snap or visible dislocation may be induced with reproduction of this mechanism on physical examination.
   - If diagnosed early, long-arm cast immobilization (or Muenster splint) with the wrist held in pronation and slight radial deviation can be attempted.
   - Chronic cases require either direct repair or reconstruction of the overlying extensor retinaculum, often accompanied by deepening of the ulnar groove.
   - Wrist arthroscopy reveals concurrent triangular fibrocartilage complex (TFCC) tears in ~50% of cases.

VI. DISTAL RADIOULNAR JOINT, TRIANGULAR FIBROCARTILAGE COMPLEX, AND WRIST ARTHROSCOPY

A. Anatomy

1. Radius rotates about a fixed ulna at the DRUJ.
2. Ulnar variance measures the distance in millimeters between the distal aspect of the ulnar head and the articular surface of the distal radius (Figure 7-31).

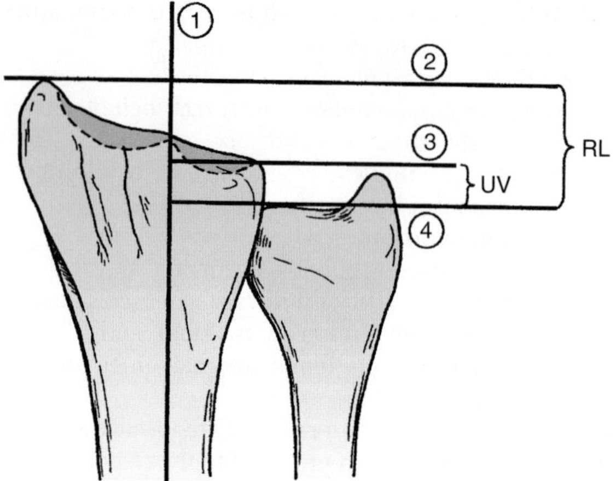

Figure 7-31 **The relative length (RL) of the radius and ulna can be determined by measuring the distance from the tip of the radial styloid *(line 2)* drawn perpendicular to the long axis of the radius *(line 1)* and the distal end of the ulnar articular surface *(line 4)*. The ulnar variance (UV) is the distance between line 4 and *line 3,* the dense cortical line along the ulnar border of the distal radius articular surface.** (From Trumble TE: Distal radioulnar joint and triangular fibrocartilage complex. In Trumble TE, editor: *Principles of hand surgery and therapy,* Philadelphia, 2000, WB Saunders.)

- Determined on posteroanterior radiograph of wrist with forearm in neutral
- There is relative positive ulnar variance with forearm in pronation and negative ulnar variance with forearm in supination.

3. The TFCC stabilizes the DRUJ and transmits 20% of axial load at the wrist (neutral ulnar variance).

Table 7-6 Class I: Traumatic TFCC Injuries

Class	Characteristics	Treatment
IA	Central perforation or tear	Resection of an unstable flap back to a stable rim
IB	Ulnar avulsion with or without ulnar styloid fracture	Repair of the rim to its origin at the ulnar styloid
IC	Distal avulsion (origins of UL and UT ligaments)	Advancement of the distal volar rim to the triquetrum (bone anchor)
ID	Radial avulsion (involving the dorsal and/or volar radioulnar ligaments)	Direct repair to the radius to preserve the TFCC contribution to DRUJ stability

DRUJ, distal radioulnar joint; TFCC, triangular fibrocartilage complex; UL, ulnolunate; UT, ulnotriquetral.

4. **Components of the TFCC include the dorsal and volar radioulnar ligaments, the articular disc, a meniscus homologue, the ECU subsheath, and the origins of the ulnolunate and ulnotriquetral ligaments.**
5. Periphery is well vascularized, whereas the radial central portion is relatively avascular (Figure 7-32).
6. TFCC is composed of superficial and deep limbs.
   - Deep fibers inserting into the distal ulna fovea termed "ligamentum subcruentum."

B. **TFCC tears**

1. Classified as traumatic (class I) or degenerative (class II)
2. Further divided by Palmer into subtypes based on the specific location within the complex (Tables 7-6 and 7-7)
3. Class and location of the tear have important implications for treatment.

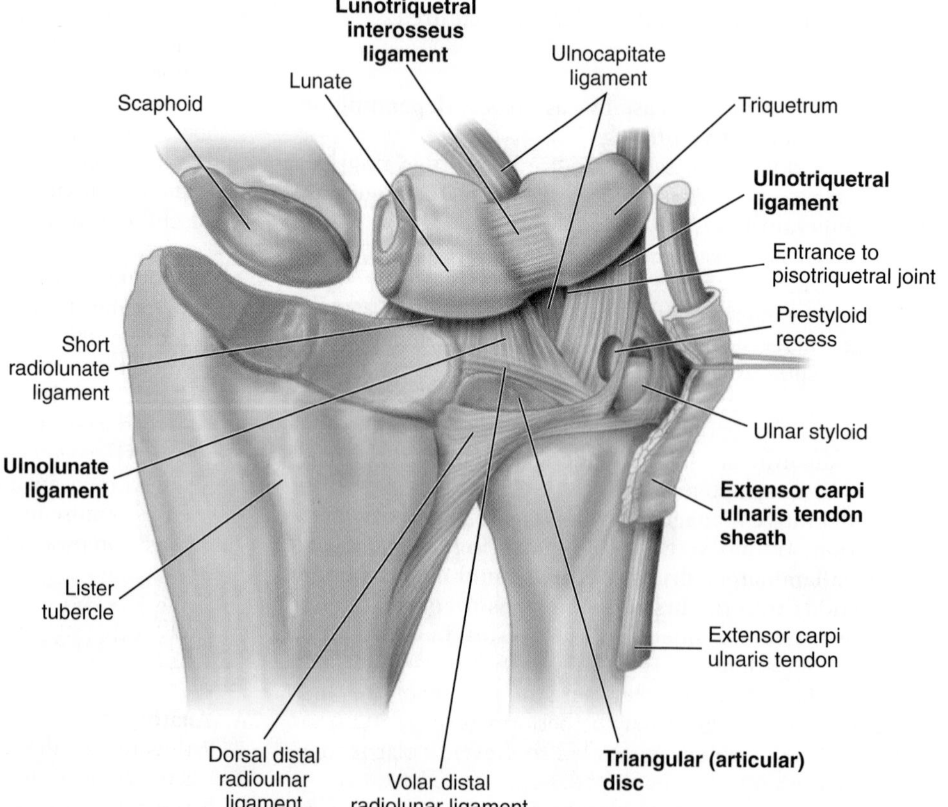

Figure 7-32 **Anatomy of the triangular fibrocartilage complex.** (From Cooney WP, et al: *The wrist: diagnosis and operative treatment,* St Louis, 1998, Mosby.)

Table 7-7 Class II: Degenerative TFCC Tears (Ulnocarpal Impaction Syndrome)

Class	Characteristics
IIA	TFCC wear (thinning)
IIB	IIA + lunate and/or ulnar chondromalacia
IIC	TFCC perforation + lunate and/or ulnar chondromalacia
IID	IIC + LT ligament disruption
IIE	IID + ulnocarpal and DRUJ arthritis

DRUJ, distal radioulnar joint; LT, lunotriquetral; TFCC, triangular fibrocartilage complex.

4. Value of MRI is increasing with regard to overall detection and localization of TFCC pathology.
5. All acute traumatic TFCC injuries are initially managed with immobilization and NSAIDs.
6. When nonoperative management fails to relieve persistent symptoms, wrist arthroscopy and/or open repair is indicated.
7. Arthroscopic trampoline test is performed to assess TFCC resiliency by balloting central portion with small probe.
   - Class I
     - Central class IA tears are inherently stable and may simply be débrided when persistently symptomatic.
       - A 2-mm peripheral rim must be maintained.
     - Peripheral class IB tears are amenable to arthroscopic or open repair.
       - Concurrent fractures of ulnar styloid with persistent instability are either excised or internally fixed.
     - Rare class IC tears are managed by either arthroscopic or open repair.
     - Class ID tears are frequently associated with distal radius fractures and often respond to reduction of radius.
     - Patients who undergo repair of a traumatic TFCC tear within 3 months of injury should expect to regain 80% of wrist range of motion and grip strength.
   - Class II
     - Degenerative class II tears are associated with positive ulnar variance, increased ulnocarpal loading, and **ulnocarpal impaction syndrome** from abutment of the ulnar head into the proximal carpal row.
     - Patients present with chronic ulnar-sided wrist pain, increased with forearm rotation and grip.
     - Pain with loading wrist in extension and ulnar deviation
     - In addition to detectable TFCC pathology, MRI may demonstrate focal increased signal in lunate and/or ulnar head at point of chronic impaction.
     - When conservative management fails, the goal of surgery is reduction of ulnocarpal loading.
       - **In the absence of DRUJ arthrosis, the most commonly performed procedure is an ulnar-shortening osteotomy.**
       - Alternatively, a simple wafer resection of the ulnar head dome has been described.
       - Coexisting TFCC pathology is addressed by arthroscopic or open débridement.

C. DRUJ instability and post-traumatic osteoarthritis

1. Instability
   - Acute dislocation of DRUJ can occur alone or in combination with ulnar styloid (base), radial shaft (Galeazzi), or Essex-Lopresti injuries.
   - Isolated dislocations may be treated by closed reduction and immobilization.
   - Closed reduction may be impeded by interposition of the ECU tendon.
   - Concurrent distal ulna fractures and TFCC tears may require open or arthroscopic treatment.
   - In a Galeazzi injury, ORIF of the radial shaft is followed by assessment of DRUJ stability.
     - An unstable DRUJ may require TFCC repair and/or temporary radioulnar pinning proximal to the joint with the forearm immobilized in relative supination.
   - Chronic DRUJ instability may result from distal radius malunion, ulnar styloid nonunion, or large TFCC/ligamentous disruptions.
     - Subtle chronic instability of the DRUJ may be evaluated on sequential CT scans with the forearm held in a neutral position, full supination, and full pronation and compared with the contralateral side (>50% translation is abnormal).
     - When chronic instability results from soft tissue incompetence, TFCC repair or ligament reconstruction (Adams) with a palmaris tendon autograft may be indicated.
     - A severely angulated distal radius malunion necessitates corrective osteotomy and appropriate treatment of resulting positive ulnar variance.
2. Post-traumatic DRUJ osteoarthritis
   - Maximize nonoperative management.
   - Surgical options
     - Distal ulna resection (the Darrach procedure) is typically reserved for low-demand, elderly patients and may lead to painful proximal ulna stump instability.
     - **Hemiresection or interposition arthroplasty maintains the ulnar insertion of the TFCC and prevents radioulnar impingement by soft tissue (ECU tendon or capsular flap) interposition.**
     - Fusion of the DRUJ with creation of a proximal pseudarthrosis at the ulnar neck is termed the Sauve-Kapandji procedure.
     - Early results of metallic ulnar head prosthetic replacement are promising, but no long-term studies have been performed to date.
     - Creation of a one-bone forearm eliminates forearm rotation altogether and remains the ultimate salvage operation for persistent pain or other complications.

D. Wrist arthroscopy

1. Indicated for the diagnosis of unexplained wrist pain
2. Indications
   - TFCC tears
   - Osteochondral injuries
   - Loose bodies
   - Partial intracarpal ligament injuries
   - Ganglions
3. May assist in the treatment of distal radius and scaphoid fractures
4. Traction tower, 2.7-mm 30-degree arthroscope

5. Arthroscopic portals (Figure 7-33)
6. Radiocarpal and midcarpal joint inspected systematically
7. Injury to superficial sensory nerves is most common complication.

VII. NAIL AND FINGERTIP INJURIES

A. Introduction

1. Fingertip injuries are most common hand injuries seen in emergency departments.
2. Long finger is most commonly involved digit.
3. These injuries may be broadly classified as those with and those without soft tissue loss.
4. Crush injuries without extensive soft tissue loss may result in nail plate avulsions, nail matrix lacerations, and distal phalanx (tuft) fractures.
5. Distal phalanx fractures are typically reduced when the nail bed is repaired, but large, displaced fragments may require percutaneous pinning.

B. Nail structure

1. Nail plate is composed of keratin and originates from germinal matrix proximal to nail fold.
2. Sterile matrix lies directly beneath nail plate and contributes keratin to increase plate thickness.
3. Crescent-shaped white lunula is seen through proximal nail plate at junction of sterile and germinal matrices.
4. Hyponychium lies between distal nail bed and skin of fingertip, serving as a barrier to microorganisms.
5. The eponychium, also called the cuticle, is at distal margin of proximal nail fold.
6. The paronychium forms the lateral margins (Figure 7-34).

C. Nail bed injury

1. A small subungual hematoma constituting less than 50% of nail area may be treated without nail plate removal.
   - Nail plate should be perforated with a sterile needle.
2. Subungual hematomas greater than 50% of nail area require nail plate removal for repair of underlying nail matrix lacerations.
   - Acute repair offers best results.
   - Tetanus prophylaxis and antibiotics given

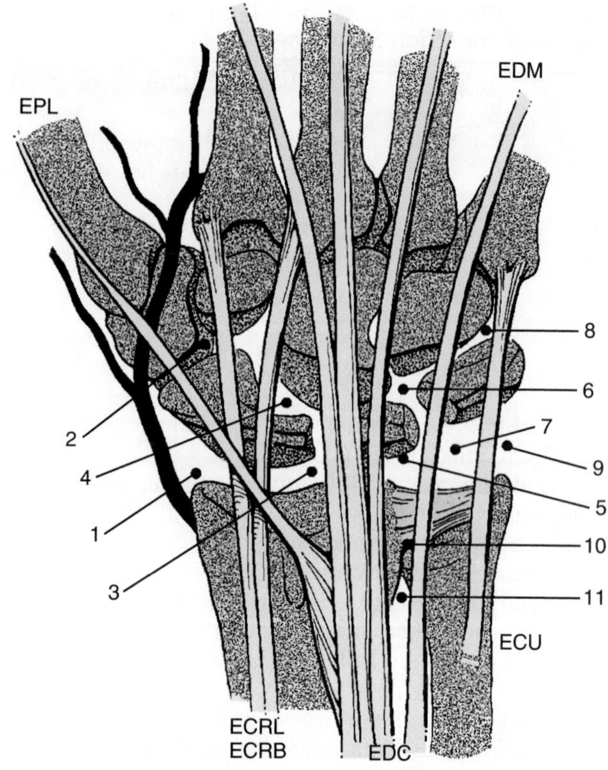

Figure 7-33 Diagram illustrating the six extensor (dorsal) compartments of the wrist and their relationship to the underlying carpal bones. DRUJ, distal radioulnar joint; ECRB, extensor carpi radialis brevis; ECRL, extensor carpi radialis longus; ECU, extensor carpi ulnaris; EDC, extensor digitorum communis; EDM, extensor digiti minimi; EPL, extensor pollicis longus; RMC, radial midcarpal; STT, scaphotrapeziotrapezoid; UMC, ulnar midcarpal. (Modified from Green DP, et al, editors: *Green's operative hand surgery,* ed 5, Philadelphia, 2005, Churchill Livingstone, p 770.)

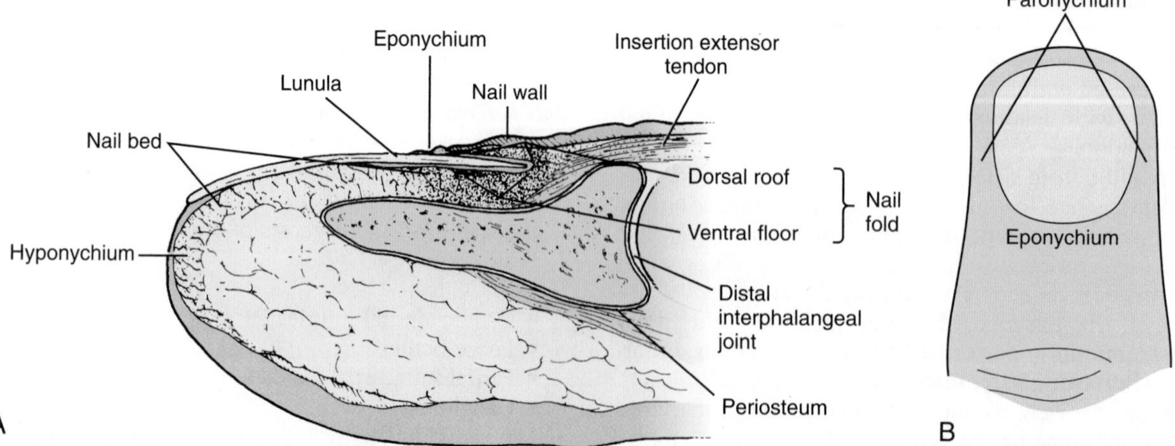

Figure 7-34 A, The anatomy of the nail bed is shown in sagittal section. **B,** The perionychium includes the paronychium, eponychium, hyponychium, and nail matrix. (From Green DP, et al, editors: *Green's operative hand surgery,* ed 5, Philadelphia, 2005, Churchill Livingstone.)

- A digital block should be administered, and a Penrose drain may be used as a temporary finger tourniquet.
- If it is still available, the nail plate is removed and soaked in Betadine.
- The wound is débrided and thoroughly irrigated.
- Sterile and/or germinal matrix repaired with 6-0 or smaller absorbable suture under loupe magnification
- The eponychial fold is then splinted open with the Betadine-soaked nail plate, piece of aluminum foil, or nonadherent gauze to allow new nail plate to grow distally from germinal matrix.
- **A single-institution, randomized controlled trial has demonstrated faster healing using 2-octylcyanoacrylate (Dermabond) compared to suture repair.**

3. If significant nail matrix has been lost, options include a split-thickness matrix graft from an adjacent injured finger or transfer of the nail matrix from second toe.
4. Nail plate deformities, especially nail ridging, are very common after crush injuries and nail bed repair.
5. A hook nail may result from a tight nail bed repair, distal advancement of the matrix, or loss of underlying bony support.
6. Patients should be counseled about high incidence of fingertip hypersensitivity and/or cold intolerance for up to 1 year.
7. Complete growth of a new nail plate takes 3 to 6 months, depending on the age of the patient.

D. Fingertip injuries with tissue loss

1. Treatment of these injuries may be time intensive and challenging.
2. The general principles of treatment include preservation of digit length, maintenance of sensate fingertip pulp, prevention of joint contracture, and eventual pain-free use of digit.
3. **The correct characterization of the injury is critical and guides treatment.**
   - Fingertip injuries without exposed bone
     - These may be allowed to heal by secondary intention if less than 1 cm^2 of the tip or pulp is involved.
     - Otherwise, skin or composite grafts may be required.
     - Full-thickness skin grafts are best for the fingertip because they provide better durability, minimal contraction, and superior sensibility compared with the split-thickness variety.
   - Fingertip injuries with exposed bone
     - Characterized by the orientation of tissue loss
       - **Volar oblique injury**
         - **Cross-finger flap**
           - Dorsal skin and subcutaneous tissue elevated superficial to the paratenon from adjacent digit to create a bed for the injured fingertip
           - Donor site is covered with a split-thickness skin graft.
           - The flap is split during a separate procedure 2 to 3 weeks later (Figure 7-35).
         - Thenar flap
           - **Best reserved for volar oblique injuries to the index or long digits**
           - Flap is lifted parallel to the proximal thumb crease and split after 2 to 3 weeks (Figure 7-36).

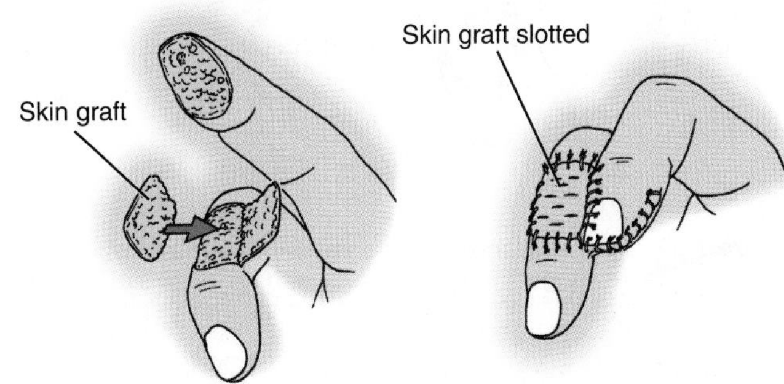

Figure 7-35 A cross-finger flap provides soft tissue coverage for the volar aspect of the adjacent finger or thumb, but a skin graft is required for the donor site. (From Trumble TE, editor: *Principles of hand surgery and therapy,* Philadelphia, 2000, WB Saunders.)

           - Potential complications include donor site tenderness and PIP contracture (especially in older patients).
         - Homodigital island flap
           - Raised on digital artery of involved finger and may maintain sensory innervation to the fingertip
         - Heterodigital island flap
           - Raised on ulnar aspect of the long or ring finger and typically tunneled in the palm to provide coverage to the thumb
         - Other possible donor sites
           - Include distant flaps in the chest, abdomen, and groin, although they may be cumbersome and too bulky for the fingertip
       - Transverse or dorsal oblique digit injury
         - V-Y advancement
           - May be performed to preserve length and cover transverse or dorsal oblique fingertip injuries
           - A wide volar flap is lifted off the distal phalanx, with a tapered base created at the level of the DIP flexion crease.
           - Flap is advanced over the fingertip toward the dorsal side, and a tension-free closure is made (Figure 7-37).

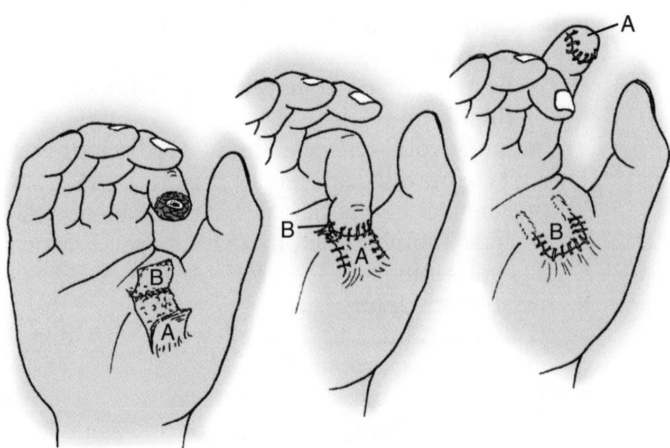

Figure 7-36 A thenar flap provides soft tissue coverage for the index and middle fingers without requiring a skin graft for the donor site. (From Trumble TE, editor: *Principles of hand surgery and therapy,* Philadelphia, 2000, WB Saunders.)

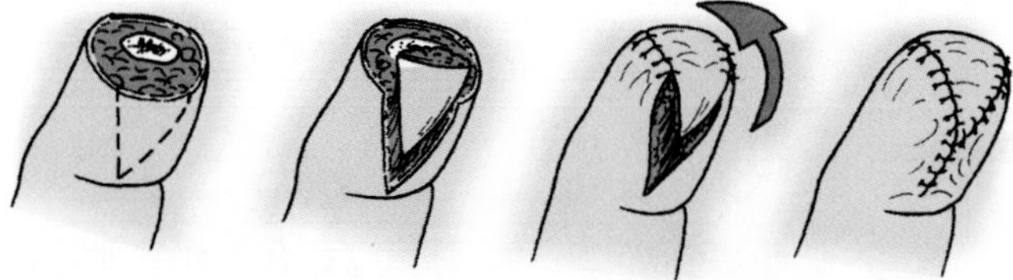

Figure 7-37 **A V-Y advancement flap provides sensate soft tissue coverage for the fingertip in small central deficits.** (From Trumble TE, editor: *Principles of hand surgery and therapy,* Philadelphia, 2000, WB Saunders.)

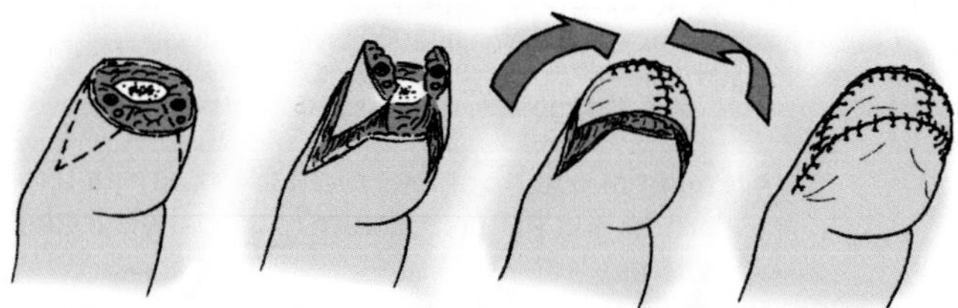

Figure 7-38 **A Kutler flap provides sensate soft tissue coverage for the fingertip in small central defects.** (From Trumble TE, editor: *Principles of hand surgery and therapy,* Philadelphia, 2000, WB Saunders.)

- Kutler popularized two separate smaller V-Y advancements from the lateral aspects of the digit to cover transverse fingertip injuries (Figure 7-38).
- Alternatively, these injuries are treated by bone shortening and conversion to a volar coverage option.
- **Shortening and closing an injury that acutely violates the FDP insertion may result in a lumbrical-plus finger.**
    - **FDP tendon retracts and creates tension on the extensor mechanism through its lumbrical, causing paradoxical interphalangeal joint extension with active finger flexion.**
    - **Treated with release of the radial lateral band**

- Transverse or volar oblique thumb injury
    - **Moberg advancement flap**
        - **Best used for transverse or volar oblique thumb injuries**
        - Entire volar surface of thumb is advanced with its neurovascular bundles (Figure 7-39).
        - Potential complications include flap necrosis and thumb interphalangeal joint flexion contracture.
- Dorsal thumb injury
    - This injury may be covered with a first dorsal metacarpal artery kite flap.
- Pediatric distal fingertip amputation
    - Composite flaps (reattachment of amputated tissue without vascular repair) for distal fingertip amputations may be attempted in patients younger than 6 years old, but parents must be willing to see it fail.

VIII. SOFT TISSUE COVERAGE AND MICROSURGERY

A. Upper extremity wounds

1. Introduction
    - Management begins with thorough assessment of wound, including size, location, involvement of deep structures, and presence of contamination.
    - Standard of care involves early débridement and administration of antibiotics.
    - Complex wounds may require several surgical débridements to remove nonviable tissue.
    - A clean wound bed is essential before any definitive coverage procedure.
    - Infection rates increase dramatically if coverage is delayed longer than 1 week after injury.
2. Reconstructive ladder
    - Goals of soft tissue reconstruction
        - Provide coverage of deep structures (e.g., bone, cartilage, tendons, nerves, blood vessels)
        - Create a barrier to microorganisms, restore dynamic function of the limb, and prevent joint contracture
        - Cosmetic appearance is secondary priority.
    - Options for soft tissue reconstruction
        - Primary closure
        - Secondary intention
        - Skin grafting
        - Flaps

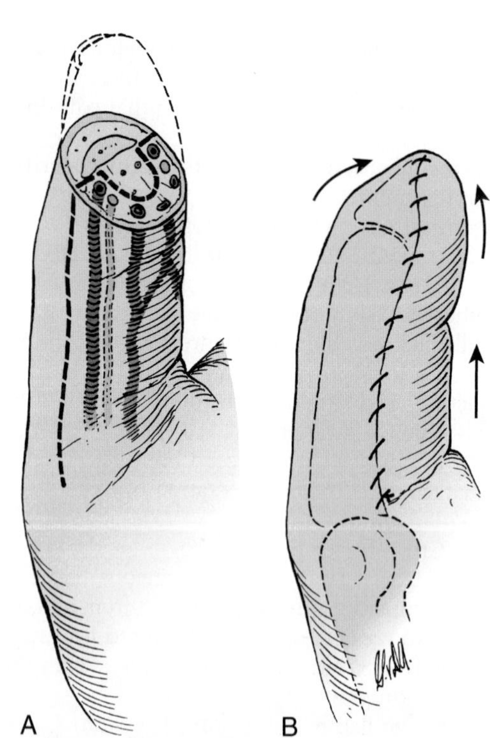

Figure 7-39 **A Moberg advancement flap. A, Most useful for amputations distal to the thumb interphalangeal joint, the Moberg advancement flap is composed of the entire volar skin of the thumb, including the neurovascular bundles. B, Flexion of the interphalangeal joint assists in coverage of the defect by the advancement flap.** (Modified from Lister GD: The theory of the transposition flap and its practical application in the hand, *Clin Plast Surg* 8:115-128, 1981.)

- Choice of definitive procedure is guided by wound characteristics and patient factors.
- Primary closure of a traumatic wound is generally not advised unless the wound is minimally contaminated and can be closed within 6 hours of injury.
- Wounds may be allowed to heal by secondary intention, a process involving wound granulation, epithelialization, and contraction.
  - Bone, nerve, vessel, tendon must not be exposed.
  - Regular dressing changes or vacuum-assisted closure (VAC) devices necessary to promote this type of healing
- Skin grafts
  - Autografts may be either split-thickness skin grafts or full-thickness skin grafts.
  - Both types require clean wound bed without exposed bone or tendon.
  - Skin grafts are prone to early failure from shear stress and hematoma formation.
  - Split-thickness skin grafts
    - Preferred for dorsal hand wounds
    - Meshed grafts provide a greater surface area and typically have better "take" because of a lower incidence of hematoma formation and infection.
    - Anterolateral thigh is common donor site.
  - Full-thickness skin grafts
    - **Preferred for volar hand and fingertip wounds**
    - **More durable, contract less, and provide better sensibility**
    - Less contraction with higher total percentage of dermis grafted, early grafting, and pressure application during remodeling phase
    - Proximal forearm, medial arm and hypothenar aspect of the hand are common donor sites.
  - Allografts may be used as temporary measure to prepare a wound bed for later autografting.
  - Xenografts are occasionally used as biologic dressings.
- Flaps
  - A flap is a unit of tissue supported by blood vessels and moved from a donor site to a recipient site to cover a defect.
  - This unit may be composed of one tissue type or a composite of several tissue types that may include skin, fascia, muscle, tendon, nerve, or bone.
  - Transfer of vascularized tissue promotes healing and lowers the secondary infection rate.
  - Flap reconstruction indicated when wound has exposed bone (stripped of periosteum), tendon (stripped of paratenon), cartilage, or an orthopaedic implant
  - Flaps may be classified by their vascular supply, tissue type, donor site, and method of transfer.
    - Flap classification by blood supply
      - Axial-pattern flaps
        - Single named arteriovenous pedicle
        - More predictable blood supply
        - Greater resistance to infection
        - Raised on their pedicle and transferred locally or pedicle can be divided and transferred to a distant site as a free flap
      - Random-pattern flaps
        - No single named arteriovenous pedicle
        - Depend on microcirculation
        - Examples are cross-finger and thenar flaps.
    - Flap classification by tissue type
      - Single
        - Fascia
          - Lateral arm
        - Muscle
          - Lattissimus, gastrocnemius
        - Bone
          - Medial femoral condyle
      - Composite
        - Cutaneous flaps include skin and subcutaneous tissue.
          - Thenar flap
        - Fasciocutaneous flaps include fascia with overlying skin and subcutaneous tissue.
          - Radial forearm flap
        - Musculocutaneous flaps include muscle with the overlying skin, subcutaneous tissue, and fascia.
          - Gracilis
        - Osteocutaneous flap composed of a portion of bone with overlying soft tissue
          - Fibular, iliac crest
      - Innervated flaps preserve the nerve supply with the tissue unit.
        - Either motor or sensory nerves may be preserved, depending on their anatomic location and the choice of flap to be transferred.
    - Flap classification by donor site
      - Local flap—provided by tissue adjacent to or near the defect
        - Transposition flaps are geometric in design and may be either axial or random pattern with regard to blood supply.
          - **One example is Z-plasty.**
          - **Limbs should always be equal, but the flap cut angles may vary to change the amount of desired lengthening.**
          - **Theoretically 30 degrees, 45 degrees, 60 degrees yields 25%, 50%, 75% lengthening, respectively, along the line of the central limb (Figure 7-40).**
        - Rotation flaps are not geometric and are universally random pattern with regard to blood supply.
          - Length of rotated flap should not exceed the width of its base, for doing so will exceed the

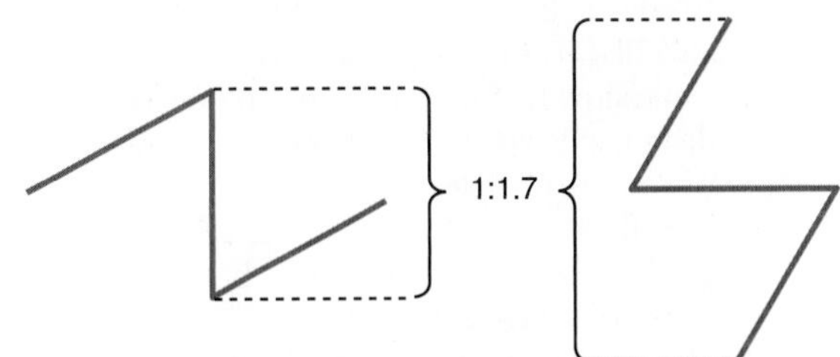

Figure 7-40 Standard 60-degree Z-plasty. Here all limbs of the Z-plasty are of equal length, and the angles between the limbs are 60 degrees. When the flaps are transposed, the lengthening that is achieved along the line of the central limb is 70% to 75% of its original length. (From Green DP, et al, editors: *Green's operative hand surgery,* ed 5, Philadelphia, 2005, Churchill Livingstone, p 1655.)

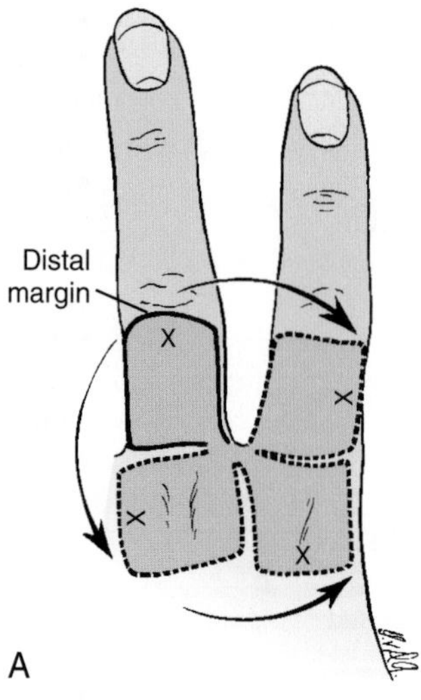

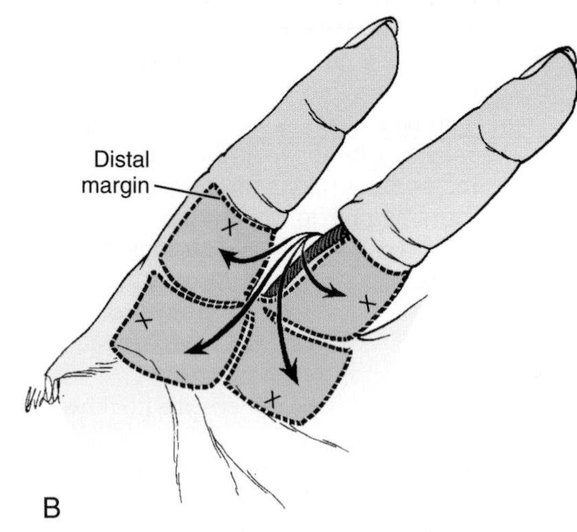

Figure 7-41 A, An axial flag flap raised on the dorsum of the middle finger can be rotated to cover defects on the proximal phalanx of the index finger or over the MCP joint of either of those two digits. **B,** By carrying the flap through the web space, it can reach defects on the volar surface of the MCP joint of either the index or the middle finger. (Modified from Lister GD: The theory of the transposition flap and its practical application in the hand, *Clin Plast Surg* 8:115-128, 1981.)

capacity of the microcirculation to maintain tissue viability.

- Advancement flaps such as V-Y and Moberg types proceed in straight line to fill defect.
- Axial flag flaps are based on the dorsal digital artery (Figure 7-41).
  - Homodigital
  - Heterodigital
- Fillet flap, taken from an amputated digit, occasionally salvaged for initial coverage of a mangled hand

- Distant flap
  - Used when local flaps are either inadequate or unavailable for soft tissue coverage
  - For example, a degloved or burned hand may be placed in a raised pocket of tissue in the abdomen or groin.
    - Several weeks later, the flap is divided and the donor site either skin grafted or allowed to heal by secondary intention.
    - Alternatively, the defect site may be dissected away from the distant pocket of skin. In this case the donor site is primarily closed, and the defect may require a split-thickness skin graft over the vascularized granulation tissue.

- Flap classification by method of transfer
  - Flap reconstruction may be performed in a single stage or in two stages, like the previously mentioned abdominal or groin pocket flap.
  - In most instances, the donor tissue remains attached to the native vasculature.
  - Alternatively, free flaps (free tissue transfer) are distant axial-pattern flaps raised on a named arteriovenous pedicle.
  - Free flaps are then divided and reanastomosed to donor vessels near the defect but away from the zone of injury.
  - Most frequently used donors for use in the upper extremity include
    - Gracilis (medial femoral circumflex artery)
    - Latissimus dorsi (thoracodorsal artery)
    - Serratus anterior (the serratus branch of the subscapular artery)
    - Anterolateral thigh (descending branch of lateral femoral circumflex artery)
    - Lateral arm (posterior branch of radial collateral artery)
  - Patients typically monitored postoperatively in intensive care unit
  - The room is kept warm for vasodilation.
  - Main cause of free-flap failure is inadequate arterial blood flow.
  - Persistent vasospasm may lead to thrombosis at the anastomosis.
  - Hypotension must be avoided and the patient kept well hydrated.
  - Vasoconstrictive agents such as nicotine and caffeine are restricted.
  - Seroma or hematoma formation can also lead to flap demise.

B. Traumatic upper extremity amputation

1. Indications and contraindications
   - Primary indications to attempt replantation
     - Thumb
     - Multiple digits
     - Wrist level or proximal
     - Any amputation in child
   - Relative indication is a level distal to the FDS insertion (zone I).
   - Primary contraindications to replantation
     - Single digit amputation, especially index
     - Crushed or mangled amputated parts
     - Prolonged ischemia
     - Segmental amputations
     - **Level of amputation within zone II flexor tendon sheath**
   - Patients with multisystem traumatic injuries and those with multiple medical comorbidities or disabling psychiatric conditions may be poor candidates for attempted replantation.
2. Care of the amputated part
   - Part should be wrapped in moist gauze (normal saline or lactated Ringer solution) and placed within a sealed plastic bag, which is then placed in an ice-water bath.
   - Although controversial, replantation is not recommended if warm ischemia time is more than 6 hours for

an amputation level proximal to the carpus or more than 12 hours for an amputated digit.
- Cold ischemia times of less than 12 hours for an amputation level proximal to the carpus or less than 24 hours for an amputated digit may still permit successful replantation, highlighting the importance of appropriate cooling of the amputated part.

3. Operative sequence of replantation
   - Bone stabilization, usually with shortening
   - Extensor tendon repair
   - Flexor tendon(s) repair
   - Arterial reanastomosis
   - Venous reanastomosis
   - Nerve repair
   - Skin approximation (loose)
     - If multiple digits, priority sequence is thumb, long, ring, small, and index.
     - **Structure-by-structure technique faster and yields higher viability rate**
     - Surgeon preference and level of amputation may lead to variation in operative sequence.
4. Postoperative care
   - Warm environment (~80° F)
   - Adequate hydration
   - Aspirin
   - Dextran/heparin controversial
   - Thorazine acts as both vasodilator and anxiolytic (especially good for children).
   - Prohibit nicotine, caffeine, other vasoconstricting agents.
5. Replantation monitoring
   - Most reliable methods are close observation of color, capillary refill, and tissue turgor.
   - Measuring oxygen saturation by pulse oximetry and measuring skin surface temperature are safe, noninvasive, reproducible monitoring methods.
     - **Either a drop in temperature of more than 2° C in 1 hour or a temperature of less than 30° C indicates decreased digital perfusion.**
   - Others advocate placement of implantable venous Doppler probe.
   - Flap monitoring may be discontinued after day 4 to 5.
6. Complications
   - **Most frequent cause of early (within 12 hours) replantation failure is arterial thrombosis from persistent vasospasm.**
     - **Arterial insufficiency suggested by pale skin color, decreased or absent capillary refill, loss of Doppler-measurable signal.**
     - **Consider releasing constricting bandages, place extremity in dependent position, administer heparin, perform stellate ganglion block.**
     - If these measures fail, exploration and attempt at reanastomosis warranted
   - Failure after 12 hours is typically secondary to venous congestion or thrombosis.
     - Venous insufficiency suggested by ruborous skin color, increased capillary refill, tissue engorgement
     - May subsequently diminish arterial inflow
     - Remove dressings and elevate extremity.
     - Heparin-soaked pledgets
     - Medicinal leeches (*Hirudo medicinalis*)
       - Produce the anticoagulant hirudin, yield 8 to 12 hours of sustained bleeding
       - May be required for up to 5 to 7 days
       - *Aeromonas hydrophila* infection is risk, prophylactic antibiotics such as ceftriaxone or ciprofloxacin warranted during leech therapy
     - Revision of venous anastomosis is last resort.
   - Late complications include tendon adhesions, bone nonunion, and neuroma formation.
     - **Tenolysis is the most commonly performed secondary procedure following successful replantation.**
7. Results
   - **Factor most predictive of digit survival after replantation is mechanism of injury.**
   - Next most important factor is probably ischemia time.
   - Clean, transverse amputations with cold ischemia time less than 8 hours survive replantation in more than 90% of cases.
   - After 8 hours, the success rate drops to approximately 75%.
   - Replanted digits typically regain 50% total active motion and static two-point discrimination of approximately 10 mm.
   - Long-term cold intolerance almost universal, regardless of whether amputated digit is replanted or revised
8. Forearm and arm replantation
   - Arterial inflow established before skeletal stabilization with the use of shunts, if necessary, to minimize ischemia time
   - Post replantation fasciotomies performed to prevent reperfusion-induced compartment syndrome
   - Muscle necrosis may lead to myoglobinuria and life-threatening renal failure.
   - Elevated postoperative serum potassium level may be prognostic of replantation failure.
   - Late complications include infection, Volkmann ischemic contracture, and insignificant functional recovery.
9. Hand allotransplantation
   - Controversial procedure that introduces potentially life-threatening complications from postoperative immunosuppression for a condition that is not itself life threatening
   - Occurring around the world with more frequency, including the United States, at specialized centers with abundant resources
   - Bilateral transplants have been performed with good survivorship, including one above the elbow.
   - Newer immunosuppressive protocols are less toxic and may lead to less long-term morbidity.
   - Still debatable whether this tremendously expensive endeavor is superior to an upper limb prosthetic

C. Ring avulsion injuries

1. Forceful avulsion of overlying soft tissues from skeletal structures
2. Classified by Urbaniak
   - Class I—adequate circulation, digit salvage with standard soft tissue treatment
   - Class II—circulation compromised and inadequate, revascularization recommended if no accompanying severe bone or tendon injury
   - Class III—complete degloving treated with completion amputation

D. Thumb reconstruction
1. Traumatic thumb loss devastating to overall hand function
2. Amputation through middle to proximal third of proximal phalanx
   - First web space deepening
   - Metacarpal lengthening with distraction external fixator
     - Average 3-cm gain
3. More proximal amputation level
   - Index pollicization
   - Great or second toe transfer by microvascular reconstruction

IX. VASCULAR DISORDERS

A. Anatomy
1. The hand is supplied by the radial and ulnar arteries.
2. The ulnar artery is the main contributor to the superficial palmar arch.
3. The radial artery is the main contributor to the deep palmar arch and the thumb via the princeps pollicis artery.
4. A complete arch, present in more than 80% of hands, provides arterial branches to all five digits, and if either the radial or ulnar artery is injured proximally, sufficient digital perfusion remains through the uninjured artery and the complete arch.
5. Individuals with an incomplete arch (~20%) may have significant compromise of perfusion if the dominant artery is injured (Figure 7-42).
6. Presence of an incomplete arch can be detected by an Allen test.
7. In some studies up to 15% have a persistent median artery.
   - Associated with high median nerve division or bifid nerve

B. Evaluation of vascular dysfunction
1. Allen test
   - Compress both radial and ulnar arteries at distal forearm, and ask patient to squeeze and release hand several times.
   - In sequential tests, one artery is released while the other remains compressed.
   - A positive test denotes absent arterial filling of the digits when either the compressed radial or ulnar artery is released at the wrist.
   - May also be performed with aid of Doppler probe
2. Cold-stimulation testing
   - May demonstrate autonomic vascular dysfunction
   - Patients with arterial disease require more than 20 minutes to return to preexposure temperatures when submersed in ice water for 20 seconds, compared with normal subjects, who require approximately 10 minutes.
3. Digital brachial index
   - Comparison of blood pressure between arm and digit
   - Less than 0.7 is abnormal for a digit.
4. Color duplex ultrasonography
   - Excellent noninvasive study to help detect many forms of vessel pathology, with rates of sensitivity and

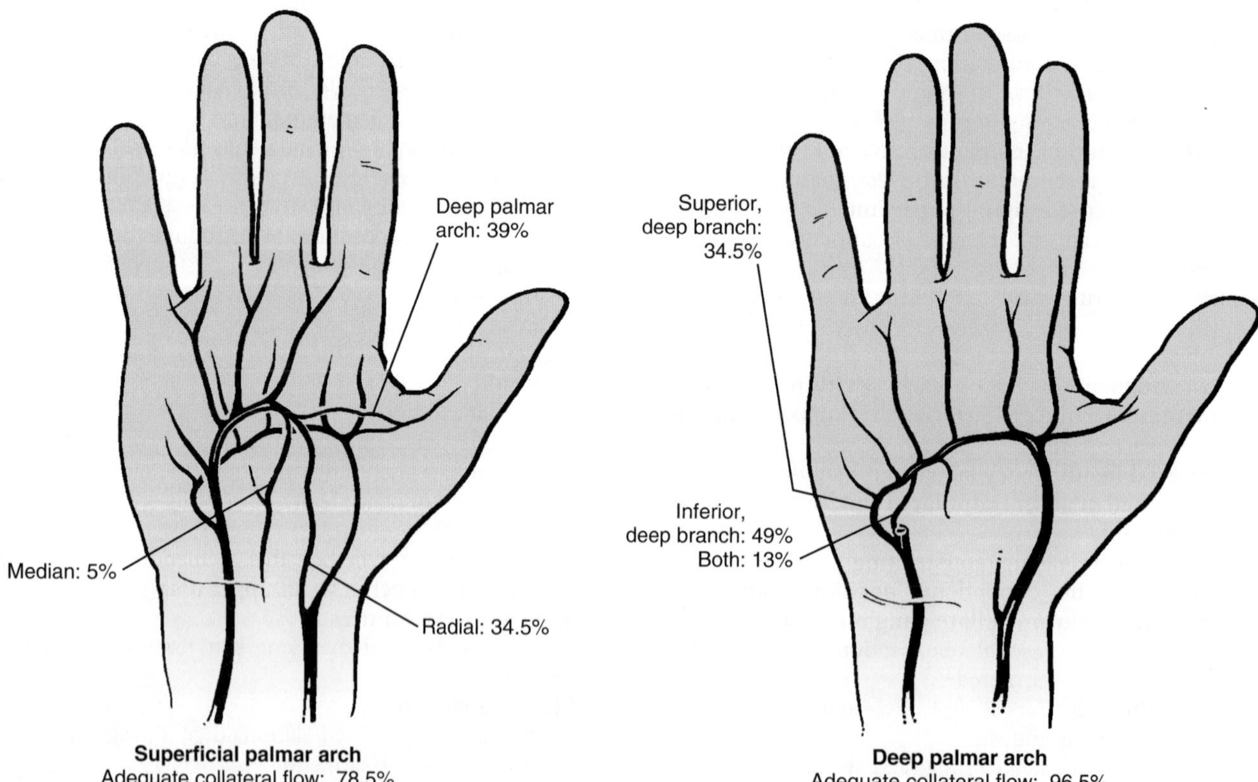

Figure 7-42 The superficial palmar arch is completed by branches from the deep palmar arch, radial artery, or median artery in 78.5% of patients; the remaining 21.5% are "incomplete." The deep palmar arch is completed by the superior branch of the ulnar artery, the inferior branch of the ulnar artery, or both in 96.5% of patients. (Modified from Koman LA, Urbaniak JR: Ulnar artery thrombosis. In Brunelli G, editor: *Textbook of microsurgery,* Milan, 1988, Masson, pp 75-83, with permission.)

specificity similar to those in arteriography (with experienced operators)

5. Photoplethysmography (pulse volume recordings)
   - Demonstrates arterial insufficiency when there is loss of the dicrotic notch or a decreased rate of rise in the systolic peak
6. Three-phase bone scan
   - May be useful adjunctive test in certain clinical scenarios
     - Phase 1 images taken 2 minutes after radiotracer injection provide information similar to arteriography.
     - Arterial occlusion, arteriovenous malformations, and vascular tumors can be detected during this phase.
     - After 5 to 10 minutes, phase II (soft tissue) images may show decreased perfusion when vasospastic disorders are present.
     - Delayed phase III (skeletal) images are obtained 2 to 3 hours after injection but are not particularly helpful in vascular disorders.
7. Arteriography
   - Gold standard for elucidating the nature and extent of thrombotic and embolic disease of the hand vasculature
   - Provides a road map for surgical intervention

C. Occlusive vascular disease

1. Etiologies include blunt or penetrating arterial trauma, atherosclerosis, aneurysm formation, emboli, and a variety of systemic diseases.
2. Often presents with unilateral claudication (ischemic pain), paresthesias, and/or cold intolerance
3. Ulcerations and gangrene are late findings of unrecognized vascular compromise.
   - Hypothenar hammer syndrome
     - Most common post-traumatic vascular occlusive condition of the upper extremity
     - Thrombosis or aneurysm formation of the distal ulnar artery occurs from blunt trauma to the hypothenar eminence (roofers, carpenters, etc.).
     - Clinical findings may include localized tenderness, cold intolerance, ischemic pain, and accompanying compression neuropathy of the ulnar nerve in the Guyon canal.
     - Noninvasive vascular studies or arteriography may help confirm the diagnosis.
     - Treatment may involve resection and ligation of the thrombosed ulnar artery or reconstruction with a reversed interposition vein graft.
   - Small-vessel occlusive disease
     - May be seen in connective tissue diseases such as scleroderma, systemic lupus erythematosus, rheumatoid arthritis (RA), Sjögren syndrome, and dermatomyositis
     - Buerger disease is small vessel arteritis, which affects predominantly male heavy smokers.
     - These conditions are often progressive despite treatments such as calcium channel blockers and periarterial sympathectomy.
   - Embolic disease
     - Majority of upper extremity emboli are of cardiac origin.
     - Another subset of emboli originate from the subclavian system in cases of vascular thoracic outlet syndrome.
     - Emergency embolectomy is performed when feasible and followed by anticoagulation.
     - Smaller vessels are treated with thrombolytic agents such as tissue plasminogen activator, streptokinase, or urokinase if the diagnosis is made within 36 hours of occlusion.
     - Warfarin is given for 3 to 6 months.

D. Vasospastic disease

1. Periodic digital ischemia may be induced by cold temperature or other sympathetic stimuli, such as pain or emotional stress.
2. Digits initially turn white from vasospasm and cessation of flow, then blue from cyanosis and venous stasis, and finally red from rebound hyperemia.
3. Last stage is often accompanied by dysesthesia.
4. Vasospastic disease with a known underlying cause (Box 7-1) is termed the Raynaud phenomenon (Table 7-8).

Box 7-1

Causes of Secondary Vasospastic Disorder

- Connective tissue disease: scleroderma (incidence of Raynaud disease, 80%-90%), SLE (incidence, 18%-26%), dermatomyositis (incidence, 30%), RA (incidence, 11%)
- Occlusive arterial disease
- Neurovascular compression: thoracic outlet syndrome
- Hematologic abnormalities: cryoproteinemia, polycythemia, paraproteinemia
- Occupational trauma: percussion and vibratory tool workers
- Drugs and toxins: sympathomimetics, ergot compounds, β-adrenergic blockers
- CNS disease: syringomyelia, poliomyelitis, tumors/infarcts
- Miscellaneous: RSD, malignant disease

CNS, central nervous system; RA, rheumatoid arthritis; RSD, reflex sympathetic dystrophy; SLE, systemic lupus erythematosus.

Table 7-8 Raynaud Disease versus Raynaud Phenomenon

Characteristic	Disease	Phenomenon
History		
Triphasic color change	Yes	Yes
Age >40 years	No	Yes
Progression rapid	No	Yes
Underlying disease	No	Yes
Female predominance	Frequent	Occasional
Physical examination		
Trophic findings (ulcer, gangrene)	Infrequent	Frequent
Abnormal Allen test	No	Common
Asymmetric findings	Infrequent	Frequent
Laboratory testing		
Blood chemistry	Normal	Frequently abnormal
Microangiology	Normal	Frequently abnormal
Angiography	Normal	Frequently abnormal

From Green DP, et al, editors: *Green's operative hand surgery,* ed 5, Philadelphia, 2005, Churchill Livingstone, p 2304.

- Some degree of vascular occlusive disease is always present, giving a combined clinical picture.
- Symptoms are usually asymmetric, and peripheral pulses are often absent.
- Trophic changes may occur.
- Treatment is focused on the underlying disease.

5. When no underlying cause is present, the clinical condition is known as Raynaud disease (see Table 7-8).
   - Most commonly affected group is premenopausal women.
   - Symptoms are usually bilateral, and peripheral pulses often present.
   - Calcium channel blockers may provide transient relief of symptoms.
   - Biofeedback techniques may also be beneficial.
   - Digital sympathectomy is considered in severe cases.
6. Smoking cessation and avoidance of cold exposure are imperative in both the Raynaud phenomenon and Raynaud disease.
7. Recent interest in use of botulinum toxin type A for treatment of vasospastic digital ischemia

E. Acute compartment syndrome

1. Surgical emergency resulting from increased pressure within a closed anatomic space, leading to reduced capillary blood flow below the threshold for local tissue perfusion and oxygen delivery
2. Prolonged ischemia secondary to a missed or delayed diagnosis may result in irreversible muscle or nerve damage within a compartment.
3. Forearm compartments (3)
   - Mobile wad of three (brachioradialis, ECRL, and ECRB)
   - Dorsal
   - Volar (deep muscles incur highest pressure)
4. Hand compartments (10)
   - Thenar
   - Hypothenar
   - Adductor pollicis
   - Four dorsal interosseous
   - Three volar interosseous
5. Compartment syndrome is a clinical diagnosis, and a high index of suspicion is critical after crush injuries and limb reperfusion.
6. The most common cause in children is a supracondylar humerus fracture.
7. Compartment pressures should be measured in equivocal cases or in unresponsive patients.
8. Compartment monitoring is also imperative after animal bites, high-energy trauma, and burn injuries.
9. Increased pain with passive stretch of the affected compartment is most sensitive finding on physical examination.
10. Paresthesias, pallor, pulselessness, and paralysis are late findings.
11. Treatment is emergency fasciotomy of affected compartments.
    - Forearm fasciotomies require three skin incisions over the three compartments.
    - Hand fasciotomies may be accomplished through five skin incisions.
      - Two dorsal incisions to release five interossei and the adductor pollicis
      - Separate incisions over the thenar and hypothenar musculature (Figure 7-43)
      - Carpal tunnel release often done in same setting
    - Delayed wound closure and/or skin grafting recommended
12. Most important prognostic factor is time between tissue compromise and surgical intervention
13. Long-term sequelae of unrecognized and untreated acute compartment syndrome include muscle fibrosis and Volkmann ischemic contracture.

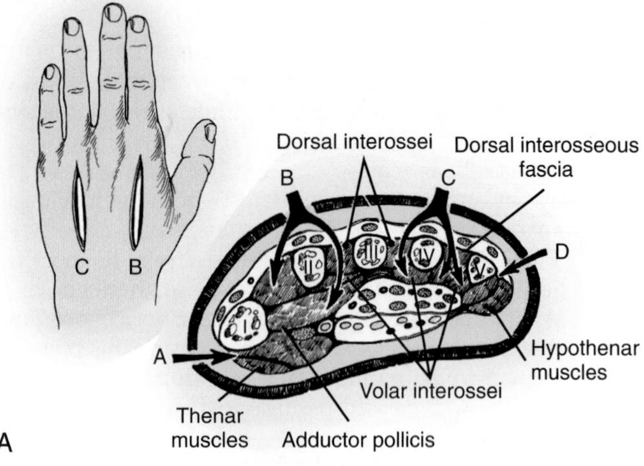

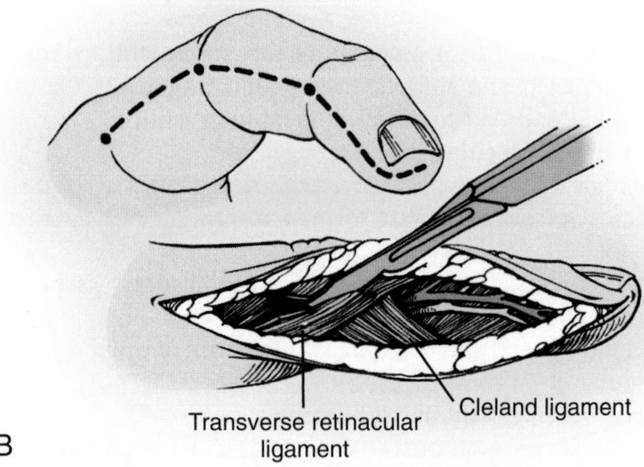

Figure 7-43 **A,** Both dorsal and volar interosseous compartments and the adductor compartment to the thumb can be released through two longitudinal incisions over the second and third metacarpals (*B* and *C*). The thenar and hypothenar compartments are opened through separate incisions (*A* and *D*). **B,** Correct placement of a midaxial incision in the finger. A flexion contracture of the finger may occur if the incision is placed too far volar. (From Green DP, et al, editors: *Green's operative hand surgery,* ed 5, Philadelphia, 2005, Churchill Livingstone, p 1993.)

F. Volkmann ischemic contracture

1. Classical sequela of untreated acute compartment syndrome developing from advanced myonecrosis and muscle fibrosis in the forearm
2. FDP and FPL muscles are most vulnerable.

3. Mild, moderate, and severe forms have been described.
4. The mild form is manifested as mild DIP flexion contractures, but patients often have normal strength and sensibility.
5. Progressively worsening contractures and sensorimotor deficits are seen in the moderate and severe forms.
6. Chronic pain and significant hand dysfunction are common.
7. Patients with the severe form often have an insensate hand with an intrinsic-minus ("claw hand") deformity.
8. Contracture releases and tendon transfers are performed to help improve function, although the success of these procedures may be limited in severe cases.
9. Nerve decompression may be necessary in patients with chronic neuropathic pain, especially when muscle fibrosis causes extrinsic compression on intrinsically compromised peripheral nerves.
10. Free innervated gracilis muscle transfer in severe cases

G. Frostbite

1. Damage to tissue from prolonged exposure to subfreezing temperatures
2. Ice crystals form within extracellular fluid, causing subsequent intracellular dehydration and cell death.
3. Increased wind chill, skin contact with metal or ice, and alcohol intoxication exacerbate frostbite.
4. After initial resuscitative management, rapid rewarming of the affected body part is performed in a water bath kept at 40° to 42° C.
5. Intravenous analgesics or conscious sedation is usually necessary during this exquisitely painful process.
6. Repeated freeze-thaw cycles are avoided.
7. Local wound management with topical aloe vera, limb elevation, splinting, and early therapy are routine aspects of care.
8. Surgical débridement and amputation should be delayed until unequivocal tissue demarcation occurs (1 to 3 months), although escharotomy is required for constrictive, circumferential digital involvement.
9. Bone scan used to evaluate severity of injury as early as day 3
   - Intravenous TPA recommended if no digital blood flow
10. Chronic cold intolerance, neuropathy, and articular cartilage degradation are common.
11. Calcium channel blockers or surgical sympathectomy may be required for late, persistent vasospastic disease.
12. Children may have premature growth plate closure.

X. COMPRESSION NEUROPATHY

A. Introduction

1. Chronic condition with sensory, motor, or mixed involvement
2. First sensory perceptions to be lost are those of light touch, pressure, and vibration, and last to be impaired are pain and temperature.
3. Paresthesias result from early microvascular compression and neural ischemia.
   - Intraneural edema increases over time and exacerbates microvascular compression.
   - Pressure and vibratory thresholds are increased.

Box 7–2

Nerve Compression Etiology

SYSTEMIC	ANATOMIC
Diabetes	Synovial fibrosis
Alcoholism	Lumbrical encroachment
Renal failure	Anomalous tendon
Raynaud	Median artery
INFLAMMATORY	Fracture deformity
Rheumatoid arthritis	**MASS**
Infection	Ganglion
Gout	Lipoma
Tenosynovitis	Hematoma
FLUID IMBALANCE	
Pregnancy	
Obesity	

4. Continued compression may lead to structural changes such as demyelination, fibrosis, and axonal loss.
   - These changes may cause weakness or paralysis of the motor nerve.
   - Abnormal two-point discrimination may also be evident after prolonged compression.
5. Patient history may reveal night symptoms, dropping of objects, clumsiness, or weakness.
6. If onset of symptoms was preceded by viral illness and shoulder pain, consider Parsonage-Turner syndrome, a self-limiting inflammatory brachial neuritis or plexopathy.
7. Changes in skin color, temperature, texture, and moisture may result from sympathetic nervous system dysfunction.
8. Other clues may indicate an associated systemic disease, such as diabetes, thyroid disease, inflammatory arthropathy, and vitamin deficiency (Box 7-2).
9. Examine individual muscle strength (grades 0 to 5), pinch strength, and grip strength in cases of long-standing compression with complaints of weakness.
10. Neurosensory testing performed in context of both dermatomal and peripheral nerve distributions
    - Semmes-Weinstein monofilaments measure the cutaneous pressure threshold, a function of large nerve fibers (the first to be affected in compression neuropathy).
      - Sensing 2.83 monofilament is normal.
    - Two-point discrimination should be performed with patient's eyes closed.
      - Inability to perceive a difference between points greater than 6 mm apart is considered abnormal and constitutes a late finding in compression neuropathy.
    - Pertinent provocative maneuvers are described for each nerve compression syndrome below.
11. Electrodiagnostic testing
    - Sensory and motor nerve function tested by electromyography (EMG) and nerve conduction studies (NCSs)

Table 7-9 Compression Neuropathy

Phase	Symptoms	NCV	EMG	Pathology	Treatment
Early	Intermittent	Normal or ↑ sensory latency	Normal	Edema	Nonoperative
Intermediate	Constant	+	±	Edema	Surgery
Late	Sensory and motor deficit	+	+	Fibrosis and axonal loss	Surgery—less predictable outcome

EMG, electromyography; NCV, nerve conduction velocity; ↑, increased.

- Operator dependent but may provide only objective evidence of neuropathic condition
- Most helpful in localizing point of compromise and distinguishing between several differential diagnoses in equivocal cases
- High false-negative rate especially in early disease
- NCSs measure nerve conduction velocity, distal latency, and amplitude.
  - Demyelination decreases conduction velocity (sensory fibers before motor fibers) and increases distal latency.
  - Decreased sensory and/or motor potential amplitude with axonal loss
- EMG measures electrical activity of muscle during voluntary contraction.
  - With muscle denervation, EMG abnormalities include fibrillations, positive sharp waves, and fasciculations.

12. Compression neuropathy is characterized by phases of disease (Table 7-9).
    - Treatment decisions guided by history, physical examination, sensory threshold testing, and electrodiagnostic testing.
13. Double-crush phenomenon
    - Normal axonal function is dependent on factors synthesized in the nerve cell body.
    - Blockage of axonal transport at one point makes the entire axon more susceptible to compression elsewhere.
    - Cervical radiculopathy or proximal nerve entrapment may coexist with distal nerve compression in double-crush syndrome.
    - Outcome of surgical decompression may be disappointing unless all points of compression are addressed.
    - Logical to start with less complex distal releases first.

B. Median nerve

1. Carpal tunnel syndrome (CTS)
   - Most common compressive neuropathy in the upper extremity
     - Approximately 500,000 cases per year in United States
   - Anatomy of the carpal tunnel
     - Volar boundary is TCL.
       - Attaches to scaphoid tubercle/trapezium radially and to pisiform/hook of hamate ulnarly
     - Dorsal boundary (floor) formed by proximal carpal row and deep extrinsic volar carpal ligaments.
     - Carpal tunnel contains the median nerve, flexor pollicis longus tendon, four FDS tendons, and four FDP tendons.
     - Normal pressure approximately 2.5 mm Hg
     - When pressure exceeds 20 mm Hg, epineural blood flow decreases and nerve becomes edematous.
     - When pressure exceeds 30 mm Hg, nerve conduction decreases.
   - Forms of CTS
     - Idiopathic form most common in adults
       - **Mucopolysaccharidosis is the most common cause in children.**
     - May also be anatomic variation
       - Persistent median artery, small carpal canal, anomalous muscles, extrinsic mass effect
     - Common systemic risk factors include obesity, pregnancy, diabetes, thyroid disease, chronic renal failure, inflammatory arthropathy, storage diseases, vitamin deficiency, alcoholism, advanced age, and vibratory exposure during occupational activity.
     - Direct relationship between repetitive work activities, such as keyboarding, and CTS has never been established.
     - Acute CTS occurs in the setting of high-energy trauma, hemorrhage, or infection.
       - Evolving paresthesias become severely intense.
       - Requires emergency decompression
     - Diagnosis
     - Paresthesias and pain (often at night) in volar aspect of radial 3½ digits (thumb, index, long and radial half of ring)
     - Most sensitive provocative test is carpal tunnel compression test (Durkan test).
       - Other provocative tests include Tinel and Phalen.
     - Large sensory fibers (light touch, vibration) are affected before small fibers (pain and temperature).
     - Semmes-Weinstein monofilament testing is sensitive for diagnosing early CTS.
     - Weakness, loss of fine motor control, and abnormal two-point discrimination are later findings.
     - Thenar atrophy may be present in severe denervation.
     - Electrodiagnostic tests are not necessary for the diagnosis of CTS but may help confirm diagnosis in equivocal cases.
       - Distal sensory latencies of more than 3.5 msec or motor latencies of more than 4.5 msec are abnormal.
       - Decreased conduction velocity and decreased peak amplitude are less specific.
       - EMG may show increased insertional activity, positive sharp waves, fibrillation, and/or abductor pollicis brevis fasciculation.
     - Differential diagnoses include cervical radiculopathy, brachial plexopathy, thoracic outlet syndrome,

pronator syndrome, ulnar neuropathy with Martin-Gruber anastomoses, and peripheral neuropathy of multiple etiologies.

- Treatment
  - Nonoperative treatment includes activity modification, night splints, and NSAIDs.
  - **Single corticosteroid injection yields transient relief in approximately 80% after 6 weeks, but only 20% are symptom free by 1 year.**
    - Failure to improve after corticosteroid injection is poor prognostic sign and surgery is less successful in these cases.
  - Operative treatment options include open, mini-open, or endoscopic release of the TCL.
    - No additional benefit gained from internal median neurolysis or flexor tenosynovectomy
    - Ulnar neurovascular structures within Guyon canal can be injured if incision and approach are too ulnar.
    - Risk to recurrent motor branch of the median nerve increased if incision and approach too radial (Figure 7-44)
      - Three main variations of the recurrent motor branch (Figure 7-45):
        - Extraligamentous—approximately 50%
        - Subligamentous—approximately 30%
        - Transligamentous—approximately 20%
    - Endoscopic carpal tunnel release may be associated with less early scar tenderness, improved short-term grip/pinch strength, and better patient satisfaction scores in some studies.
      - Long-term results compared to open release are largely equivalent.
      - May have slightly higher complication rate
        - Most common is incomplete TCL division.
        - Reports of neurapraxia slightly higher than open approaches
  - After standard open release, pinch strength returns to the preoperative level in 6 weeks and grip strength in 3 months.
  - Pillar pain adjacent to incision common for 3 to 4 months after open carpal tunnel release
  - Persistent symptoms after carpal tunnel release may be secondary to incomplete release of the TCL, iatrogenic median nerve injury, a missed double-crush phenomenon, concomitant peripheral neuropathy, or a space-occupying lesion.
  - Preoperative symptom severity negatively impacts the degree of symptom relief after carpal tunnel release.
    - Depression and poor coping mechanisms shown to predict patient dissatisfaction.
    - Pain catastrophizing also prolongs return to work.
  - In elderly patients with chronic compression
    - Full sensory and motor function rarely recovered
    - Relief of nocturnal paresthesias more consistent
    - Improved activities of daily living, work performance, and overall hand function
    - Over 90% satisfied with outcome
  - The success of revision carpal tunnel release relies on identifying the underlying cause of the failure.
    - Hypothenar or inguinal fat pad graft

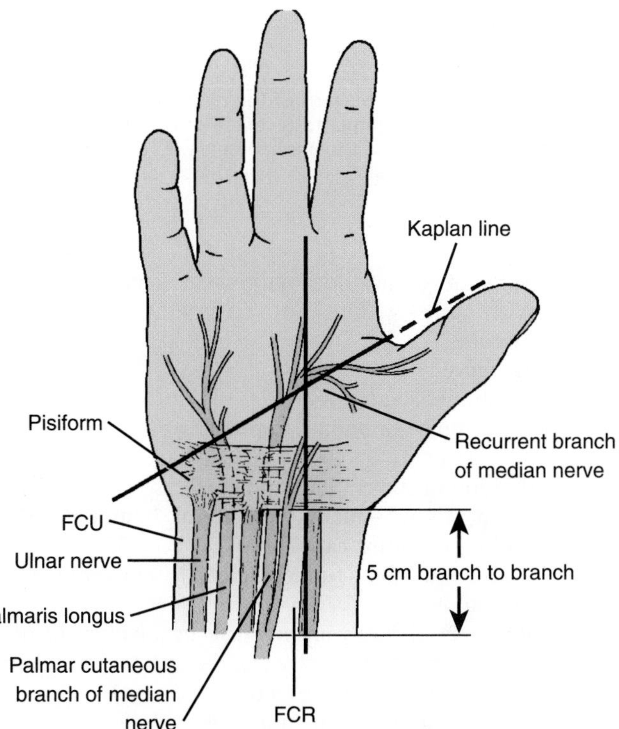

Figure 7-44 **The Kaplan line is drawn along the ulnar border of the abducted thumb. The motor branch is identified as the intersection of the Kaplan line and a line drawn longitudinally in the web space of the index and middle fingers. FCR, flexor carpi radialis; FCU, flexor carpi ulnaris.** (From Trumble TE, et al, editors: *Core knowledge in orthopaedics: hand, elbow, and shoulder,* Philadelphia, 2006, Mosby.)

2. Pronator syndrome
   - Compression of the median nerve in the arm/forearm
   - Potential offending structures include (Figure 7-46)
     - Supracondylar process (anterior distal humerus seen on lateral radiograph), occurs in approximately 1% of the population
     - **Ligament of Struthers (courses between the supracondylar process and medial epicondyle)**
     - Bicipital aponeurosis (lacertus fibrosis)
     - Between the two heads of pronator teres muscle
     - FDS aponeurotic arch
   - Pronator syndrome differentiated from CTS by proximal volar forearm pain and sensory disturbances in distribution of palmar cutaneous branch of the median nerve
   - Test resisted elbow flexion with the forearm supinated (bicipital aponeurosis), resisted forearm pronation with the elbow extended (pronator teres), and resisted long finger PIP joint flexion (FDS).
   - Electrodiagnostic tests usually unrevealing
   - Nonoperative treatment consists of activity modification, splints, and NSAIDs.
   - When nonoperative management fails, surgery must address all potential sites of compression.
   - Success rate of approximately 80% in most series
   - Pronator syndrome is associated with medial epicondylitis and improves with its treatment.
3. Anterior interosseous nerve syndrome

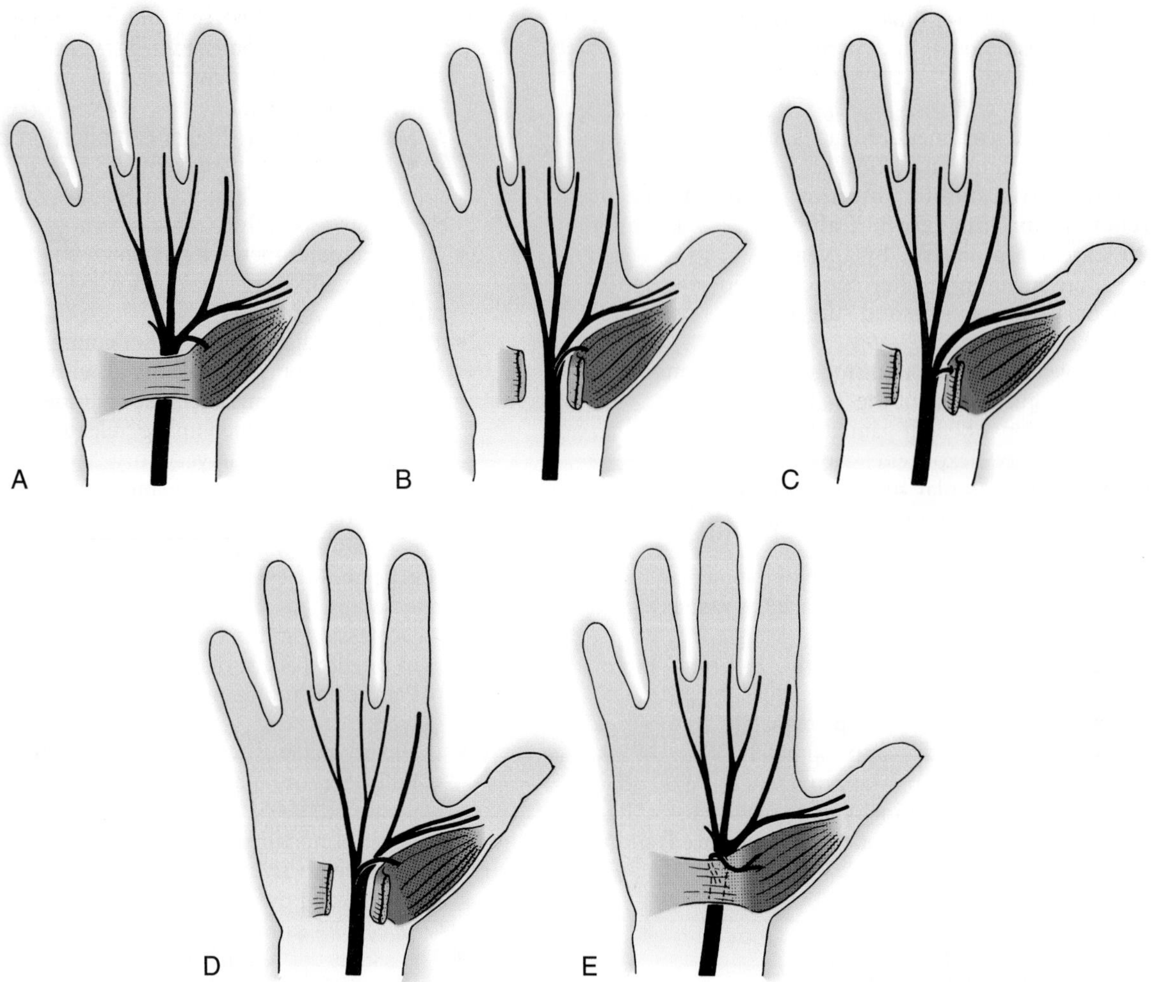

Figure 7-45 Variations in median nerve anatomy in the carpal tunnel. **A,** The most common pattern of the motor branch is extraligamentous and recurrent. **B,** Subligamentous branching of a recurrent median nerve. **C,** Transligamentous course of the recurrent branch of the median nerve. **D,** The motor branch can uncommonly originate from the ulnar border of the median nerve. **E,** The motor branch can lie on top of the transverse carpal ligament. (From Lanz U: Anatomical variations of the median nerve in the carpal tunnel, *J Hand Surg Am* 2:44-53, 1977.)

- **Involves motor loss of FPL, index +/– long FDP, and pronator quadratus**
- **No sensory disturbance**
- Index FDP and thumb FPL tested by asking patient to make an "OK" sign (precision pinch)
- Pronator quadratus involvement is tested by resisted pronation with the elbow maximally flexed.
- Transient anterior interosseous nerve palsy is associated with Parsonage-Turner syndrome (viral brachial neuritis), especially if motor loss was preceded by intense shoulder pain.
- Electrodiagnostic tests may be helpful.
- Important to rule out isolated tendon disruption, such as FPL rupture in patients with RA (Mannerfelt syndrome)
- Apart from aforementioned sites in pronator syndrome, additional sites of compression include
  - Enlarged bicipital bursa
  - Gantzer muscle (accessory head of the FPL)
- Vast majority of patients recover with observation.
- Nonoperative treatment involves activity modification and elbow splinting in 90 degrees of flexion.
- Results of surgical decompression generally satisfactory if done within 3 to 6 months after onset of symptoms.

C. **Ulnar nerve**

1. Cubital tunnel syndrome
   - Second most common compression neuropathy of the upper extremity
   - Definition of the cubital tunnel
     - **Deep (floor)—medial collateral ligament (MCL) and elbow joint capsule**
     - Walls of the tunnel—medial epicondyle and olecranon
     - Roof—FCU fascia and arcuate ligament of Osborne (fibrous band that traverses the cubital tunnel from the medial epicondyle to the olecranon)
   - Sites of compression include (Figure 7-47)
     - Arcade of Struthers (fascial thickening at hiatus of medial intermuscular septum as the ulnar nerve passes from anterior to posterior compartment 8 cm proximal to the medial epicondyle)
     - Medial head of triceps
     - Medial intermuscular septum

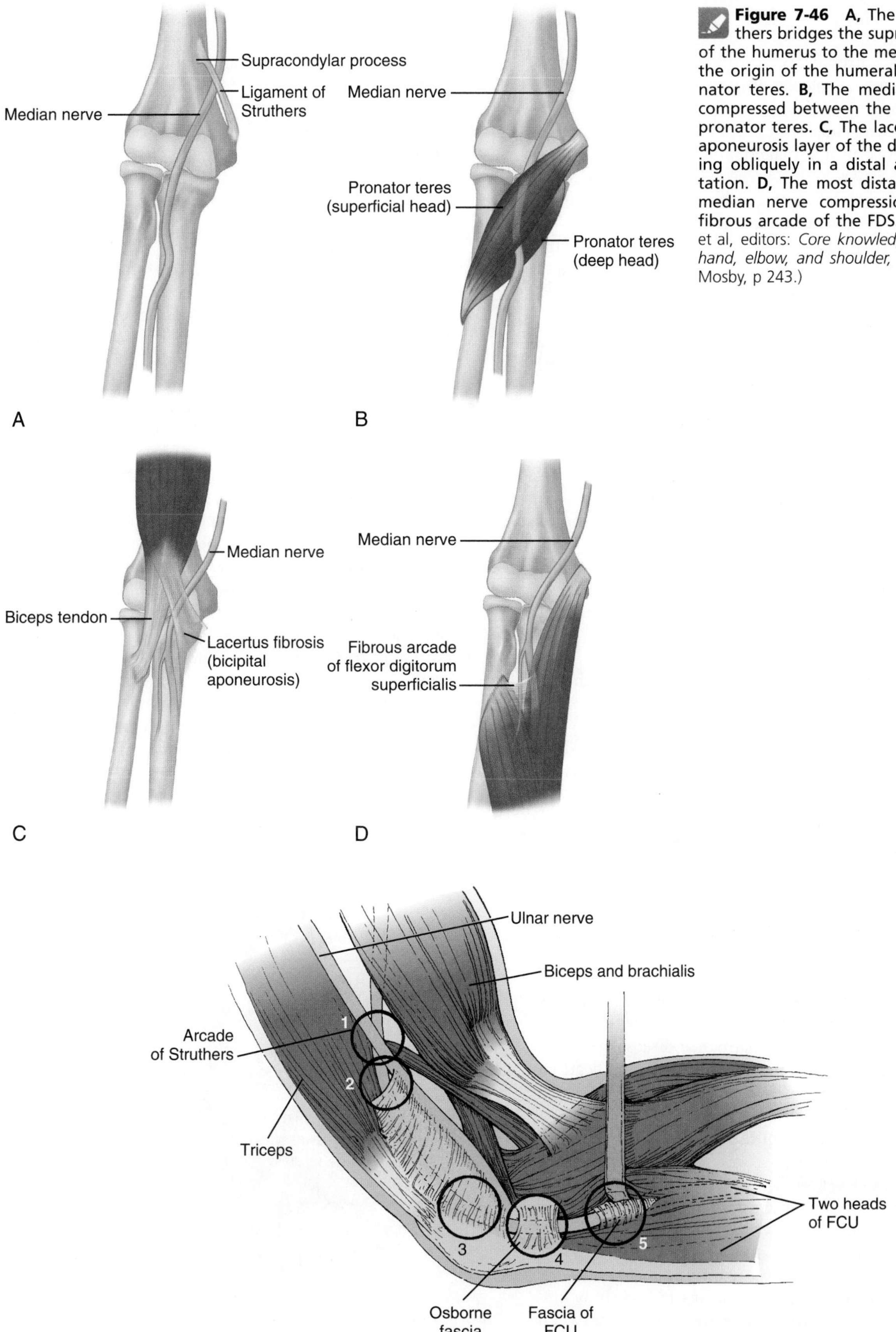

Figure 7-46 **A,** The ligament of Struthers bridges the supracondylar process of the humerus to the medial epicondyle or the origin of the humeral head of the pronator teres. **B,** The median nerve may be compressed between the two heads of the pronator teres. **C,** The lacertus fibrosis is an aponeurosis layer of the distal biceps, coursing obliquely in a distal and medial orientation. **D,** The most distal site of proximal median nerve compression occurs at the fibrous arcade of the FDS. (From Trumble TE, et al, editors: *Core knowledge in orthopaedics: hand, elbow, and shoulder,* Philadelphia, 2006, Mosby, p 243.)

Figure 7-47 Sites of ulnar entrapment. The nerve may be entrapped by (1) the arcade of Struthers, (2) the medial intermuscular septum, (3) the distal transverse fibers of the arcade of Struthers, (4) the Osborne ligament, and/or (5) the fascia (aponeurosis) of the flexor carpi ulnaris (FCU) and fascial bands within the FCU. (From Miller MD, et al: *Surgical atlas of sports medicine,* Philadelphia, 2003, WB Saunders, p 402.)

- Osborne ligament (cubital tunnel roof or retinaculum)
- Anconeus epitrochlearis (anomalous muscle originating from medial olecranon and inserting on medial epicondyle)
- Between two heads of FCU muscle/aponeurosis
- Aponeurosis of proximal edge of FDS

- Other potential external sources of compression include tumors, ganglions, osteophytes, heterotopic ossification, and medial epicondyle nonunion.
- Burns, cubitus varus or valgus deformities, medial epicondylitis, and repetitive elbow flexion/valgus stress during occupational or athletic activities are other associations.
- **Symptoms include paresthesias of the ulnar 1½ digits (ulnar half of ring finger and small finger) and ulnar dorsal hand.**
- Provocative tests include direct cubital tunnel compression, Tinel sign, and elbow hyperflexion, all of which may reproduce or intensify paresthesias.
- Check for subluxation of ulnar nerve over medial epicondyle during elbow flexion-extension arc.
- Classical examination findings secondary to motor weakness
  - Froment sign
    - Compensatory thumb interphalangeal joint flexion (FPL) during key pinch due to weak adductor pollicis
  - Jeanne sign
    - Hyperextension of thumb MCP with key pinch due to weak adductor pollicis
  - Wartenberg sign
    - Persistent abduction and extension of small digit during attempted adduction due to weak third volar interosseous and small finger lumbrical
  - Masse sign
    - Flattening of palmar arch and loss of ulnar hand elevation due to weak opponens digiti quinti and decreased small digit MCP flexion
  - Interosseous and/or first web space atrophy
  - Ring and small digit clawing
- Electrodiagnostic tests are helpful for diagnosis and prognosis.
  - Conduction velocity of less than 50 m/sec across elbow typical threshold for diagnosis; larger decreases in conduction velocity signal worse disease
- Nonoperative treatment includes activity modification, night splints (elbow held in relative extension), and NSAIDs.
- Numerous surgical techniques described
  - In situ decompression
  - Anterior transposition
    - Subcutaneous
    - Submuscular
    - Intramuscular
  - Medial epicondylectomy
- **Recent meta-analyses of techniques fail to show statistically significant difference in outcome between simple decompression and transposition.**
- Higher rate of recurrence than after carpal tunnel release
- Surgery should be performed before motor denervation.
- No long-term clinical data for endoscopic techniques.
- Persistent postoperative medial/posterior elbow pain may be secondary to neuroma formation from iatrogenic injury to branches of the medial antebrachial cutaneous nerve.

2. Ulnar tunnel syndrome
   - Compression neuropathy of ulnar nerve in the Guyon canal
   - Most common cause of ulnar tunnel syndrome is ganglion cyst (80% of nontraumatic cases).
     - Other causative factors may include hook-of-hamate nonunion, ulnar artery thrombosis, ganglion, lipoma, palmaris brevis hypertrophy, or other anomalous muscles.
   - Borders of the Guyon canal are the volar carpal ligament (roof), the transverse carpal ligament (floor), the hook of hamate (radial), and the pisiform and abductor digiti minimi muscle belly (ulnar) (Figure 7-48).
   - Ulnar tunnel divided into three zones
     - Zone I is proximal to bifurcation of ulnar nerve and associated with mixed motor/sensory symptoms.
     - Zone II includes the deep motor branch and is associated with pure motor symptoms.
     - Zone III includes the distal sensory branches and is associated with pure sensory symptoms.
   - Useful adjunctive tests include CT for hamate hook fracture, MRI for ganglion cyst or other space-occupying lesion, and Doppler ultrasonography for ulnar artery thrombosis.
   - Success of treatment depends on identifying the cause.
   - Nonoperative treatment includes activity modification, splints, and NSAIDs.
   - Operative treatment involves decompressing the ulnar nerve by addressing underlying cause.

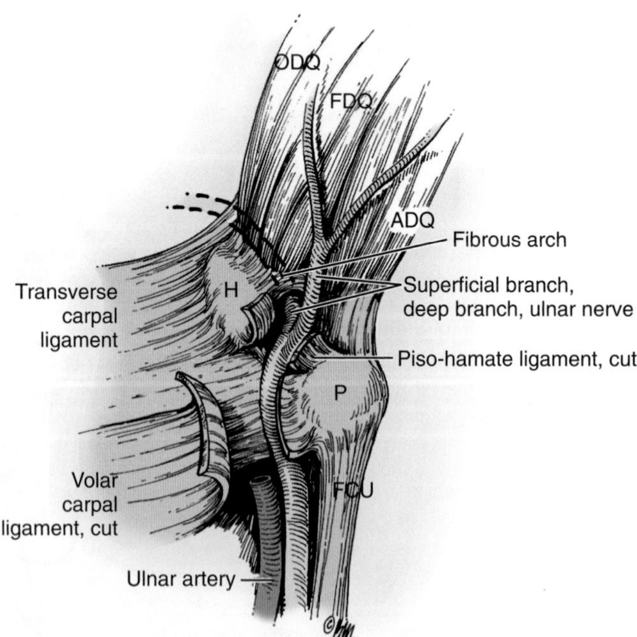

Figure 7-48 The ulnar nerve courses through the Guyon canal between the volar carpal ligament and the transverse carpal ligament. ADQ, abductor digiti quinti; FCU, flexor carpi ulnaris; FDQ, flexor digiti quinti; H, hamate; ODQ, opponens digiti quinti; P, pisiform. (From Green DP, et al, editors: *Green's operative hand surgery,* ed 5, New York, 2005, Churchill Livingstone, p. 1023.)

- Guyon canal is adequately decompressed by release of the transverse carpal ligament when concurrent CTS exists.

D. Radial nerve

1. Proper radial nerve
   - Rarely compressed by lateral head of triceps, typically compromised in setting of humerus trauma or related surgical approaches
   - "Saturday night palsy"—Intoxicated patient passes out with arm hanging over chair, wakes up with wrist drop.
   - Clinical findings include weakness of proper radial nerve–innervated muscles such as triceps, brachioradialis, and ECRL plus muscles innervated by the PIN.
   - Sensory deficits may be present in distribution of superficial sensory branch.
   - EMG may be helpful.
   - May be initially observed but may be explored if no significant recovery after 3 months
2. Posterior interosseous nerve compression syndrome
   - **Symptoms include lateral elbow pain and distal muscle weakness.**
   - **Radial deviation with active wrist extension because ECRL innervated by proper radial nerve more proximally.**
   - **PIN innervates the ECRB, supinator, EIP, ECU, extensor digitorum communis (EDC), extensor digiti minimi, APL, EPB, and EPL.**
   - Patients may also have dorsal wrist pain, where the terminal nerve fibers provide sensory innervation to the dorsal wrist capsule.
     - Terminal branch is located on the floor of the fourth extensor compartment.
   - EMG may be helpful.
   - Anatomic sites of compression include (Figure 7-49)
     - Fascial band at the radial head
     - Recurrent leash of Henry
     - Edge of the ECRB
     - Arcade of Frohse (the most common site, proximal edge of the supinator)
     - Distal edge of the supinator (see Figure 7-49)
   - Unusual causes include chronic radial head dislocation, Monteggia fracture-dislocation, radiocapitellar rheumatoid synovitis, and space-occupying elbow mass (e.g., lipoma)
   - PIN palsy is differentiated from extensor tendon rupture by a normal wrist tenodesis test.
   - Nonoperative treatment includes activity modification, splinting, and NSAIDs.
   - Operative intervention warranted if no recovery by 3 months
   - Surgical decompression of anatomic sites of compression provides good to excellent results for 85% of patients.
3. Radial tunnel syndrome
   - Characterized by lateral elbow and radial forearm pain without motor or sensory dysfunction
   - Provocative tests include resisted long-finger extension (positive if resistance reproduces pain at the radial tunnel) and resisted supination
   - Lateral epicondylitis coexists in a small percentage of patients.

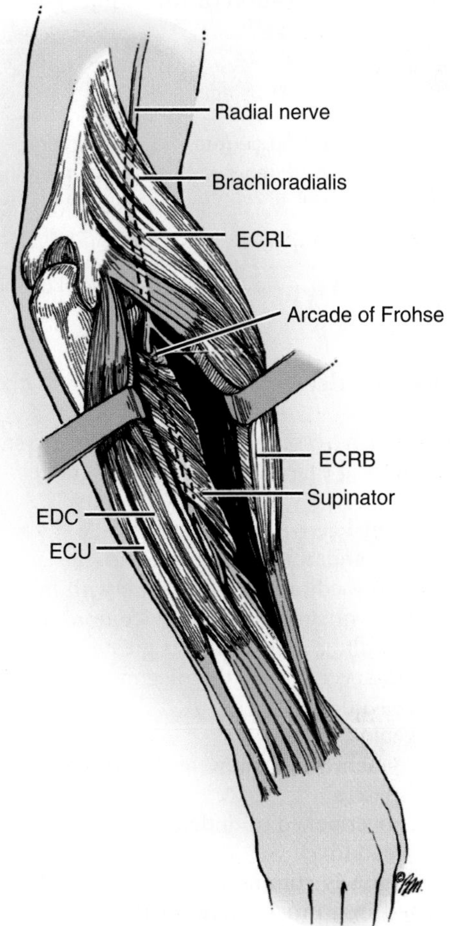

Figure 7-49 Extension of the dorsal Thompson approach to the radial tunnel. ECRB, extensor carpi radialis brevis; ECRL, extensor carpi radialis longus; ECU, extensor carpi ulnaris; EDC, extensor digitorum communis. (From Green DP, et al, editors: *Green's operative hand surgery,* ed 5, Philadelphia, 2005, Churchill Livingstone, p 1039.)

   - The point of maximum point tenderness is anterior and distal to the lateral epicondyle.
   - Despite affecting the same nerve (PIN) and sites of compression, electrodiagnostic tests are typically normal.
   - Prolonged nonoperative treatment for up to 1 year with activity modification, splints, NSAIDs, and local modalities.
   - Success of surgical decompression less predictable than for PIN syndrome, with good to excellent results in only 50% to 80% after prolonged postoperative recovery
4. Cheiralgia paresthetica (Wartenberg syndrome)
   - Compressive neuropathy of superficial sensory branch of the radial nerve
   - Compressed between brachioradialis and ECRL with forearm pronation (by a scissor-like action between the tendons)
   - Symptoms include pain, numbness, and paresthesias over the dorsoradial hand.
   - Provocative tests include forceful forearm pronation for 60 seconds and a Tinel sign over the nerve.
   - Initially treated by activity modification, splinting, and NSAIDs
   - Surgical decompression warranted if 6-month trial of nonoperative treatment fails.

Table 7-10 Classification of Nerve Injury

CLASSIFICATION			
Seddon	Sunderland	Injury	Prognosis
Neurapraxia	First degree	Demyelination injury	Temporary conduction block; resolves in 1-2 days
Axonotmesis	Second degree	Axonal injury	Regeneration is usually complete but may take several weeks or months
	Third degree	Endoneurium injured	Regeneration occurs but is not satisfactory
	Fourth degree	Perineurium injured	Spontaneous regeneration is unsatisfactory, resulting in neuroma in continuity
Neurotmesis	Fifth degree	Severed nerve trunk	Spontaneous regeneration is not possible without surgery

From Trumble TE, et al, editors: *Core knowledge in orthopaedics: hand, elbow, and shoulder,* Philadelphia, 2006, Mosby, p 227.

E. Thoracic outlet syndrome

1. Vascular
   - Subclavian vessel compression or aneurysm diagnosed by physical examination and angiography
   - Adson test
     - Patient keeps the arm at the side, hyperextends the neck, and rotates the head to the affected side. A diminished radial artery pulse with inhalation is suggestive of subclavian artery compromise.
   - Duplex ultrasonography has greater than 90% sensitivity and specificity in the diagnosis of vascular thoracic outlet syndrome.
2. Neurogenic
   - Entrapment neuropathy of the lower trunk of the brachial plexus
   - Often overlooked or undetected on history and physical examination
     - **Fatigue is common, particularly when the arm is used in a provocative position.**
     - **Paresthesias are most common initial complaint and are present in 95% of patients. However, they are nonspecific.**
   - Electrodiagnostic studies rarely helpful
   - Sensory disturbance of medial brachial and antebrachial cutaneous nerves may differentiate the condition from cubital tunnel syndrome.
   - Roos sign
     - Indicates heaviness or paresthesias in the hands after holding them above the head for at least 1 minute
   - Cervical and chest radiographs obtained to rule out cervical rib or Pancoast tumor
   - Physical therapy focuses on shoulder girdle strengthening and proper posture and relaxation techniques.
   - Transaxillary first rib resection (thoracic surgeon) yields good to excellent results when cervical rib is cause.
     - Combined approach with anterior and middle scalenectomy also described

XI. NERVE INJURIES AND TENDON TRANSFERS

A. Peripheral nerve injuries

1. Introduction
   - Peripheral nerve function may be compromised by compression, stretch, blast, crush, avulsion, transection, and tumor invasion.
   - Evaluation and treatment of traumatic peripheral nerve dysfunction are guided by mechanism of injury and presence of other injuries.
   - Most important prognostic factor for nerve recovery is age.
   - Prognosis also better in stretch injuries, clean wounds, and after direct surgical repair.
   - Conversely, poor outcome expected in crush or blast injuries, infected or scarred wounds, and delayed surgical repair.
2. Classification
   - Seddon and Sunderland (Table 7-10)
     - Neurapraxia
       - Mild nerve stretch or contusion
       - Focal conduction block
       - No wallerian degeneration
       - Disruption of myelin sheath
       - Epineurium, perineurium, endoneurium intact
       - Prognosis excellent, recovery expected
     - Axonotmesis
       - Incomplete nerve injury
       - Focal conduction block
       - Wallerian degeneration distal to injury
       - Disruption of axons
       - Sequential loss of axon, endoneurium, perineurium (Sunderland class 2, 3, and 4)
       - May develop neuroma-in-continuity
       - Recovery unpredictable
     - Neurotmesis
       - Complete nerve injury
       - Focal conduction block
       - Wallerian degeneration distal to injury
       - Disruption of all layers, including epineurium
       - Proximal nerve end forms neuroma
       - Distal end forms glioma
       - Worst prognosis
   - In axonotmesis and neurotmesis, the distal nerve segment undergoes wallerian degeneration.
     - The degradation products are removed by phagocytosis.
   - Myelin-producing Schwann cells proliferate and align themselves along the basement membrane, forming a tube that will receive regenerating axons.
   - Nerve cell body enlarges as the rate of structural protein production increases.
   - Each proximal axon forms multiple sprouts that connect to the distal stump and migrate at a rate of 1 mm/day.
3. Surgical repair
   - Best results achieved when performed within 10 to 14 days of injury
   - Repair must be free of tension.

- Repair must be within clean, well-vascularized wound bed.
- Nerve length may be gained by neurolysis or transposition.
- Repair techniques
  - Epineurial
  - Individual fascicular
  - Group fascicular
- No technique deemed superior
- **Use of nerve conduits has gained popularity for digital nerve gaps greater than 8 mm (polyglycolic acid and collagen based).**
- Larger gaps, especially of mixed nerves, require grafting.
  - Autogenous (e.g., sural, medial/lateral antebrachial cutaneous, terminal/PIN)
  - Vascularized
- Limited data available on decellularized nerve allografts
- Growth factor augmentation (e.g., insulin-like, fibroblast) studied in animal models and shown to promote nerve regeneration
- Chronic peripheral nerve injuries may be treated with neurotization and/or tendon transfers.
  - Use of nerve transfers for high radial and ulnar nerve injuries gaining popularity

B. Traumatic brachial plexus injury

1. Knowledge of brachial plexus anatomy is critical for understanding the evaluation and diagnosis of brachial plexus lesions (Figure 7-50).
2. High-energy mechanisms are associated with more severe lesions, such as nerve root avulsions and rupture of entire segments of the plexus.
   - Diagnosis
     - Location and severity of injury
     - Comprehensive motor and sensory evaluation
     - Supraclavicular versus infraclavicular
     - **Preganglionic (nerve root avulsions) have worst prognosis.**
     - Signs of severe injury
       - Complete sensory loss
       - Global motor dysfunction
       - Neuropathic pain
       - **Horner sign—ptosis, miosis, anhidrosis**
     - Complete radiographic series should include cervical spine, chest, and shoulder girdle.
       - Inspiratory and expiratory chest radiographs may demonstrate a paralyzed hemidiaphragm, indicating a severe upper root injury.
       - Root avulsions may be indicated by the presence of corresponding fractures of transverse spinal processes.
       - Scapulothoracic dissociation is often linked to multiple root avulsions and major vascular injury.
     - MRI and CT myelography
     - EMG and NCSs to monitor recovery
     - Somatosensory evoked potentials
3. Timing of surgical treatment
   - Modern series reveal reverse relationship between time from injury to operative intervention and clinical outcome.
   - Immediate surgical exploration may be indicated in certain cases of penetrating trauma or iatrogenic injury.
   - On the other hand, one study showed that many patients with gunshot wounds to the plexus improved over time without surgical exploration.

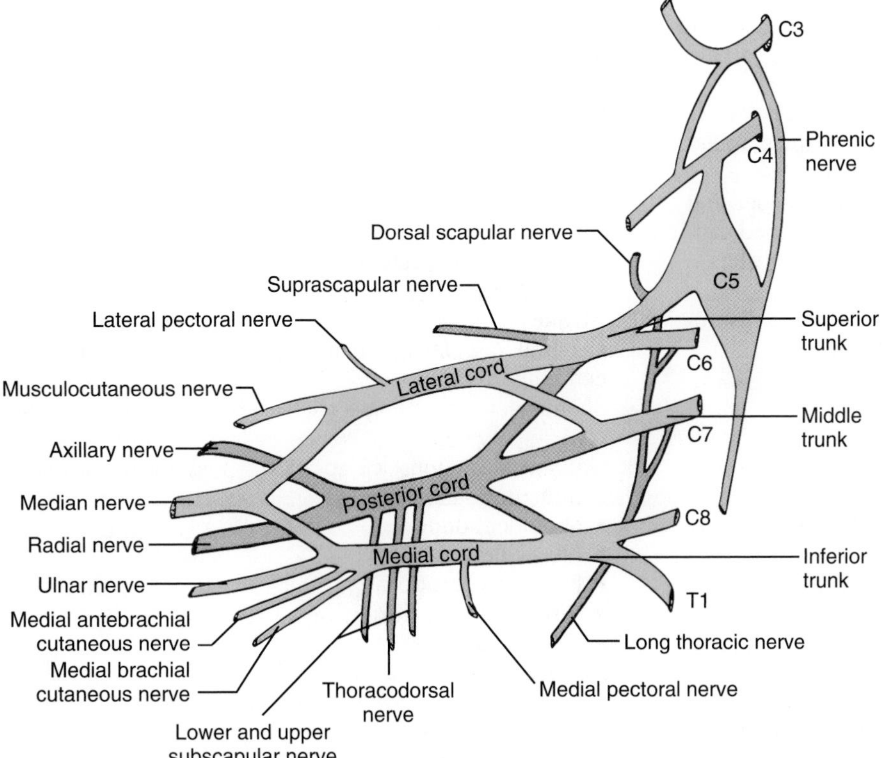

Figure 7-50 Brachial plexus anatomy. (From Brushart TM, Wilgus EF: Brachial plexus and shoulder girdle injuries. In Browner BD, Jupiter JB, editors: *Skeletal trauma,* ed 2, Philadelphia, 1998, WB Saunders, p 1696.)

- Reasonable to observe these patients for 3 months in the absence of major vascular injury
- Early surgical intervention (3 weeks to 3 months after injury) is indicated in patients with complete or near-complete injuries resulting from a high-energy mechanism.
- Patients with brachial plexus palsy resulting from low-energy mechanisms, especially in those with an incomplete upper plexus lesion, are best observed for at least 3 to 6 months for spontaneous recovery.
- Surgery may be warranted if recovery plateaus early.
- Nerve repair or reconstruction beyond 6 months from the time of injury has a less predictable clinical outcome.
- Most reliable clinical sign of nerve regeneration and recovery is an advancing Tinel sign.
- Muscle fibrosis occurs after 18 to 24 months.

4. Tendon/nerve transfers
   - An isolated C8 to T1 injury best treated with early tendon transfers
     - Full recovery unlikely because of distance between lesion and intrinsic muscles of hand
   - For other lesions, nerve repair or reconstruction prioritized
     - Elbow flexion
     - Shoulder stabilization
     - Hand function
   - Direct repair often compromised by excessive tension
     - Neuroma excision and nerve cable grafting favored methods
     - Donor sites include sural, medial brachial cutaneous, and medial antebrachial cutaneous nerves.
     - Best outcomes obtained in young patients treated within 3 months of injury
   - Nerve transfers indicated when insufficient number of proximal axons available, such as occurs in multiple root avulsions
     - Oberlin transfer—ulnar nerve branch (fascicle) to the FCU transferred to musculocutaneous nerve to help restore elbow flexion
     - Descending branch of the spinal accessory nerve (cranial nerve [CN] XI) transferred to suprascapular nerve to help restore shoulder abduction
   - Patients without meaningful recovery of shoulder and elbow function after 6 to 12 months may be good candidates for shoulder arthrodesis and tendon transfers.

C. Obstetric brachial plexopathy

1. Associated with high birth weight, cephalopelvic disproportion, shoulder dystocia, and forceps delivery
2. Muscle grading system
   - M0—no contraction
   - M1—contraction without movement
   - M2—contraction with slight movement
   - M3—complete movement
3. Complete recovery possible if biceps and deltoid are M1 by 2 months
4. Incomplete recovery expected if biceps and deltoid do not contract within 3 to 6 months
5. Surgery usually not recommended if biceps contraction evident by 6 months (some advocate sooner)
6. Results of nerve grafting better in infants than adults, and reinnervation of the hand intrinsic muscles is possible

D. Cerebral palsy

1. Introduction
   - Nonprogressive central nervous system injury
   - Upper extremity deformities
     - Thumb-in-palm
     - Clenched fist
     - Wrist flexion
     - Forearm pronation
     - Elbow flexion
     - Shoulder internal rotation
2. Nonoperative treatment
   - Initially involves physical therapy and nighttime static splinting
   - Antispasticity medications such as diazepam, baclofen, tizanidine, and dantrolene
   - Intrathecal baclofen infusion pump
   - Botulinum toxin A is transiently effective (3 to 6 months) and may be used periodically for severe spasticity.
3. Operative treatment
   - Best performed on children with higher IQs (over 50 to 70), voluntary muscle control, and good sensibility
     - **Voluntary muscle control is the most important predictor of success.**
   - A thumb-in-palm deformity is corrected by release or lengthening of the adductor pollicis, first dorsal interosseous, flexor pollicis brevis, and FPL muscles, combined with first web space Z-plasty and tendon transfers to augment thumb extension and abduction.
   - Fractional or Z-lengthening of tendon with or without ulnar motor neurectomy may improve digital flexor tightness and intrinsic spasticity in patients with a clenched fist.
   - Wrist flexion deformity may be treated early by FCU to ECRB tendon transfer or wrist arthrodesis for fixed contractures in late stages.
     - Concomitant proximal row carpectomy may improve wrist positioning and help rebalance severe digital flexor tightness.
   - Mild elbow contractures may be improved by musculocutaneous neurectomy.
   - Severe contractures addressed by biceps and brachialis muscle lengthening combined with anterior joint capsulotomy.
   - Shoulder contractures may be addressed with derotational humeral osteotomy, lengthening of the subscapularis and pectoralis major muscles, or shoulder arthrodesis.

E. Stroke

1. Cerebral vascular accident may lead to significant upper extremity disability.
2. Spontaneous neurologic recovery 6 to 12 months after CVA
3. Uncontrolled muscle spasticity may lead to joint contracture.
   - Shoulder adduction
   - Elbow flexion
   - Forearm pronation
   - Wrist and digit flexion
   - Thumb-in-palm
4. Contracture release and/or tendon transfers for functional positioning

F. Tendon transfers

1. Indications

- Replace irreparably injured tendons/muscles
- Substitute for function of a paralyzed muscle
- Restore balance to a deformed hand

2. Timing of tendon transfers is controversial and depends on age, indication, and prognosis.
3. Tendon transfers are generally deferred until tissue equilibrium is achieved and passive joint mobility is restored.
   - Sometimes over 12 months after brachial plexus injury or until spasticity resolves in a tetraplegic hand
4. Key concepts
   - Force is proportional to the cross-sectional area of the muscle.
     - The greatest force of contraction is exerted when the muscle is at its resting length.
   - Amplitude or excursion is proportional to the length of the muscle.
     - Smith 3-5-7 rule estimates the excursion of the wrist flexors/extensors (3 cm), MCP extensors (5 cm), and the FDP (7 cm).
   - Work capacity is force times length (F × L).
   - Power is the amount of work performed in a unit of time.
5. Selection of a transfer
   - What function is missing?
   - What muscle-tendon units are available?
   - What are the options for transfer?
6. Basic tenets
   - **Donor must be expendable.**
   - **Donor must be of similar excursion and power.**
   - **One transfer should perform one function.**
   - **Synergistic transfers are easier to rehabilitate.**
   - **A straight line of pull is optimal.**
   - **One grade of motor strength will be lost after transfer.**
7. Classical transfers outlined in Table 7-11
8. Most common complication of tendon transfer is development of motion-limiting adhesions, requiring aggressive hand therapy and possible secondary tenolysis if minimal improvement.

XII. ARTHRITIS

A. Osteoarthritis

1. Primary idiopathic degenerative joint disease
2. Commonly affects DIP joints and trapeziometacarpal joint of thumb

Table 7-11 Classical Tendon Transfers

Palsy	Loss	Transfer
Radial	Wrist extension	Pronator teres to ECRB
	Finger extension	FCU to EDC II-V, FCR to EDC II-V FDS III to EPL and EIP, FDS IV to EDC III-V
	Thumb extension	Palmaris longus to EPL FDS to radial lateral band
Low ulnar	Hand intrinsics (interosseous and ulnar lumbricals)	ECRL to lateral band EDQ EIP to lateral band FCR + graft to lateral band Metacarpal phalangeal capsulodesis
	Thumb adduction	ECRL + graft to adductor pollicis Brachioradialis + graft to adductor pollicis
	Index abduction	EIP to first dorsal interosseous Abductor pollicis longus to first dorsal interosseous ECRL to first dorsal interosseous
High ulnar	Low problems + FDP Ring and small fingers	Suture to functioning FDP index and long index and long finger
Low median	Opposition	FDS ring to abductor pollicis brevis (FCU pulley) EIP to thumb proximal phalanx (routed around the ulna for line of pull) Abductor digiti quinti to abductor pollicis brevis Palmaris longus to abductor pollicis brevis
High median	Thumb IP flexion	Brachioradialis to flexor pollicis longus
	Index- and long-finger flexion	Suture to functioning FDP ring and small finger or ECRL to FDP index and long finger if additional power is needed
Low median and ulnar	Thumb adduction	ECRB + graft to adductor tubercle of thumb
	Index abduction	Abductor pollicis longus to first dorsal interosseous
	Opposition	EIP to abductor pollicis brevis
	Clawed fingers	Brachioradialis + four-tailed free graft to the A2 pulley
	Volar sensibility	Neurovascular island flap from back of hand
High median and ulnar	Thumb adduction	ECRB + graft to adductor tubercle of thumb
	Thumb IP flexion	Brachioradialis to FPL
	Thumb abduction	EIP to abductor pollicis brevis
	Index abduction	Abductor pollicis longus to first dorsal interosseous
	Finger flexion	ECRL to FDP
	Clawed fingers	Tenodesis of all metaphalangeal joints, with free-tendon graft from dorsal carpal ligament routed deep to transverse metacarpal ligament to extensor apparatus
	Wrist flexion	ECU to FCU
	Volar sensibility	Neurovascular island flap from back of hand

ECRB, extensor carpi radialis brevis; ECRL, extensor carpi radialis longus; ECU, extensor carpi ulnaris; EDC, extensor digitorum communis; EDQ, extensor digiti quinti; EIP, extensor indicis proprius; EPL, extensor pollicis longus; FCR, flexor carpi radialis; FCU, flexor carpi ulnaris; FDP, flexor digitorum profundus; FDS, flexor digitorum superficialis; FPL, flexor pollicis longus; IP, interphalangeal.

3. Erosive form more commonly affects PIP joints.
4. MCP joints not typically involved
5. Osteoarthritis of wrist is usually post-traumatic.
6. Hallmark symptoms of osteoarthritis are pain, swelling, and decreased motion.
7. Classical radiographic findings are joint space narrowing, osteophytes, subchondral sclerosis, and subchondral cyst formation.
8. Nonoperative management includes activity modification, NSAIDs, and intraarticular corticosteroid injections.
9. Specific joint findings and treatment
   - DIP joint
     - Often asymptomatic despite radiographic changes
     - Heberden nodes from marginal osteophytes
     - **May be associated with symptomatic mucous cyst**
       - **The cyst may be excised, along with any accompanying osteophytes, for symptomatic relief.**
       - **Occasionally, skin coverage with a local rotational flap is necessary after cyst excision.**
     - Definitive surgery may be warranted for unremitting pain, instability, or deformity.
       - Arthrodesis with Kirschner wires or headless cannulated screw with joint in 5 to 10 degrees of flexion
   - PIP joint
     - Bouchard nodes from marginal osteophytes
     - Surgical options include arthrodesis and arthroplasty.
       - Arthrodesis provides more predictable outcome for the index PIP joint, where the lateral stresses associated with pinch may compromise the durability of arthroplasty.
       - If arthrodesis is chosen, the joint should be fused in increasing degrees of flexion from radial to ulnar.
         - Index—40 degrees
         - Long—45 degrees
         - Ring—50 degrees
         - Small—55 degrees
       - PIP arthroplasty is better reserved for the long, ring, and small digits, which are involved in power grasp.
         - Dorsal and volar approaches described
         - Silicone and pyrocarbon implants available
           - Use of pyrocarbon requires competent collateral ligaments to prevent instability.
         - Postoperative motion is most dependent on preoperative motion.
   - MCP joint
     - Primary cases rare
     - May be involved in patients with hemochromatosis
     - Silicone or pyrocarbon implants are preferred treatment.
     - Arthrodesis severely limits hand function, but may be necessary in setting of failed arthroplasty or septic arthritis.
       - Index—25 degrees
       - Long—30 degrees
       - Ring—35 degrees
       - Small—40 degrees
   - Thumb MCP joint
     - Wide variability in range of motion depending on metacarpal head morphology
     - Rarely involved in primary osteoarthritis
     - Pain is reliably relieved by arthrodesis, with the joint placed in 10 to 20 degrees of flexion.

Table 7-12 Eaton Radiographic Stages of Trapeziometacarpal Osteoarthritis

Stage	Description
I	Normal joint with the exception of possible widening from synovitis
II	Joint space narrowing, with debris and osteophytes <2 mm
III	Joint space narrowing, with debris and osteophytes >2 mm
IV	Involvement of scaphotrapezial joint space in addition to narrowing of the trapeziometacarpal joint

From Trumble TE, et al, editors: *Core knowledge in orthopaedics: hand, elbow, and shoulder,* Philadelphia, 2006, Mosby, p 330.

   - Thumb trapeziometacarpal joint
     - Also termed basal joint or CMC joint
     - Theorized by Pellegrini to result from anterior oblique ligament ("beak" ligament) attenuation
       - Leads to instability, dorsoradial subluxation, and abnormal articular cartilage degeneration
     - Pain and/or crepitus may be elicited with the axial grind test, using combined axial compression and circumduction.
     - Metacarpal adduction, first web space contracture, and compensatory MCP hyperextension are late findings.
     - Up to 50% of patients with thumb CMC osteoarthritis also have carpal tunnel syndrome.
     - Eaton and Littler staging (Table 7-12)
     - **Many treatment alternatives exist, but all share at least partial excision of trapezium.**
     - Young laborers treated with arthrodesis
       - 20 degrees of radial abduction and 40 degrees of palmar abduction
     - Arthroscopic hemitrapeziectomy recently described for early stage disease
     - Most commonly performed procedure for advanced thumb CMC osteoarthritis is trapezium excision with ligament reconstruction and tendon interposition.
       - FCR and APL common choices for tendon graft
       - Status of scaphotrapezoidal joint assessed intraoperatively and treated accordingly
       - Thumb MCP hyperextension is addressed with either volar capsulodesis or arthrodesis.
       - Proximal migration ("settling") of first metacarpal during pinch does not seem to correlate with clinical outcome in most series.
     - There is evidence to support simple trapeziectomy alone for lowest complication rate and similar clinical outcome to more complex procedures.
     - Interposition of synthetic or allograft materials, as well as prosthetic arthroplasty have been described but to date do not offer superior outcome to traditional procedures.
     - Past use of silicone arthroplasty resulted in unacceptably high failure rate from silicone synovitis or instability.
     - **Use of off-label hyaluronic acid injection has not demonstrated a difference between placebo or corticosteroid injection.**

B. Rheumatoid arthritis

1. Overview
   - Systemic autoimmune inflammatory disease that primarily affects the synovium surrounding small joints of hand and wrist
   - Arthritis of hand joints lasting longer than 6 weeks is one of seven diagnostic criteria used by American College of Rheumatology.
   - In contrast to osteoarthritis, the DIP joints are usually spared in RA.
   - Emergence of more effective disease-modifying antirheumatic drugs (DMARDs) has dramatically reduced the frequency of surgical intervention for these patients.
2. Diagnosis
   - Symmetric complaints of pain, morning stiffness, hand swelling
   - Tenosynovitis and tendon rupture are common.
     - Digit triggering treated by tenosynovectomy in addition to A1 pulley release.
     - May require ulnar FDS slip excision or debulking of flexor tendon to relieve triggering
   - Tendon ruptures often require tendon transfer.
   - Serologic studies may be positive (rheumatoid factor in 70% to 90% of patients) within several months of disease onset.
   - Classical radiographic features, including diffuse osteopenia, periarticular erosion, and joint subluxation, may not appear for several years (Figure 7-51).
   - MRI with intravenous contrast more sensitive for detecting early disease, with findings of enhanced synovial proliferation, bone marrow edema, and periarticular erosion
   - Disability may be diminished by early diagnosis, referral to rheumatologist, and aggressive medical management with DMARDs and/or oral corticosteroids.

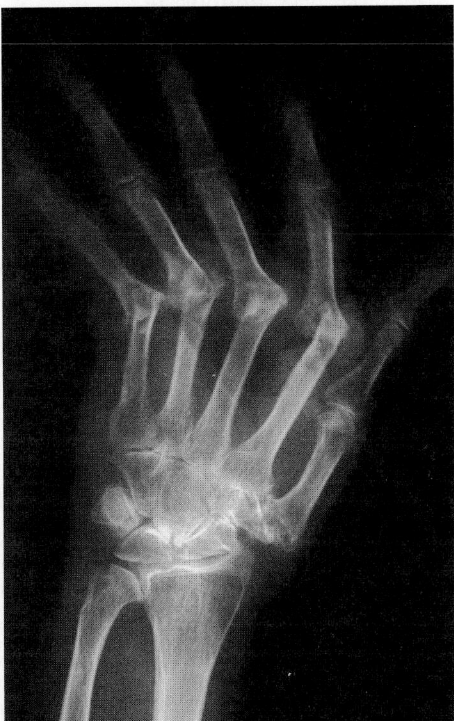

Figure 7-51 Radiograph showing distal radioulnar joint arthritis, ulnar translocation of the carpus, radial deviation of the metacarpals, and ulnar deviation and subluxation of the proximal phalanges. (From Trumble TE, et al, editors: *Core knowledge in orthopaedics: hand, elbow, and shoulder,* Philadelphia, 2006, Mosby, p 347.)

3. Treatment
   - Rheumatoid nodules
     - Subcutaneous masses consisting of chronic inflammatory cells surrounded by collagenous capsule
     - Most common extraarticular manifestation of the disease
     - Occur over bony prominences on extensor surfaces
     - May erode through skin and cause chronic draining sinus
     - Excision may be indicated for diagnostic biopsy, pain relief, or improved cosmesis.
   - Tenosynovitis
     - Hyperplasia and inflammatory cell infiltration of synovium-lined tendon sheaths that may precede joint manifestations
     - May involve flexor and/or extensor tendons of hand/wrist
     - Nonoperative management with rest, activity modification, splinting, and anti-inflammatory medication is attempted for 4 to 6 months.
     - Tenosynovectomy reserved for cases that fail conservative treatment or when impending tendon rupture evident
   - Tendon rupture
     - May occur secondary to chronic tenosynovitis or mechanical abrasion over bony prominences
     - **Vaughan-Jackson syndrome describes progressive rupture of extensor tendons, starting with extensor digiti minimi and continuing radially, from attrition over a prominent distal ulnar head (caput ulnae syndrome).**
     - EPL may rupture from same process at the Lister tubercle.
     - **Mannerfelt syndrome results in FPL and/or index FDP rupture secondary to attrition over a volar STT joint osteophyte.**
     - Direct repair prone to failure, so tendon transfer is preferred method of treatment (Figure 7-52)
   - Caput ulnae syndrome
     - End-stage finding of DRUJ instability from chronic synovitis and surrounding capsular and ligamentous laxity
     - As the ECU subsheath stretches, the ECU tendon subluxes in ulnar and volar direction.
     - Subsequently, the carpus supinates on radius and further stretches the dorsal restraints.
     - Ulnar head subluxes dorsally ("piano-key sign").
     - Attritional rupture of extensor tendons (see earlier discussion of Vaughan-Jackson syndrome)
     - Treatment options include Darrach distal ulna resection, Sauve-Kapandji procedure, resection hemiarthroplasty, and ulnar head prosthetic replacement.
   - Rheumatoid wrist
     - Extensive synovitis and pannus formation weakens the capsular and ligamentous structures that stabilize the radiocarpal joint and DRUJ.
     - Carpus subluxes in volar and ulnar direction.

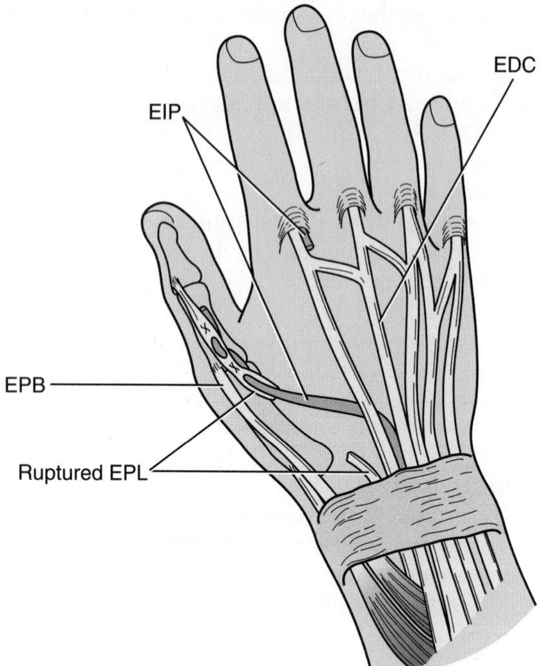

Figure 7-52 **Transfer of the extensor indicis proprius (EIP) for an extensor pollicis longus (EPL) rupture. EDC, extensor digitorum communis; EPB, extensor pollicis brevis.** (From Trumble TE, et al, editors: *Core knowledge in orthopaedics: hand, elbow, and shoulder,* Philadelphia, 2006, Mosby, p 365.)

  - Chronic scapholunate ligament disruption can lead to rotatory subluxation of the scaphoid and progressive carpal collapse.
  - Early synovectomy may delay severe joint destruction and deformity in some cases.
  - Intermediate-stage disease may benefit from radiolunate arthrodesis (Chamay), which centralizes the lunate and diminishes further carpal subluxation and ulnar translocation (preserves midcarpal motion).
  - Total wrist arthrodesis remains gold standard for advanced radiocarpal destruction.
    - For bilateral procedures, fuse one wrist in slight extension and the other in slight flexion.
  - Total wrist arthroplasty is an option in low-demand patients with adequate bone stock, minimal deformity, and intact extensor tendon function.
    - Newer-generation metal/polyethylene combination implants are helping decrease the historically high rate of complications associated with total wrist arthroplasty.
  - Both total wrist arthrodesis and total wrist arthroplasty have been deemed cost-effective procedures for the treatment of rheumatoid wrist.
  - It may be reasonable to consider an arthroplasty of the dominant wrist and a fusion of the nondominant wrist in select patients.
- MCP joint involvement
  - Characteristic deformity pattern of ulnar deviation and volar subluxation
    - **Initial presentation may be an extension lag.**
  - **Synovitis and pannus formation stretch the weaker radial sagittal bands, and extensor tendons subluxate ulnarly.**
  - Concurrent loss of volar plate and collateral ligament integrity
  - Contracture of the intrinsic muscle tendons leads to ulnar deviation of fingers.
  - Simultaneous wrist involvement leads to Z-deformity.
    - Ulnar translocation and supination of carpus
    - Radial deviation of metacarpals
    - Ulnar deviation of digits
  - **Early treatment with synovectomy and recentralization of the extensor tendons provides temporary solution.**
  - Silicone MCP arthroplasty most common definitive treatment to relieve pain and improve cosmesis
    - Ultimate function less predictable
    - Complications may include infection, implant failure, and recurrent deformity.
    - Concomitant correction of wrist deformity is paramount to the success of MCP arthroplasty.
- PIP joint involvement
  - Synovitis leads to attenuation of stabilizing structures, and characteristic deformities.
    - Boutonniere—Attenuation of central slip leads to volar subluxation of lateral bands and consequent PIP hyperflexion and DIP hyperextension.
    - Swan neck—Attenuation of volar plate leads to dorsal subluxation of lateral bands and consequent PIP hyperextension and DIP hyperflexion.
  - Rheumatoid thumb
    - Classified into six types by Nalebuff (Table 7-13)
    - Most common deformity is type I boutonniere.
    - Treatment dictated by deformity with options including synovectomy, soft tissue reconstruction, arthrodesis, and arthroplasty

C. **Juvenile rheumatoid arthritis**

1. Age of onset before 16 years
2. Other rheumatic diseases must be excluded.
3. A classical difference between juvenile rheumatoid arthritis (JRA) and adult form is radial deviation of the MCP joints and ulnar deviation of the wrist.
4. Nonoperative treatment favored to avoid damage to growing physes
5. Three disease types—systemic (20%), polyarticular (40%), and pauciarticular (40%)
   - Systemic form (Still disease)
     - May be associated with transient arthritis in the setting of fever, anemia, hepatosplenomegaly, uveitis, and lymphadenitis

Table 7-13 Nalebuff Classification of Rheumatoid Thumb Deformities

Type	Description
I	Boutonniere
II	Boutonniere with carpometacarpal involvement
III	Swan neck deformity
IV	Gamekeeper's deformity
V	Swan neck deformity with no metacarpal adduction or carpometacarpal changes
VI	Skeletal collapse with loss of bone substance (arthritis mutilans)

From Trumble TE, et al, editors: *Core knowledge in orthopaedics: hand, elbow, and shoulder,* Philadelphia, 2006, Mosby, p 368.

  - Rheumatoid factor is negative.
  - Only one fourth of patients develop chronic, disabling arthritis.
- Polyarticular form
  - Symmetric form affecting at least five joints
  - Small percentage have positive rheumatoid factor.
  - More closely resembles adult form
  - Chronic progression likely
- Pauciarticular form
  - Asymmetric form affecting less than five joints
  - Produces more large-joint and lower extremity involvement
  - Female patients typically have earlier disease onset and may have positive antinuclear antibody.
  - An association with human leukocyte antigen (HLA)-B27 and sacroilitis is more common in male patients.

D. Psoriatic arthritis

1. Seronegative spondyloarthropathy affects approximately 20% of patients with psoriasis.
2. Skin involvement precedes joint manifestations by several years.
3. Classical clinical findings include nail pitting and sausage digits.
4. PIP flexion and MCP extension contractures
5. Radiographs may show DIP joint "pencil-in-cup" deformity.
6. Operative treatment with DIP arthrodesis

E. Systemic lupus erythematosus

1. Most often affects young women between ages 15 and 25 years
2. Majority have rheumatoid-like presentation of inflammatory small joint hand and wrist arthritis.
3. Swan neck more common than boutonniere deformity in systemic lupus erythematosus
4. MCP joints have characteristic ulnar deviation and volar subluxation.
5. Other potential findings in systemic lupus erythematosus include marked joint laxity, Raynaud phenomenon, facial butterfly rash, positive antinuclear antibody, and anti-DNA antibodies.
6. Radiographs largely normal
7. DMARDs are mainstay of treatment.
8. When medical management is maximized, arthrodesis of affected joints is more reliable than arthroplasty.

F. Scleroderma (systemic sclerosis)

1. Hand manifestations include Raynaud phenomenon, PIP flexion contractures, skin ulceration, fingertip pulp atrophy, and calcific deposits within digits (calcinosis cutis).
2. Absorption of distal phalangeal tufts may be seen radiographically.
3. Periadventitial digital sympathectomy may be necessary for refractory cases of Raynaud phenomenon with unremitting ischemic pain or signs of distal tissue ulceration or necrosis.
   - Results of sympathectomy better for scleroderma than for atherosclerotic disease.
4. Arthrodesis is used for fixed PIP flexion contractures.
5. Symptomatic calcific deposits may be excised.
6. Fingertip ulcerations/necrosis are best treated with débridement and possible amputation.

G. Gout

1. Caused by precipitation of monosodium urate crystals, which deposit in joints and other tissues
2. Ninety percent of cases occur in men.
3. Elevated uric acid levels do not necessarily correlate with the prevalence of gouty attacks.
4. Gout may be associated with any state of high metabolic turnover.
5. Radiographs may show periarticular erosions and soft tissue tophi in chronic cases.
6. Aspiration yields negatively birefringent monosodium urate crystals.
7. Acute attacks treated with high dose NSAIDs, oral steroids, or colchicine.
8. Allopurinol used for chronic prophylaxis against further attacks

H. Calcium pyrophosphate deposition disease (pseudogout)

1. Causes an acute monoarticular arthritis that mimics septic arthritis
2. Wrist is second most commonly affected joint (knee).
3. Aspiration yields positively birefringent calcium pyrophosphate dihydrate crystals.
4. Radiographs may show chondrocalcinosis of the TFCC and/or other wrist ligaments.
5. Treat acute attacks with high-dose NSAIDs.
6. Chronic arthritis (scaphotrapeziotrapezoid, SLAC patterns) treated according to stage of disease

XIII. IDIOPATHIC OSTEONECROSIS OF THE CARPUS

A. Kienböck disease (idiopathic osteonecrosis of the lunate)

1. Overview
   - Progressive, often debilitating disease
   - Characterized by fragmentation and collapse of lunate
   - Most common in men between ages of 20 and 40
   - Rare in children but better prognosis
   - Rarely bilateral
   - Multifactorial etiology postulated
     - Lunate geometry
     - Anatomic variability of lunate blood supply
       - Single arterial supply, limited intraosseous branching most susceptible
     - Increased intraosseous pressure from venous stasis
     - Negative ulnar variance
       - Increased shear stress on marginally perfused lunate
     - Decreased radial inclination
2. Diagnosis
   - Dorsal wrist pain, mild swelling, limited motion, weakness
   - Ulnar variance determined with wrist posteroanterior in neutral rotation
   - Radiographs may be initially normal or show a linear fracture.
     - **Subsequent involvement demonstrates lunate sclerosis followed by lunate collapse.**
   - **Unexplained, persistent, non–activity-related dorsal wrist pain in young adult with negative ulnar variance should prompt MRI evaluation.**
   - MRI findings in early Kienböck disease include diffuse low-signal intensity throughout lunate on T1- and

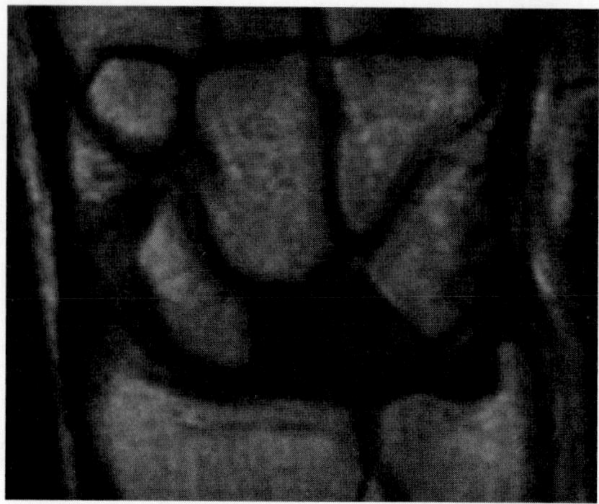

Figure 7-53 **T1-weighted magnetic resonance image of the carpus revealing decreased signal within the lunate.** (From Trumble TE, et al, editors: *Core knowledge in orthopaedics: hand, elbow, and shoulder,* Philadelphia, 2006, Mosby, p 179.)

T2-weighted images (Figure 7-53); increased signal intensity on T2-weighted images may indicate revascularization.

- Lichtman classification (Table 7-14)
  - Modification of using radioscaphoid angle greater than 60 degrees to distinguish between Stage IIIA and B increases interobserver reliability (Goldfarb).

3. Treatment
   - Based on Lichtman stage and ulnar variance
   - A 3-month trial of cast immobilization is appropriate for stage I disease, but the long-term success of nonoperative treatment is limited.
   - Operative treatment is indicated for patients who present with radiographic abnormalities (stage II or higher) or those who fail a trial of immobilization.
   - **First line of surgical treatment is a joint-leveling procedure.**
     - **In patients with ulnar-negative variance, radial-shortening osteotomy is preferred over ulnar lengthening with bone grafting (goal is neutral or 1-mm positive).**
     - Capitate shortening with capitohamate fusion is used for patients with ulnar-positive variance.
   - **Core decompression of the radius and ulna has been described.**
   - **Thought to incite local vascular healing response**
   - Vascularized bone grafting has been used for stages I to IIIA.
     - Preferred pedicle is from the fourth plus fifth extra compartmental artery (4+5 ECA).
     - May be combined with scaphocapitate pinning and/or external fixation to "unload" the lunate temporarily
     - Pedicled vascularized transfers from pisiform and index metacarpal have also been described, as well as free transfers from remote sites.
   - There is little evidence to support one procedure over another for the treatment of stage I to IIIA disease.
   - Treatment of stage IIIB Kienböck disease must address the associated carpal instability.
     - Options include scaphoid-trapezium-trapezoid fusion, scaphocapitate fusion, and proximal row carpectomy.
     - Stage IV disease with radiocarpal and/or midcarpal osteoarthrosis typically requires either proximal row carpectomy or wrist fusion.

Table 7-14 Stages of Kienböck Disease

Stage	Description
I	Normal radiographs or linear fracture, abnormal but nonspecific bone scan, diagnostic appearance on magnetic resonance imaging (lunate shows low signal intensity on T1-weighted images; lunate may show high or low signal intensity on T2-weighted images, depending on extent of disease process)
II	Lunate sclerosis, one or more fracture lines with possible early collapse of lunate on radial border
III	Lunate collapse
A	Normal carpal alignment and height
B	Fixed scaphoid rotation (ring sign), carpal height decreased, capitate migrates proximally
IV	Severe lunate collapse with intraarticular degenerative changes at midcarpal joint, radiocarpal joint, or both

From Allan CH, et al: Kienböck's disease: diagnosis and treatment, *J Am Acad Orthop Surg* 9:128-136, 2001.

B. Preiser disease (idiopathic osteonecrosis of the scaphoid)

1. Rare diagnosis based on radiographic evidence of sclerosis and fragmentation of the scaphoid without evidence of prior fracture
2. Predisposing vascular patterns have not been determined.
3. Average age at onset is 45 years.
4. Patients present with insidious dorsoradial wrist pain.
5. Four-stage radiographic classification similar to Kienböck disease
6. Preiser disease may also be simply classified into complete and partial involvement by MRI.
7. Initially treated with cast immobilization
8. Operative treatment may include core decompression, curettage, allograft replacement, vascularized bone grafting, proximal row carpectomy, scaphoid excision and four-corner fusion, or total wrist fusion.

XIV. DUPUYTREN DISEASE

A. Introduction

1. Dupuytren disease is a benign fibroproliferative disorder of unclear etiology.
2. Typically begins as a nodule in the palmar fascia and progresses insidiously to form diseased cords and finally digital flexion contractures, beginning at the MCP joint and progressing distally
3. Predominantly in Caucasian male patients of northern European descent
4. **Although an autosomal dominant inheritance pattern with variable penetrance is suspected, the offending gene has not been isolated, and sporadic cases are still more common.**
5. Dupuytren disease has been associated with tobacco and alcohol use, diabetes, epilepsy, chronic pulmonary disease,

tuberculosis, and human immunodeficiency virus/acquired immunodeficiency syndrome (HIV/AIDS).

6. No association with occupation has been determined.

B. **Myofibroblast formation**

1. Cytokine-mediated transformation of normal fibroblasts into myofibroblasts has been implicated.
2. **Myofibroblasts are predominant cell type found histologically in Dupuytren fascia, and their contractile properties are abnormal and exaggerated.**
3. Increase in ratio of type III to type I collagen as well as an increase in free radical formation in the palm
4. Three stages of disease are recognized.
   - Proliferative, involutional, and residual

C. **Structural anomalies**

1. Normal fascial structures that become involved (Figure 7-54)
   - Pretendinous band
   - Natatory band
   - Spiral band
   - Retrovascular band
   - Grayson ligament
   - Lateral digital sheet
2. **Cleland ligaments are not involved.**
3. Normal bands become diseased cords (Figure 7-55).
   - Spiral cord
     - Contributions from the pretendinous band, spiral band, lateral digital sheet, and Grayson ligament

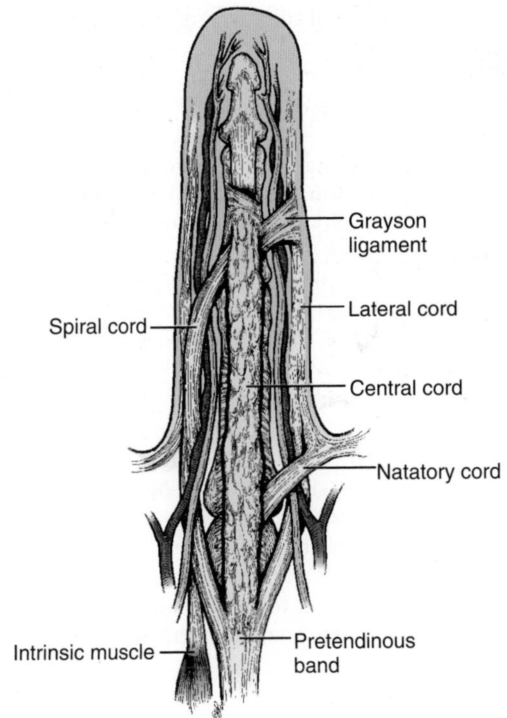

Figure 7-55 The change in the normal fascia bands to diseased cords. (From Green DP, et al, editors: *Green's operative hand surgery*, ed 5, New York, 2005, Churchill Livingstone, p.164. Courtesy of Dr. R. M. McFarlane.)

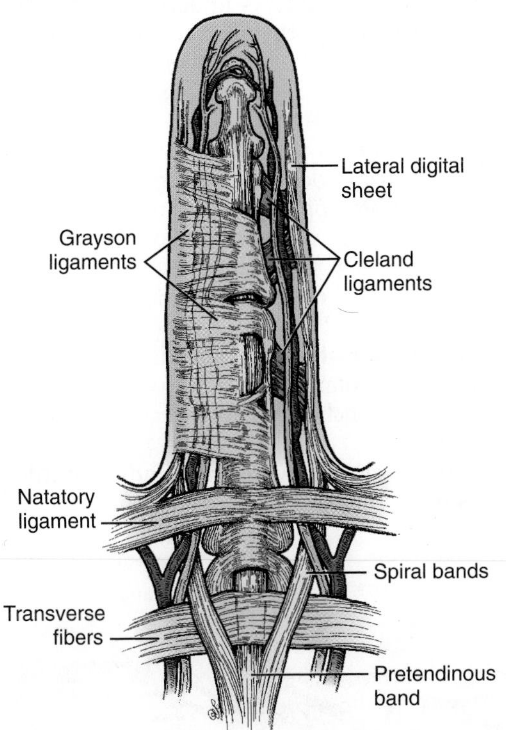

Figure 7-54 Parts of the normal digital fascia that become diseased. The Grayson ligament, *shown on the left,* is an almost continuous sheet of thin fascia in the same plane as the natatory ligament. Cleland ligaments, *shown on the right,* do not become diseased. The lateral digital sheet receives fibers from the natatory ligament and the spiral bands. The spiral bands pass on either side of the metacarpophalangeal joint, deep to the neurovascular bundles, to reach the side of the finger. (From McFarlane RM: Patterns of the diseased fascia in the fingers in Dupuytren's contracture, *Plast Reconstr Surg* 54:31-44, 1974.)

     - Leads to PIP contracture
     - **Put neurovascular bundle at risk during surgery by displacing it more centrally and superficially**
   - Central cord
   - Lateral cord
   - Retrovascular cord
   - Abductor digiti minimi cord
   - Intercommissural cord of first web space

D. **Diagnosis**

1. May present early with tender palmar nodule or later with flexion contractures that impair simple activities of daily living
2. Distributions of digit involvement, in decreasing order of frequency, are the ring, small, long, thumb, and index digits.
3. Dupuytren diathesis describes patients with early disease onset and rapid progression of joint contractures, often bilateral and including more radial digits.
4. Additional extrapalmar locations may be involved, such as the dorsum of the PIP joint (Garrod knuckle pads), penis (Peyronie disease), and plantar surface of the foot (Ledderhose disease).
   - Suggests more aggressive form of disease
5. Patients with Dupuytren diathesis should be counseled about flare reactions and higher recurrence rates after surgical intervention.

E. **Treatment**

1. Nonoperative
   - Largely unsuccessful
   - Emerging collagenase injections (derived from *Clostridium hystolyticum*) are promising but not without side

effects and potential complications such as flexor tendon rupture.
  - Early clinical results better for MCP joints and those with contractures less than 50 degrees
2. Operative
  - **Indications include inability to place hand flat on tabletop (Hueston test), MCP flexion contracture greater than 30 degrees, or any PIP flexion contracture.**
  - Procedure of choice is typically open limited fasciectomy.
    - Iatrogenic digital nerve injury in up to 7% of cases in some series
    - Tourniquet should be deflated to assess digital perfusion after large contracture releases.
  - Percutaneous aponeurotomy gaining acceptance in some clinical scenarios such as mild contractures or elderly patient with low demands.
  - Total palmar fasciectomy no longer favored because of high complication rate.
  - Open-palm McCash technique may still be used to reduce hematoma formation, decrease edema, and allow early motion.
  - Dermofasciectomy generally reserved for Dupuytren diathesis or recurrent cases
  - Skin deficits after contracture release may be addressed with Z-plasty, V-Y advancement, full-thickness skin grafting, or healing by secondary intention.
3. Complications and postoperative care
  - Most common complication after operative treatment is recurrence, with long-term rates around 50% (higher in Dupuytren diathesis).
  - Judicious postoperative therapy with active range of motion and static splinting to maintain extension correction is critical for improved outcomes and the prevention or delay of recurrence.
  - Early postoperative "flare reactions" are more common in women and may be treated with short courses of oral steroids or NSAIDs.
  - Other potential complications include infection, digital neurovascular injury, complex regional pain syndrome, hematoma, skin loss, and amputation.

XV. HAND TUMORS

A. Benign soft tissue tumors

1. Ganglion
  - Most common soft tissue mass of the hand and wrist
  - Contains either joint or tendon sheath fluid
  - Encapsulating tissue does not have true epithelial lining.
  - These masses often fluctuate in size over time.
  - A traumatic etiology is suspected in many cases.
  - Ganglions are often firm and well-circumscribed and may transilluminate on physical examination.
  - **Seventy percent of cases occur at the dorsal wrist, usually originating from the scapholunate articulation** (Figure 7-56).
    - Small (occult) dorsal ganglions may be more symptomatic than larger ones.
  - Majority of volar wrist ganglions originate from the radioscaphoid or scaphotrapezial joints (Figure 7-57).

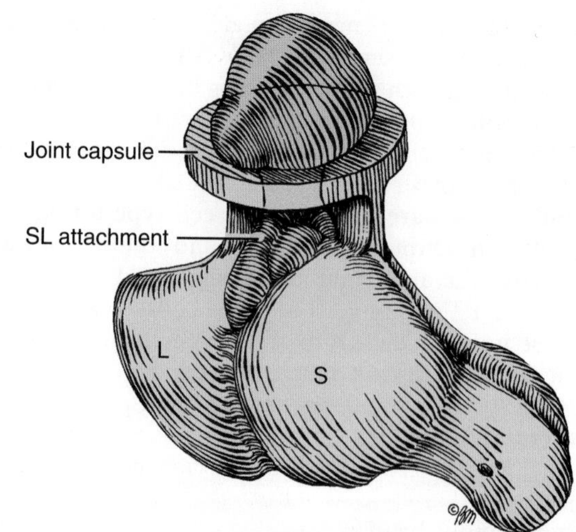

Figure 7-56 The ganglion and scapholunate (SL) attachments are isolated from the remaining, uninvolved joint capsule (not shown). L, lunate; S, scaphoid. (From Green DP, et al, editors: *Green's operative hand surgery,* ed 5, Philadelphia, 2005, Churchill Livingstone, p 2229)

    - These emerge in close proximity to radial artery and its branches.
    - Higher recurrence rate compared to dorsal ganglions
  - **Mucous cysts occur at dorsum of DIP joint in patients with osteoarthritis.**
    - **Surgery must address underlying osteophytes.**
  - Retinacular cysts form from herniated tendon sheath fluid.
  - Overall recurrence rate after aspiration of ganglions is approximately 50%.
  - Open excision is the surgical procedure of choice, although many dorsal ganglions can be effectively removed arthroscopically.
    - The cyst stalk and portion of capsule should be removed.
  - A brief period of immobilization is recommended postoperatively.
2. **Giant cell tumor of tendon sheath**
  - Second most common soft tissue mass of the hand
  - Other names include xanthoma and localized nodular synovitis.
  - **Presents as slow-growing, nontender, multilobulated mass on the volar aspect of a digit.**

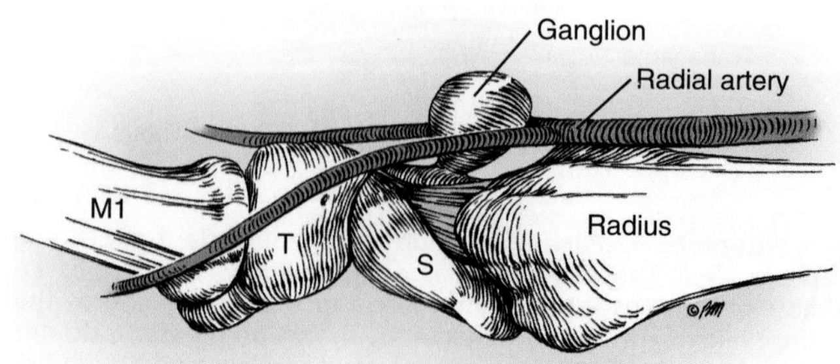

Figure 7-57 The usual relationship of the ganglion to the radial artery and volar joint capsule. M1, first metacarpal; S, scaphoid; T, trapezium. (From Green DP, et al, editors: *Green's operative hand surgery,* ed 5, Philadelphia, 2005, Churchill Livingstone, p 2232.)

- Contains multinucleated giant cells, xanthoma cells, and hemosiderin deposits (histology similar to pigmented villonodular synovitis)
- **Treatment is marginal excision.**
- Lesions with multiple discrete tumors associated with higher recurrence rate (~50% in some series)

3. Lipoma
   - Extremely common tumor of adipose cell origin
   - Though usually painless, they may reach substantial size over time.
   - Lipomas in the palm may compress the carpal tunnel or the Guyon canal, leading to neurologic deficits.
   - MRI may be helpful for preoperative planning in these cases.
   - Lesions have same bright signal characteristics as subcutaneous fat on T1-weighted images.
   - Treatment is either observation or marginal excision.
   - Low recurrence rate
4. Epidermal inclusion cyst
   - Common, painless, slow-growing mass arising after penetrating injury that drives keratinizing epithelium into subcutaneous tissue
   - Curative treatment is marginal excision.
5. Neurilemoma (schwannoma)
   - Most common peripheral nerve tumor of the upper extremity
   - Typically painless mass that may have positive Tinel sign
   - Cell of origin is the myelin-forming Schwann cell.
     - The tumor is composed of Antoni A (cellular) and Antoni B (matrix) regions.
   - Treatment is marginal excision.
   - Because these tumors are eccentric and encapsulated, they can be shelled out of nerve without disrupting axons.
   - Neurologic injury in less than 5% of cases
   - Low recurrence rate
6. Neurofibroma
   - Slow-growing, painless mass arising from nerve fascicle
   - May be solitary in hand and wrist (no history of neurofibromatosis)
   - Portion of nerve usually sacrificed during excision, and grafting may be necessary
7. Glomus tumor
   - Smooth muscle tumor of perivascular temperature-regulating bodies
   - Usually occurs in subungual region and may cause nail ridging and erosions of the distal phalanx
   - Also reported in palm
   - Characterized by exquisite pain and cold intolerance
   - MRI with gadolinium is helpful adjunctive diagnostic study.
   - Treatment is marginal excision.
   - Low recurrence rate
8. Hemangioma
   - Vascular proliferations divided into capillary (superficial) and cavernous (deep) lesions
   - **Many infantile hemangiomas become involuted by age 7, and those that arise during childhood are observed.**
   - Kasabach-Merritt syndrome is a rare complication resulting from entrapped platelets and a potentially fatal coagulopathy.
   - In adults, MRI with gadolinium may help distinguish these benign vascular tumors from arteriovenous malformations and angiosarcomas.
   - **Small and accessible lesions treated with marginal excision**
   - **Embolization may be more feasible alternative for larger lesions.**
9. Pyogenic granuloma (lobular capillary hemangioma)
   - Rapidly growing, pedunculated cutaneous lesion with friable tissue that bleeds easily
   - Vascular tumor with lobules of endothelial cells and luminal structures in edematous stroma histologically
   - Occurs in all ages
   - Many methods of treatment described, all with high recurrence rates
   - Some evidence to support simple silver nitrate cauterization

B. Malignant soft tissue tumors

1. **Squamous cell carcinoma**
   - **Most common malignancy of the hand**
   - Usually seen in elderly men with premalignant conditions such as actinokeratosis or chronic osteomyelitis
     - Dorsum of hand is high-risk lesion.
   - Primary risk factor is excessive exposure to ultraviolet radiation.
   - Also most common subungual malignancy
   - Higher metastatic potential than basal cell carcinoma
   - Consultation with dermatologist recommended
   - Mohs micrographic surgery has highest cure rate (highest for all nonmelanotic skin cancers).
   - Excision of aggressive lesions that are poorly differentiated or greater than 2.5 cm requires at least 6-mm margin.
   - Lymph node biopsy may be necessary.
   - Adjuvant radiation for tumor recurrence, lesions over 2 cm wide and/or 4 mm deep, perineural invasion, lymph node metastases
2. Sarcoma
   - **Most common sarcomas are epithelioid and synovial.**
   - Other common sarcomas of the upper extremity include liposarcoma and malignant fibrous histiocytoma.
   - Evaluated by MRI
   - Most soft tissue sarcomas metastasize to the lungs.
   - Lymph nodes are the second most common area.
     - Epithelioid sarcoma
       - Firm, slow-growing mass presenting in young to middle-age adults
       - Locations include digits, palm, or forearm
       - May eventually ulcerate and drain
       - Commonly spreads to regional lymph nodes
       - Composed of malignant epithelial cells and central areas of necrosis
       - Treatment is wide or radical excision accompanied by sentinel lymph node biopsy.
       - Adjuvant chemotherapy or radiation therapy may be considered but is controversial for this tumor.
     - Synovial sarcoma
       - Firm, slow-growing mass presenting in young to middle-age adults
       - Usually forms adjacent to the carpus

- Composed of epithelial and spindle cells with multiple histologic patterns
- Treatment is wide or radical excision, with 5-year survival rates of approximately 80%.
- More recently, adjuvant chemotherapy and external beam radiation have proven successful in reducing local recurrence rates.

C. **Benign bone tumors**

1. Enchondroma
   - Most common benign bone tumor of the upper extremity
   - Typically occurs in second to fourth decades
   - Most cases asymptomatic and discovered incidentally
   - Arises from metaphyseal medullary canal and spreads to diaphysis
   - Usually involves proximal phalanx or metacarpal (Figure 7-58)
   - Symmetric fusiform expansion of bone with endosteal scalloping and intramedullary calcifications
   - May present as pathologic fracture
   - Hand enchondromas are distinguished histologically by their high cellularity.
     - Presence of mitotic figures may signal low-grade chondrosarcoma.
   - Treatment is curettage.
     - Bone grafting not shown to affect outcome
2. Osteochondroma

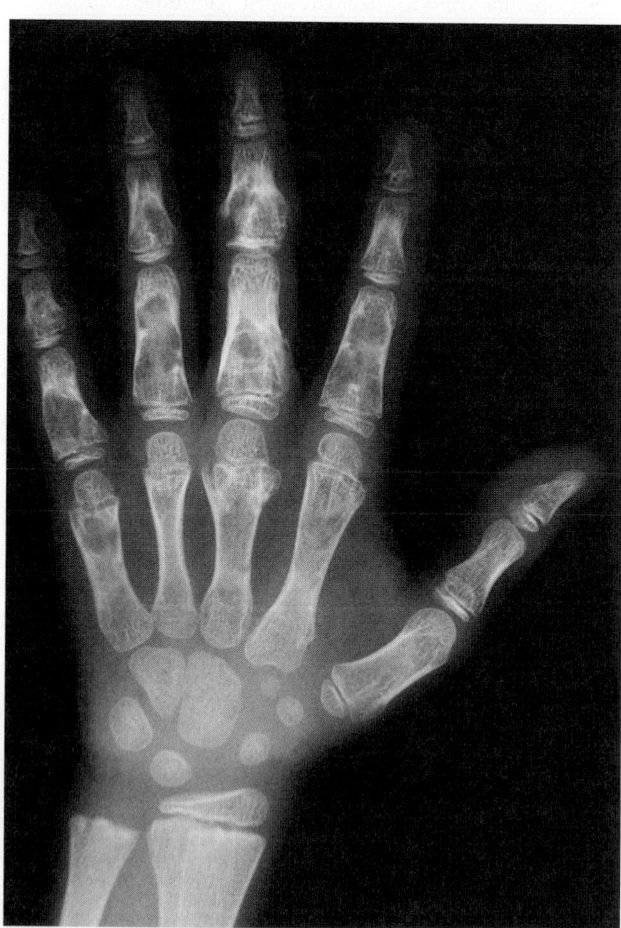

Figure 7-58 Multiple enchondromas (Ollier disease). (From Green DP, et al, editors: *Green's operative hand surgery,* ed 5, Philadelphia, 2005, Churchill Livingstone, p 2250.)

   - Benign tumor characterized by a bony surface outgrowth capped by cartilage
   - Rarely seen in the hand, except in multiple hereditary exostosis
   - Distal aspect of P1 is most common location in hand.
   - May be seen near DRUJ or arising from shafts of radius/ulna
   - Low chance of malignant transformation
   - Asymptomatic lesions observed
   - Symptomatic lesions may have associated bursitis/periostitis and are excised with low recurrence rate.
3. Osteoid osteoma
   - May present with swelling without pain in the hand
   - Usually found in carpus (scaphoid) or proximal phalanx
   - Radiolucent nidus within sclerotic lesion
   - Nonoperative management with immobilization/NSAIDs
   - Excision of nidus is curative.
   - Radiofrequency ablation also effective
4. Unicameral bone cyst
   - Common tumor in children
   - Occasionally seen in metacarpals, phalanges, or metaphyseal portion of distal radius
   - Most resolve spontaneously.
   - Treatment with aspiration and injection of methylprednisolone acetate
5. Giant cell tumor
   - Characterized as benign but may be locally aggressive
   - More common in young to middle-age women
   - Presents with pain, swelling, and/or pathologic fracture
   - Distal radius is most common location.
   - An eccentric, lytic lesion is seen in metaphysis and epiphysis.
   - May cause cortical destruction and associated soft tissue mass
   - Osteoclast-like, multinucleated giant cells and stromal cells with matching nuclei histologically
   - Treatment is wide excision (curettage alone yields high local recurrence rate).
   - Packing the lesion with polymethylmethacrylate (PMMA) has been successful.
   - Occasionally requires reconstruction with allograft or vascularized free fibula

D. **Malignant bone tumors**

1. Most common hand malignancy is metastatic lung carcinoma, usually involving distal phalanx.
2. Breast and kidney metastases also reported
3. Acral metastasis is poor prognostic sign, with less than 6-month survival expected at time of discovery.
4. The three most common primary malignant bone tumors of the hand
   - Chondrosarcoma
   - Osteosarcoma
   - Ewing sarcoma
5. Location is usually metacarpals or phalanges.
6. Treatment for each tumor is same as elsewhere in the body.

XVI. HAND INFECTIONS

A. **Introduction**

1. Hand infections can involve any tissue type and a variety of pathogens (Table 7-15).
2. *Staphylococcus aureus* is overall most common pathogen.

Table 7-15 Hand Infections

Type	Location	Pathogen	Antibiotic	Comment
Paronychia	Eponychium	*Staphylococcus aureus*	Dicloxacillin or clindamycin PO Nafcillin IV	Release eponychial fold May require nail removal
Felon	Pulp space	*S. aureus*	Dicloxacillin or clindamycin PO Nafcillin IV	Release all septa Volar incision preferred
Human bite	MCP and PIP	*Streptococcus* sp. *S. aureus* *Eikenella corrodens*	Ampicillin/sulbactam IV Penicillin for *E. corrodens*	Treatment failure with cephalosporins usually due to *E. corrodens*
Dog and cat bites	Varied	α-Hemolytic streptococci (46%) *Pasteurella multocida* (26%) *S. aureus* (13%) Anaerobes (41%)	Ampicillin/sulbactam IV or amoxicillin/clavulanate PO	Failure of oral treatment common
Necrotizing fasciitis	Varied	Clostridia Group A β-streptococci	Broad-spectrum triple antibiotic—penicillin, clindamycin, gentamicin	High mortality Amputations frequent
Fungal	Cutaneous	*Candida albicans*	Topical antifungal	Common in diabetic patients with chronic paronychia
	Nail	*Trichophyton rubrum*	Ketoconazole or itraconazole PO	Pulse dosing 1 week per month
	Subcutaneous	*Sporothrix schenckii* *Mycoplasma* sp.	Based on culture	

IV, intravenously; MCP, metacarpophalangeal; PIP, proximal interphalangeal; PO, orally.

3. *Streptococcus* organisms are second most common.
4. **Gram-negative and anaerobic bacteria are seen in intravenous drug abusers (IVDA), diabetic patients, and after farmyard injuries or bite wounds.**
5. Community-acquired, methicillin-resistant *S. aureus* (MRSA) is becoming more prevalent, especially in urban communities.
   - Risk factors include antibiotic use in previous year, close and crowded living conditions, compromised skin integrity, shared items (towels, whirlpools, fitness equipment).
   - Risk groups include IVDA, homeless, children in daycare, prison inmates, military recruits, athletes in contact sports.
   - High complication rate in diabetic patients
   - Intravenous treatment with vancomycin or clindamycin, outpatient treatment with oral trimethoprim-sulfamethoxazole or clindamycin

B. Paronychia/eponychia

1. Infections involving the nail fold are most common in hand.
2. Typically *S. aureus*
3. Treated by incision and drainage, partial or total nail plate removal, oral antibiotics, soaks, and dressing changes
4. Important to preserve eponychial fold (cuticle) if possible
5. Chronic paronychia unresponsive to oral antibiotic therapy often secondary to fungal infection (*Candida albicans*)
6. In rare cases, marsupialization (excision of the dorsal eponychium) may be required to eradicate the infection.

C. Felon

1. Infection of the septated fingertip pulp
2. *S. aureus* is most common pathogen.
3. Treated by incision and drainage through a central or midlateral incision
   - Important to break up the septae to adequately decompress the fingertip
   - Midlateral digital incisions are usually placed ulnarly, except for the thumb and small digit, where they are placed radially (Figure 7-59).

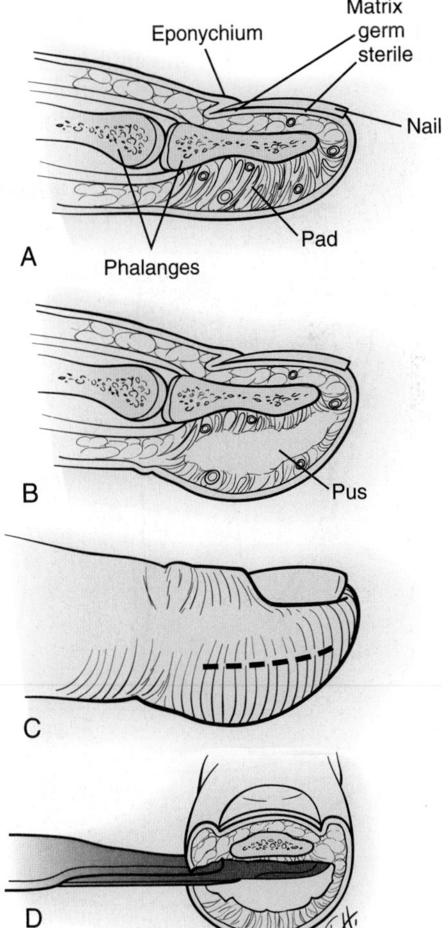

Figure 7-59 **A,** Cross-section of the distal fingertip showing the septated anatomy of the pad. **B,** Collection of pus within the finger pulp space. **C,** Incision for drainage of felon. **D,** The incision should include all of the involved septal compartments. (From Green DP, et al, editors: *Green's operative hand surgery,* ed 5, Philadelphia, 2005, Churchill Livingstone, p 61.)

- Incision should be left open to heal by secondary intention.
- Delayed treatment may lead to concurrent flexor tenosynovitis, osteomyelitis, or digital tip necrosis.

D. Human bite

1. Potentially serious infection treated promptly with incision and drainage, especially if joint or tendon sheath is violated
2. Most commonly involves the third or fourth MCP joint (fight bite)
3. Most frequently isolated organisms are group A streptococcus, *S. aureus, Eikenella corrodens,* and *Bacteroides* species.
4. Empiric antibiotics of choice are intravenous ampicillin/sulbactam and oral amoxicillin/clavulanate.

E. Dog and cat bites

1. More than two million cases per year in the United States
2. Vast majority are dog bites, with low rate of serious infection.
   - More likely to avulse or crush soft tissue but often amenable to local wound care
3. **Minority are cat bites, but with high rate of serious infection.**
   - Higher depth of penetrance and longer time to initiation of treatment
4. If patient presents immediately after bite, nonoperative treatment
   - Splinting, elevation, soaks, and antibiotics, followed by aggressive therapy once infection controlled
5. Delayed treatment may lead to abscess formation and need for operative incision and drainage.
   - Further delay could lead to septic tenosynovitis, septic arthritis, and/or osteomyelitis.
6. Ampicillin/sulbactam and amoxicillin/clavulanate are empiric antibiotics of choice (ciprofloxacin, doxycycline, or tetracycline if penicillin allergic).
   - Covers *Pasteurella multocida* (part of animal oral flora), *S. aureus,* and *Streptococcus* species

F. Pyogenic flexor tenosynovitis (FTS)

1. Infection of flexor tendon sheath
2. May occur in delayed fashion after penetrating trauma
3. *S. aureus* is most common pathogen.
4. **Kanavel signs (four)**
   - **Flexed, resting posture of digit**
   - **Fusiform swelling of the digit**
   - **Tenderness of flexor tendon sheath**
   - **Pain with passive digit extension**
5. **If infection recognized early, patient should be admitted and treated with splinting, intravenous antibiotics, and close observation.**
   - **If signs improve within first 24 hours, surgery may be avoided.**
6. **Otherwise, the treatment of choice is incision and drainage of flexor tendon sheath.**
   - May be accomplished either by full open exposure using long midaxial or Bruner incision or with two small incisions placed distally (open A5 pulley) and proximally (open A1 pulley) using an angiocatheter (Figure 7-60)
   - Continuous-drip irrigation with an indwelling catheter carries a risk for extreme digit swelling.

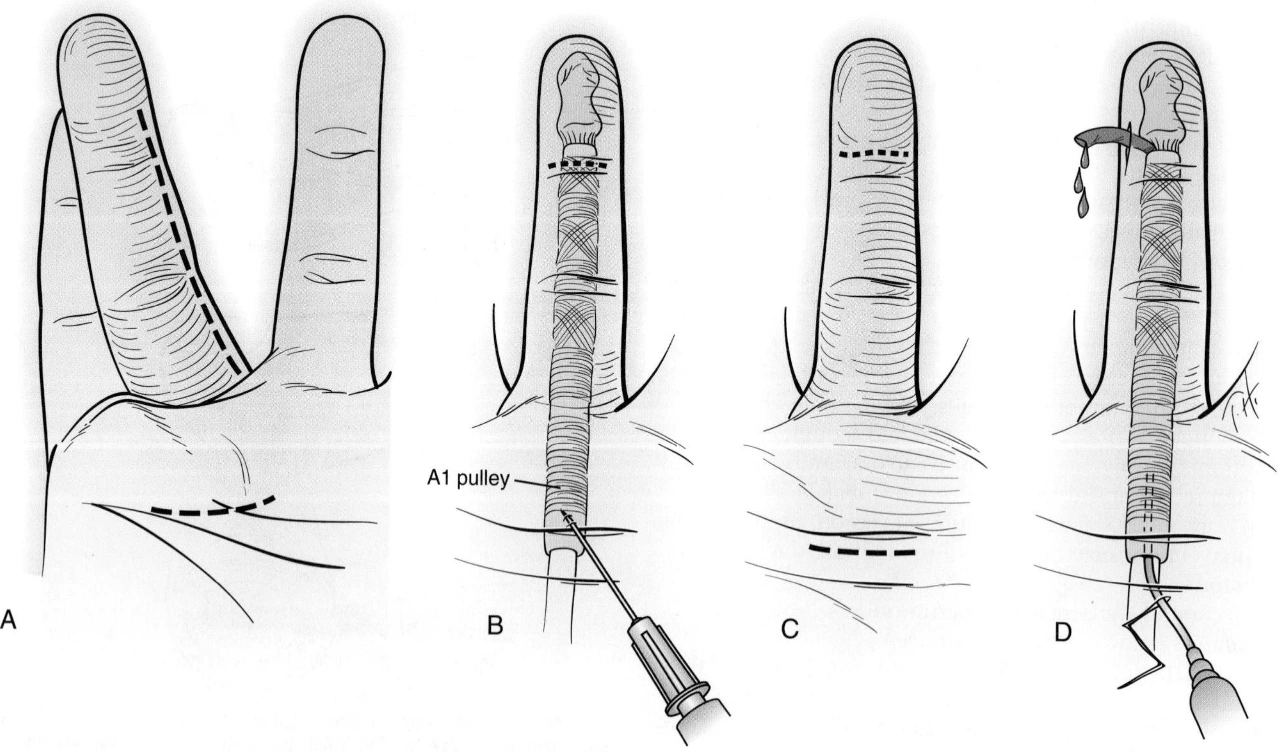

Figure 7-60 Incision for drainage of flexor tendon sheath infections. **A,** Open drainage incisions through the midaxial approach. **B,** Sheath irrigation with distal opening of the sheath and proximal syringe irrigation. **C,** Incisions for intermittent through-and-through irrigation. **D,** Technique for closed tendon sheath irrigation. (From Green DP, et al, editors: *Green's operative hand surgery,* ed 5, Philadelphia, 2005, Churchill Livingstone, p 67.)

7. Index and thumb FTS can spread to deep thenar space.
8. Long, ring, and small finger FTS can spread to the midpalmar space.
   - Small finger FTS can also spread to the ulnar bursa.
   - Classical "horseshoe abscess" is based on proximal communication between the thumb and small finger flexor tendon sheaths in the Parona space, a potential space between the pronator quadratus and FDP tendons.
   - Aggressive postoperative hand therapy is paramount, because tendon adhesions and digital stiffness are likely.
9. Herpetic whitlow
   - Caused by herpes simplex virus (HSV) type 1
   - **Dental hygienists, health care workers, and toddlers at risk**
   - Presents with digit pain and erythema, followed by formation of small vesicles that may coalesce into bullae
   - May be accompanied by fever, malaise, and lymphadenitis
   - Diagnosis confirmed by Tzanck smear and antibody titers
   - Self-limiting, usually resolves within 7 to 10 days
   - **Incision and drainage are not recommended because the rates of secondary bacterial infection are high.**
   - Treatment with acyclovir may shorten the duration of symptoms.
   - Recurrence may be stimulated by fever, stress, and/or sun exposure.
10. Deep potential-space infections
   - A collar button abscess occurs in the web space between digits.
     - Treated by incision and drainage with volar and dorsal incisions (avoiding the skin in the web itself) and intravenous antibiotics
   - Midpalmar space infections are rare.
     - Clinically, there is loss of midline contour of the hand.
     - Palmar pain elicited with flexion of the long, ring, and small fingers
   - Thenar and hypothenar space infections are also rare.
     - Present with pain and swelling over respective areas, exacerbated by flexion of the thumb or small finger
   - Incision and drainage and intravenous antibiotics are required for all of these deep potential-space infections (Figure 7-61).

G. **Necrotizing fasciitis**

1. Severe infection with devastating outcomes and potential death when treatment delayed
2. Group A β-hemolytic streptococcus is the most common organism.
3. Groups at risk include immunocompromised patients (those with diabetes, cancer, or AIDS) as well as alcoholics and IVDA.
4. Requires emergency, radical débridement, and broad-spectrum intravenous antibiotic coverage
5. Intraoperative findings may include liquefied subcutaneous fat, dishwater pus, muscle necrosis, and venous thrombosis.
6. Hemodynamic monitoring is urgent.
7. Amputation may be necessary when life threatening.

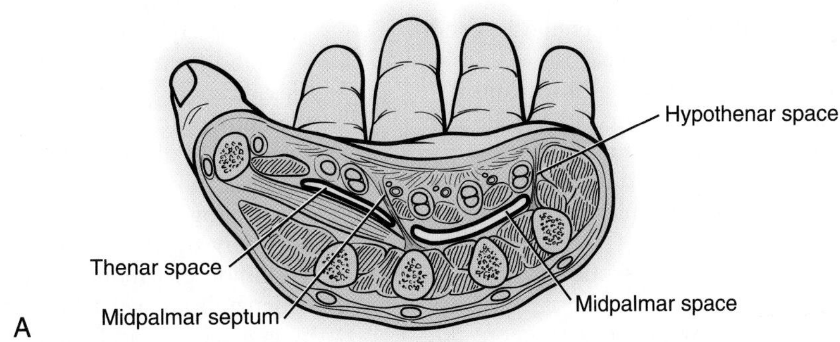

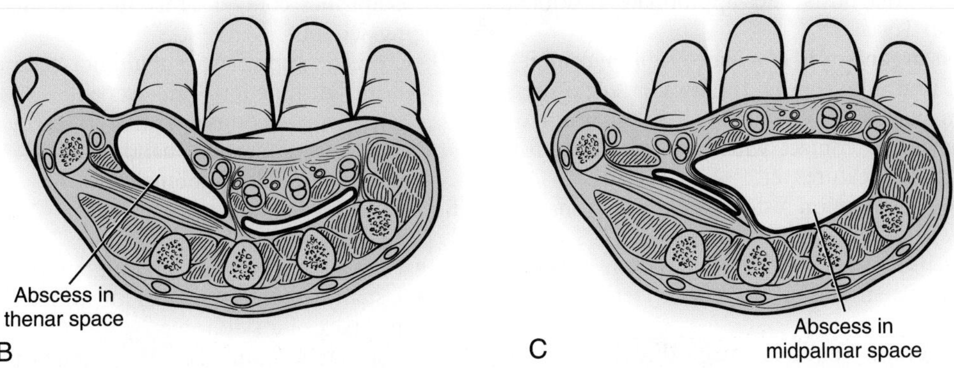

Figure 7-61 Deep palmar spaces. **A,** Potential spaces of the midpalm. **B,** Thenar space abscess. **C,** Midpalmar space abscess. (From Green DP, et al, editors: *Green's operative hand surgery,* ed 5, Philadelphia, 2005, Churchill Livingstone, p 71.)

8. Mortality rate is high and correlates with time to initiation of treatment.

H. Gas gangrene

1. Caused by *Clostridium perfringens* and other *Clostridium* species (gram-positive rods)
2. Condition occurs in devitalized, contaminated wounds and leads to myonecrosis.
3. Extensive surgical débridement is necessary to prevent systemic infection.

I. Fungal infection

1. Serious infection usually seen in immunocompromised patients
2. Divided into cutaneous, subcutaneous, and deep locations
   - Cutaneous infection
     - Chronic paronychia usually caused by *C. albicans* and treated with topical or oral antifungal agents and nail marsupialization
     - Onychomycosis is a destructive, deforming infection of the nail plate that is usually caused by *Trichophyton rubrum* and treated with topical or oral antifungal agents.
   - Subcutaneous infection
     - Usually caused by *Sporothrix schenckii*, following penetrating injury while handling plants or soil (the rose thorn is the classical vehicle of transmission)
     - Starts with papule at site of inoculation with subsequent lesions developing along the lymphatic vessels
     - Treatment is with potassium iodine solution.
   - Deep infection
     - Several forms of deep infection exist, including tenosynovitis, septic arthritis, and osteomyelitis.
     - Treatment involves surgical débridement and culture-specific antifungal agents.
     - Endemic pathogens include histoplasmosis, blastomycosis, and coccidioidomycosis.
     - Opportunistic infections include aspergillosis, candidiasis, mucormycosis, and cryptococcosis.

J. Atypical nontuberculous mycobacterial infections

1. These organisms are widely distributed in the environment but are infrequent human pathogens.
2. Often indolent and fail to respond to usual treatments
3. Musculoskeletal manifestations (papules, ulcers, nodules) involve hand in majority of cases.
4. May progress to tenosynovitis, septic arthritis, or osteomyelitis
5. Average incubation period 2 weeks, can be more than 6 months
6. Average time to diagnosis and appropriate treatment often more than 1 year
7. **Most common organism is *Mycobacterium marinum*.**
   - Proliferates in freshwater and saltwater enclosures, especially in stagnant environment (e.g., aquarium)
   - Patients come into contact with infected water, fish hooks, spiny sea creatures, etc.
8. Granulomas are common on histopathology; they may or may not show acid-fast bacilli.
9. Cultures and sensitivities are critical and require a special medium (Lowenstein-Jensen) at exact temperatures (32° C).
10. **Treatment generally requires surgical débridement and oral antibiotics such as ethambutol, trimethoprim-sulfamethoxazole, clarithromycin, azithromycin, or tetracycline.**
    - Combination of agents often used
    - Rifampin added for bone involvement
    - Oral therapy continued 3 to 6 months

K. Injection injury

1. **High-pressure injection injuries can be devastating.**
2. **High rate of digital amputation**
   - **Organic solvents more toxic to tissue**
   - **Oil-based paint worse than latex, water-based**
3. **Emergency wide surgical débridement recommended**

XVII. CONGENITAL HAND DIFFERENCES

A. Introduction

1. Limb bud appears during fourth week of gestation.
2. Hand begins as paddle with digital separation occurring between 47 and 54 days.
3. Development of lower limb lags behind by 48 hours.
4. All limb structures present by end of embryogenesis at 8 weeks.
   - Most congenital anomalies occur by this time.
5. Signaling centers that control limb development
   - **Apical ectodermal ridge**
     - **Mediates proximal-to-distal growth**
       - Fibroblast growth factor important
   - Zone of polarizing activity formation
     - Mediates anterior-to-posterior growth (e.g., index versus small digit sides of a limb)
       - Sonic hedgehog gene important
   - Wingless-type pathway
     - Mediates dorsoventral axis (flexor versus extensor side of limb)
6. Congenital hand anomalies occur at a rate of 1 in 600 live births
   - Three most common types
     - Polydactyly (1 in 600)
     - Syndactyly (1 in 2000)
     - Bifid thumb (radial polydactyly) (1 in 3000)
7. Classification
   - Failure of formation
   - Failure of differentiation
   - Duplication
   - Overgrowth
   - Undergrowth
   - Amnion disruption sequence
   - Generalized skeletal abnormalities
8. In general, surgical intervention to address congenital hand differences should be performed before the child establishes compensatory mechanisms and before starting school.
9. Cosmetic appearance should not be improved at the cost of further functional impairment.
10. Early genetic counseling is a critical part of the care of a child with congenital hand differences in the setting of other extraskeletal anomalies.

B. Failure of formation

1. Transverse absence
   - Also termed congenital amputations
   - Usually occur at proximal forearm level and are typically not part of a syndrome
   - Majority are unilateral and thought to be result of vascular insult to apical ectodermal ridge.
   - Amputation through proximal third of forearm most common

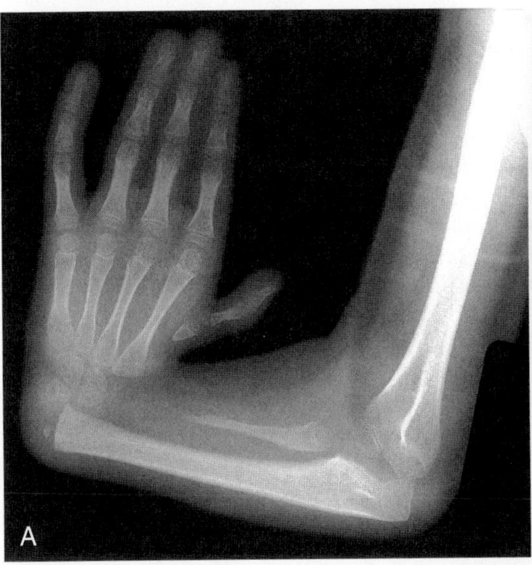

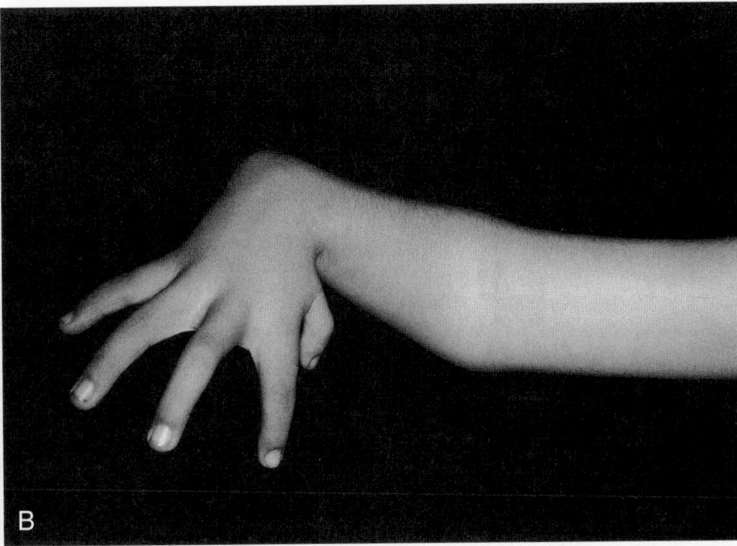

Figure 7-62 **An 8-year-old child with Holt-Oram syndrome whose cardiac problems precluded earlier surgery. A and B, The deformity from his type III radius deficiency was too severe for single-stage centralization.** (From Green DP, et al, editors: *Green's operative hand surgery,* ed 5, Philadelphia, 2005, Churchill Livingstone, p 1473.)

- End of limb may have nubbins or dimpling.
- Early prosthetic fitting before age 2 years is treatment of choice.

2. Longitudinal absence
   - Radial dysplasia (radial clubhand)
     - Characterized by deficiency of the radius and radial carpal structures (Figure 7-62)
     - Thumb dysplasia is included in the spectrum of presentation (see the section Undergrowth).
     - Both extremities are affected in over 50% of cases.
     - Associated systemic syndromes
       - Thrombocytopenia with absent radius (TAR)
       - VACTERL syndrome (**v**ertebral, **a**nal, **c**ardiac, **t**racheal, **e**sophageal, **r**enal, and limb anomalies)
       - Holt-Oram syndrome
       - **Fanconi anemia**
         - **Life threatening; treated with bone marrow transplant**
     - Four types recognized
       - Type I—short radius
       - Type II—hypoplastic radius
       - Type III—partially absent radius
       - Type IV—completely absent radius
     - Early therapy to preserve passive range of motion is critical.
     - A centralization procedure to realign the carpus on the distal ulna may be attempted when the child is between 6 and 12 months of age.
       - **Inadequate elbow range of motion is a contraindication to a centralization procedure.**
   - Ulnar dysplasia (ulnar clubhand)
     - Characterized by deficiency of the ulna or ulnar carpal structures
     - This type of dysplasia is tenfold less common than its radial counterpart and is not associated with systemic syndromes.
     - Additional hand anomalies, however, such as a digit absence and syndactyly, are prevalent.
     - Elbow abnormalities are frequently evident.
     - Other musculoskeletal anomalies, including proximal femoral focal deficiency, fibula deficiency, phocomelia, and scoliosis, are also common.
     - Five types recognized
       - Type 0—deficiencies of hand/carpus only
       - Type I—small ulna with both physes present
       - Type II—partially absent ulna
       - Type III—completely absent ulna
       - Type IV—radiohumeral synostosis
     - General clinical considerations include the position of the hand, function of the thumb, stability of the elbow, and presence of syndactyly.
     - The condition of the thumb is the most important determinant of surgical intervention in ulnar dysplasia.
   - Cleft hand
     - Also known as split hand-foot malformation
     - Often bilateral and familial, involves the feet, and has associated absent metacarpals, differentiating it from symbrachydactyly
     - Severity of this anomaly varies widely from a cleft between the middle and ring fingers to absent radial digits and syndactyly of the ulnar digits.
     - Cleft closure and thumb web construction are the top priorities.
     - Syndactyly should be released early.
     - Thumb reconstruction may require web space deepening, tendon transfer, rotational osteotomy, and/or toe-to-hand transfer.
       - Web deepening should not precede cleft closure because it may compromise the flaps for cleft closure.
     - Transverse bones should be removed because they widen the cleft as the child grows.

C. **Failure of differentiation**

1. Radioulnar synostosis
   - Bony bridge between proximal radius and ulna
   - Bilateral in over 60%

- **Associated with chromosomal abnormalities, particularly duplication of sex chromosomes**
- **Examination reveals a fixed pronation deformity.**
- Radius is wide and bowed, whereas the ulna is narrow and straight.
- If significant pronation deformity exists, a rotational osteotomy may be done at approximately age 5 for better hand positioning.

2. Symphalangism (congenital digital stiffness)
   - Hereditary symphalangism is autosomal dominant and associated with correctable hearing loss.
     - More common in ulnar digits
   - Nonhereditary symphalangism is seen in conjunction with syndactyly, Apert syndrome, and Poland syndrome.
   - Appearance and function of the digits may be improved by angular osteotomies toward the end of adolescent growth.
3. Camptodactyly (congenital digital flexion deformity)
   - Classically occurs at small-finger PIP joint
     - Type I seen in infancy and affects the sexes equally
       - Responds to splinting and stretching
     - Type II seen in adolescent girls
       - Deformity results from either abnormal lumbrical insertion or an abnormal FDS origin and/or insertion.
       - If full PIP extension can be achieved actively with the MCP held in flexion, the digit can be explored and the abnormal tendon transferred to the radial lateral band.
     - Type III involves multiple digits with more severe flexion contractures and is usually associated with a syndrome.
   - In general, nonoperative treatment is favored for all three types.
   - If functional deficit exists after skeletal maturity, corrective osteotomy may improve alignment and function.
4. Clinodactyly (congenital curvature of the digit in the radioulnar plane)
   - Small finger most common
   - Type I—most common, minor angulation, normal digit length
   - Type II—present in 25% of children with Down syndrome, minor angulation, short middle phalanx
   - Type III—marked angulation and a delta phalanx
     - C-shaped epiphysis and longitudinally bracketed diaphysis
     - Early excision is performed when the delta phalanx is a separate bone and involved digit is excessively long.
     - Otherwise, opening wedge osteotomy to correct angulation
5. Flexed thumb
   - Two main causes are pediatric trigger thumb and congenital clasped thumb.
     - Pediatric trigger thumb
       - Common developmental condition
       - Mechanical catching/locking of thumb, may progress to fixed flexion deformity at interphalangeal joint
       - Postural hyperextension of MCP joint
       - Some cases respond to early splinting or may resolve spontaneously.
       - May be surgically treated with A1 pulley release (similar to adult) with low recurrence rate
         - Thumb radial digital nerve in jeopardy as it crosses more centrally near MCP joint flexion crease
     - Congenital clasped thumb
       - Flexion-adduction thumb deformity at MCP joint
       - Typically caused by absent or hypoplastic EPB
       - Supple deformities may be treated by splinting or long/ring FDS tendon transfer to EPB.
       - Rigid variety associated with hypoplastic extensors, MCP joint contractures, UCL deficiency, thenar muscle hypoplasia, and first web space skin deficiency
       - Complex cases may require release of MCP capsule; release of adductor pollicis, flexor pollicis brevis, or first dorsal interosseous; Z-lengthening of the FPL; extensor or opposition tendon transfer; and/or deepening of the first web space.
6. Arthrogryposis (congenital curved joints)
   - Results from defect in the motor unit and may be either neurogenic (90%) or myopathic (10%)
   - Immobility in the womb results in symmetric joint contractures.
   - Three types
     - Type I—single localized deformity such as fixed forearm pronation or complex clasped thumb, which may be surgically corrected in usual fashion
     - Type II—full expression with absence of shoulder musculature, tubular limbs, elbow extension contractures, wrist flexion and ulnar deviation contractures, finger flexion contractures, and thumb adduction contractures
     - Type III—type II contractures plus polydactyly and other organ system involvement
   - Types II and III are treated with a combination of splinting, serial casts, and therapy to decrease the severity of joint contractures.
   - Once passive joint mobility is restored, tendon transfers may be performed.
   - An attempt is made to provide child with functional elbows and wrists; however, arthrodesis may provide improved ability to perform activities of daily living in certain cases.
7. Syndactyly
   - This common congenital hand anomaly (1 in 2500 live births) results from failure of apoptosis to separate digits.
   - Classified based on absence (simple) or presence (complex) of bony connections between the involved digits and whether the bony connections are complete or incomplete (Figure 7-63)
   - Acrosyndactyly refers to fusion between more distal portions of the digit, often seen in constriction ring syndrome.
   - Pure syndactyly is autosomal dominant, with reduced penetrance and variable expression that yield a positive family history in 10% to 40% of cases.
   - Distribution of digit involvement
     - Long-ring—50%
     - Ring-small—30%
     - Index-long—15%
     - Thumb-index—5%

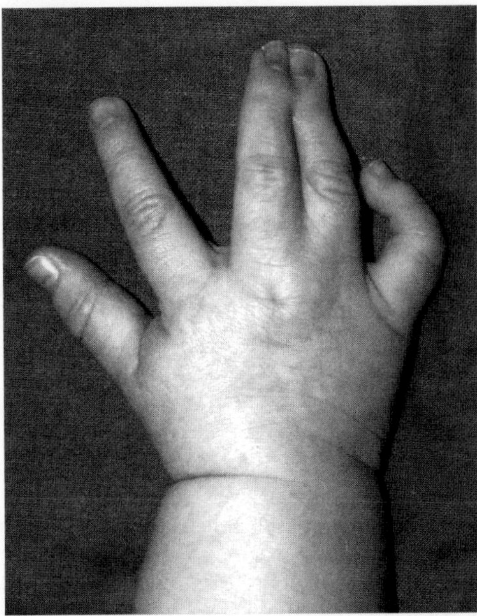

Figure 7-63 Simple and complete syndactyly between third and fourth rays. (From Green DP, et al, editors: *Green's operative hand surgery,* ed 5, Philadelphia, 2005, Churchill Livingstone, p 1382.)

- Release performed at approximately 1 year of age
- Rays of unequal length should be released before 6 months.
- Acrosyndactyly requires distal release in neonatal period.
- Multiple digit syndactyly releases are performed in two stages, with only one side of the digit released during one operation, in order to reliably preserve circulation of digit.
- Full-thickness skin grafting invariably required
- Possible complications include web creep and nail deformities.
- **Poland and Apert syndromes are commonly tested conditions with associated syndactyly.**

D. Duplication

1. Preaxial polydactyly (thumb duplication)
   - Classified by Wassel (Table 7-16)
     - Type IV is the most common (43%), characterized by duplicated proximal phalanx (Figure 7-64).
   - Thumb duplication usually unilateral, sporadic, and not associated with a syndrome except in type VII
     - Type VII associations include Holt-Oram syndrome, Fanconi anemia, Blackfan-Diamond anemia, hypoplastic anemia, imperforate anus, cleft palate and tibial defects.
   - Best possible thumb is reconstructed from the available anatomic structures.
   - **If duplicate thumbs of equal size, preserve ulnar thumb to retain ulnar collateral ligament for pinch.**
     - **Soft tissue from ablated thumb should be preserved and used to augment retained thumb.**
   - Most reconstructed thumbs have satisfactory length and girth, but nail deformity and interphalangeal joint angulation are reported problems.

Table 7-16 Preaxial Polydactyly Thumb Classification

Type	Description	Frequency
I	Bifid distal phalanx	2%
II	Duplicated distal phalanx	15%
III	Bifid proximal phalanx	6%
IV	Duplicated proximal phalanx	43% (most common)
V	Bifid metacarpal	10%
VI	Duplicated metacarpal	4%
VII	Triphalangia	20%

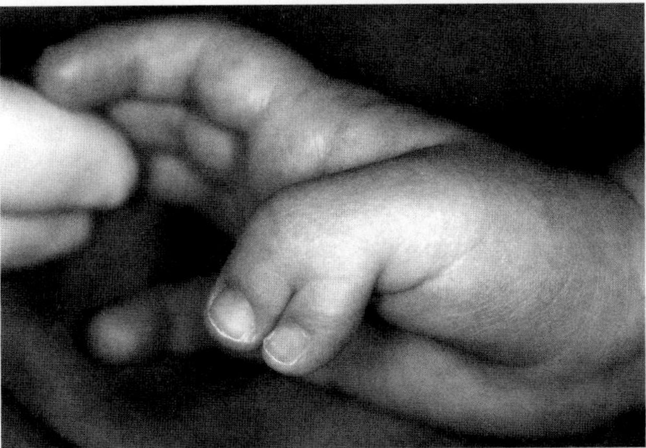

Figure 7-64 Type IV duplication with duplicated proximal and distal phalanges that articulate with a bifid metacarpal head. (Courtesy of Shriners Hospitals for Children, Philadelphia.)

2. **Postaxial polydactyly (small-finger duplication)**
   - **Ten times more common in African Americans (1 in 143 live births) than whites (1 in 1339 live births)**
     - **Autosomal dominant inheritance**
     - **More extensive genetic workup mandatory in whites because of multiple known chromosomal abnormalities**
   - Type A is a well-formed duplicated digit.
     - Ulnar digit removed
   - Type B is a rudimentary skin tag.
     - May be tied off shortly after birth
3. Central polydactyly
   - Usually associated with syndactyly
   - Early surgery indicated to prevent angular deformity with growth
   - Impaired motion may result from interposed digits or symphalangism of adjacent digits.
   - Tendons, nerves, and vessels may be shared to the point that only one finger from three skeletons may be obtainable.
   - Angular deviation may require ligament reconstruction and/or osteotomy.

E. Overgrowth

1. Macrodactyly
   - Characterized by nonhereditary congenital digital enlargement
   - Ninety percent of cases are unilateral, and 70% of cases involve multiple digits.
   - Adult analogue is lipofibromatous hamartoma of the median or other peripheral nerves.

Table 7-17 Blauth Classification of Thumb Hypoplasia

Type	Characteristics
I	Minor hypoplasia, all structures present, small thumb
II	Adduction contracture, MCP joint ulnar collateral ligament instability, thenar hypoplasia, normal skeleton with respect to articulations
IIIA	Extensive intrinsic and extrinsic musculotendinous deficiencies, intact CMC joint
IIIB	Extensive intrinsic and extrinsic musculotendinous deficiencies, basal metacarpal aplasia, CMC joint not intact
IV	Total or subtotal aplasia of the metacarpal, rudimentary phalanges, thumb attached to hand by a skin bridge (pouce flottant)
V	Complete absence of thumb

CMC, carpometacarpal; MCP, metacarpophalangeal.

- Angular deviation, joint stiffness, and nerve compression syndromes also occur.
- Static macrodactyly is present at birth, and growth is linear with the adjacent digits.
- Progressive macrodactyly is not always evident at birth, but exponential growth occurs thereafter.
- Most favorable outcome for severely affected single digit is amputation.
- **When the thumb or multiple digits are involved, the following procedures may offer improvement.**
  - **Epiphyseal ablation, angular and/or shortening osteotomies, longitudinal narrowing osteotomies, nerve stripping, and debulking**
- Stiffness and neurovascular compromise are common.

F. **Undergrowth**

1. Thumb hypoplasia
   - Classified by Blauth (Table 7-17)
   - **Critical structure is CMC joint.**
     - **Separates type IIIA from type IIIB**
     - **Determines whether the thumb is reconstructable (II, IIIA) or whether it requires pollicization (IIIB, IV, V)**
   - Type I—Small thumb with slender bones and normal thenar musculature typically requires no treatment.
   - Types II and IIIA are treated with stabilization of the MCP joint UCL, web deepening, and extrinsic extensor tendon reconstruction.
   - Types IIIB to V are best treated with index pollicization.

G. **Amnion disruption sequence (constriction ring syndrome)**

1. Sporadic occurrence with no evidence of hereditary predisposition
2. Manifested in four ways
   - Simple constriction rings
   - Rings with distal deformity, with or without lymphedema
   - Acrosyndactyly
   - Amputation
3. Neonatal surgery is indicated when edema jeopardizes digital circulation.
4. Release accomplished by multiple circumferential Z-plasties

H. **Generalized skeletal abnormalities**

1. Congenital dislocation of the radial head
   - May be distinguished from traumatic origin by bilateral involvement, other congenital anomalies (60%), and familial occurrence
   - Typically irreducible by closed means
   - Some helpful radiographic clues include
     - Hypoplastic capitellum
     - Short ulna with long radius
     - Convex radial head
   - Surgical indications include pain, limited motion, and cosmetic dissatisfaction.
     - Radial head excision performed at skeletal maturity
2. Madelung deformity
   - Disruption of volar ulnar physis of distal radius
     - Implicated tethering structure is the Vickers ligament.
   - As child grows, the distal radius exhibits excessive radial inclination and volar tilt (spectrum of abnormality seen).
   - **Hypothesized to be due to an X-linked dominant disorder, Leri-Weill dyschondrosteosis, which is a mutation in the short-stature homebox-containing (SHOX) gene**
   - Early release of Vickers ligament advocated by some
   - Often asymptomatic and found incidentally in adulthood after minor wrist injury prompts radiographic examination
   - Symptoms arise from ulnocarpal impaction, restricted forearm rotation, and median nerve compression.
     - Corrective osteotomy of the radius with or without distal ulna resection

XVIII. ELBOW

A. **Articular anatomy**

1. Ulnohumeral, radiocapitellar, and proximal radioulnar joints
2. Articular surface of distal humerus angled 30 degrees anterior to humeral shaft axis
3. Distal humerus consists of medial and lateral columns.
4. Normal range of elbow flexion/extension—0 to 150 degrees
5. Normal forearm pronosupination (rotation)—80 to 85 degrees each direction
6. Functional range of motion—30 to 130 degrees flexion/extension and 50 degrees pronosupination
7. Normal valgus carrying angle of the elbow is 5 to 10 degrees for men and 10 to 15 degrees for women.
8. In full extension, 60% of axial load is transmitted through the radiocapitellar joint.

B. **Ligamentous anatomy**

1. Medial (ulnar) collateral ligament (MCL)
   - Anterior, posterior, and transverse bundles (Figure 7-65)
   - **Anterior bundle is primary restraint to valgus stress within functional elbow range of motion (secondary restraint is radial head).**
   - Originates on posterior medial epicondyle, inserts on sublime tubercle of medial coronoid process
   - Posterior bundle is primary restraint to valgus stress with elbow in maximal flexion.
   - Stability in full extension is provided by MCL, joint capsule and ulnohumeral articulation.
2. Lateral collateral ligament (LCL) complex

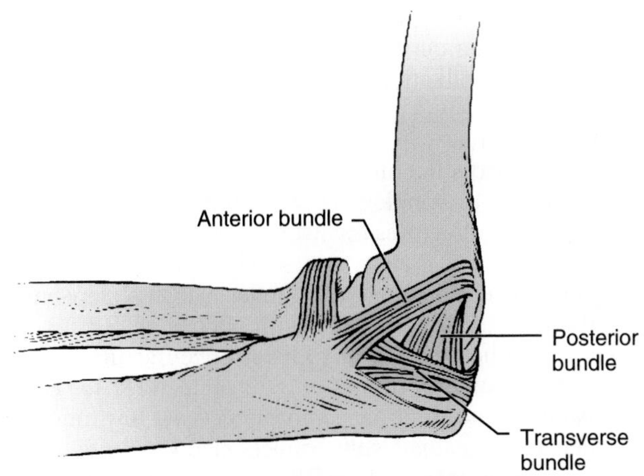

Figure 7-65 Medial collateral ligament complex. (From Trumble TE, et al, editors: *Core knowledge in orthopaedics: hand, elbow, and shoulder,* Philadelphia, 2006, Mosby, p 484.)

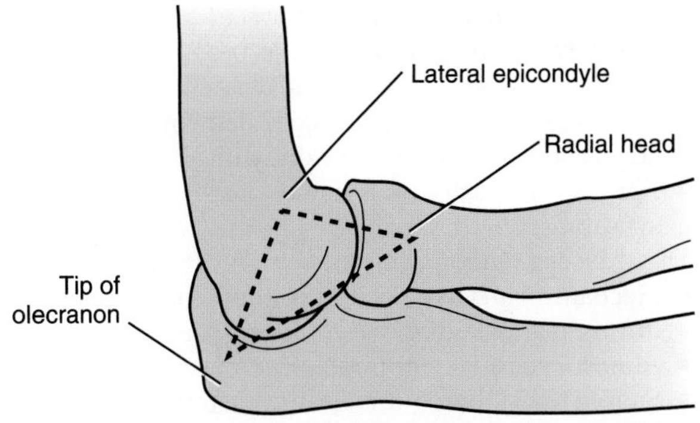

Figure 7-67 The anconeal soft spot (lateral infracondylar recess) is the most sensitive area in which to detect a joint effusion. This triangular area located on the lateral aspect of the elbow is outlined by the radial head, tip of the olecranon, and lateral epicondyle. (From Trumble TE, et al, editors: *Core knowledge in orthopaedics: hand, elbow, and shoulder,* Philadelphia, 2006, Mosby, p 489.)

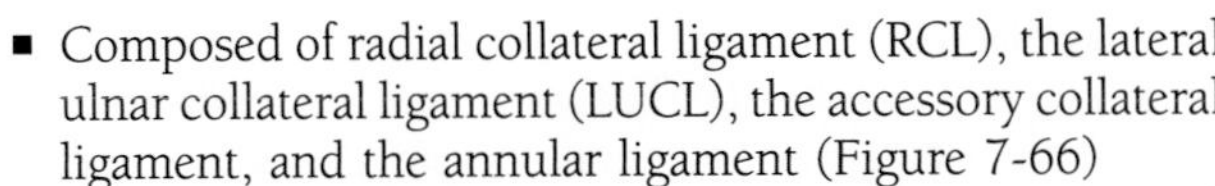

- Composed of radial collateral ligament (RCL), the lateral ulnar collateral ligament (LUCL), the accessory collateral ligament, and the annular ligament (Figure 7-66)
- LUCL originates on posterior lateral epicondyle and inserts on crista supinatoris of the proximal ulna.
- LUCL is primary restraint to varus and external rotational stress throughout elbow motion.

C. **Joint aspiration or injection**

1. Best performed through anconeal soft spot laterally
2. Between triangle of bony landmarks (Figure 7-67)
   - Radial head
   - Lateral epicondyle
   - Tip of olecranon
3. Therapeutic aspiration of hemarthrosis after trauma

D. **Elbow imaging**

1. Plain radiographs—anteroposterior, lateral, and oblique views
2. CT—provides superior bony detail
   - Complex fractures of the distal humerus, radial head and coronoid process; ossified loose bodies, heterotopic ossification

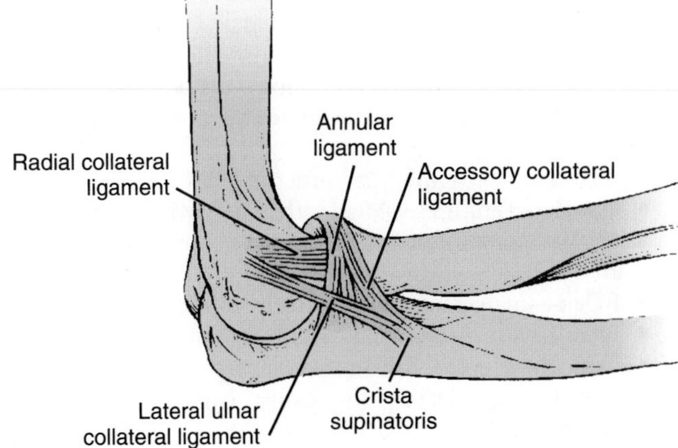

Figure 7-66 Lateral collateral ligament complex. (From Trumble TE, et al, editors: *Core knowledge in orthopaedics: hand, elbow, and shoulder,* Philadelphia, 2006, Mosby, p 484.)

3. MRI—provides superior soft tissue detail
   - Ligamentous injuries, occult fractures, osteochondritis dissecans, nonossified loose bodies, tendinous injury, and soft tissue masses

E. **Tendon disorders**

1. Lateral epicondylitis (tennis elbow)
   - **Common tendinopathy of ECRB origin**
   - **Degenerative rather than inflammatory process**
     - Histologic examination—angiofibroblastic hyperplasia
   - Repetitive wrist extension and forearm rotation
   - Related to vocation more often than racket-sport play
   - Lateral elbow pain, exacerbated by resisted wrist extension
   - Positive chair lift-off test
   - Grip strength diminished with elbow extended as compared to elbow flexed to 90 degrees
   - Treatment
     - Nonoperative with avoidance of aggravating activity, anti-inflammatories, counterforce bracing, occupational therapy for local modalities (ice, heat, ultrasonography, iontophoresis), corticosteroid injection
     - Efficacy of corticosteroid injection recently debated
       - Prospective, double-blind, randomized clinical trial showed no more efficacy than placebo (pain, grip strength, Disabilities of the Arm, Shoulder, and Hand [DASH] score)
       - Depression and ineffective coping skills strongest predictors of perceived arm-specific disability
     - Extracorporeal shock wave therapy trials show no difference at 6 months compared to placebo.
     - Platelet-rich plasma injection of recent interest
     - May take 6 to 12 months, usually self-limited
     - Surgical intervention may be open or arthroscopic.
     - ECRB tendon débridement with or without lateral epicondylectomy
     - Nirschl scratch test—degenerative, friable tendon
     - Avoid iatrogenic injury to LUCL.
     - Watertight deep closure to avoid synovial fistula
     - Other causes of lateral elbow pain if surgery fails—LUCL injury, osteochondritis dissecans, radiocapitellar osteoarthrosis

2. Medial epicondylitis (golfer's elbow)
   - Common tendinopathy of flexor-pronator mass origin
   - Prolonged conservative management recommended because success of surgical débridement is less predictable than it is in lateral epicondylitis
   - Always evaluate for associated cubital tunnel syndrome.
3. Distal biceps tendon injury
   - Mechanism—eccentric loading of the flexed elbow during manual labor, weight lifting, or other activity
   - Almost exclusively in middle-age males
   - Steroid and tobacco use are risk factors.
   - Patients may experience a painful "pop" and pain felt deep to antecubital fossa.
   - **Supination strength is diminished more than flexion strength (biceps is main forearm supinator, brachialis is main elbow flexor).**
     - **If left untreated, only approximately 50% supination strength versus approximately 70% flexion strength regained by 1 year.**
   - Biceps muscle belly unlikely to be proximally retracted if lacertus fibrosis (bicipital aponeurosis) remains intact
   - Abnormal hook test
   - MRI may help distinguish partial from complete injuries in equivocal cases.
     - May see associated bicipitoradial bursitis in chronic tendinopathy
     - **Partial ruptures primarily occur on the radial side of the tuberosity footprint, owing to its function as a supinator.**
   - **Partial injuries initially treated nonoperatively with rest, NSAIDs and therapy, slow recovery—may eventually require detachment, débridement, and reattachment**
   - Surgical reattachment to radial tuberosity recommended in active individuals with complete rupture to regain strength
   - Single- and two-incision techniques described
     - **Single-incision—risk for neurologic injury (lateral antebrachial cutaneous nerve and PIN).**
     - Two-incision—risk for radioulnar synostosis
   - Bone trough/drill holes, suture anchors, interference screw, Endobutton all described fixation methods
     - Studies have shown Endobutton to have superior strength.
   - Chronic injuries for longer than 6 weeks may require tendon autograft or allograft augmentation; strength recovery diminished as compared to acute reattachment with native tendon
   - Avoid strengthening for approximately 8 weeks postoperatively.
4. Distal triceps tendon injury
   - Less common injury caused by direct blow to posterior elbow or sudden forceful flexion of extended elbow
   - Patients describe posterior elbow pain and swelling; they may have palpable defect proximal to olecranon tip.
   - Diminished elbow extension strength, although active extension possible through intact anconeus
     - As many as 50% of these injuries are initially missed.
   - Rupture may occur at musculotendinous junction or olecranon insertion.
   - May also be assessed by MRI
   - Surgical repair/reattachment for high-grade partial (>50% of tendon width) and complete tears
   - Slow rehabilitation with progressive elbow flexion recovery

F. Elbow trauma

1. Distal humerus fractures
   - Anatomic morphology is two columns with a spool.
   - Most adult fractures involve both columns and articular surface.
   - High-energy trauma in younger patients, low-energy trauma in elderly patients with poor bone quality
   - CT scan helpful to better characterize fracture pattern
   - Nonoperative treatment only recommended for elderly patients with multiple comorbidities and low functional demands; goal is a stiff, painless elbow
   - Vast majority treated by ORIF
   - Approaches include triceps-splitting, triceps-sparing, and olecranon osteotomy.
   - Articular surface reconstructed with headless compression screws and/or lag screws across spool
   - Anatomically precontoured column locking plates available
   - Plates may be applied orthogonally (90-90—direct medial and posterolateral) or parallel with interdigitation of screw threads
   - Healthy, active elderly patients with severe articular comminution may be better served by semiconstrained total elbow arthroplasty (TEA) to allow early rehabilitation but are restricted to 10-pound weight-lifting limit for life.
     - In patients over age 65, higher Mayo Elbow Performance Score (MEPS) at 2-year follow-up for those randomized to TEA compared to ORIF
2. Radial head fracture
   - Lateral elbow pain and swelling after trauma, may be occult on initial plain radiographs (check for fat pad sign)
   - May require aspiration of hemarthrosis and injection of local anesthetic to assess for mechanical block to forearm rotation
   - Classified by Mason, modified by Hotchkiss (Figure 7-68)
     - Type I—nondisplaced or minimally displaced, no mechanical block
     - Type II—less than 2 mm of articular displacement, with or without mechanical block
     - Type III—comminuted
     - Type IV—associated with elbow dislocation
   - Often difficult to characterize by plain radiographs alone
     - CT may be helpful in borderline cases.
   - Associated injuries—MCL, other periarticular fractures
   - Always assess forearm and wrist for Essex-Lopresti injury.
   - Type I—managed nonoperatively with early motion
   - Type II with mechanical block—may require ORIF
   - Type III—either ORIF, or metallic replacement
   - Overstuffing leads to early capitellar wear/late instability.
   - Excision contraindicated with incompetent MCL/interosseous membrane
3. Essex-Lopresti injury

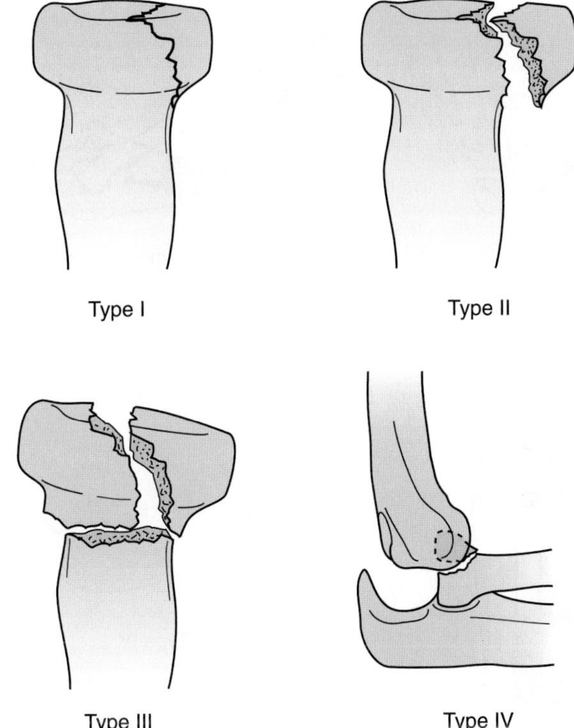

Figure 7-68 Radial head fracture classification. (From Trumble TE, et al, editors: *Core knowledge in orthopaedics: hand, elbow, and shoulder,* Philadelphia, 2006, Mosby, p 526.)

- Longitudinal radioulnar instability caused by sequential injury to the DRUJ, interosseous membrane, and radial head
- Radial head injury must either be internally fixed or replaced to prevent proximal migration of radius, ulnocarpal impaction.
- Treat TFCC pathology concurrently.
- Notoriously difficult injury to treat
- Reconstruction of interosseous membrane described but long-term results unknown

4. Coronoid fractures
   - Occur most often in setting of elbow dislocation
   - Divided into types I to III based on size of fragment
   - **Even small fractures may contribute to persistent elbow instability, owing to involvement of the sublime tubercle.**
     - **Insertion point of anterior bundle of MCL**
   - Treat with ORIF.
     - Suture, screw, and miniplate fixation all described
5. Olecranon fractures
   - Typically result from direct blow to proximal forearm
   - Proximal fragment displaced by triceps pull
   - Treatment depends on displacement and articular congruity.
   - Tension band constructs work well for simple transverse fracture patterns but associated with high rate of symptomatic hardware (>50%)
   - Comminuted fractures with articular displacement best treated with ORIF using plate-and-screw construct
   - Elderly patients with severely comminuted fractures may benefit from excision of the proximal fragment and reattachment of triceps tendon adjacent to the joint line.
6. Elbow dislocation
   - Most commonly posterolateral
   - Simple or complex (with associated fractures)
   - Closed reduction performed promptly after assessment of neurovascular status
   - Test elbow stability through flexion-extension arc after reduction; immobilize initially at 90 degrees with forearm pronation.
   - Simple dislocations treated with early range of motion within 3 weeks of injury
   - Persistent instability within 30 degrees of full extension may be indication for acute ligamentous repair.
     - Lateral ligamentous complex always repaired, followed by MCL if instability persists
   - **Loss of terminal extension is the most common complication after closed treatment of a simple elbow dislocation.**
   - "Terrible triad" injury consists of
     - Elbow dislocation
     - Radial head fracture
     - Coronoid process fracture
     - Almost always treated with ORIF of coronoid process, ORIF or prosthetic radial head replacement, and lateral and/or medial ligamentous repair
     - Persistent instability may require hinged external fixator or transarticular ulnohumeral pinning.
     - Early range of motion starting with intraoperative arc of stability
       - LCL-repaired and MCL-intact elbow kept in forearm pronation to increase stability
       - LCL-repaired but MCL-deficient elbow kept in forearm supination to increase stability
       - LCL- and MCL-repaired elbow kept in neutral
7. Monteggia fracture-dislocations
   - Proximal one-third ulna fracture accompanied by radial head subluxation/dislocation
   - Bado classification types I to IV (Figure 7-69)
   - Anatomic reduction of the proximal ulna usually reduces the radial head.
   - **Persistent proximal radioulnar instability may require annular ligament reconstruction.**

G. Elbow instability

1. Posterolateral rotatory instability
   - **Caused by incompetence of the LUCL** (Figure 7-70)
   - Patients relate history of previous elbow dislocation treated nonoperatively.
   - Pain and subjective instability
   - LCL-deficient elbow more stable in forearm pronation
   - Lateral pivot shift test
     - Reproduces instability with combination of supination, axial compression, and valgus loading as the elbow is brought from full extension to 40 degrees of flexion
     - The ulna rotates externally on trochlea and produces posterior radial head subluxation.
     - With increasing flexion, the triceps becomes taut and the radial head reduces with palpable clunk.
     - Patient apprehension is common, and either intraarticular local anesthetic or examination under general anesthesia may be necessary to confirm diagnosis
   - MRI shows LUCL pathology in approximately 50% of cases.

Figure 7-69 **Classification of Monteggia fracture-dislocations.** (From Reckling FW, Cordell LD: Unstable fracture-dislocations of the forearm, *Arch Surg* 96:1004, 1968; reprinted by permission. Copyright 1968 American Medical Association.)

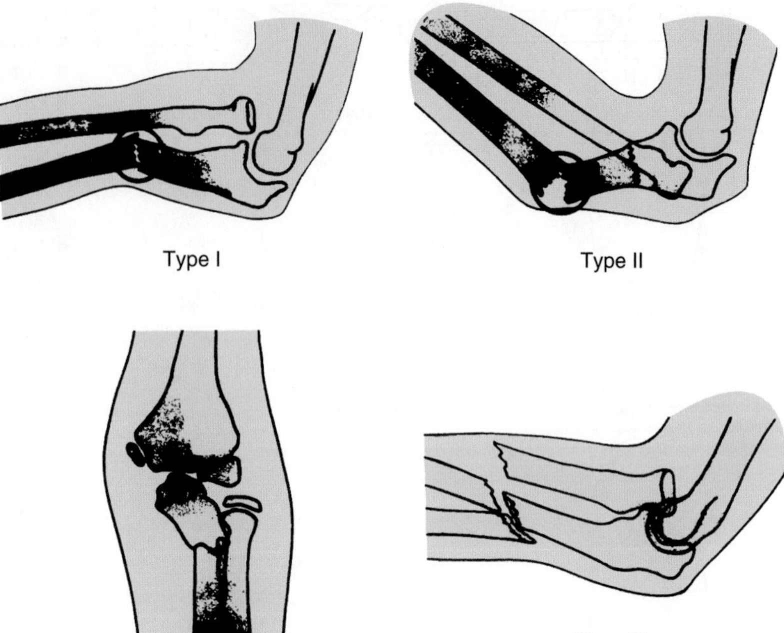

Type IV

Type III

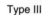

Figure 7-70 Mechanism of deforming torsional forces. With active triceps contraction *(solid straight arrow)* while extension is being resisted, the deforming forces and moments cause a medial pull and external rotation torsion on the ulna about its long axis *(small curved arrow)*. This not only moves the ulna into external rotation but also causes the radial head to rotate posterolaterally off the capitellum *(straight dashed arrow)*. These represent the initial kinematic displacements of posterolateral rotatory subluxation *(large curved arrow)*. Over time, these chronic forces cause attenuation of the lateral collateral ligament complex, including the important ulnar portion, leading to frank posterolateral rotatory subluxation. (From O'Driscoll SW, et al: Tardy posterolateral rotatory instability of the elbow due to cubitus varus, *J Bone Joint Surg Am* 83:1358-1369, 2001. Reproduced with permission from Mayo Foundation.)

- Chronic instability may require reconstruction of the LUCL with tendon autograft.

2. Varus posteromedial rotatory instability
   - Increasingly recognized but poorly understood entity
   - **Results from fracture of anteromedial coronoid process**
   - Treatment requires ORIF of coronoid.
3. Valgus instability
   - May be acute after elbow trauma or chronic from repetitive loading and attenuation of the MCL
     - **In baseball, the late cocking phase of throwing places the highest stress on the MCL.**
   - Primary ligamentous repair or reattachment with suture anchors only possible in acute setting
   - Chronic instability and dysfunction common in overhead-throwing athletes such as baseball pitchers or javelin throwers
     - **Valgus extension overload**
       - Pain during deceleration phase as elbow reaches terminal extension
       - **Osteophytes of the posteromedial olecranon process block full extension.**
   - FCU is primary dynamic stabilizer to valgus stress, and FDS is a secondary stabilizer.
   - May attempt gradual rehabilitation with symptomatic treatment, maintenance of elbow motion, local modalities, and return to throwing protocol
   - MRI to evaluate MCL, flexor-pronator mass, adjacent bone
   - Ulnar neuritis/cubital tunnel syndrome may also be present.
   - MCL reconstruction with tendon autograft may be indicated in competitive athletes (Tommy John surgery) who fail nonoperative treatment.

- Unrecognized or untreated MCL insufficiency may lead to capitellar wear, posteromedial impingement, olecranon osteophyte formation, and loose-body formation (valgus overload syndrome).
- Arthroscopic débridement of osteophytes and loose-body removal may be effective.

H. Elbow contracture

1. Stiffness and loss of motion frequent complications after elbow injury
2. Aggressive motion recovery started as soon as possible
3. Loss of 30 degrees terminal extension well tolerated in general population
4. Loss of flexion interferes with activities of daily living (<130 degrees).
5. Intrinsic factors
   - Articular incongruity, loose bodies, synovitis
6. Extrinsic factors
   - Heterotopic ossification, muscle fibrosis, and ligamentous contracture
7. Aggressive therapy
8. Dynamic/static progressive splinting
9. Arthroscopic versus open treatment

I. Elbow arthritis

1. Rheumatoid arthritis (RA)
   - Most prevalent type of elbow arthritis
   - Elbow affected in up to 50% of patients with RA
   - Chronic inflammation and synovitis lead to ligament attenuation, periarticular osteopenia, and joint contracture.
   - Medical management is mainstay.
   - Synovectomy and radial head resection is historically good short-term.
   - Semiconstrained total elbow arthroplasty for more permanent pain relief and preserved function
     - □ Complication rate must be considered.
       - Infection rate
       - Implant failure requiring revision
       - Periprosthetic fracture
2. Post-traumatic ulnotrochlear/radiocapitellar arthritis
   - Second most common type of elbow arthritis
   - Typically young, active patients treated by
     - □ Arthroscopic or open débridement of osteophytes, abrasion chondroplasty, and removal of loose bodies
     - □ Interposition arthroplasty with autograft or allograft
3. Primary osteoarthritis
   - Uncommon form of elbow arthritis
   - Typically affects middle-age male laborers
   - Pain at extremes of motion
   - Osteophyte formation may lead to mechanical block of motion.
   - Open or arthroscopic débridement to delay arthroplasty
   - Postoperative continuous passive motion not shown to add benefit postoperatively
4. TEA
   - **Indications**
     - □ **Refractory RA**
     - □ **Advanced osteoarthritis (primary and post-traumatic)**
     - □ **Chronic instability**
     - □ **Complex distal humerus fractures in elderly patients**
   - TEA is contraindicated in setting of infection, in which primary arthrodesis is favored.
   - Patients have lifelong weight-lifting restriction of 10 pounds.
   - Two primary types:
     - □ Unconstrained (unlinked) and semiconstrained (linked)
     - □ Unconstrained TEA is used in osteoarthritis with competent collateral ligaments and good bone quality.
     - □ Semiconstrained TEA acts as "sloppy hinge" with limited rotational and coronal plane motion.
       - Best for RA, chronic instability, and distal humerus fractures in elderly patients
   - Each prosthetic design has demonstrated reliable pain relief.
   - Surgical approaches may split or spare triceps; ulnar nerve transposed anteriorly; radial head often resected
   - Repair of triceps mechanism is of paramount importance for good postoperative function.
   - Complications of TEA include infection, nerve injury, instability, periprosthetic fracture, and implant loosening from polyethylene wear.
   - Staged reimplantation after infection has a poor salvage rate.

TESTABLE CONCEPTS

I. Anatomy

- Flexor tendon nutrition is via direct vascular supply and synovial diffusion.
  - Vascular supply is via the vincular system.
- The carpal tunnel contains the median nerve and nine flexor tendons.
  - One flexor pollicis longus (FPL), four flexor digitorum superficialis (FDS), and four flexor digitorum profundus (FDP) tendons; FPL is most radial, whereas the long and ring FDS tendons are volar to index and small FDS
- Lumbrical muscles originate on radial aspect of FDP tendons and pass volar to transverse metacarpal ligaments to insert on the radial aspect of the extensor hood lateral bands.
- Intrinsic tightness commonly occurs in cerebral palsy, rheumatoid arthritis (RA), and following trauma. The intrinsic tightness test demonstrates decreased proximal interphalangeal (PIP) flexion with the metacarpophalangeal (MCP) held in extension.

II. Distal Radius Fractures

- Examination of a patient with a distal radius fracture should include evaluation for concurrent ulnar-sided and anatomic snuffbox tenderness, as well as assessment of median and ulnar nerve function.
  - Acute carpal tunnel syndrome requires emergency release.
- Radiographic evaluation follows the 11-22-11 guide.
  - Radial height, 11 mm; radial inclination, 22 degrees; volar tilt, 11 degrees
  - Assess ulnar variance, because the load sharing across the radius and ulna is significantly altered in either ulnar-positive (more force across ulna) or ulnar-negative (less force across ulna) variance.
  - Distal radioulnar joint (DRUJ) involvement should be evaluated on a true lateral radiograph.
- Acceptable reduction parameters
  - Radial shortening less than 3 mm
  - Dorsal articular tilt less than 10 degrees
  - Intraarticular step-off less than 2 mm
- Closed treatment is indicated for minimally displaced injuries. Wrist and digit stiffness, muscle atrophy, and disuse osteopenia may result from prolonged immobilization. However, formal physical therapy compared to home exercise demonstrates no significant difference.
- Open reduction with internal fixation (ORIF) via a dorsal approach is best for dorsally displaced fractures with dorsal bony defects. Direct visualization of the articular surface is best from the dorsal exposure.
- The most common complication after distal radius fracture is median nerve dysfunction.
- Extensor pollicis longus (EPL) tendon rupture most commonly occurs as a late complication following closed treatment due to attritional wear and/or vascular insufficiency near the Lister tubercle. It typically presents as a painless, acute loss of thumb IP joint extension.
  - Treat with palmaris longus (PL) intercalary autograft or extensor indicis proprius (EIP)-to-EPL tendon transfer, because primary repair often is not possible.
- FPL rupture is the most common rupture after volar locking plating. EPL is the most common extensor tendon injured.

III. Carpal Fractures and Instability

- Scaphoid fractures most commonly occur in forced hyperextension and radial deviation. The scaphoid is locked in the scaphoid fossa in this position. There is force transmission through the radioscaphoid articulation, and the radioscaphocapitate ligament acts as fulcrum against which the distal pole of the scaphoid palmar flexes on impact.
  - Operative indications include more than 1 mm displacement, intrascaphoid angle greater than 35 degrees (humpback deformity), and trans-scaphoid perilunate dislocation. Proximal pole fracture is a relative indication.
  - Minimally displaced fractures may be treated with percutaneous internal fixation, commonly performed via a dorsal approach. Direct visualization of the screw via a limited incision is recommended to ensure seating of the screw in subchondral bone. This results in faster radiographic union and return to activity.
  - Formal ORIF with headless compression screw is used for displaced injuries. Guide pin placement should be along the central axis of both the proximal and distal fragments.
  - Volar approach potentially avoids disruption to the blood supply of the scaphoid and is the most commonly employed approach.
- Scaphoid nonunion that is early stage may be treated with ORIF and bone grafting.
  - Untreated, chronic scaphoid nonunion may lead to post-traumatic osteoarthrosis. This is termed scaphoid nonunion advanced collapse (SNAC) wrist.
  - The radioscaphoid joint is affected first, followed by the scaphocapitate and then the lunocapitate.
- Hook-of-hamate fractures are due to blunt trauma to the palm and associated with golf, baseball, hockey, and racquet sports. A carpal tunnel view or computed tomographic (CT) scan is diagnostic. Failure of cast immobilization can be salvaged with fragment excision.
- Carpal instability can be broadly classified into four types
  - Carpal instability dissociative
    - Dorsal intercalated segmental instability (DISI)
    - Volar intercalated segmental instability (VISI)
  - Carpal instability nondissociative
  - Carpal instability adaptive
  - Carpal instability complex
- DISI is the most common form of carpal instability.
  - Scapholunate ligament disruption
    - Dorsal portion strongest
    - Chronic static instability may result in scapholunate advanced collapse (SLAC) wrist.
- VISI is the second most common.

- Lunotriquetral ligament disruption
  - Volar portion strongest
- Perilunate dislocations are classified as carpal instability complex.
  - The Mayfield four stages of ligamentous disruptions
    - I—Scapholunate
    - II—Scaphocapitate
    - III—Lunotriquetral
    - IV—Circumferential
  - Prompt treatment with closed reduction (especially if acute carpal tunnel syndrome)
  - ORIF with dorsal +/– volar approach

IV. Metacarpal and Phalangeal Injuries

- The majority of metacarpal and phalangeal injuries can be treated nonoperatively. General guidelines for operative intervention: displaced and unstable fractures, intraarticular fractures, digit malrotation, open injuries and multiple fractures
- Bennett fracture is an intraarticular fracture-dislocation of the thumb metacarpal base. Abductor pollicis longus (APL) and thumb extensors cause proximal, dorsal and radial displacement of the metacarpal shaft. The "beak" ligament keeps the volar-ulnar base fragment *reduced* to the trapezium.
- Skier's or gamekeeper's thumb is an injury to the thumb metacarpophalangeal (MCP) joint ulnar collateral ligament (UCL).
  - Stress joint with radial deviation both at neutral and 30 degrees of flexion. Instability in 30 degrees of flexion indicates injury to proper UCL.
  - In over 85% of cases, a complete injury is accompanied by a Stener lesion, in which the adductor pollicis aponeurosis is interposed between the avulsed UCL and its insertion site on the base of the proximal phalanx.
- PIP dislocation is typically dorsal and represents injury to the volar plate.
  - Volar dislocation is an injury to the central slip and must be splinted in full extension. Failure of adequate treatment will result in a boutonniere deformity.
  - Rotatory dislocation occurs when one of the phalangeal condyles is buttonholed between the central slip and lateral band.
- PIP fracture-dislocations are classified based on the amount of middle phalanx (P2) articular surface involvement. In general, a volar fragment with less than 40% involvement acts as dorsal dislocation and can be treated nonoperatively.
  - The two most important factors in treatment are joint congruity and stability. Unstable injuries often require some type of open treatment.
- Irreducible distal interphalangeal (DIP) dislocations are typically due to interposition of the volar plate; treatment is via open reduction and extraction of the volar plate.

V. Tendon Injuries and Overuse Syndromes

- Mallet finger is treated with DIP extension splinting if detected within 12 weeks of injury. A relative surgical indication is a displaced bony mallet injury with significant volar subluxation of distal phalanx (P3).
- Injury over the PIP of a digit often results in central slip involvement.
  - An acute boutonniere deformity results from central slip disruption and volar subluxation of the lateral bands, resulting in DIP hyperextension.
  - Chronic boutonniere deformity requires central slip reconstruction.
- Partial flexor tendon lacerations may be trimmed if there is triggering under the pulley system. More than 60% involvement necessitates core and epitendinous repair.
- Fundamental principles of flexor tendon repair
  - Strength of repair proportional to number of suture strands that cross repair site
  - High-caliber (e.g., 5-0 instead of 6-0) suture material decreases gap formation and increases strength and stiffness.
  - A locking-loop configuration decreases gap formation.
  - Epitendinous repair decreases gap size and increases overall strength by 10% to 50%.
  - Repair of the flexor tendon sheath has no effect on flexor tendon repair.
  - Purchase should be 0.7 to 1.2 cm.
  - Dorsally placed core sutures are stronger.
- In general, early protected range of motion is advocated to increase tendon excursion, decrease adhesion formation, and increase repair strength. However, use of an active flexion protocol postoperatively requires a minimum four-strand repair with epitendinous suture.
  - Young children cannot comply with protected motion protocols and require cast immobilization for 4 weeks.
- Closed flexor tendon injury in zone I is termed a "jersey" finger and is a closed FDP avulsion occurring distal to the FDS insertion. The mechanism of injury is forced extension of the DIP joint during grasping.
  - Profundus advancement of 1 cm or more carries a risk of DIP joint flexion contracture or quadriga.
    - Quadriga occurs because the FDP tendons share a common muscle belly, and distal advancement of one tendon will compromise flexion of the adjacent digits, resulting in forearm pain.
- Adult trigger finger that has failed conservative management should be treated surgically with release of A1 pulley. Preserve A2 pulley in fingers and oblique fibers in thumb.
- Pediatric trigger thumb is more common than trigger finger. It presents with fixed flexion deformity of the interphalangeal joint and generally requires release of the annular pulley.
  - Pediatric trigger finger etiology is unknown, and A1 release may not fully resolve triggering.
- de Quervain tenosynovitis often affects middle-age women, new mothers, and golfers. Corticosteroid injection into the first dorsal extensor compartment is successful in more than 80% of patients.
- Intersection syndrome is a tenosynovitis and/or bursitis occurring at the junction between first and second extensor compartments. It commonly affects rowers and is generally treated nonoperatively.

Continued

VI. Distal Radioulnar Joint, Triangular Fibrocartilage Complex, and Wrist Arthroscopy

- Components of the triangular fibrocartilage complex (TFCC) include the dorsal and volar radioulnar ligaments, the articular disc, a meniscus homologue, the extensor carpi ulnaris (ECU) subsheath, and the origins of the ulnolunate and ulnotriquetral ligaments.
- Degenerative (class II) tears are associated with positive ulnar variance and ulnocarpal impaction syndrome. In the absence of DRUJ arthrosis, the most commonly performed procedure is an ulnar-shortening osteotomy.
- Post-traumatic DRUJ osteoarthritis may be treated with hemiresection or interposition arthroplasty. This maintains the ulnar insertion of the TFCC and prevents radioulnar impingement by soft tissue interposition (e.g., ECU tendon or a capsular flap).

VII. Nail and Fingertip Injuries

- Nail bed injuries less than 50% may be treated without nail plate removal. Those greater than 50% require removal and repair of underlying matrix lacerations. Recent data suggest that 2-octylcanoacrylate (Dermabond) has faster healing than suture repair.
- Fingertip injury treatment requires correct characterization to guide treatment.
  - Without exposed bone—secondary intention if less than 1 cm^2 of tip involved
  - Exposed bone
    - Volar oblique injury—cross-finger flap or thenar flap (index or long digits)
    - Transverse or dorsal oblique injury—V-Y advancement (finger), Moberg advancement flap (thumb)
  - Shortening and closing an injury that acutely violates the FDP insertion may result in a lumbrical-plus finger. FDP tendon retracts and creates tension on the extensor mechanism through its lumbrical, causing paradoxical interphalangeal joint extension with active finger flexion. Treated with release of the radial lateral band

VIII. Soft Tissue Coverage and Microsurgery

- Full-thickness skin grafts are preferred for volar hand and fingertip wounds, because they are more durable, contract less, and provide better sensibility.
- Primary contraindications to replantation
  - Level of amputation within zone II flexor tendon sheath, single digit amputation (except thumb), segmental, crush, or prolonged ischemia
- The operative sequence of replantation—(BEFAVNS) bone, extensor tendon, flexor tendon, artery, vein, nerve, skin
  - A structure-by-structure technique in multiple digit amputations is faster and improves outcomes.
- Replantation monitoring includes observation of color, capillary refill, and tissue turgor. A drop in temperature more than 2° C in 1 hour or a temperature below 30° C indicates decreased digital perfusion.
- Factor most predictive of digit survival after replantation is mechanism of injury.
- Most frequent cause of early (within 12 hours) replantation failure is arterial thrombosis from persistent vasospasm. Arterial insufficiency suggested by pale skin color, decreased or absent capillary refill, and loss of Doppler-measurable signal.
  - Consider releasing constricting bandages, place extremity in dependent position, administer heparin, and perform stellate ganglion block.
- Failure after 12 hours is typically due to venous congestion or thrombosis.
- Late complications include tendon adhesions, bone nonunion, and neuroma formation. Tenolysis is the most commonly performed secondary procedure following successful replantation.

IX. Vascular Disorders

- Allen test is used to determine the presence or absence of a complete arch in the palm. Approximately 20% of people have an incomplete arch.
- Hypothenar hammer syndrome is the most common post-traumatic vascular occlusive condition of the upper extremity, involving the ulnar artery in the proximal palm. Treatment may include resenction of the thrombosed segment and interposition vein grafting.
- Vasospastic disease with a known underlying cause is termed *Raynaud phenomenon*. When no cause can be determined, the entity is otherwise known as *Raynaud disease*.
- There are 10 hand compartments: thenar, hypothenar, adductor pollicis, four dorsal interosseous, and three volar interosseous.
- The FDP and FPL muscles are most vulnerable in Volkmann ischemic contracture.

X. Compression Neuropathy

Median Nerve

- Carpal tunnel syndrome is most commonly idiopathic in adults, but mucopolysaccharidosis is the most common cause in children.
  - Single corticosteroid injection yields transient relief in approximately 80% after 6 weeks, but only 20% are symptom free by 1 year.
  - Endoscopic carpal tunnel release may be associated with less early scar tenderness, improved short-term grip/pinch strength, and better patient satisfaction scores in some studies. Long-term results compared to open release are largely equivalent.
- Pronator syndrome is a compression of the median nerve in the arm/forearm.
  - Five potential sites of compression—supracondylar process, ligament of Struthers (courses between the supracondylar process and medial epicondyle), lacertus fibrosis, between the two heads of pronator teres muscle, FDS aponeurotic arch
- Anterior interosseous nerve syndrome
  - Involves motor loss of FPL, index +/– long FDP, and pronator quadratus; no sensory disturbance

Ulnar Nerve

- The floor of the cubital tunnel is defined by the medial collateral ligament and elbow joint capsule. The roof is the flexor carpi ulnaris (FCU) fascia and arcuate ligament of Osborne.

- Cubital tunnel syndrome symptoms include paresthesias of the ulnar 1½ digits (ulnar half of ring finger and small finger) and ulnar dorsal hand.
  - Recent meta-analyses of techniques fail to show statistically significant difference in outcome between simple decompression and transposition.

Radial Nerve

- Posterior interosseous nerve (PIN) compression syndrome symptoms include lateral elbow pain and distal muscle weakness.
  - Radial deviation with active wrist extension because extensor carpi radialis longus (ECRL) innervated by proper radial nerve more proximally
    - PIN innervates the extensor carpi radialis brevis (ECRB), supinator, EIP, ECU, extensor digitorum communis (EDC), extensor digiti minimi, APL, extensor pollicis brevis (EPB), and EPL.
- Proper radial nerve palsy ("Saturday night palsy") is differentiated from PIN compression by additional weakness of proper radial nerve–innervated muscles, such as triceps, brachioradialis, and ECRL. Radial tunnel syndrome is marked by lateral proximal forearm pain rather than distal motor weakness.

Thoracic Outlet

- Paresthesias are most common initial complaint and are present in 95% of patients. However, they are nonspecific. Fatigue is common, particularly when the arm is used in a provocative position.

XI. Nerve Injuries and Tendon Transfers

- The Seddon classification divides nerve injury into neurapraxia, axonotmesis, and neurotmesis.
- Preganglionic traumatic brachial plexus injuries have the worst prognosis.
- Six basic tenets of tendon transfers
  - Donor must be expendable.
  - Donor must be of similar excursion and power.
  - One transfer should perform one function.
  - Synergistic transfers are easier to rehabilitate.
  - A straight line of pull is optimal.
  - One grade of motor strength will be lost after transfer.
- Radial nerve palsy
  - Wrist extension—pronator teres to ECRB
  - Finger extension—FCU or FCR EDC II-V
  - Thumb extension—PL to EPL

XII. Arthritis

- Osteoarthritis commonly affects the DIP joint and presents as a mucous cyst. The cyst may be excised, along with any accompanying osteophytes, for symptomatic relief. Occasionally, skin coverage with a local rotational flap is necessary after cyst excision.
- Thumb CMC joint osteoarthritis (basal joint arthritis) is theorized to result from anterior oblique ligament attenuation. Many treatment alternatives exist, with ligament reconstruction and tendon interposition most common. All share at least partial excision of trapezium.
- Rheumatoid arthritis is a systemic disease of synovial tissue.
  - Tenosynovitis most commonly involves the dorsal wrist, volar wrist, and volar digits.
  - Vaughan-Jackson syndrome describes progressive rupture of extensor tendons, starting with extensor digiti minimi and continuing radially, from attrition over a prominent distal ulnar head (caput ulnae).
  - Mannerfelt syndrome describes rupture of FPL and/or index FDP secondary to attrition over a volar scaphoid osteophyte.
  - The classical MCP joint involvement is ulnar deviation and volar subluxation.
- Synovitis and pannus formation stretch the weaker radial sagittal bands, and extensor tendons subluxate ulnarly.
- Initial presentation may be an extension lag.
- Early treatment with synovectomy and recentralization of the extensor tendons provides temporary solution. Silicone MCP arthroplasty most common definitive treatment

XIII. Idiopathic Osteonecrosis of the Carpus

- Kienböck disease (idiopathic osteonecrosis of the lunate) is most common in young men and presents with dorsal wrist pain and decreased grip strength.
- Unexplained, persistent, non–activity-related dorsal wrist pain in young adult with negative ulnar variance should prompt magnetic resonance imaging (MRI) evaluation.
  - The Lichtman classification can be used to direct treatment, particularly between stage IIIA (lunate collapse with normal carpal alignment and height) and stage IIIB (fixed scaphoid rotation with decreased carpal height and proximal migration of capitate).
- First line of surgical treatment is a joint-leveling procedure.
  - In patients with ulnar-negative variance, radial-shortening osteotomy is preferred over ulnar lengthening with bone grafting (goal is neutral or 1 mm positive).
- Treatment of stage IIIB must address associated carpal instability (partial wrist fusion or proximal row carpectomy).

XIV. Dupuytren Disease

- Benign fibroproliferative disorder of unclear etiology; autosomal dominant inheritance pattern with variable penetrance; sporadic cases more common
- Myofibroblasts are predominant cell type found histologically in Dupuytren fascia, and their contractile properties are abnormal and exaggerated.
- Cleland ligaments are not involved.
- The spiral cord is clinically most important and leads to PIP contracture. It puts the neurovascular bundle at risk during surgery by displacing it more centrally and superficially.
- Surgical indications include inability to place hand flat on tabletop (Hueston test), MCP flexion contracture greater than 30 degrees, or any PIP flexion contracture.

Continued

- Open limited fasciectomy is generally the preferred technique. The open-palm McCash technique may still be used to reduce hematoma formation, decrease edema, and allow early motion.

XV. Hand Tumors

- Ganglions are the most common soft tissue mass of the hand and wrist.
  - Dorsal wrist—scapholunate articulation
  - Volar wrist—radioscaphoid or scaphotrapezial joint
  - Dorsal digit DIP joint—osteophyte
  - Distal palm–flexor tendon sheath
- Giant cell tumor of tendon sheath presents as a slow-growing firm mass on the volar aspect of a digit.
  - Treatment is marginal excision.
- Infantile hemangiomas typically become involuted by age 7, and those arising during childhood are observed.
  - Small and accessible lesions treated with marginal excision
  - Embolization may be more feasible alternative for larger lesions.
- Most common tumors
  - Most common malignancy—squamous cell carcinoma
  - Most common sarcomas—epithelioid and synovial
  - Most common benign bone tumor—enchondroma
  - Most common malignant bone tumor—metastatic lung carcinoma
  - Most common malignant primary bone tumor—chondrosarcoma, osteosarcoma, Ewing sarcoma

XVI. Hand Infections

- *Staphylococcus aureus* is the most common pathogen. Gram-negative and anaerobic bacteria are seen in intravenous drug abusers (IVDAs), diabetic patients, and after farmyard injuries or bite wounds.
- Human bites are a potentially serious infection treated promptly with incision and drainage, especially if joint or tendon sheath is violated.
  - Most frequently isolated organisms are group A streptococcus, *S. aureus, Eikenella corrodens,* and *Bacteroides* species.
- Dog bites are more common than cat bites, but cat bites more commonly result in serious infection.
  - α-Hemolytic streptococci, *Pasteurella multocida,* and *S. aureus* are the most common pathogens.
  - Ampicillin/sulbactam and amoxicillin/clavulanate are empiric antibiotics of choice (ciprofloxacin, doxycycline, or tetracycline if penicillin allergic).
- Pyogenic flexor tenosynovitis is an infection of the flexor tendon sheath.
  - Kanavel signs—flexed, resting posture of digit; fusiform swelling of the digit; tenderness of flexor tendon sheath; pain with passive digit extension
  - If recognized early, patient should be admitted and treated with splinting, intravenous antibiotics, and close observation.
    - If signs improve within first 24 hours, surgery may be avoided.
  - Otherwise, the treatment of choice is incision and drainage of flexor tendon sheath.
- A herpetic whitlow is commonly seen in toddlers, dental hygienists, and health care workers. Incision and drainage are not recommended because the rates of secondary bacterial infection are high.
- Atypical mycobacterial infections commonly involve the hand. The most common organism is *Mycobacterium marinum.*
  - Treatment generally requires surgical débridement and oral antibiotics such as ethambutol, trimethoprim-sulfamethoxazole, clarithromycin, azithromycin, or tetracycline.
- High-pressure injection injuries can be devastating with a high rate of digital amputation.
  - Organic solvents more toxic to tissue, and oil-based paint worse than latex or water-based.
  - Emergency wide surgical débridement recommended

XVII. Congenital Hand Differences

- The three signaling centers that control limb development are the apical ectodermal ridge, zone of polarizing activity formation, and wingless-type pathway.
  - The apical ectodermal ridge controls proximal-to-distal growth, zone of polarizing activity formation controls anterior-to-posterior growth, and wingless type controls dorsoventral growth.
- Radial clubhand is associated with a variety of systemic problems, including thrombocytopenia with absent radius (TAR) syndrome, VACTERL syndrome (**v**ertebral, **a**nal, **c**ardiac, **t**racheal, **e**sophageal, **r**enal, and **l**imb anomalies) and life-threatening Fanconi anemia. Early therapy is used to preserve range of motion. Centralization may be attempted only if there is adequate elbow range of motion.
- Radioulnar synostosis is associated with duplication of sex chromosomes. Examination reveals a fixed pronation deformity. Treatment is conservative unless significant pronation deformity exists.
- Duplication can be preaxial (radial or tibial side) or postaxial (ulnar or fibular side).
- Syndactyly results from failure of apoptosis to separate digits. Poland syndrome (absent pectoralis major and chest wall abnormalities) and Apert syndrome (acrosyndactyly and mental retardation) are commonly associated.
- Preaxial polydactyly (thumb duplication) is most commonly a type IV with duplicate proximal phalanx. It is reconstructed using the best possible structures. If there are thumbs of equal size, preserve the ulnar thumb to retain the ulnar collateral ligament for pinch. Retain the soft tissue from the ablated thumb for augmentation.
- Postaxial polydactyly (small-finger duplication) is 10 times more common in African Americans than whites and follows an autosomal dominant inheritance. Genetic workup is warranted in whites because of multiple associated chromosomal abnormalities.
- Macrodactyly is a nonhereditary digital enlargement. Severely affected single digit should be amputated for the most favorable outcome. Thumb or multiple digit involvement can be treated with epiphyseal ablation, angular and/or shortening osteotomies, longitudinal narrowing osteotomies, and debulking.

- Thumb hypoplasia treatment is based on the carpometacarpal (CMC) joint (separates type IIIA from IIIB). If the CMC joint is intact, reconstruction may be performed. If not intact, pollicization is performed.

XVIII. Elbow

- The anterior bundle of the medial (ulnar) collateral ligament is the primary restraint to valgus stress. The lateral ulnar collateral ligament (LUCL) is the primary restraint to varus and external rotational stress.
- Lateral epicondylitis is a degenerative process of the ECRB origin. Histologic examination demonstrates angiofibroblastic hyperplasia.
- Distal biceps rupture results in diminished supination strength more than flexion strength. If left untreated, only approximately 50% supination strength versus approximately 70% flexion strength is regained by 1 year.
  - Partial ruptures primarily occur on the radial side of the tuberosity footprint, owing to its function as a supinator.
  - Partial injuries initially treated nonoperatively with rest, nonsteroidal anti-inflammatory drugs (NSAIDs), and therapy; slow recovery—may eventually require detachment, débridement, and reattachment
  - Single-incision technique risks the PIN and lateral antebrachial cutaneous nerve.
  - Two-incision technique risks radioulnar synostosis.
- Posterolateral rotatory instability results from incompetence of the LUCL. Varus posteromedial rotatory instability typically results from fracture of the anteromedial coronoid process.
- Valgus extension overload is an overuse syndrome due to repetitive valgus loading of the MCL leading to microtears of the ligament. The midsubstance of the anterior bundle is most commonly involved.
  - Untreated, there is increased contact pressure over the posteromedial aspect of the elbow, leading to posteromedial osteophytes and impingement. There is increased compressive force across the radiocapitellar joint, predisposing to cartilage injury.
- Indications for total elbow arthroplasty
  - Refractory RA
  - Advanced osteoarthritis (primary and post-traumatic)
  - Chronic instability
  - Complex distal humerus fractures in elderly patients

SELECTED BIBLIOGRAPHY

The selected bibliography for this chapter can be found on www.expertconsult.com.

Chapter 8

SPINE

William C. Lauerman and Clark C. Baumbusch

CONTENTS

I. INTRODUCTION

A. Anatomy (see Chapter 2, Anatomy)

B. History and physical examination (Table 8-1; Figure 8-1)

1. Localized pain (tumor, infection)
2. Mechanical pain (instability, discogenic disease)
3. Radicular pain (herniated nucleus pulposus [HNP], stenosis), night pain (tumor)
4. Systemic symptoms such as fever or unexplained weight loss (infection, tumor)
5. The physical examination must evaluate both the spine and the neurologic function of the extremities (Table 8-2).
6. Localized hip and shoulder pathology may simulate spine disease and must also be evaluated.

C. Objective tests

1. **Plain radiographs** should be obtained 4 to 6 weeks after onset of symptoms; add flexion-extension views for suspected instability.
2. **Magnetic resonance imaging** (MRI) is excellent for further imaging of HNP, stenosis, soft tissue, tumor, and infection.
3. **Computed tomography** (CT) with fine cuts ± myelographic dye is used to examine bony anatomy after previous surgery and the quality of fusion.
4. **Bone scan** is helpful in evaluating metastatic disease and may be negative with multiple myeloma.
5. **Laboratory evaluation** consists of C-reactive protein and erythrocyte sedimentation rate for infection, metabolic screening, serum/urine protein electrophoresis for myeloma, and a complete blood cell count (there is often a high-normal white blood cell count with infection or anemia with myeloma).

D. Workup of back pain—Complaint of back pain is second only to upper respiratory tract infection as a cause of office visits, with 60% to 80% lifetime prevalence. Standard workup begins with a history (most important) and progresses to physical examination (see Table 8-1). Radiographic and laboratory studies rarely help in acute cases. The following considerations in the evaluation of back pain are important:

1. Age at onset
   - Children may be affected by congenital or, more often, developmental disorders or infection.
   - Young adults are more likely to suffer from disc disease, spondylolisthesis, or acute fractures.
   - Complaints from older adults, including spinal stenosis, metastatic disease, and osteopenic compression fractures are more common.
2. Radicular signs and symptoms
   - Often associated with disc herniation or spinal stenosis
   - Intraspinal pathologic conditions or other entities associated with cord or root impingement may be responsible.
   - Herpes zoster is a rare cause of lumbar radiculopathy, with pain preceding the skin eruption.
3. Systemic symptoms—Careful history-taking can help guide diagnosis of systemic conditions with associated spine pathology.
   - Metabolic disease
   - Rheumatologic conditions
     - Polyarticular involvement (rheumatoid arthritis)
     - Ophthalmologic symptoms (spondyloarthropathies)
   - Metastatic disease
     - Age older than 50
     - Cancer history
     - Rest pain
     - Weight loss
   - Infection (confirmed by laboratory studies)
     - Indwelling catheters (hemodialysis)
   - Chronic back pain is often refractory to localized treatment in many patients with fibromyalgia.
   - Fibromyalgia (multiple associations)
     - Sleep disturbance
     - Irritable bowel syndrome
     - Dysmenorrhea
     - Hallmark physical finding: excessive generalized tenderness on both sides of the midline
     - More common in women
4. Sources of referred back pain
   - Viscerogenic
     - Peptic ulcer disease
     - Cholecystitis
     - Nephrolithiasis

Table 8-1 Examination of Patients with Disorders of the Spine

Component	Features
Inspection	Overall alignment in sagittal and coronal planes (sciatic scoliosis)
Gait	Wide-based (myelopathy), forward-leaning (stenosis), antalgic
Palpation	Localized posterior swelling (trauma), acute gibbus deformity, tenderness
Range of motion	Flexion/extension, lateral bend, full versus limited
Neurologic function	Motor, sensory, reflexes, assessment of long-tract signs (see also Table 8-7)
Special tests	Straight-leg raise, Spurling test, Waddell signs of inorganic pathology

- Pancreatitis
- Pelvic inflammatory disease
- Vascular
  - Abdominal aortic aneurysm
- Distant musculoskeletal areas
  - Hip arthritis, trochanteric bursitis

5. Psychogenic pain—may play important role in some patients with chronic low back disorders
   - Evidence of secondary gain
   - Workers' compensation or litigation
   - Inappropriate physical findings (Waddell) signs, symptoms, and maneuvers
   - Thorough evaluation of real pathologic conditions is essential.
6. Chronic back pain—Risk factors for development include:
   - Frequent disabling episodes
   - Availability of workers' compensation
   - History of smoking
   - Age older than 30
   - Declining incidence of disabling pain after age 60

II. CERVICAL SPINE

A. Cervical spondylosis—Chronic disc degeneration and associated facet arthropathy result in three clinical entities:

- Discogenic neck pain (axial pain)
- Radiculopathy (root compromise)
- Myelopathy (cord compression) and combinations of these conditions

1. Epidemiology
   - Peak between ages of 40 and 50
   - Men affected more than women
   - Occurs at C5-C6 level most frequently
     - C6-C7 level next most common
   - Risk factors
     - Frequent lifting
     - Cigarette smoking
     - History of excessive driving
2. Pathoanatomy—Cervical spondylosis involves the intervertebral disc and four other articulations (Figure 8-2):
   - Two uncovertebral joints (of Luschka)
   - Two facet joints—Facet joint capsules are known to have sensory receptors that may play a role in pain and proprioceptive sensation in the cervical spine.
   - Cord compromise as canal diameter decreases
     - Normal 17 mm
     - Concern when diameter less than 13 mm
       - Measured on plain lateral radiograph
   - Progressive collapse of the cervical discs, resulting in loss of normal lordosis of the cervical spine and chronic anterior cord compression across the kyphotic spine/anterior chondroosseous spurs
   - Spondylotic changes in the foramina, primarily from chondroosseous spurs of the joints of Luschka, may restrict motion and lead to nerve root compression.
   - Soft disc herniation
     - Usually posterolateral, between the posterior edge of the uncinate process and the lateral edge of the posterior longitudinal ligament, it may result in acute radiculopathy.
     - Anterior herniation may cause dysphagia (rare).
     - Myelopathy may be seen with large central herniation or spondylotic bars with a congenitally narrow canal.
   - Ossification of the posterior longitudinal ligament
     - Results in cervical stenosis and myelopathy
     - Common in Asians but may also be seen in non-Asians
   - Neck extension: Cord is compressed between the degenerative disc and spondylotic bar anteriorly and the hypertrophic facets and infolded ligamentum flavum posteriorly.
   - Neck flexion results in slight increase in canal diameter and relief of cord compression.
3. Signs and symptoms—Degenerative discogenic neck pain may present as the insidious onset of neck pain without neurologic signs or symptoms, exacerbated by excess vertebral motion.
   - Occipital headache common
   - Radiculopathy
     - Can involve one or multiple roots
     - Neck, shoulder, and arm pain; paresthesias; and numbness

Table 8-2 Findings in Nerve Root Compression

Level	Root	Muscles Affected	Sensory Loss	Reflex
C3-C4	C4	Scapular	Lateral neck, shoulder	None
C4-C5	C5	Deltoid, biceps	Lateral arm	Biceps
C5-C6*	C6	Wrist extensors, biceps, triceps (supination)	Radial forearm	Brachioradialis
C6-C7	C7	Triceps, wrist flexors (pronation)	Middle finger	Triceps
C7-C8	C8	Finger flexors, interossei	Ulnar hand	None
C8-T1	T1	Interossei	Ulnar forearm	None

*Most common level.

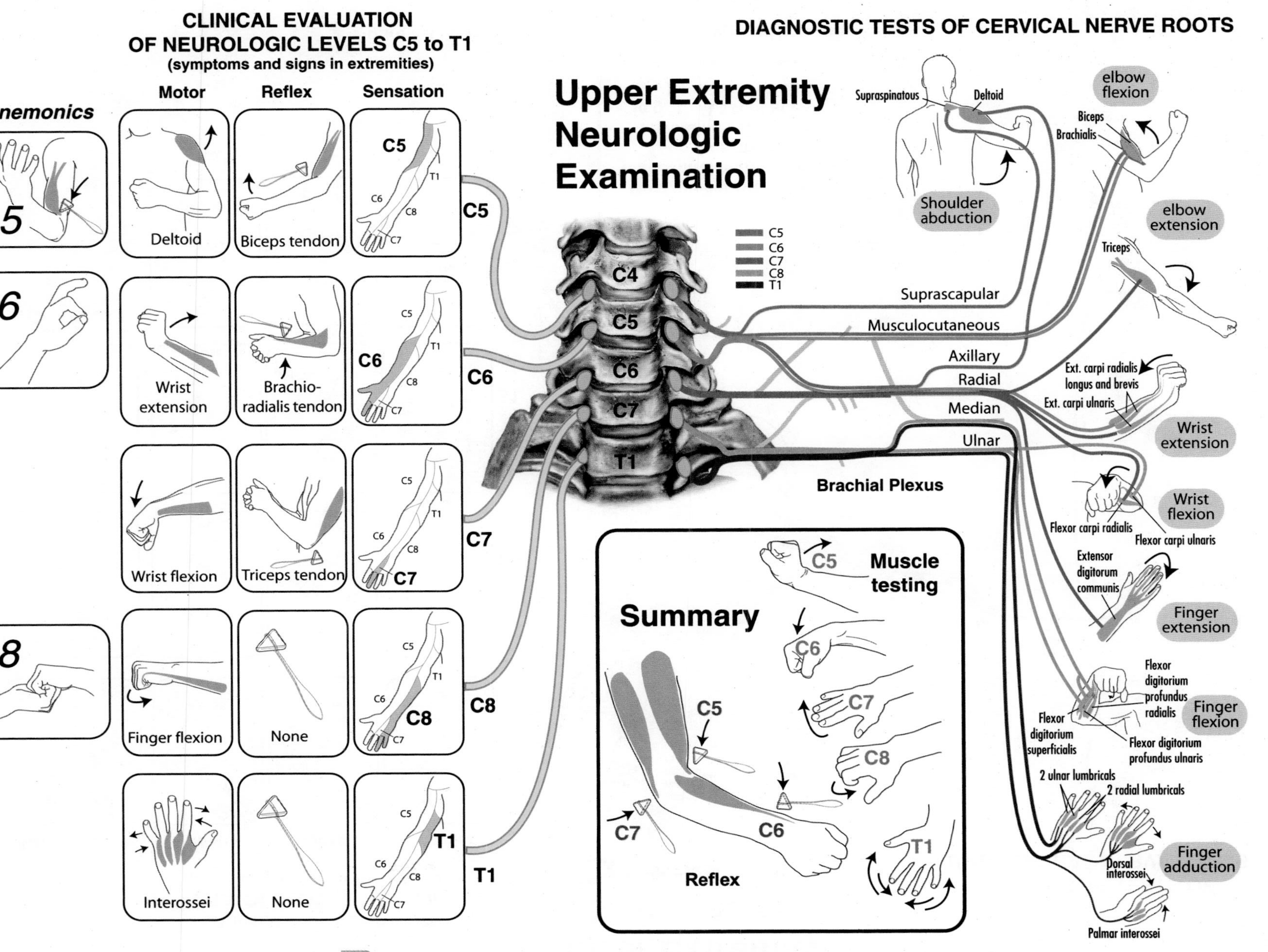

Figure 8-1 Upper and lower extremity neurologic examination.

Continued

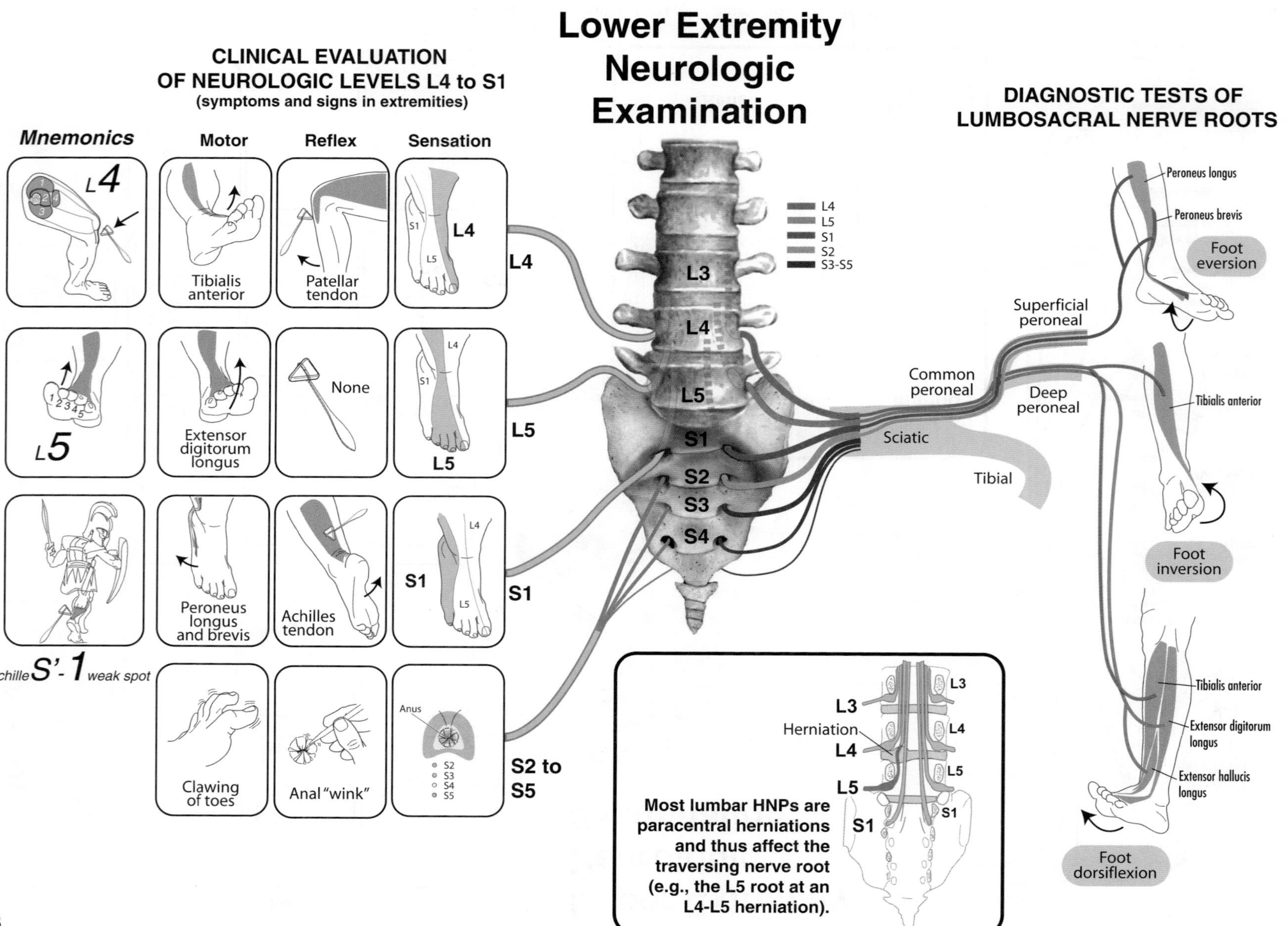
Lower Extremity Neurologic Examination
CLINICAL EVALUATION OF NEUROLOGIC LEVELS L4 to S1
(symptoms and signs in extremities)
Mnemonics
Motor
Reflex
Sensation
L4
Tibialis anterior
Patellar tendon
L4
L5
Extensor digitorum longus
None
L5
achille S'-1 weak spot
Peroneus longus and brevis
Achilles tendon
S1
Clawing of toes
Anal "wink"
Anus
S2
S3
S4
S5
S2 to S5
L4
L5
S1
S2
S3-S5
L3
L4
L5
S1
S2
S3
S4
Common peroneal
Sciatic
Tibial
Superficial peroneal
Deep peroneal
DIAGNOSTIC TESTS OF LUMBOSACRAL NERVE ROOTS
Peroneus longus
Peroneus brevis
Foot eversion
Tibialis anterior
Foot inversion
Tibialis anterior
Extensor digitorum longus
Extensor hallucis longus
Foot dorsiflexion
Herniation
Most lumbar HNPs are paracentral herniations and thus affect the traversing nerve root (e.g., the L5 root at an L4-L5 herniation).
B

Figure 8-1, Cont'd Upper and lower extremity neurologic examination.

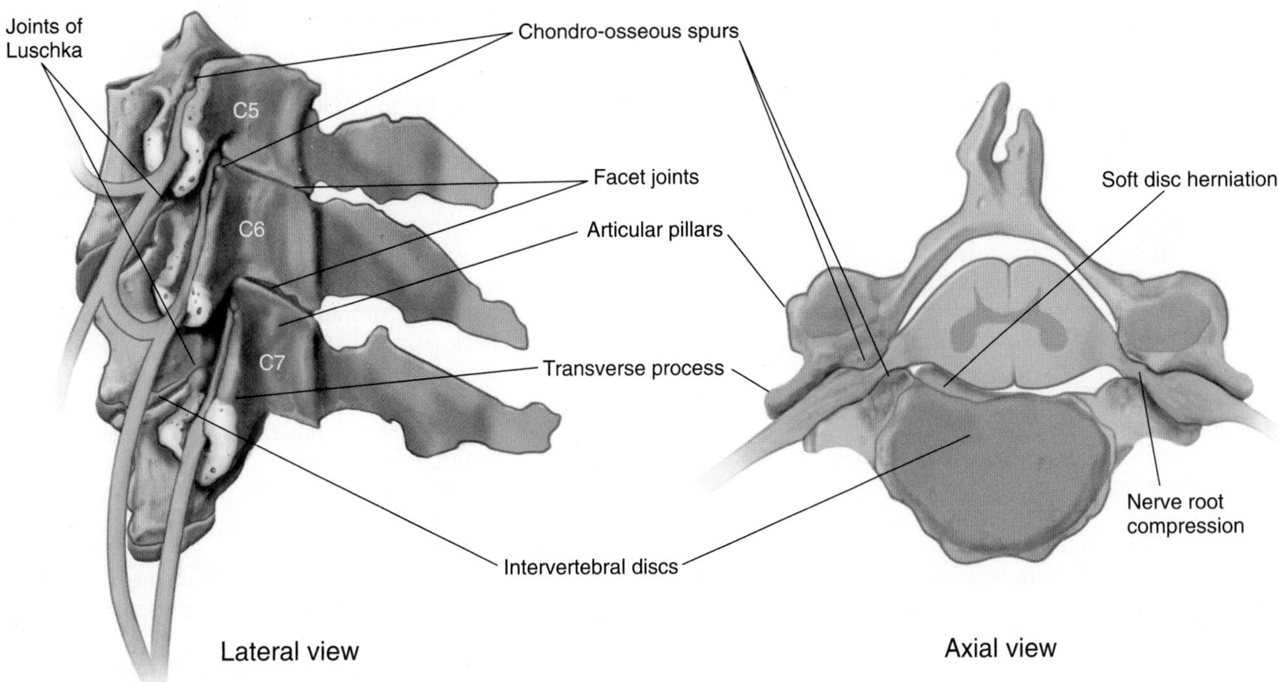

Figure 8-2 Cervical root impingement due to cervical spondylosis.

   - Overlapping findings because of intraneural intersegmental connections of sensory nerve roots
   - Symptoms are exacerbated by mechanical stress such as excessive vertebral motion, in particular rotation and lateral bend with a vertical compressive force (Spurling test).
   - Relief of radicular pain with shoulder abduction is suggestive of a cervical etiology.
   - Caudal nerve root at a given level is usually affected (see Table 8-2).
     - Cervical nerve roots exit above their corresponding vertebrae (e.g., C5 exits at the C4-C5 neural foramen).
     - Consequently, disc herniation at C5-C6 involves the C6 nerve root.
 - Myelopathy is characterized by:
   - Weakness (upper more than lower extremity)
     - Lower extremity weakness (corticospinal tracts)—associated with worse prognosis
   - Decreased manual dexterity
     - Buttoning buttons, use of chopsticks
   - Gait disturbances—ataxic broad-based, shuffling gait
   - Sensory changes
   - Spasticity
   - Urinary retention (rare)
     - Additional complaints of urinary urgency or frequency
   - **The natural history of cervical spondylotic myelopathy is characterized by stepwise deterioration in symptomatology followed by a period of stability.**

4. Physical examination findings
   - Upper motor neuron findings in myelopathy
     - "Myelopathy hand" and the "finger escape sign" (small finger spontaneously abducts because of weak intrinsic muscles)
     - Hyperreflexia
     - Hoffmann sign
     - Inverted radial reflex (ipsilateral finger flexion when eliciting the brachioradialis reflex)
     - Clonus or Babinski sign
     - Upper extremities may have radicular (lower motor neuron) signs along with evidence of distal myelopathy.
     - Upper motor neuron findings are not always present in all patients.
   - Funicular pain—central burning and stinging with or without the Lhermitte sign (radiating lightning-like sensations down the back with neck flexion)
5. Diagnostic testing
   - Imaging
     - Plain radiographs
       - Anteroposterior, lateral, and oblique views
       - Assess for arthrosis
         - Facet joints
         - Uncovertebral joints
       - Osteophytes (bars)
       - Malalignment
       - Sagittal canal diameter
       - Low specificity of plain radiographs
         - By age 65, 95% of men and 70% of women have degenerative changes.
     - CT myelography or MRI
       - Effectively demonstrates neural compressive pathology
       - False-positive MRIs are common:
         - Twenty-five percent of asymptomatic patients older than age 40 will have findings of either HNP or foraminal stenosis on cervical MRI.
         - Correlation with history and physical examination is critical.

- MRI is also useful for detecting intrinsic changes in the spinal cord and disc degeneration.
  - Myelomalacia—area of bright signal in the cord on T2-weighted imaging
- Discography
  - Controversial and rarely used for cervical spine disorders
- Electrodiagnostic studies
  - Have a high false-negative rate
  - Are useful for differentiating peripheral nerve compression from radiculopathy and for detecting systemic neurologic disorders such as amyotrophic lateral sclerosis

6. Treatment
   - Nonsurgical treatment
     - Nonsteroidal anti-inflammatory drugs (NSAIDs)
     - Extraforaminal cervical nerve blocks
     - Moist heat
     - Cervical isometric exercises
     - Temporary collar immobilization
     - Traction
     - Pain clinic modalities are helpful in most cases of discogenic neck pain and radiculopathy
     - Extraforaminal nerve blocks have been shown to be safe in large series of patients, with a less than 2% rate of minor complications
   - Surgical treatment
     - Indications
       - Myelopathy with motor/gait impairment
       - Radiculopathy with persistent, disabling pain and weakness
       - Surgery for discogenic neck pain is less rewarding.
     - Procedures
       - Combined anterior (cervical) Smith-Robinson discectomy and fusion (ACDF)
         - Involves excision of osteophytes and corpectomy with a strut graft fusion with or without instrumentation
         - Anterior plating may increase the fusion rate in multilevel discectomies with fusion and will protect a strut graft in multilevel corpectomies.
         - Adjunctive posterior plating may be considered in cases involving prior laminectomy, multilevel corpectomy and strut grafting, or three-level ACDF.
         - Early postoperative complications:
           - Dysphagia from esophageal retraction (9.5%)
           - Surgical site hematoma with airway compromise (1%-11%)
           - **Recurrent laryngeal nerve injury**
             - Higher incidence from right-sided approach (controversial)
         - Late postoperative complications:
           - Nonunion
             - Single level: 5%
             - Two levels: 6%
             - Three levels: 10%
             - **Treatment of a nonunion should be posterior fusion.**
           - Adjacent segment disease
             - Symptomatic disease in 25% at 10 years after ACDF
       - Posterior foraminotomy
         - Useful for single-level radiculopathy
       - Canal expansive laminoplasty
         - Used for multilevel spondylosis and myelopathy and ossification of posterior longitudinal ligament (OPLL)
         - Allows for more extensive decompression
         - Lower incidence of instability compared with multilevel laminectomies
         - **Contraindicated in setting of fixed kyphosis**
         - Relative contraindication in preexisting axial neck pain
         - Nerve root palsy at C5 of 5% to 7%
           - Motor deficit more prevalent
       - Laminectomy and posterior plating/fusion
         - Multiple-level stenosis
         - Appropriate when spine can be extended into lordosis
       - Total disc arthroplasty
         - Theoretical advantage of eliminating compressive pathologic process while preserving motion segments
         - Two-year follow-up available at present
         - Used for radiculopathy or myelopathy from single-level degenerative disc disease occurring at C3 to C7

B. Cervical stenosis

1. Congenital versus acquired (traumatic, degenerative)
2. Absolute stenosis (anteroposterior canal diameter <10 mm)
3. Relative stenosis (anteroposterior canal diameter 10 to 13 mm)
4. Pavlov (Torg) ratio (canal/vertebral body width) should be 1.0.
   - Ratio of less than 0.80 or a sagittal diameter of less than 13 mm is considered a significant risk factor for later neurologic involvement.
5. Minor trauma such as hyperextension may lead to a central cord syndrome, even without overt skeletal injury.
6. Surgery may serve a prophylactic function but is usually reserved for patients who develop myelopathy or radiculopathy.

C. Rheumatoid spondylitis

1. Overview
   - Cervical spine involvement is common in rheumatoid arthritis (occurring in up to 90% of patients) and is more common with long-standing disease and multiple joint involvement.
   - Presenting complaints
     - Axial neck pain
     - Stiffness
     - Occipital headaches
       - Compression of greater occipital branch of C2
   - Neurologic impairment (weakness, decreased sensation, hyperreflexia) in patients with rheumatoid arthritis usually occurs gradually and is often overlooked or attributed to other joint disease.
   - Neurologic impairment with rheumatoid arthritis has been classified by Ranawat (Table 8-3).
   - Surgery may not reverse significant neurologic deterioration, especially if a tight spinal canal is present, but it can stabilize it.
   - Look for subtle signs of neurologic involvement.

Table 8-3 Ranawat Classification of Neurologic Impairment in Rheumatoid Arthritis

Grade	Characteristics
I	Subjective paresthesias, pain
II	Subjective weakness; upper motor neuron findings
III	Objective weakness; upper motor neuron findings
IIIA	Ambulatory
IIIB	Nonambulatory

- Assess the radiographic markers for impending neural compression (Figure 8-3).
  - Space available for the cord
    - Lower cervical spine
  - Posterior atlanto–dens interval (PADI)
    - Upper cervical spine
- Indications for surgical stabilization:
  - Instability
  - Pain
  - Neurologic deficit owing to neural compression
  - Impending neurologic deficit (based on objective studies)
    - PADI less than 14 mm
    - Cervicomedullary angle less than 135 degrees
- Patients with rheumatoid arthritis should have flexion/extension films before elective surgery.

2. Atlantoaxial subluxation—occurs in 50% to 80% of cases of rheumatoid arthritis and is often the result of pannus formation at synovial joints between the dens and the ring of C1, resulting in destruction of transverse ligament, dens, or both
   - Diagnosis
     - Anterior subluxation of C1 on C2 is the most common finding, but posterior and lateral subluxation can also occur.
     - Findings on examination may include limitation of motion, upper motor neuron signs, and weakness.

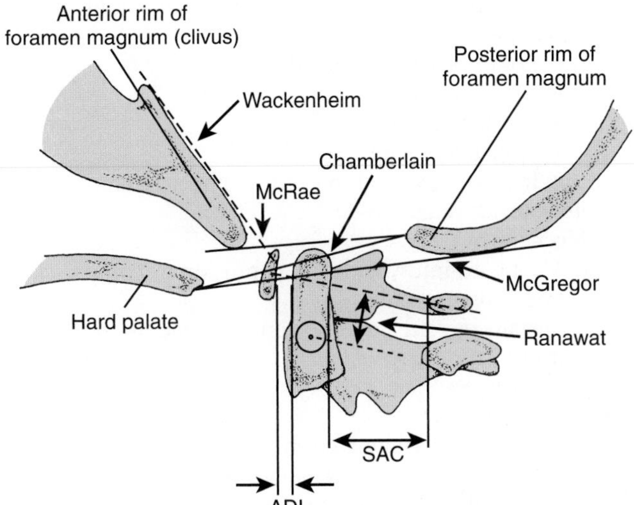

Figure 8-3 Common measurements in C1 to C2 disorders. ADI, atlanto–dens interval; SAC, space available for the cord.

     - Plain radiographs that include patient-controlled flexion and extension views are evaluated to determine the **anterior atlanto–dens interval** as well as the PADI.
     - Instability is present with motion of more than 3.5 mm on flexion and extension views, although radiographic instability in rheumatoid arthritis is common and not necessarily an indication for surgery.
     - C1-C2 motion of more than 9 to 10 mm or a **PADI of less than 14 mm is associated with an increased risk of neurologic injury and usually requires surgical treatment.**
     - Myelopathy, progressive neurologic impairment, and progressive instability are also indications for surgical stabilization, usually a posterior C1-C2 fusion.
   - Treatment
     - Transarticular screw fixation (Magerl) across C1-C2 eliminates the need for halo immobilization associated with wiring alone.
       - Necessary to obtain preoperative CT to evaluate the position of the vertebral arteries
     - Nonreducible atlantoaxial subluxation
       - Remove posterior arch of C1 to decompress cord.
       - Fuse occiput to C2.
     - Anterior cord compression because of pannus often resolves after posterior spinal fusion.
     - Odontoidectomy should be reserved as a secondary procedure.
     - Surgery is less successful in Ranawat grade IIIB patients but should be considered.
     - Complications include pseudarthrosis (10%-20%) and adjacent segment involvement on long-term follow-up.
       - Extension of the fusion to the occiput lessens the nonunion rate.
       - PADI of less than 14 mm is a relative indication for prophylactic fusion, even in absence of myelopathy.

3. Cranial settling (basilar invagination)
   - The second most common manifestation of rheumatoid arthritis in cervical spine
     - Forty percent of patients with rheumatoid arthritis
     - Cranial migration of the dens from erosion and bone loss between the occiput and C1-C2
     - Often seen in combination with fixed atlantoaxial subluxation
     - Measurements are shown in Figure 8-3.
       - Landmarks may be difficult to identify.
       - Ranawat line is most reproducible.
     - Progressive cranial migration or neurologic compromise may require operative intervention (occiput to C2 fusion).
     - Cervicomedullary angle less than 135 degrees (on MRI) suggests impending neurologic impairment.
       - Consider surgery.
     - Transoral or retropharyngeal dens resection for brainstem compression
       - Vertical nystagmus on examination
     - If there is any suggestion of cranial settling in cases of atlantoaxial subluxation, occipitocervical fusion is the conservative approach.

4. Subaxial subluxation
   - Occurs in 20% of cases of rheumatoid arthritis
   - Seen in combination with upper cervical spine instability
   - Pathoanatomy
     - Pannus formation in uncovertebral joints (joints of Luschka) and facet joints
     - Subluxation may occur at multiple levels.
   - Radiographic markers of instability
     - Subaxial subluxation of greater than 4 mm or more than 20% of the body is indicative of cord compression.
     - A cervical height index (cervical body height/width) of less than 2.00 approaches 100% sensitivity and specificity in predicting neurologic compromise.
   - Posterior spinal fusion may be required for subluxation greater than 4 mm with intractable pain and neurologic compromise.

D. Cervical spine and cord injuries—See Chapter 11, Trauma, for classification and treatment of cervical spine injuries.

1. Epidemiology
   - Young males
   - Motor vehicle accidents
   - Falls
   - Diving accidents
   - Gunshot wounds are an increasing cause.
   - The findings may be subtle; the significant morbidity and mortality rates associated with missed injuries have led to the current emphasis on cervical spine protection after polytrauma.
   - Missed cervical spine injuries are the most common in the presence of a decreased level of consciousness, alcohol/drug intoxication, and head injury and in patients with multiple injuries.
2. Progression of injury
   - Spinal shock
     - Spinal shock usually involves a 24- to 72-hour period of paralysis, hypotonia, and areflexia.
     - **Return of the bulbocavernosus reflex (anal sphincter contraction in response to squeezing the glans penis or tugging on the Foley catheter) signifies the end of spinal shock.**
       - Injuries below the thoracolumbar level (conus or cauda equina) may permanently interrupt the bulbocavernosus reflex.
     - After the conclusion of spinal shock, spasticity, hyperreflexia, and clonus progress over days to weeks.
     - In complete injuries, further neurologic improvement is minimal.
   - Neurogenic shock
     - **Neurogenic shock (secondary to loss of sympathetic tone) can be differentiated from hypovolemic shock based on the presence of relative bradycardia in neurogenic shock.**
       - Selective vasopressors are effective in neurogenic shock.
   - Hypovolemic shock
     - The physiologic state of loss of intravascular volume leading to hypotension and tachycardia
       - Swan-Ganz monitoring is helpful in the setting of spine trauma because neurogenic and hypovolemic shock often occur concurrently.
       - Hypovolemic shock is treated with fluid resuscitation.
3. Physical and neurologic examination
   - Secondary survey
     - Facial injuries, hypotension, and localized tenderness or spasm should be investigated.
     - Careful neurologic examination to document the lowest remaining functional level and to assess the patient for the possibility of sacral sparing (sparing of posterior column function, indicating an incomplete spinal cord injury) is essential (see Figure 8-1).
       - The neurologic level, as defined by the standards of the American Spine Association, is the most cephalad level with normal bilateral motor and sensory function.
4. Radiographic evaluation
   - Radiographs
     - Complete cervical spine series (C1-T1)
       - Multiple-level injuries occur in 10% to 20% of cases.
       - Assess radiographic lines for continuity.
         - Anterior spinal line
         - Posterior spinal line
         - Spinolaminar line
         - Anterior soft tissue shadows
           - At C2: 6 mm
           - At C6: 20 mm
     - Oblique views to investigate facet subluxation, dislocations, or fractures
   - CT
     - Replacing plain radiography as the initial imaging study in most trauma centers
     - Highly sensitive and more easily obtained than appropriate cervical spine radiographs in most cases
       - Sagittal views detect 85% of cervical spine fractures.
     - CT is useful for evaluating C1 fractures and assessing bone in the canal but may miss an axial plane fracture (type II odontoid).
   - MRI
     - Has advantages for demonstrating soft tissue abnormalities:
       - Posterior ligamentous disruption
       - Disc herniation
       - Canal compromise
       - Spinal cord trauma
       - Increasingly used in cervical spine "clearance"
5. Cord injuries (Figure 8-4)
   - Mechanism
     - Most cord injury is due to contusion or compression, not transection.
     - Sustained cord compression can lead to secondary injury and may result in more limited functional recovery.
   - Complete
     - No function below a given level
     - With complete injuries, an improvement of one nerve root level can be expected in 80% of the patients, and approximately 20% recover two functioning root levels.

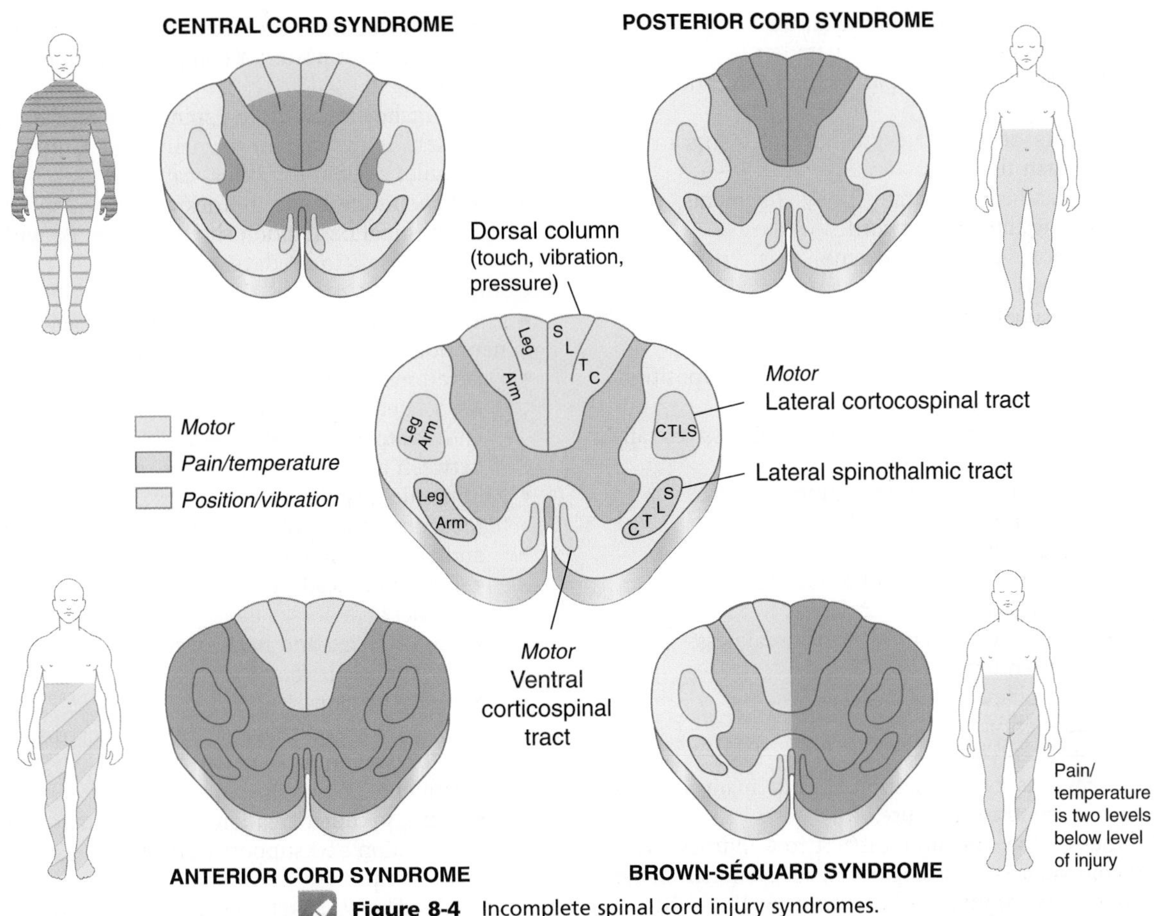

Figure 8-4 Incomplete spinal cord injury syndromes.

- Incomplete
  - Defined as some sparing of distal motor or sensory function
  - Three important generalizations regarding prognosis:
    - The greater the sparing, the greater recovery.
    - The more rapid the recovery, the greater recovery.
    - When recovery plateaus, no further recovery will happen.
  - Anatomic classification of incomplete spinal cord injury (Table 8-4)
    - **Central cord syndrome**
      - Most common
      - Presents as upper greater than lower extremity motor and sensory loss
      - Often seen in patients with preexisting cervical spondylosis who sustain a hyperextension injury
      - Cord is compressed anteriorly by osteophytes and posteriorly by the infolded ligamentum flavum.
      - Cord is injured in the central gray matter, resulting in proportionately greater loss of motor function to the upper extremities than to the lower extremities.
      - Variable sensory sparing
      - Independent ambulation is regained in approximately half of elderly patients and almost always in young patients.
    - Anterior cord syndrome
      - The second most common incomplete cord injury

Table 8-4 Spinal Cord Injury Syndromes

Syndrome	Pathology	Characteristics	Prognosis
Central	Age >50, extension injuries	Affects upper >lower extremities; motor and sensory loss	Fair
Anterior	Flexion-compression	Incomplete motor and some sensory loss	Poor
Brown-Séquard	Penetrating trauma	Loss of ipsilateral motor function, contralateral pain, and temperature sensation	Best
Root	Foramina compression/herniated nucleus pulposus	Based on level (weakness)	Good
Complete	Burst/canal compression	No function below injury level	Poor

  - Damage is primarily in the anterior two thirds of the cord.
  - Posterior columns spared (proprioception and vibratory sensation)
  - Patients demonstrate greater motor loss in the legs than the arms.
  - CT may demonstrate bony fragments compressing the anterior cord.
  - Anterior cord syndrome has the worst prognosis.
- Brown-Séquard syndrome
  - Damage to half of the cord
  - Ipsilateral motor loss, loss of position/proprioception
  - Contralateral pain and temperature loss (usually two levels below the insult)
  - Usually the result of penetrating trauma
  - Best prognosis
- Single-root lesions
  - Can occur at the level of a fracture
  - Typically at the C5 or C6 level
    - Leading to deltoid or biceps weakness
  - Most often unilateral

6. Treatment—See Chapter 11, Trauma.
   - Medical treatment
     - High-dose methylprednisolone
       - Efficacy has been questioned, and many centers have discontinued its use.
       - Indicated for cord injuries (not root injuries) with accompanying neurologic deficit (National Acute Spinal Cord Injury Studies [NASCIS] II and III)
         - Relative contraindications
           - Pregnancy
           - Age younger than 13 years
           - Concomitant infection
           - Penetrating spinal wounds
           - Uncontrolled diabetes
         - Gastrointestinal prophylaxis should be given.
   - Other treatment
     - Immobilization
       - Stable, nondisplaced fractures
         - Hard collar
       - Unstable, displaced fractures
         - Skeletal traction
         - Halo vest
         - Surgery for unstable fractures
     - Skeletal traction
       - Used acutely to realign the spine in the presence of a displaced fracture with or without neurologic injury
       - Requires the placement of Gardner-Wells tongs
         - Pins parallel to the external auditory meatus
         - Addition of 5 to 10 pounds initially
         - 5 to 7 additional pounds per cervical level up to body weight
         - Sequential radiographs after weight added
     - Surgery
       - Anterior decompression for incomplete injuries with persistent cord compression can lead to improvement of one to three levels, even with complete injuries. Also, stabilization may be indicated.
       - Late decompression for up to 1 year may be effective in improving root return.
       - Laminectomies are contraindicated except in the rare case of posterior compression from a fractured lamina.
       - Gunshot injury to the spine is treated surgically if there is progression of neurologic injury or if the bullet rests in the spinal canal.
       - Penetrating spine injuries accompanied by gastrointestinal perforation should be treated with antibiotics for 7 to 14 days.
7. Complications
   - Potentially negative outcomes are numerous and include neurologic injury, nonunion, and malunion.
   - Delayed instability
     - Associated with greater than 3.5 mm of subluxation and greater than 11 degrees of difference in angulation between adjacent motion segments
   - Autonomic dysreflexia
     - Most commonly follows spinal cord injuries above T6 and encompasses a constellation of symptoms
       - Pounding headache (from severe hypertension)
       - Anxiety
       - Profuse head and neck sweating
       - Nasal obstruction
       - Blurred vision
     - Most commonly triggered by bladder distension or fecal impaction
     - Treatment
       - Urinary catheterization or amelioration of rectal impaction and supportive treatment usually relieve the symptoms.
8. Prognosis—The Frankel classification is useful when assessing functional recovery from spinal cord injury (Table 8-5).

E. Sports-related cervical spine injuries

1. Burner (stinger) syndrome
   - Commonly associated with stretching of the upper brachial plexus by bending the neck away from the depressed shoulder or neck extension toward the painful shoulder in the setting of foraminal stenosis (root irritation)
   - Symptoms include burning dysesthesia and weakness in the involved extremity.
   - Fracture or acute HNP should be ruled out.
   - The athlete with a neck injury should be further evaluated for cervical pain, tenderness, or persisting neurologic symptoms.
2. Transient quadriplegia
   - Usually seen after axial load injury (spearing) but may also be seen after forced hyperextension or hyperflexion

Table 8-5 Frankel Classification of Cervical Spine Injuries

Frankel Grade	Function
A	Complete paralysis
B	Sensory function only below injury level
C	Incomplete motor function (grades 1-2 of 5) below injury level
D	Fair to good (useful) motor function (grades 3-4 of 5) below injury level
E	Normal function (grade 5 of 5)

- Presents as bilateral burning paresthesia and weakness or paralysis
- Risk factors
  - Cervical stenosis
  - Torg ratio less than 0.8
  - Preexisting instability
  - HNP
  - Congenital fusions
- The third and fourth cervical levels are the most commonly affected.
- It has no definitive association with future permanent neurologic injury.
- Patients with concurrent pathologic conditions, including instability, HNP, degenerative changes, and symptoms that last more than 36 hours, should be prohibited from participating in contact sports.

F. Other cervical spine disorders

1. Ankylosing spondylitis
   - Patients must be carefully evaluated for occult fracture because of the problem of pseudarthrosis and progressive kyphotic deformity.
   - Chin-on-chest deformity
     - Inability to look straight ahead
     - Associated with severe hip flexion contractures
     - Flexion deformity of the lumbar spine
   - Treatment
     - Correction of hip and lumbar disorder first
     - May require cervicothoracic laminectomy, osteotomy, and fusion for correction of the neck deformity
       - Procedure performed under local anesthesia with brief general anesthesia
       - Postoperative immobilization is carried out in a halo cast.

III. THORACIC/LUMBAR SPINE

A. Differential diagnosis—The physical examination, imaging studies, and laboratory tests assist with the differential diagnosis (Table 8-6).

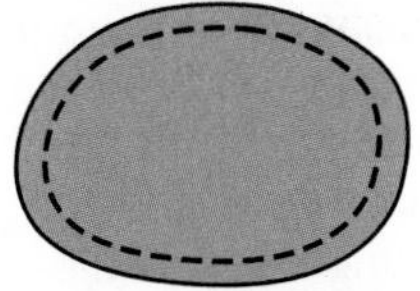

A **Diffuse Disc Bulge**

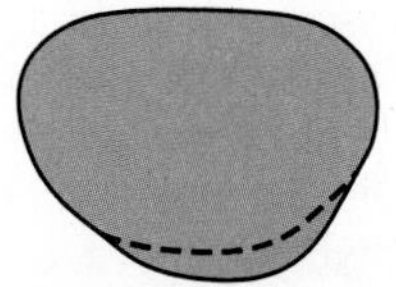

B **Broad-Based Protrusion** (or focal disc bulge)

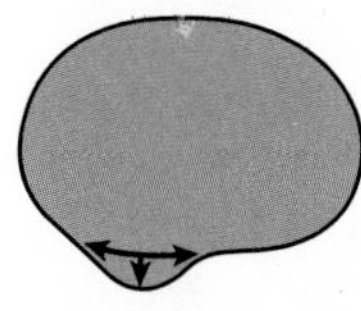

C **Focal Disc Protrusion** AP < Mediolateral dimension

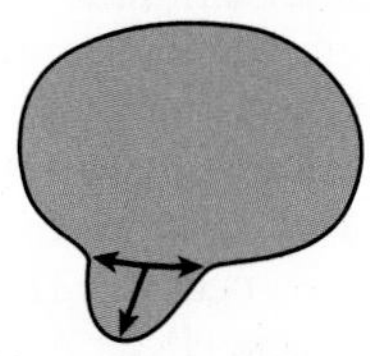

D **Disc Extrusion** AP ≥ Mediolateral dimension

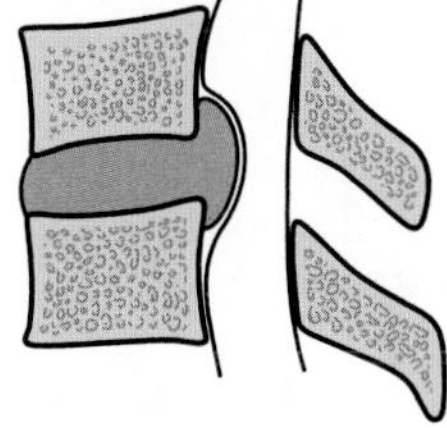

E **Disc Extrusion** Disc migrates above and/or below parent disc, maintaining continuity with it

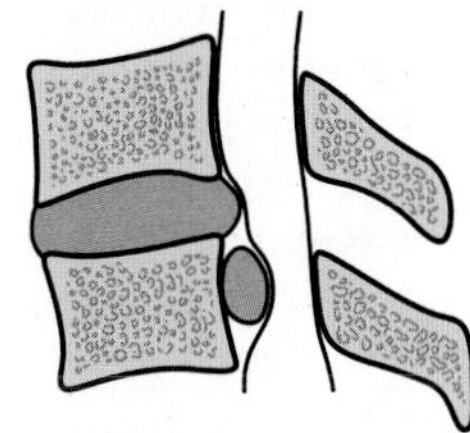

F **Sequestered Disc** Separate from parent disc

Figure 8-5 Types of disc herniation.

B. Herniated nucleus pulposus (HNP)

1. Pathophysiology
   - Disc degeneration
     - Aging results in loss of water content
     - Tearing of the annulus
     - Myxomatous changes, resulting in herniation of nuclear material
   - Disc herniation (Figure 8-5)

Table 8-6 Differential Diagnosis of Disorders in the Lumbar Spine

	DISORDER						
Parameter	HNP	Spinal Stenosis	Spondylolisthesis/ Instability	Tumor	Spondyloarthropathy	Metabolic Abnormality	Infection
Predominant pain (leg vs. back)	Leg	Leg	Back	Back	Back	Back	Back
Constitutional symptoms				+	+		+
Tension sign	+						
Neurologic examination		+	+ After stress				
Plain radiographic studies		+	+	±	+	+	±
Lateral motion radiographic studies				+			
CT	+	+		+			+
Myelogram	+	+					
Bone scan				+	+	+	+
ESR				+	+		+
Ca/P/alk phos				+			

Modified from Weinstein JN, Wiesel SW: *The lumbar spine,* Philadelphia, 1990, WB Saunders, 1990, p 360.

Ca/P/alk phos, calcium, phosphorus, alkaline phosphatase; CT, computed tomography; ESR, erythrocyte sedimentation rate; HNP, herniated nucleus pulposus; +, present; ±, present or absent.

- Discs can protrude (bulging nucleus, intact annulus).
- Disc extrusion (through the annulus but confined by the posterior longitudinal ligament)
- Disc sequestration (disc material free in canal).
- HNP usually a disease of young and middle-aged adults; in older patients the nucleus desiccates and is less likely to herniate

2. Thoracic disc disease
   - Epidemiology
     - Relatively uncommon (1% of all surgical HNPs)
     - Typically involves the middle to lower thoracic levels
       - Most herniations occur at T11 to T12.
       - 75% occur at T8 to T12.
     - Thoracic HNP can be divided into central, posterolateral, and lateral herniations.
     - Underlying Scheuermann disease may predispose patients to develop HNP.
   - Diagnosis
     - Presents as the onset of back or chest pain
     - May include radicular symptoms
       - Bandlike chest or abdominal discomfort, numbness, paresthesias, leg pain
     - Myelopathy may be present.
       - Sensory changes, paraparesis, bowel/bladder/sexual dysfunction
     - Physical findings may be difficult to elicit
       - Localized tenderness
       - Dermatomal sensory changes
       - Upper motor neuron signs with leg hyperreflexia, weakness, and normal upper extremity findings
       - Abnormal rectal examination
     - Imaging
       - Radiographs may show disc narrowing and calcification or osteophytic lipping.
       - CT myelography or MRI should demonstrate thoracic HNP.
       - MRI is useful for ruling out cord disorder, but there is a high false-positive rate, requiring close clinical correlation (Figure 8-6).

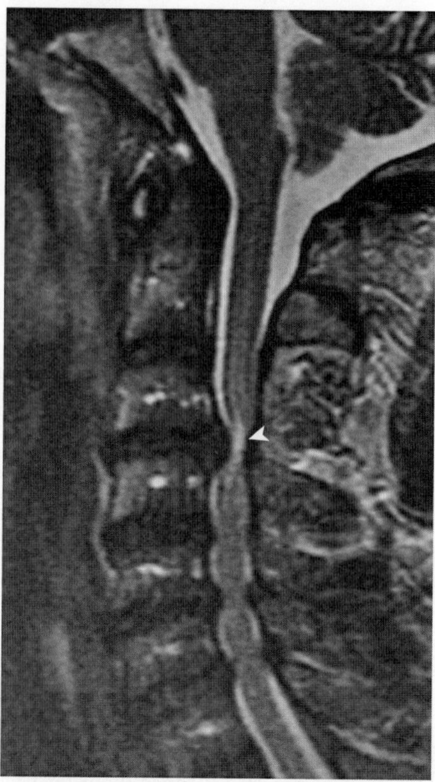

Figure 8-6 Disc-related myelopathy. Fast T2-weighted sagittal image of the cervical spine. The C3-C4 disc is protruding into the spinal canal, and there is compression of the cord with high signal within it *(arrowhead)*. The cord abnormality is the result of cord ischemia with myelomalacia. The discs are protruding to a lesser extent at lower levels, causing multilevel canal stenosis.

   - Treatment
     - Immobilization, analgesics, and nerve blocks are sometimes helpful for radiculopathy.
     - Surgery
       - Usually performed through an anterior transthoracic approach for midline or central HNP (including anterior discectomy and hemicorpectomy as needed)
       - Transpedicular approach for lateral HNP
       - Indicated in the presence of myelopathy or persistent, unremitting radicular pain
       - Thoracoscopic discectomy can also be employed.
       - Posterior approach (laminectomy)
         - Contraindicated because of the high rate of neurologic injury

3. Lumbar disc disease
   - Introduction—A major cause of morbidity with a major financial impact in the United States, this disc disease:
     - Usually involves the L4 to L5 disc (the "backache disc"), followed closely by L5 to S1.
     - Most herniations are posterolateral (where the posterior longitudinal ligament is the weakest) and may present as back pain and nerve root pain/sciatica involving the lower nerve root at that level (L5 at the L4-L5 level).
       - Herniations lateral to the neural foramen involve the upper nerve root.
     - Central prolapse is often associated with back pain only; however, acute insults may precipitate a cauda equina compression syndrome (Figure 8-7).

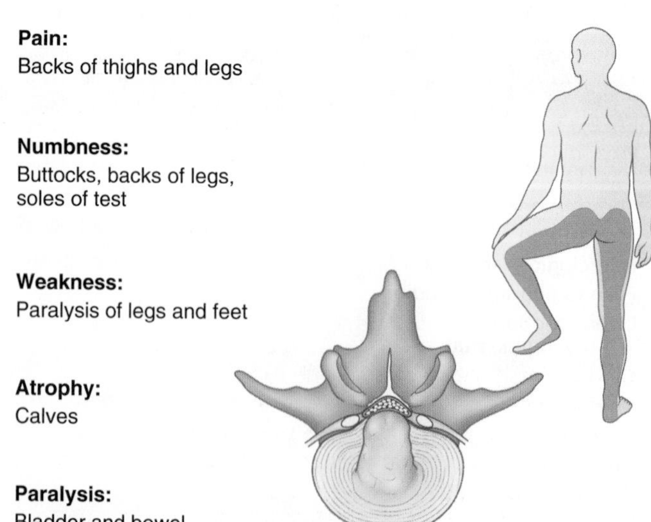

Figure 8-7 Cauda equina syndrome. (From Herkowitz HW, et al: *Rothman-Simeone the spine*, ed 6, Philadelphia, 2011, Elsevier.)

Table 8-7 Findings in Lumbar Disc Disease

Level	Nerve Root	Sensory Loss	Motor Loss	Reflex Loss
L1-L3	L2, L3	Anterior thigh	Hip flexors	None
L3-L4	L4	Medial calf	Quadriceps, tibialis anterior	Knee jerk
L4-L5	L5	Lateral calf, dorsal foot	EDL, EHL	None
L5-S1	S1	Posterior calf, plantar foot	Gastrocnemius/soleus	Ankle jerk
S2-S4	S2, S3, S4	Perianal	Bowel/bladder	Cremasteric

EDL, extensor digitorum longus; EHL, extensor hallucis longus.

- This syndrome is a surgical emergency that usually presents as bilateral buttock and lower extremity pain as well as bowel or bladder dysfunction (usually urinary retention), saddle anesthesia, and varying degrees of loss of lower extremity motor or sensory function.
- Digital rectal examination and evaluation of perianal sensation are important for the immediate diagnosis.
- Immediate MRI and surgery (if the test results are positive) are indicated to arrest progression of neurologic loss.
- Although the prognosis for recovery is guarded in most cases, surgical decompression within the first 48 hours was reported to lead to best outcomes.

- Patient history
  - History of an acute injury or precipitating event should be investigated.
  - Location of symptoms (especially pain radiating to the extremity)
  - Character of pain—referred pain in mesodermal tissues of the same embryologic origin
    - Localizes to buttocks or posterior thighs
    - Must be differentiated from true radicular pain due to nerve root impingement (typically distal to the knee)
  - Postural effects
    - Disc pathology leads to pain in flexion or sitting.
      - Flexion holding weight is worst.
    - Usually pain relieved in extension
      - Supine is best.
  - Complete review of symptoms (including psychiatric history)
    - The finding of an "inverted-**V**" triad of hysteria, hypochondriasis, and depression on the Minnesota Multiphasic Personality Inventory has been identified as a significant adverse risk factor for lumbar disc surgery.
    - Psychosocial evaluation, pain drawings, and psychological testing are helpful in some cases.
  - Occupational risks
    - Jobs requiring prolonged sitting and repetitive lifting
- Physical examination
  - Physical examination should include:
    - Observation (change in posture, gait)
    - Palpation of the posterior spine (spasm, localized tenderness)
    - Measurement of range of motion (decreased flexion)
    - Hip examination
    - Vascular evaluation (distal pulses)
    - Abdominal (bruits and pulsatile masses) and rectal examination
    - Neurologic evaluation (see Figure 8-1)
      - Tension signs such as straight-leg raising or the bowstring sign (L4-L5 or L5-S1) and the femoral nerve stretch test (L2-L3 or L3-L4) are critical findings that suggest HNP and are important when discectomy is considered.
      - A positive contralateral straight-leg raising test (pain in the affected buttock/leg when the opposite leg is raised) is the most specific test for HNP.
      - A large central disc herniation at one level may impinge on more than one nerve root.
      - Specific findings by level are presented in Table 8-7.
    - Inappropriate signs and symptoms (Waddell) are also important to note.
      - Pain at the tip of the "tailbone"
      - Pain plus numbness
      - Giving way of the whole leg
    - Nonorganic physical signs
      - Tenderness with light touch in nonanatomic areas
      - Simulation (light axial loading)
      - Distraction testing
      - Pain with pelvic rotation
      - Negative sitting (and positive supine) straight-leg raising test
      - Regional nonanatomic disturbances (e.g., a stocking-glove distribution)
      - Overreaction
- Diagnostic tests
  - Plain radiography
    - **Indicated before proceeding with special tests to rule out other disorders, such as isthmic defects.**
    - **However, most plain radiographic findings are nonspecific and plain radiography can usually be deferred for 6 weeks.**
      - **"Red flag" symptoms warrant immediate radiographs.**
  - CT and myelography
    - These are effective when used as confirmatory studies.
    - CT is noninvasive and helpful for demonstrating bony stenosis and identifying lateral pathologic conditions.
    - Imaging of neural compression may be improved if combined with myelography.
  - MRI
    - As the neuroradiographic test of choice in most cases, it is superior for identifying cord disorders, neural tumors, and disc disorders.

        - Multiplanar views allow imaging of central, foraminal, and extraforaminal stenosis.
        - It can demonstrate the state of hydration of the discs and visualize the marrow of the vertebral bodies, thus representing an excellent modality to screen for tumor or infection.
        - False-positive findings are common (occurring in 35% of those younger than 40 years old and in 93% of those older than 60 years old) and therefore require correlation with the history and physical examination.
        - MRI with gadolinium is the best study for a recurrent HNP.
    - Other testing
        - Electromyography and nerve conduction velocity testing (which demonstrate fibrillations 3 weeks after nerve root pressure) are not usually helpful and rarely provide more information than a good physical examination.
- Treatment
    - Nonoperative treatment
        - More than half of the patients who seek treatment for low back pain recover in 1 week, and 90% recover within 1 to 3 months.
        - Half of the patients with sciatica recover in 1 month.
        - Activity modification
            - Instruction should include avoiding rotation and flexion to avoid the increased disc pressure associated with these activities.
            - Progressive ambulation is successful in returning most patients to their normal function.
            - Bed rest is shown to be no more effective than continued normal activity in terms of patient improvement.
        - NSAIDs
        - Moist heat
        - This treatment is followed by back rehabilitation and a fitness program.
        - Aerobic conditioning and education are the most important factors in avoiding missed workdays due to disc disease and returning patients to work.
        - Failure of nonoperative therapy
            - If patients fail to improve within 6 weeks of conservative care, further evaluation is indicated.
            - Those patients with predominantly low back pain may require bone scan, MRI, and medical workup to rule out spinal tumors or infection.
                - If these study results are normal, back rehabilitation will continue.
            - In patients who have predominantly leg pain (sciatica) and in whom conservative therapy fails, a trial of lumbar epidural steroids may be helpful in 40% to 60% of patients.
            - Additional studies (MRI) are performed in patients who after 6 to 12 weeks continue to be symptomatic with pain, neurologic deficits, and positive nerve tension signs.
            - As a rule, these studies are preoperative tests and should be done to confirm clinical suspicions.
    - Surgical discectomy
        - Patients with positive study results, neurologic findings, tension signs, and predominantly sciatic symptoms without mitigating psychosocial factors are the best candidates for surgical discectomy.
        - Standard partial laminotomy and discectomy are the most commonly performed surgical procedures.
        - Operative positioning requires the abdomen to be free to decrease pressure on the inferior vena cava and consequently on the epidural veins.
    - Outcomes **(SPORT trial)**
        - At 2-year follow-up there were no significant differences in primary outcome measures for operative compared with nonoperative groups.
            - SF-36 Bodily Pain and Physical Function
            - Oswestry Disability Index
        - Trends favoring surgical intervention in primary outcome measures
        - Statistically significant improvement in secondary outcome measures for surgical intervention
            - Sciatica bothersomeness
            - Self-rated improvement
        - Patient prognosis depends on the anatomy of the disc at surgery, with recurrence rates being higher for patients with massive posterior annulus loss or without a contained defect (20%-40%).
        - Contained disc defects or disc fissuring correlates with better clinical outcomes and lower recurrence of symptoms (1%-10%).
        - Workers' compensation patients are more likely to continue to receive disability compensation and have worse symptoms, functional status, and satisfaction outcomes.
    - Minimally invasive surgical treatment
        - Percutaneous discectomy currently has limited indications in the treatment of lumbar disc disease, with no long-term follow-up studies proving its efficacy.
            - It is contraindicated in the presence of a sequestered fragment or spinal stenosis.
        - Endoscopic discectomy does allow direct visualization and can address sequestered fragments and lateral recess stenosis.
        - Intradiscal enzyme therapy has fallen out of favor because of its questionable efficacy and serious complications.
            - Anaphylaxis and transverse myelitis
- Complications—fortunately rare, but can be devastating
    - Vascular injury—may occur during attempts at disc removal if curets are allowed to penetrate the anterior longitudinal ligament
        - Intraoperative pulsatile bleeding due to deep penetration is treated with rapid wound closure, intravenous administration of fluids and blood, repositioning the patient, and a transabdominal approach to find and stop the source of bleeding.
        - Mortality may exceed 50%.
        - Late sequelae of vascular injuries may include delayed hemorrhage, pseudoaneurysm, and arteriovenous fistula formation.
    - Nerve root injury—more common with anomalous nerve roots
    - Failed back syndrome—often the result of poor patient selection; other causes include:

- Recurrent herniation (usually acute recurrence of signs/symptoms after a 6- to 12-month pain-free interval)
- Herniation at another level
- Unrecognized lateral stenosis (may be the most common)
- Vertebral instability
- Epidural fibrosis occurs at about 3 months postoperatively and may be associated with back or leg pain.
  - It responds poorly to re-exploration.
  - Scarring can be differentiated from recurrent HNP with a gadolinium-enhanced MRI.
- Dural tear—1% to 4% incidence
  - Primary repair necessary to avoid the development of a pseudomeningocele or spinal fluid fistula
  - More common during revision surgery
  - Fibrin adhesive sealant may be a useful adjunct for effecting dural closure.
  - Bed rest and subarachnoid drain placement are advocated if cerebrospinal fluid leak is suspected postoperatively.
  - If tear is adequately repaired, clinical outcomes are generally unaffected.
- **Wound infection (approximately 1% in open discectomy)**
  - **Increased risk in diabetics**
- Discitis (3-6 weeks postoperatively, with rapid onset of severe back pain)
  - MRI best diagnostic modality
  - Needle biopsy followed by empiric use of antibiotics
  - Surgery usually not needed
- Cauda equina syndrome—secondary to extruded disc, surgical trauma, and hematoma
  - It should be suspected with postoperative urinary retention.
  - Digital rectal examination is used for the initial diagnosis.

C. **Discogenic back pain**

1. Diagnosis
   - Paucity of physical findings
   - Back pain greater than leg pain
   - No radiculopathy
     - Negative tension signs
   - Radiographs are negative for instability but may show disc space narrowing or other stigmata of spondylosis.
   - MRI reveals decreased signal intensity in the disc space on T2 weighting (dark disc).
   - Discography is a useful preoperative study to correlate MRI findings with a clinically significant pain generator.
     - The study should be performed at multiple levels to include all abnormal levels and one or more normal levels on MRI.
     - To be considered reliably positive, the procedure should elicit pain after injection similar to that usually described by the patient (concordant pain) and should involve at least one minimally painful, nonconcordant level.
2. Treatment
   - Conservative treatment
     - **NSAIDs, physical therapy, and conditioning**
   - Interbody fusion
     - If extended nonoperative treatment has failed and the patient has a positive MRI and discogram, interbody fusion can be performed from either an anterior or a retroperitoneal approach or through a posterior midline (posterior lumbar) or posterior transforaminal lumbar interbody fusion approach.
     - Fusion is performed with structural constructs (femoral ring allografts or interbody fusion cages) in the disc space.
   - Intradiscal electrothermy—involves percutaneously heating the fibers of the annulus fibrosus to reconfigure the collagen fibers, thus restoring the mechanical integrity of the disc.
     - This may be effective in early conditions (<50% loss of disc height) but not in more advanced disease
     - Long-term follow-up suggests that symptomatic improvement often lasts less than 1 year, and this procedure has been largely abandoned.
   - Total disc arthroplasty
     - Another surgical option for patients with degenerative disc disease at a single level (L4-S1) in the lumbar spine with the absence of spondylolisthesis and no relief from 6 months of nonoperative therapy
     - In direct comparison with anterior interbody fusion, total disc arthroplasty showed equivalent clinical results and no catastrophic failures at 2-year follow-up.
     - Significant concerns include long-term results, design issues, cost, and the safety of revision procedures.

D. **Lumbar segmental instability—present when normal loads produce abnormal spinal motion**

1. Diagnosis
   - The most common symptom is mechanical back pain, although "dynamic" stenosis can occur, leading to radicular symptoms.
   - The most consistent clinical sign is the "instability catch" (sudden, painful catch with extension from a flexed position).
   - Degenerative lumbar disc disease is indicated by disc space narrowing.
   - A combination of annulus damage and disc space narrowing may reduce the disc's ability to resist rotatory forces.
   - Continuing degeneration or facet subluxation may then lead to instability.
   - Radiographic findings
     - Traction spurs (horizontal and below disc margin),
     - Angular changes greater than 10 degrees (20 degrees at L5-S1) on flexion films
     - Translational motion greater than 3-4 mm (6 mm at L5-S1) with flexion-extension views are characteristic of lumbar instability but are difficult to quantify and may not correlate with clinical symptoms.
     - Progressive subluxation or deformity after decompressive surgery can occur after removal of one or more facet joints.
2. Treatment
   - Surgical treatment options do not have clearly defined indications, but posterolateral fusion is the standard treatment.

- The use of pedicle screw instrumentation is well established, with fusion rates approaching 90% in nonsmokers for one- or two-level fusions.
- The anatomic landmark for pedicle screw insertion in the lumbar spine is the junction of the transverse process, pars intra-articularis, and lateral aspect of the superior articular facet.
- Pseudarthrosis (5%-35%)
- Adjacent-level degeneration can occur in these patients.
  - In large studies, the rates of symptomatic degeneration at an adjacent spinal level are 15% at 5 years and about 40% at 10 years, with no correlation with the number of levels fused or preoperative degeneration.
- In achieving fusion, a posterior iliac crest bone graft is the gold standard and is associated with a significantly lower risk of postoperative complications than an anterior iliac crest bone graft.
  - Up to 30% of patients have persistent postoperative pain at the graft site.
  - Graft alternatives:
    - BMP2 (Infuse)—U.S. Food and Drug Administration–approved indication is in single-level anterior interbody fusion.
    - Several studies have shown equivalent fusion rates between BMP2 and an iliac crest bone graft in instrumented posterolateral fusions.
- The use of NSAIDs, including aspirin and ketorolac (Toradol) has been shown to decrease spinal fusion rates.
  - Cyclooxygenase-2 inhibitors have not been shown to have the same inhibitory effect.
- **The use of alendronate has been shown to decrease spinal fusion rates in animal models**
  - Administration should be held in the postoperative period.

E. **Spinal stenosis (Figure 8-8)**

1. Introduction—Spinal stenosis is narrowing of the spinal canal or neural foramina, producing nerve root compression, root ischemia, and a variable syndrome of back and leg pain.
   - Central stenosis—thecal sac compression
     - The central canal is defined as the space posterior to the posterior longitudinal ligament, anterior to the ligamentum flavum and laminae, and bordered laterally by the medial border of the superior articular process.
     - Soft tissue structures, including the hypertrophied ligamentum flavum, facet capsule, and bulging disc, may contribute as much as 40% to thecal sac compression.
     - *Absolute stenosis* is defined as a cross-sectional area of less than 100 mm^2 or less than 10 mm of anteroposterior diameter as seen on CT cross section.
     - Central stenosis is more common in men because their spinal canal is smaller at the L3 to L5 levels than in women
     - It affects an older population more than lateral recess stenosis does.
   - Lateral recess stenosis—nerve root compression
     - The lateral recess is defined by the superior articular facet posteriorly, the thecal sac medially, the pedicle laterally, and the posterolateral vertebral body anteriorly.
     - It comprises compression of individual nerve roots by the medial overgrowth of the superior articular facet at a given facet joint.
   - Foraminal stenosis—nerve root compression
     - The intervertebral foramen is bordered superiorly and inferiorly by the adjacent level pedicles, posteriorly by the facet joint and lateral extensions of the ligamentum flavum, and anteriorly by the adjacent vertebral bodies and disc.
     - Normal foraminal height is 20 to 30 mm; superior width is 8 to 10 mm.
   - Stenosis usually is not symptomatic until patients reach late middle age; men are affected somewhat more often than women.
   - "Tandem stenosis" is the occurrence of both cervical and lumbar stenosis that often presents as both neurogenic claudication and myelopathy.
2. Central stenosis
   - Etiology—congenital versus acquired
     - Congenital (idiopathic or developmental in achondroplastic dwarfs)
     - Acquired stenosis (most common) is usually:
       - Degenerative owing to enlargement of osteoarthritic facets with medial encroachment
       - Degenerative due to spondylolisthesis
       - Post-traumatic
       - Iatrogenic (postsurgical)
       - Secondary to systemic disease processes
         - Paget disease
         - Ankylosing spondylitis
         - Acromegaly
         - Fluorosis
   - Patient history and physical examination
     - Symptoms include insidious pain and paresthesias with ambulation or prolonged standing and are relieved by sitting or with flexion of the spine.
     - Patients commonly complain of lower extremity pain, usually in the buttock and thigh, with numbness or "giving way."
     - Although typical with HNP, a history of radiating leg pain in a true dermatomal distribution is relatively uncommon in those with spinal stenosis.
     - Neurogenic claudication
       - Occurs in about 50% of patients
       - To differentiate from vascular claudication
         - Pain starts proximal (buttock) and extends distal.
         - Pain relieved only when sitting, not with standing
         - Normal vascular examination
     - Physical examination
       - Limited extension is primary finding.
         - May exacerbate pain
       - Normal extremity perfusion and pulses
       - Few neurologic findings
         - Abnormal neurologic examination is found in fewer than 50%.
         - Tension signs are rarely positive.

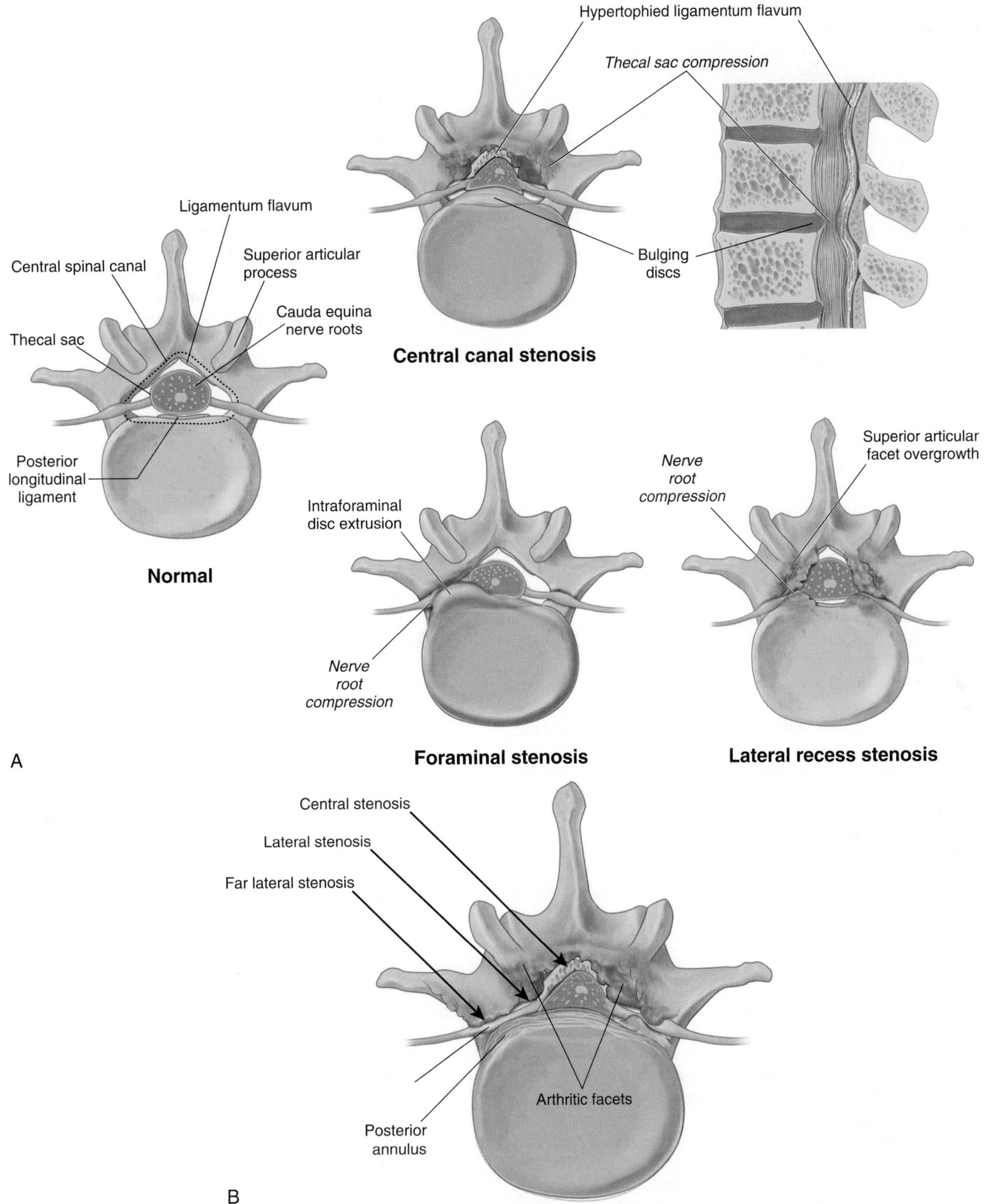

Figure 8-8 Pathoanatomy of spinal stenosis. Comparison of central, lateral/foraminal, and far lateral/lateral recess stenosis.

Table 8-8 Findings on Treadmill Tests in Neurogenic Claudication

	FINDING	
Activity	Vascular Claudication	Neurogenic Claudication
Walking	Distal-proximal pain, calf pain	Proximal-distal thigh pain
Uphill walking	Symptoms develop sooner	Symptoms develop later
Rest	Relief with sitting or bending	
Bicycling	Symptoms develop	Symptoms do not develop
Lying flat	Relief	May exacerbate symptoms

  - ▫ Standing treadmill tests can be a sensitive (>90%) provocative evaluation of neurogenic claudication (Table 8-8).
- ▪ Imaging—Further workup may include:
  - ▫ Plain radiographs
    - ▪ Interspace narrowing due to disc degeneration
    - ▪ Medially placed facets
    - ▪ Flattening of the lordotic curve
    - ▪ Subluxation and degenerative changes of the facet joints may also be seen.
  - ▫ Plain CT
    - ▪ Osteophyte formation
    - ▪ Axial of axial canal morphology
  - ▫ MRI (test of choice)
    - ▪ Hypertrophy of ligamentum flavum
    - ▪ Foraminal stenosis and nerve root entrapment
    - ▪ Evaluation for malignancy
  - ▫ Electromyography/nerve conduction velocity testing may be used.
    - ▪ Sensitivity is variable and depends on the examiner.
    - ▪ Nerve conduction velocity testing is sometimes helpful in differentiating radiculopathy from peripheral neuropathy.
- ▪ Treatment
  - ▫ Nonoperative
    - ▪ Rest
    - ▪ Williams flexion exercises
    - ▪ NSAIDs
    - ▪ Weight reduction
    - ▪ Lumbar epidural steroids
      - ▫ Helpful for short-term relief but have shown variable results in controlled studies
      - ▫ Transforaminal nerve block can be effective when the involved roots can be identified and should be considered in most cases before moving to surgery.
  - ▫ Surgery
    - ▪ Indications
      - ▫ Positive study results and a persistent, unacceptably impaired quality of life.
    - ▪ Techniques
      - ▫ **Adequate decompression of the identified disorder typically includes laminectomy and partial medial facetectomy, which can usually be done without destabilizing the spine, thus avoiding fusion.**
      - ▫ Residual foraminal stenosis is a common reason for persistent radicular pain after laminectomy
      - ▫ Indications for fusion
        - ▪ Surgical instability (removal of one facet or more)
        - ▪ Pars defects (including those that are postsurgical) with disc disease
        - ▪ Symptomatic radiographic instability
        - ▪ Degenerative or isthmic spondylolisthesis
        - ▪ Degenerative scoliosis
    - ▫ Outcomes **(SPORT trial)**
      - ▪ **At 4-year follow-up, significant improvement in primary outcome measures for operative compared with nonoperative groups**
        - ▫ SF-36 Bodily Pain and Physical Function
        - ▫ Oswestry Disability Index
      - ▪ Both operative and nonoperative groups had improvement from baseline.

3. Lateral recess stenosis
   - ▪ Etiology
     - ▫ Impingement of nerve roots lateral to the thecal sac as they pass through the lateral recess and into the neural foramen
     - ▫ Associated with facet joint arthropathy (superior articular process enlargement) and disc disease (Figure 8-8, *B*)
     - ▫ Subarticular compression consists of compression between the medial aspect of a hypertrophic superior articular facet and the posterior aspect of the vertebral body and disc.
       - ▪ Affects the traversing (lower) nerve root (L5 root at L4-L5)
     - ▫ Hypertrophy of the ligamentum flavum and/or ventral facet joint capsule and vertebral body osteophyte/disc exacerbates the stenosis.
   - ▪ Treatment
     - ▫ **After failure of nonoperative treatment, decompression of the hypertrophied lamina and ligamentum flavum and partial facetectomy are usually successful.**
     - ▫ Fusion may be necessary if instability is present or created.
     - ▫ Nerve root compression can occur at more than one level and must be completely decompressed to relieve the symptoms.
4. Foraminal stenosis
   - ▪ Etiology
     - ▫ Intraforaminal disc protrusion
     - ▫ Impingement of the tip of the superior facet
     - ▫ Uncinate spurring
     - ▫ Lower lumbar areas are usually involved because the foramina decrease in size as the size of the nerve root increases.
     - ▫ Foraminal stenosis affects the exiting (upper) root (L4 at L4-L5) at a motion segment.
     - ▫ Pain may be the result of intraneural edema and demyelination.
       - ▪ Substance P may be released as a response to irritation of the spinal nerve root.

F. Spondylolysis and spondylolisthesis

1. Spondylolysis—defect in the pars interarticularis

- One of the most common causes of low back pain in children and adolescents
- Fatigue fracture from repetitive hyperextension stresses
  - Most common in gymnasts and football linemen
  - Probable hereditary predisposition
- Imaging
  - Plain lateral radiographs demonstrate 80% of the lesions.
  - Another 15% are visible on oblique radiographs, which show a defect in the neck of the "Scottie dog."
  - CT, bone scanning, and (more recently) **single-photon emission computed tomography** (SPECT) may be helpful in identifying subtle defects.
    - Increased uptake on SPECT is more compatible with acute lesions that have the potential to heal.
- Treatment
  - Usually aimed at symptomatic relief rather than fracture healing in spondylolysis without spondylolisthesis
    - Activity restriction
    - Flexion exercises
    - Bracing.
    - Nonunion is common and may not show on scans.
- Prognosis
  - **Unilateral defects almost never progress to olisthesis.**

2. Spondylolisthesis—forward slippage of one vertebra on another
   - Etiology—six types (Newman, Wiltse, McNab) (Table 8-9; Figures 8-9 and 8-10)
   - Classification

Table 8-9 Types of Spondylolisthesis

Type	Age	Pathology/Other
I—Dysplastic	Child	Congenital dysplasia of S1 superior facet
II—Isthmic*	5-50 yr	Predisposition leading to elongation/fracture of pars (L5-S1)
III—Degenerative	>40 yr	Facet arthrosis leading to subluxation (L4-L5)
IV—Traumatic	Any age	Acute fracture other than pars
V—Pathologic	Any age	Incompetence of bony elements
VI—Postsurgical	Adult	Excessive resection of neural arches/facets

*Most common type.

- Severity—five grades according to severity (Meyerding); the severity of the slip is based on the amount or degree (compared with S1 width) (Figure 8-11)
  - Grade I: 0%-25%
  - Grade II: 25%-50%
  - Grade III: 50%-75%
  - Grade IV: greater than 75%
  - Grade V: greater than 100% (spondyloptosis)
- Other relevant measurements (see Figure 8-11)
  - Sacral inclination (normally >30 degrees)
  - Slip angle (normally <0 degrees, signifying lordosis at the L5-S1 disc)
    - Means for quantifying lumbopelvic deformity
    - Predicts intervention and affects cosmesis as well as prognosis
  - Pelvic incidence (normally 50 degrees)

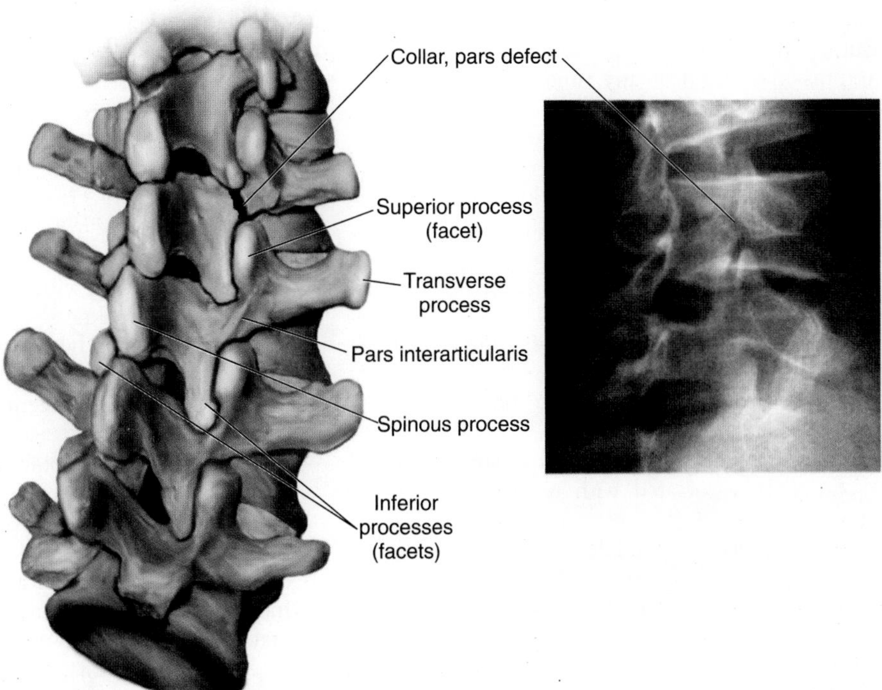

Figure 8-9 Spondylolysis. Note disruption of the neck of the "Scottie dog."

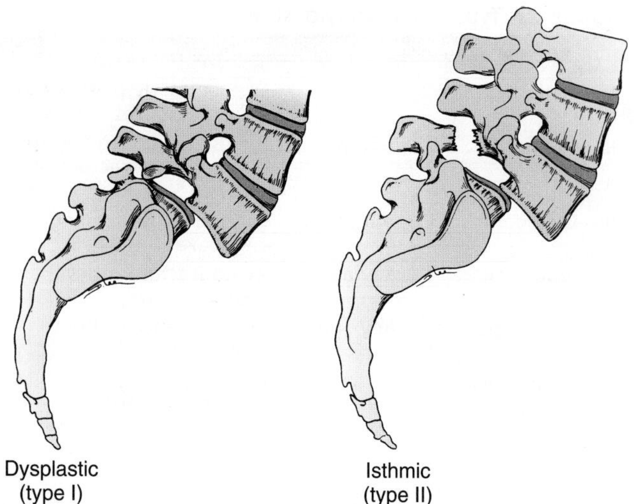

Figure 8-10 Comparison of dysplastic versus isthmic spondylolisthesis. (Adapted from Rothman RH, Simeone FA: *The spine,* ed 2, Philadelphia, 1982, WB Saunders, p 264.)

- The natural history of the disorder is that unilateral pars defects almost never slip and that the progression of spondylolisthesis slows over time.
- However, in adulthood, degeneration and narrowing of the disc (usually L5-S1) are common and lead to narrowing of the neural foramen and compression of the exiting (L5) root that causes the radicular symptoms.

3. Childhood spondylolisthesis
   - Presentation
     - Back pain (instability)
       - Patients with a greater than 25% slip, or with L4-L5 or L3-L4 spondylolisthesis have a higher risk of low back pain than the general population.
     - Hamstring tightness
     - Palpable step-off
     - Alteration in gait ("pelvic waddle")
     - Although symptoms may begin at any time in life, screening studies identify the slippage as occurring most commonly at age 4 to 6 years.
     - Severe slips are rare and may be associated with radicular findings (L5), cauda equina dysfunction, kyphosis of the lumbosacral junction, and "heart-shaped" buttocks.
   - Epidemiology
     - Usually at L5-S1 and typically grade II
     - Occurs most often in whites, boys, and children who participate in hyperextension activities
     - Remarkably frequent in some Eskimo tribes (>50%)
   - Etiology
     - It is thought to result from shear stress at the pars interarticularis and to be associated with repetitive hyperextension.
     - Patients with type I or dysplastic spondylolisthesis are at a higher risk for slip progression and the development of cauda equina dysfunction because the neural arch is intact.
     - Spina bifida occulta, thoracic hyperkyphosis, and Scheuermann disease have been associated with spondylolisthesis.
   - Treatment
     - Low-grade disease (<50% slip)
       - **Usually responds to nonoperative treatment consisting of activity modification and exercise**
         - Adolescents with a grade I slip may return to normal activities, including contact sports, once asymptomatic.
         - Those with asymptomatic grade II spondylolisthesis are restricted from activities such as gymnastics or football.
       - Risk factors for progression:
         - Young age at presentation
         - Female gender, a slip angle of greater than 10 degrees
         - High-grade slip
         - Dome-shaped or significantly inclined sacrum (>30 degrees beyond vertical position)
       - Surgery for patients with a low-grade slip generally consists of L5-S1 posterolateral fusion in situ and is usually reserved for those with intractable pain in whom nonoperative treatment has failed or those demonstrating progressive slippage.
       - Wiltse has popularized a paraspinal muscle–splitting approach to the lumbar transverse process and sacral alae that is frequently used in this setting.
       - L5 radiculopathy is uncommon in children with low-grade slips and rarely if ever requires decompression.
       - Repair of the pars defect with the use of a lag screw (Buck) or tension band wiring (Bradford) with bone grafting has been reported.
         - Indicated in young patients with slippage less than 10% and a pars defect at L4 or above
     - High-grade disease (grades III through V)
       - These commonly cause neurologic abnormalities.
       - L5-S1 isthmic spondylolisthesis causes an L5 radiculopathy (contrast to S1 radiculopathy in L5-S1 HNP).
       - Prophylactic fusion is recommended in growing children with slippage of more than 50%.
         - It often requires in situ bilateral posterolateral fusion, usually at L4 to S1 (L5 is too far anterior to effect L5-S1 fusion) with or without instrumentation.
         - Nerve root exploration is controversial but usually limited to children with clear-cut radicular pain or significant weakness.
         - Reduction of spondylolisthesis has been associated with a 20% to 30% incidence of L5 root injuries (most are transient) and should be used cautiously.
         - A cosmetically unacceptable deformity and L5-S1 kyphosis so severe that the posterior fusion mass from L4 to the sacrum would be under tension without reversal of the kyphosis are the most commonly cited indications.
         - In situ fusion leaves a patient with a high-grade slip and lumbosacral kyphosis with such severe compensatory hyperlordosis above the fusion that long-term problems frequently ensue.

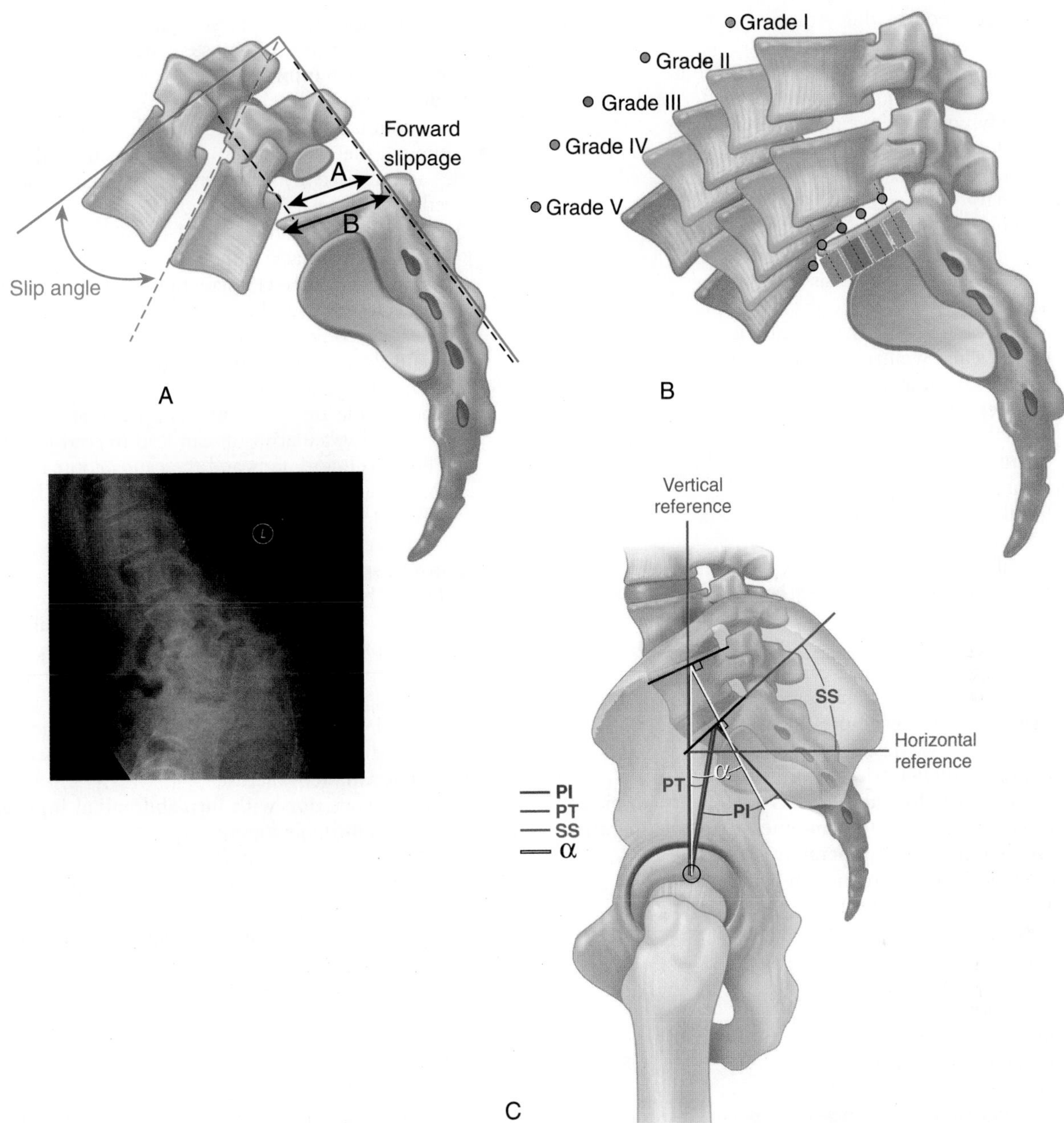

Figure 8-11 Spondylolisthesis. **A, Slip angle** and percentage of forward slippage. The slip angle is measured from the superior border of L5 and a perpendicular line from the posterior edge of the sacrum. **B, Meyerding grades I to V.** The grade of spondylolisthesis is determined by dividing the sacral body into four segments, with grade V as spondyloptosis. **C, Pelvic incidence (PI).** A line perpendicular to the midpoint of the sacral end-plate is drawn. A second line connecting the same sacral midpoint and the center of the femoral heads is drawn. The angle subtended by these lines is the pelvic incidence. Should the femoral heads not be superimposed, the center of each femoral head is marked, and the point halfway between the two centers serves as the femoral head center. **Pelvic tilt (PT).** A line from the midpoint of the sacral end-plate is drawn to the center of the femoral heads. The angle subtended between this line and the vertical reference line is the pelvic tilt. **Sacral slope (SS).** A line parallel to the sacral end-plate is drawn. The angle subtended between this line and the horizontal reference line is the sacral slope. **α angle—L5 incidence.** A line from the midpoint of the upper end-plate of L5 is connected to the center of the femoral heads. A second line perpendicular to the upper L5 end-plate is drawn from the midpoint of the end-plate. The angle subtended by these two lines (α) is the L5 incidence. (Modified from Herring J: *Tachdjian's pediatric orthopaedics*, ed 4, Philadelphia, 2007, Elsevier.)

- Reduction in this setting is gaining widespread acceptance.
- Close neurologic monitoring is needed during the procedure and for several days afterward to identify postoperative neuropathy.
- Posterior decompression, fibular interbody fusion, and posterolateral fusion without reduction have been reported, with excellent long-term results (Bohlman).
- Vertebrectomy and fusion for spondyloptosis

4. Degenerative spondylolisthesis
   - Epidemiology
     - More common in African Americans, persons with diabetes and women older than age 40
     - Most frequent at the L4-L5 level
     - It is reported to be more common in patients with transitional (sacralized) L5 vertebrae and sagittally oriented facet joints.
   - Presentation
     - Results in central and lateral recess stenosis with **L5 radiculopathy** owing to root compression in the lateral recess between the hypertrophic and subluxated inferior facet of L4 and the posterosuperior body of L5
   - Treatment
     - Nonoperative—same as for stenosis
     - The operative treatment for degenerative spondylolisthesis involves decompression of the nerve roots and stabilization by posterolateral fusion.
   - Outcomes **(SPORT trial)**
     - **At 4-year follow-up there is significant improvement in primary outcome measures for operative compared with nonoperative groups.**
       - SF-36 Bodily Pain and Physical Function
       - Oswestry Disability Index
     - Both operative and nonoperative groups had improvement from baseline.
5. Adult isthmic spondylolisthesis
   - Presentation
     - Low back pain
     - L5 radicular pain
   - Etiology
     - **Associated with an increased pelvic incidence**
       - As pelvic incidence increases, sacral slope increases, necessitating an increasing in lumbar lordosis to maintain sagittal balance
       - Normal subjects have a pelvic incidence of 50 to 55 degrees, whereas patients with spondylolisthesis have 70 to 80 degrees.
       - Pelvic incidence, however, does not predict progression of listhesis.
     - Pars defect
     - L5 radiculopathy
       - L5-S1 slips are most common, causing compression of exiting L5 nerve root by fibrous repair tissue at the site of the defect.
   - Treatment
     - Nonoperative
       - Hamstring stretching, core strengthening, lumbar flexion exercises
       - NSAIDs
     - Operative
       - Foraminal decompression
       - In situ L4 or L5-S1 posterolateral fusion

G. Thoracolumbar injuries

1. Introduction
   - Most common site for vertebral column injuries
   - Although the classification and treatment of these injuries is included in Chapter 11, Trauma, some points need to be emphasized here.
   - Anatomic considerations
     - The upper thoracic spine (T1 to T10) is stabilized by the ribs and the facet orientation as well as the sternum and is less susceptible to trauma.
     - The thoracolumbar junction is a transitional area from relatively rigid motion segments to relatively mobile segments.
     - The middle thoracic spine is a vascular "watershed" area, and vascular insult can lead to cord ischemia.
     - The spinal cord ends and the cauda equina begins at the level of L1-L2, so lesions below the L1 level have a better prognosis because the nerve roots (not the cord) are affected.
   - Gunshot spine fractures
     - **Typically stable injuries** and rarely require surgery
     - Patients with neurologic injury in cervical or thoracic spine do not benefit from operative decompression; lumbar deficits may benefit from bullet removal.
     - Surgical indications: acute lead intoxication, new-onset neurologic deficit, or intracanal copper bullet
   - **Pediatric Chance fractures**
     - **High association with intraabdominal injuries**
2. Stable versus unstable injuries
   - The three-column system (Denis) has been proposed for evaluating spinal injuries and determining which are stable and which unstable.
     - Anterior column—anterior longitudinal ligament and the anterior two thirds of the annulus and vertebral body
     - Middle column—posterior third of the body and annulus and the posterior longitudinal ligament
     - Posterior column—the pedicles, facets, spinous processes, and posterior ligamentous complex
       - Posterior ligamentous column includes interspinous and supraspinous ligaments, ligamentum flavum, and facet capsules.
   - There is only moderate reliability and repeatability of the Denis classification of spinal fractures.
   - Disruption of the middle column (seen as widening of the interpedicular distances on anteroposterior radiographs or a change in height of the posterior cortex of the body on lateral views) suggests an unstable injury that may require operative fixation.
   - In a lumbar burst fracture, the anterior and middle columns are compromised, potentially resulting in canal stenosis.
     - The burst fracture is a dynamic event, with maximum canal occlusion and neural element compression during the moment of impact.
     - In addition, disruption of the posterior ligamentous complex in the presence of anterior fracture or dislocation is a strong indication of instability and the potential need for surgical stabilization.

- Exceptions may include the upper thoracic spine, which is inherently more stable, and bony Chance fractures.
- Nonpathologic compression fractures of three sequential vertebrae lead to an increased risk of post-traumatic kyphosis.

3. Treatment
   - Nonoperative
     - **Fractures with less than 20 to 30 degrees of kyphosis, less than 50% loss of vertebral height, an intact posterior ligamentous column, and no neurologic compromise are usually treated nonoperatively.**
       - **Thoracolumbar orthosis or casting with serial radiographs to confirm maintenance of acceptable alignment**
     - Stable burst fractures are best treated nonoperatively.
     - The goals of surgery include stabilization of the fracture and preservation or improvement of neural function in all patients as well as more rapid entry into rehabilitation and a shorter hospital stay for patients with complete injuries.
     - Rehabilitation after spinal cord injury is discussed more fully in Chapter 10, Rehabilitation: Gait, Amputations, Prostheses, Orthoses, and Neurologic Injury.
   - Operative
     - Surgery is indicated in unstable fractures.
     - There is also increasing suggestion that some stable fractures should be fixed in the setting of polytrauma and neurologic injury.
       - Allows for early mobilization
       - Prevention of subsequent neurologic injury
     - **Operative intervention includes decompression for progressive neurologic deficit (emergency) or incomplete neurologic deficit.**
       - Accomplished anteriorly via vertebrectomy and stabilization or posteriorly via a transpedicular route
       - Historically, posterior instrumentation and fusion have extended three levels above and two levels below the injury to stabilize the fracture.
4. Complications
   - Short term
     - Respiratory failure is a significant problem for the multiply injured patient with a thoracolumbar fracture.
       - Multifactorial risks
       - Only independent risk factor under the surgeon's control is interval before surgery, which ideally is less than 48 hours.
   - Long-term complications of a thoracolumbar fracture, treated with or without surgery, are:
     - Chronic pain
       - The relationships among chronic pain, "stability," deformity, pseudarthrosis, and many other factors are unclear.
       - Post-traumatic syringomyelia (also results in progressive neurologic deterioration)
     - Post-traumatic deformity
       - Progressive kyphosis (common in unrecognized posterior ligamentous injury)
       - Symptomatic flat back of the lumbar spine results in a forward-flexed posture and easy fatigue (occurs with uncontoured distraction instrumentation).
       - Late development of a neuropathic spine (Charcot), with gross bony destruction and bony spicules in the soft tissue, has also been described.

H. Other thoracolumbar disorders

1. Destructive spondyloarthropathy
   - Seen in hemodialysis patients with chronic renal failure
   - Typically involves three adjacent vertebrae and two intervening discs
   - Changes include subluxation, degeneration, and narrowing of the disc height.
   - Although the process may resemble infection, it probably represents crystal or amyloid deposition.
2. **Diffuse idiopathic skeletal hyperostosis** (DISH)—also known as Forestier disease (Figure 8-12)
   - DISH is defined by the presence of **nonmarginal syndesmophytes** (differentiated from ankylosing spondylitis, which has marginal syndesmophytes) at three successive levels.
     - Syndesmophytes are vertical outgrowths that extend across the disc space and represent calcification of the anulus fibrosus and anterior and posterior longitudinal ligaments.
   - DISH can occur anywhere in the spine but usually in the thoracic region and is more often seen on the right side.
   - DISH is associated with chronic low back pain and is more common in patients with diabetes and gout.
   - The prevalence of DISH has been found to be as high as 28% in autopsy specimens.
   - DISH is associated with extraspinal ossification at several joints, including an increased risk of heterotopic ossification after total hip surgery.
3. Ankylosing spondylitis (see Figure 8-12)
   - 95% of patients with ankylosing spondylitis are positive for human leukocyte antigen–B27 (HLA-B27)
   - Usually young men present with the insidious onset of back and hip pain during the third or fourth decade of life.
   - Sacroiliac joint obliteration (iliac side affected first) and marginal syndesmophytes allow radiographic differentiation from DISH.
     - ***Bamboo spine*** is the descriptive term applied to multiple vertebral levels ankylosed by marginal syndesmophytes.
   - **May result in fixed kyphotic deformities leading to sagittal imbalance**
     - Extension osteotomy and fusion of the lumbar spine with compression instrumentation can successfully balance the head over the sacrum.
     - Assessment of the patient for hip flexion contractures or cervicothoracic kyphosis is mandatory.
     - The cervical spine may be corrected by a C7 to T1 osteotomy and fusion under local anesthesia.
     - The complications of osteotomy include nonunion, loss of correction, and neurologic and aortic injury.
   - It has multiple medical associations:
     - Anterior uveitis
     - Restrictive lung disease and pulmonary fibrosis
     - Aortic regurgitation and stenosis
     - Ileitis or colitis
4. Adult scoliosis

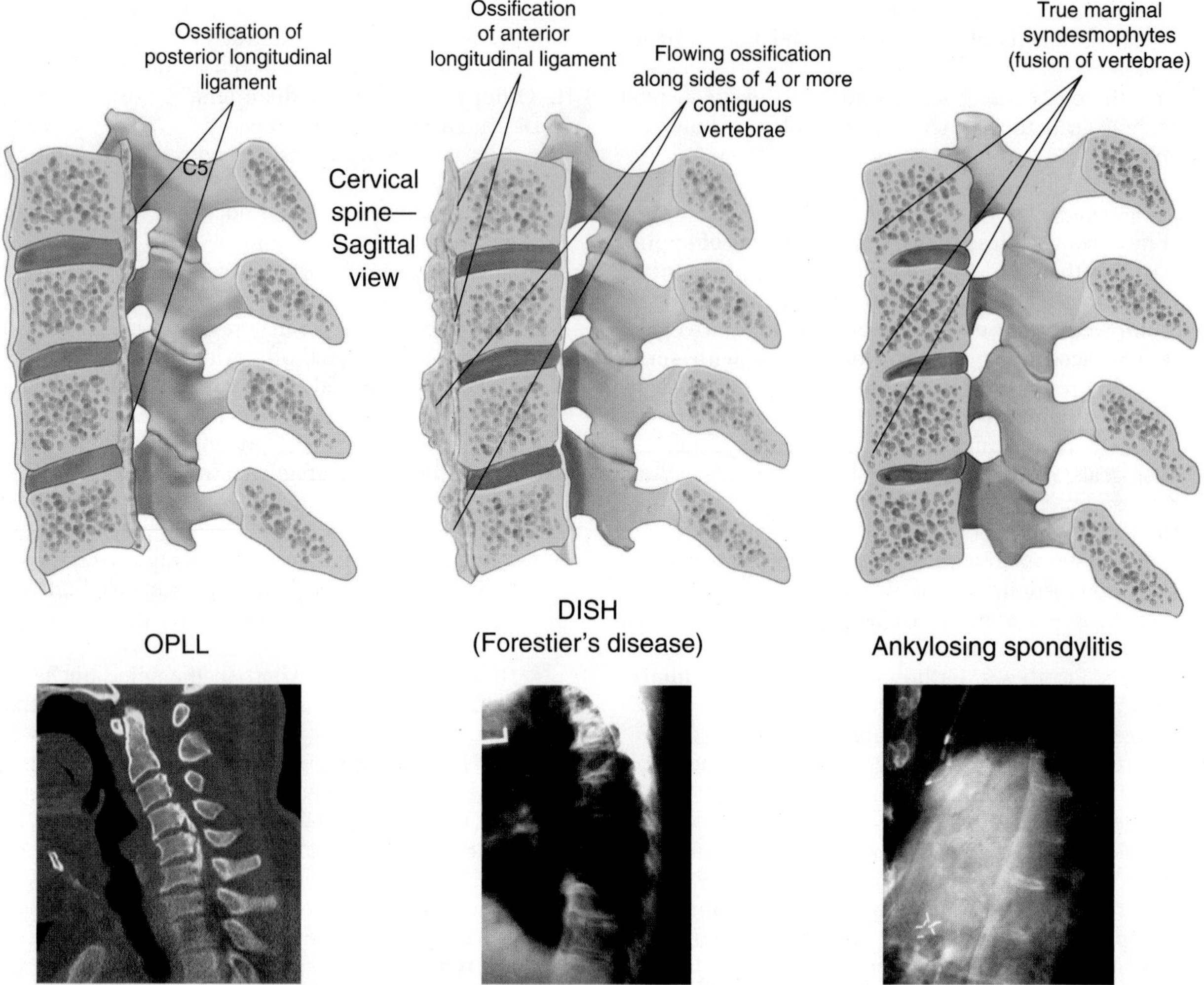

Figure 8-12 Radiographic appearance of ossification of the posterior longitudinal ligament (OPLL), the diffuse idiopathic skeletal hyperostosis (DISH), and ankylosing spondylitis.

- Usually defined as scoliosis in patients older than age 20, it is more symptomatic than its childhood counterpart (see Chapter 3, Pediatric Orthopaedics).
- Classification
  - Idiopathic—progression of untreated adolescent scoliosis
  - De novo
    - Neuromuscular
    - Degenerative (secondary to degenerative disc disease or osteoporosis)
    - Post-traumatic
    - Iatrogenic
  - The curves are usually thoracic (secondary to unrecognized adolescent scoliosis) or lumbar/thoracolumbar (most common in adults).
- Diagnosis
  - Association between pain and scoliosis in the adult is controversial.
  - Progression of symptoms to side of curve convexity indicates poor prognosis.
  - Lumbar stenosis, in particular in the concavity of the curve
  - Cosmetic deformity may be present.
  - Cardiopulmonary problems (thoracic curves >60 to 65 degrees may alter pulmonary function tests; curves >90 degrees may affect mortality)
  - Myelography with CT or MRI is useful for the evaluation of nerve root compression in stenosis.
  - MRI, facet injections, and/or discography may be used to evaluate symptoms in the lumbar spine.
- Curve progression
  - There is no demonstrated association between curve progression and pregnancy.
  - Progression is unlikely in curves of less than 30 degrees.
  - Right thoracic curves of greater than 50 degrees are at the highest risk for progression (usually 1 degree/yr), followed by right lumbar curves.
- Treatment
  - Nonoperative treatment
    - Uncertain correlation between adult scoliosis and back pain makes conservative management essential.
    - Nonoperative treatment includes NSAIDs, weight reduction, therapy, muscle strengthening, facet jointinjections, and orthoses (used with activity).

- ▫ Operative treatment
  - ▪ Indications
    - ▫ Young adults (<30 years) with curves of greater than 50 to 60 degrees
    - ▫ Older patients with refractory pain
    - ▫ Sagittal plane imbalance is a strong predictor of disability.
    - ▫ Progressive curves
      - ▪ Cardiopulmonary compromise (worsening pulmonary function tests in severe curves)
      - ▪ Refractory spinal stenosis
  - ▪ Techniques
    - ▫ Selective posterior fusions for flexible thoracic curves
    - ▫ Combined anterior release and fusion and posterior fusion and instrumentation may be beneficial for large (>70 degree), more rigid curves (as determined on side-bending films) or curves in the lumbar spine.
    - ▫ Fusion to L5
      - ▪ **Associated with development of L5-S1 degenerative disc disease and progressive sagittal imbalance**
    - ▫ Fusion to sacrum
      - ▪ Increases stability of long lumbar fusion
      - ▪ Increased incidence of pseudarthrosis and potential for postoperative gait disturbances
    - ▫ Fixation to ilium
      - ▪ Indicated in lumbosacral fusions involving more than three levels
        - ▫ Potential for prominent hardware
    - ▫ Anterior interbody fusion
      - ▪ Increases stability of long fusions including L5-S1
      - ▪ Helps maintain corrections of sagittal and coronal deformities
- ▪ Outcomes
  - ▫ Nonsurgically treated adults with late-onset idiopathic scoliosis are highly productive at 50-year follow-up, with a slightly increased risk of shortness of breath with activity and chief complaints of back pain and poor cosmesis.
  - ▫ Operative risk for these patients is high (up to a 25% complication rate in older patients).
  - ▫ Complications
    - ▪ Pseudarthrosis (15% with posterior fusion only; the highest risk at the thoracolumbar junction and at L5-S1)
    - ▪ Urinary tract infection, instrumentation problems, infection (up to 5%), and neurologic deficits
    - ▪ Preservation of normal sagittal alignment with fusion is critical.

5. Postlaminectomy deformity
   - ▪ Progressive deformity (usually kyphosis) resulting from a prior wide laminectomy
   - ▪ In children this procedure is followed by a high risk (90%) of deformity.
   - ▪ Fusion plus internal fixation may be considered prophylactic for young patients who require extensive decompression.
   - ▪ Fusion using pedicular screw fixation is best for reconstruction in the adult lumbar spine.

I. Kyphosis

1. Introduction
   - ▪ Etiology
     - ▫ Idiopathic (old Scheuermann disease [since adolescence])
     - ▫ Post-traumatic (missed posterior ligamentous complex injury)
     - ▫ Ankylosing spondylitis
     - ▫ Metabolic bone disease
       - ▪ Progressive kyphosis secondary to multiple osteoporotic compression fractures is usually treated with exercise, bracing, and medical management of the underlying bone disease.
2. Nontraumatic adult kyphosis
   - ▪ Severe idiopathic or congenital kyphosis may be a source of back pain in the adult, particularly when it is present in the thoracolumbar or lumbar spine.
   - ▪ When the symptoms fail to respond to nonoperative management (see the preceding discussion on adult scoliosis), posterior instrumentation and fusion of the entire kyphotic segment with a compression implant may be indicated.
   - ▪ Anterior fusion is considered for curves not correcting to 55 degrees or less on hyperextension lateral radiographs.
3. Post-traumatic kyphosis
   - ▪ Present after fractures of the thoracolumbar spine treated without surgery, particularly in setting of posterior ligamentous complex injury
   - ▪ Fractures treated by laminectomy without fusion and also fractures for which fusion has been performed unsuccessfully
   - ▪ Progressive kyphosis may produce pain at the fracture site, with radiating leg pain and/or neurologic dysfunction if there is associated neural compression.
   - ▪ Operative options
     - ▫ Posterior fusion with compression instrumentation for milder deformities
     - ▫ Combined anterior and posterior osteotomies, instrumentation, and fusion for more severe deformities
       - ▪ Pedicle subtraction osteotomy
         - ▫ Thirty degrees of sagittal plane correction
       - ▪ Smith-Peterson osteotomy
     - ▫ Anterior spinal cord or cauda equina decompression combined with posterior instrumentation and fusion for cases involving neurologic dysfunction.
4. Metabolic bone disease
   - ▪ Treatment
     - ▫ An underlying malignancy as a cause of the osteopenia should be considered; evaluation with MRI is sensitive for determining the presence of tumor.
     - ▫ Prevention of compression fractures has been successful with bisphosphonate treatment, with a decreased incidence of vertebral fractures of 65% at 1 year and 40% at 3 years.
     - ▫ Surgical attempts at correction and stabilization are marked by a high complication rate.
     - ▫ Vertebroplasty and kyphoplasty

- Percutaneous techniques designed to relieve pain and correct deformity (kyphoplasty)
- Indicated for subacute injuries, although precise indications are poorly defined
- To respond to either technique, a fracture must still be in the active healing phase, which is best demonstrated on MRI (spin tau inversion recovery sequences)
  - A patient with a painful but healed fracture is unlikely to improve.
- Kyphoplasty has also been proposed to correct deformity.
- Improvement in pain and quality of life has been questioned in recent studies.

- Complications
  - Hypotensive reaction to cement
  - Extravasation of cement into canal resulting in compression of neural elements

IV. SACRUM AND COCCYX

A. Sacroiliac joint pain

1. Diagnosis
   - Gaenslen test
     - Elicited with the patient lying on the affected side without support
   - FABER test
     - Flexion, abduction, and external rotation of involved extremity
   - Direct compression with reproduction of symptoms or with the flexion, abduction, and external rotation (FABER) test of the involved extremity
2. Treatment
   - Local injections may have diagnostic and therapeutic roles.
   - Orthotic management (trochanteric cinch) can be helpful.
   - Fusion is not indicated unless an infection is present.

B. Idiopathic coccygodynia

1. Diagnosis
   - Pain and point tenderness over the coccyx
   - More common in women and may occur after pregnancy or minor trauma or idiopathically
   - Occasionally associated with a fracture
2. Treatment
   - The symptoms may last 1 to 2 years but are almost always self-limiting.
   - Treatment should be conservative and may include a sitting donut, NSAIDs, stretching exercises, and local injection.
   - Surgery is associated with a high failure rate and significant risk of complications.

C. Sacral insufficiency fracture

1. Diagnosis
   - Occurs in older patients with osteopenia
   - Often without a history of trauma
   - Complaints include low back and groin pain
   - This fracture is diagnosed with a technetium bone scan (H-shaped uptake pattern is diagnostic) or with CT.
2. Treatment
   - Nonoperative: rest, analgesic medication, and ambulatory aids until the symptoms resolve

V. TUMORS AND INFECTIONS OF THE SPINE

A. Introduction—The spine is a frequent site of metastasis, and certain tumors with a predilection for the spine have unique manifestations in vertebrae.

1. Tumors of the vertebral body
   - Histiocytosis X
   - Giant cell tumor
   - Chordoma
   - Osteosarcoma
   - Hemangioma
   - Metastatic disease
   - Marrow cell tumors
2. Tumors of the posterior elements include
   - Aneurysmal bone cysts
   - Osteoblastoma
   - Osteoid osteoma
3. Radiographic changes include
   - Absent pedicle (winking owl sign on anteroposterior radiograph)
   - Cortical erosion or expansion
   - Vertebral collapse
   - Bone scans can be helpful in cases of protracted back pain or night pain
   - MRI is the diagnostic test of choice.
     - Malignant tumors have decreased T1 and increased T2 signal intensity.
     - Sensitivity of MRI is increased with the use of gadolinium.
   - Malignant tumors occur more frequently in the lower (lumbar > thoracic > cervical) spinal levels and in the vertebral body.
4. Treatment
   - Complete surgical excision is difficult and usually consists of tumor debulking and stabilization.
     - Corpectomy, anterior cage, posterior fusion
   - Adjuvant therapy (chemotherapy, external beam radiation therapy) is essential
   - For more details on these tumors, refer to Chapter 9, Orthopaedic Pathology.

B. Metastasis—the most common tumors of the spine, spreading to the vertebral body first and later to the pedicles

1. Diagnosis
   - **Red flags for possible spinal metastasis**
     - **History of cancer**
       - Breast, lung, and prostate metastases are the most common, the latter of which are blastic.
     - Recent unexplained weight loss
     - Night pain
     - Age older than 50 years
   - Radiographic workup
     - Most tumors are osteolytic and not demonstrated on plain films until over 30% destruction of the vertebral body has occurred.
     - CT-guided needle biopsy is often possible, and surgery for diagnosis can be avoided.
2. Treatment
   - A poor prognosis is associated with neurologic dysfunction, proximal lesions, long duration of symptoms, and rapid growth of the metastasis.
   - Nonsurgical treatment

- Radiation therapy and chemotherapy have traditionally been the mainstays of treatment unless the tumor is destabilizing and progressive or causes spinal cord or cauda equina dysfunction.
- In the case of epidural spinal cord compression, radiation therapy should be combined with direct surgical decompression for the best clinical outcomes.
- Radiosensitivity varies among primary tumor types.
  - Prostate and lymphoid tumors are radiosensitive.
  - Breast cancer is 70% sensitive and 30% resistant.
  - Gastrointestinal and renal cell tumors are radioresistant.

- Surgical treatment
  - Indications
    - Progressive neurologic dysfunction that is unresponsive to radiation therapy
    - Persistent pain despite radiation therapy
    - Need for an open diagnostic biopsy
    - Pathologic instability
    - Radioresistant tumor
    - Life expectancy should play an important role with regard to whether surgical treatment is performed.
  - Techniques
    - Vertebroplasty is gaining favor in cases of metastatic disease of the spine (myeloma, breast) without instability or neurologic compromise and represents a minimally invasive alternative to open surgery.
    - In cases of neurologic deficit and/or spinal instability, anterior decompression and stabilization (preserving intact posterior structures) may result in recovery of neurologic function.
    - Posterior stabilization or a circumferential approach is indicated in cases of multiple levels of destruction, involvement of both the anterior and posterior columns, or translational instability.
      - Also allows immediate stability and early mobilization
    - Methylmethacrylate may be useful as an anterior strut but should be used only as an adjunct because of the high complication rate.
    - Bone grafting is preferred if life expectancy is more than 6 months.
    - Metastatic renal cell carcinoma requires preoperative arteriography and embolism.

C. Primary tumors

1. Osteoid osteoma and osteoblastoma
   - Diagnosis
     - Common in the spine
     - May present with painful scoliosis in a child
     - Pain is typically relieved by aspirin.
     - Bone scan can help localize the level.
     - Thin-cut CT can direct surgical excision.
     - Osteoblastomas typically occur in the posterior elements in older patients, with neurologic involvement in more than half.
   - Treatment
     - Scoliosis (the lesion is typically at the apex of the convexity) resolves with early resection (within 18 months) in a child younger than age 11 years.
     - If there is no scoliosis, NSAIDs are the mainstay of treatment.
     - Surgery is done if nonoperative treatment fails.
       - Resection and posterior fusion
2. Aneurysmal bone cyst
   - Diagnosis
     - May represent degeneration of more aggressive tumors
     - Presents during the second decade of life
     - Arises in the posterior elements but possibly also involving the anterior elements
   - Treatment
     - Excision and/or radiation therapy
3. Hemangioma
   - Diagnosis
     - Typically seen in asymptomatic patients
     - Symptomatic patients older than age 40 years may seek treatment after small spinal fractures
     - The classic patient with hemangioma has "jailhouse striations" on plain films and "spikes of bone" demonstrated on CT.
     - Vertebrae are typically of normal size and not expanded (as in Paget disease).
   - Treatment
     - Observation or radiation therapy in cases of persistent pain after pathologic fracture
     - Anterior resection and fusion are reserved for refractory cases or pathologic collapse and neural compression, but massive bleeding may be encountered.
4. Eosinophilic granuloma
   - Diagnosis
     - Usually seen in children younger than age 10 years
     - More common in the thoracic spine
     - May present with progressive back pain
     - Classically results in vertebral flattening (vertebra plana [Calvé disease]) seen on lateral radiographs.
     - Biopsy may be required for diagnosis unless the radiographic picture is classic.
   - Treatment
     - Symptoms are usually self-limiting.
     - Chemotherapy is useful for the systemic form.
     - Bracing may be indicated in children to prevent progressive kyphosis.
     - Low-dose radiation therapy may be indicated in the presence of neurologic deficits.
     - At least 50% reconstitution of vertebral height may be expected.
5. Giant cell tumor
   - Diagnosis
     - Usually seen in the fourth and fifth decades of life
     - Destruction of the vertebral body in an expansile fashion
   - Treatment
     - Surgical excision and bone grafting
     - High recurrence rate is reported.
     - Radiation therapy should be avoided because of the possibility of malignant degeneration of the tumor.
6. Plasmacytoma/multiple myeloma
   - Diagnosis
     - Shown as osteopenic, lytic lesions on radiographs
     - Workup includes skeletal survey.
       - Lesions are cold on bone scans.

- Pain secondary to pathologic fractures
- Increased calcium level and decreased hematocrit levels as well as abnormal protein studies are common.

- Treatment
  - Radiation therapy (3000-4000 cGy) with or without chemotherapy
  - Surgery is reserved for patients with spinal instability and those with refractory neurologic symptoms.

7. Chordoma
   - Diagnosis
     - Slow-growing lytic lesion in the midline of the anterior sacrum or the base of the skull
     - It may occur in other vertebrae (cervical spine most common).
     - Patients with these tumors may present with intra-abdominal complaints and a presacral mass.
     - Physaliferous cells on biopsy specimens
   - Treatment
     - Radiation therapy and surgery are preferred.
     - Surgical excision can include up to half of the sacral roots (i.e., all roots on one side) and the patient still maintains bowel and bladder function.
     - High recurrence rate
     - Aggressive attempts at surgical excision are indicated.
     - Although a complete cure is rare, patients typically survive 10 to 15 years after diagnosis.
8. Osteochondroma
   - Arises in the posterior elements and is frequently seen in the cervical spine
   - Treatment is by excision, which may be necessary to rule out sarcomatous changes.
9. Neurofibroma
   - Can present with enlarged intervertebral foramina seen on oblique radiographs
10. Malignant primary skeletal lesions
    - Diagnosis
      - Osteosarcoma, Ewing sarcoma, and chondrosarcoma are uncommon in the spine.
      - When they occur they are associated with a poor prognosis.
    - Treatment
      - Chemotherapy and irradiation are the mainstays of treatment, but aggressive surgical excision may have a role.
      - The lesions may actually be metastases, which are treated palliatively
11. Lymphoma
    - Can present as "ivory" vertebrae
    - Usually associated with a systemic disease, lymphoma is treated after histologic diagnosis by irradiation and/or chemotherapy.
12. Fibrous dysplasia
    - At least 60% of patients with polyostotic fibrous dysplasia will have spinal involvement, mostly in the posterior elements.
    - There is a strong correlation between the presence of a lesion and scoliosis, making scoliosis screening very important in the population with polyostotic disease.

D. Spinal infections

1. Disc space infection
   - Introduction
     - Bloodborne infection can primarily invade the disc space in children.
     - *Staphylococcus aureus* is the most common offender, but gram-negative organisms are common in older patients.
   - Diagnosis
     - Although all age groups are affected, children (mean age, 7 years) are affected more often.
     - Presentation
       - Inability to walk, stand, or sit
       - Back pain/tenderness
       - Restricted range of motion
     - Laboratory studies
       - Elevated erythrocyte sedimentation rate, C-reactive protein, and white blood cell count (often high normal or mildly elevated)
     - Radiographic findings
       - Loss of normal lumbar lordosis is earliest finding.
       - Disc space narrowing
       - End plate erosion
       - Findings do not occur until 10 days to 3 weeks after onset and their absence is unreliable.
       - MRI is the diagnostic test of choice, although a bone scan is also useful in the diagnosis.
   - Treatment
     - Bed rest, immobilization, and antibiotics
2. Pyogenic vertebral osteomyelitis
   - Introduction
     - Seen with increasing frequency but still associated with a significant (6- to 12-week) delay in diagnosis
   - Diagnosis
     - Patient history and physical examination
       - Older, debilitated patients
       - Intravenous drug users are at increased risk
       - More common in patients with a history of pneumonia, urinary tract infection, skin infection, or immunologic compromise (transplant, rheumatoid arthritis, diabetes mellitus, human immunodeficiency virus [CD4+ >200])
     - Organism usually hematogenous (*S. aureus*, 50%-75% of cases)
     - Fungal spondylitis can be seen in patients with immunologic compromise.
     - A history of unremitting spinal pain at any level is characteristic, and tenderness, spasm, and loss of motion are seen.
     - Forty percent of neurologic deficits are seen in older patients, patients with infections at more cephalic levels of the spine, patients with debilitating systemic illnesses such as diabetes or rheumatoid arthritis, and those with delayed diagnoses.
     - Imaging
       - Plain radiographic findings
         - Osteopenia
         - Paraspinous soft tissue swelling (loss of a psoas shadow)
         - Erosion of the vertebral end plates
         - Disc destruction (disc space preserved in metastatic disease)
       - Bone scanning is sensitive for a destructive process.
       - MRI

- Sensitive for detecting infection and specific in differentiating infection from tumor
- Gadolinium enhances the sensitivity.
- Tissue diagnosis via blood cultures or aspirate of the infection is mandatory.
- Treatment
  - After tissue diagnosis, 6 to 12 weeks of intravenous antibiotics is the treatment of choice.
  - Bracing may be used adjunctively.
  - Open biopsy is indicated when a tissue diagnosis has not been made
  - Anterior débridement and strut grafting are reserved for refractory cases that are typically associated with abscess formation or cases involving neurologic deterioration, extensive bony destruction, or marked deformity.
  - Posterior surgery is usually ineffective for débridement; posterior stabilization is only occasionally required after anterior débridement and strut grafting.

3. Epidural abscess
   - Introduction
     - Bacterial infection that results in the accumulation of purulent material within the epidural space
     - Most located posteriorly in the thoracic and lumbar spine
   - Diagnosis
     - Back pain is the most common presenting symptom, followed by neurologic deficit and fever. Nevertheless, diagnosis is delayed in half of patients
     - Risk factors include intravenous drug abuse, diabetes and multiple medical problems.
     - Erythrocyte sedimentation rate and C-reactive protein values are elevated.
     - MRI is the modality of choice, and supplementation with gadolinium allows differentiation between the epidural abscess and cerebrospinal fluid.
       - Abscess and cerebrospinal fluid have high signal intensity on T2-weighted images.
       - Gadolinium enhances the pus on T1-weighted images, whereas the cerebrospinal fluid remains low signal.
   - Management
     - Urgent evaluation and treatment
     - If diagnosis is made prior to neurologic deficits, a trial of intravenous antibiotics may be attempted. Failure to improve in 24 to 48 hours warrants surgical intervention.
     - Laminectomy is performed because the pus is predominately posterior. If there is concomitant vertebral osteomyelitis, anterior and posterior decompression is performed.
4. Spinal tuberculosis (Figure 8-13)
   - Introduction
     - The most common extrapulmonary location of tuberculosis
     - It may be seen in the human immunodeficiency virus–positive population with a CD4+ count of 50 to 200.
     - Originates in the metaphysis of the vertebral body and spreads under the anterior longitudinal ligament
       - This leads to destruction of several contiguous levels or results in skip lesions (15%) or abscess formation (50%).
   - Diagnosis
     - On early plain radiographs, anterior vertebral body destruction, with preservation of the disc, distinguishes tuberculosis from pyogenic infection.

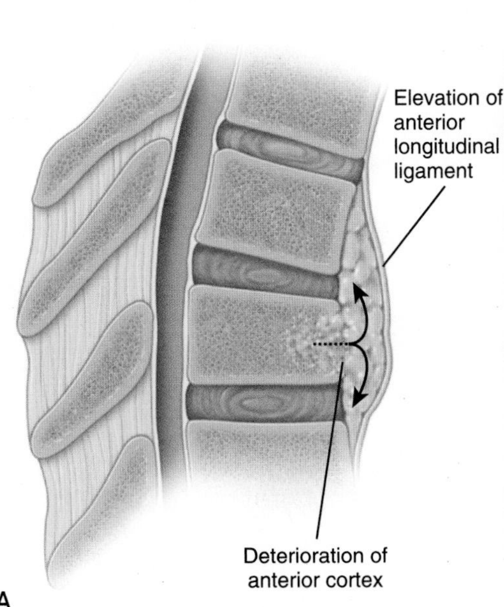

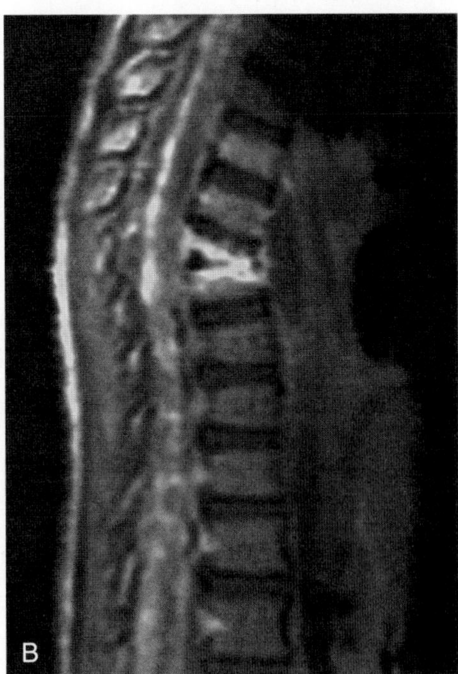

Figure 8-13 Pathogenesis of spinal tuberculosis. (From Herring JA: *Tachdjian's pediatric orthopaedics,* ed 3, Philadelphia, 2002, WB Saunders, p 1832.)

- About two thirds of patients have abnormal chest radiographs, and 20% have a negative test for purified protein derivative of tuberculin or are anergic.
- Severe kyphosis, sinus formation, and (Pott) paraplegia are late sequelae.
- Spinal cord injury may occur secondary to direct pressure from the abscess, bony sequestra (good prognosis), or (rarely) meningomyelitis (poor prognosis).

- Treatment
  - Chemotherapy is the mainstay of treatment.
  - Surgical indications:
    - Neurologic deficit
    - Spinal instability
    - Progressive kyphosis
    - Advanced disease with caseation, fibrosis, and avascularity that limits antibiotic penetration
  - Radical anterior débridement of the infection followed by uninstrumented autogenous strut grafting (Hong Kong procedure) is the accepted surgical treatment.
  - Advantages include less progressive kyphosis, earlier healing, and a decrease in sinus formation.
  - Adjuvant chemotherapy beginning 10 days before surgery is recommended.

TESTABLE CONCEPTS

II. CERVICAL SPINE

- Cervical spondylosis most commonly occurs at C5-C6.
  - Cervical nerve roots exit above their corresponding vertebrae (e.g., C5 exits at the C4-C5 neural foramen). Consequently, disc herniation at C5-C6 involves the C6 nerve root.
  - The natural history of cervical spondylotic myelopathy is characterized by stepwise deterioration in symptomatology followed by a period of stability.
  - False-positive MR images are common with 25% of asymptomatic patients older than age 40 years demonstrating a herniated nucleus pulposus or foraminal stenosis.
  - Operative indications include myelopathy with motor/gait impairment and radiculopathy with persistent, disabling pain that has failed nonoperative measures
  - Anterior cervical discectomy and fusion complications include recurrent laryngeal nerve injury, dysphagia, airway obstruction, nonunion and adjacent segment disease. Nonunion should be treated with posterior fusion.
  - Canal expansive laminoplasty is used for multilevel spondylosis, congenital cervical stenosis and ossification of posterior longitudinal ligament. It is contraindicated in the setting of fixed kyphosis.
- In cervical stenosis, a Pavlov (Torg) ratio of less than 0.80 or a sagittal diameter of less than 13 mm is considered a significant risk factor for later neurologic involvement. Absolute stenosis is defined as an anteroposterior canal diameter less than 10 mm.
- Rheumatoid spondylitis most commonly presents as an occipital headache due to compression of the greater occipital branch of C2.
  - Progressive cervical instability secondary to pannus formation and erosion of the joints and capsular structures occurs in up to 90% of patients. This can manifest as (1) atlantoaxial instability, (2) cranial settling (basilar invagination), and (3) subaxial subluxation.
  - Atlantoaxial subluxation is most common. A posterior atlanto–dens interval less than 14 mm is associated with an increased risk of neurologic injury and usually requires surgical treatment. Transarticular screw fixation (Magerl) across C1-C2 eliminates the need for halo immobilization associated with wiring alone. Surgery is less successful in Ranawat grade IIIB patients but should be considered.
  - Always obtain flexion/extension films before elective surgery in patients with rheumatoid arthritis.
- Cervical spine injury can be associated with spinal shock and/or neurogenic shock.
  - Spinal shock is over when the bulbocavernosus reflex returns.
  - Neurogenic shock is secondary to loss of sympathetic tone and can be recognized by relative bradycardia.
- Incomplete spinal cord syndromes are anatomically classified and all involve some sparing of distal function.
  - Central cord syndrome is most common, affecting elderly patients with a spondylotic cervical spine. It presents as upper greater than lower extremity motor and sensory loss. It has the best prognosis. Independent ambulation is regained in approximately half of elderly patients and almost always in young patients.
  - Anterior cord syndrome is the second most common and has the worst prognosis. It presents as greater motor loss in the legs than in the arms.
  - Brown-Séquard syndrome presents as motor weakness on the side of injury and contralateral loss of pain and temperature.
- Autonomic dysreflexia is a syndrome of uncontrolled sympathetic nervous output occurring in patients with a spinal cord injury above T6. It presents as hypertension, pupillary dilation, headache, pallor and reflex bradycardia. Treat with urinary catheterization, fecal disimpaction, antihypertensives and atropine in severe cases.

III. THORACIC/LUMBAR SPINE

- Thoracic HNP is typically treated via an anterior transthoracic approach for midline or central herniations. Anterior discectomy and hemicorpectomy are performed as needed. A transpedicular approach is used for a lateral herniation.
  - Posterior approach and laminectomy are contraindicated because of an inability to retract the spinal cord and high rate of neurologic injury.
- The differential diagnosis of thoracolumbar disease can be (over)simplified based on whether leg pain or back pain are predominant and whether the pain is worse with flexion or extension:
  - Back pain predominant
    - Worse with flexion → discogenic back pain
    - Worse with extension → spondylolisthesis or facet arthropathy
  - Leg pain predominant
    - Worse with flexion → lumbar disc disease
    - Worse with extension → spinal stenosis

Lumbar Disc Disease

- Most herniations are posterolateral (where the posterior longitudinal ligament is the weakest) and may present as back pain and nerve root pain/sciatica involving the lower nerve root at that level (L5 at the L4-L5 level).
  - Far lateral herniation or foraminal stenosis involves the exiting nerve root (L4 at the L4-5 level).
- A positive contralateral straight-leg raising test (pain in the affected buttock/leg when the opposite leg is raised) is the most specific test for HNP.
- More than half of the patients who seek treatment for low back pain recover in 1 week, and 90% recover within 1 to 3 months. Half of the patients with sciatica recover in 1 month. Conservative treatment is with NSAIDs and physical therapy.
- Failure to improve within 6 weeks warrants further investigation. Radiographs are generally performed at this point.
- Standard partial laminotomy and discectomy are the most commonly performed surgical procedures.

Continued

- Outcomes from the SPORT trial (2-year follow-up):
  - No significant differences in primary outcome measures for operative compared with nonoperative groups
  - However, trends favoring surgical intervention in primary outcome measures
  - Statistically significant improvement in secondary outcome measures for surgical intervention: sciatica bothersomeness, self-rated improvement
- Workers' compensation patients are more likely to continue to receive disability compensation and have worse symptoms, functional status, and satisfaction outcomes.
- Complications include vascular injury, nerve root injury, infection (1% but increased in diabetics), discitis, cauda equina syndrome, and dural tear.
  - Treatment of a dural tear includes bed rest and subarachnoid drain placement. If adequately repaired, clinical outcomes are generally unaffected.

Spinal Stenosis

- Spinal stenosis can be classified anatomically into central, lateral recess, and foraminal stenosis. Tandem stenosis is said to occur when there is both cervical and lumbar stenosis.
  - Central → narrowing of central spinal canal from one edge of dural tube to the other
  - Lateral → narrowing of subarticular recess, bounded by takeoff of nerve root from dural tube to the medial border of the pedicle
  - Foraminal → narrowing of neural foramen, bounded by disc anteriorly, pars articularis posteriorly, and pedicles superiorly and inferiorly
- Central stenosis that fails nonoperative management should be treated with laminectomy and partial medial facetectomy. Surgical instability (via removal of a facet), a pars defect, spondylolisthesis (degenerative or isthmic), degenerative scoliosis and radiographic instability are indications for fusion.
  - Residual foraminal stenosis is a common reason for persistent radicular pain after laminectomy
  - Outcomes from the SPORT trial (4-year follow-up):
    - Significant improvement in pain and function for operative compared with nonoperative groups
- Lateral recess stenosis that fails nonoperative management should be treated with decompression of the hypertrophied lamina and ligamentum flavum and partial facetectomy.
- The use of alendronate has been shown to decrease spinal fusion rates in animal models. Administration should be held in the postoperative period.

Spondylosis and Spondylolisthesis

- Spondylosis is a defect in the pars interarticularis. Unilateral defects almost never progress to olisthesis.
- Spondylolisthesis is divided into six types. The most common is isthmic (L5-S1 level), followed by degenerative (L4-L5 level).
- Isthmic spondylolisthesis can present in childhood or in adults.
  - Pediatric
    - Low-grade disease (<50% slip) typically responds to nonoperative treatment.
    - High-grade disease should be treated with prophylactic fusion. This often requires in situ bilateral posterolateral fusion from L4-S1.
  - Adult
    - Associated with an increased pelvic incidence.
    - Operative treatment includes in situ L4 or L5-S1 posterolateral fusion.
- Degenerative spondylolisthesis is four to five times more common in women and more common in African Americans and diabetics.
  - It presents as symptoms of central and lateral recess spinal stenosis.
  - Operative treatment for degenerative spondylolisthesis involves decompression of the nerve roots and stabilization by posterolateral fusion.
  - Outcomes from the SPORT trial (4-year follow-up):
    - Significant improvement in pain and function for operative compared with nonoperative groups

Thoracolumbar Injuries (see Chapter 11, Trauma)

- Gunshot spine fractures are typically stable injuries that rarely require surgery. Patients in whom bullets have passed through the gastrointestinal tract should be treated with broad-spectrum intravenous antibiotics for 7 to 10 days.
- Pediatric Chance fractures have a high association with intra-abdominal injuries.

Adult Deformity

- Adult scoliosis is typically lumbar/thoracolumbar and more symptomatic than its childhood counterpart.
- Right thoracic curves of greater than 50 degrees are at the highest risk for progression (usually 1 degree/yr), followed by right lumbar curves.
- Sagittal plane imbalance is a strong predictor of disability, and preservation of normal sagittal alignment with fusion is critical.
- Whether to end a fusion at L5 or S1 is controversial. Fusion to L5 is associated with development of L5-S1 degenerative disc disease and progressive sagittal imbalance. Fusion to the sacrum is associated with increased incidence of pseudarthrosis and gait disturbance.

Inflammatory and Other Disorders

- Ankylosing spondylitis is associated with HLA-B27. However, only 2% of patients with HLA-B27 have ankylosing spondylitis; therefore, it is not used in the diagnosis.
  - Sacroiliac joint obliteration (iliac side affected first) and marginal syndesmophytes allow radiographic differentiation from diffuse idiopathic skeletal hyperostosis.
  - The spine often becomes fused in kyphosis. Posterior extension osteotomies are performed followed by posterior fusion.
- Diffuse idiopathic skeletal hyperostosis is typically seen in older patients and more common in the thoracic spine. It is differentiated on radiographs by undulating "nonmarginal syndesmophytes."

V. TUMORS AND INFECTIONS OF THE SPINE

- Metastatic disease is the most common malignancy of the spine and most commonly involves the vertebral body.
- "Red flags" for metastatic disease include a history of cancer, unexplained weight loss, night pain, and age older than 50.
- Wide excision is typically performed for primary bone tumors without known metastases and solitary metastases with likelihood of prolonged survival.
- Decompressive surgery techniques:
  - Upper cervical spine → posterior approach
  - Posterior element tumor of lower cervical, thoracic, or lumbar spine → posterior approach
  - Majority of lower cervical, thoracic or lumbar spine → anterior approach, because most tumors are located in the body
  - Multilevel involvement or en bloc spondylectomy → combined anterior/posterior approach
- Discitis most commonly presents as pain and elevated erythrocyte sedimentation rate and C-reactive protein level.
  - Radiographs are often negative, with loss of lumbar lordosis and disc space narrowing the earliest findings
  - Treatment is with intravenous antibiotics and C-reactive protein should be used to monitor response.
  - Anterior débridement and strut grafting are reserved for refractory cases. Laminectomy is generally avoided.
- Tuberculosis spondylitis differs from pyogenic infections in four ways:
  - Originates in metaphysis of vertebral body and spreads under the anterior longitudinal ligament
  - Large anterior abscesses
  - Discs are preserved.
  - Severe kyphosis more common

SELECTED BIBLIOGRAPHY

The selected bibliography for this chapter can be found on www.expertconsult.com.

Chapter 9

ORTHOPAEDIC PATHOLOGY

Frank J. Frassica, Deborah A. Frassica, and Edward F. McCarthy

CONTENTS

SECTION 1 INTRODUCTION

I. STAGING

Staging systems may be useful for developing evaluation strategies, planning treatment, and predicting prognosis. For musculoskeletal lesions, the staging systems of the Musculoskeletal Tumor Society (also called the *Enneking system*) and the **American Joint Commission on Cancer** (AJCC) are the most popular. Enneking system is based on knowing the histologic grade of the lesion (low or high), the anatomic features (intracompartmental or extracompartmental), and the absence (M_0) or presence (M_1) of metastases.

A. Enneking system: This staging system can be synthesized into six distinct stages (Table 9-1).

B. Variables of AJCC system: The most recent edition of the AJCC system has become more popular than Enneking's system among medical oncologists and many orthopaedic oncologists. A working knowledge of both systems is necessary for examinations. To use this system, the clinician must know the grade, the size, the presence or absence of discontinuous tumor (skip metastases), and the absence or presence of systemic metastases. The various stages are listed in Table 9-2. The order of importance for the variables of the AJCC staging system is as follows: stage (takes into account all factors), presence of metastases, discontinuous tumor, grade, and size.

II. GRADING

Grading can be difficult and is based on nuclear anaplasia (degree of loss of structural differentiation), pleomorphism (variations in size and shape), and nuclear hyperchromasia (increased nuclear staining). Grading of tumors covers a morphologic range.

A. Most grading systems are based on three grades:
1. Grade I: well differentiated
2. Grade II: moderately differentiated
3. Grade III: poorly differentiated

B. The grade of the tumor is most strongly correlated with the potential for metastasis:
1. Grade I (low grade): less than 10% potential
2. Grade II (intermediate grade): 10% to 30% potential
3. Grade III (high grade): greater than 50% potential

C. Most malignant lesions are high grade (Enneking grade G_2); low-grade malignant (Enneking grade G_1) lesions are less common. Commonly graded lesions are shown in Table 9-3.

III. TUMOR SITE

The plain radiographs and special studies, such as computed tomographic (CT) scan and magnetic resonance imaging (MRI), are used to determine how the tumor is situated:

Table 9-1 Staging System of the Musculoskeletal Tumor Society (Enneking System)

Stage	Grade, Tumor Size, and Metastasis Status	Description
IA	$G_1T_1M_0$	Low grade Intracompartmental No metastases
IB	$G_1T_2M_0$	Low grade Extracompartmental No metastases
IIA	$G_2T_1M_0$	High grade Intracompartmental No metastases
IIB	$G_2T_2M_0$	High grade Extracompartmental No metastases
IIIA	$G_{1/2}T_1M_1$	Any grade Intracompartmental With metastases
IIIB	$G_{1/2}T_2M_1$	Any grade Extracompartmental With metastases

High-grade (G_2) lesions are intermediate between low-grade (G_1), well-differentiated tumors and high-grade, undifferentiated tumors. The size of the tumor is determined through specialized procedures, including radiography, tomography, nuclear studies, computed tomography (CT), and magnetic resonance imaging (MRI). Compartments are specified to describe the tumor site. These compartments are usually easily defined on the basis of fascial borders in the extremities. Of note, the skin and subcutaneous tissues are classified as a compartment, and the potential periosseous space between cortical bone and muscle is often considered a compartment as well. T_0 lesions are confined within the capsule and within its compartment of origin. T_1 tumors have extracapsular extension into the reactive zone around it, but both the tumor and the reactive zone are confined within the compartment of origin. T_2 lesions extend beyond the anatomic compartment of origin by direct extension or some other means (e.g., trauma, surgical seeding). Tumors that involve major neurovascular bundles are almost always classified as T_2 lesions. Both regional and distal metastases have ominous prognoses; therefore, the distinction is simply between the absence of metastases (M_0) and the presence of metastases (M_1).

A. Within the bone compartment (intracompartmental, or T1)

B. Extending beyond the confines of the bone (extracompartmental, or T2)

Preoperative MRI scans are used to determine the anatomic features of the tumor and plan surgical margins. A T1-weighted coronal MRI is obtained to determine the intramedullary extent of the tumor and detect skip metastases (discontinuous tumor).

IV. METASTASES

A. Chest radiograph and CT scan of the chest are obtained to search for pulmonary lesions.

B. Technetium-labeled bone scan is obtained to exclude the presence of other bone lesions.

V. EVALUATION

A. Clinical presentation: Most patients with bone tumors present with musculoskeletal pain. However, the most common presentation of a benign bone tumor in childhood is as an incidental finding.

Table 9-2 American Joint Committee on Cancer Staging System for Primary Malignant Tumors of Bone for Those Tumors Diagnosed on or after January 1, 2003

Stage	Tumor	Lymph Node	Metastases	Grade
IA	T1	N0	M0	G1 or G2
IB	T2	N0	M0	G1 or G2
IIA	T1	N0	M0	G3 or G4
IIB	T2	N0	M0	G3 or G4
III	T3	N0	M0	Any G
IVA	Any T	N0	M1a	Any G
IVB	Any T	N1	Any M	Any G
	Any T	Any N	M1b	Any G

From American Joint Committee on Cancer: Bone. In Greene FL, et al, editor: *AJCC cancer staging manual,* New York, 2002, Springer-Verlag, pp 213-219.

G1, well differentiated (low grade); G2, moderately differentiated (low grade); G3, poorly differentiated (high grade); G4, undifferentiated (high grade); M0, no distant metastasis; M1a, metastasis to lung; M1b, metastasis to other distant sites; N0, no regional lymph node metastases; N1, regional lymph node metastasis; primary tumor cannot be assessed; T0, no evidence of primary tumor; T1, tumor 8 cm or less in greatest dimension; T2, tumor more than 8 cm in greatest dimension; T3, discontinuous tumors in the primary bone.

1. Pain is typically deep-seated and may resemble a that of a toothache.
2. Pain may initially be intermittent and related to activity, a work injury, or a sporting injury.
3. Pain usually progresses in intensity and becomes constant.
4. Patients experience pain at night.
5. Pain progresses, and it is not relieved by **nonsteroidal anti-inflammatory drugs** (NSAIDs) or weaker narcotics (such as acetaminophen [Tylenol] with codeine).
6. Patients with a high-grade sarcoma present with a 1- to 3-month history of pain.
7. With low-grade tumors, such as chondrosarcoma, adamantinoma, and chordoma, there may be a long history of mild to moderate pain (6 to 24 months).

Table 9-3 Typical Low- and High-Grade Bone and Soft Tissue Tumors

Low-Grade Tumors	High-Grade Tumors
Bone	
Parosteal osteosarcoma	Intramedullary (classic) osteosarcoma
Primary chondrosarcoma	Postradiation sarcoma
Secondary chondrosarcoma	Paget sarcoma
Hemangioendothelioma	Fibrosarcoma
Chordoma	Malignant fibrous histiocytoma
Adamantinoma	
Soft Tissue	
Myxoid liposarcoma	Malignant fibrous histiocytoma
Lipoma-like liposarcoma	Pleomorphic liposarcoma
Angiomatoid malignant fibrous histiocytoma	Synovial sarcoma
Rhabdomyosarcoma	Alveolar cell sarcoma

B. Physical examination: Patients with suspected bone tumors should be examined carefully.

1. Site is inspected for soft tissue masses, overlying skin changes, adenopathy, and general musculoskeletal condition.
2. When metastatic disease is suspected, the thyroid gland, abdomen, prostate, and breasts should be examined, as appropriate.

C. Imaging studies: Radiographs in two planes are the first imaging studies to be performed. When the clinician suspects malignancy but the radiographs are normal, selected studies may follow.

1. Technetium-labeled bone scan is an excellent modality to search for occult bone involvement. In patients with myeloma for whom scan results may be negative, a skeletal survey is more sensitive.
2. MRI is an excellent modality for screening the spine for occult metastases, myeloma, or lymphoma.
3. A chest radiograph should be obtained for patients of any age when the clinician suspects a malignant lesion.
4. The radiographs must be carefully inspected to formulate a working diagnosis. The working diagnosis then guides the clinician during further evaluation and treatment. Formulation of the differential diagnosis is based on several clinical and radiographic parameters:
   - **Age of the patient: Knowledge of common diseases in defined age groups is the first step. Certain diseases are uncommon in particular age groups** (Table 9-4).
   - Number of bone lesions: Is the process monostotic or polyostotic? If there are multiple destructive lesions in middle-aged and older patients (ages 40 to 80 years), the most likely diagnosis is metastatic bone disease, multiple myeloma, or lymphoma. In young patients (ages 15 to 40 years), multiple lytic and oval lesions in the same extremity are probably vascular tumors (hemangioendothelioma). In children younger than 5 years, multiple destructive lesions may represent metastatic disease such as neuroblastoma or Wilms tumor. Histiocytosis X (**Langerhans cell histiocytosis** [LCH]) may also lead to multiple lesions in the young patient. Fibrous dysplasia and Paget disease may manifest with multiple lesions in all age groups.
   - Anatomic location within bone: Certain lesions have a predilection for occurring within a certain bone or a particular part of the bone (Figure 9-1; Table 9-5).

Table 9-4 Age at Occurrence of Various Bone Lesions

	TYPE OF LESION	
Age	Malignant	Benign
Birth to 5 yr	Leukemia Metastatic neuroblastoma Metastatic rhabdomyosarcoma	Osteomyelitis Osteofibrous dysplasia
10-25 yr	Osteosarcoma Ewing tumor Leukemia	Eosinophilic granuloma Osteomyelitis Enchondroma Fibrous dysplasia
40-80 yr	Metastatic bone disease Myeloma Lymphoma Chondrosarcoma Malignant fibrous histiocytoma Paget sarcoma Postradiation sarcoma	Hyperparathyroidism Paget disease Mastocytosis Enchondroma Bone infarct

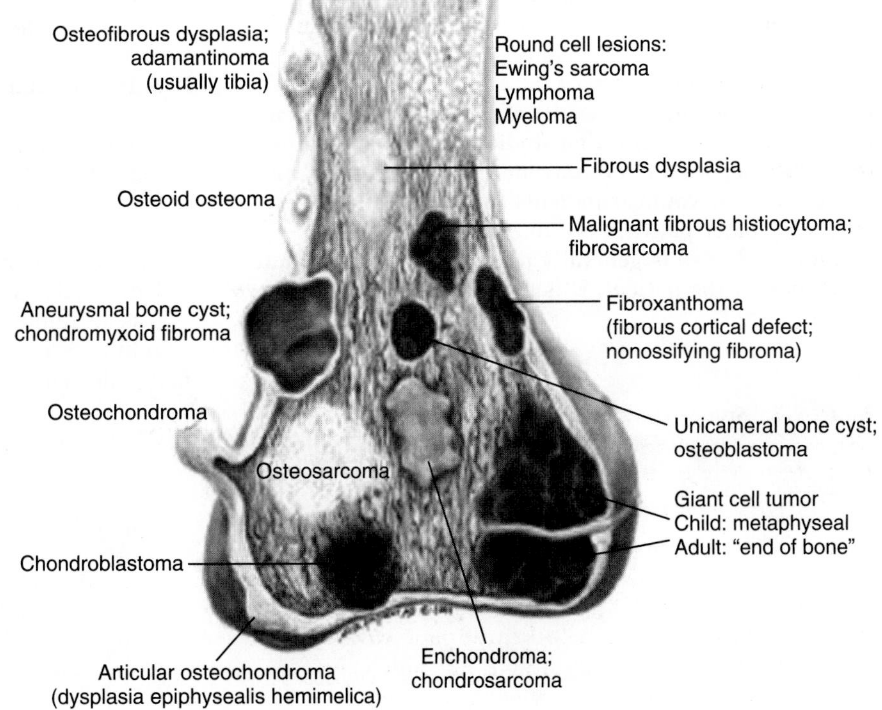

Figure 9-1 Map of neoplasms. Typical locations for both benign and malignant neoplasms. (From Wodajo FM, et al: *Visual guide to musculoskeletal tumors,* Philadelphia, 2010, Elsevier.)

Table 9-5 Most Common Musculoskeletal Tumors

Tumor Type	Tumor Name
Soft tissue tumor (children)	Hemangioma
Soft tissue tumor (adults)	Lipoma
Malignant soft tissue tumor (children)	Rhabdomyosarcoma
Malignant soft tissue tumor (adults)	Malignant fibrous histiocytoma
Primary benign bone tumor	Osteochondroma
Primary malignant bone tumor	Osteosarcoma
Secondary benign lesion	Aneurysmal bone cyst
Secondary malignancies	Malignant fibrous histiocytoma Osteosarcoma Fibrosarcoma
Phalangeal tumor	Enchondroma
Sarcoma of the hand and wrist	Epithelioid sarcoma
Sarcoma of the foot and ankle	Synovial sarcoma

Courtesy of Luke S. Choi, MD, Resident, Department of Orthopaedic Surgery, University of Virginia.

- Typical neoplasms of whole bone:
  - Tibia: adamantinoma, osteofibrous dysplasia
  - Posterior cortex distal femur: parosteal osteosarcoma, periosteal desmoid (also known as cortical desmoid, avulsive cortical irregularity)
- Typical neoplasms of part of bone (Table 9-6):
  - Epiphysis: giant cell tumor, chondroblastoma, aneurysmal bone cyst, osteomyelitis (tuberculosis, fungus)
    - Giant cell tumor typically begins in the metaphysis and extends through the epiphysis to lie just below the cartilage.
  - Metaphysis: metaphyseal fibrous defect (nonossifying fibroma), aneurysmal bone cyst, giant cell tumor, osteosarcoma
  - Diaphysis: Ewing sarcoma, fibrous dysplasia, eosinophilic granuloma (histiocytosis), multiple myeloma

D. Laboratory studies: Results of blood tests are often nonspecific. A set of routine studies should be obtained when the diagnosis is not obvious. Certain studies are appropriate for younger patients (up to age 40) and others for older patients (40 to 80 years; Box 9-1).

E. Biopsy: Biopsy is generally performed after complete evaluation of the patient. It is of great benefit to both the pathologist and the surgeon to have a narrow working diagnosis because it allows accurate interpretation of the frozen-section analysis, and definitive treatment of some lesions can be based on the frozen section. Clinicians must follow several surgical principles:

1. The orientation and location of the biopsy tract are critical. If the lesion proves to be malignant, the entire biopsy tract must be removed with the underlying lesion. **Transverse incisions should be avoided.**
2. The surgeon must maintain **meticulous hemostasis** to prevent hematoma formation and subcutaneous hemorrhage. When possible, **biopsy incisions are made through muscles** so that the muscle layer can be closed tightly. **Neurovascular structures should be avoided.** Tourniquets are used to obtain tissue in a bloodless field and then are released so that bleeding points can be controlled. Avitene, Gelfoam, and Thrombostat sprays are used as necessary. If hemostasis cannot be achieved, **a small drain should be placed at the corner of the wound to prevent hematoma formation.** A compression dressing is routinely used on the extremities.
3. A **frozen-section analysis is performed on all biopsy samples to ensure that adequate diagnostic tissue is obtained.** Before biopsy, the surgeon should review the radiographs with the pathologist to plan the biopsy site. When possible, the soft tissue component rather than the bony component should be sampled.
4. All biopsy samples **should be submitted for bacteriologic analysis** if the frozen section does not reveal a neoplasm. Antibiotics should not be delivered until the cultures are obtained.
5. Needle biopsy is an excellent method for achieving a tissue diagnosis and providing minimum tissue disruption. Careful correlation of the small tissue sample with the radiographs often yields the correct diagnosis. When the nature of the lesion is obvious on the basis of the radiographic features and when adequate tissue can be obtained with a needle, the needle biopsy technique is safe to use. The pathologist must be experienced and comfortable with the small sample of tissue. When the diagnoses of needle biopsy and imaging studies are not concordant, an open biopsy should be performed to establish the diagnosis. Open biopsy is often necessary with low-grade tumors and

Box 9-1

Laboratory Evaluations for Younger and Older Patients

AGES 5 TO 40 YEARS
Complete blood cell count with differential
Peripheral blood smear
Erythrocyte sedimentation rate

AGES 40 TO 80 YEARS
Complete blood cell count with differential
Erythrocyte sedimentation rate
Chemistry profiles: calcium and phosphate
Serum or urine protein electrophoresis
Urinalysis

Table 9-6 Spinal Tumors

Anterior Spine	Posterior Spine
Giant cell tumor	Aneurysmal bone cyst
Hemangioma	Osteoid osteoma
Eosinophilic granuloma	Osteoblastoma
Metastases	
Chordoma	
Multiple myeloma	

Courtesy of Luke S. Choi, MD, Resident, Department of Orthopaedic Surgery, University of Virginia.

Table 9-7 Tumor Immunostains

Tumor	Immunostain
Langerhans cell histiocytosis	S100, +CD1A
Lymphoma	+CD20
Ewing sarcoma	+CD99
Chordoma	Keratin, S100
Myeloma	+CD138
Adamantinoma	Keratin

Courtesy of Luke S. Choi, MD, Resident, Department of Orthopaedic Surgery, University of Virginia.

when the needle biopsy does not provide a definitive diagnosis. Immunostains are helpful in diagnosis (Table 9-7).

VI. TREATMENT

A. Surgical procedures: The goal of the treatment of malignant bone tumors is to remove the lesion with minimal risk of local recurrence.

1. **Limb salvage is performed when two essential criteria are met:**
   - **Local control of the lesion must be at least equal to that of amputation surgery.**
   - **The limb that has been saved must be functional. A wide-margin surgical resection (excising a cuff of normal tissue around the tumor) is the operative goal.**
2. **Surgical margins are graded according to the system of the Musculoskeletal Tumor Society** (Figure 9-2).

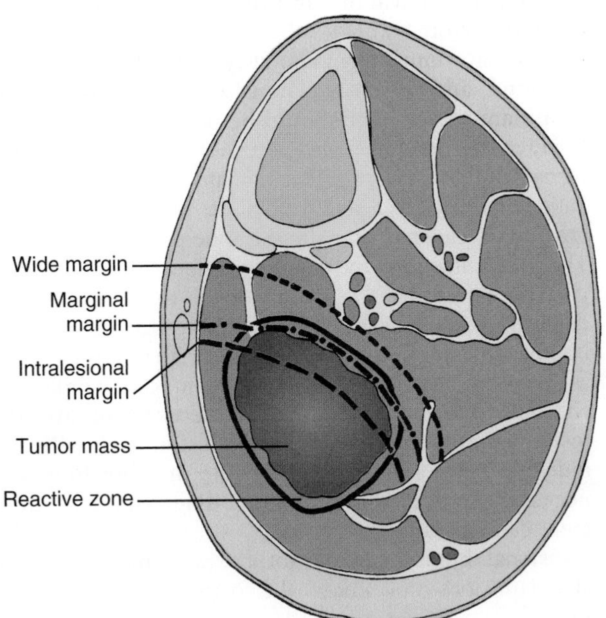

Figure 9-2 Types of surgical margins. An intralesional line of resection enters the substance of the tumor. A marginal line of resection travels through the reactive zone of the tumor. Wide-margin surgical resection removes the tumor, along with a cuff of normal tissue. (From Sim FH, et al: Soft tissue tumors: diagnosis, evaluation and management, *Am Acad Orthop Surg* 2:209, 1994. ©1994 American Academy of Orthopaedic Surgeons. Reprinted with permission.)

- Intralesional margin: The plane of dissection goes directly through the tumor. When the surgery involves malignant mesenchymal tumors, an intralesional margin results in 100% local recurrence.
- Marginal margin: A marginal line of resection goes through the reactive zone of the tumor; the reactive zone contains inflammatory cells, edema, fibrous tissue, and satellites of tumor cells. When malignant mesenchymal tumors are resected, a plane of dissection through the reactive zone probably results in a local recurrence rate of 25% to 50%. A marginal margin may be safe and effective if the response to preoperative chemotherapy has been excellent (95% to 100% tumor necrosis).
- Wide margin: A wide line of surgical resection is accomplished when the entire tumor is removed with a cuff of normal tissue. The local recurrence rate drops below 10% when such a surgical margin is achieved.
- Radical margin: A radical margin is achieved when the entire tumor and its compartment (all surrounding muscles, ligaments, and connective tissues) are removed.

B. Adjuvant therapy

1. **Chemotherapy**
   - **Multiagent chemotherapy has a significant effect on both the efficacy of limb salvage and disease-free survival for osteogenic sarcoma and Ewing tumor.**
   - The common mechanism of action of drugs is the induction of programmed cell death (apoptosis).
   - Most protocols entail preoperative regimens (neoadjuvant chemotherapy) for 8 to 24 weeks. The tumor is then restaged and, if appropriate, limb salvage is performed.
   - Patients undergo maintenance chemotherapy for 6 to 12 months.
   - Patients with localized osteosarcoma or Ewing tumor have up to a 60% to 70% chance for long-term disease-free survival with the combination of multiagent chemotherapy and surgery.
   - The role of chemotherapy for soft tissue sarcoma remains more controversial.
2. Radiation therapy
   - **External beam irradiation is used in the following scenarios:**
     - **For local control of Ewing tumor, lymphoma, myeloma, and metastatic bone disease**
     - As an adjunct in the treatment of soft tissue sarcomas, in which it is used in combination with surgery.
     - For their mechanism of action, which is the production of free radicals and direct genetic damage. There are several complications of radiation therapy:
       - Postirradiation sarcoma: This is a devastating complication in which a spindle sarcoma occurs within the field of irradiation for a previous malignancy (e.g., Ewing tumor, breast cancer, Hodgkin disease). The histologic features are usually those of an osteosarcoma, a fibrosarcoma, or a malignant fibrous histiocytoma. Postirradiation sarcomas are probably more frequent in patients who undergo intensive chemotherapy (especially with alkylating agents) and irradiation.

- **Late stress fractures: These also may occur in weight-bearing bones to which high-dose irradiation has been applied. The subtrochanteric region and the diaphysis of the femur are common sites.**

VII. MOLECULAR BIOLOGY

Several bone and soft tissue neoplasms have been associated with tumor suppressor genes or specific genetic defects. For osteosarcoma, the associations are the retinoblastoma tumor suppressor gene. For Ewing tumor, there is a balanced translocation of chromosomes 11 and 22. There is a gene fusion product from this balanced translocation: EWS-FLI1 (Table 9-8).

Table 9-8 Common Tumor-Associated Genetic Translocations

Tumor Type	Genetic Translocation
Myxoid liposarcoma	t(12;16)
Ewing sarcoma	t(11;22)
Synovial sarcoma	t(X;18)
Myxoid chondrosarcoma	t(9;22)
Rhabdomyosarcoma	t(1;13) or t(2;13)

Courtesy of Luke S. Choi, MD, Fellow, Orthopaedic Sports Medicine, Massachusetts General Hospital.

SECTION 2 SOFT TISSUE TUMORS

I. INTRODUCTION

Soft tissue tumors are common. They may appear as small lumps or large masses.

A. Classification: Soft tissue tumors can be broadly classified as benign or malignant (sarcoma) or characterized by reactive tumor-like conditions (Box 9-2). Lesions are classified according to the direction of differentiation of the lesion: the tumor tends to produce collagen (fibrous lesion), fat, or cartilage.

1. Benign soft tissue tumors: These tumors may occur in all age groups. The biologic behavior of these lesions varies from asymptomatic and self-limiting to growing and symptomatic. On occasion, benign lesions grow rapidly and invade adjacent tissues.
2. Malignant soft tissue tumors (sarcomas): Sarcomas are rare tumors of mesenchymal origin. In the United States, there are approximately 9000 new cases of soft tissue sarcoma each year.
   - Diagnosis: **Patients often experience an enlarging painless or painful soft tissue mass, which is the most common reason for seeking medical attention.**
     - Most sarcomas are large (>5 cm), deep, and firm.
     - In some instances, they are small and may be present for a long time before they are recognized as tumors (synovial sarcoma, rhabdomyosarcoma, epithelioid sarcoma, and clear cell sarcoma).
     - Initial radiographic evaluation begins with radiographs in two planes.
     - MRI is the best imaging modality for defining the anatomy and helping characterize the lesion. When a mass is judged to be indeterminate, an open incisional or needle biopsy is performed. A definitive histologic diagnosis must be established before treatment is planned.
     - **CT scan of the chest is required in order to evaluate for metastasis. CT scan of the abdomen and pelvis is obtained for liposarcoma because of synchronous retroperitoneal liposarcoma.**
   - Treatment: Radiation therapy is an important adjunct to surgery in the treatment of soft tissue sarcomas.
     - Ionizing radiation can be delivered preoperatively, perioperatively with brachytherapy after loading tubes, or postoperatively.
     - Treatment regimens are often designed to use combinations of the three types of preoperative, postoperative, and external beam irradiation. Poor prognostic factors include the presence of metastases, high grade, size greater than 5 cm, and location below the deep fascia.

B. Diagnosis: The evaluation of patients with soft tissue tumors must be systematic to avoid errors.

1. **Unplanned removal of a soft tissue sarcoma is the most common error.**
   - **Residual tumor may exist at the site of the operative wound, and repeat excision for all patients with an unplanned removal should be performed.**
2. Delay in diagnosis may also occur if the clinician does not recognize that the lesion is malignant.
3. Patients who have a new soft tissue mass or one that is growing or causing pain should undergo MRI.
4. The MRI scan should be carefully reviewed with a radiologist to characterize the nature of the mass. If it can be determined that the lesion is a benign process such as a lipoma, ganglionic cyst, or muscle tear, then it is classified as a *determinate lesion,* and treatment can be planned without a biopsy. **In contrast, if the exact nature of a lesion cannot be determined, the lesion is classified as *indeterminate,* and either a needle or open biopsy is necessary to determine the exact diagnosis.** Then treatment can be planned.
5. Excisional biopsy should not be performed when the clinician does not know the origin of a soft tissue tumor.

C. Metastasis: Most soft tissue sarcomas metastasize to the lung.

1. **Lymph node metastasis occurs with 5% of soft tissue sarcomas. Rhabdomyosarcoma, clear cell sarcoma, epithelioid sarcoma, and synovial sarcoma are the tumors that most commonly metastasize via the lymphatic vessels.**

Box 9-2

Classification of Soft Tissue Tumors

TUMORS AND TUMOR-LIKE LESIONS OF FIBROUS TISSUE

Benign
- Fibroma
- Nodular fasciitis
- Proliferative fasciitis

Fibromatoses
- Superficial fibromatoses
- Palmar and plantar fibromatoses
- Knuckle pads
- Deep fibromatoses (extra-abdominal fibromatoses)

Malignant
- Adult fibrosarcoma
- Postirradiation fibrosarcoma

FIBROHISTIOCYTIC TUMORS

Benign
- Fibrous histiocytoma
- Atypical fibroxanthoma

Intermediate
- Dermatofibrosarcoma protuberans

Malignant (malignant histiocytoma)
- Storiform-pleomorphic
- Myxoid (myxofibrosarcoma)
- Giant cell (malignant giant cell tumor of soft parts)
- Inflammatory (malignant xanthogranuloma, xanthosarcoma)

TUMORS AND TUMOR-LIKE CONDITIONS OF ADIPOSE TISSUE

Benign
- Lipoma (cutaneous, deep, and multiple)
- Angiolipoma
- Spindle cell and pleomorphic lipoma
- Lipoblastoma and lipoblastomatosis
- Intramuscular and intermuscular lipoma
- Hibernoma

Malignant
- Liposarcoma
- Well-differentiated (lipoma-like, sclerosing, inflammatory)
- Myxoid
- Round cell (poorly differentiated myxoid)
- Pleomorphic
- Dedifferentiated

TUMORS OF MUSCLE TISSUE

Smooth Muscle

Benign
- Leiomyoma (cutaneous and deep)
- Angiomyoma (vascular leiomyoma)

Malignant
- Leiomyosarcoma

Striated Muscle

Benign
- Adult rhabdomyoma

Malignant
- Rhabdomyosarcoma: predominantly embryonal (including botryoid), alveolar, pleomorphic, and mixed

TUMORS OF LYMPH VESSELS

Benign (lymphangioma)
- Cavernous
- Cystic (cystic hygroma)

Malignant
- Lymphangiosarcoma
- Postmastectomy lymphangiosarcoma

TUMORS AND TUMOR-LIKE LESIONS OF SYNOVIAL TISSUE

Benign
- Giant cell tumor of tendon sheath
- Localized (nodular tenosynovitis)
- Diffuse (florid synovitis)

Malignant
- Synovial sarcoma (malignant synovioma), predominantly biphasic or monophasic (either fibrous or epithelial)
- Malignant giant cell tumor of tendon sheath

TUMORS AND TUMOR-LIKE LESIONS OF PERIPHERAL NERVES

Benign
- Traumatic neuroma
- Morton neuroma
- Neurilemoma (benign schwannoma)
- Neurofibroma, solitary
- Neurofibromatosis (von Recklinghausen disease)
- Localized
- Plexiform
- Diffuse

Malignant
- Malignant schwannoma
- Peripheral tumors of primitive neuroectodermal tissues

TUMORS AND TUMOR-LIKE LESIONS OF CARTILAGE AND BONE-FORMING TISSUES

Benign
- Panniculitis ossificans
- Myositis ossificans
- Fibrodysplasia (myositis) ossificans progressiva
- Extraskeletal chondroma
- Extraskeletal osteoma

Malignant
- Extraskeletal chondrosarcoma
- Well-differentiated
- Myxoid (choroid sarcoma)
- Mesenchymal
- Extraskeletal osteosarcoma

TUMORS AND TUMOR-LIKE LESIONS OF PLURIPOTENTIAL MESENCHYME
- Benign mesenchymoma
- Malignant mesenchymoma

TUMORS AND TUMOR-LIKE CONDITIONS OF BLOOD VESSELS

Benign
- Hemangioma
- Deep hemangioma (intramuscular, synovial, perineural)
- Glomus tumor

Intermediate
- Hemangioendothelioma

Malignant
- Hemangiosarcoma
- Malignant hemangiopericytoma

TUMORS AND TUMOR-LIKE CONDITIONS OF DISPUTED OR UNCERTAIN HISTOGENESIS

Benign
- Tumoral calcinosis
- Myxoma (cutaneous and intramuscular)

Malignant
- Alveolar soft-part sarcoma
- Epithelioid sarcoma
- Clear cell sarcoma of tendons and aponeuroses
- Extraskeletal Ewing sarcoma

UNCLASSIFIED SOFT TISSUE TUMORS AND TUMOR-LIKE LESIONS

II. TUMORS OF FIBROUS TISSUE

Fibrous tumors are common, and their characteristics range widely, from small, self-limiting, benign conditions to aggressive, invasive, benign tumors. The malignant fibrous tumors are fibrosarcoma and malignant fibrous histiocytoma.

A. Calcifying aponeurotic fibroma

1. Manifests as a slow-growing, painless mass in the hands and feet in children and young adults 3 to 30 years of age.
2. Radiographs may reveal a faint mass with stippling.
3. Histologic examination reveals a fibrous tumor with centrally located areas of calcification and cartilage formation.
4. After local excision, the tumor often recurs (in up to 50% of cases); however, the condition appears to resolve with maturity.

B. Fibromatosis

1. Palmar (Dupuytren) and plantar (Ledderhose) fibromatosis: These disorders consist of firm nodules of fibroblasts and collagen that develop in the palmar and plantar fascia. The nodules and fascia become hypertrophic, producing contractures.
2. Extraabdominal desmoid tumor
   - Most locally invasive of all benign soft tissue tumors.
   - Commonly occurs in adolescents and young adults.
     - **Patients with Gardner syndrome (familial adenomatous polyposis) have colonic polyps and a 10,000-fold increased risk of developing desmoid tumors.**
   - **On palpation, the tumor has a distinctive "rock-hard" character.**
   - Multiple lesions may be present in the same extremity (10% to 25%).
   - Histologically, the tumor consists of well-differentiated fibroblasts and abundant collagen. The lesion infiltrates adjacent tissues. **Immunohistochemistry study reveals positivity for estrogen receptor β, and inhibitors have been used for treatment.**
   - Surgical treatment is aimed at resecting the tumor with a wide margin.
   - Local recurrence is common.
   - Radiotherapy has been used as an adjunctive treatment to prevent recurrence and progression.
   - Behavior of the tumor is capricious: Recurrent nodules may remain dormant for years or grow rapidly for some time and then stop growing.

C. Nodular fasciitis

1. **A common reactive lesion that manifests as a painful, *rapidly enlarging* mass in a young person (15 to 35 years of age).**
2. Half of these lesions occur in the upper extremity.
3. Short, irregular bundles and fascicles; a dense reticulum network; and only small amounts of mature collagen characterize the lesion histologically. Mitotic figures are common, but atypical mitoses are not a feature.
4. Treatment consists of excision with a marginal line of resection.

D. Malignant fibrous soft tissue tumors: Malignant fibrous histiocytoma and fibrosarcoma are the two malignant fibrous lesions.

1. Diagnosis
   - Similar clinical and radiographic manifestations; treatment methods are similar
   - Patients are generally between the ages of 30 and 80 years.
   - Most common manifestation is an enlarging, generally painless mass.
   - **MRI often shows a deep-seated, inhomogeneous mass that has a low signal on T1-weighted images and a high signal on T2-weighted images**. The two lesions may be similar histologically, but there are distinctive features:
     - *Malignant fibrous histiocytoma:* The spindle and histiocytic cells are arranged in a storiform (cartwheel) pattern. Short fascicles of cells and fibrous tissue appear to radiate about a common center around slit-like vessels. Chronic inflammatory cells may also be present.
     - *Fibrosarcoma:* There is a fasciculated growth pattern, with fusiform or spindle-shaped cells, scanty cytoplasm, and indistinct borders, and the cells are separated by interwoven collagen fibers. In some cases, the tissue is organized into a herringbone pattern, which consists of intersecting fascicles in which the nuclei in one fascicle are viewed transversely but in an adjacent fascicle are viewed longitudinally.
   - Treatment is by wide-margin local excision. Radiation therapy is employed in many cases when the size of the tumor exceeds 5 cm.
   - A common scenario is to deliver radiation preoperatively (5000 cGy), followed by resection of the lesion. A final radiation boost (1400 to 2000 cGy) is then administered postoperatively or with brachytherapy afterloading tubes if the margins are very close or positive.
   - **Postoperative external beam irradiation (6300 to 6600 cGy) yields equal local control rates, with a lower postoperative wound complication rate but a higher incidence of postoperative fibrosis.**

E. Dermatofibrosarcoma protuberans

1. Rare, nodular, cutaneous tumor that occurs in early to middle adulthood
2. Low grade, with a tendency to recur locally, but it only rarely metastasizes (often after repeated local recurrence)
3. In 40% of the cases, it occurs on the upper or lower extremities. The tumor grows slowly but progressively.
4. The central portion of the nodules shows uniform fibroblasts arranged in a storiform pattern around an inconspicuous vasculature.
5. Wide-margin surgical resection is the best form of treatment.

III. TUMORS OF FATTY TISSUE

There is a wide spectrum of benign and malignant tumors of fat origin. Each has a particular biologic behavior that guides evaluation and treatment.

A. Lipomas: common benign tumors of mature fat

1. Occur in a subcutaneous, intramuscular, or intermuscular location
2. History of a mass is long, but sometimes the mass was only recently discovered.
3. Not painful

4. Radiographs may show a radiolucent lesion in the soft tissues if the lipoma is deep within the muscle or between the muscle and bone.
5. **CT scan or MRI shows a well-demarcated lesion with the same signal characteristics as those of mature fat on all sequences. On fat suppression sequences, the lipoma has a uniformly low signal. If the patient experiences no symptoms and the radiographic features are diagnostic of lipoma, no treatment is necessary.**
6. **If the mass is growing or causing symptoms, excision with a marginal line of resection or an intralesional margin is all that is necessary.**
7. Local recurrence is uncommon.
8. Several variants:
   - Spindle cell lipoma
     - Commonly occurs in men (45 to 65 years of age)
     - Manifests as a solitary, painless, growing, firm nodule
     - Histologically characterized by a mixture of mature fat cells and spindle cells. There is a mucoid matrix with a varying number of birefringent collagen fibers.
     - Treatment is excision with a marginal margin.
   - Pleomorphic lipoma
     - Occurs in middle-aged patients
     - Manifests as a slow-growing mass
     - Histologically characterized by lipocytes; spindle cells; and scattered, bizarre giant cells
     - May be confused with different types of liposarcoma
     - Treatment is by excision with a marginal margin.
   - Angiolipoma
     - The only lipoma that is very painful when palpated.
     - Manifests with small nodules in the upper extremity that are intensely painful
     - MRI may show a small, fatty nodule or completely normal appearance.
     - Consists of mature fat cells (as in a typical lipoma) and nests of small arborizing vessels

B. Liposarcomas

1. Type of sarcoma; direction of differentiation is toward fatty tissue
2. Heterogeneous group of tumors, having in common the presence of lipoblasts (signet ring–shaped cells) in the tissue
3. **Liposarcomas virtually never occur in the subcutaneous tissues.**
4. They are classified into the following types:
   - Well-differentiated liposarcoma (low grade)
     - Lipoma-like
     - Sclerosing
     - Inflammatory
   - Myxoid liposarcoma (intermediate grade)
   - Dedifferentiated (high grade)
   - Round-cell liposarcoma (high grade)
   - Pleomorphic liposarcoma (high grade)
5. Liposarcomas metastasize according to the grade of the lesion:
   - Well-differentiated liposarcomas have a very low rate of metastasis (<10%)
   - The metastasis rate of intermediate-grade liposarcomas is 10% to 30%.
   - The metastasis rate of high-grade liposarcomas is more than 50%.

IV. TUMORS OF NEURAL TISSUE

The two benign neural tumors are neurilemoma and neurofibroma. Their malignant counterpart is neurofibrosarcoma.

A. Neurilemoma (benign schwannoma)

1. Benign nerve sheath tumor
2. Occurs in young to middle-aged adults (20 to 50 years of age)
3. Patients have no symptoms except for the presence of the mass.
4. Tumor grows slowly and may wax and wane in size (cystic changes).
5. MRI studies may demonstrate an eccentric mass arising from a peripheral nerve, or they may show only an indeterminate soft tissue mass (low signal on T1-weighted images and high signal on T2-weighted images).
6. Histologically, the lesion is composed of Antoni A and B areas.
   - Antoni A area:
     - Compact spindle cells usually having twisted nuclei; indistinct cytoplasm; and occasionally clear, intranuclear vacuoles
     - There may be nuclear palisading, whorling of cells, and Verocay bodies.
     - When the lesion is predominantly cellular (Antoni A), the tumor may be confused with a sarcoma.
     - Treatment: removing the eccentric mass while leaving the nerve intact
   - Antoni'a B area:
     - Less orderly and cellular
     - Arranged haphazardly in the loosely textured matrix (with microcystic changes, inflammatory cells, and delicate collagen fibers)
     - Vessels are large and irregularly spaced.

B. Neurofibroma

1. Solitary or multiple (neurofibromatosis)
2. Superficial, slow-growing, and painless
3. When they involve a major nerve, they may expand it in a fusiform manner.
4. **Histologic study shows interlacing bundles of elongated cells with wavy, dark-staining nuclei.**
5. **Cells are associated with wirelike strands of collagen.**
6. Small to moderate amounts of mucoid material separate the cells and collagen
7. Treatment: excision with a marginal margin.

C. Neurofibromatosis (von Recklinghausen disease)

1. Autosomal dominant trait (both peripheral and central forms)
2. **Café au lait spots (smooth) and Lisch nodules (melanocytic hamartomas in the iris)**
3. Variable skeletal abnormalities (metaphyseal fibrous defect [nonossifying fibroma], scoliosis, and long-bone bowing)
4. Malignant changes occur in 5% to 30% of affected patients.
5. Pain and an enlarging soft tissue mass may herald conversion to a sarcoma.

D. Neurofibrosarcoma

1. Rare tumor that arises in a de novo manner or in the setting of neurofibromatosis
2. High-grade sarcoma; treated in a manner similar to that for other high-grade sarcomas

V. TUMORS OF MUSCLE TISSUE

A. Leiomyosarcoma

1. Manifests as a small nodule or a large extremity mass
2. May or may not be associated with blood vessels
3. Low or high grade

B. Rhabdomyosarcoma

1. **The most common sarcoma in young patients; may grow rapidly**
2. Composed of spindle cells in parallel bundles, multinucleated giant cells, and racquet-shaped cells
3. Cross-striations within the tumor cells (rhabdomyoblasts)
4. Rhabdomyosarcomas are sensitive to multiagent chemotherapy and wide-margin surgical resection after induction of chemotherapy. External beam irradiation plays a prominent role in treatment.

VI. VASCULAR TUMORS

A. Hemangioma

1. Commonly seen in children and adults
2. Cutaneous, subcutaneous, or intramuscular location
3. Large tumors have signs of vascular engorgement (aching, heaviness, swelling).
4. MRI scans demonstrate a heterogeneous lesion with numerous small blood vessels and fatty infiltration.
5. It is important to examine the patient in both the supine and standing positions. (The lower extremity often fills with blood after several minutes).
6. **Radiographs may reveal small phleboliths**.
7. Nonoperative treatment: NSAIDs, vascular stockings, and activity modification if local measures adequately control discomfort
8. Can be treated by application of a sclerosing agent such as alcohol

B. Angiosarcoma

1. Cells resemble the endothelium of blood vessels.
2. Highly malignant
3. Infiltrative; with local excision, the rate of failure is high.
4. Amputation may be necessary to achieve local control.
5. Pulmonary metastases are common.

VII. SYNOVIAL DISORDERS

A. Ganglia

1. Out-pouching of the synovial lining of an adjacent joint
2. Common locations include the wrist, foot, and knee.
3. Filled with gelatinous, mucoid material
4. Paucicellular connective tissue without a true epithelial lining
5. MRI: homogeneously low signal on T1-weighted images and a very bright signal on T2-weighted images; contrast agent such as gadolinium is useful in differentiating a cyst from a solid neoplasm because cysts do not enhance (except for a small rim at the periphery) but active neoplasms usually do.

B. Pigmented villonodular synovitis (PVNS)

1. Reactive condition (not a true neoplasm) characterized by an exuberant proliferation of synovial villi and nodules
2. May occur locally (within a joint) or diffusely
3. **The knee is affected most often, followed in frequency by the hip and shoulder.**
4. Manifests with pain and swelling in the affected joint
5. Recurrent, atraumatic hemarthrosis is the hallmark (arthrocentesis demonstrates a bloody effusion).
6. **Cystic erosions may occur on both sides of the joint.**
7. **Highly vascular villi are lined with plump, hyperplastic synovial cells; hemosiderin-stained, multinucleated giant cells; and chronic inflammatory cells.**
8. **Treatment is aimed at complete synovectomy by arthroscopy for resection of all the intraarticular disease, followed by open posterior synovectomy to remove the posterior extraarticular extension.**
   - **The local form of PVNS may be treated with partial synovectomy.**
9. Local recurrence is common (30% to 50% of cases) despite complete synovectomy.
10. External beam irradiation (3500 to 4000 cGy) can reduce the rate of local recurrence to 10% to 20%.

C. Giant cell tumor of tendon sheath

1. Benign nodular tumor occurs along the tendon sheaths (hands/feet).
2. Moderately cellular (sheets of rounded or polygonal cells) zones; hypocellular, collagenized zones; multinucleated giant cells are common, as are xanthoma cells.
3. Treatment: resection with a marginal margin
4. Local recurrence is common (usually treated with repeat excision).

D. Synovial chondromatosis

1. Synovial proliferative disorder that occurs within joints or bursae, ranging in appearance from metaplasia of the synovial tissue to firm nodules of cartilage
2. Typically affects young adults, who present with pain, stiffness, and swelling
3. The knee is the most common location.
4. **Radiographs may demonstrate fine, stippled calcification.**
5. Treatment: removal of the loose bodies and synovectomy

E. Synovial sarcoma

1. Highly malignant, high-grade tumor that occurs near joints, most commonly around the knee
2. **Although the name implies that it arises from synovial cells, it rarely arises from an intraarticular location.**
   - **Typically manifests between the ages of 15 and 40 years**
3. May be present for years or may manifest as a rapidly enlarging mass
4. Lymph nodes may be involved.
5. **Most common synovial sarcoma is in the foot.**
6. **Radiographs or CT scans may show mineralization within the lesion in up to 25% of cases (spotty mineralization may even resemble the peripheral mineralization seen in heterotopic ossification).**
   - Irregular contour differentiates these lesions from hemangioma.
7. The tumor is often biphasic, with both epithelial and spindle cell components.
   - The epithelial component may show epithelial cells that form glands or nests, or they may line cystlike spaces.
9. The tumor may also be composed of a single type of cell (monophasic); the monophasic fibrous type is much more common than the monophasic epithelial type.

10. **Translocation between chromosome 18 and the X chromosome—t(X;18)—is always present in tumor cells, and staining of the tumor cells yields positive results for keratin and epithelial membrane antigen.**
11. **The balanced translocation results in gene fusion products. The two most common are SYT-SSX1 and SYT-SSX2.**
12. Wide-margin surgical resection with adjuvant radiotherapy is the most common method of treatment.
13. Metastases develop in 30% to 60% of cases.
14. Larger tumors (>5 to 10 cm) are more prone to distant spread.

VIII. OTHER RARE SARCOMAS

A. Epithelioid sarcoma

1. Rare nodular tumor that commonly occurs in the upper extremities of young adults
2. May also occur about the buttock/thigh, knee, and foot
3. The most common sarcoma of the hand
4. May ulcerate and mimic a granuloma or rheumatoid nodule
5. Lymph node metastases are common.
6. Cells range in shape from ovoid to polygonal, with deeply eosinophilic cytoplasm (cellular pleomorphism is minimal).
7. Often misdiagnosed as benign processes.
8. Wide-margin surgical resection is necessary to prevent local recurrence.

B. Clear cell sarcoma

1. Manifests as a slow-growing mass in association with tendons or aponeuroses
2. Usually occurs about the foot and ankle but may also involve the knee, thigh, and hand
3. Characterized by compact nests or fascicles of rounded or fusiform cells with clear cytoplasm; multinucleated giant cells are common
4. Wide-margin surgical resection with adjuvant irradiation is the treatment of choice.

C. Alveolar cell sarcoma

1. Manifests as a slow-growing, painless mass in young adults (15 to 35 years of age)
2. Occurs in the anterior thigh
3. Dense, fibrous trabeculae dividing the tumor into an organoid or nestlike arrangement; cells are large and rounded and contain one or more vesicular nuclei with small nucleoli
4. Treatment: wide-margin surgical resection with adjuvant irradiation in selected cases

IX. POST-TRAUMATIC CONDITIONS

A. Hematoma

1. Hematoma may occur after trauma to the extremity.
2. Organizes and resolves with time
3. **Sarcomas may spontaneously hemorrhage into the body of the tumor or after minor trauma and masquerade as a benign process. A lack of fascial plane tracking and subcutaneous ecchymosis suggests that the bleeding is contained by a pseudocapsule; this is an important physical examination finding.**
4. Clinicians should monitor patients with hematomas at 6-week intervals until the mass resolves.
5. MRI scanning is often not able to distinguish a simple hematoma from a sarcoma with spontaneous hemorrhage.

B. Myositis ossificans (heterotopic ossification)

1. Develops after single or repetitive episodes of trauma (occasionally, patients cannot recall the traumatic episode)
2. Most common locations are over the diaphyseal segment of long bones (in the middle aspect of the muscle bellies).
3. As maturation progresses, radiographs show peripheral mineralization with a central lucent area.
4. Lesion is not attached to the underlying bone, but in some cases, it may become fixed to the periosteal surface.
5. Zonal pattern, with mature, trabecular bone at the periphery and immature tissue in the center
6. Nonoperative treatment is all the management that is necessary.

SECTION 3 BONE TUMORS

I. NOMENCLATURE

A common classification system for bone tumors is shown in Table 9-9.

A. Sarcomas

1. Malignant neoplasms of connective tissue (mesenchymal) origin
2. Exhibit rapid growth in a centripetal manner and invade adjacent normal tissues
3. Each year in the United States, about 2800 new bone sarcomas are diagnosed.
   - **Malignant bone tumors manifest most commonly with pain. This is in contrast to soft tissue tumors, which most commonly manifest as a painless mass.**
4. High-grade, malignant bone tumors tend to destroy the overlying cortex and spread into the soft tissues.
5. Low-grade tumors are generally contained within the cortex or the surrounding periosteal rim.
6. Bone sarcomas metastasize primarily via the hematogenous route; the lungs are the most common site.
7. Osteosarcoma and Ewing sarcoma may also metastasize to other bone sites either at the initial manifestation or later in the disease.

B. Benign bone tumors

1. These may be small and have a limited growth potential, or they may be large and destructive.

C. Tumor simulators and reactive conditions

1. These processes occur in bone but are not true neoplasms (e.g., osteomyelitis, aneurysmal bone cyst, bone island).

Table 9-9 Classification of Primary Tumors of Bone*

Histologic Type	Benign	Malignant
Hematopoietic		Myeloma Lymphoma
Chondrogenic	Osteochondroma Chondroma Chondroblastoma Chondromyxoid fibroma	Primary chondrosarcoma Secondary chondrosarcoma Dedifferentiated chondrosarcoma Mesenchymal chondrosarcoma Clear cell chondrosarcoma
Osteogenic	Osteoid osteoma Osteoblastoma	Osteosarcoma Parosteal osteosarcoma Periosteal osteosarcoma
Unknown origin	Giant cell tumor (fibrous) histiocytoma	Ewing tumor Malignant giant cell tumor Adamantinoma
Fibrogenic	Fibroma Desmoplastic fibroma	Fibrosarcoma Malignant fibrous histiocytoma
Notochordal		Chordoma
Vascular	Hemangioma	Hemangioendothelioma Hemangiopericytoma
Lipogenic	Lipoma	
Neurogenic	Neurilemoma	

*Classification is based on that advocated by Lichtenstein L: Classification of primary tumors of bone, *Cancer* 4:335-341, 1951.

II. BONE-PRODUCING LESIONS

There are three lesions in which the tumor cells produce osteoid: osteoid osteoma, osteoblastoma, and osteosarcoma.

A. Osteoid osteoma

Self-limiting benign bone lesion produces pain in young patients (5 to 30 years of age)

1. Diagnosis
   - Pain that increases with time, pain at night
     - **Classically relieved by salicylates and other NSAIDs**
   - Pain may be referred to an adjacent joint, and when the lesion is intracapsular, it may simulate arthritis.
   - May produce painful nonstructural scoliosis, growth disturbances, and flexion contractures
     - **Scoliosis caused by an osteoid osteoma results in a curve with the lesion on the concave side. This is thought to result fromj marked paravertebral muscle spasm.**
   - Common locations include the proximal femur, tibial diaphysis, and spine (Figure 9-3).
   - Radiographs usually show intensely reactive bone and a radiolucent nidus (Figure 9-4). **It may be possible to detect the lesion only with tomograms, CT scans, or MRI scans, because of the intense sclerosis.**
   - The nidus is, by definition, always less than 1.5 cm in diameter, although the area of reactive bone sclerosis may be long.
   - Technetium-labeled bone scans always yield positive findings and show intense focal uptake.
   - **CT scans are superior to MRI scans in detecting and characterizing osteoid osteomas because the CT scans provide better contrast between the lucent nidus and the reactive bone than the MRI scan does.**
   - There is a distinct demarcation between the nidus and the reactive bone (nidus consists of an interlacing network of osteoid trabeculae with variable mineralization), trabecular organization is haphazard, and the greatest degree of mineralization is in the center of the lesion.
2. Patients can be treated with three different methods: NSAIDs, CT scan–guided radiofrequency ablation, and open surgical removal.
   - In about 50% of patients treated with NSAIDs, the lesions burn out, with no further medical or surgical treatment necessary.
   - **CT scan–guided radiofrequency ablation has become the dominant method of treatment.**
     - A radiofrequency probe is placed into the lesion, and the nidus is heated to 80° C.
     - In about 90% of selected patients, the tumor is successfully treated with one or two sessions of radiofrequency ablation.

B. Osteoblastoma

1. Rare bone-producing tumor that can attain a large size and is not self-limiting

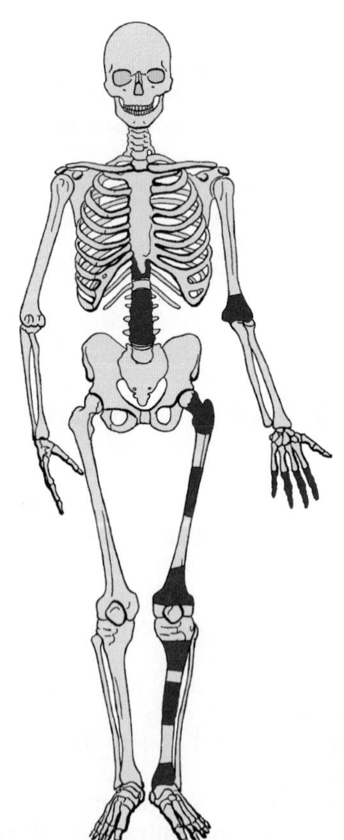

Figure 9-3 Skeletal distribution of the most common sites of osteoid osteoma. (From McCarthy EF, Frassica FJ: *Pathology of bone and joint disorders,* Philadelphia, 1998, WB Saunders.)

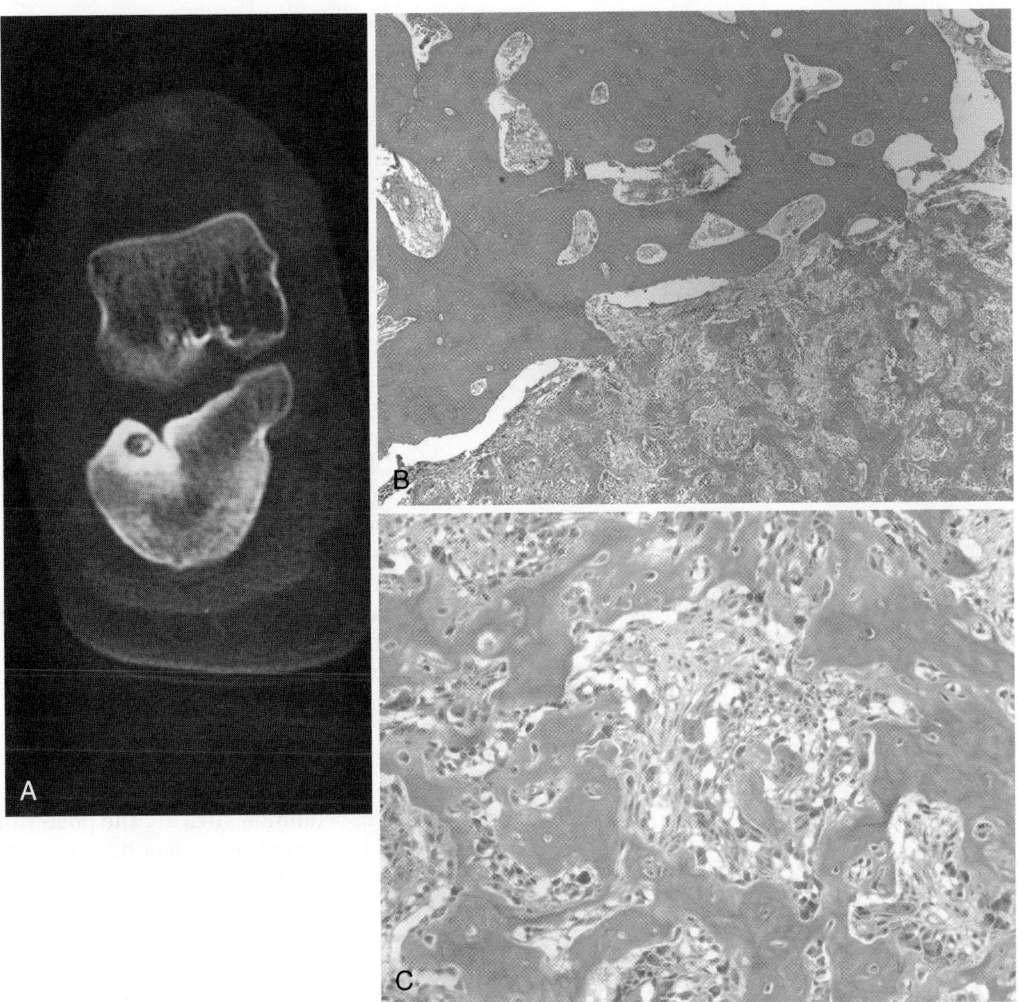

Figure 9-4 Osteoid osteoma of the calcaneus. **A,** Radiograph shows a well-circumscribed lytic lesion with dense surrounding bone and a central nidus. **B,** Low-power photomicrograph (×25) shows the nidus. **C,** Higher-power photomicrograph (×160) shows mineralizing new bone with a loose fibrovascular stroma.

2. Manifests with pain, and when the lesion involves the spine, neurologic symptoms may be present
3. Common locations include the spine, proximal humerus, and hip (Figure 9-5).
4. Causes bone destruction, with or without the characteristic reactive bone formation in osteoid osteoma
5. Area of bone destruction occasionally has a moth-eaten or permeative appearance simulating a malignancy.
6. Lesions show regularly shaped nuclei containing little chromatin but abundant cytoplasm (tissue is loosely arranged, with numerous blood vessels).
7. Tumor does not permeate the normal trabecular bone but instead merges with it.
8. Treatment: curettage or excision with a marginal line of resection

C. Osteosarcoma

1. Spindle cell neoplasms that produce osteoid are arbitrarily classified as osteosarcoma.
2. There are many types of osteosarcoma (Box 9-3 and Figure 9-6).
3. **Lesions that must be recognized include high-grade intramedullary osteosarcoma (ordinary or classic osteosarcoma), parosteal osteosarcoma, periosteal osteosarcoma, telangiectatic osteosarcoma, osteosarcoma occurring with Paget disease, and osteosarcoma after irradiation.**
4. Historically, osteosarcoma was treated by amputation; long-term studies demonstrated a survival rate of only 10% to 20%, the pulmonary system being the most common site of failure.

Box 9-3

Classification of Osteosarcoma

High-grade central osteosarcoma
Low-grade central osteosarcoma
Telangiectatic osteosarcoma
Surface osteosarcoma
Parosteal osteosarcoma
Periosteal osteosarcoma
High-grade surface osteosarcoma
Osteosarcoma of the jaw
Multicentric osteosarcoma
Secondary osteosarcoma
- Osteosarcoma in Paget disease
- Postradiation osteosarcoma

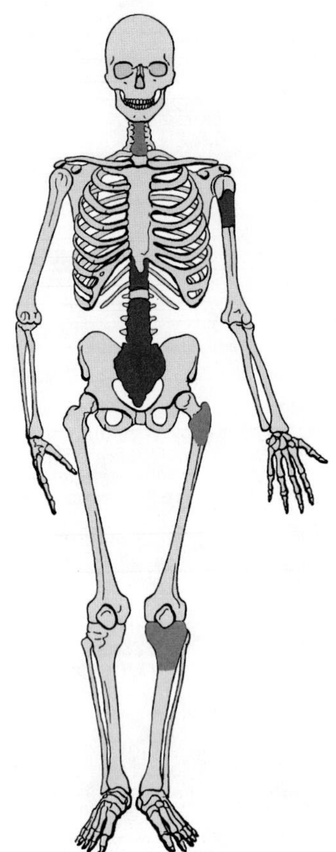

Figure 9-5 Skeletal distribution of the most common sites of osteoblastoma. (From McCarthy EF, Frassica FJ: *Pathology of bone and joint disorders,* Philadelphia, 1998, WB Saunders.)

5. Multiagent chemotherapy has dramatically improved long-term survival and the potential for limb salvage.
   - **Doxorubicin (cardiac toxicity)**
   - Methotrexate (for cases of myelosuppression, also administer leucovorin)
6. **Chemotherapy both kills the micrometastases that are present in 80% to 90% of the patients at presentation and sterilizes the reactive zone around the tumor.**
7. Preoperative chemotherapy is delivered for 8 to 12 weeks, followed by resection of the tumor.
   - **Osteosarcoma metastasizes most commonly to the lung and next most commonly to bone.**
8. **Rate of long-term survival is approximately 60% to 70%.**
9. Prognostic factors that adversely affect survival include (1) expression of P-glycoprotein, high serum level of alkaline phosphatase, high lactic dehydrogenase level, vascular invasion, and no alteration of DNA ploidy after chemotherapy and (2) the absence of anti–shock protein-90 antibodies after chemotherapy.
10. **Osteosarcoma is associated with an abnormality in the tumor suppressor genes Rb (retinoblastoma) and p53 (Li-Fraumeni syndrome).**
    - High-grade intramedullary osteosarcoma
      - Also called "ordinary" or "classic" osteosarcoma, this neoplasm is the most common type of osteosarcoma and **usually occurs about the knee in children and young adults** (Figure 9-7), **but its incidence has a second peak in late adulthood.**
      - Other common sites include the proximal humerus, proximal femur, and pelvis.
      - Patients present primarily with pain.
      - More than 90% of intramedullary osteosarcomas are high-grade and penetrate the cortex early to form a soft tissue mass (stage IIB lesion).
      - About 10% to 20% of affected patients have pulmonary metastases at presentation.
      - Radiographs demonstrate a lesion in which there is bone destruction and bone formation (Figure 9-8). On occasion, the lesion is purely sclerotic or lytic. MRI and CT scans are useful for defining the anatomy of the lesion with regard to intramedullary extension, involvement of neurovascular structures, and muscle invasion.
      - Diagnosis depends on two histologic criteria: (1) the tumor cells produce osteoid and (2) the stromal cells are frankly malignant.
      - **Treatment: neoadjuvant chemotherapy (i.e., before surgery), followed by wide-margin surgical resection and adjuvant chemotherapy (i.e., after surgery)**
    - Parosteal osteosarcoma
      - Low-grade osteosarcoma that occurs on the surface of the metaphysis of long bones
      - Affected patients often present with a painless mass.
      - **Most common sites are the posterior aspect of the distal femur,** proximal tibia, and proximal humerus (Figure 9-9).
      - Characteristic radiographic appearance: a heavily ossified, often lobulated mass arising from the cortex (Figure 9-10)
      - **Most prominent feature is regularly arranged osseous trabeculae; between the nearly normal trabeculae are slightly atypical spindle cells, which typically invade skeletal muscle found at the periphery of the tumor.**
      - **Treatment: resection with a wide margin, which is usually curative**
    - **Low-grade lesion: chemotherapy *not* required**
      - Of the lesions that appear radiographically to be parosteal osteosarcoma, approximately 17% are high-grade malignancies (dedifferentiated parosteal osteosarcoma).
    - Periosteal osteosarcoma
      - Rare surface form of osteosarcoma occurs most often in the diaphysis of long bones (typically the femur or tibia; Figure 9-11).
      - Radiographic appearance is fairly constant: a sunburst-type lesion rests on a saucerized cortical depression (Figure 9-12).
      - Histologic characteristics: The lesion is predominantly chondroblastic, and the grade of the lesion is intermediate (grade II). Highly anaplastic regions are not found.
      - The prognosis for periosteal osteosarcoma is intermediate between those of very low-grade parosteal osteosarcoma and high-grade intramedullary osteosarcoma. Preoperative chemotherapy, resection, and maintenance chemotherapy constitute the preferred

Text continued on page 641

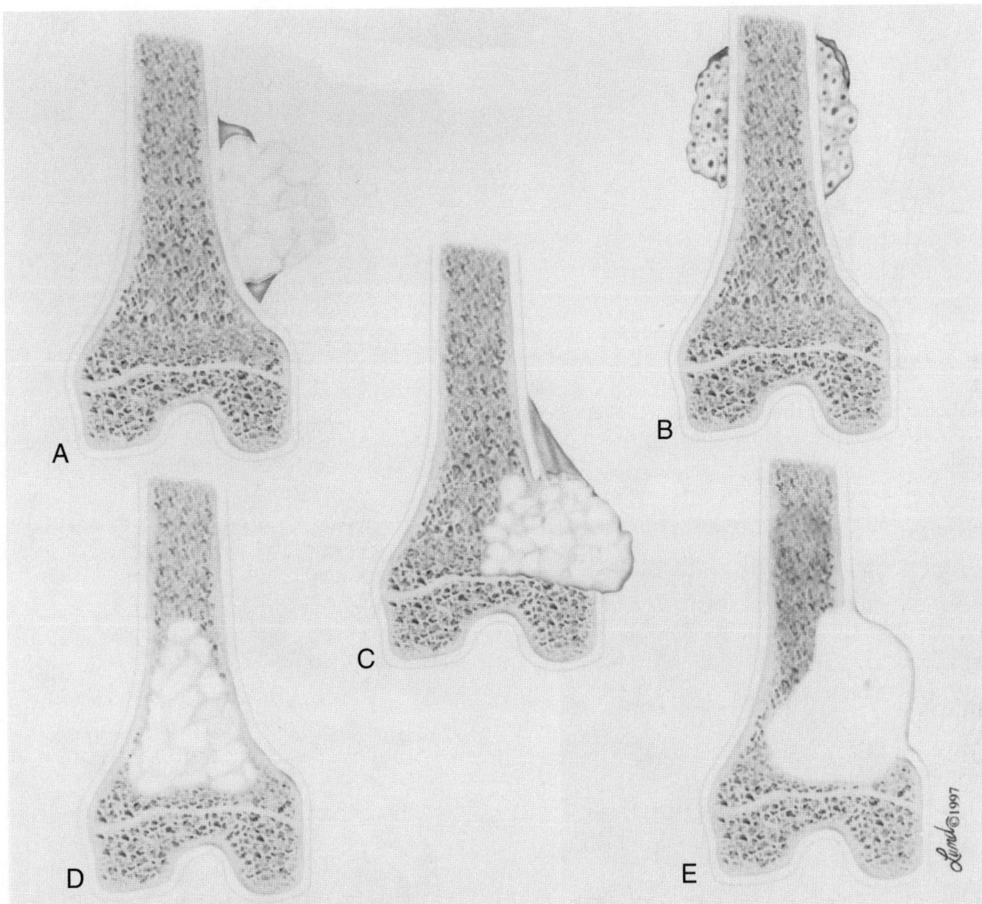

Figure 9-6 **A,** Parosteal osteosarcoma arises from the surface of the bone with broad cortical attachment. The tumor grows in a lobulated manner. **B,** Periosteal osteosarcoma. Poorly mineralized lesion on the surface of the bone. **C,** High-grade intramedullary osteosarcoma. The cortical bone destruction and extension into the soft tissues is typical. **D,** Well-differentiated intramedullary osteosarcoma stays within the medullary cavity and usually does not break through the cortex. **E,** Telangiectatic osteosarcoma, a destructive lytic lesion with no bone production. The overlying cortex has been destroyed, with extension into the soft tissue. (From McCarthy EF, Frassica FJ: *Pathology of bone and joint disorders,* Philadelphia, 1998, WB Saunders.)

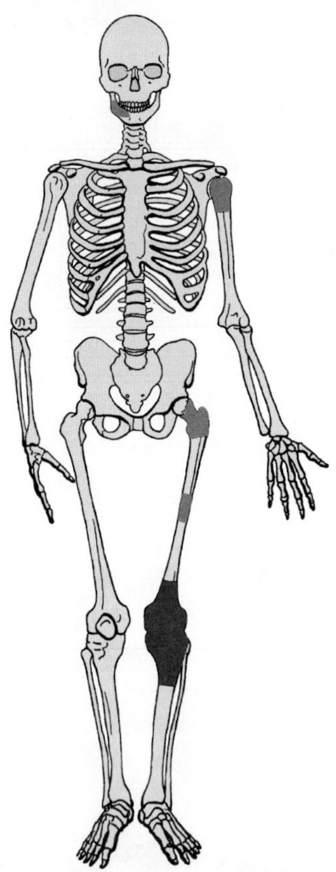

Figure 9-7 Skeletal distribution of the locations of conventional osteosarcoma. (From McCarthy EF, Frassica FJ: *Pathology of bone and joint disorders,* Philadelphia, 1998, WB Saunders.)

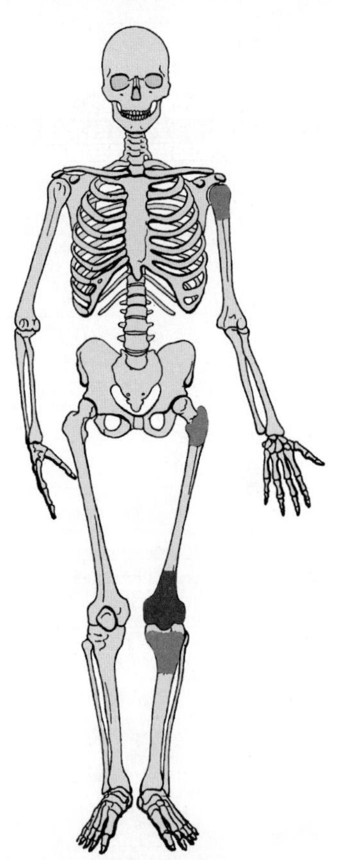

Figure 9-9 Skeletal distribution of the most common sites of parosteal osteosarcoma. (From McCarthy EF, Frassica FJ: *Pathology of bone and joint disorders,* Philadelphia, 1998, WB Saunders.)

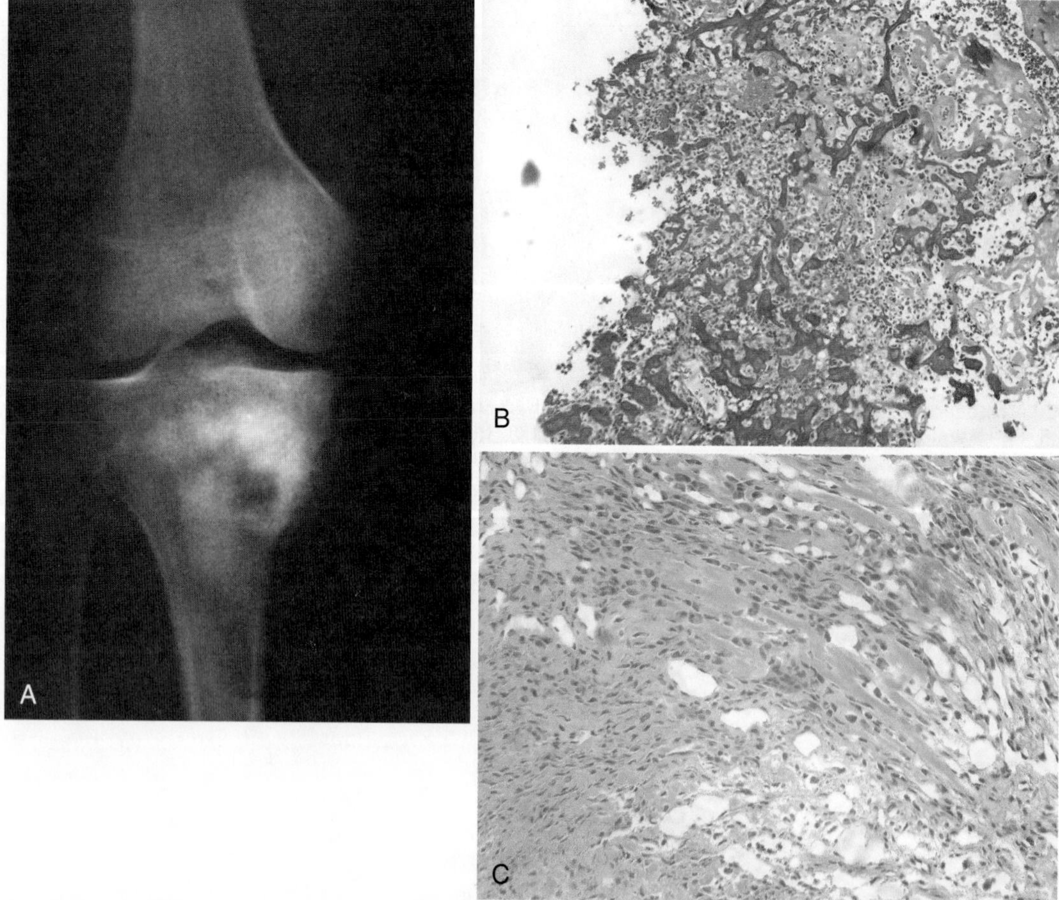

Figure 9-8 Conventional osteoblastic osteosarcoma of the proximal tibia. **A,** Radiograph shows a poorly defined osteoblastic lesion in the proximal tibial metaphysis. **B,** Low-power photomicrograph (×160) shows lacelike mineralizing osteoid surrounding atypical osteoblasts. **C,** Higher-power photomicrograph (×400) shows pleomorphism and bone formation.

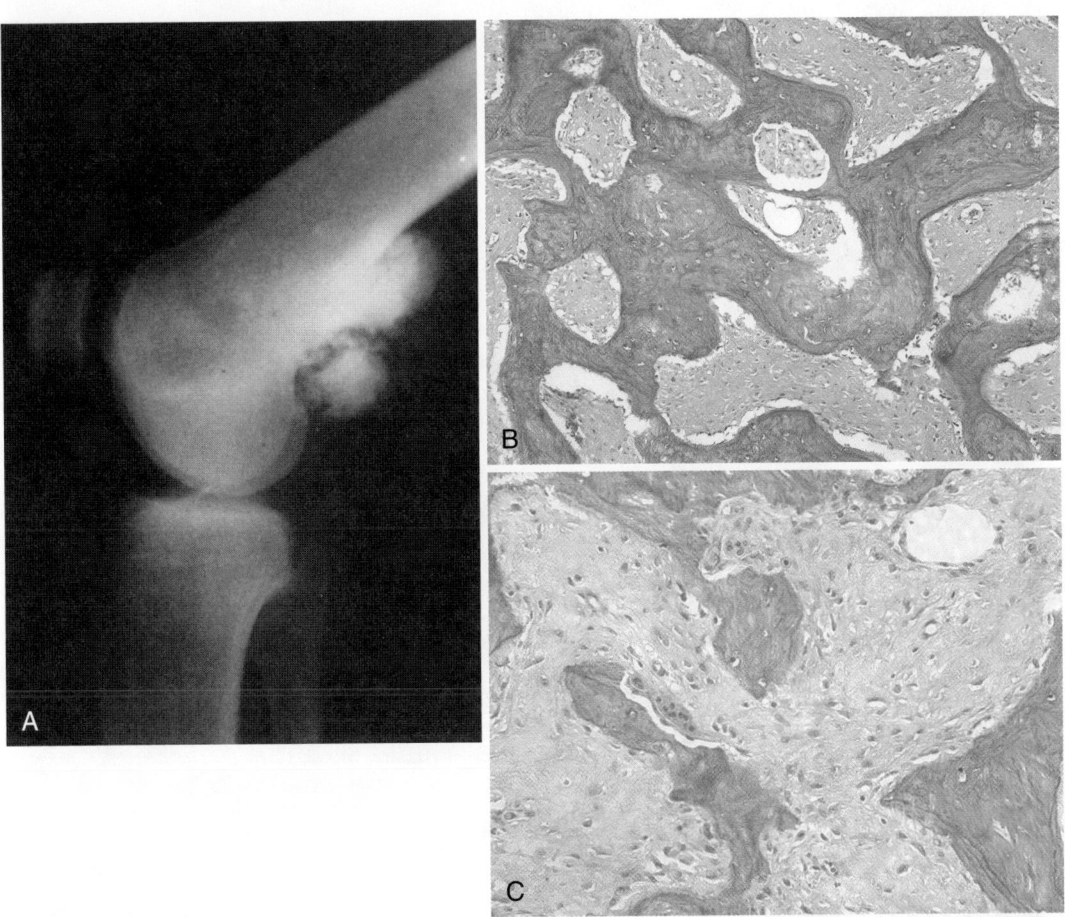

Figure 9-10 Parosteal osteosarcoma of the distal femur. **A,** Radiograph shows an exophytic, bony mass in the posterior distal femur. **B,** Low-power photomicrograph (×160) shows plates of new bone in a fibrous matrix. **C,** Higher-power photomicrograph (×400) shows a fibrous stroma with atypical cells.

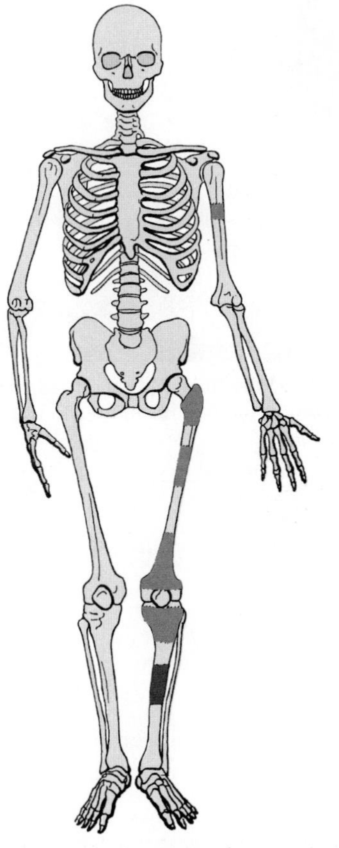

Figure 9-11 Skeletal distribution of the most common sites of periosteal osteosarcoma. (From McCarthy EF, Frassica FJ: *Pathology of bone and joint disorders,* Philadelphia, 1998, WB Saunders.)

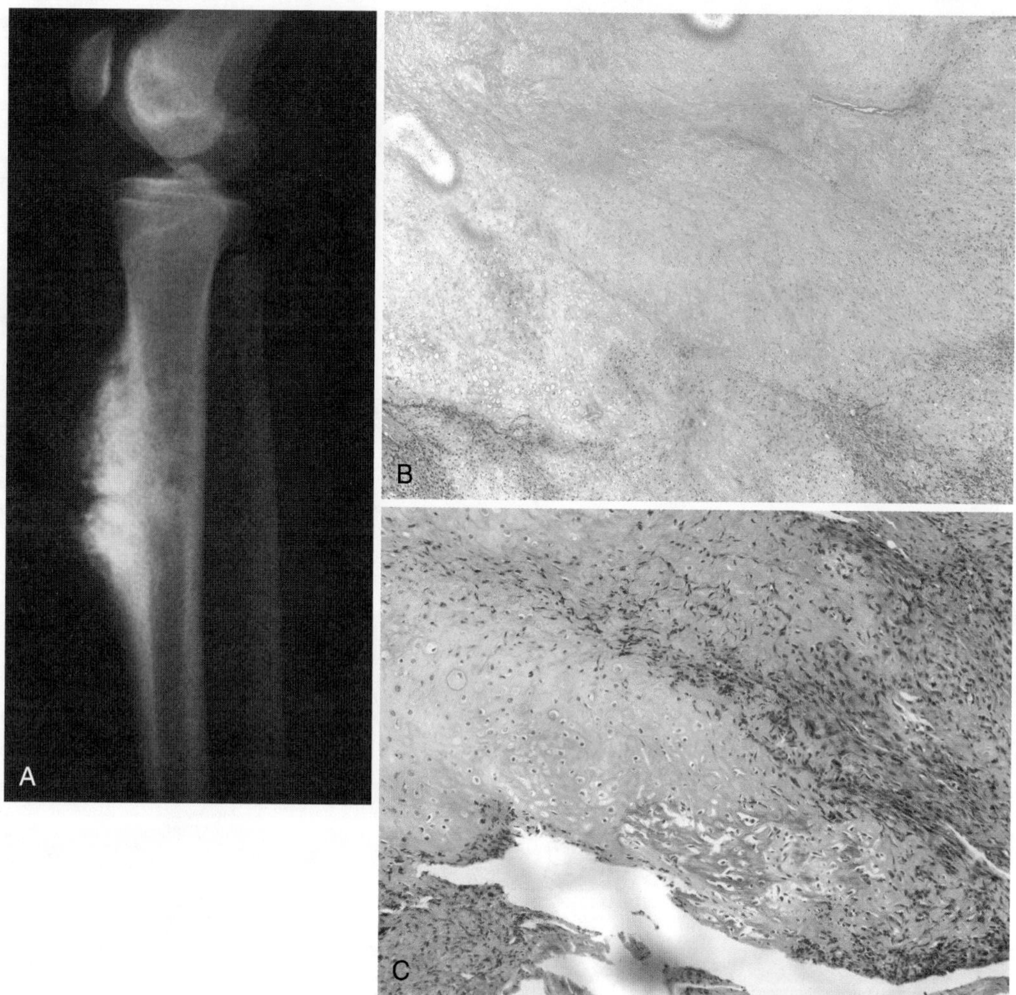

Figure 9-12 Periosteal osteosarcoma of the diaphysis of the tibia. **A,** Lateral radiograph showing a surface lesion with bone formation. **B,** Low-power photomicrograph (×160) showing cartilage and bone formation. **C,** Higher-power photomicrograph showing pleomorphism and direct production of osteoid by the tumor cells.

treatment. The risk of pulmonary metastasis is 10% to 15%.

- Telangiectatic osteosarcoma
  - The tissue of the lesion can be described as a bag of blood with few cellular elements.
  - The radiographic features of telangiectatic osteosarcoma are those of a destructive, lytic, expansile lesion. Telangiectatic osteosarcomas occur in the same locations as aneurysmal bone cysts (Figure 9-13), and the radiographic appearances of both can be confused.

III. CHONDROGENIC LESIONS

Appearances of these lesions are shown in Figure 9-14.

A. Chondroma

1. Histologic and radiographic features
   - **When benign cartilage tumors occur on the surface of the bone, they are called *periosteal chondroma***
   - They occur on the surfaces of the distal femur, proximal humerus, and proximal femur (Figure 9-15).
   - Appearance: usually a well-demarcated, shallow cortical defect and a slight periosteal chondroma
     - Buttress of cortical bone at the edges of the lesion
     - One third of the periosteal chondromas exhibit a mineralized cartilaginous matrix on the radiograph (Figure 9-16), whereas two thirds have no apparent radiographic mineralization.
   - In the medullary cavity in the metaphysis of long bones, especially the proximal femur and humerus and the distal femur, they are called *enchondromas* (Figure 9-17).
   - Enchondromas are also common in the hand, where they usually occur in the diaphysis and metaphysis. Lesions in the hand may be hypercellular and display

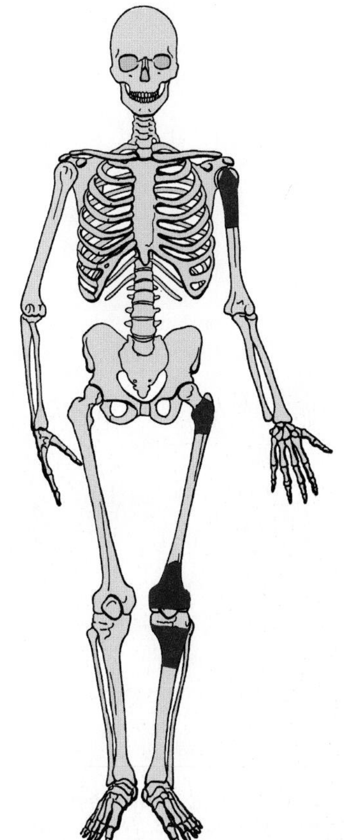

Figure 9-13 Skeletal distribution of the locations of telangiectatic osteosarcoma. (From McCarthy EF, Frassica FJ: *Pathology of bone and joint disorders,* Philadelphia, 1998, WB Saunders.)

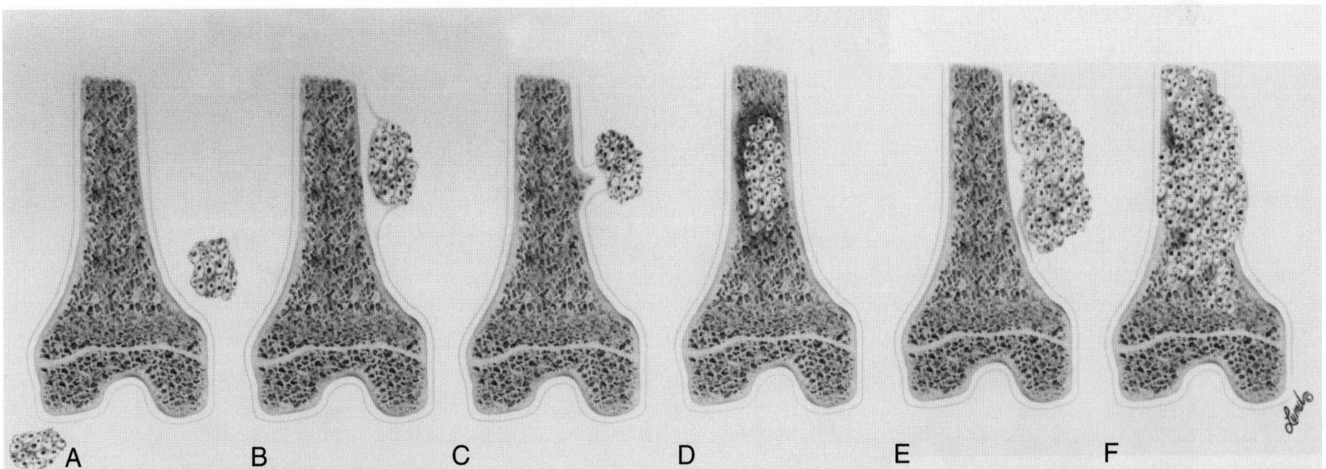

Figure 9-14 The common types of cartilage tumors. **A,** Lobular pattern of cartilage in synovial chondromatosis. **B,** Surface tumor of bone composed of mature cartilage that sits in a saucer-shaped depression on the bone's surface. These lesions are called *periosteal chondromas.* **C,** Surface tumor in which the cortices are continuous between the surface lesion and the host cortex. On top of the bone sits a thin (1- to 3-mm) rim of cartilage. This lesion is called an *osteochondroma* and is one of the most common benign cartilage tumors. **D,** Enchondroma. Notice that this benign cartilage tumor sits in the medullary cavity in a quiescent manner. There are no cortical changes, such as erosions, cortical thickening, or cortical bone destruction. **E,** Surface chondrosarcoma is a rare malignant bone tumor in the form of a malignant cartilage mass on the surface of the bone. **F,** In medullary chondrosarcoma with active growth, there may be destruction of the cortex and extension into the soft tissues. In this instance the cartilage is growing and destroying the bone rather than being quiescent. (From McCarthy EF, Frassica FJ: *Pathology of bone and joint disorders,* Philadelphia, 1998, WB Saunders.)

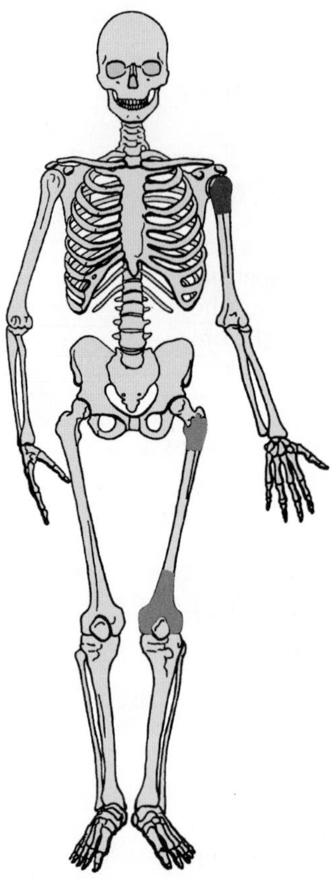

Figure 9-15 Skeletal distribution of the most common sites of periosteal chondroma. (From McCarthy EF, Frassica FJ: *Pathology of bone and joint disorders,* Philadelphia, 1998, WB Saunders.)

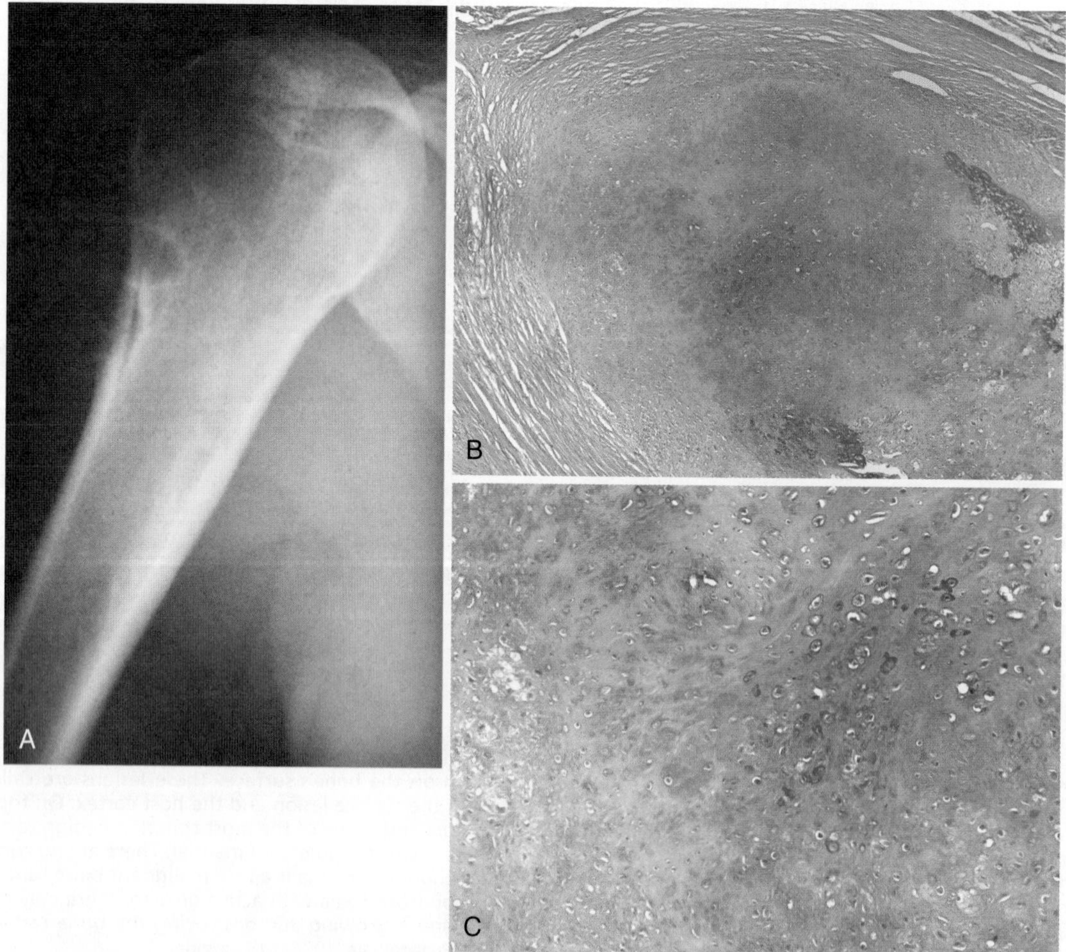

Figure 9-16 Periosteal chondroma of the proximal humerus. **A,** Radiograph shows surface lesion with stippled calcifications scalloping the cortex. **B,** Low-power photomicrograph (×100) shows bland hyaline cartilage. **C,** Higher-power photomicrograph (× 250) shows cartilage cells and matrix.

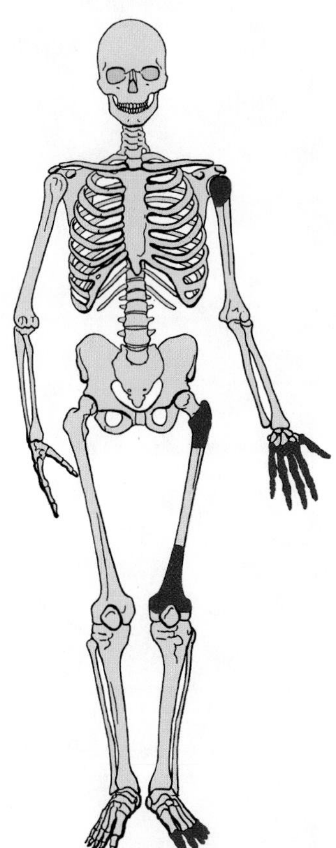

Figure 9-17 **Skeletal distribution of the most common sites of enchondromas. Note the common location in the phalanges of the hand, the proximal humerus, and the distal femur.** (From McCarthy EF, Frassica FJ: *Pathology of bone and joint disorders,* Philadelphia, 1998, WB Saunders.)

worrisome histologic features, and pathologic fractures in the hand are common.

- Most enchondromas in long bones are asymptomatic.
- **Radiographically there may be a prominent stippled or mottled calcified appearance** (Figure 9-18).
- Tumor is composed of small cells that lie in lacunar spaces; it is hypocellular, and the cells have a bland appearance (no pleomorphism, anaplasia, or hyperchromasia).
- When lesions are not causing pain, serial radiographs are obtained to ensure that the lesions are inactive (not growing). Radiographs are obtained every 3 to 6 months for 1 to 2 years and then annually as necessary.
- **Enchondroma can be distinguished from low-grade chondrosarcoma on serial plain radiographs**. (10)In low-grade chondrosarcomas, cortical bone changes (large erosions [>50%] of the cortex, cortical thickening, and destruction) or lysis of the previously mineralized cartilage is visible.

2. Ollier disease/Maffucci syndrome
   - When there are many lesions, the involved bones are dysplastic, and the lesions tend toward unilaterality, the diagnosis is multiple enchondromatosis, or Ollier disease.
   - Inheritance pattern is sporadic.
   - If soft tissue angiomas are also present, the diagnosis is Maffucci syndrome.
   - **Patients with multiple enchondromatosis are at increased risk of malignancy (in Ollier disease, 30%; in Maffucci syndrome, 100%).**
   - Patients with Maffucci syndrome also have a markedly increased risk of visceral malignancies, such as astrocytomas and gastrointestinal malignancies.
   - **For most enchondromas, no treatment other than observation is required.** When surgical treatment is necessary, enchondromas are treated by curettage and bone grafting. Periosteal chondromas are usually excised with a marginal margin.

B. **Osteochondroma**

1. Features
   - Benign surface lesions probably arise secondary to aberrant cartilage (from the perichondrial ring) on the surface of bone.
   - They manifest with a painless mass after trauma, or the mass is discovered incidentally.
   - Osteochondromas usually occur about the knee, proximal femur, and proximal humerus (Figure 9-19).
   - **Characteristic appearance: a surface lesion in which the cortex of the lesion and the underlying cortex are continuous and the medullary cavity of the host bone also flows into (is continuous with) the osteochondroma** (Figure 9-20).
   - Osteochondromas may have a narrow stalk (pedunculated) or a broad base (sessile).
   - They typically occur at the site of tendon insertions, and the affected bone is abnormally wide.
   - Underlying cortex is covered by a thin cap of cartilage (usually only 2 to 3 mm thick;. in a growing child, the cap thickness may exceed 1 to 2 cm).
   - Chondrocytes are arranged in linear clusters, with an appearance resembling that of the normal physis.
   - **When asymptomatic, these lesions are treated with observation only.**
   - Patients may experience pain secondary to muscle irritation, mechanical trauma (contusions), or an inflamed bursa over the lesion. In this scenario, excision is a logical alternative.
2. Malignant transformation
   - Pain in the absence of mechanical factors is a warning sign of malignant change.
   - The development of a sarcoma in an osteochondroma is rare, occurring in far fewer than 1% of cases.
   - Destruction of the subchondral bone, mineralization of a soft tissue mass, and an inhomogeneous appearance are radiographic changes of malignant transformation.
   - A low-grade chondrosarcoma is usually present, although a dedifferentiated chondrosarcoma may occur in rare cases.
   - The lesion is termed a "secondary chondrosarcoma."
   - The prognosis is usually excellent; these low-grade tumors seldom metastasize.
3. Multiple hereditary exostoses
   - The osteochondromas are often sessile and large. This is an autosomal dominant condition with mutations in the *EXT1* and *EXT2* gene loci. **Approximately 10% of patients with multiple exostoses develop a secondary chondrosarcoma. The *EXT1* mutation is associated with a greater burden of disease and higher risk of malignancy.**

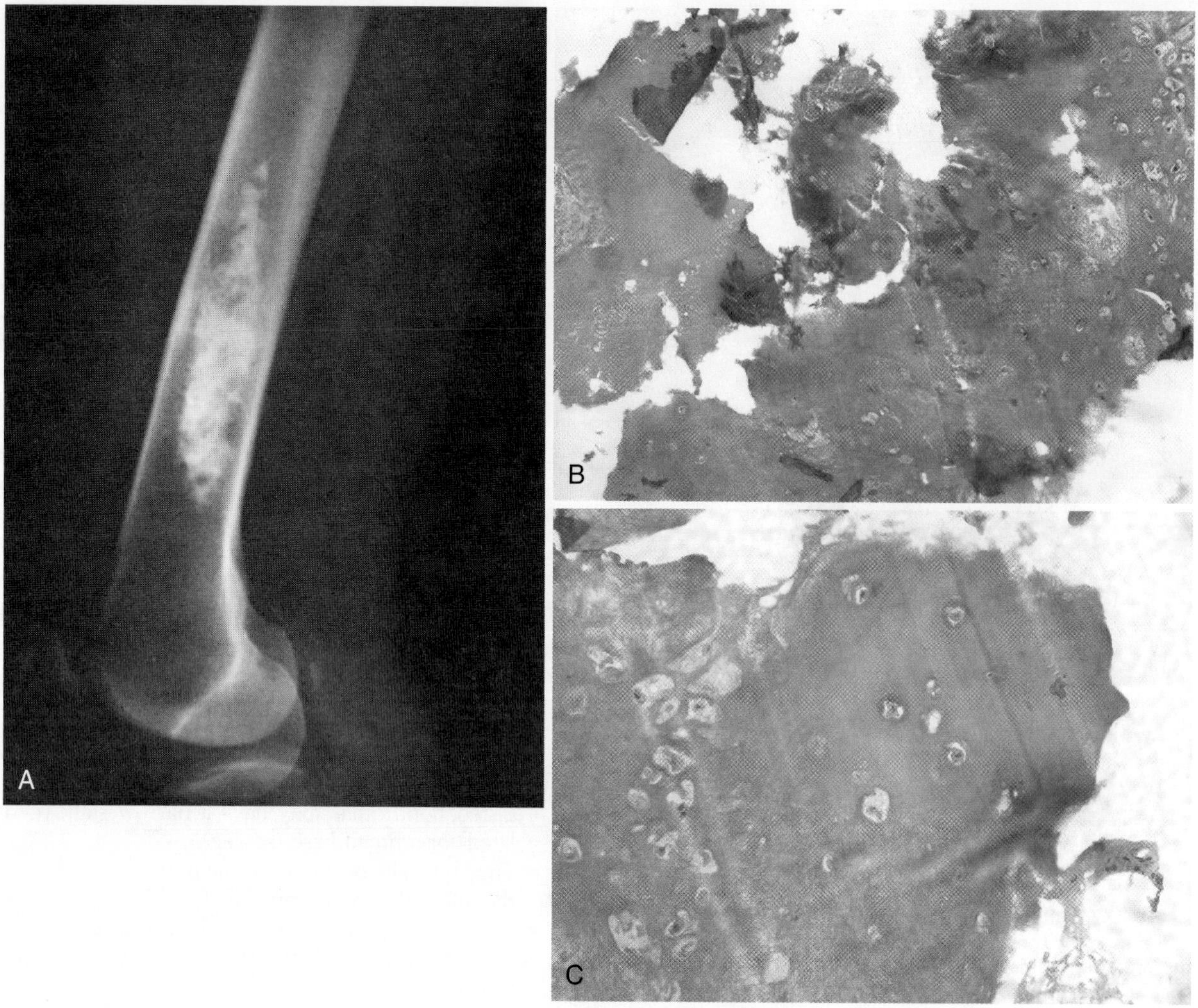

Figure 9-18 Enchondroma of the distal femur. **A,** Radiograph shows densely mineralized medullary lesion. **B,** Low-power (×160) photomicrograph shows mineralized hyaline cartilage. **C,** Higher-power (×250) photomicrograph shows bland chondrocytes in lacunae.

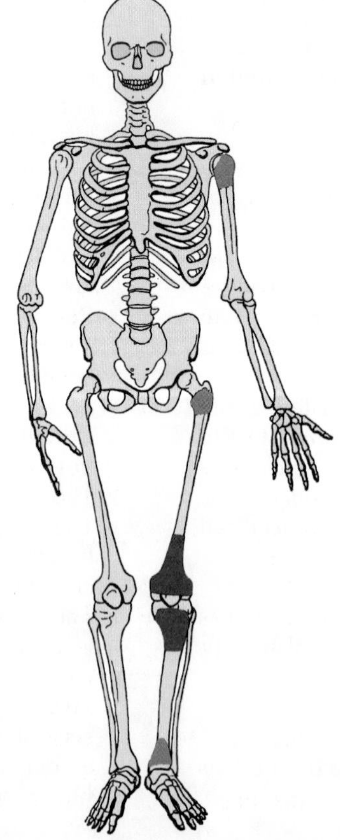

Figure 9-19 Skeletal distribution of the most common sites of osteochondromas. (From McCarthy EF, Frassica FJ: *Pathology of bone and joint disorders,* Philadelphia, 1998, WB Saunders.)

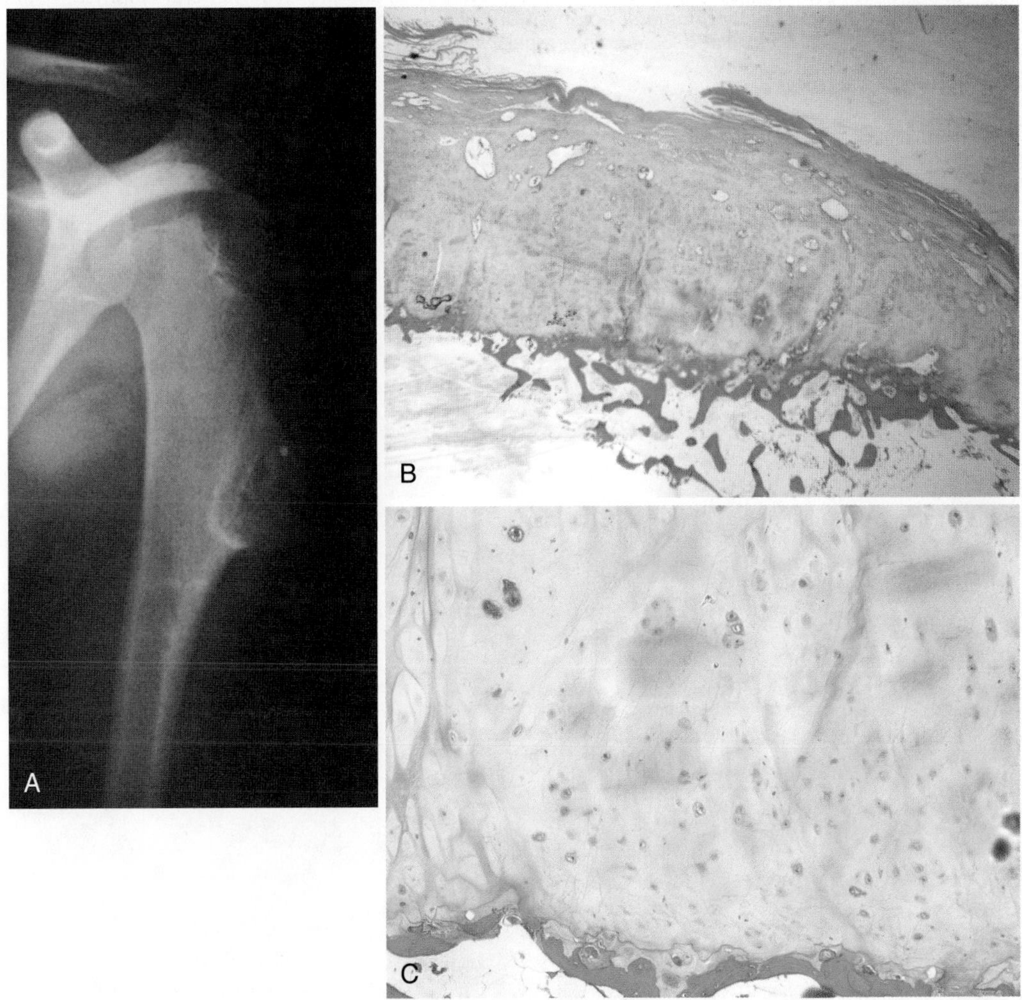

Figure 9-20 Osteochondroma of the proximal humerus. **A,** Radiograph shows sessile osteochondroma of the proximal humerus. **B,** Photomicrograph (×6) shows the osteochondroma with a cartilaginous cap. **C,** Higher-power photomicrograph (×25) is a closeup view of the cartilage cap, which is undergoing endochondral ossification.

C. Chondroblastoma

1. **Centered in the epiphysis in young patients, usually with open physes**
2. The most common locations are the distal femur, proximal tibia, and proximal humerus (Figure 9-21).
3. Lesion is usually in the epiphysis; it may also occur in an apophysis.
4. Manifests with pain referable to the involved joint.
5. **It causes a central region of bone destruction that is usually sharply demarcated from the normal medullary cavity by a thin rim of sclerotic bone** (Figure 9-22).
6. Mineralization may or may not occur within the lesion.
7. The basic proliferating cells are thought to be chondroblasts.
   - Scattered multinucleated giant cells are found throughout the lesion.
   - Zones of chondroid substance are present.
   - Mitotic figures may be found.
8. **Treatment: curettage (intralesional margin) and bone grafting**
9. Of benign chondroblastomas, 2% metastasize to the lungs.

D. Chondromyxoid fibroma

1. Rare, benign cartilage tumors that contain variable amounts of chondroid, fibromatoid, and myxoid elements
2. More common in boys and men
3. Tend to involve long bones (especially the tibia); the pelvis and distal femur are other common locations (Figure 9-23)
4. Manifest with pain of variable duration (months to years).
5. There is a lytic, destructive lesion that is eccentric and sharply demarcated from the adjacent normal bone (Figure 9-24).
6. It grows in lobules, and there is often a condensation of cells at the periphery of the lobules (concentration of chondroid element may vary from light to heavy).
7. Treatment: curettage and grafting

E. Chondrosarcoma

1. Intramedullary chondrosarcoma
   - This malignant neoplasm of cartilage occurs in older adults.
   - Most common locations include the shoulder and pelvic girdles, knee, and spine.
   - Patients may have pain or a mass.

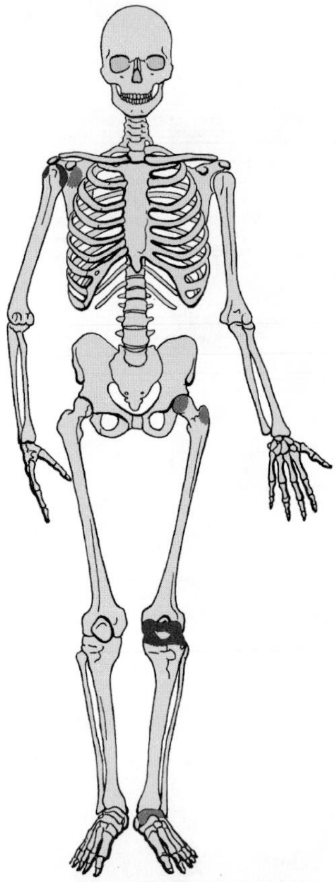

Figure 9-21 Skeletal distribution of the most common sites of chondroblastomas. Chondroblastomas begin in either the epiphysis or apophysis. They commonly occur in the distal femur, proximal tibia, femoral head, greater trochanteric apophysis, and proximal humeral epiphysis. Chondroblastomas in the proximal humeral epiphysis are called *Codman tumor.* (From McCarthy EF, Frassica FJ: *Pathology of bone and joint disorders,* Philadelphia, 1998, WB Saunders.)

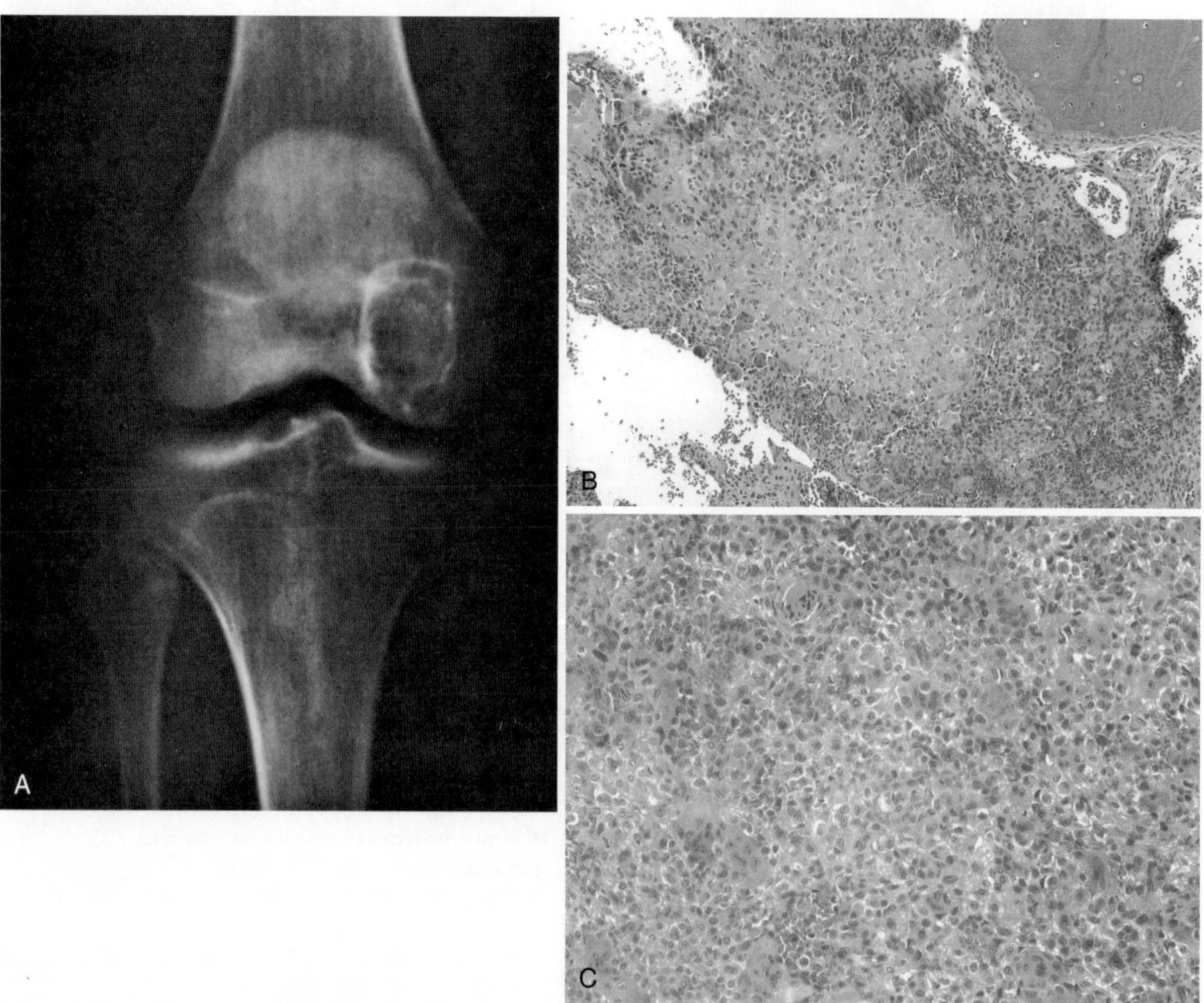

Figure 9-22 Chondroblastoma of the distal femur. **A,** Radiograph shows a well-circumscribed lytic lesion with a sclerotic rim in the distal femoral epiphysis. **B,** Low-power photomicrograph (×160) shows cellular stroma in a chondroid matrix. **C,** Higher-power photomicrograph (×400) shows rounded stromal cells with multinucleated giant cells.

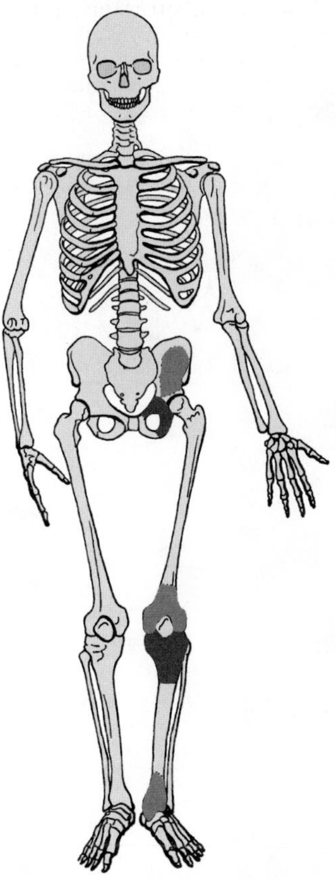

Figure 9-23 Skeletal distribution of the most common sites of chondromyxoid fibroma. The tibia, pelvis, and distal femur are common locations. (From McCarthy EF, Frassica FJ: *Pathology of bone and joint disorders,* Philadelphia, 1998, WB Saunders.)

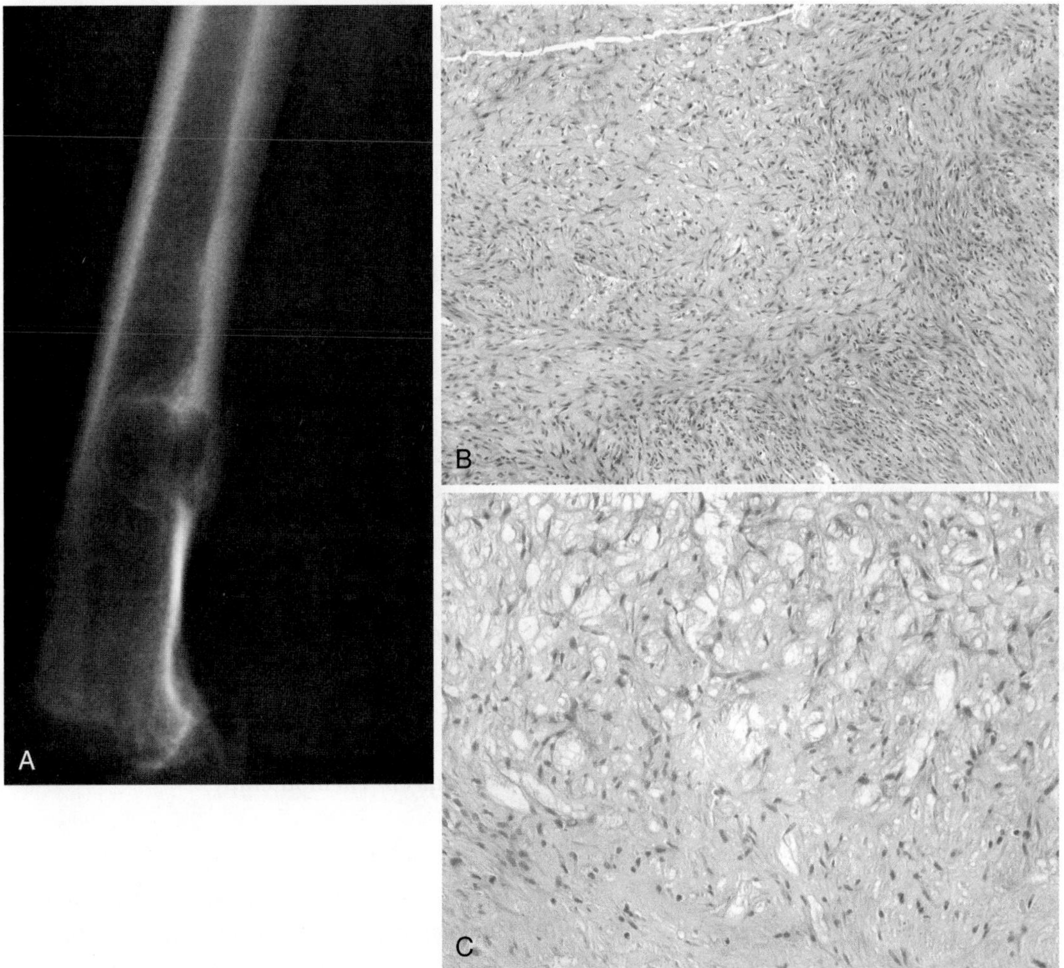

Figure 9-24 Chondromyxoid fibroma of the femur. **A,** Radiograph shows a well-circumscribed lytic lesion in the distal femur, with a rim of sclerotic bone. **B,** Low-power photomicrograph (×100) shows lobules of fibromyxoid tissue. **C,** Higher-power photomicrograph (× 250) shows myxoid stroma with stellate cells.

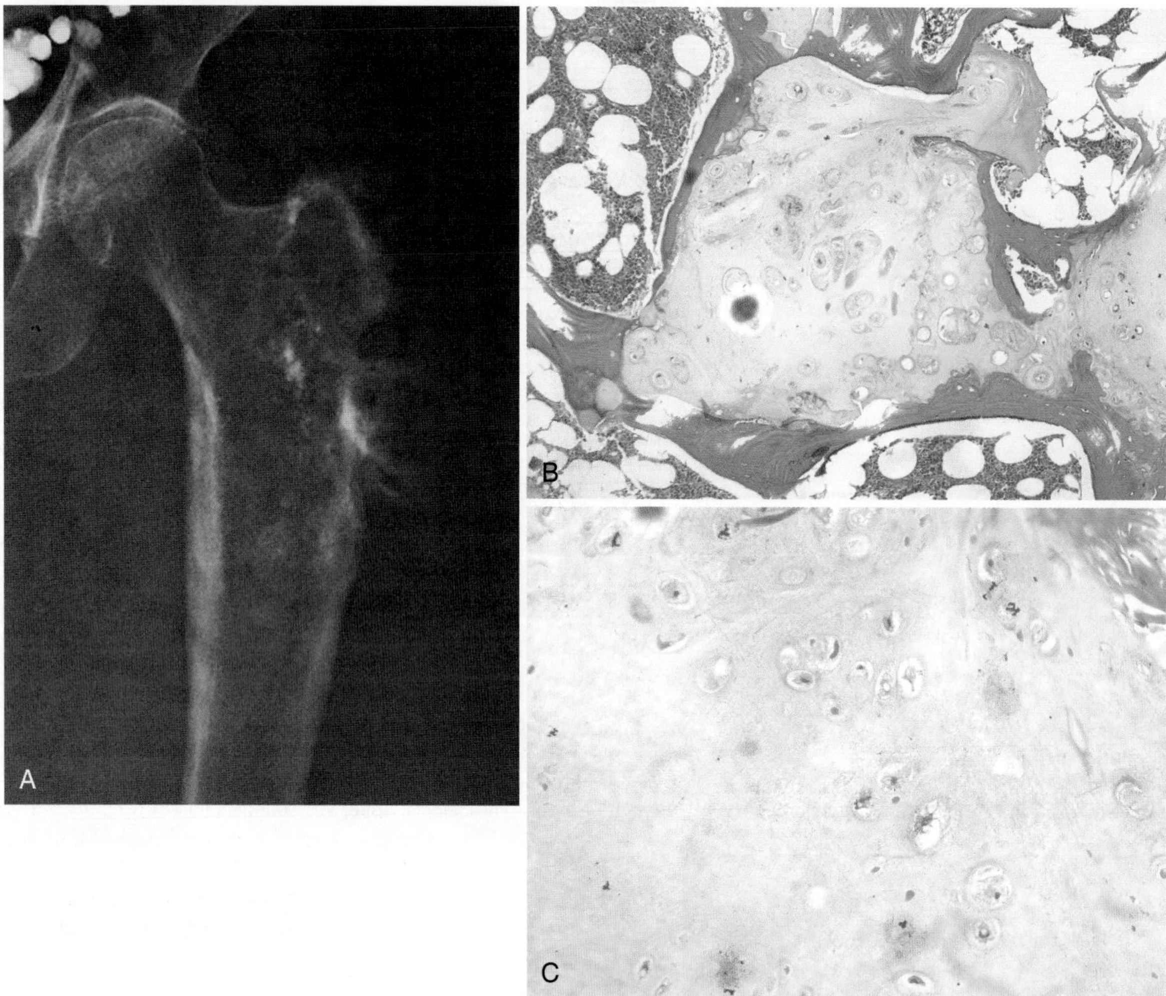

Figure 9-25 Central (intramedullary) chondrosarcoma of the proximal femur. **A,** Radiograph shows an expansile lytic lesion in the proximal femur with stippled calcifications. **B,** Low-power photomicrograph (×40) shows cartilage with a permeative growth pattern. **C,** Higher-power photomicrograph (×250) shows cellular cartilage.

- Radiographs usually show diagnostic findings, with bone destruction, thickening of the cortex, and mineralization consistent with cartilage within the lesion (Figure 9-25).
- Prominent cortical changes are present in 85% of affected patients.
- **Differentiating malignant cartilage may be extremely difficult on the basis of histologic features alone.**
- **The clinical, radiographic, and histologic features of a particular lesion must be considered in combination to avoid incorrect diagnosis.** The criteria for the diagnosis of malignancy include the following:
  - Many cells with plump nuclei
  - More than an occasional cell with two such nuclei
  - Especially large cartilage cells with large single or multiple nuclei containing clumps of chromatin
  - Infiltration of the bone trabeculae
- Chondromas of the hand (enchondromas)—the lesions in patients with Ollier disease and Maffucci syndrome—and periosteal chondromas may have atypical histopathologic features (Figure 9-26).
- **Treatment: wide-margin surgical resection.**
  - **Chemotherapy has not been shown to improve survival.**

2. **Dedifferentiated chondrosarcoma**
   - Most malignant cartilage tumor
   - Most common locations include the distal and proximal femur and the proximal humerus (Figure 9-27).
   - **Bimorphic histologic and radiographic appearances**
   - **Low-grade cartilage component that is intimately associated with a high-grade spindle cell sarcoma (osteosarcoma, fibrosarcoma, malignant fibrous histiocytoma)**
   - More than 80% of the lesions are typical chondrosarcomas with a superimposed, highly destructive area (Figure 9-28).
   - Manifestations are similar to those of low-grade chondrosarcoma, including pain and decreased function.
   - Prognosis is poor, and rate of long-term survival is less than 10%.
   - **Treatment: wide-margin surgical resection and multiagent chemotherapy**

IV. FIBROUS LESIONS

A. Metaphyseal fibrous defect (also known as *nonossifying fibroma, nonosteogenic fibroma,* and *xanthoma*)

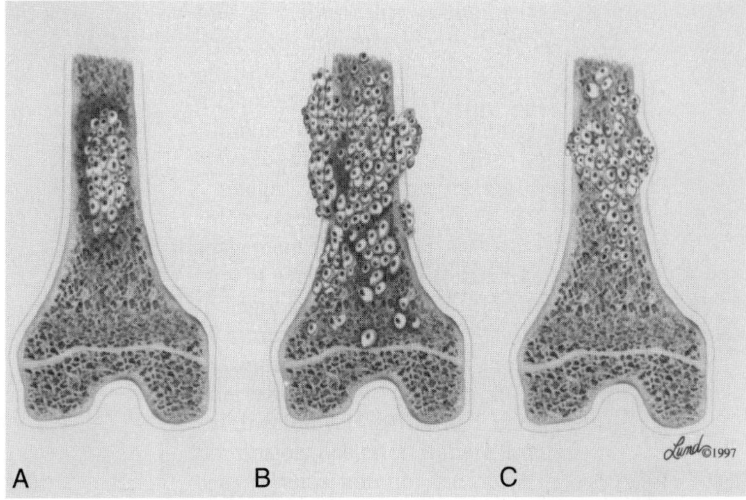

Figure 9-26 The three types of intramedullary cartilage tumors. **A**, Enchondromas are inactive intramedullary tumors of the hyaline cartilage. Note that the cortices are not involved. There is no cortical erosion, thickening, expansion, or breakthrough. **B**, In contrast, high-grade chondrosarcomas cause destruction of the cortex and extend into the soft tissues. **C**, Low-grade chondrosarcomas cause cortical erosion, with expansion into the cortex but no breakthrough. (From McCarthy EF, Frassica FJ: *Pathology of bone and joint disorders,* Philadelphia, 1998, WB Saunders.)

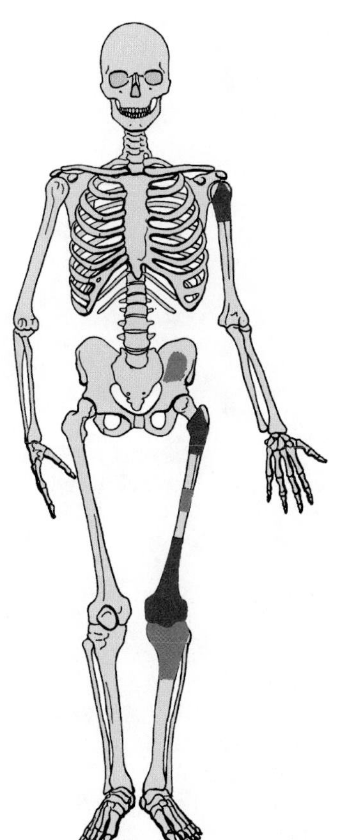

Figure 9-27 Skeletal distribution of the most common sites of dedifferentiated chondrosarcoma. **The femur and proximal humerus are the most common sites.** (From McCarthy EF, Frassica FJ: *Pathology of bone and joint disorders,* Philadelphia, 1998, WB Saunders.)

1. Occurs in young patients
2. Most such lesions resolve spontaneously and are probably not true neoplasms.
3. Most common locations are the distal femur, distal tibia, and proximal tibia.
4. These lesions are usually asymptomatic and discovered incidentally.
5. **Characteristic radiographic appearance: a lucent lesion that is metaphyseal, eccentric, and surrounded by a sclerotic rim** (Figure 9-29). **The overlying cortex may be slightly expanded and thinned.**
6. Cellular, fibroblastic connective tissue background, with the cells arranged in whorled bundles **(numerous giant cells,** lipophages, and various amounts of hemosiderin pigmentation).
7. **Treatment: observation if the radiographic appearance is characteristic and the risk of pathologic fracture is not excessive.**
8. If more than 50% to 75% of the cortex is involved and the patient has symptoms, curettage and bone grafting are performed.

B. **Desmoplastic fibroma**

1. Rare and low-grade but aggressive fibrous tumor of bone
2. Lesion is purely lytic.
3. When process is low grade, residual or reactive trabeculated (or corrugated) bone is often present.
4. Lesion is composed of abundant collagen and mature fibroblasts with no cellular atypia.
5. With wide-margin surgical resection, the risk of local recurrence is lowest, but the joint must be removed in young patients.

C. **Fibrosarcoma**

1. Presentation and localization are similar to those of osteosarcoma.
2. This tumor affects primarily older persons but does occur during all decades of life.
3. Lytic bone destruction is often in permeative pattern (Figure 9-30).
4. Spindle cells, variable collagen production, and a herringbone pattern
5. Treatment: wide-margin surgical resection

V. MALIGNANT FIBROUS HISTIOCYTOMA

A. Most common locations include the distal femur, proximal tibia, proximal femur, ilium, and proximal humerus (Figure 9-31).

B. Malignant bone tumors that have proliferating cells with a histiocytic quality

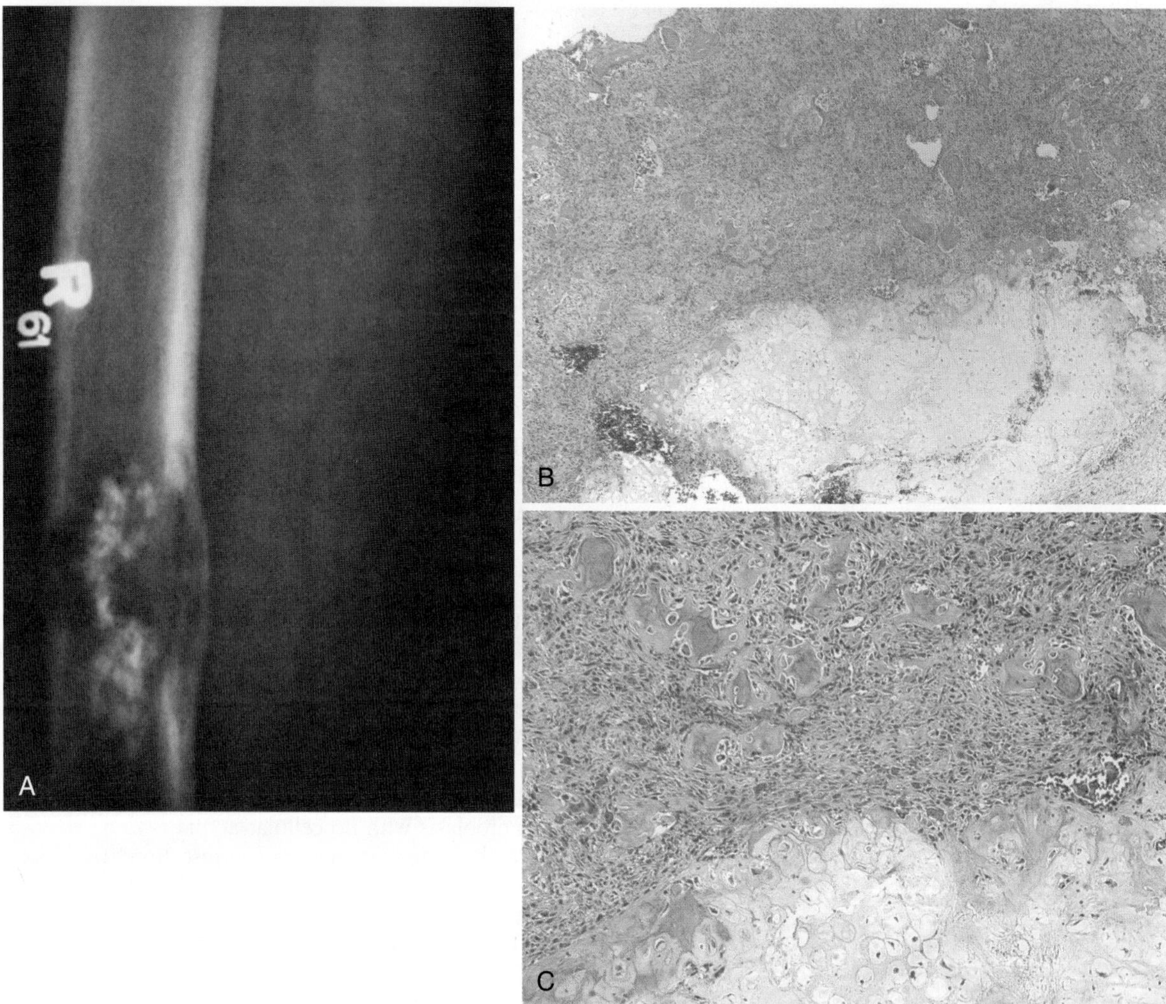

Figure 9-28 Dedifferentiated chondrosarcoma of the femur. **A,** Radiograph shows focal dense mineralization surrounded by a poorly defined lytic lesion. **B,** Low-power photomicrograph (×100) shows an island of hyaline cartilage surrounded by a cellular neoplasm. **C,** Higher-power photomicrograph (×250) shows hyaline cartilage adjacent to pleomorphic rounded cells.

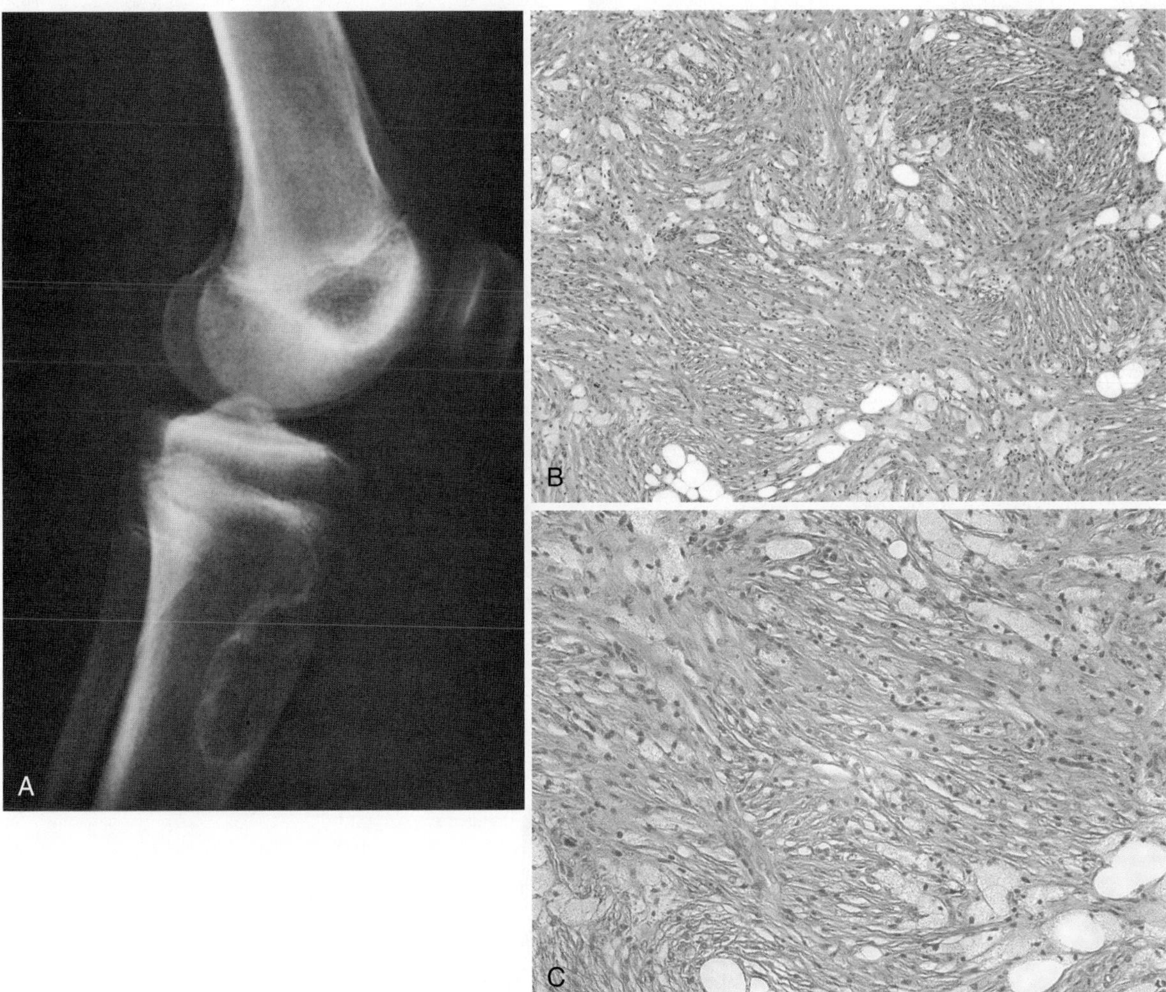

Figure 9-29 Metaphyseal fibrous defect (nonossifying fibroma) of the proximal tibia. **A,** Radiograph shows a scalloped, well-circumscribed lesion with a sclerotic rim in the proximal tibial metaphysis. **B,** Low-power photomicrograph (×160) shows spindle cells in a storiform pattern and occasional multinucleated giant cells. **C,** Higher-power photomicrograph (×250) of photomicrograph **(B)**.

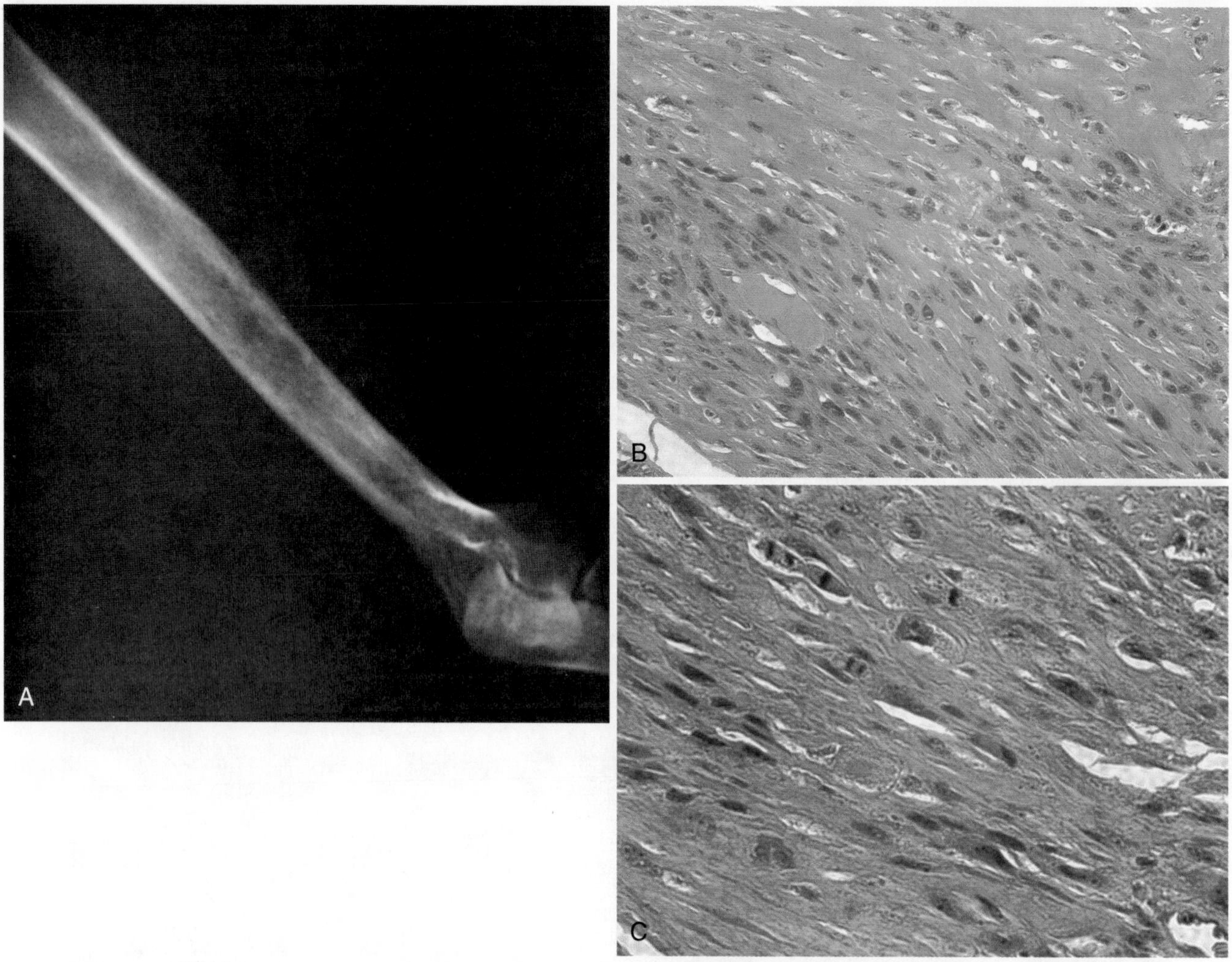

Figure 9-30 Fibrosarcoma of the humerus. **A,** Radiograph shows a permeative lesion in the midshaft of the humerus. **B,** Low-power photomicrograph (×250) shows atypical spindle cells. **C,** Higher-power photomicrograph (×400).

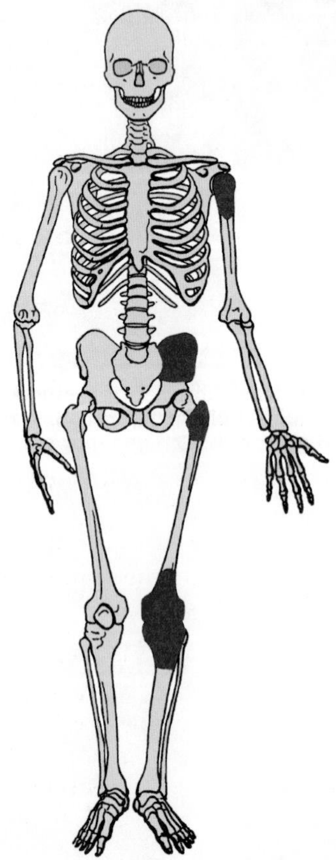

Figure 9-31 Skeletal distribution of the most common sites of malignant fibrous histiocytoma. (From McCarthy EF, Frassica FJ: *Pathology of bone and joint disorders,* Philadelphia, 1998, WB Saunders.)

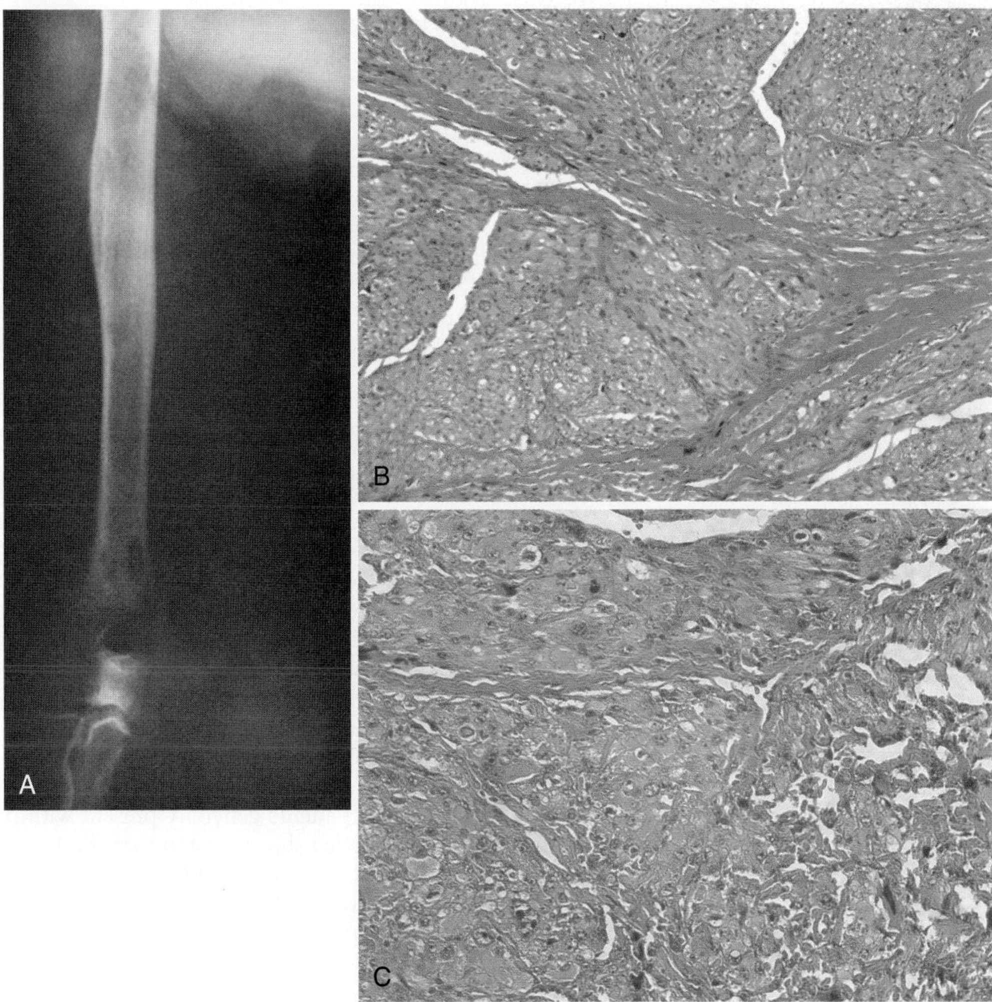

Figure 9-32 Malignant fibrous histiocytoma of the humerus. **A,** Radiograph shows poorly defined lytic lesions in the proximal and distal humerus. **B,** Low-power photomicrograph (×200) shows spindle cells arranged in a storiform pattern. **C,** Higher-power photomicrograph (×400) shows a uniform population of pleomorphic cells.

C. Nuclei are often indented, the cytoplasm is usually abundant and may be slightly foamy, the nucleoli are often large, and multinucleated giant cells are usually a prominent feature.
D. Variable amounts of fibrous tissue found within the lesion, and the fibrogenic areas have a storiform appearance
E. Patients present with pain and swelling.
F. This lesion is destructive, with either purely lytic bone destruction or a mixed pattern of bone destruction and formation (Figure 9-32).
G. Treatment: wide-margin surgical excision

VI. NOTOCHORDAL TISSUE

A. Chordoma is a malignant neoplasm in which the cell of origin is derived from primitive notochordal tissue.
B. Occurs predominantly at the ends of the vertebral column (sacrococcygeal; Figure 9-33)
C. About 10% of chordomas occur in the vertebral bodies (cervical, thoracic, and lumbar regions).
D. Patients present with an insidious onset of pain. Lesions in the sacrum may manifest as pelvic pain, low-back pain, or hip pain or with primarily gastrointestinal symptoms (obstipation, constipation, loss of rectal tone). When vertebral bodies are involved, neurologic symptoms may vary widely because of nerve compression.
E. Radiographs often do not reveal the true extent of sacrococcygeal chordomas. The sacrum is difficult to evaluate on plain radiographs because of overlying bowel gas and fecal material and the angulation of the sacrum away from the x-ray beam on the anteroposterior view. In addition, the anteroposterior pelvic view reveals bone destruction only at the sacral cortical margins and neural foramina; these areas are not typically involved early.
F. CT scans show midline bone destruction and a soft tissue mass (Figure 9-34).
G. MRI is an excellent modality for both detecting a chordoma and defining the anatomic features of the tumor.

1. Low signal on T1-weighted images
2. Very bright signal on T2-weighted images
3. Sacrum is often expanded, and the soft tissue mass may exhibit irregular mineralization.

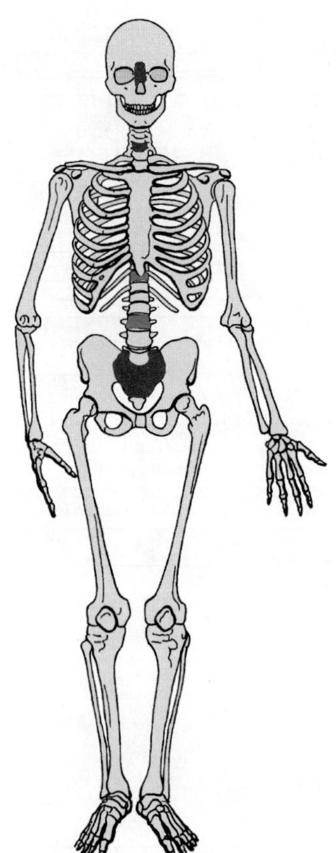

Figure 9-33 Skeletal distribution of the most common sites of chordoma. Chordomas occur exclusively in the spine; 50% are sacrococcygeal, 40% occur in the spheno-occipital region, and 10% occur in the vertebra. (From McCarthy EF, Frassica FJ: *Pathology of bone and joint disorders,* Philadelphia, 1998, WB Saunders.)

4. In the vertebral bodies, areas of lytic bone destruction or a mixed pattern of both bone formation and bone destruction are often observed.

H. The tumor grows in distinct lobules.

1. Chordoma cells sometimes have a vacuolated appearance and are called *physaliferous* cells.
2. Often arrayed in strands in a mass of mucus
3. Treatment: wide-margin surgical resection
4. Radiation therapy may be added if a wide margin is not achieved.

J. Chordomas metastasize late in the course of the disease, and local extension can be fatal.

VII. VASCULAR TUMORS

A. Hemangioma (Figure 9-35)

1. These tumors usually occur in vertebral bodies.
2. Patients may present with pain or pathologic fracture (often asymptomatic).
3. Vertebral hemangiomas have a characteristic appearance, with lytic destruction and vertical striations or a coarsened honeycomb appearance. On occasion, more than one bone is involved.
4. There are numerous blood channels. Most lesions are cavernous, although some may be a mixture of capillary and cavernous blood spaces.

B. Hemangioendothelioma

1. May occur in any age group, and affected patients present with pain
2. Multifocal involvement of the bones of the same extremity is common
3. Predominantly oval lytic lesion with no reactive bone formation
4. The tumor cells form vascular spaces. The lesions range in structure from very well differentiated (easily recognizable vascular spaces) to very undifferentiated (difficult to recognize their vasoformative quality).
5. Low-grade multifocal lesions may be treated with radiation alone.

VIII. HEMATOPOIETIC TUMORS

A. Lymphoma

1. Lymphoma of bone is uncommon and occurs in three scenarios:
   - As a solitary focus (primary lymphoma of bone)
   - In association with other osseous sites and nonosseous sites (nodal disease and soft tissue masses)
   - As metastatic foci
2. The most common locations include the distal femur, proximal tibia, pelvis, proximal femur, vertebra, and shoulder girdle (Figure 9-36).
3. Occurs at all ages
4. Affected patients generally present with pain.
5. Images often show a lesion that involves a large portion of the bone (long lesion; Figure 9-37).
   - Bone destruction is common and often has a mottled appearance.
   - Reactive bone formation admixed with bone destruction is often observed. The cortex may be thickened.
6. A mixed cellular infiltrate is usually present. Most lymphomas of bone are diffuse, large B-cell lymphomas.
7. Treatment generally combines multiagent chemotherapy and consolidative irradiation.
8. Surgery is generally used only to stabilize fractures.

B. Myeloma

Plasma cell dyscrasias represent a wide range of conditions from **monoclonal gammopathy of undetermined significance** (MGUS; Kyle disease) to multiple myeloma. There are three plasma cell dyscrasias with which orthopaedists must be familiar: multiple myeloma, solitary plasmacytoma of bone, and osteosclerotic myeloma.

1. Multiple myeloma
   - Malignant plasma cell disorder that commonly occurs in patients between 50 and 80 years of age
   - Manifests with bone pain, usually in the spine and ribs, or a pathologic fracture
   - Fatigue is a common complaint secondary to the associated anemia.
   - Symptoms may be related to complications such as renal insufficiency, hypercalcemia, and the deposition of amyloid.
   - Serum creatinine levels are elevated in about 50% of affected patients.
   - Hypercalcemia is present in about 33% of affected patients.
   - Radiographic appearance is of punched-out, lytic lesions (Figure 9-38), which may show expansion and a

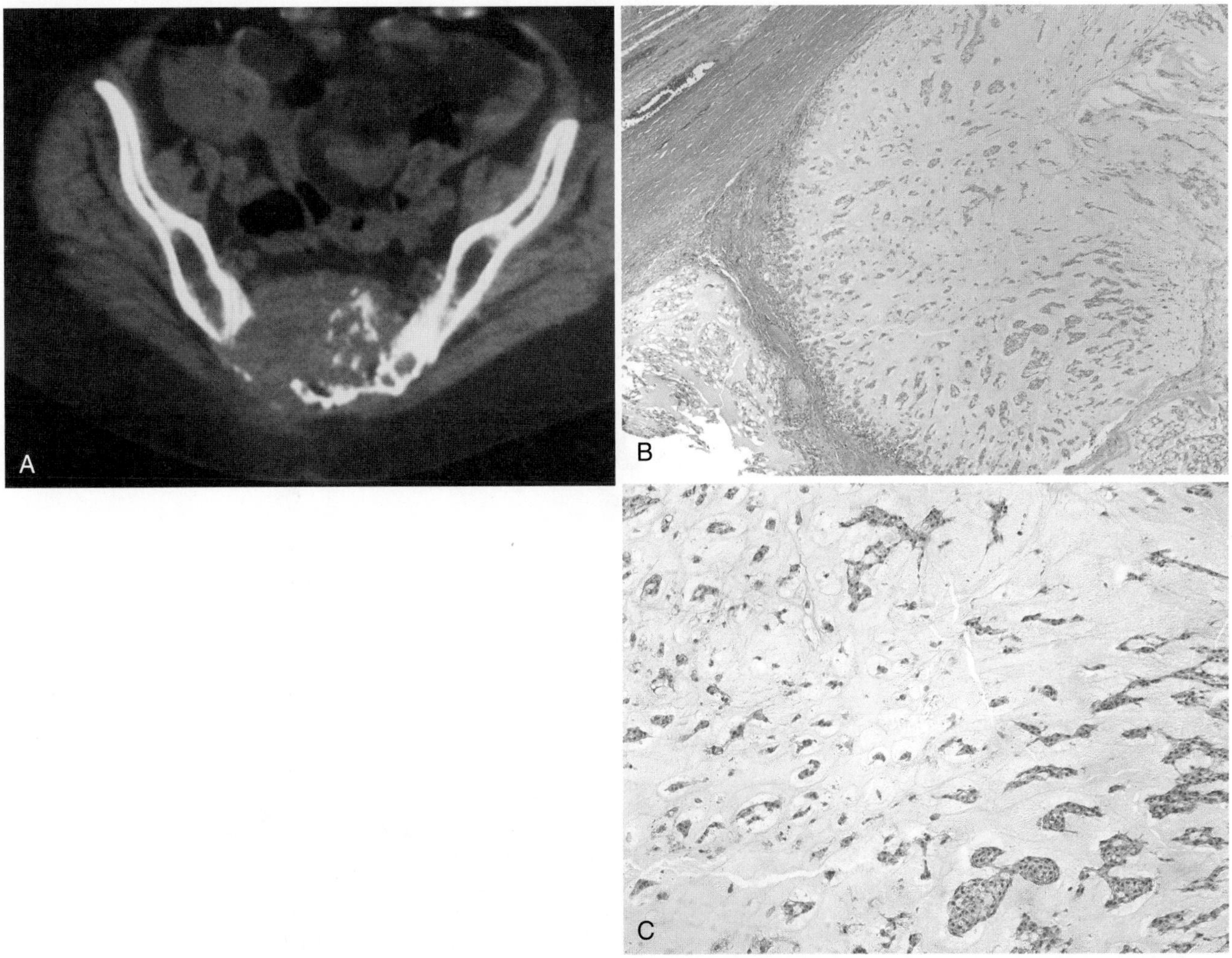

Figure 9-34 Chordoma of the sacrum. **A,** Computed tomographic scan shows a destructive lesion in the sacrum. **B,** Low-power photomicrograph (×100) shows a lobular arrangement of tissue. **C,** Higher-power photomicrograph (× 250) shows nests of physaliferous cells.

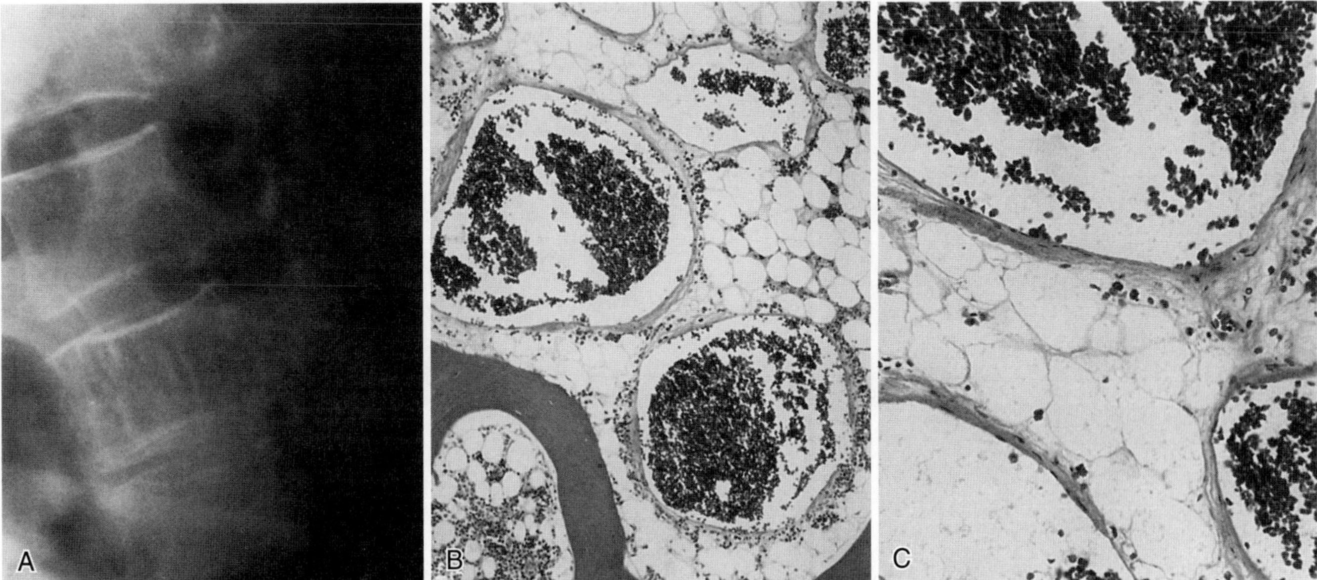

Figure 9-35 Hemangioma of the vertebra. **A,** Radiographic view shows vertical strictions. **B,** Low-power photomicrograph shows dilated vascular spaces in the marrow (×50). **C,** Higher-power photomicrograph (×100) shows endothelium-lined spaces.

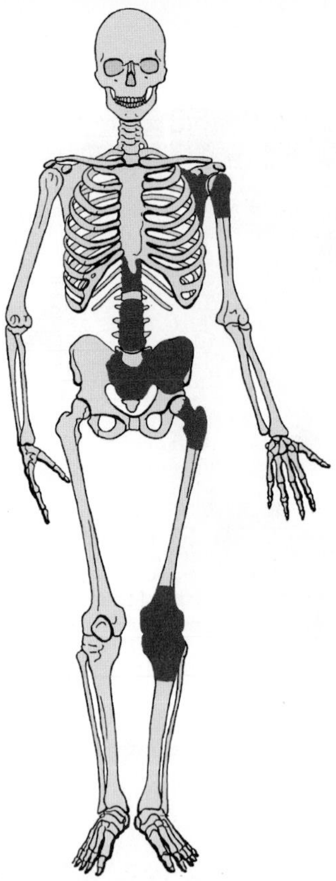

Figure 9-36 Skeletal distribution of the most common sites of lymphoma of the bone. The knee, pelvis, and vertebra are common sites. (From McCarthy EF, Frassica FJ: *Pathology of bone and joint disorders,* Philadelphia, 1998, WB Saunders.)

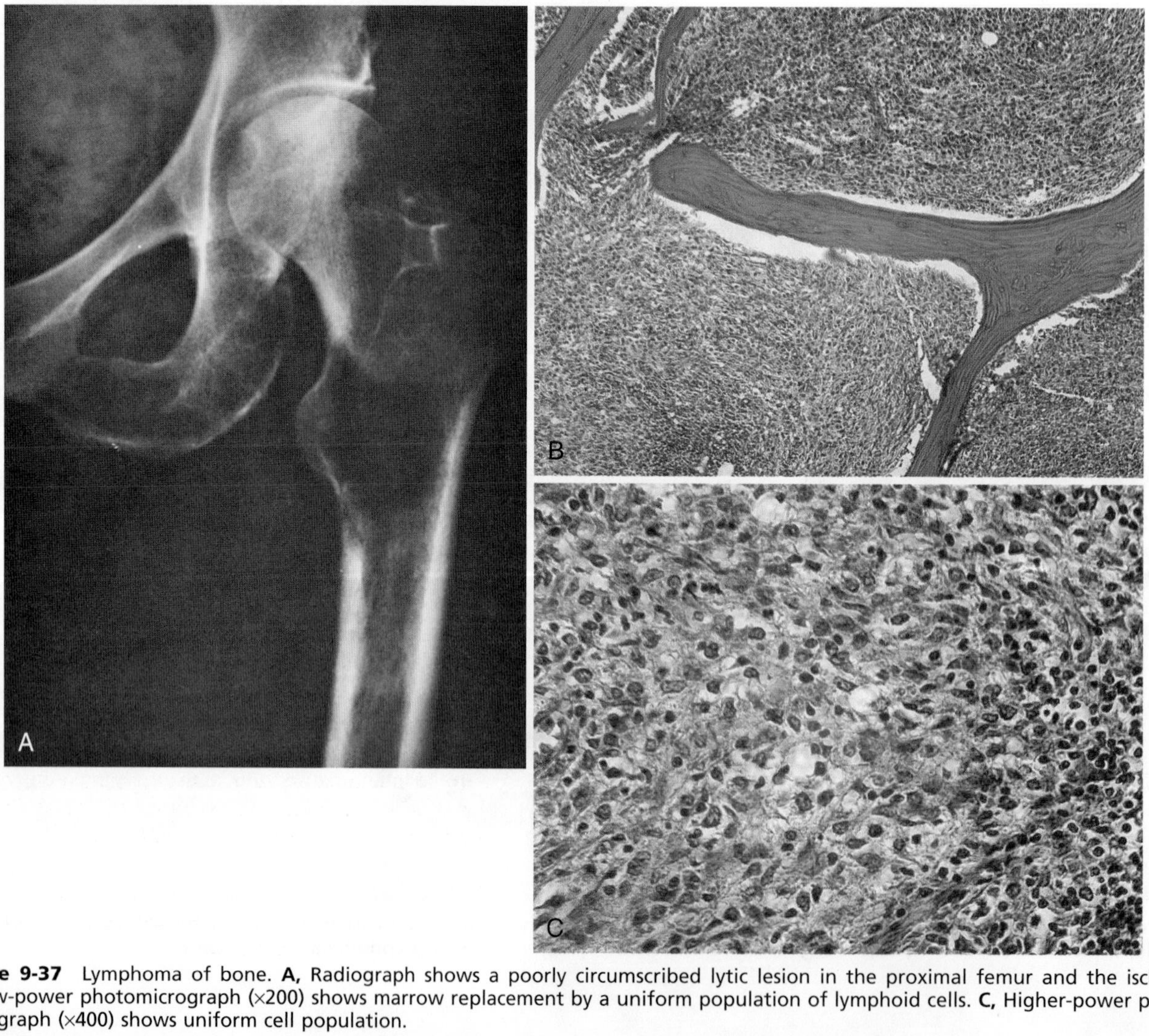

Figure 9-37 Lymphoma of bone. **A,** Radiograph shows a poorly circumscribed lytic lesion in the proximal femur and the ischium. **B,** Low-power photomicrograph (×200) shows marrow replacement by a uniform population of lymphoid cells. **C,** Higher-power photomicrograph (×400) shows uniform cell population.

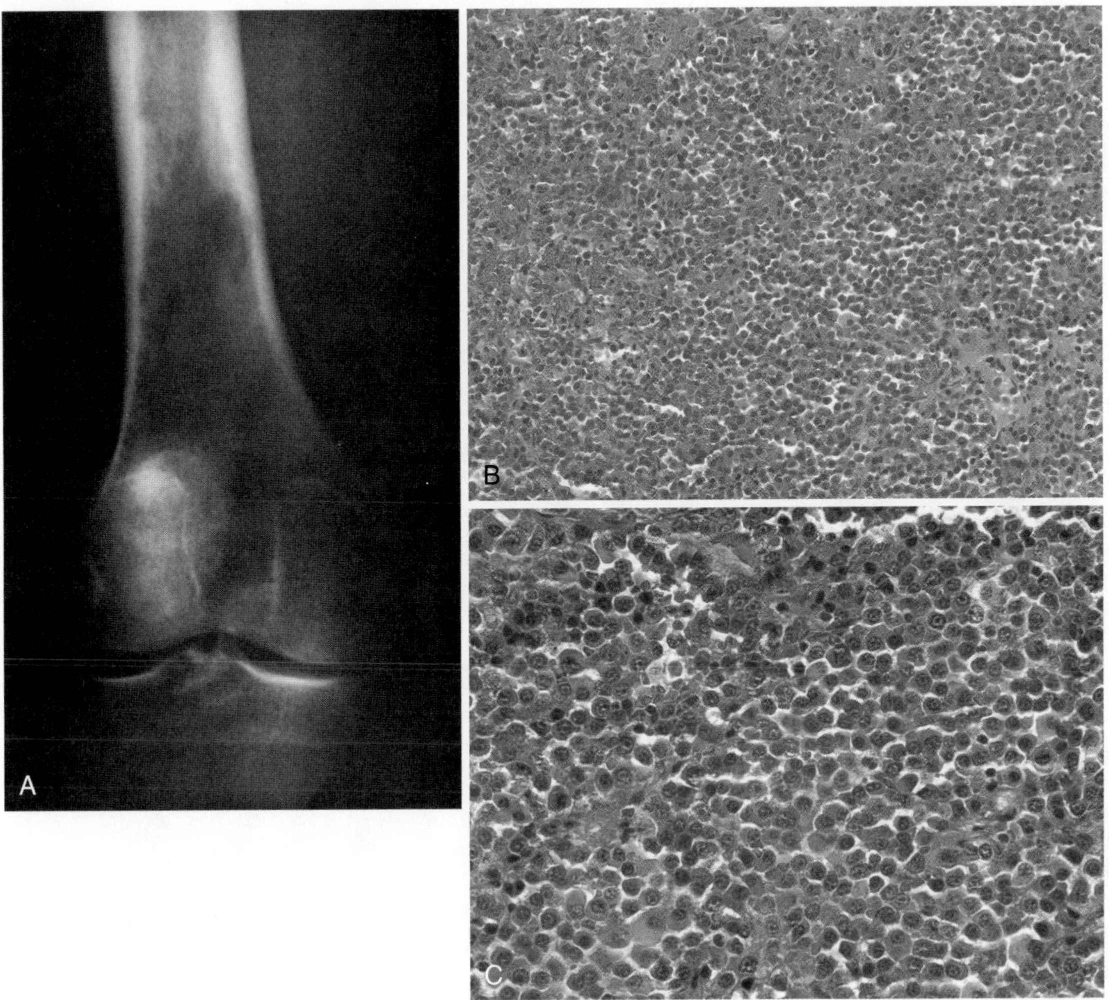

Figure 9-38 Multiple myeloma in the femur. **A,** Radiograph shows a poorly circumscribed lytic lesion in the distal femur. **B,** Low-power micrograph shows marrow replacement by a uniform population of cells. **C,** Higher-power photomicrograph (× 400) shows sheets of atypical plasma cells.

"ballooned" appearance. Osteopenia may be the only laboratory finding.

- Classic histologic appearance: sheets of plasma cells that appear monoclonal with immunostaining.
  - Well-differentiated plasma cells have an eccentric nucleus and a peripherally clumped, chromatic "clock face" (Figure 9-39).
  - There is a perinuclear clear zone (halo) that represents the Golgi apparatus.
- Treatment:
  - Systemic therapy and bisphosphonates
  - Surgical stabilization with irradiation is used for impending and complete fractures.
  - Radiotherapy is also used for palliation of pain and treatment of neurologic symptoms.
- The prognosis is related to the stage of disease; the overall median survival time is 18 to 24 months.

2. Solitary plasmacytoma of bone

It is important to differentiate solitary myeloma from multiple myeloma because of the more favorable prognosis in patients with the solitary form. Diagnostic criteria include the following:

- A solitary lesion on skeletal survey
- Histologic confirmation of plasmacytoma
- Bone marrow plasmacyte count of 10% or less
- Patients with serum protein abnormalities and Bence Jones proteinuria (protein levels of less than 1 g/24 hr) at presentation are not excluded if they meet the aforementioned criteria.
- Treatment:
  - External beam irradiation of the lesion (4500 to 5000 cGy)
  - When necessary, prophylactic internal fixation
- In approximately 50% to 75% of affected patients, solitary myeloma progresses to multiple myeloma.

3. Osteosclerotic myeloma
   - Rare variant in which bone lesions are associated with a chronic inflammatory demyelinating polyneuropathy.
   - Diagnosis of osteosclerotic myeloma is not generally made until the polyneuropathy is recognized and evaluated.
   - Sensory symptoms (tingling, pins and needles, coldness) are noted first, followed by motor weakness.
     - Sensory and motor changes begin distally, are symmetric, and proceed proximally.

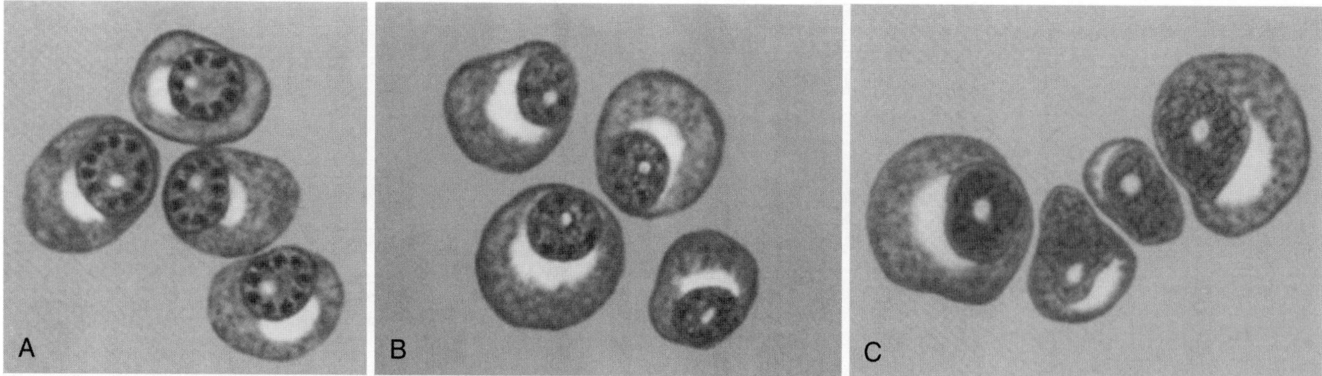

Figure 9-39 Myeloma cells. **A,** Plasma cells from a well-differentiated case of myeloma. They resemble the plasma cells seen in benign inflammatory cases. **B,** Plasma cells of intermediate maturity. **C,** Plasma cells that are immature and less well differentiated. (From Frassica FJ, et al: Myeloma of bone. In Stauffer RN, editor: *Advances in operative orthopaedics,* vol 2, St. Louis, 1994, Mosby–Year Book, p 362.)

- Severe weakness is common, but bone pain is not characteristic.
- Radiographs may show a spectrum from pure sclerosis to a mixed pattern of lysis and sclerosis. The lesions usually involve the spine, pelvic bones, and ribs; the extremities are generally spared.
- Affected patients may have abnormalities outside the nervous system and have a constellation of findings termed the *POEMS* syndrome (**p**olyneuropathy, **o**rganomegaly, **e**ndocrinopathy, **M**-protein, and **s**kin changes). Treatment is with a combination of chemotherapy, radiotherapy, and plasmapheresis. The neurologic changes may not improve with treatment.

IX. TUMORS OF UNKNOWN ORIGIN

A. Giant cell tumor

1. Benign form
   - Distinctive neoplasm that has poorly differentiated cells
   - Benign but aggressive
   - **Confusion in diagnosis results from the fact that in rare cases (<2%), this benign tumor metastasizes to the lungs (benign metastasizing giant cell tumor).**
   - Most common in the epiphysis and metaphysis of long bones, and about 50% of lesions occur about the knee; the vertebra, sacrum, and distal radius are involved in about 10% of cases (Figure 9-40).
   - **The sacrum is the most common axial location of giant cell tumors of bone.**
   - Unlike most bone tumors, which occur more often in boys and men, giant cell tumors are more common in girls and women.
   - They are uncommon in children with open physes.
   - **Manifest with pain that is usually referable to the joint involved**
   - **A purely lytic destructive lesion in the metaphysis that extends into the epiphysis and often borders the subchondral bone** (Figure 9-41)
   - Early in the symptomatic phase, the radiographs may appear normal; a small lytic focus is difficult to detect.
   - **Basic proliferating cell has a round to oval or even spindle-shaped nucleus (giant cells appear to have the same nuclei as the proliferating mononuclear cells).** Mitotic figures may be numerous.

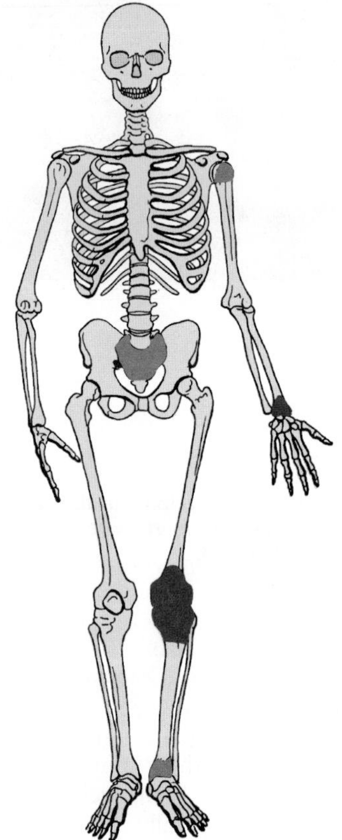

Figure 9-40 Skeletal distribution of the most common sites of giant cell tumor of the bone, which are the knee, distal radius, proximal humerus, and sacrum. (From McCarthy EF, Frassica FJ: *Pathology of bone and joint disorders,* Philadelphia, 1998, WB Saunders.)

   - Giant cell tumors may undergo a number of secondary degenerative changes, such as aneurysmal bone cyst formation, necrosis, fibrous repair, foam cell formation, and reactive new bone (Figure 9-42).
   - **Treatment is aimed at removing the lesion, with preservation of the involved joint.**
     - **Extensive exteriorization (removal of a large cortical window over the lesion)**
     - **Curettage with manual and power instruments**

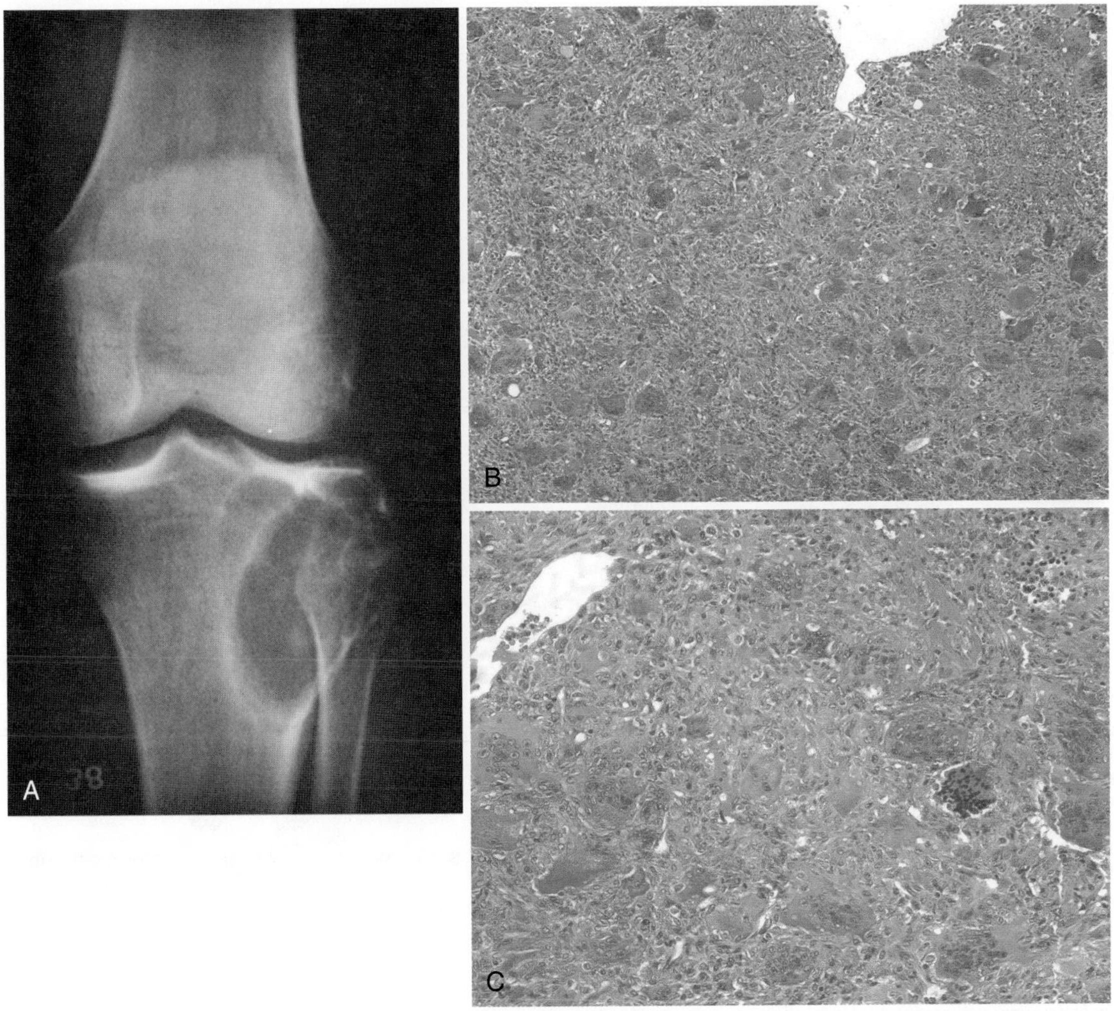

Figure 9-41 Giant cell tumor of the proximal tibia. **A,** Radiograph shows a well-circumscribed lytic lesion involving both the epiphysis and the metaphysis. **B,** Low-power photomicrograph (×160) shows sheets of multinucleated giant cells. **C,** Higher-power photomicrograph (×300) shows giant cells and mononucleic cells.

- **Chemical cauterization with phenol**
- **Area of defect is usually reconstructed with subchondral bone grafts, methylmethacrylate, or both.**
- **Local control with this treatment regimen has a success rate of 85% to 90%.**

2. Malignant forms: primary and secondary malignant giant cell tumors
   - With primary malignant giant cell tumor of bone, a benign giant cell tumor coexists with a high-grade sarcoma (occurs with about 1% of giant cell tumors).
   - Secondary malignant giant cell tumor occurs after irradiation to treat a giant cell tumor or after multiple local recurrences

B. Ewing tumor

1. Diagnosis
   - **Distinctive small, round cell sarcoma that occurs most often in children and young adults; most affected children are older than 5 years**
   - When a small blue cell tumor is found in a child younger than 5 years, metastatic neuroblastoma and leukemia should be confirmed or ruled out. In patients older than 30 years, metastatic carcinoma must be confirmed or ruled out (Table 9-10).
   - Most common locations include the pelvis, distal femur, proximal tibia, femoral diaphysis, and proximal humerus (Figure 9-43).
   - Manifests with pain, and fever may be present.
   - Affected patients may exhibit an elevated erythrocyte sedimentation rate, leukocytosis, anemia, and an elevated white blood cell count.
   - Radiographs often show a large, destructive lesion that involves the metaphysis and diaphysis.

Table 9-10 Small, Round Blue Cell Tumors

Children
Ewing sarcoma
Neuroblastoma
Adult
Plasmacytoma/multiple myeloma
Lymphoma
Small round cell carcinoma

Courtesy of Luke S. Choi, MD, Resident, Department of Orthopaedic Surgery, University of Virginia.

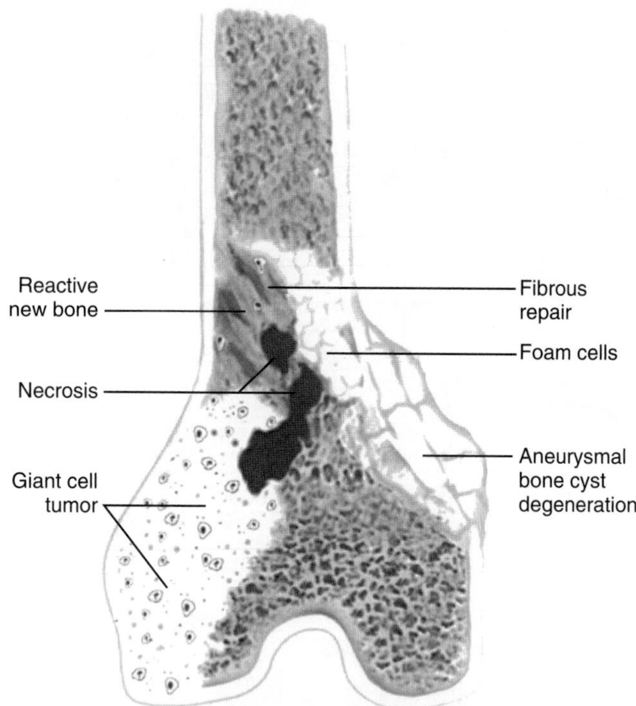

Figure 9-42 The secondary changes seen in giant cell tumor of the bone. This tumor may undergo many secondary changes, including aneurysmal bone cyst formation, in which the tumor causes marked expansion of the bone with resulting ballooning out of the cortex. Necrosis, cyst formation, fibrous repair, reactive new bone, and foam cells are also often found. (From McCarthy EF, Frassica FJ: *Pathology of bone and joint disorders,* Philadelphia, 1998, WB Saunders.)

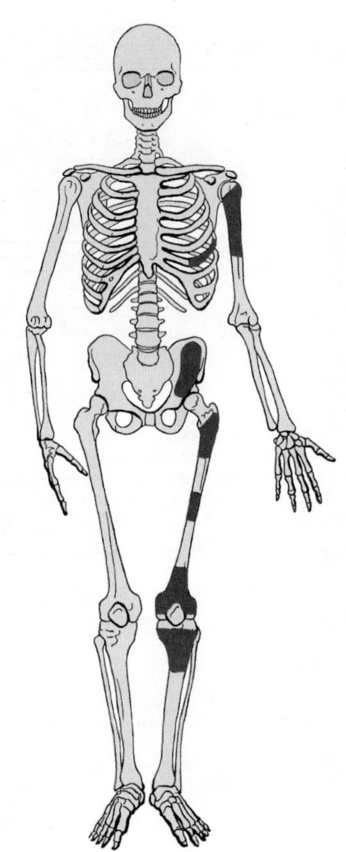

Figure 9-43 Skeletal distribution of the most common sites of Ewing tumor of the bone. The femur, pelvis, ribs, and humerus are common sites. (From McCarthy EF, Frassica FJ: *Pathology of bone and joint disorders,* Philadelphia, 1998, WB Saunders.)

    - The lesion may be purely lytic or may have variable amounts of reactive new bone formation (Figure 9-44).
    - The periosteum may be lifted off in multiple layers, which produces a characteristic but uncommon onionskin appearance.
    - The soft tissue component is often large.
  - **Immunohistochemistry studies reveal CD99 positivity.**
  - **Bone marrow biopsy is performed for staging purposes.**
2. Treatment: a multimodality approach with multiagent chemotherapy, irradiation, and surgical resection
  - **Most lesions have traditionally been treated with chemotherapy and irradiation, but the role of surgery is evolving.**
  - In some centers, chemotherapy and surgery are the major forms of treatment, whereas in others, traditional chemotherapy and external beam irradiation are preferred.
  - Major benefits of wide-margin surgical resection are a decrease in the risk of local recurrence and the avoidance of the potential for postirradiation sarcoma.
3. Survival:
  - The rate of long-term survival with multimodality treatment may be as high as 60% to 70%.
    - **There is a consistent chromosomal translocation (11;22) with the formation of a fusion protein (EWS-FLI 1).**
    - **Metastatic disease involves the lungs (50%), bone (25%), and bone marrow (20%).**
  - Poor prognostic factors include the following:
    - Spine and pelvic tumors
    - Tumors larger than 100 cm^3 in diameter
    - A poor response to chemotherapy (less than 90% tumor cell necrosis)
    - Elevated lactic dehydrogenase levels (Temple)
    - The *P53* mutation and gene fusion products other than EWS-FLI 1

C. Adamantinoma

1. Rare low-grade, malignant tumor of long bones that contains epithelium-like islands of cells
2. The tibia is the most common site, although other long bones are infrequently involved (fibula, femur, ulna, radius; Figure 9-45).
3. Affected patients are young adults and experience pain over months to years.
4. Radiographic appearance: multiple, sharply circumscribed, lucent defects of different sizes, with sclerotic bone interspersed between the zones and extending above and below the lucent zones (Figure 9-46; one of the lesions in the midshaft is the largest and is associated with cortical bone destruction).
5. The cells have an epithelial quality and are arranged in a palisading or glandular pattern; the epithelial cells occur in a fibrous stroma.
6. Treatment: wide-margin surgical resection

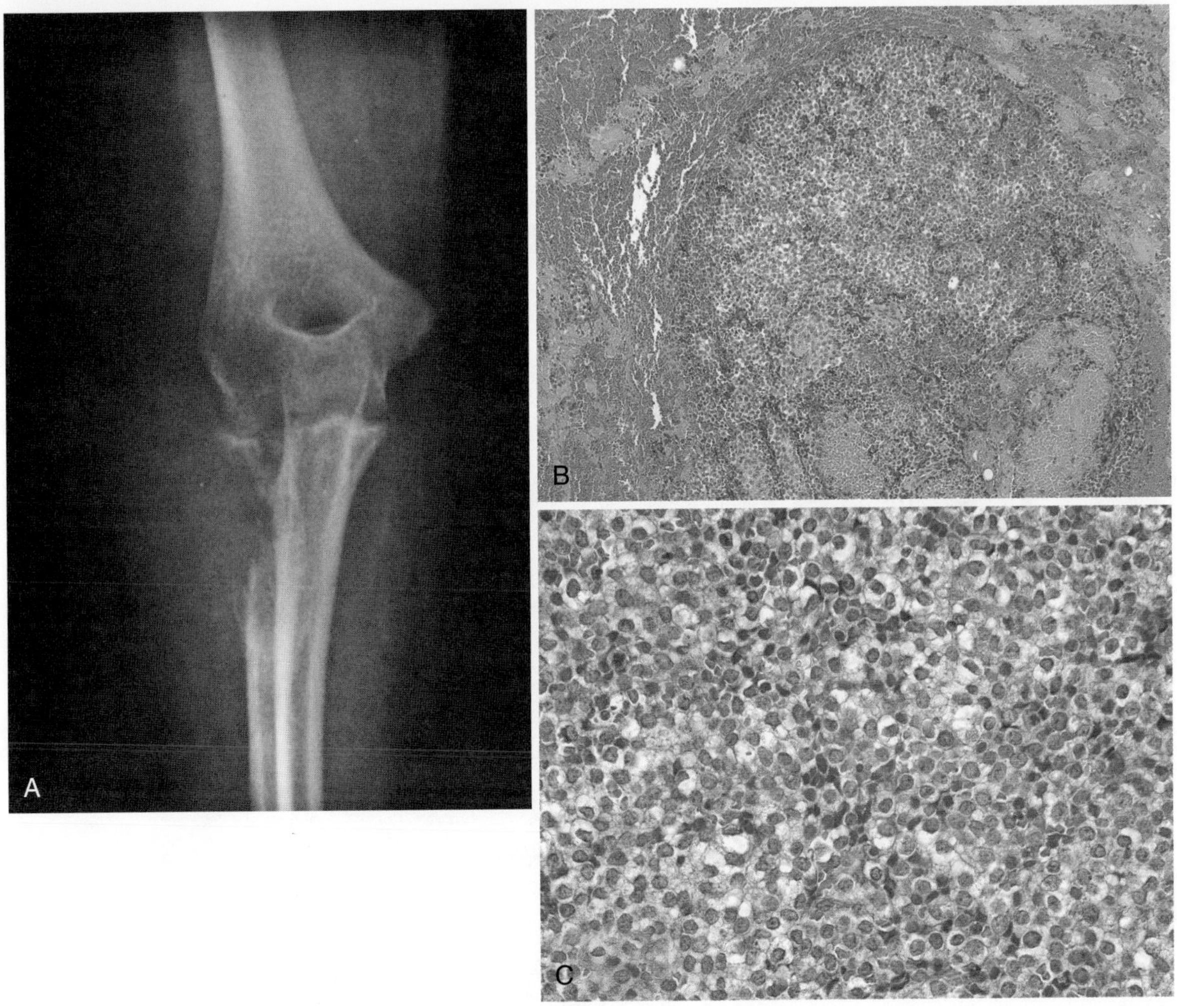

Figure 9-44 Ewing sarcoma of the proximal radius. **A,** Radiograph shows a destructive expansile lesion in the proximal radius. **B,** Low-power photomicrograph (×100) shows bone surrounded by a highly cellular neoplasm. **C,** Higher-power photomicrograph (×400) shows sheets of rounded cells.

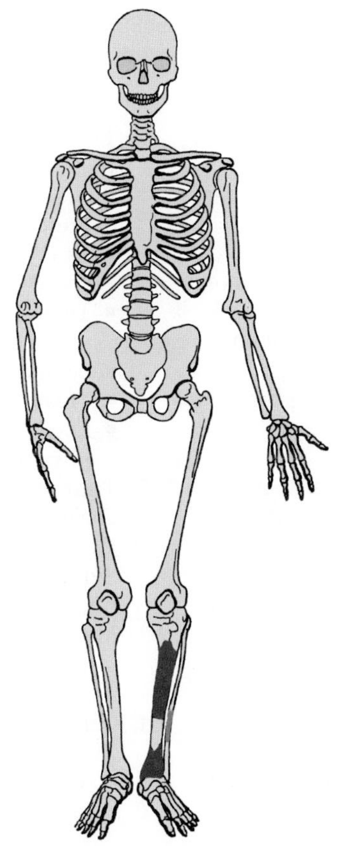

Figure 9-45 Skeletal distribution of the most common sites of adamantinoma. This peculiar tumor most often affects the tibia. (From McCarthy EF, Frassica FJ: *Pathology of bone and joint disorders,* Philadelphia, 1998, WB Saunders.)

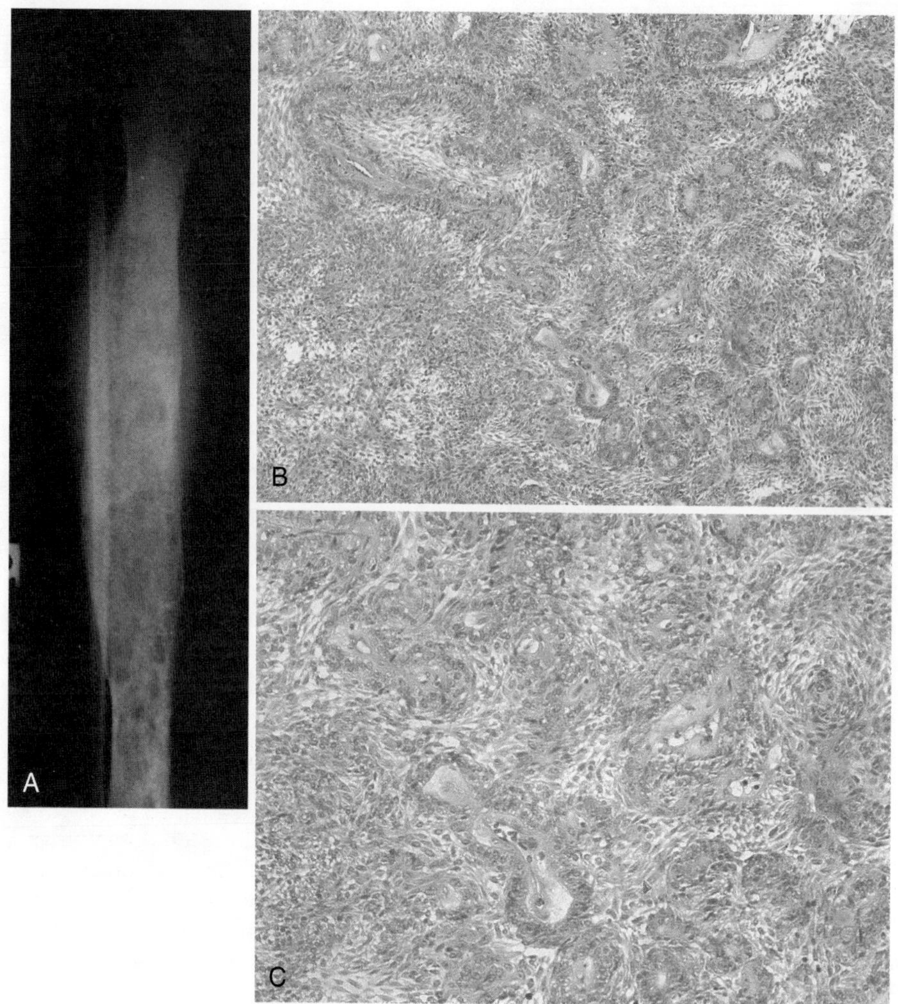

Figure 9-46 Adamantinoma of the tibia. **A,** Radiograph shows a bubbly, symmetric lytic lesion in the tibial diaphysis. **B,** Low-power photomicrograph (×250) shows biphasic differentiation, with spindle cells and epithelioid cells. **C,** Higher-power photomicrograph (×400) shows epithelial cells forming glands and spindle cells.

7. Tumor may metastasize either early or after multiple failed attempts at local control.

X. TUMOR-LIKE CONDITIONS

There are many lesions that simulate primary bone tumors and must be considered in the differential diagnosis (Box 9-4). These lesions range from metastases to reactive conditions.

A. Aneurysmal bone cyst

1. Nonneoplastic reactive condition that may be aggressive in its ability to destroy normal bone and extend into the soft tissues
2. May arise primarily in bone or be found in association with other tumors, such as giant cell tumor, chondroblastoma, chondromyxoid fibroma, and fibrous dysplasia
3. Of the patients with an aneurysmal bone cyst, 75% are younger than 20 years.
4. Affected patients experience pain and swelling.
5. **Characteristic radiographic finding: an eccentric, lytic, expansile area of bone destruction in the metaphysis**
6. In classical cases, there is a thin rim of periosteal new bone surrounding the lesion (Figure 9-47).
7. Radiograph may demonstrate the periosteal bone if it is mineralized.
8. MRI scan usually shows the periosteal layer surrounding the lesion.
   - **Fluid-fluid levels visible on T2-weighted MRI scans are characteristic of aneurysmal bone cysts.**
   - Essential histologic feature: cavernous blood-filled spaces without an endothelial lining.
   - There are thin strands of bone present in the fibrous tissue of the septa.
   - Benign giant cells may be numerous.
   - **Treatment: careful curettage and bone grafting**
   - **Local recurrence is common in children with open physes.**

B. Unicameral bone cyst (a.k.a., simple bone cyst)

1. Occurs most often in the proximal humerus; other sites are the proximal femur and distal tibia
2. **Symmetric cystic expansion with thinning of the involved cortices**
3. **Manifests with pain, usually after a fracture caused by minor trauma (e.g., sporting event, throwing a baseball, wrestling)**
4. Central lytic area and symmetric thinning of the cortices (Figure 9-48)
   - Affected bone is often expanded; however, the bone is generally no wider than the physis.

Box 9-4

Tumor-like Conditions (Tumor Simulators)

YOUNG PATIENT
Eosinophilic granuloma
Osteomyelitis
Avulsion fractures
Aneurysmal bone cyst
Fibrous dysplasia
Osteofibrous dysplasia
Heterotopic ossification
Unicameral bone cyst
Giant cell reparative granuloma
Exuberant callus

ADULT
Synovial chondromatosis
Pigmented villonodular synovitis
Stress fracture
Heterotopic ossification
Ganglionic cyst

OLDER ADULT
Mastocytosis
Hyperparathyroidism
Paget disease
Bone infarcts
Bone islands
Ganglionic cyst
Cyst secondary to joint disease
Epidermoid cyst

- Often appears trabeculated
- When the cyst abuts the physeal plate, the process is called *active;* when normal bone intervenes, the cyst is termed *latent.*
- Thin, fibrous lining contains fibrous tissue, giant cells, hemosiderin pigment, and a few chronic inflammatory cells.
- Treatment: aspiration to confirm the diagnosis, followed by methylprednisolone acetate injection
- Unicameral bone cysts of the proximal femur are often treated with curettage, grafting, and internal fixation to avoid fracture and osteonecrosis.

C. Histiocytosis X (Langerhans cell histiocytosis)

1. Lichtenstein originally divided this disorder into three entities: eosinophilic granuloma (monostotic bone disease), Hand-Schüller-Christian disease (multiple bone lesions and visceral disease), and Letterer-Siwe disease (a fulminating condition in young children).
2. This disorder is now usually referred to as *LCH.*
3. The cellular abnormality is a proliferation of the Langerhans cells of the dendritic system.
4. Eosinophilic granuloma of bone is analogous to monostotic LCH, whereas Hand-Schüller-Christian disease could be called *polyostotic LCH with visceral involvement.*
   - Eosinophilic granuloma of bone is the most common manifestation; only a single bone or, on occasion, multiple bones are involved.
   - Patients present with pain and swelling.
   - The lesion is highly destructive and has well-defined margins (Figure 9-49).
   - Cortex may be destroyed and a periosteal reaction with a soft tissue mass simulating a malignant bone tumor may be present.
   - Often different amounts of bone destruction of the involved cortices, resulting in the appearance of a bone within a bone
   - There may be expansion of the involved bone.
   - Any bone may be involved.
   - The proliferating Langerhans cell, with an indented or grooved nucleus, is the characteristic cell.
     - Cytoplasm is eosinophilic.
     - Nuclear membrane has a crisp border.
     - Mitotic figures may be common.
     - Bilobed eosinophils with bright, granular, eosinophilic cytoplasm are present in large numbers.
   - Treatment:
     - Eosinophilic granuloma is a self-limiting process.
     - Treatments such as corticosteroid injection, low-dose irradiation (600 to 800 cGy), curettage and bone grafting, and observation have been successful.
     - If the articular surface is in jeopardy or an impending fracture is a possibility, concomitant curettage and bone grafting is a logical treatment.
     - Low-dose irradiation is effective for most lesions that cannot be injected and is associated with low rates of morbidity.
5. Hand-Schüller-Christian disease:
   - Bone lesions and visceral involvement
   - Classic triad, which occurs in fewer than one fourth of patients, includes exophthalmos, diabetes insipidus, and lytic skull lesions
   - Multifocal disease is usually treated with chemotherapy.
6. Letterer-Siwe disease occurs in young children and is usually fatal.

D. Fibrous dysplasia

1. Developmental abnormality of bone that is characterized by monostotic or polyostotic involvement
2. Yellow or brown patches of skin (café au lait spots with irregular borders) may accompany the bone lesions
3. Failure of the production of normal lamellar bone
4. **Genetic mutation is an activating mutation of the GSα surface protein**
   - Increased production of **cyclic adenosine monophosphate** (cAMP)
5. **When endocrine abnormalities (especially precocious puberty) accompany multiple bone lesions and skin abnormalities, the condition is called *McCune-Albright syndrome.***
6. Any bone may be involved; the proximal femur is the most commonly affected.
7. Variable appearance (looks highly lytic or like ground glass; Figure 9-50)
   - Well-defined rim of sclerotic bone
   - Proliferation of fibroblasts (produces a dense collagenous matrix)
   - Trabeculae of osteoid and bone within the fibrous stroma
   - Cartilage may be present in variable amounts.
   - **Bone fragments are present in a disorganized manner, and their appearance has been likened to "alphabet soup" and "Chinese letters."**

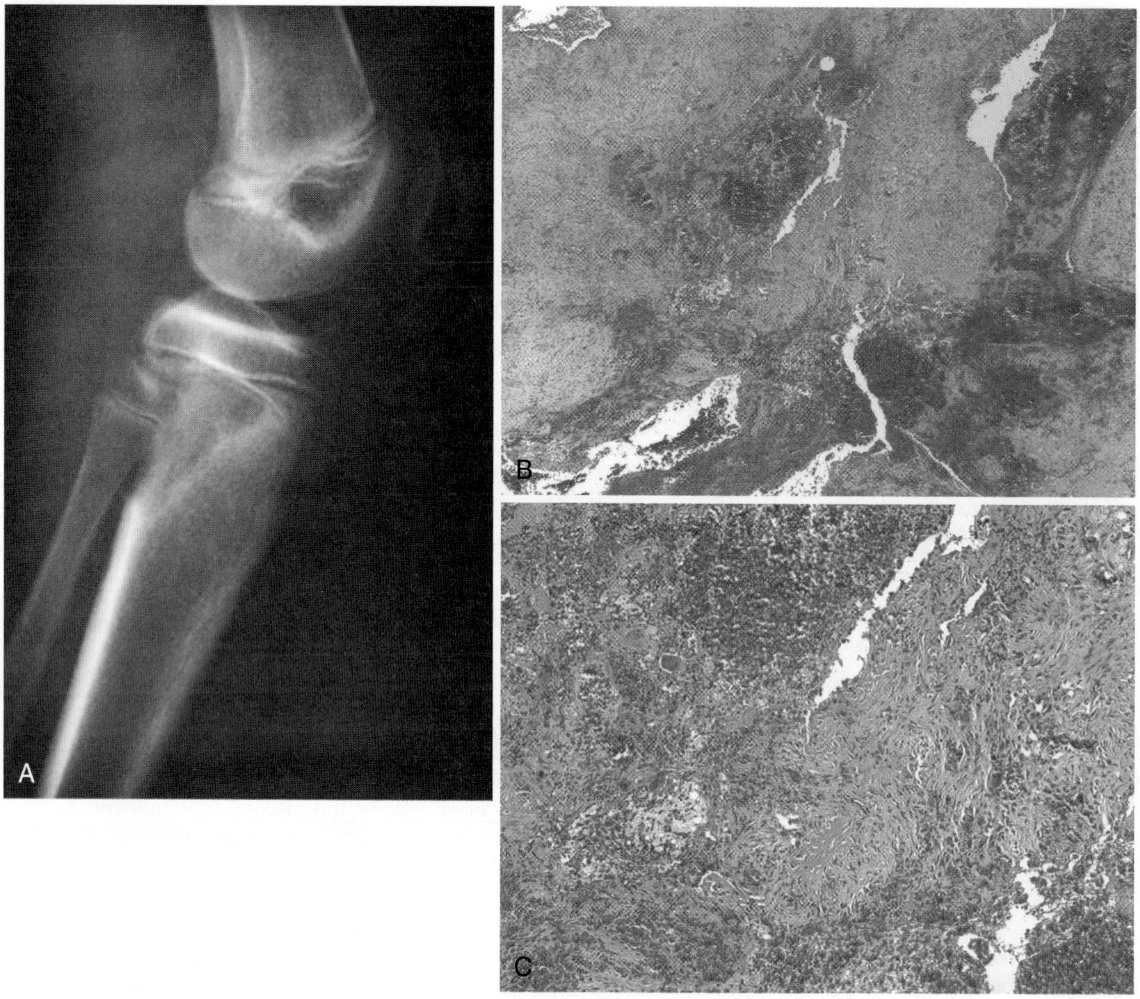

Figure 9-47 Aneurysmal bone cyst of the proximal tibia. **A,** Radiograph shows a well-defined lytic lesion in the posterior tibial metaphysis. **B,** Low-power photomicrograph (×25) shows blood-filled lakes. **C,** Higher-power photomicrograph (×50) shows the wall of the cyst, with fibroblasts and occasional multinucleated giant cells.

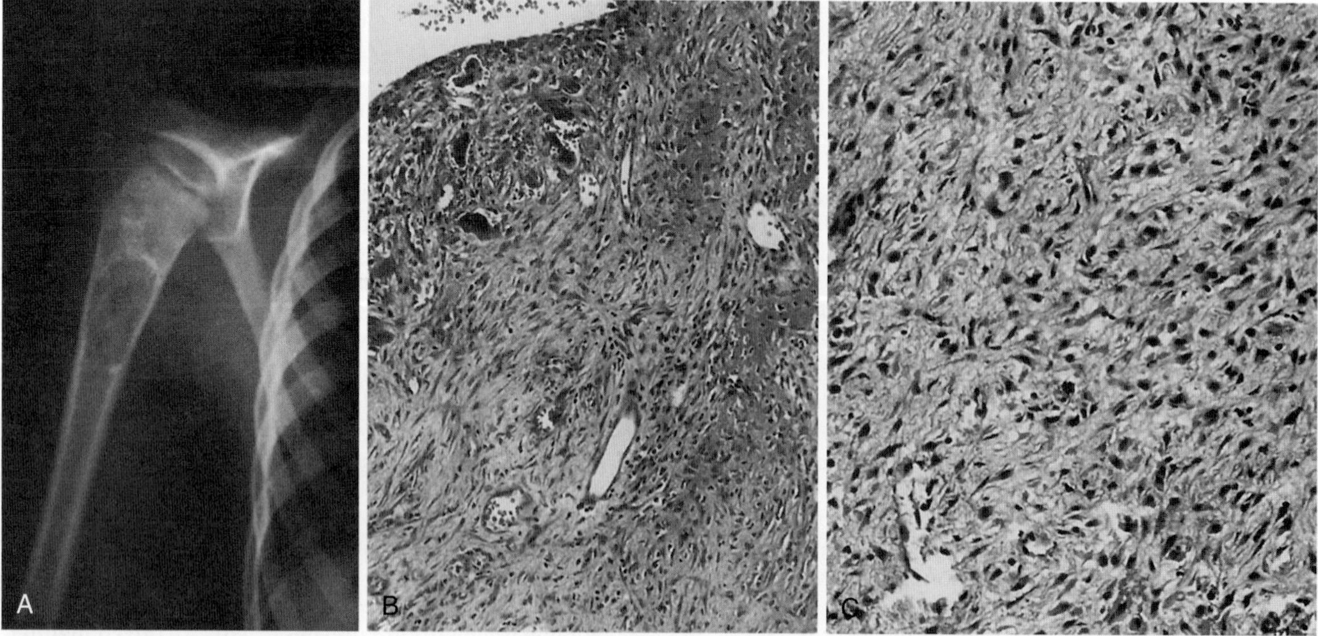

Figure 9-48 Unicameral bone cyst of the humerus. **A,** Radiograph shows a symmetric, midline, well-circumscribed lytic lesion in the humeral metaphysis. **B,** Low-power photomicrograph (×160) shows the fibrous tissue membrane, with reactive bone and occasional multinucleated giant cells. **C,** High-power photomicrograph shows a uniform population of spindle cells without nuclear atypia.

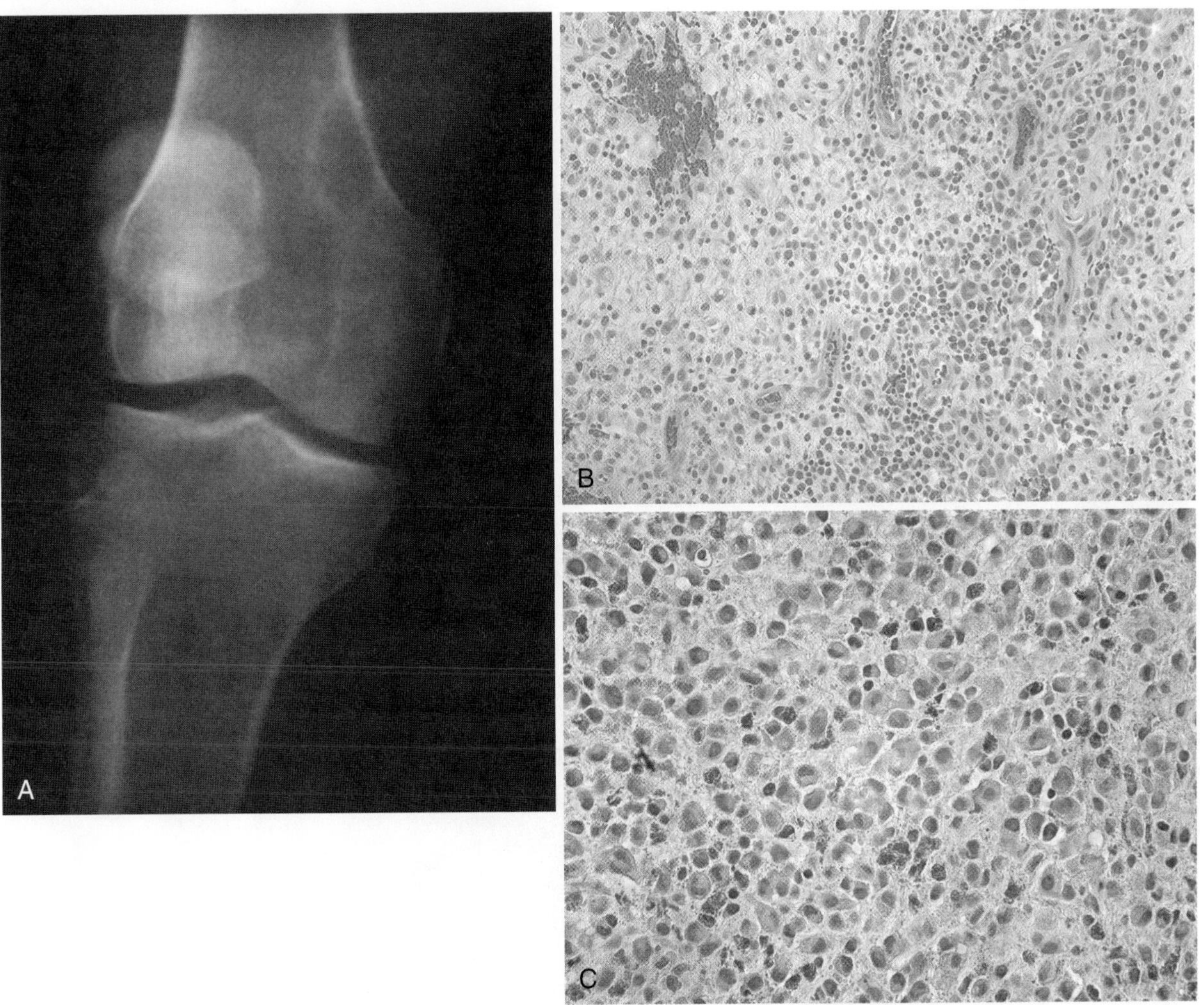

Figure 9-49 Eosinophilic granuloma of the distal femur. **A,** Radiograph shows a well-circumscribed lesion with a sclerotic rim in the femoral metaphysis. **B,** Low-power photomicrograph (×160) shows a heterogeneous population of inflammatory cells, with an aggregation of histiocytes. **C,** Higher-power photomicrograph (×400) shows nests of Langerhans histiocytes.

- Treatment: predicated on the presence of symptoms and the risk of fracture
  - Internal fixation and bone grafting are used in areas of high stress in which nonoperative treatment would not be effective.
  - Most affected patients do not need surgical treatment.
  - **Autogenous cancellous bone grafting is never used because the transplanted bone is quickly transformed into the woven bone of fibrous dysplasia.**
  - Cortical or cancellous allografts are usually used.
  - Diphosphonate therapy has been shown to be effective in decreasing pain and reducing bone turnover in patients with polyostotic fibrous dysplasia.

E. Osteofibrous dysplasia (also called *ossifying fibroma* or *Campanacci lesion*)

1. **Primarily involves the tibia and is usually confined to the anterior tibial cortex.**
2. Bowing is very common, and affected children may develop pathologic fractures.
3. **Lesion typically manifests in children younger than 10 years.**
4. Biopsy is not necessary.
5. Biopsy, when performed, reveals fibrous tissue stroma and a background of bone trabeculae with osteoblastic rimming.
6. Nonoperative treatment is preferred until the child reaches maturity.
7. These lesions usually regress and do not cause problems in adults.

F. Paget disease

1. **Characterized by abnormal bone remodeling**
2. Usually diagnosed during the fifth decade of life
3. Monostotic or polyostotic
4. Radiographs demonstrate coarsened trabeculae and remodeled cortices.
5. Coarsened trabeculae give the bone a blastic appearance.
6. Characteristic features: irregular, broad trabeculae; reversal or cement lines; osteoclastic activity; and fibrous vascular tissue between the trabeculae
7. Manifests with pain
8. Medical treatment: aimed at retarding the activity of the osteoclasts
9. **Agents used include diphosphonates and calcitonin (pamidronate and zometa).**

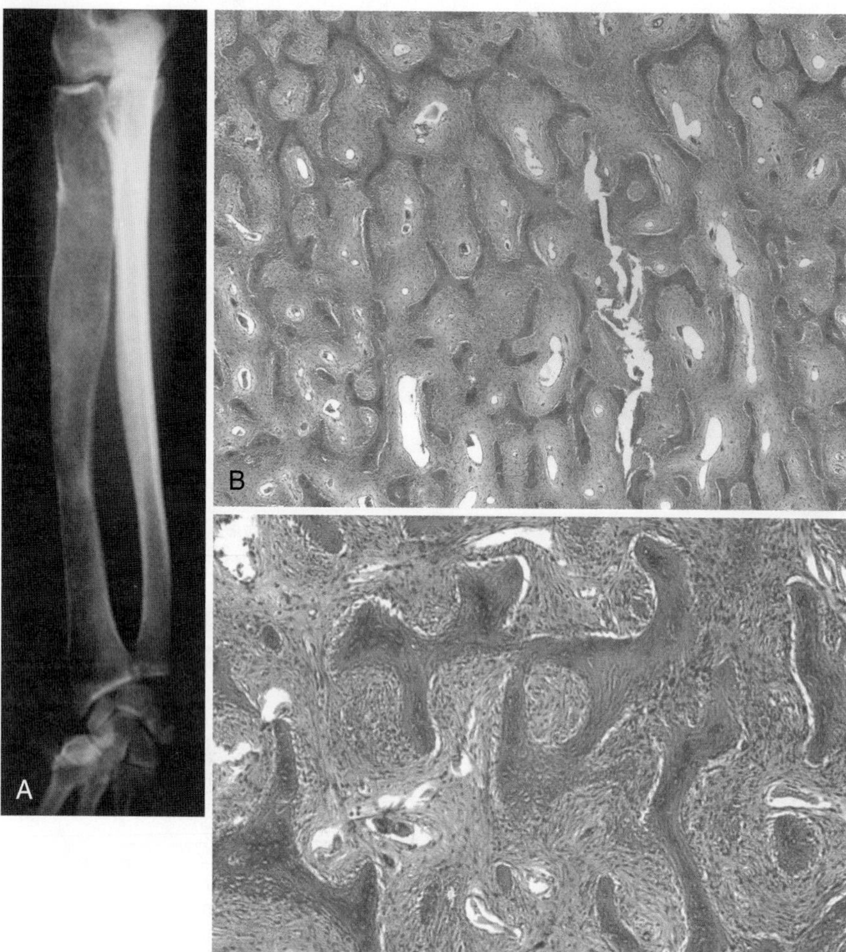

Figure 9-50 Fibrous dysplasia of the radius. **A,** Radiograph shows a long, symmetric lytic lesion of the radius with a ground-glass appearance. **B,** Low-power photomicrograph (×50) shows seams of osteoid in a fibrous background. **C,** Higher-power photomicrograph (×160) shows osteoid surrounded by bland fibrous tissue.

10. Affected patients may present with degenerative joint disease, fracture, or neurologic encroachment; joint degeneration is common in the hip and knee.
11. Patients undergoing arthroplasty should be treated with diphosphonates to decrease bleeding at the time of surgery.
12. **Fewer than 1% of patients with Paget disease develop malignant degeneration with the formation of a sarcoma within a focus of a Paget lesion.**
    - Symptoms of Paget sarcoma are the abrupt onset of pain and swelling.
    - Radiographs usually demonstrate cortical bone destruction and the presence of a soft tissue mass.
    - **Paget sarcoma is a deadly tumor with a poor prognosis (rate of long-term survival is <20%).**

G. Osteomyelitis

1. Bone infections that often simulate primary tumors
2. Occult infections may occur in all age groups.
3. Affected patients may present with fever, chills, bone pain, or a combination of these symptoms.
4. Affected patients usually present with bone pain but without systemic symptoms.
5. The radiograph findings may be nonspecific:
    - Bone destruction and formation are the characteristic findings of chronic infections.
    - Acute infections often produce cortical bone destruction and periosteal elevation.
    - Serpiginous tracts and irregular areas of bone destruction are suggestive of infection rather than neoplasm.
    - The lesion is usually apparent with the following:
        - Edema of the granulation tissue
        - Numerous new blood vessels
        - A mixed-cell population of inflammatory cells, plasma cells, polymorphonuclear leukocytes, eosinophils, lymphocytes, and histiocytes
6. A chronic infection with long-standing wound drainage is occasionally complicated by a squamous cell carcinoma.
7. Material that has been sent for culture should be subjected to biopsy, and material that has been sent for biopsy should be subjected to culture.
8. Treatment: removal of all dead tissue and appropriate antibiotic therapy

XI. METASTATIC BONE DISEASE

A. Most common entity that destroys the skeleton in older patients

B. When a destructive bone lesion is found in a patient older than 40 years, metastases must be considered first.

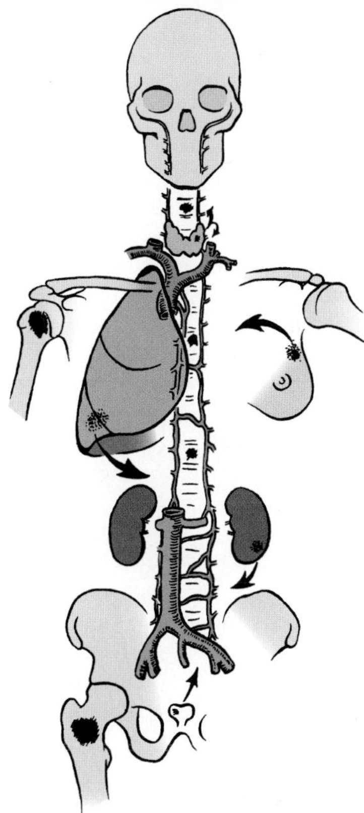

Figure 9-51 Batson venous plexus. This plexus is longitudinal and valveless and extends from the sacrum to the skull. The breast, lung, kidney, prostate, and thyroid glands connect to this system. Tumor cells can enter this system and spread to the vertebrae, ribs, pelvis, and proximal limb girdle. (From McCarthy EF, Frassica FJ: *Pathology of bone and joint disorders,* Philadelphia, 1998, WB Saunders.)

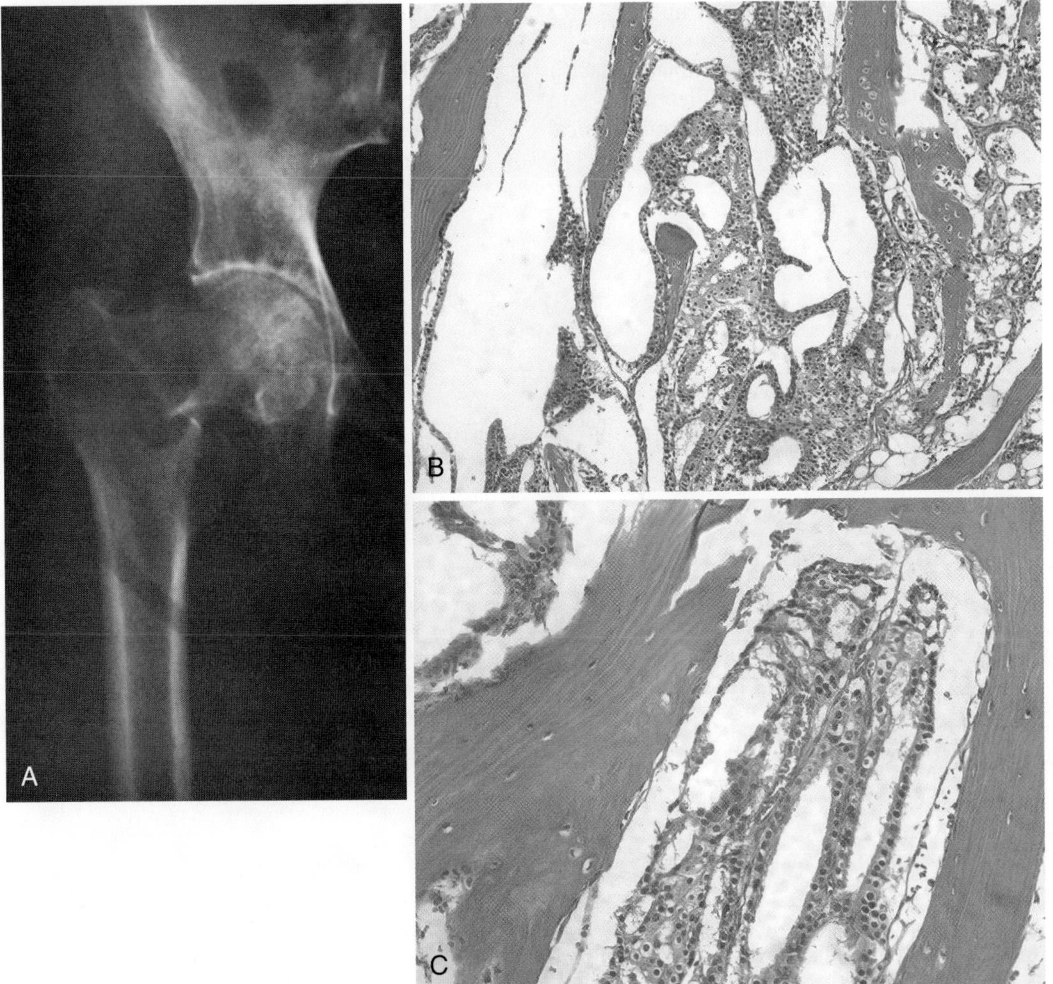

Figure 9-52 Metastatic carcinoma. **A,** Radiograph shows a lytic lesion in the femoral neck and the ilium. **B,** Low-power photomicrograph (×100) shows the glandular arrangement of cells in the marrow space. **C,** Higher-power photomicrograph (×400) shows epithelial cells in an organoid pattern.

C. The five carcinomas that are most likely to metastasize to bone are those of the breast, lung, prostate, kidney, and thyroid. (Mnemonic: "BLT and a Kosher Pickle")

D. Most common locations of metastasis are the pelvis, vertebral bodies, ribs, and proximal limb girdles.

1. **Pathologic fractures secondary to metastatic disease occur most commonly in the proximal femur.**

E. The pathogenesis is probably related to Batson vertebral vein plexus.

1. Venous flow from the breast, lung, prostate, kidney, and thyroid drains into the vertebral vein plexus (Figure 9-51).
2. The plexus has intimate connections to the vertebral bodies, pelvis, skull, and proximal limb girdles.

F. Radiographs demonstrate a destructive lesion that may be purely lytic, may have a mixed pattern of bone destruction and formation, or may be purely sclerotic (Figure 9-52).

G. Histologic hallmark: appearance of epithelial cells in a fibrous stroma; the epithelial cells are often arranged in a glandular pattern

H. The bone destruction is caused not by the tumor cells themselves but by activation of osteoclasts (Figure 9-53).

1. **Tumor cells secrete parathyroid hormone–related peptide (PTHrP), which stimulates the release of the receptor activator for nuclear factor κB ligand (RANKL) from the osteoblasts and marrow stromal cells.**
2. RANKL attaches to the receptor activator for nuclear factor κ (RANK) receptor on the osteoclast precursor cells.
3. In the presence of granulocyte colony–stimulating factor (G-CSF), the osteoclast precursor cells differentiate into active osteoclasts that resorb the trabecular and cortical bone.
4. With bone resorption, transforming growth factor-β, insulin-like growth factor-1, and calcium are released, and these factors stimulate the tumor cells to multiply and release more PTHrP.
5. This process has been termed as the "vicious cycle" of metastatic bone disease.
6. To combat the osteoclastic bone destruction, many patients are now treated with antiresorptive agents (diphosphonates) such as intravenous pamidronate and zoledronic acid.
7. Treatment: aimed at controlling pain and maintaining the independence of the patient
8. Prophylactic internal fixation is performed when impending fracture is deemed likely.
   - In comparison with treatment of completed pathologic fractures, prophylactic fixation results in less blood loss, shorter hospital stays, greater likelihood of discharge to home, and greater likelihood of independent ambulation.
9. There are many suggested criteria for fixation. The following conditions put the patient most at risk for fracture:
   - More than 50% destruction of the diaphyseal cortices
   - Permeative destruction of the subtrochanteric femoral region
   - More than 50% to 75% destruction of the metaphysis
   - Persistent pain after irradiation
   - Pain on weight bearing (especially in lower extremity with every footstep)

I. Treatment of pathologic fractures is almost always surgical, inasmuch as these fractures rarely have the potential to heal.

J. Surgical procedures should not rely on bony healing.

1. **Most proximal femur fractures should be treated with cemented endoprosthesis.** To protect the femoral shaft in

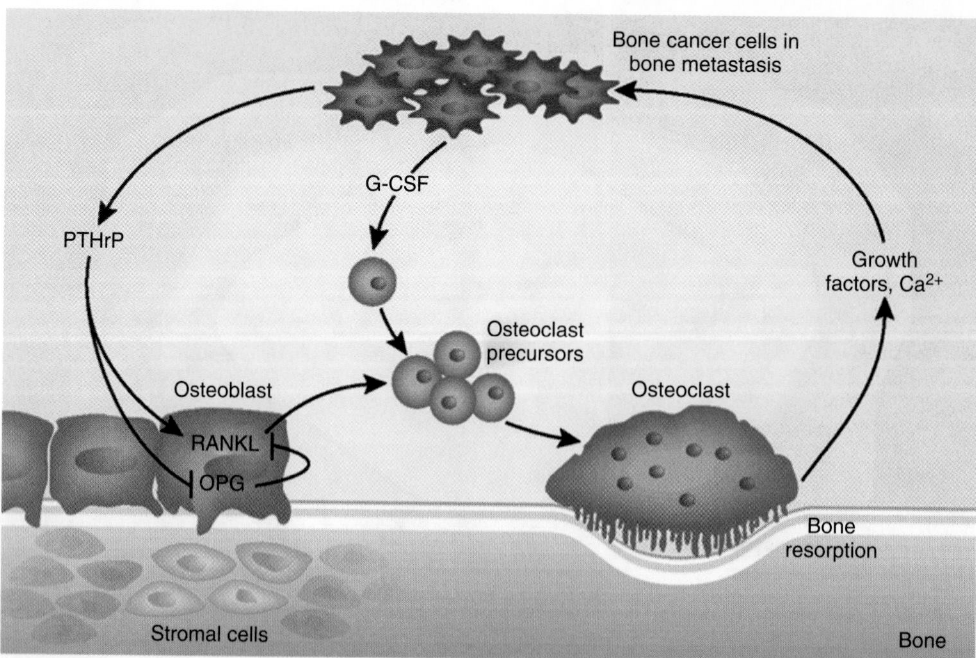

Figure 9-53 Breast cancer cells produce factors such as parathyroid hormone–related peptide (PTHrP) and granulocyte colony–stimulating factor (G-CSF), which enhance the formation of osteoclasts. OPG, osteoprotegerin; RANKL, receptor activator for nuclear factor κB ligand. (From Roodman GD: Bone breaking cancer treatment, *Nat Med* 13:25-26, 2007, Figure 1.)

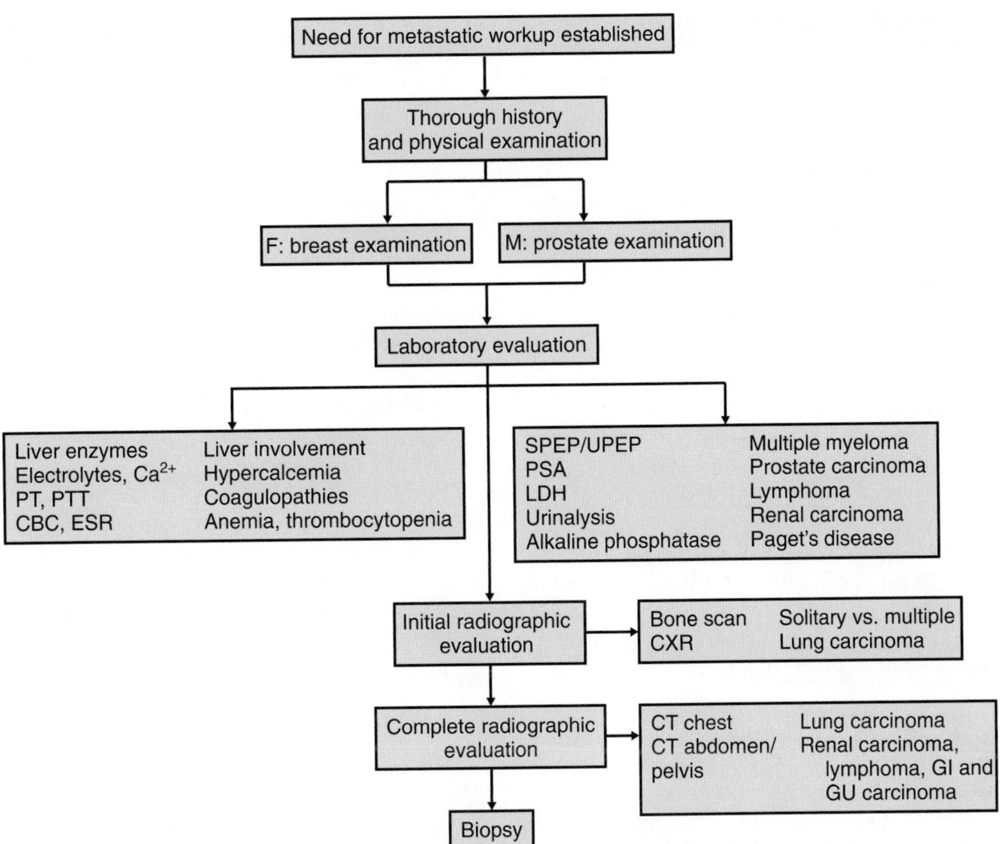

Figure 9-54 Algorithm showing the evaluation of the older patient with a single bone lesion and suspected metastases of unknown origin. CBC, complete blood cell count; CT, computed tomography; CXR, chest radiograph; ESR, erythrocyte sedimentation rate; F, female patient; GI, gastrointestinal; GU, genitourinary; LDH, lactate dehydrogenase; M, male patient; PSA, prostate-specific antigen; PT, prothrombin time; PTT, partial thromboplastin time; SPEP, serum protein electrophoresis; UPEP; urine protein electrophoresis. (From Damron TA: *Orthopaedic surgery essentials, oncology and basic science,* Philadelphia, 2008, Lippincott Williams & Wilkins, p 233.)

patients with relatively long life expectancy, consideration should be given to using a long stem.

2. Risk factors for sudden death during insertion of a long-stem prosthesis: presence of breast cancer, hypovolemia, reduced pulmonary function

K. In patients older than 40 years with a single destructive bone lesion but without a known primary tumor, metastatic disease must be considered present. Simon outlined a diagnostic strategy that identifies the primary lesion in up to 80% to 90% of patients (Figure 9-54).

L. Histologically confirmed metastatic cancer for which a definitive primary site is not identified after a detailed medical examination is known as a *carcinoma, unknown primary* (CUP).

TESTABLE CONCEPTS

SECTION 1 INTRODUCTION

- Grading of a tumor is based on pathologic determination of anaplasia, pleomorphism, and nuclear hyperchromasia. The grade of the tumor is most strongly correlated with the potential for metastasis. High-grade tumors have more than a 50% likelihood of metastasizing. Staging is clinical and based on histologic grade, anatomic features, and presence of metastasis.
- Benign bone tumors in children are most commonly an incidental finding.
- Different lesions occur in typical age ranges. Classic age associations are as follows:
  - Birth to age 5 years: rhabdomyosarcoma, osteofibrous dysplasia, leukemia
  - Ages 10 to 20 years: metaphyseal fibrous defect (nonossifying fibroma), enchondroma, unicameral bone cyst, osteosarcoma, Ewing sarcoma, osteoid osteoma, chondroblastoma, fibrous dysplasia
  - Ages 20 to 30 years: giant cell tumor
  - Ages 30 to 50 years: metastatic bone disease, fibrosarcoma, malignant fibrous histiocytoma
  - Older than 50 years: metastatic bone disease, myeloma, lymphoma, chondrosarcoma, malignant fibrous histiocytoma, Paget disease
- Some lesions have classic anatomic locations:
  - Anterior cortex of tibia: adamantinoma, osteofibrous dysplasia
  - Posterior cortex of the distal femur: parosteal osteosarcoma, periosteal desmoid
  - Epiphysis: giant cell tumor, chondroblastoma, aneurysmal bone cyst, osteomyelitis, dysplasia epiphysealis hemimelica (Trevor disease)
  - Metaphysis: metaphyseal fibrous defect (nonossifying fibroma), aneurysmal bone cyst, giant cell tumor, osteosarcoma
  - Diaphysis: Ewing sarcoma, fibrous dysplasia, eosinophilic granuloma (histiocytosis), multiple myeloma
- Principles of biopsy:
  - Use longitudinal incisions and excise biopsy tracts if the lesion is malignant.
  - Approach lesions through muscles wherever possible. However, avoid functionally important structures and neurovascular structures.
  - Maintain meticulous hemostasis, and—only in rare cases—use a small drain at the corner of the wound to prevent hematoma formation.
  - Frozen-section analysis should be performed intraoperatively to ensure that adequate diagnostic tissue is obtained.
  - Samples should be sent for bacteriologic analysis.
- There are four surgical margins of tumor excision: intralesional, marginal (through reactive zone), wide (including a cuff of normal tissue), and radical (entire tumor and its compartment, including surrounding muscles, ligaments, and connective tissues).
- Two essential criteria for limb salvage surgery: local control is at least equal to that of amputation; limb must be functional.
- Chemotherapy has a significant effect in osteosarcoma and Ewing tumor; for chemotherapy combined with surgery, long-term survival rates are 60% to 70%.
- Radiation therapy is used for local control of Ewing tumor, lymphoma, myeloma, and metastatic bone disease. It can be used as an adjunct treatment of soft tissue sarcoma. Radiation therapy is associated with late stress fractures and postirradiation sarcoma.
- Common tumor-associated genetic associations:
  - Osteosarcoma: tumor suppressor genes Rb (retinoblastoma) and p53 (Li-Fraumeni syndrome)
  - Ewing sarcoma: t(11;22); gene product is EWS-FLI1
  - Synovial sarcoma: t(X;18); gene products are SYT-SSX1 and SYT-SSX2
  - Myxoid liposarcoma: t(12;16); gene product is FUS-CHOP
  - Alveolar rhabdomyosarcoma: t(2;13); gene product is PAX3-FKHR
  - Fibrous dysplasia: activating mutation of the GSα surface protein

SECTION 2 SOFT TISSUE TUMORS

I. Introduction

- The most common manifestation of a soft tissue sarcoma is an enlarging painful or painless soft tissue mass.
- On MRI, most soft tissue malignancies are well defined (pseudocapsule) and heterogenous. Any large (>5 cm) soft tissue mass deep to fascia should be considered a sarcoma.
- Metastatic workup for includes CT scan of the chest. For liposarcoma, a CT scan of the abdomen and pelvis is required because of synchronous retroperitoneal liposarcoma.
- Unplanned removal of a soft tissue sarcoma is the most common error. Residual tumor may exist, and repeat excision should be performed.
- Most soft tissue sarcomas metastasize to the lung. Lymphatic metastasis occurs in 5% of cases; metastases of rhabdomyosarcoma, clear cell sarcoma, epithelioid sarcoma and synovial sarcoma are the most common.

II. Tumors of Fibrous Tissue

- Extraabdominal desmoid tumors are "rock-hard." Patients with Gardner syndrome (familial adenomatous polyposis) have a 10,000-fold increased risk for such tumors. Estrogen receptor β inhibitors can be used for treatment. Wide-margin surgical resection is recommended, but local recurrence is common.
- Modular fasciitis is a painful, rapidly enlarging mass in a person 15 to 35 years of age. Perform a resection with a marginal margin.
- Malignant fibrous histiocytoma is the most common malignant sarcoma of soft tissue in adults. It appears on MRI as a deep-seated, inhomogeneous mass that has a low signal on T1-weighted images and a high signal on T2-weighted images. Treatment is with wide-margin local excision and adjuvant radiotherapy. Postoperative external beam irradiation yields equal local control rates, with

a lower rate of postoperative wound complications but a higher incidence of postoperative fibrosis.

III. Tumors of Fatty Tissue

- Lipomas appear on MRI as well-demarcated lesions with the same signal characteristics as those of mature fat on all sequences. On fat-suppression sequences, the lipoma has a uniformly low signal. Treatment of asymptomatic lesions is observation, whereas that for expanding or symptomatic lesions is marginal excision.
- Liposarcoma is the second most common soft tissue sarcoma in adults. It virtually never occurs in the subcutaneous tissues. MRI demonstrates thicker and more irregular septa than for lipomas, which also appear bright on T2-weighted images.

IV. Tumors of Neural Tissue

- Histologic characteristics of neurofibroma are interlacing bundles of elongated cells with wavy, dark-staining nuclei. Cells are associated with wirelike strands of collagen.
- Neurofibromatosis can manifest with more than one neurofibroma or one plexiform neurofibroma, with café au lait spots, with Lisch nodules (melanocytic hamartomas in the iris), and with anterolateral tibial bowing.

V. Tumors of Muscle Tissue

- Rhabdomyosarcoma is the most common soft tissue sarcoma in children. It most commonly manifests in the head and neck, genitourinary tract, and retroperitoneum. Extremity involvement is associated with the alveolar subtype; it involves a translocation of chromosomes 2 and 13, and the gene product is PAX3-FKHR.
- Rhabdomyosarcomas are sensitive to multiagent chemotherapy. Wide-margin surgical resection and irradiation are also important.

VI. Vascular Tumors

- Hemangiomas are common in children and adults. Radiographs may reveal phleboliths. Multiple hemangiomas are associated with Maffucci syndrome.

VII. Synovial Disorders

- PVNS most commonly affects the knee, followed by the hip and shoulder. Recurrent, atraumatic hemarthrosis with associated pain is the most common manifestation. Radiographs may show cystic erosions on both sides of the joint. Histologic study reveals highly vascular villi lined with plump, hyperplastic synovial cells; hemosiderin-stained, multinucleated giant cells; and chronic inflammatory cells.
- On both T1- and T2-weighted MRI sequences, PVNS appears as low-signal lesions.
- Treatment of PVNS is complete synovectomy except in highly localized forms of PVNS.
- Synovial sarcoma rarely arises from an intraarticular location. It most commonly occurs about the knee and is the most common sarcoma of the foot. Spotty mineralization on radiographs is highly characteristic.
- Histologic study of synovial sarcoma reveals a biphasic pattern: epithelial cells (resembling carcinoma) and spindle cells (resembling fibrosarcoma).
- All cells of synovial sarcomas have a translocation between chromosome 18 and the X chromosome that produces two gene fusion products (SYT-SSX1 and SYT-SSX2). Staining of tumor cells yield appearances positive for keratin and epithelial membrane antigen.

VIII. Other Rare Sarcomas

- Epithelioid sarcoma is the most common sarcoma of the hand. Lymph node metastases are common.
- Clear cell sarcoma is a melanin-producing lesion, but its cells have a t(12;22) translocation not present in melanoma cells.

IX. Post-Traumatic Conditions

- Sarcomas may spontaneously hemorrhage. On advanced imaging, the appearance of "hematomas" that do not have fascial plane tracking or subcutaneous ecchymosis suggests that the bleeding is contained by a pseudocapsule, and this finding is suspect for a sarcoma.
- For myositis ossificans, radiography reveals peripheral mineralization with a central lucent area.

SECTION 3 BONE TUMORS

I. Nomenclature

- Malignant bone tumors manifest most commonly with pain. This is in contrast to soft tissue tumors, which most commonly manifest as painless masses.
- Bone sarcomas metastasize primarily via the hematogenous route. The lung is the most common site of metastasis.
- Osteosarcoma and Ewing sarcoma commonly metastasize to other bone sites.

II. Bone-Producing Lesions

Osteoid Osteoma

- Classically manifests with increasing pain that is relieved by salicylates and other NSAIDs
- Radiographs show intensely reactive bone and a radiolucent nidus. CT scans provide better contrast between the lucent nidus and the reactive bone than does MRI.
- This lesion may produce a painful nonstructural scoliosis. This results in a curve with the osteoid osteoma on the concave side and is thought to result from marked paravertebral muscle spasm.
- CT scan–guided radiofrequency ablation has become the dominant method of treatment; however, in 50% of patients treated with NSAIDs alone, the symptoms resolve.

Osteosarcoma

- There are many types of osteosarcoma. The most commonly recognized are high-grade intramedullary osteosarcoma (ordinary or classic osteosarcoma), parosteal osteosarcoma, periosteal osteosarcoma, telangiectatic osteosarcoma, osteosarcoma occurring with Paget disease, and osteosarcoma that occurs after irradiation.
- Classic high-grade intramedullary osteosarcoma is the most common type and usually occurs about the knee in children and young adults, but its incidence has a second peak in late adulthood.

Continued

- Treated with neoadjuvant chemotherapy, followed by resection of the tumor and adjuvant chemotherapy.
- Chemotherapy both kills the micrometastases that are present in 80% to 90% of affected patients at presentation and sterilizes the reactive zone around the tumor.
- The rate of long-term survival is approximately 60% to 70%.
- Parosteal osteosarcoma is a low-grade osteosarcoma. It most commonly arises on the posterior aspect of the distal femur.
  - Histologic study reveals regularly arranged osseous trabeculae. Between the nearly normal trabeculae are slightly atypical spindle cells, which typically invade skeletal muscle found at the periphery of the tumor.
  - Treatment is by wide-margin surgical resection. Because this lesion is low grade, chemotherapy is not required.
- Periosteal osteosarcoma is a surface form that appears radiographically as a sunburst-type lesion resting on a saucerized cortical depression.
- Telangiectatic osteosarcoma is described as a "bag of blood." Radiographic features are similar to those of aneurysmal bone cysts.

III. Chondrogenic Lesions

Chondroma

- Benign cartilage tumors on the surface of bone are called *periosteal chondromas.* When they are in the medullary cavity, they are called *enchondromas.*
- Enchondromas appear radiographically as areas of stippled calcifications. However, the radiographic distinction between low-grade chondrosarcoma and enchondromas can be difficult. Serial plain radiographs show cortical bone changes or lysis of the previously mineralized cartilage in chondrosarcoma.
- Most enchondromas necessitate no treatment.
- Syndromes of multiple enchondromas include Ollier disease and Maffucci syndrome.
  - Ollier disease:
    Multiple enchondromas
    Dysplastic bones (particularly a shortened ulna)
    A 30% risk of transformation to chondrosarcoma
    Random spontaneous mutation
  - Maffucci syndrome:
    Multiple enchondromas and soft tissue hemangiomas
    A 100% risk of malignancy

Osteochondroma

- Characteristic appearance is a surface lesion in which the cortex of the lesion and the underlying cortex are continuous and the medullary cavity of the host bone also flows into (is continuous with) the osteochondroma.
- When asymptomatic, these lesions are monitored with observation only.
- Malignant transformation into a secondary chondrosarcoma is rare, occurring in far fewer than 1% of cases. Thickness of the cartilage cap (>2 cm) may increase the risk of malignancy.
- Multiple hereditary exostosis is an autosomal disorder manifesting in childhood with multiple osteochondromas. Mutations are found in the *EXT1*, *EXT2*, and *EXT3* gene loci; the *EXT1* mutation is associated with a greater burden of disease and higher risk of malignancy. Approximately 5% to 10% of affected patients develop a secondary chondrosarcoma.

Chondroblastoma

- Centered in the epiphysis in young patients, usually with open physes
- Radiographs show a central region of bone destruction that is usually sharply demarcated from the normal medullary cavity by a thin rim of sclerotic bone.
- Treatment is with curettage and bone grafting.

Chondrosarcoma

- Typically occurs in older persons, and the pelvis is the most common location.
- It may be extremely difficult to differentiate malignant cartilage on the basis of histologic features alone. The clinical, radiographic, and histologic features of a particular lesion must be considered in combination to avoid incorrect diagnosis.
- Treatment consists of wide-margin surgical resection. Chemotherapy has not been shown to improve survival rates. Recurrence is common.
- Dedifferentiated chondrosarcoma is the most malignant cartilage tumor and has a bimorphic histologic and radiographic appearance. In typical cases, a high-grade spindle cell carcinoma is intimately associated with the low-grade cartilage component. Treatment is with wide-margin surgical resection and chemotherapy.

IV. Fibrous Lesions

- Metaphyseal fibrous defect (nonossifying fibroma) is an extraordinarily common lesion, occurring in approximately 30% to 40% of children. The characteristic radiographic appearance is of a lucent lesion that is metaphyseal, eccentric, and surrounded by a sclerotic rim. The overlying cortex may be slightly expanded and thinned.
- Histologic study reveals a cellular, fibroblastic connective tissue background, with the cells arranged in whorled bundles. Numerous giant cells and hemosiderin deposits are visible.
- Treatment is with observation. Curettage and bone grafting are indicated in symptomatic lesions with more than 50% of cortical involvement.

VI. Notochordal Tissue

- Chordoma is a malignant neoplasm that arises from primitive notochordal tissue.
- The most common location is the sacrococcygeal, and second most common is the spheno-occipital region.
- CT scans show midline bone destruction.

VIII. Hematopoietic Tumors

- Multiple myeloma is the most common primary tumor of bone.
- Light-chain subunits of immunoglobulins G and A are found in the urine.
- Radiographic appearance of multiple myeloma is punched-out lytic lesions.

- The classical histologic appearance of is sheets of plasma cells that appear monoclonal with immunostaining. Well-differentiated plasma cells have an eccentric nucleus and a peripherally clumped, chromatic "clock face."
- Treatment is multimodal and includes chemotherapy, radiation therapy, and surgery.

IX. Tumors of Unknown Origin

Giant Cell Tumor

- This is a benign but aggressive neoplasm that in rare cases metastasizes to the lung.
- It most commonly occurs about the knee and sacrum. Pain is referred to the involved joint.
- Radiographs demonstrate a purely lytic destructive lesion in the metaphysis that extends into the epiphysis and often borders the subchondral bone.
- Treatment is aimed at removal of the lesion with preservation of the involved joint. Curettage and subsequent reconstruction with subchondral bone grafts or methylmethacrylate is frequently performed.

Ewing Tumor

- This distinctive small, round cell sarcoma occurs most often in children and young adults; most affected children are older than 5 years.
- Radiographs show a large destructive lesion that involves the metaphysis and diaphysis. Periosteum may be lifted off in multiple layers, which results in a characteristic but uncommon onionskin appearance.
- Immunohistochemistry studies reveal CD99 positivity. There is a consistent chromosomal translocation—t(11;22)—with the formation of a fusion protein (EWS-FLI1).
- Bone marrow biopsy is performed for staging purposes.
- Most lesions have traditionally been treated with chemotherapy and irradiation, but the role of surgery is evolving.
- Metastatic disease occurs in the lung (50%), bone (25%), and bone marrow (20%).

Adamantinoma

- Adamantinoma is rare tumor that classically manifests in the anterior cortex of the tibial diaphysis. Treatment is with wide-margin surgical resection.

X. Tumor-like Conditions

Aneurysmal Bone Cyst

- This lesion is nonneoplastic but aggressive in its ability to destroy normal bone and extend into the soft tissues.
- Characteristic radiographic finding is an eccentric, lytic, expansile area of bone destruction in the metaphysis. Fluid-fluid levels are characteristically visible on T2-weighted MRI scans.
- Treatment is with curettage and bone grafting. Local recurrence is common in children.

Unicameral Bone Cyst (Simple Bone Cyst)

- These most commonly involve the proximal humerus and manifest either with pain or with a pathologic fracture.
- Characteristic radiographic finding is symmetric cystic expansion with thinning of the involved cortices.
- Aneurysmal bone cyst in comparison with unicameral bone cyst (simplified):
  - Aneurysmal bone cyst manifests with pain and swelling. Unicameral bone cyst manifests with pathologic fracture and pain.
  - Aneurysmal bone cyst commonly occurs in the distal femur and proximal tibia. Unicameral bone cyst occurs in proximal humerus and proximal femur.
  - Aneurysmal bone cyst is eccentric and can expand wider than the growth plate. Unicameral bone cyst is central and does not expand wider than the growth plate.

Histiocytosis X (Langerhans Cell Histiocytosis)

- This lesion manifests as entities:
  - Eosinophilic granuloma
    - Monostotic
    - Highly destructive lesion with well defined margin
    - Self-limiting
  - Hand-Schüller-Christian disease
    - Multiple bone lesions and visceral disease (skull defects, exophthalmos, and diabetes insipidus)
  - Letterer-Siwe disease (a fulminating condition in young children)
    - Typically fatal

Fibrous Dysplasia

- This condition is caused by a genetic activating mutation of the GSα surface protein, which results in increased production of cAMP.
- Its radiographic appearance is variable but classically referred to as "ground glass."
- Its histologic appearance has been likened to "alphabet soup" and "Chinese letters."
- Autogenous cancellous bone grafting is never used for this disorder because the transplanted bone is quickly transformed into the woven bone of fibrous dysplasia.
- Polyostotic fibrous dysplasia is less common but more symptomatic and diagnosed earlier (before the age of 10 years) than monostotic fibrous dysplasia.
- Polyostotic fibrous dysplasia with endocrinopathy is termed *McCune-Albright syndrome* (café au lait spots, precocious puberty, and polyostotic fibrous dysplasia).

Osteofibrous Dysplasia

- This condition manifests in a similar manner but in children younger than 10 years.

Paget Disease

- This disorder is characterized by abnormal bone remodeling, which results in coarsened trabeculae and remodeled cortices.
- Medical treatment of Paget disease is aimed at retarding the activity of the osteoclasts. Agents used include diphosphonates and calcitonin.
- Fewer than 1% of patients with Paget disease develop malignant degeneration with the formation of a sarcoma within a focus of Paget disease.

Continued

- Paget sarcomas are deadly tumors with a poor prognosis (the rate of long-term survival is <20%).

XI. Metastatic Bone Disease

- Patients older than 40 with a destructive bone lesion should be presumed to have metastatic disease.
- The five carcinomas that are most likely to metastasize to bone are those of the breast, lung, prostate, kidney, and thyroid.
- Pathologic fractures secondary to metastatic disease occur most commonly in the proximal femur.
- Histologic hallmark is the appearance of epithelial cells in a fibrous stroma; the epithelial cells are often arranged in a glandular pattern.
- Bone destruction in metastatic disease results from activation of osteoclasts. Tumor cells secrete PTHrP, which stimulates RANKL release and results in activation of osteoclasts.

SELECTED BIBLIOGRAPHY

The selected bibliography for this chapter can be found on www.expertconsult.com.

Chapter 10

REHABILITATION: GAIT, AMPUTATIONS, PROSTHESES, ORTHOSES, AND NEUROLOGIC INJURY

Frank A. Gottschalk

CONTENTS

SECTION 1 GAIT

I. WALKING

A. Definitions

1. **Walking** is the repetitive process of sequential lower limb motion to move the body from one location to another while maintaining upright stability.
2. Walking is a cyclic, energy-efficient activity: one foot must be in contact with the ground at all times (single-limb support), with a period when both limbs are in contact with the ground (double-limb support) (Figure 10-1).
3. The **step** is the distance between initial swing and initial contact of the same limb.

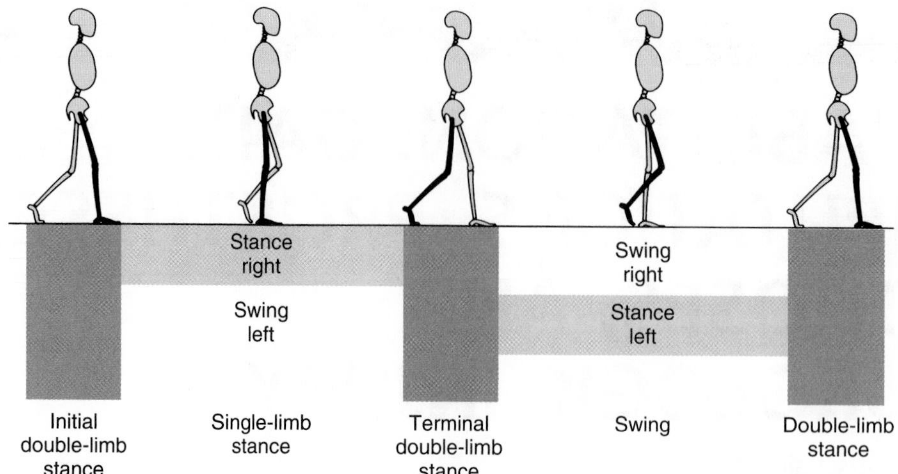

Figure 10-1 **Subdivisions of gait and their relationships to the pattern of bilateral floor contact.** (Adapted from Perry J: *Gait analysis: normal and pathological function,* New York, 1992, Slack Inc.)

4. **Stride** is the period from initial contact to initial contact of the same limb (i.e., each stride comprises two steps) (Figure 10-2).
5. **Velocity** is a function of cadence (steps per unit of time) and stride length.
6. **Running** involves a period when neither limb is in contact with the ground.

B. Phases: Prerequisites for normal gait include stance-phase stability, swing-phase ground clearance, the correct position of the foot before initial contact, and energy-efficient step length and speed.

1. The stance phase occupies 60% of the cycle.
   - Five parts of stance phase:
     - Initial contact
     - Loading response
     - Midstance
     - Terminal stance
     - Preswing
2. The swing phase is 40% of the cycle.
   - Starts at initial swing (toe-off) and proceeds with limb acceleration to midswing, when the limb decelerates at terminal swing before the next cycle (Figure 10-3)
   - During initial swing, the hip and knee flex, and the ankle begins to dorsiflex.
3. Important characteristics of gait cycle:
   - During stance phase, 12% of time is spent in double-limb support.

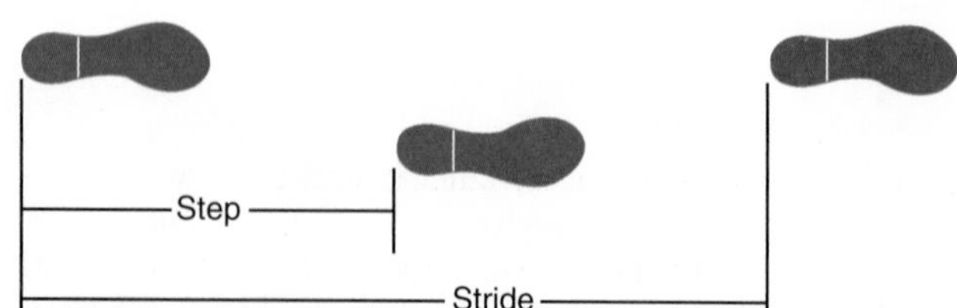

Figure 10-2 **Step versus stride.** (Adapted from Perry J: *Gait analysis: normal and pathological function,* New York, 1992, Slack Inc.)

   - Thirty-eight percent of stance is spent in single-limb support.
   - The body's center of gravity, while being propelled forward, is also subject to vertical and lateral displacement.
     - From a sagittal viewpoint, the vertical displacement follows a sinusoidal curve. The amplitude of this curve is 5 cm.
     - Lateral displacement also follows a sinusoidal curve, with an amplitude of 6 cm.

II. GAIT DYNAMICS

A. The combined phases of gait contribute to an energy-efficient process by lessening excursion of the center of body mass.

B. The head, neck, trunk, and arms account for 70% of body weight.

C. The trunk center of gravity of body mass is located just anterior to T10, which is 33 cm above the hip joints in an individual of average height (184 cm).

D. The body's line of gravity is anterior to S2 and provides a reference for the moment arm to the center of the joint under consideration. The resulting gait pattern resembles a sinusoidal curve.

III. DETERMINANTS OF GAIT (MOTION PATTERNS)

In mechanical terms, there are six independent degrees of freedom (Figure 10-4):

A. Pelvic rotation: The pelvis rotates horizontally about a vertical axis, alternately to the left and right of the line of progression, lessening the center-of-mass deviation in the horizontal plane and reducing the impact at initial floor contact.

B. Pelvic list: The non–weight-bearing, contralateral side drops 5 degrees, reducing superior deviation.

C. Knee flexion at loading: The stance-phase limb is flexed 15 degrees to dampen the impact of initial loading.

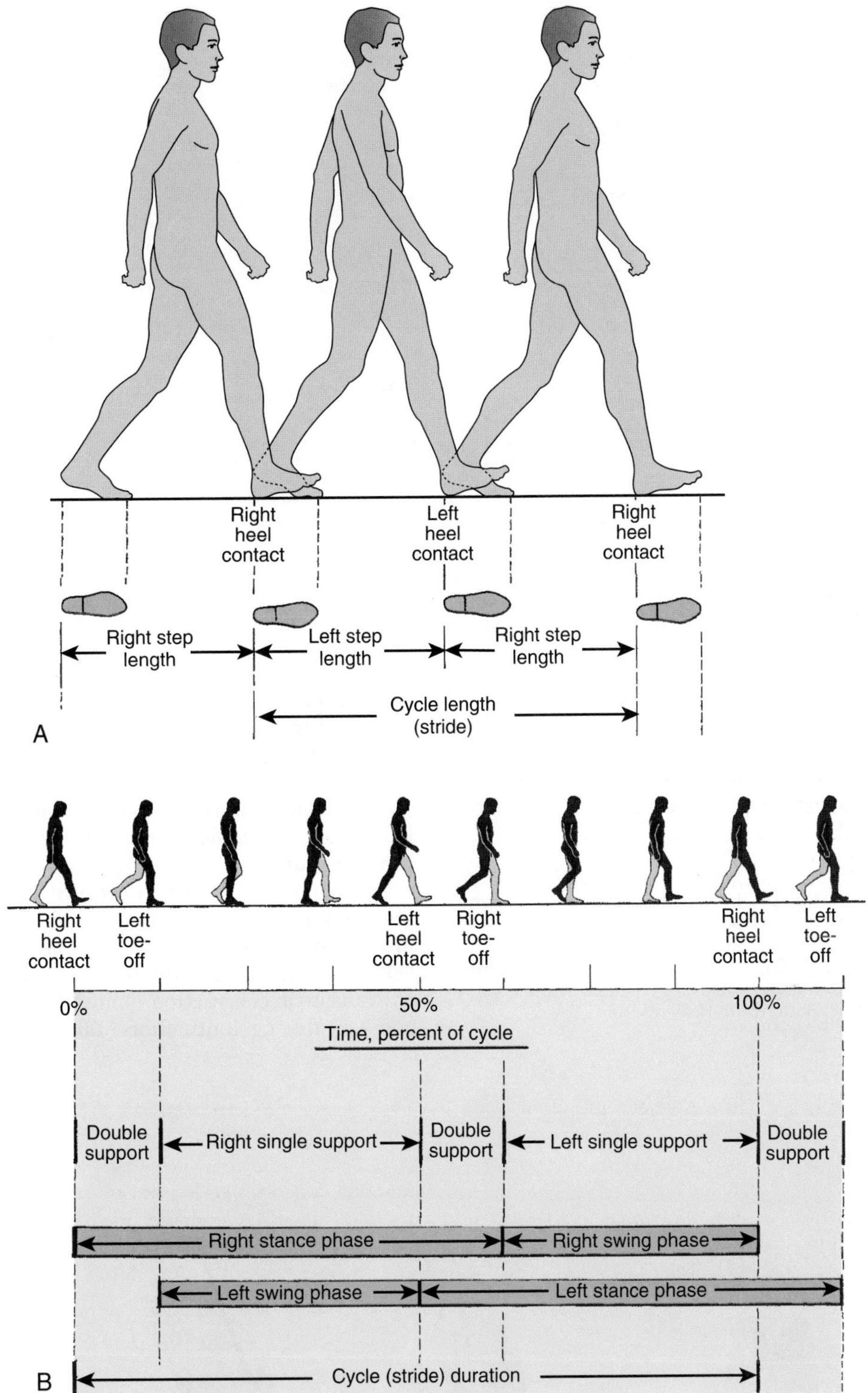

Figure 10-3 Dimensions of the walking cycle: distance **(A)** and time (duration) **(B)**. (From Inman VT, et al: *Human walking,* Baltimore, 1982, Williams & Wilkins, p 26.)

D. Foot and ankle motion: Through the subtalar joint, damping of the loading response occurs, leading to stability during midstance and efficiency of propulsion at push-off.
E. Knee motion: The knee works together with the foot and ankle to decrease necessary limb motion. The knee flexes at initial contact and extends at midstance.
F. Lateral pelvic displacement: This relates to the transfer of body weight onto the limb. The length of motion is 5 cm over the weight-bearing limb, narrowing the base of support and increasing stance-phase stability.

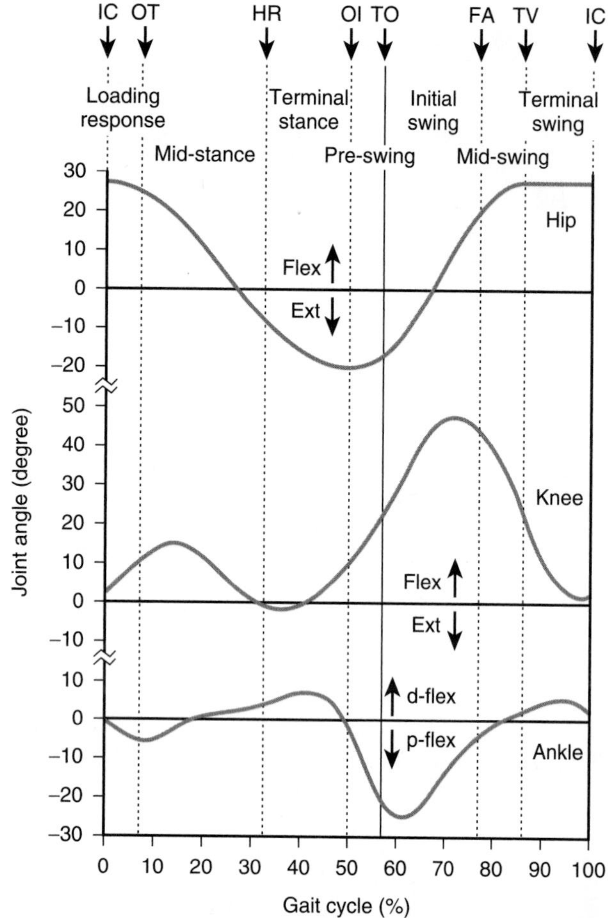

Figure 10-4 Sagittal plane joint angles (degrees) during a single gait cycle of right hip (flexion positive), knee (flexion positive) and ankle (dorsiflexion positive). d-flex, dorsiflexion; Ext, extension; FA, feet adjacent; Flex, flexion; HR, heel rise; IC, initial contact; OI, opposite initial contact; OT, opposite toe off; p-flex, plantar flexion; TO, toe off; TV, tibia vertical. (From Whittle MW: *Gait analysis,* ed 4, Edinburgh, 2007, Butterworth-Heinemann.)

Table 10-1 Muscle Action and Function

Muscle	Action	Function
Gluteus medius	Eccentric	Controls pelvic tilt (midstance)
Gluteus maximus	Concentric	Powers hip extension
Iliopsoas	Concentric	Powers hip flexion
Hip adductors	Eccentric	Control lateral sway (late stance)
Hip abductors	Eccentric	Control pelvic tilt (midstance)
Quadriceps	Eccentric	Stabilizes knee at heel-strike
Hamstrings	Eccentric	Control rate of knee extension (stance)
Tibialis anterior	Concentric Eccentric*	Dorsiflexes ankle at swing Slows plantar flexion rate (heel-strike)
Gastrocnemius-soleus	Eccentric	Slows dorsiflexion rate (stance)

*Predominant role.

IV. MUSCLE ACTION

A. Agonist and antagonist muscle groups work in concert during the gait cycle to effectively advance the limb through space.

B. The hip flexors advance the limb forward during the swing phase and are opposed during terminal swing, before initial contact by the decelerating action of the hip extensors.

C. Most muscle activity is eccentric, which is muscle lengthening while it contracts, and allows an antagonist muscle to dampen the activity of an agonist and act as a "shock absorber" (Figure 10-5).

D. Isocentric contraction is muscle length's remaining constant during contraction (Table 10-1).

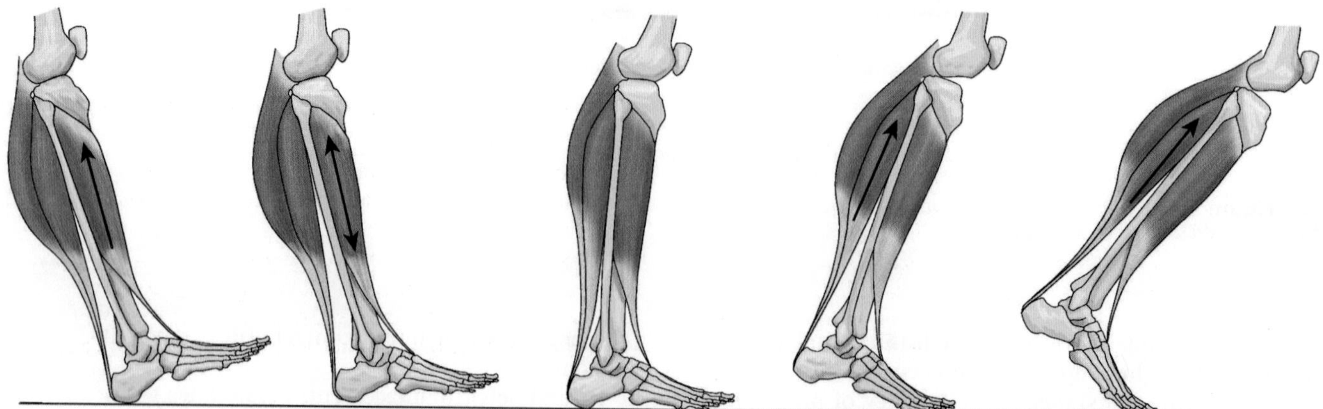

Figure 10-5 Effect of ankle motion, controlled by muscle action, on the pathway of the knee. The smooth and flattened pathway of the knee during the stance phase is achieved by forces acting from the leg on the foot. Foot slap is restrained during initial lowering of the foot; afterward, the plantar flexors raise the heel. (From Inman VT, et al: *Human walking,* Baltimore, 1982, Williams & Wilkins, p 11.)

Table 10-2 Gait Abnormalities Caused by Muscle Weakness

Weak Muscle	Phase	Direction	Type of Abnormal Gait	Treatment
Gluteus medius	Stance	Lateral	Abductor lurch	Cane
Gluteus maximus	Stance	Backward	Lurch (hip hyperextension)	
Quadriceps	Stance	Forward	Lurch/back knee gait	AFO
Swing	Forward	Abnormal hip rotation		
Gastrocnemius/soleus	Stance	Forward	Flatfoot (calcaneal) gait	±AFO
Swing	Forward	Delayed heel rise		
Tibialis anterior	Stance	Forward	Foot drop/slap	AFO
Swing	Forward	Steppage gait		

±, with or without.
AFO, ankle-foot orthosis.

E. Some muscle activity can be concentric, in which the muscle shortens to move a joint through space.

V. PATHOLOGIC GAIT

Abnormal gait patterns are caused by the following factors:

A. Muscle weakness or paralysis: decreases the ability to normally move a joint through space. A walking pattern develops on the basis of the specific muscle or muscle group involved and the ability of the individual to acquire a substitution pattern to replace that muscle's action (Table 10-2).

B. Neurologic conditions: may alter gait by producing muscle weakness, loss of balance, reduced coordination between agonist and antagonist muscle groups (i.e., spasticity), and joint contracture.

1. **Hip scissoring** is associated with overactive adductors, and knee flexion contracture may be caused by hamstring spasticity.
2. **Equinus deformity** of the foot and ankle may result in a steppage gait and backwards setting of the knee.

C. Pain in a limb: creates an antalgic gait pattern, in which the individual shortens the stance phase to lessen the time that the painful limb is loaded. The contralateral swing phase is more rapid.

D. Joint abnormalities: alter gait by changing the range of motion of that joint or producing pain

1. A hip and knee with **arthritis** may have joint contractures and reduced range of motion.
2. An **anterior cruciate–deficient knee** has quadriceps-avoidance gait, which is a net quadriceps moment during midstance that is lower than normal.

E. Hemiplegia: characterized by prolongation of stance and double-limb support

1. Gait impairment may be excessive plantar flexion, weakness, and balance problems.
2. Associated problems are ankle equinus, limitation of knee flexion, and increased hip flexion.
3. Equinus deformity is surgically corrected 1 year after onset.

F. Crutches and canes: devices that ameliorate instability and pain, respectively

1. Crutches increase stability by providing two additional loading points.
2. A cane helps shift the center of gravity to the affected side when the cane is used in the opposite hand. This decreases the joint reaction forces of the lower limb and reduces pain.

G. Arthritis: Forces across the knee may be four to seven times those of body weight; 70% of the load across the knee occurs through the medial compartment.

H. Water walking: There is a significant decrease in joint and total joint contact forces as a result of the effect of buoyancy.

SECTION 2 AMPUTATIONS

I. INTRODUCTION

A. All or part of a limb may be amputated to treat peripheral vascular disease, trauma, tumor, infection, or a congenital anomaly.

B. It is often an alternative to limb salvage and should be considered a reconstructive procedure.

C. Because of the psychologic implications and the alteration of body self-image, a multidisciplinary-team approach should be instituted to help the patient.

II. METABOLIC COST OF AMPUTEE GAIT

A. The metabolic cost of walking is increased with proximal-level amputations and is inversely proportional to the length of the residual limb and the number of functional joints preserved.

B. With a proximal amputation, patients have a decreased self-selected, maximum walking speed.

C. The higher the level of amputation (or the shorter the stump), the higher the oxygen consumption; thus, the transfemoral amputee with peripheral vascular disease uses close to maximum energy expenditure during normal walking at self-selected velocity (Table 10-3).

D. Of note is that the required increase in energy expenditure for ambulation in bilateral transtibial amputation (41%) is less than that of unilateral transfemoral amputation (65%).

Table 10-3 Energy Expenditure for Ambulation

Amputation Level	Energy Above Baseline (%)	Speed (m/min)	O_2 Cost (mL/kg/m)
Long transtibial	10	70	0.17
Average transtibial	25	60	0.20
Short transtibial	40	50	0.20
Bilateral transtibial	41	50	0.20
Transfemoral	65	40	0.28
Wheelchair	0-8	70	0.16

III. LOAD TRANSFER

A. The soft tissue envelope acts as an interface between the bone of the residual limb and the prosthetic socket.

1. Ideally, it is composed of a mobile, securely attached muscle mass covering the bone end and full-thickness skin that tolerates the direct pressures and "pistoning" (mobility) within the prosthetic socket.
2. It is rare for the prosthetic socket to achieve a perfect, intimate fit. A nonadherent soft tissue envelope allows some degree of mobility of the skin and muscle, thus eliminating the shear forces that produce tissue breakdown and ulceration.

B. Load transfer (i.e., weight bearing) occurs either directly or indirectly.

1. **Direct load transfer** (i.e., terminal weight bearing) occurs in knee or ankle disarticulation (Syme amputation). For direct load transfer, intimacy of the prosthetic socket is necessary only for suspension.
2. When the amputation is performed through a long bone (i.e., transfemoral or transtibial), the end of the stump does not take all the weight, and the load is transferred indirectly by the total contact method.
   - This process requires an intimate fit of the prosthetic socket, 7 to 10 degrees of flexion of the knee for transtibial amputation, and 5 to 10 degrees of adduction and flexion of the femur for transfemoral amputation (Figure 10-6).

IV. AMPUTATION WOUND HEALING

The healing of amputation wounds depends on several factors, which include **vascular supply, nutrition,** and an **adequate immune status.** Transcutaneous partial pressure of oxygen is the factor that is most predictive of whether wound healing will be successful.

A. Nutrition and immune status:

1. Patients with malnutrition or immune deficiency have a high rate of wound failure or infection. A serum albumin level of less than 3.5 g/dL indicates that a patient is malnourished. An absolute lymphocyte count of less than 1500/mm^3 is a sign of immune deficiency.
2. If possible, amputation surgery should be delayed in patients with stable gangrene until these values can be improved by nutritional support, usually in the form of oral hyperalimentation.
3. In severely affected patients, nasogastric or percutaneous gastric feeding tubes are sometimes essential.
4. When infection or severe ischemic pain necessitates urgent surgery, open amputation at the most distal, viable level, followed by open-wound management, can be accomplished until wound healing can be optimized.

B. Vascular supply: Oxygenated blood is a prerequisite for wound healing, and a hemoglobin concentration of more than 10 g/dL is necessary. Amputation wounds generally heal by collateral flow; thus, arteriography is rarely useful for predicting the success of wound healing.

1. Standard Doppler ultrasonography helps measure arterial pressure and has been used as the measure of vascular inflow to predict the success of wound healing in the ischemic limb.
   - An absolute Doppler pressure of 70 mm Hg was originally described as the minimum inflow pressure to support wound healing.
   - The **ischemic index** is the ratio of the Doppler pressure at the level being tested to the brachial systolic pressure. It is generally accepted that patients require an ischemic

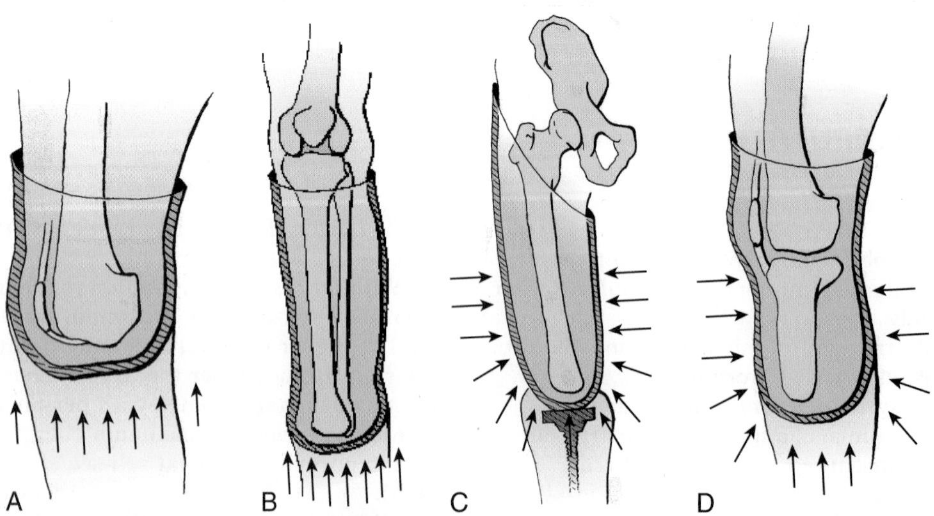

Figure 10-6 Direct load transfer is accomplished in the through-knee **(A)** and Syme ankle disarticulation **(B)** amputations. Load distribution is achieved in transfemoral amputations with either a standard quadrilateral socket or a narrow mediolateral socket **(C).** The transtibial amputation **(D)** transfers weight with the knee flexed approximately 10 degrees. (From Pinzur M: New concepts in lower limb amputation and prosthetic management, *Instr Course Lect* 39:361, 1990.)

index of 0.5 or greater at the surgical level to support wound healing. The ischemic index at the ankle (i.e., the ankle-brachial index) is the most accepted method for assessing adequate inflow to the ischemic limb.
- In the normal limb, the area under the Doppler waveform tracing is a measure of flow. In at least 15% of patients with diabetes and peripheral vascular disease, those values are falsely elevated and not predictive because of the incompressibility and loss of compliance of calcified peripheral arteries. The ischemic index for toe pressure is more accurate in such patients and, if greater than 0.45, is usually predictive of adequate blood flow.

2. **Transcutaneous partial pressure of oxygen** is the current "gold standard" for measurement of vascular inflow. It reflects the oxygen-delivering capacity of the vascular system to the level of contemplated surgery.
   - Values higher than 40 mm Hg are correlated with acceptable wound-healing rates without the false-positive values seen in noncompliant, diseased peripheral vascular vessels.
   - Pressures lower than 20 mm Hg are predictive of poor healing potential.

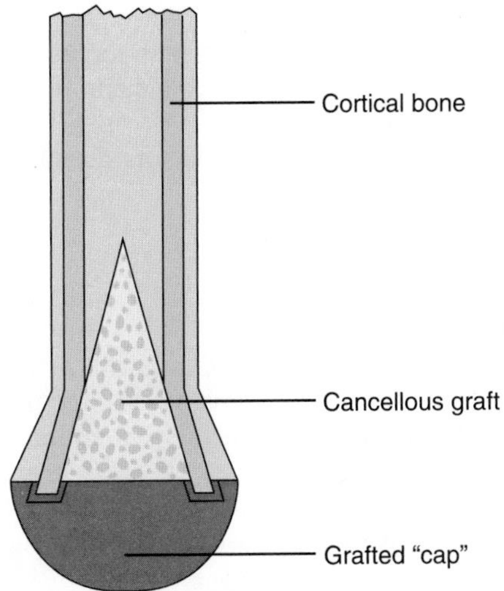

Figure 10-7 Diagram of the stump-capping procedure. The bone end has been split longitudinally. (Adapted from Bernd L, et al: The autologous stump plasty: treatment for bony overgrowth in juvenile amputees, *J Bone Joint Surg Br* 73:203-206, 1991.)

V. PEDIATRIC AMPUTATION

A. Pediatric amputations are usually undertaken because of congenital limb deficiencies, trauma, or tumors.
B. Congenital amputations are the result of failure of formation.
C. The current classification system is based on the original work of the 1975 Conference of the International Society for Prosthetics and Orthotics (ISPO) and the subsequent standard developed by the International Organization for Standardization (ISO).
D. Deficiencies are either longitudinal or transverse, with the potential for intercalary deficits.
E. Amputation is rarely indicated in congenital upper limb deficiency; even rudimentary appendages can be functionally useful. In the lower limb, amputation of an unstable segment may allow direct load transfer and enhanced walking (e.g., Syme amputation for fibular hemimelia).
F. In a growing child, disarticulations should be performed only when it is possible to maintain maximum residual limb length and prevent terminal bony overgrowth.
- Such overgrowth usually occurs in the humerus, fibula, tibia, and femur, in that order; it is typical in diaphyseal amputations.
- Numerous surgical procedures have been described to resolve this problem, but the best method is surgical revision of the residual limb with adequate resection of bone or autogenous osteochondral stump capping (Figure 10-7).

VI. AMPUTATION AFTER TRAUMA

The grading scales for evaluating mangled extremities are not absolute predictors but provide reasonable guidelines for determining whether salvage is appropriate.

A. Indications
1. The absolute indication for amputation after trauma is an ischemic limb with a vascular injury that cannot be repaired.
2. The guidelines for immediate or early amputation of mangled upper limbs differ from those for mangled lower limbs.
3. Early amputation in appropriate scenarios may prevent emotional, marital, financial, and addiction problems.
4. Most grades IIIB and IIIC tibia fractures occur in young men who are laborers and may be more likely to return to gainful employment after amputation and prosthetic fitting.
5. Sensation is not as crucial in the lower limb as in the upper limb, and current prostheses more closely approximate normal function.
6. Disadvantages of limb salvage:
   - Severe open tibia fractures that are managed by limb salvage rather than amputation are often associated with **high rates of mortality and morbidity** as a result of infection, increased energy expenditure for ambulation, and decreased potential to return to work.
   - Limb salvage for Gustillo-Anderson grades IIIB and IIIC open fractures of the tibia and fibula generally has poor functional outcomes and multiple complications, and multiple surgical procedures may be needed.
   - The salvaged lower extremity with an insensate plantar weight-bearing surface (loss of posterior tibial nerve), with associated major functional muscle and bone loss, is unlikely to provide a durable limb for stable walking and is a potential source of early or late sepsis.

B. Contraindications
1. Upper limb
   - When a salvaged upper limb remains sensate and has prehensile function, it will often function better than an amputated limb with prosthetic replacement.
   - Maintaining as much length as possible is the key to subsequent prosthetic use.

2. Lower limb
   - Lack of plantar sensation is not an indication to amputate because it may result from neurapraxia that can resolve.
   - In the absence of other major factors, amputation should not be performed.

VII. RISK FACTORS

A. Cognitive deficits

1. In order for patients to learn to walk with a prosthesis and care for their stumps and prostheses, they must possess certain cognitive capacities: memory, attention, concentration, and organization.
   - Patients with cognitive deficits or psychiatric disorders have a low likelihood of using prostheses successfully.

B. Diabetes

1. A majority of patients who undergo amputation are diabetic, with inherent immune deficiency.
2. The most important risk factors in amputation in diabetic patients are the **presence of peripheral neuropathy** and development of deformity and infection.

C. Peripheral vascular disease

1. Most of the other patients who undergo amputation are malnourished patients with peripheral vascular disease of sufficient magnitude to necessitate amputation, and their coronary and cerebral arteries are diseased.
2. Appropriate consultation with physical therapy, social work, and psychology departments is important to determine **rehabilitation potential.**
3. Medical consultation helps determine cardiopulmonary reserve. The vascular surgeon should determine whether vascular reconstruction is feasible or appropriate.
4. The **biologic amputation level** is the most distal functional amputation level with a high probability of supporting wound healing.
   - This level is determined by the presence of adequate, viable local tissue to construct a residual limb capable of supporting weight bearing; an adequate vascular inflow; and serum albumin level and a total lymphocyte count sufficient to aid surgical wound healing.
   - The selection of an appropriate amputation level is determined by combining the biologic amputation level with the rehabilitation potential in order to choose the level that maximizes ultimate functional independence.
5. Morbidity and mortality rates have remained unchanged for several decades. Thirty percent of patients with peripheral vascular disease die in the first 3 months after amputation, and nearly 50% die within the first year. The overall rate of prosthetic use is 43%.

VIII. MUSCULOSKELETAL TUMORS

A. Goal of surgery: to remove the tumor with adequate surgical margins.

B. Amputation versus limb salvage:

1. Advances in chemotherapy and allograft or prosthetic reconstruction have made limb salvage a viable option in extremity sarcomas.
2. If adequate margins can be achieved with limb salvage, the decision can then be based on **expected functional outcome.**
3. The advantage of limb salvage over amputation—with regard to energy expenditure to ambulate, quality-of-life measures, and function with activities of daily living—is controversial in the literature.
4. Expected functional outcome should include the psychosocial and body-image values associated with limb salvage.
   - These concerns should be balanced with improved task performance and lesser concern for late mechanical injury associated with amputation and fitting of prosthetic limbs.

IX. TECHNICAL CONSIDERATIONS

A. Skin flaps should be of full thickness, and dissection between tissue planes should be avoided.

B. Periosteal stripping should be sufficient to allow for bone transection; this minimizes regenerative bone overgrowth.

C. Wounds should not be sutured under tension. Muscles are best secured directly to bone at resting tension (myodesis) rather than to antagonist muscle (myoplasty).

D. Stable residual limb muscle mass can improve function by reducing atrophy and providing a stable soft tissue envelope over the end of the bone.

E. All transected nerves form neuromata. The nerve end should come to lie deep in a soft tissue envelope, away from potential pressure areas. Crushing the nerve may contribute to postoperative phantom or limb pain.

F. Rigid dressings (postoperative) help reduce swelling, decrease pain, and protect the stump from trauma.

G. Early prosthetic fitting is done within 5 to 21 days after surgery in selected patients.

X. COMPLICATIONS

A. Pain

1. **Phantom limb sensation**—the feeling that all or part of the amputated limb is present—occurs in almost all adults who have undergone amputation. It usually decreases with time.
2. **Phantom pain** is a burning, painful sensation in the part having undergone amputation. It is diminished by prosthetic use, physical therapy, compression, and transcutaneous nerve stimulation.
3. A common cause of residual pain is **complex regional pain syndrome** (reflex sympathetic dystrophy) or causalgia. Amputation should not be performed for this condition.
4. **Localized stump pain** is often related to bony or soft tissue problems.
5. **Pain referred to the limb** occurs in a frequent number of cases.

B. Edema

1. Postoperative edema occurs after amputation. It may impede wound healing and place significant tension on the tissues.
2. Rigid dressings and soft compression help reduce the problem.
3. Swelling occurring after stump maturation is usually caused by poor socket fit, medical problems, or trauma.

4. Persistence of chronic swelling may lead to **verrucous hyperplasia,** a wartlike overgrowth of skin with pigmentation and serous discharge.
   - It should be treated by a total-contact cast, which is changed regularly to accommodate the reduced edema.

C. **Joint contractures**

1. These complications are usually noted as hip and knee flexion contractures, which can be produced at the time of surgery by anchoring of the respective muscles with the joints in a flexed position.
2. They can be avoided by correct positioning of the amputated limb.

D. **Wound failure to heal**

1. This outcome occurs most often in patients with diabetes and those with vascular disease.
2. If the wound is not amenable to local care, wedge excision of soft tissue and bone, with closure and without tension, is the preferred treatment.

XI. UPPER LIMB AMPUTATIONS (FIGURE 10-8)

A. **Wrist disarticulation**

1. Advantages
   - Wrist disarticulation has two advantages over transradial amputation:
     - Preservation of more forearm rotation because of preservation of the distal radioulnar joint
     - Improved prosthetic suspension because of the flare of the distal radius
   - Effective function can be obtained at this level of amputation. Forearm rotation and strength are directly related to the length of the transradial (below-elbow) residual limb.
2. Disadvantages
   - Wrist disarticulation provides challenges to the prosthetist that may outweigh its benefits.
   - Cosmetic disadvantage
     - The prosthetic limb is longer than the contralateral limb.
     - If myoelectric components are used, the motor and battery cannot be hidden within the prosthetic shank.

B. **Transradial amputation or elbow disarticulation**

1. Complete brachial plexus injury and a nonfunctioning hand and forearm may be best treated by a transradial amputation or elbow disarticulation, which can be fitted with a prosthesis.
2. The optimal length of the residual limb is at the junction of the middle and distal thirds of the forearm, where the soft tissue envelope can be repaired by myodesis and the components of a myoelectric prosthesis can be hidden within the prosthetic shank.
3. Because the patient can maintain function at this level prosthetically only by being able to open and close the terminal device, retention of the elbow joint is essential.

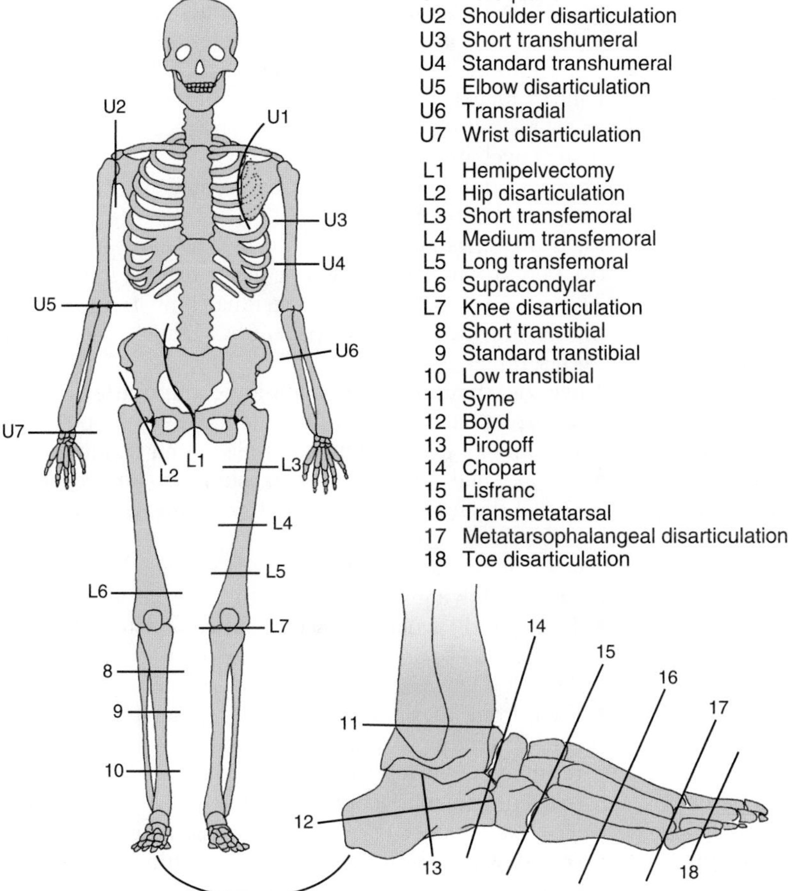

Figure 10-8 Composite illustration of common amputation levels.

4. The length and shape of elbow disarticulation provides improved suspension and lever-arm capacity.
5. To enhance suspension and reduce the need for shoulder harnessing, a 45- to 60-degree distal humeral osteotomy is performed.
6. Gangrene of the upper limb, when it is not due to Raynaud or Buerger disease, represents end-stage disease, especially in diabetic patients. Such patients usually do not survive beyond 24 months.
   - Localized finger amputations are unlikely to heal. When surgery becomes necessary, amputation should be performed at the transradial level to achieve wound healing during the final months of the patient's life.

XII. LOWER LIMB AMPUTATIONS (SEE FIGURE 10-8)

A. Toe and ray amputation

1. Patients with ischemia generally ambulate with a propulsive gait pattern, so they suffer little disability from toe amputation.
2. Patients with traumatic amputions lose some stability after toe amputation in the late-stance phase.
3. The great toe should be amputated distal to the insertion of the flexor hallucis brevis.
4. Isolated second-toe amputation should be performed just distal to the proximal phalanx metaphyseal flare, leaving the stump to act as a buttress and prevent late hallux valgus.
5. Patients who undergo single outer (first or fifth) ray resections function well in standard shoes.
6. Resection of more than one ray leaves the forefoot narrow, which is difficult to fit in shoes, and often results in a late equinus deformity.
7. Central ray resections are complicated by prolonged wound healing and rarely achieve better results than does midfoot amputation.

B. Transmetatarsal and Lisfranc tarsal-metatarsal amputation

1. There is little functional difference in the outcomes of these two procedures. The long plantar flap acts as a myocutaneous flap and is preferred to fish-mouth dorsal-plantar flaps.
2. Transmetatarsal amputation should be performed through the proximal metaphyses to prevent late plantar pressure ulcers under the residual bone ends.
3. Percutaneous Achilles tendon lengthening should be performed with transmetatarsal and Lisfranc amputations to prevent the late development of equinus or equinovarus deformity.
4. Late varus deformity can be corrected with the transfer of the tibialis anterior tendon to the neck of the talus.
   - The second tarsometatarsal joint should be osteotomized in order to preserve midfoot stability.
   - The soft tissue at the fifth metatarsal base should be preserved because this represents the insertion site of peroneus brevis and tertius, which act as antagonists to the posterior tibial tendon.
     - Failure to preserve these tissues results in inversion during gait.
5. Some authors have reported reasonable functional outcomes with hindfoot amputation (i.e., Chopart or Boyd amputations), but most experts recommend avoiding amputation at these levels if possible in patients with diabetes or vascular disease.
6. Although children have been reported to function reasonably well, adults retain an inadequate lever arm and are prone to experience fixed equinus deformity of the heel if Achilles tendon lengthening and tibialis anterior tendon transfer are not performed.

C. Ankle disarticulation (Syme amputation)

1. Often performed for forefoot trauma, this amputation allows direct load transfer and is rarely complicated by late residual limb ulcers or tissue breakdown.
2. It provides a stable gait pattern that rarely necessitates prosthetic gait training after surgery.
3. The outcome is more energy efficient than that of a midfoot amputation, despite the fact that it is a more proximal level.
4. Surgery should be performed in one stage, even in ischemic limbs with insensate heel pads.
5. The posterior tibial artery must be patent to ensure healing.
6. The malleoli and metaphyseal flares should be removed from the tibia and fibula, but the remaining tibial articular surface should be retained to provide a resilient residual limb.
7. The heel pad should be secured to the tibia either anteriorly through drill holes or posteriorly by securing the Achilles tendon.

D. Transtibial (below-knee) amputation

1. A long posterior myocutaneous flap is the preferred method of creating a soft tissue envelope, especially in patients with vascular disease, inasmuch as the direction of blood flow is from posterior to anterior.
2. The optimum bone length is at least 12 cm below the knee joint or longer if adequate amounts of the gastrocnemius or soleus muscle can be used to construct a durable soft tissue envelope.
3. The posterior muscle should be secured to the beveled anterior tibia by myodesis.
4. Rigid dressings are preferred during the early postoperative period, and early prosthetic fitting may be started 5 to 21 days after surgery if the residual limb is capable of transferring load and if the patient has a satisfactory physical reserve.

E. Knee disarticulation (through-knee amputation)

1. The current technique involves the use of a long posterior flap, with the gastrocnemius muscle as end padding.
   - The alternative is to use sagittal skin flaps and cover the end of the femur with the gastrocnemius muscle to act as a soft tissue envelope end pad.
2. The patella tendon is sutured to the cruciate ligaments in the notch, leaving the patella on the anterior femur.
   - This level is generally used in nonambulatory patients who can support wound healing at the transtibial or distal level.
   - Data from the Lower Extremity Assessment Project (LEAP) study have demonstrated this amputation to result in the slowest walking speed and produce the least self-reported satisfaction.
3. Knee disarticulation is muscle balanced and provides an excellent weight-bearing platform for sitting and a lever arm for bed to chair transfer. When this amputation is

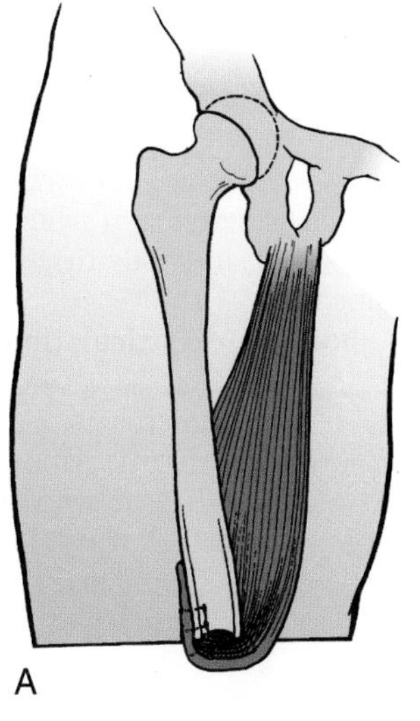

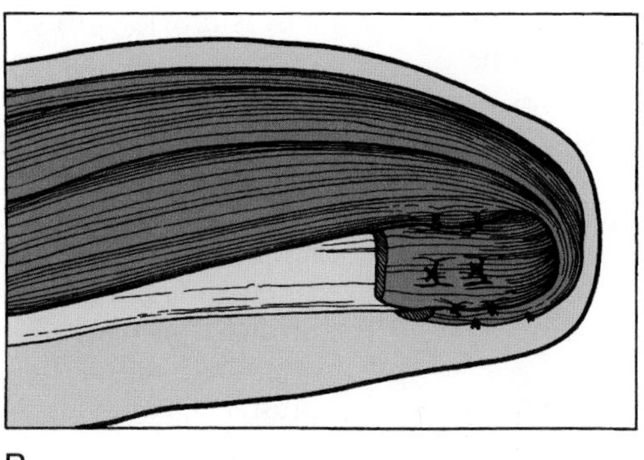

Figure 10-9 **A,** Diagram showing attachment of the adductor magnus to the lateral part of the femur. **B,** Diagram depicting attachment of the quadriceps over the adductor magnus. (From Gottschalk F: Transfemoral amputation. In Bowker J, Michael J, editors: *Atlas of limb prosthetics,* St. Louis, 1992, Mosby–Year Book, pp 479-486.)

performed in a potential walker, it provides a residual limb for direct bed to chair transfer (end bearing).

F. **Transfemoral (above-knee) amputation**

1. This amputation increases the energy cost for walking.
2. Patients with transfemoral amputations who have peripheral vascular disease are unlikely to become efficient walkers; thus, salvaging the limb at the knee disarticulation (transtibial level) is crucial for maintaining functional walking independence.
3. With greater femoral length, the lever arm, suspension, and limb advancement are optimized. The optimum transfemoral bone length is 12 cm above the knee joint to accommodate the prosthetic knee.
4. Adductor myodesis is important for maintaining femoral adduction during the stance phase in order to allow optimal prosthetic function (Figure 10-9).
5. The major deforming force is toward abduction and flexion. Adductor myodesis at normal muscle tension eliminates the problem of adductor roll in the groin. Transecting the adductor magnus results in a loss of 70% of the adductor pull (Figure 10-10).
6. Rigid dressings are difficult to apply and maintain at this level. Elastic compression dressings are used and may be suspended about the opposite iliac crest.

G. **Hip disarticulation**

1. This procedure is infrequently performed, and of the patients who undergo this amputation, only a few make meaningful use of prostheses because of the high energy requirements for walking.
2. Patients who have suffered trauma or who have tumors occasionally use the prosthesis for limited activity. These patients sit in their prostheses and must use the torso in order to achieve momentum for "throwing" the limb forward to advance it.

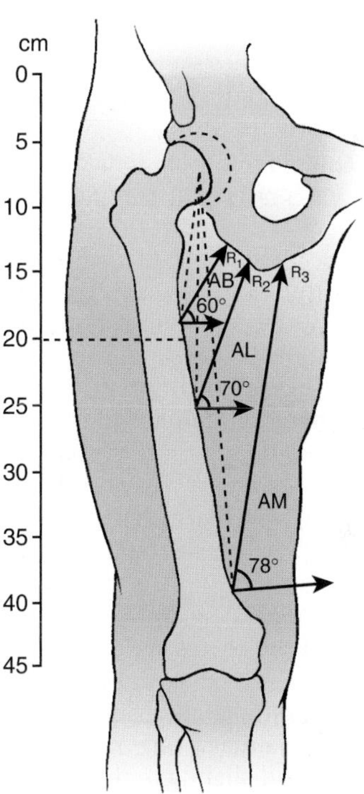

Figure 10-10 Diagram of moment arms of the three adductor muscles. Loss of the distal attachment of the adductor magnus (AM) will result in a loss of 70% of the adductor pull. AB, adductor brevis; AL, adductor longus. (From Gottschalk FA, et al: Does socket configuration influence the position of the femur in above-knee amputation? *J Prosthet Orthot* 2:94-102, 1989.)

SECTION 3 PROSTHESES

I. UPPER LIMB

A. Upper limb biomechanics

1. The shoulder provides the center of the radius of the functional sphere of the upper limb. The elbow acts as the caliper to position the hand at a workable distance from that center in order to perform its tasks.
2. In a normal arm, tasks performed with the use of multiple joint segments usually occur simultaneously, whereas upper limb prostheses perform these same tasks sequentially; thus, joint- and residual-limb-length salvage is directly correlated with functional outcome.
3. Motion at the retained joints is essential for maximizing that function.
4. Residual limb length is important for suspending the prosthetic socket and providing the lever arm necessary to "drive" the prosthesis through space.

B. Benefits of limb salvage

1. Limb salvage is more important for the upper limb, where sensation is crucial for function.
   - An insensate prosthesis provides less function than a partially sensate, partially functional salvaged limb.

C. Timing of prosthetic fitting

1. Prosthetic fitting should be undertaken as soon as possible after amputation, even before complete wound healing has occurred.
2. For transradial amputation, the outcomes for prosthetic limb use vary from 70% to 85% when prosthetic fitting occurs within 30 days of amputation, in contrast to less than 30% when the fitting starts later.

D. Types of prostheses for different levels of amputation

1. **Midlength transradial amputation**:
   - Myoelectric prostheses provide good cosmesis and are used for sedentary work. They can be used in any position, including overhead activity, and are the most successful for patients with midlength transradial amputations, for whom only the terminal device needs to be activated.
   - Body-powered prostheses are used for heavy labor. The terminal device is activated by shoulder flexion and abduction. For optimal mechanical efficiency of figure-8 harnesses, the harness ring must be at the spinous process of C7 and slightly to the nonamputated side.
2. **Elbow disarticulation and transhumeral (above-elbow) amputations**
   - When the residual forearm is so short that it precludes an adequate lever arm for driving the prosthesis through space, **supracondylar suspension (Munster socket)** and **step-up hinges** can be used to augment function.
   - In elbow disarticulation and transhumeral (above-elbow) amputations, two motions are needed to develop prehension; thus, these levels of amputation have significantly less efficient outcomes, and the prostheses are heavier than they are for amputation at the transradial level.
   - Elbow flexion and extension are controlled by shoulder extension and depression. Amputations at these levels provide minimal function because the patient must sequentially control two joints and a terminal device.
   - The best function with the least weight at the lowest cost is provided by hybrid prosthetic systems in which myoelectric, traditional body-powered, and body-driven switch components are combined.
3. **Proximal transhumeral and shoulder disarticulation amputations**
   - When the lever-arm capacity of the humerus is lost in proximal transhumeral or shoulder disarticulation amputations, limited function can be achieved with a manual universal shoulder joint positioned with the opposite hand and combined with lightweight hybrid prosthetic components.

II. LOWER LIMB

A. Prosthetic feet: Several designs are available and divided into five classes.

1. **Single-axis foot**
   - The single-axis foot is based on an ankle hinge that provides dorsiflexion and plantar flexion.
   - The disadvantages of the single-axis foot include poor durability and cosmesis.
2. **Solid-ankle, cushioned-heel (SACH) foot**
   - This has been the standard for decades and was appropriate for general use in patients with low levels of activity.
   - It may lead to overload problems on the nonamputated foot, and its use is being discontinued.
3. **Dynamic-response foot**
   - The selection of the correct dynamic prosthetic foot depends on the patient's height, weight, activity level, access for maintenance, cosmesis, and funding.
   - The dynamic-response foot prostheses, including the Seattle foot, Carbon Copy II/III, and Flex Foot, allow amputees to undertake most normal activities (Figure 10-11).
   - Dynamic-response foot prostheses may be grouped into articulated and nonarticulated.
     - **Articulated dynamic-response foot**
       - These allow inversion/eversion and rotation of the foot and are useful for activities on uneven surfaces.
       - They may absorb loads and decrease shear forces to the residual limb.
       - Most dynamic-response feet have a **flexible keel** and are the standard for general use (Figure 10-12). The keel deforms under load, becoming a spring and allowing dorsiflexion and thereby decreasing the loading on the normal side and providing a springlike response for push-off.
       - Posterior projection of the keel provides a response at heel-strike for smooth transition through the stance phase. A sagittal split allows for moderate inversion or eversion.
     - **Nonarticulated dynamic-response foot**
       - These can have short or long keels. Shortened keels are not as responsive and are indicated for the moderate-activity ambulator, whereas long keels are for very-high-demand activities.

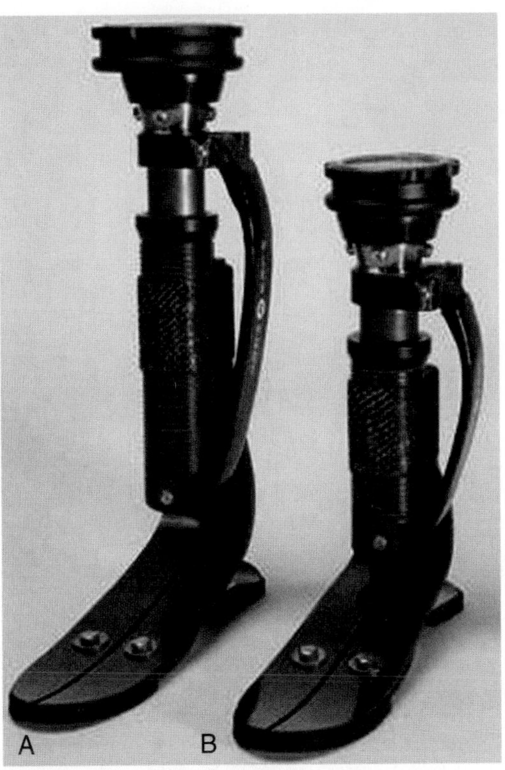

Figure 10-11 **A,** Flex Foot with carbon-fiber leaf and posterior projection of the keel for heel-strike. **B,** Flex Foot with split-toe configuration and spring-leaf design. (Courtesy of Flex Foot, Inc, Aliso Viejo, California.)

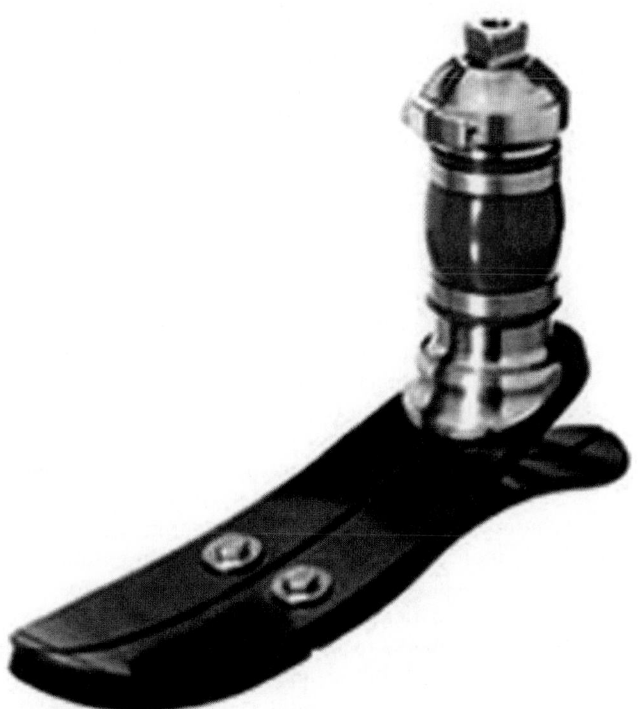

Figure 10-12 Ceterus prosthetic foot with leaf spring and shock absorber. (Courtesy of Ossur Americas, Aliso Viejo, California.)

Table 10-4 Characteristics of Various Prosthetic Knees

	CHARACTERISTICS		
Knee Type	Action	Advantages	Disadvantages
Constant-friction	Limits flexion	Durable, long resistance	Decreased stability
Variable-friction	Varies with flexion	Variable cadence	Poor durability
Stance-control	Friction brake	Stability during stance	Poor durability, difficult to use on stairs
Polycentric	Instant center moves	Stable, increased flexion	Poor durability, heavy
Manual locking	Must unlock to sit	Maximum stability	Abnormal gait
Fluid-control	Deceleration in swing	Variable cadence	Weight, cost

- Separate prosthetic feet for running and lower-demand activities may be indicated.

B. **Prosthetic shanks**

1. These shanks provide the structural link between or among prosthetic components.
2. Two varieties exist: **endoskeletal,** with a soft exterior and load-bearing tubing inside (the most common), and **exoskeletal,** with a hard load-bearing exterior shell.
3. **Rotator units** are sometimes added for patients involved in twisting activities (e.g., golf) or for sitting.

C. **Prosthetic knees (Table 10-4)**

1. Prosthetic knees provide controlled knee motion in the prosthesis.
2. These components are used in transfemoral and knee disarticulation and are chosen on the basis of the patient's needs.
3. **Alignment stability** (the position of the prosthetic knee in relation to the patient's line of weight bearing) is important in the design and fitting of prosthetic knees. Placing the knee center of rotation posterior to the line of weight bearing allows control in the stance phase but makes flexion difficult. Alternatively, with the knee center of rotation anterior to the line of weight bearing, flexion is made easier but at the expense of control.
4. Only the **polycentric knee component** offers the possibility of both options by having a variable center of rotation. Six basic types of knees are available:
   - **Polycentric (four-bar linkage) knee:** This prosthesis has a moving instant center of rotation that provides for different stability characteristics during the gait cycle and may allow increased flexion for sitting. It is recommended for patients with transfemoral amputations, those with knee disarticulations, and those with bilateral amputations (Figure 10-13).
   - **Stance-phase control (weight-activated [safety]) knee:** This knee functions like a constant-friction knee during the swing phase but "freezes" by application of high-friction housing when weight is applied to the limb. Its use is reserved primarily for older patients, those with very proximal amputations, or those walking on uneven terrain.
   - **Fluid-control (hydraulic and pneumatic) knee:** This knee allows adjustment of cadence response by

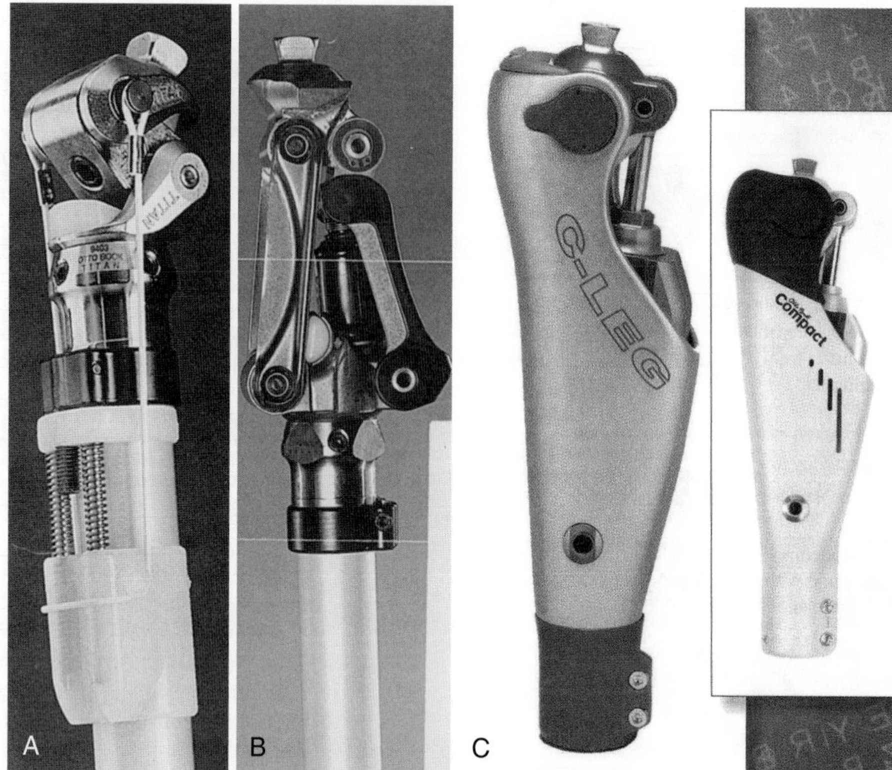

Figure 10-13 **A,** Stance-phase control unit for transfemoral prosthesis. **B,** Modular endoskeletal four-bar knee with hydraulic swing-phase control unit. **C,** Microprocessor knee unit. (Courtesy of Otto Bock Orthopaedic Industries, Minneapolis.)

changing resistance to knee flexion by means of a piston mechanism. The design prevents excessive flexion and is extended earlier in the gait cycle, allowing a more fluid gait. The knee is best used in active patients who prefer greater utility and variability at the expense of more weight.

- **Constant-friction knee:** This knee prosthesis is essentially a hinge that is designed to dampen knee swing by a screw or rubber pad that applies friction to the knee bolt. It is designed for general utility and may be used on uneven terrain. It is the most common knee prosthesis for children. Its major disadvantages are that it allows only single-speed walking and relies solely on alignment for stance-phase stability; therefore, it is not recommended for older, weaker patients.
- **Variable-friction (cadence control) knee:** This device allows resistance to knee flexion to increase as the knee extends by employing a number of staggered friction pads. This knee allows walking at different speeds but is neither durable nor available in endoskeletal systems.
- **Manual locking knee:** This knee consists of a constant-friction knee hinge with a positive lock in extension that can be unlocked to allow functioning similar to that of a constant-friction knee. The knee is often left locked in extension for more stability. It has limited indications and is used primarily in weak, unstable patients; those just learning to use prostheses; and blind amputees.

D. **Suspension systems:**

Suspension is provided in modern lower extremity prostheses primarily through **socket design** and **suspension sleeves.** Straps and belts are usually used for supplementation.

1. **Sockets** are prosthetic components designed to provide comfortable functional control and even pressure distribution on the amputated stump. Sockets can be hard (rigid or unlined) or soft (lined with a resilient material and/or flexible shell). In general, the suction-and-socket contour is the primary suspension modality used. The suction socket provides an airtight seal by means of a pressure differential between the socket and atmosphere. Total-contact support of the residual limb surface prevents edema formation. In total-contact support, different areas have different loads.
   - Transfemoral, or **quadrilateral, sockets,** in which the posterior brim provides a shelf for the ischial tuberosity, have been the classic suspension system. However, the design made it difficult to keep the femur in adduction. **Narrow mediolateral (ischial containment) transfemoral sockets** distribute the proximal and medial concentrations of forces more evenly, as well as enhance rotational control of the socket (Figure 10-14). The ischium and ramus are contained within the socket of these more anatomic, comfortable, and functional designs. Socket design for transfemoral prostheses allows for 10 degrees of adduction of the femur (to stretch the gluteus medius, allowing adequate strength for midstance stability) and 5 degrees of flexion (to stretch the gluteus maximus, allowing greater hip extension).
   - **Transtibial sockets:** Weight bearing by the patella tendon loads all areas of the residual limb that tolerate weight (i.e., patella tendon, medial tibial flare, anterior compartment, gastrocnemius muscle, and fibular shaft). Weight-intolerant areas include the tibial crest and

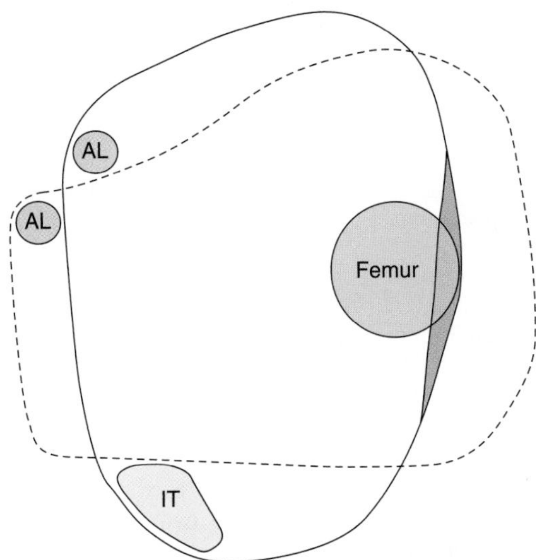

Figure 10-14 Comparison of transfemoral sockets. Note the inclusion of the ischial tuberosity (IT) and the narrow mediolateral design of newer contoured, adducted, trochanteric-controlled alignment method (CAT-CAM) socket shown by the *solid line. Dashed line* shows the outline of the quadrilateral socket brim. AL, adductor longus. (Adapted from Sabolich J: Contoured adducted trochanteric controlled alignment method, *Clin Prosthet Orthop* 9:13-17, 1985.)

tubercle, distal fibula and fibular head, peroneal nerve, and hamstring tendons. The **patella tendon–bearing supracondylar/suprapatellar socket** has proximal extensions over the distal femoral condyles and patella. Total-surface weight bearing is different from total-contact weight bearing. With total-surface weight bearing, pressure is distributed more equally across the entire surface of the transtibial residual limb, and the interface liner material in the socket is important. Urethane liners cope with multidirectional forces by easy material distortion and recovery to the original shape. Another liner is made of mineral oil gel with reinforcing fabric. These liners provide good shock absorption and reduce skin problems. The anterior wedge shape of the socket helps control rotation of the socket on the limb.

- A supracondylar suspension system is recommended when the residual limb is less than 5 cm long. The socket is designed to increase the surface area for pressure distribution by raising the medial and lateral socket brim. A wedge may be used in the soft liner.
- A supracondylar-suprapatellar suspension system encloses the patella in the socket and has a bar proximal to the patella. This design also provides mediolateral stability, and no additional cuffs or straps are required. Corset-type prostheses can lead to verrucous hyperplasia and thigh atrophy, but they reduce socket loads, control the direction of swing, and provide some additional weight support.

2. In **prosthetic sleeves,** friction and negative pressure are used for suspension. The sleeves fit snugly to the upper third of the tibial prosthesis and are made from neoprene, latex, silicone, or thermoplastic elastomers.
   - Transtibial suspension
     - **Gel-liner suspension systems with a locking pin** constitute the preferred method of suspension.
     - Liners are made from silicone, urethane, or thermoplastic elastomer.
     - The sleeve rolls onto the stump, and the locking pin is then locked into the socket (Figure 10-15).
     - The liners provide suspension through suction and friction and act as the socket interface.

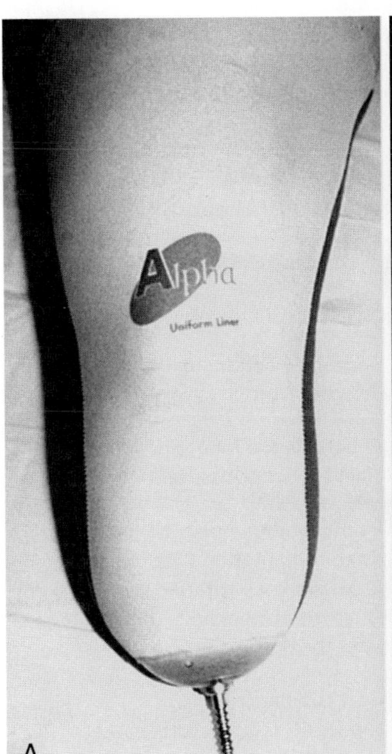

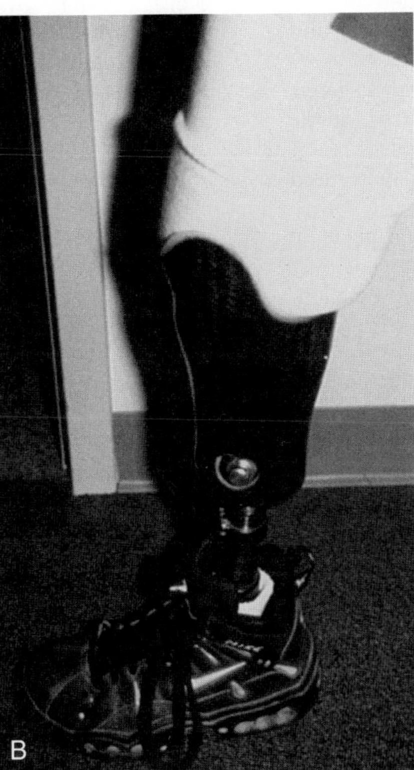

Figure 10-15 **A,** Gel liner suspension with locking pin. **B,** Transtibial prosthesis with liner locked in place.

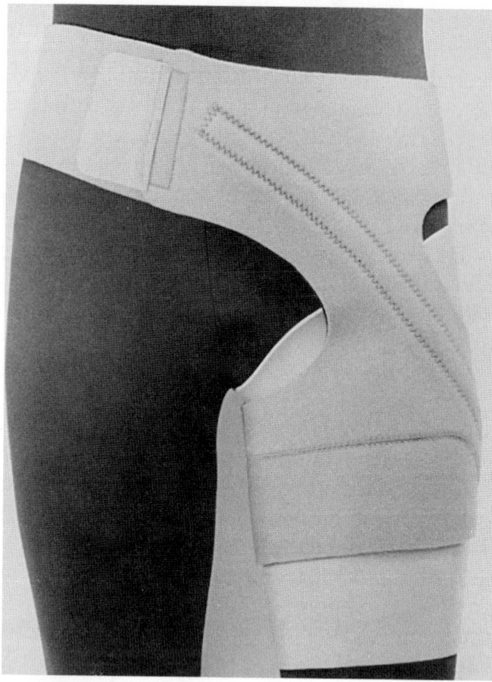

Figure 10-16 Total-elastic suspension belt for suspending a transfemoral socket. (Courtesy of Syncor Manufacturers, Green Bay, Wisconsin.)

- Prosthetic socks worn over the liner accommodate volume fluctuation.
- This suspension allows unrestricted knee flexion and minimal piston action.

- Transfemoral suspension:
  - Vacuum (suction) suspension is frequently used.
  - It relies on surface tension, negative pressure, and muscle contraction.
  - A one-way expulsion valve helps maintain negative pressure, and no belts or straps are required. Stable body weight is required for this intimate fit.
  - Roll-on silicone or thermoplastic liners may be used with or without locking pins.
  - The total-elastic suspension belt, which is made of neoprene, fastens around the waist and spreads over a larger surface area (Figure 10-16). It is an excellent auxiliary suspension.
  - Silesian belts are used to prevent socket rotation in limbs with redundant tissue. Such belts also prevent the socket from slipping off when suction sockets are fitted to short transfemoral stumps and the patient sits.

E. **Common prosthetic problems (Table 10-5)**

1. Transtibial prostheses
   - **Pistoning during the swing phase** of gait is usually caused by an ineffective suspension system.
   - **Pistoning in the stance phase** results from a poor socket fit or volume changes in the stump (a change in thickness of the stump sock may be needed).
   - **Alignment problems** are common (see Table 10-5).
   - **Pressure-related pain or redness** should be corrected, with relief of the prosthesis in the affected area.

Table 10-5 Prosthetic Foot Gait Abnormalities

Foot Position	Gait Abnormality
Inset	Varus strain, pain (proximomedial, distolateral), circumduction
Outset	Valgus strain, pain (proximolateral, distomedial), broad-based gait
Forward placement	Increased knee extension (patellar pain) but stable
Posterior placement	Increased knee flexion/instability
Dorsiflexed foot	Increased patellar pressure
Plantar-flexed foot	Drop-off, patellar pressure

   - Other problems may be **related to the foot**: Too soft a heel results in excessive knee extension, whereas too hard a heel causes knee flexion and lateral rotation of the toes.
2. Transfemoral prostheses
   - Excessive prosthetic length and weak hip abductors or flexors can lead to circumduction, vaulting, and lateral trunk bending.
   - Hip flexion contractures and insufficient anterior socket support can lead to excessive lumbar lordosis (compensatory).
   - Inadequate prosthetic knee flexion can lead to a terminal knee snap.
   - A medial whip (heel-in, heel-out) can be caused by a varus knee, excessive external rotation of the knee axis, or muscle weakness.
   - A lateral whip (heel-out, heel-in) is caused by the opposite problem: valgus knee, internal rotation at knee, or muscle weakness. Table 10-6 summarizes common transfemoral prosthetic gait problems.
3. Stair climbing
   - In general, amputees ascend stairs by leading with the normal limb and descend by leading with the prosthetic limb ("the good goes up and the bad comes down").

Table 10-6 Transfemoral Prosthetic Gait Abnormalities

Gait Abnormality	Prosthetic Problem
Lateral trunk bending	Short prosthesis, weak abductors, poor fit
Abducted gait	Poor socket fit medially
Circumducted gait	Prosthesis too long, excess knee friction
Vaulted gait	Prosthesis too long, poor suspension
Foot rotation at heel-strike	Heel too stiff, loose socket
Short stance phase	Painful stump, knee too loose
Knee instability	Knee too anterior, foot too stiff
Mediolateral whip	Excessive knee rotation, tight socket
Terminal snap	Quadriceps weakness, unsure patient
Foot slap, knee hyperextension	Heel too soft
Knee flexion	Heel too hard
Excessive lordosis	Hip flexion contracture, socket problems

SECTION 4 ORTHOSES

I. INTRODUCTION

A. The primary function of an orthosis is control of the motion of certain body segments.
B. Orthoses are used to protect long bones or unstable joints, support flexible deformities, and occasionally substitute for a functional task. They may be static, dynamic, or a combination of these.
C. With few exceptions, orthoses are not indicated for correction of fixed deformities or for spastic deformities that cannot be easily controlled manually.
D. Orthoses are named according to the joints they control and the method used to obtain/maintain that control (e.g., a short leg, below-the-knee brace is an ankle-foot orthosis [AFO]).

II. SHOES

A. Specific shoes can be used by themselves or in conjunction with foot orthoses.
B. Extra-depth shoes with a high toe box designed to dissipate local pressures over bony prominences are recommended for diabetic patients.
C. The plantar surface of an insensate foot is protected by use of a pressure-dissipating material. A paralytic or flexible foot deformity can be controlled with more rigid orthoses.
D. SACH heels absorb the shock of initial loading and lessen the transmission of force to the midfoot as the foot passes through the stance phase.
E. A rocker sole can lessen the bending forces on an arthritic or stiff midfoot during midstance, as the foot changes from accepting the weight-bearing load to pushing off. It is useful in treating metatarsalgia, hallux rigidus, and other forefoot problems. For the rocker sole to be effective, it must be rigid.
F. Medial heel out-flaring is used to treat severe flatfoot of most causes. A foot orthosis is also necessary.

III. FOOT ORTHOSES

A. Most foot orthoses are used to align and support the foot; prevent, correct, or accommodate foot deformities; and improve foot function.
B. Three main types of foot orthosis are used: rigid, semirigid, and soft.

1. Rigid foot orthoses limit joint motion and stabilize flexible deformities.
2. Semirigid orthoses have hinges and allow dorsiflexion plantar flexion of the ankle, or both.
3. Soft orthoses have the best shock-absorbing ability and are used to accommodate fixed deformities of the feet, especially neuropathic, dysvascular, and ulcerative disorders.

IV. ANKLE-FOOT ORTHOSES

A. The most commonly prescribed lower limb orthosis (AFO) is used to control the ankle joint. It may be fabricated with metal bars attached to the shoe or thermoplastic elastomer. The orthosis may be rigid, preventing ankle motion, or it can allow free or spring-assisted motion in either plane.
B. After hindfoot fusions, the primary orthotic goals are absorption of the ground reaction forces, protection of the fusion sites, and protection of the midfoot.
C. The thermoplastic foot section achieves mediolateral control with high trimlines.
D. When subtalar motion is present, an articulating AFO permits motion by a mechanical ankle joint design.
E. The primary factors in the selection of an orthotic joint include range of motion, durability, adjustability, and the biomechanical effect on the knee joint.
A posterior leaf-spring AFO provides stability in stance phase.

V. KNEE-ANKLE-FOOT ORTHOSIS

A. The knee-ankle foot orthosis (KAFO) extends from the upper thigh to the foot. It is generally used to control an unstable or paralyzed knee joint. It provides mediolateral stability with the prescribed amounts of flexion or extension control.
B. A subset of KAFOs are knee orthoses, which can be made of elastic for the treatment of patellar disease or made of metal and plastic for the treatment of an unstable anterior cruciate ligament.

VI. HIP-KNEE-ANKLE-FOOT ORTHOSIS

A. The hip-knee-ankle-foot orthosis (HKAFO) provides hip and pelvic stability but is rarely used by paraplegic adults because of the cumbersome nature of the orthosis and the magnitude of effort in achieving minimum gains.
B. In experimental studies, it is being used in conjunction with implanted electrodes and the computerized functional stimulation of paraplegic patients.
C. In children with upper-level lumbar myelomeningocele, the reciprocating gait orthoses are modified HKAFOs that can be used for standing and simulated walking.

VII. ELBOW ORTHOSES

A. Hinged-elbow orthoses provide minimum stability in the treatment of ligament instability.
B. Dynamic spring-loaded orthoses have been successfully used in the treatment of flexion and extension contractures.

VIII. WRIST-HAND ORTHOSES (WHOs)

A. The most common use of wrist and hand orthoses today is for postoperative care after injury or reconstructive surgery. These devices are static or dynamic.
B. The opponens splint is successful in prepositioning the thumb but impairs tactile sensation.

C. Wrist-driven hand orthoses are used in lower cervical quadriplegics. They may be body powered by tenodesis action or motor driven. Weight and cumbersomeness are the major limiting factors.

IX. FRACTURE BRACES

A. Fracture bracing remains a valuable treatment option for isolated fractures of the tibia and fibula.
B. Prefabricated fracture orthoses can be used in simple foot and ankle fractures, ankle sprains, and simple hand injuries.

X. PEDIATRIC ORTHOSES

A. Many dynamic orthoses are used by children to control motion without total immobilization.
B. The Pavlik harness has become the mainstay for early treatment of developmental dislocation of the hip.
C. Several dynamic orthoses have been used for containment in Perthes disease.

XI. SPINE ORTHOSES

A. Cervical spine:
1. Numerous orthoses are used to immobilize the cervical spine.
2. Effective immobilization ranges from the various types of collars, to posted orthoses that gain purchase about the shoulders and under the chin, to the halo vest, which achieves the most stability by the nature of its fixation into the skull.

B. Thoracolumbar spine:
1. Orthoses used to mechanically stabilize the back, thus reducing back pain, rely on increasing body cavity pressure.
2. Three-point orthoses achieve their control by the length of their lever arm and the subsequent limitation of motion.

SECTION 5 SURGERY FOR STROKE AND CLOSED-HEAD INJURY

I. INTRODUCTION

The orthopaedic surgeon can play a role in the early management of adult-acquired spasticity secondary to stroke or closed-head brain injury when the spasticity interferes with the rehabilitation program.

A. Nonsurgical treatment:
1. Interventional modalities may include orthotic prescription, serial casting, and motor point nerve blocks with short-acting (bupivacaine HCl) or long-acting (phenol 6% in glycerol or botulinum toxin type A [Botox]) agents.
2. Splinting a joint (e.g., the ankle) in the neutral position is not sufficient to prevent the development of a contracture (e.g., an equinus contracture).
3. When functional joint ranging is insufficient to control the deformity, intervention is often indicated.
4. Local anesthetic injection to the posterior tibial nerve or sciatic nerve before casting relieves pain and allows for maximum correction of the deformity.
5. Open nerve blocks may be warranted to avoid injecting mixed nerves with large sensory contributions.

B. Prerequisites for surgical treatment:
1. Surgical intervention in adult-acquired spasticity should be delayed until the patient achieves maximal spontaneous motor recovery (6 months for stroke and 12 to 18 months for traumatic brain injury).
2. When patients reach a plateau in functional progress or the deformity impedes further progress, intervention may be considered.
3. Invasive procedures in this population should be an adjunct to a standard functional rehabilitation program, not an alternative.
4. When surgery is considered as a method of improving function, patients should be screened for cognitive deficits, motivation, and body image awareness.
   - Patients should not be confused and must have adequate short-term memory and the capacity for new learning.
   - In addition to specific cognitive strengths, motivation is necessary for patients to use functional gains and participate in their rehabilitation program.
   - Body image awareness is essential in order for surgical intervention to become meaningful and potentially beneficial. Patients who lack the awareness of a limb or its position in space should undergo therapy directed toward ameliorating these deficits before undergoing surgical intervention.

II. LOWER LIMB

A. Balance is the best predictor of a patient's ability to ambulate after acquired brain injury. The mainstay of treatment for the dynamic ankle equinus component of this gait deviation is to achieve ankle stability in the neutral position during initial floor contact (i.e., initial contact and stance), as well as floor clearance during the swing phase.
B. An adjustable AFO with ankle dorsiflexion and a plantar flexion stop at the neutral position is often used during the recovery period, followed by a rigid AFO once the patient has reached a plateau in recovery.
C. When the dynamic equinus overcomes the holding power of the orthosis and patients are unable to keep the brace in place, motor-balancing surgery is indicated.
D. The equinus deformity is treated by percutaneous lengthening of the Achilles tendon.
E. The dynamic varus-producing force in adults is the result of out-of-phase tibialis anterior muscle activity during the stance phase. This dynamic varus deformity is corrected by either split or complete lateral transfer of the tibialis anterior muscle.

III. UPPER LIMB

There is a paucity of literature dealing with acquired spasticity in the upper limb. Invasive intervention can be considered for functional and nonfunctional goals.

A. Nonfunctional goals: Surgical release of static contracture is generally performed to complement nursing care or hygiene when the fixed contracture or spastic component results in skin maceration or breakdown.

B. Functional goals: One functional use of static contracture release is to improve upper extremity "tracking" (i.e., arm swing) during walking. Most upper extremity surgery performed in this patient population has the goal of increasing prehensile hand function. The goal may be simply to improve placement, enabling use of the hand as a "paperweight," or to achieve improved fine motor control. In patients with prehensile potential, surgery may allow the "one-handed" patient to be "two-handed" by increasing involved hand function from no function to assistive or from assistive to independent.

1. Screening: When the goal of surgery is to improve function, patients must first be screened for **cognitive capacity, motivation, and body image awareness.**
   - Patients must have the cognitive skills and learning capability to participate in their therapy after surgery and to functionally make use of their newly acquired skills at the completion of their rehabilitation program.
   - If they are not motivated, they will not participate in the prolonged effort necessary to achieve meaningful functional improvement.
   - Patients with poor stereognosis or neglect (i.e., poor body image awareness) find that the involved hand "drifts" in space and is not "available" for use if they have not been carefully trained in visual compensation techniques.
2. Grading: Once it has been determined that the patient has the potential to make functional upper extremity gains with surgery, he or she is graded on the basis of hand placement, proprioception and sensibility, and voluntary motor control. Dynamic electromyography is used when delineation of phasic motor activity is essential.
3. Methods: By means of fractional musculotendinous or step-cut methods, muscle unit lengthening of the agonist-deforming muscle units is combined with motor-balancing tendon transfers of the antagonists to achieve muscle balance and improve prehensile hand function.

SECTION 6 SPINAL CORD INJURY

I. FUNCTIONAL LEVEL

The functional level in a patient with spinal cord injury is determined by the most distal intact functional dermatome (sensory level) and the most distal motor level at which most of the muscles of that level function at least at a "fair" motor grade.

II. MOBILITY

The level at which spinal cord injury occurs determines mobility (Table 10-7).

A. Injury at C4 and higher levels necessitates high back and head support.

Table 10-7 Treatment of Spinal Cord Injury by Functional Level

Functional Level	Working	Not Working	Treatment/Mobility
Above C4	—	Diaphragm, upper extremity muscles	Respirator dependent
C4	Diaphragm/trapezius	Upper extremity muscles	Wheelchair chin/puff
C5	Elbow flexors	Below elbow	Electric wheelchair, rachet
C6	Wrist extensors	Elbow extensors	Wheelchair, flexor hinge
C7	Elbow extensor	Grasp	Wheelchair, independent
C8	Finger flexors to middle finger		
T1	Intrinsic muscles	Abdominals/lower extremity muscles	Wheelchair, independent
T2-T12	Upper extremity muscles, abdominals	Lower extremity muscles	Wheelchair, HKAFO (nonfunctional ambulation)
L1	Upper extremity muscles, abdominals, quadriceps	Lower extremity muscles	KAFO; minimum ambulation
L2	Iliopsoas	Knee/ankle	KAFO, household ambulation
L3	Quadriceps	Ankle	AFO, community ambulation
L4	Tibialis anterior	Toe, plantar flexors	AFO, community ambulation
L5	Extensor hallucis longus, extensor digitorum longus	Plantar flexors	AFO, independent
S1	Gastrocnemius/soleus	Bowel/bladder	± Metatarsal bar

±, with or without.
AFO, ankle-foot orthosis; HKAFO, hip-knee-ankle-foot orthosis; KAFO, knee-ankle-foot orthosis.

B. For injury at C5, mouth-driven accessories can control a motorized wheelchair. Various body-powered or motor-driven orthoses, such as a ratchet wrist-hand orthosis, can assist functional prehension.
C. Manual wheelchairs and the use of a flexor hinge wrist-hand orthosis can be operated by patients with injury at C6.
D. Transfers are dependent with C4-level injuries, assisted with C5-level injuries, and independent with C6-level injuries.

III. ACTIVITIES OF DAILY LIVING

A. Patients with injuries at the C6 level can groom and dress themselves.
B. Patients with injuries at the C7 level can cut meat. Bowel and bladder function can be controlled through rectal stimulation and intermittent catheterization.

IV. PSYCHOSOCIAL FACTORS

Men with spinal injuries may be impotent but can often achieve a reflex erection.

V. AUTONOMIC DYSREFLEXIA

This potentially catastrophic hypertensive event can occur with injuries above T5. It is usually caused by an obstructed urinary catheter or fecal impaction.

VI. SURGERY

A. Spinal fusion is frequently used to expedite rehabilitation and prevent the late development of pain or deformity at the fracture level. Anterior or posterior fusion, or both, with internal fixation should be performed soon after injury in order to facilitate early rehabilitation.
B. Spasticity and contracture can produce hygiene problems or the development of pressure ulcers. Percutaneous (open) motor nerve blocks with phenol can be used to treat these deformities. When the deformity is a static contracture, muscle release or disarticulation may improve sitting or transfer potential.
C. Tendon transfers can be used in the upper limb to eliminate the need for an orthosis or allow the patient to achieve function with an orthosis.

SECTION 7 POSTPOLIO SYNDROME

I. CAUSE

A. Polio is a viral disease affecting the anterior horn cells of the spinal cord. Postpolio syndrome is not a reactivation of the polio virus; it is an aging phenomenon by which more nerve cells become inactive. The syndrome occurs after middle age.
B. Affected patients use a high proportion of their capacity for normal activities of daily living. With aging and the drop-off of muscle units, they no longer have the reserves to perform their daily activities.

II. TREATMENT

A. Treatment comprises prescribed limited exercise combined with periods of rest so that muscles are maintained but not overtaxed.
B. Standard polio surgeries, combining contracture release, arthrodesis, and tendon transfer, are indicated when the deformity overcomes functional capacity.
C. The use of lightweight orthoses is important in helping patients remain functionally independent.

TESTABLE CONCEPTS

SECTION 1 GAIT

- Stance phase comprises 60% of the gait cycle; swing phase comprises 40% of the gait cycle.
- During stance phase, 12% of the time is spent in double-limb support.
- The body's center of gravity, while being propelled forward, is also subject to 5 cm vertical and 6 cm lateral displacements.
- Most muscle activity is eccentric; that is, muscle lengthens while contracting. This allows an antagonist muscle to dampen the activity of an agonist and act as a "shock absorber." Eccentric muscle contraction is the main form of muscle activity for normal daily activities.
- Antalgic gait results in decreased stance phase to lessen the time the painful limb is loaded.
- Water walking results in a significant decrease in joint moments and total joint contact forces as a result of the effect of buoyancy.

SECTION 2 AMPUTATIONS

- The metabolic cost of walking is increased with proximal-level amputations and is inversely proportional to the length of the residual limb and the number of functional joints preserved.
- The required increase in energy expenditure for ambulation in bilateral transtibial amputation (41%) is less than that of unilateral transfemoral amputation (65%).
- Transcutaneous partial pressure of oxygen is the factor that is most predictive of whether wound healing after amputation will be successful. Albumin is the most important laboratory value.
- Bony overgrowth is common in children, particularly in the humerus, fibula, tibia, and femur. Autologous stump-capping can prevent this complication.
- Percutaneous Achilles tendon lengthening should be performed with transmetatarsal and Lisfranc amputations to prevent the late development of equinus or equinovarus deformity.
- In Lisfranc amputations, the soft tissue at the fifth metatarsal base should be preserved because this represents the insertion site of peroneus brevis and tertius, which act as antagonists to the posterior tibial tendon. Failure to preserve these tissues results in inversion during gait.
- Syme amputation is more energy efficient than a midfoot amputation, despite the fact that it is at a more proximal level. The posterior tibial artery must be patent to ensure healing. The heel pad must be secured.
- Transtibial amputations should be closed with a long posterior myocutaneous flap. The optimal bone length is at least 12 cm below the knee joint.
- Knee disarticulation is generally used in nonambulatory patients, inasmuch as it is muscle balanced and provides an excellent weight-bearing platform for sitting and a lever arm for transfer from bed to chair. However, data from the LEAP trial have demonstrated this amputation to result in the slowest walking speed and produce the least self-reported satisfaction.
- Transfemoral amputation should be performed 12 cm above the knee joint to accommodate the prosthetic knee.
- In transfemoral amputation, adductor myodesis is crucial for maintaining femoral adduction during gait with a prosthesis. Transecting the adductor magnus results in a loss of 70% of the adductor pull.

SECTION 3 PROSTHESES

- Myoelectric prostheses are commonly used for midlength transradial amputation.
- Body-powered prostheses are used for heavy labor. The terminal device is activated by shoulder flexion and abduction.
- Short forearm amputations, elbow disarticulations, and above-elbow amputations necessitate supracondylar suspension (Munster socket) and step-up hinges to augment function.
- The SACH prosthetic foot is being discontinued because it results in overload problems in the nonamputated foot.
- A dynamic-response prosthetic foot can be either articulated or nonarticulated. Articulated feet are useful for uneven terrain. Nonarticulated long-keel feet are used for very high-demand activities.
- Prosthetic knees are used in transfemoral and knee disarticulations. Alignment stability is crucial.
  - Knee center of rotation posterior to line of weight bearing promotes control in stance phase, but flexion is difficult.
  - Knee center of rotation anterior to weight bearing makes flexion easier, but control is poor.
- Microprocessor knees with polycentric (four-bar linkage) configuration should be used for most ambulatory patients with transfemoral amputations.
- Stance-phase control (safety) knee prostheses are used for older patients.
- The constant-friction knee is the most common prosthetic knee in children. Its major disadvantages are that it allows only single-speed walking and relies solely on alignment for stance-phase stability; therefore, it is not recommended for older, weaker patients.
- The preferred method of suspension for transtibial prosthetic sleeves is the gel-liner with locking pin.
- Transfemoral suspension can be with or without belts and straps. Vacuum suspension requires stable body weight but avoids belts. Silesian belts prevent socket from slipping off when suction sockets are fitted to short transfemoral stumps.
- Problems are common in prosthetics. Foot placement too anterior results in increased knee extension and patellar pain. Too soft a heel results in excessive knee extension, whereas too hard a heel causes knee flexion and lateral rotation of the toes.

SECTION 4 ORTHOSES

- A rocker sole can lessen the bending forces on an arthritic or stiff midfoot during midstance, as the foot changes from accepting the weight-bearing load to pushing off.
- After hindfoot fusions, the primary orthotic goals are absorption of the ground reaction forces, protection of the fusion sites, and protection of the midfoot.
- A posterior leaf-spring AFO provides ankle stability in stance phase.

Continued

SECTION 5 SURGERY FOR STROKE AND CLOSED-HEAD INJURY

- Surgical intervention in adult-acquired spasticity should be delayed until the patient achieves maximal spontaneous motor recovery (6 months for stroke and 12 to 18 months for traumatic brain injury).
- Equinus deformity is treated by percutaneous Achilles tendon lengthening.
- Dynamic varus-producing force in adults is the result of out-of-phase tibialis anterior muscle activity during the stance phase. This dynamic varus deformity is corrected by either split or complete lateral transfer of the tibialis anterior muscle.

SECTION 6 SPINAL CORD INJURY

- The most important functional level is C6 tetraplegia. This is the highest level at which patients can function independently, including driving an adapted vehicle.
- In C7 tetraplegia, the patient retains elbow extension, and self-hygiene is relatively easy.
- L3 paraplegia (and below) allows community ambulation with an AFO.
- Autonomic dysreflexia can occur with injuries above T5.

SECTION 7 POSTPOLIO SYNDROME

- Postpolio syndrome is not a reactivation of the polio virus. It is an aging phenomenon by which more nerve cells become inactive.
- Treatment comprises prescribed limited exercise combined with periods of rest so that muscles are maintained but not overtaxed.

SELECTED BIBLIOGRAPHY

The selected bibliography for this chapter can be found on www.expertconsult.com.

Chapter 11

TRAUMA*

David B. Weiss, Matthew D. Milewski, Stephen R. Thompson, and James P. Stannard

CONTENTS

SECTION 1 CARE OF THE MULTIPLY INJURED PATIENT

I. PRINCIPLES OF TRAUMA CARE

A. Primary assessment—Assessment begins with the primary survey, which seeks to identify any life-threatening injuries. A rapid assessment of airway, breathing, and circulation (the ABCs) is performed.

1. The airway is often managed by intubation, especially in patients experiencing a great deal of pain or obtundation. The initial survey should include placement of intravenous lines and treatment of any life-threatening injuries that are encountered.

B. Fluid resuscitation

1. Aggressive fluid resuscitation should begin immediately in most cases with the placement of two large-bore intravenous cannulas.
2. Two liters of lactated Ringer solution or normal saline should be administered.
3. If the patient remains hemodynamically unstable after initial crystalloid infusion, begin infusion of blood products.
   - Typically requires greater than 30% blood loss
4. Blood products
   - Universal donor
     - Group O negative
     - Used in severe shock when specific blood products are not yet available
   - Type-specific blood
     - Crossmatched for ABO and Rh type
     - Typically available within 10 minutes
   - Fully typed and crossmatched
     - Minor antibodies are crossmatched.
     - Typically available within 60 minutes
   - Fresh frozen plasma
     - Contains coagulation factor proteins, immunoglobulins, and complement

*The Appendix at www.expertconsult.com contains the pediatric and adult trauma tables.

- Platelets
    - Typically prepared from whole blood and should be stored at 20° to 24° C with continuous gentle agitation
    - Platelets stored in the cold become activated and lose their normal discoid shape.
5. Transfusion
    - If a patient does not respond to 2 L of crystalloid, 2 units of packed red blood cells should be administered.
    - Patients become coagulopathic and, thus, require both fresh frozen plasma and platelets.
        - The amount administered is controversial.
        - **Recent literature supports administration of packed red blood cells, fresh frozen plasma, and platelets in a 1:1:1 ratio.**
            - May prevent early coagulopathy
    - The most common complication of massive transfusion is a dilutional thrombocytopenia, followed by hypothermia and metabolic alkalosis.
    - Increased citrate from packed red blood cells binds calcium directly and can cause hypocalcemia.
6. Hemodynamic instability may result from internal injury or fractures and is the most important consideration for the orthopaedic surgeon.
    - Once the airway and breathing are controlled, problems with circulation remain the biggest threat to life.
    - Rapid application of splints and reduction of fractures when possible can decrease bleeding and relieve pain.
7. The end points of adequate resuscitation are not clear; use of hemodynamic parameters is inadequate.
    - **Base deficit, as measured by lactate level, is a proxy for the amount of anaerobic metabolism by the body.**
    - **Lactate levels are frequently used in trauma to guide the adequacy of resuscitation.**
        - **In general, lactate levels less than 2.5 indicate adequate resuscitation.**
8. Shock
    - Hemorrhagic (Table 11-1)
        - Divided into four classes
        - Class III/IV requires administration of blood products.
        - **Presents as:**
            - **Increased heart rate and systemic vascular resistance**
            - **Decreased pulmonary capillary wedge pressure, central venous pressure, and mixed venous oxygen saturation**
        - Treat with fluids and blood products.
    - Neurogenic
        - Due to a loss of sympathetic tone in setting of a spinal cord injury
        - **Presents as low heart rate, low blood pressure, and warm skin**
        - Treat with dobutamine and dopamine.
    - Septic
        - Typically a hyperdynamic state with a massive loss of systemic vascular resistance
        - Cardiac index is increased and central venous pressure is decreased.
        - Treat with antibiotics and norepinephrine (causes vasoconstriction without increasing cardiac output).
    - Hemodynamic
        - Tension pneumothorax; pericardial tamponade prevents diastolic filling.
            - Pulmonary embolism
        - Adrenal insufficiency
            - Cardiovascular collapse unresponsive to fluids or pressors
9. The systemic inflammatory response syndrome (SIRS) is a generalized response to trauma characterized by an increase in cytokines, complement, and many hormones. These changes are seen in varying degrees after trauma, and there is probably a genetic predisposition to an intense form of these changes. Patients are considered to have SIRS if they have two or more of the following criteria:
    - Heart rate greater than 90 beats per minute
    - White blood cell count (WBC) less than 4/mm^3 or greater than 10/mm^3
    - Respiration greater than 20 breaths per minute, with $PaCO_2$ less than 32 mm
    - Temperature less than 36° C or greater than 38° C
10. SIRS is associated with disseminated intravascular coagulopathy, acute respiratory distress syndrome (ARDS), renal failure, shock, and multisystem organ failure.

C. Radiologic workup

1. A rapid radiologic workup that includes at a minimum anteroposterior (AP) chest, AP pelvis, and lateral cervical spine views is standard.
2. Availability and increased processing speed of computed tomographic (CT) scanners is leading to CT of cervical spine replacing lateral cervical spine radiography for trauma evaluation.
3. Care should be taken not to focus on obvious radiographic findings, such as an open-book pelvic injury, and miss other important findings, such as a widened mediastinum.

Table 11-1 Classification and Treatment of Hemorrhagic Shock

	PARAMETERS				
Class	Blood Volume Loss	Heart Rate (beats/min)	Blood Pressure	Urine Output (mL/hr)	Treatment
I	Up to 15%	<100	Normal	>30	Fluid replacement
II	15%-30%	>100	Decreased	20-30	Fluid replacement
III	30%-40%	>120	Decreased	5-15	Fluid and blood replacement
IV	>40% (emergently life threatening)	>140	Decreased	Negligible	Fluid and blood replacement

From Browner BD, on behalf of the American College of Surgeons Committee on Trauma: *Advanced trauma life support: skeletal trauma: basic science, management, and reconstruction*, ed 8, Chicago, 2008, American College of Surgeons.

4. Pelvic fractures can be life threatening. The orthopaedic surgeon may be called on to stabilize pelvic fractures in the emergency department and should be prepared to place a pelvic binder or sheet.
5. Pelvic bleeding that does not respond rapidly to pelvic compression with a sheet or binder should be evaluated by angiography and embolization, if indicated.

D. Trauma scoring systems—Numerous scoring systems seek to quantify the injury that a patient sustained (Tables 11-2 through 11-4). Although some may yield prognostic value, none is perfect. Therefore, a thorough workup is needed to identify all injuries and prioritize their management. Although it may be desirable to repair all fractures on the day of admission, it may be inherently dangerous to do so because of hemodynamic instability and the added trauma that surgery creates.

E. Damage-control orthopaedics—Principles of damage control have been applied to orthopaedic surgery and are now widely accepted. Damage-control orthopaedics involves staging the definitive care of the patient to avoid adding to the overall trauma that the patient has undergone.

1. Trauma is associated with a surge in inflammatory mediators, which peak 2 to 5 days after trauma.
2. After the initial burst of cytokines and other mediators, leukocytes are "primed" and can be activated easily with further trauma, such as surgery. This may lead to multisystem organ failure or ARDS.
3. To minimize the additional trauma that is added with surgery, traumatologists will often treat only potentially life-threatening injuries during this acute inflammatory window.
4. **In the *severely injured* polytrauma patient or one with significant chest trauma, only emergent and urgent conditions should be treated.**

Table 11-2 Glasgow Coma Scale

Response to Assessment	Score
Best Motor Response	
Obeys commands	6
Localizes pain	5
Normal withdrawal (flexion)	4
Abnormal withdrawal (flexion)—decorticate	3
Extension—decerebrate	2
None (flaccid)	1
Verbal Response	
Oriented	5
Confused conversation	4
Inappropriate words	3
Incomprehensible sounds	2
None	1
Eye Opening	
Spontaneous	4
To speech	3
To pain	2
None	1

To calculate a Glasgow Coma Scale score, add the score for Eye Opening with the scores for Best Motor Response and Verbal Response. The best possible score is 15, and the worst possible score is 3.

Table 11-3 Abbreviated Injury Score

Examples of Abbreviated Injury Score	Score
Head	
Crush of head or brain	6
Brainstem contusion	5
Epidural hematoma (small)	4
Face	
Optic nerve laceration	2
External carotid laceration (major)	3
Le Fort III fracture	3
Neck	
Crushed larynx	5
Pharynx hematoma	3
Thyroid gland contusion	1
Thorax	
Open chest wound	4
Aorta, intimal tear	4
Esophageal contusion	2
Myocardial contusion	3
Pulmonary contusion (bilateral)	4
Two or three rib fractures	2
Abdominal and Pelvic Contents	
Bladder perforation	4
Colon transaction	4
Liver laceration with >20% blood loss	3
Retroperitoneal hematoma	3
Splenic laceration—major	4
Spine	
Incomplete brachial plexus	2
Complete spinal cord, C4 or below	5
Herniated disc with radiculopathy	3
Vertebral body compression >20%	3
Upper Extremity	
Amputation	3
Elbow crush	3
Shoulder dislocation	2
Open forearm fracture	3
Lower Extremity	
Amputation	
Below knee	3
Above knee	4
Hip dislocation	2
Knee dislocation	2
Femoral shaft fracture	3
Open pelvic fracture	3
External	
Hypothermia 31° to 30° C	3
Electrical injury with myonecrosis	3
Second- to third-degree burns—20%-29% of body surface area	3

From Browner BD, et al, editors: *Skeletal trauma,* ed 3, Philadelphia, 2003, WB Saunders, p 135.

Table 11-4 Variables for the Mangled Extremity Severity Score

Component	Points
Skeletal and Soft Tissue Injury	
Low energy (stab, simple fracture, "civilian" gunshot wound)	1
Medium energy (open or multiplex fractures, dislocation)	2
High energy (close-range shotgun or "military" gunshot wound, crush injury)	3
Very high energy (same as above, plus gross contamination, soft tissue avulsion)	4
Limb Ischemia (score is doubled for ischemia >6 hr)	
Pulse reduced or absent but perfusion normal	1
Pulseless, paresthesias, diminished capillary refill	2
Cool, paralyzed, insensate (numb)	3
Shock	
Systolic blood pressure always >90 mm Hg	0
Transient hypotension	1
Persistent hypotension	2
Age (yr)	
<30	0
30-50	1
>50	2

From Johansen K, et al: Objective criteria accurately predict amputation following lower extremity trauma, *J Trauma* 30:568, 1990.

- **Compartment syndrome, fractures associated with vascular injury, unreduced dislocations, long bone fractures, open fractures, or unstable spine fractures should be stabilized acutely.**

5. **Acute stabilization is achieved primarily via external fixation.**
   - Femur fractures may be converted from an external fixator to an intramedullary (IM) nail within 3 weeks.
   - Tibia fractures should be converted within 7 to 10 days. If longer periods of time are necessary, a staged removal of the external fixator and subsequent nailing several days later is recommended.
6. The definitive treatment of pelvic and acetabular fractures is usually delayed for 7 to 10 days in polytrauma patients to allow consolidation of the pelvic hematoma and resolution of the acute inflammatory response.

F. **Care of the pregnant patient**

1. Trauma is the most common cause of death in pregnancy.
2. **Place all pregnant patients at more than 20 weeks' gestation in the left lateral decubitus position.**
   - The vena cava may be compressed by the uterus, reducing maternal cardiac output 30%.
3. Most diagnostic radiographs are below the threshold of risk to the fetus.
   - The first-trimester fetus is most at risk.

II. CARE OF INJURIES TO SPECIFIC TISSUES

A. Soft tissue injuries

1. Vascular injury—may be due to penetrating or blunt trauma
   - Diagnosis—The orthopaedic surgeon should recognize the injury and refer the patient to a vascular surgery specialist or a microsurgeon, as indicated.
     - Vascular injury can be present when pulses are palpable, and a change in pulse or a difference from the contralateral side may be the only harbinger of a serious vascular injury.
     - If pulses are not equal to the uninjured side, a workup is indicated.
     - Vascular compromise may develop over the course of hours in the case of knee dislocations and must be recognized promptly.
   - Treatment—Reduction of fractures will often restore vascularity in the case of long bone fractures.
2. Compartment syndrome
   - Diagnosis—One of the most frequently missed complications of trauma, this results when intracompartmental pressure exceeds capillary pressure, thus preventing exchange of waste and nutrients across vessel walls.
     - Unless it is treated within 4 to 6 hours, permanent injury will ensue. The diagnosis is clinical or made using a pressure monitor.
     - Clinical hallmarks are pain out of proportion to the injury and pain with passive stretching of the muscle.
       - Pulselessness, parasthesias, and pallor are late findings.
     - **Intracompartmental pressure measurement is abnormal if pressure is within 30 mm of the diastolic pressure (ΔP) *or* greater than 30 mm of the absolute pressure (the criteria are debated).**
     - **Intraoperative diastolic blood pressure during anesthesia is approximately 18 mm Hg lower than "baseline," potentially giving spurious ΔP values.**
   - Treatment—Treatment is emergent decompression via fasciotomy.
   - Sequelae—Sequelae are common and include claw toes and contractures in the hand.
3. Nerve injury
   - Cause
     - Blunt trauma—direct impact, crush injury, or shock wave from missile injury
     - Laceration—sharp edge of bone or penetrating trauma
   - The most common form is nerve palsy (neurapraxia) caused by stretching of the nerve, which will recover over time (1 mm/day).
   - Treatment
     - Nerve laceration (neurotmesis)—may be treated by repair or grafting. The results vary according to the specific nerve injured and the degree of injury to the nerve.
     - Disruption of the nerve axon with an intact epineurium (axonotmesis) that may be treated initially by observation
   - Motor recovery potential after repair
     - Excellent
       - Radial, musculocutaneous, femoral
     - Moderate
       - Median, ulnar, tibial
     - Poor
       - **Peroneal nerve**
4. Bites
   - Snake bites
     - Tend to occur in certain regions of the United States. Envenomation occurs in only 25% of cases. Venom may be neurotoxic (coral snakes) or hemotoxic (rattlesnake, cottonmouth).

   - Treatment and complications—Treatment is symptomatic and expectant: antivenom in a monitored setting, débridement of necrotic tissue, and fasciotomy. Antivenom is available for all endemic snakes, but there is a high incidence of anaphylaxis or serum sickness associated with its use.
     - Complications can include severe local tissue necrosis, compartment syndrome, coagulopathies, and arrhythmias.
 - Human and animal bites
   - Pathogens—Despite the association of certain bites with specific bacteria, *Staphylococcus* and *Streptococcus* remain the most prevalent pathogens. Other pathogens include
     - Cat bites—*Pasteurella*
     - Dog bites—*Eikenella*
     - Human bites—variable, including *Eikenella*
   - Treatment—A broad-spectrum antibiotic is commonly given, although regional variations are also common.

5. Thermal injury
   - Hypothermia
     - Cause—Injury is caused by ice crystals forming outside the cell(s).
     - Treatment—Rapid rewarming and attention to arrhythmias are the current treatments. Amputation may be necessary.
   - Burns—generally treated by burn surgeons, but extremity burns may be treated by orthopaedic surgeons. Débridement of deep dermal burns and skin grafting are the hallmarks of treatment after early, aggressive fluid resuscitation. Antibiotic prophylaxis and tetanus are routine.
6. Electrical injury—may cause bone necrosis and massive soft tissue necrosis. The extent of tissue injury may not be apparent for days after injury because the skin may not be broken despite significant injury underneath.
   - Treatment is similar to that of burns; débridement followed by reconstruction with amputation, a flap, or a skin graft is required.
7. Chemical burns—The first rule is to avoid contamination from other people and further damage to the victim.
   - Dilution with copious irrigation is the initial treatment. After initial irrigation, the degree of necrosis is assessed, with débridement of necrotic tissue. Hydrofluoric acid is extremely toxic, causing profound hypocalcemia and cardiac death with little exposure; calcium gluconate may be used to treat skin exposure.
8. High-pressure injury (water, paint, grease)—Hand injuries are the most common. There may be extensive damage to underlying soft tissues despite a small entrance wound. Wide débridement of necrotic tissue and foreign material is required.

B. Joint injuries—Joint injuries may be caused by penetrating or blunt trauma.

1. Dislocations—These orthopaedic emergencies should be reduced as soon as possible to avoid injury to the nerve and vessels and the articular cartilage; general anesthesia may be needed. Neurovascular status should be assessed and documented both before and after reduction.
2. Open joint injuries
   - Antibiotics—Penetrating trauma such as gunshot wounds may be treated with oral antibiotics if there is no debris in the joint; however, foreign matter is often carried into the joint as it is penetrated, even in "clean" gunshot wounds.
   - **Reverse arthrocentesis/saline load test**
     - Performed by injecting saline into the joint and observing the injured area for signs of extravasation
     - **At least 155 mL must be injected into the knee.**
     - This may miss a small puncture wound.
3. Fractures involving the joints—must be reduced as anatomically as possible to reduce unequal wear

Table 11-5 Classification of Open Fractures

Fracture Type	Description
I	Skin opening of ≤1 cm, quite clean; most likely from inside to outside; minimum muscle contusion; simple transverse or short oblique fractures
II	Laceration >1 cm long, with extensive soft tissue damage, flaps, or avulsion; minimum to moderate crushing component; simple transverse or short oblique fractures with minimum comminution
III	Extensive soft tissue damage, including muscles, skin, and neurovascular structures; often a high-velocity injury with severe crushing component
IIIA	Extensive soft tissue laceration, adequate bone coverage; segmental fractures, gunshot injuries
IIIB	Extensive soft tissue injury, with periosteal stripping and bone exposure; usually associated with massive contamination; requires soft tissue coverage
IIIC	Vascular injury requiring repair

From Gustilo RB, Mendoza RM, Williams DN: Problems in the management of type III (severe) open fractures: a new classification of type III open fractures, *J Trauma* 24:742, 1984.

C. Fractures

1. Open fractures
   - Classification—The Gustillo and Anderson grading system is widely used (Table 11-5). There is considerable interobserver variability, and the type may change with time.
     - Type I—no periosteal stripping, minimum soft tissue damage, small skin wound (1 cm)
     - Type II—little periosteal stripping, moderate muscle damage, skin wound (1-10 cm)
     - Type IIIA—contaminated wound (high-energy gunshot wound, farm injury, shotgun) or extensive periosteal stripping with large skin wound (>10 cm)
     - Type IIIB—same as IIIA but will require flap coverage
     - Type IIIC—same as IIIA but with vascular injury that requires repair
   - Treatment
     - Débridement—Initial treatment should consist of local wound débridement that is adequate to clean the wound and débridement of all necrotic tissue.
     - Antibiotics—usually started immediately. Antibiotic bead pouch with methylmethacrylate, tobramycin, and/or vancomycin may be used to temporize dirty wounds.
       - Types I and II—first-generation cephalosporin (cefazolin) for 24 hours
       - Type III—cephalosporin and aminoglycoside for 72 hours after last incision and drainage

- Heavily contaminated wounds and farm wounds—cephalosporin, aminoglycosides, and high-dose penicillin
- Fresh water wounds—fluoroquinolones (ciprofloxacin, levofloxacin) or third- or fourth-generation cephalosporin (ceftazidime)
- Salt water wounds—doxycycline and ceftazidime *or* a fluoroquinolone

□ Stabilization of bony injuries—will decrease further damage to soft tissue

□ **Early coverage (<5 days is the goal). However, zone of injury must be well defined before coverage.**
- Gastrocnemius flap—for proximal third tibial fractures
- Soleus flap—for middle third tibial fractures
- Fasciocutaneous flap or free-tissue transfer—for distal third fractures

□ Negative-pressure therapy is commonly used to treat wounds but is not a substitute for definitive coverage.

2. Stabilization with external fixation
   - Immediate treatment—Most fractures should be reduced and splinted promptly to avoid further soft tissue damage. External fixation may be used to treat grossly contaminated wounds and fractures that will require time for the soft tissues to heal before definitive fixation.
   - Definitive treatment—External fixation may be used definitively for periarticular fractures, articular fractures that cannot be reconstructed, and segmental fractures, but internal fixation is far more common.
3. Perioperative complications
   - Thromboembolic disease—The incidence is very high in pelvic, spine, hip, and lower extremity fractures. Pulmonary embolus develops in as many as 5% of those who have deep venous thrombosis (DVT).
     - □ Diagnosis—Diagnosis of DVT is by Doppler ultrasound, magnetic resonance venography, or D-dimer titers
     - □ Treatment—All patients with these injuries should receive some form of thromboembolic disease prophylaxis (mechanical or pharmacologic). The risks of pharmacologic prophylaxis include prolonged bleeding from surgical or traumatic wounds or a cerebral bleed.
   - Fat embolus syndrome—associated with reaming of long bones but can occur with any long bone fracture. Hypoxia, a petechial rash on the chest, and tachycardia are the hallmarks. Treatment is supportive.
   - ARDS—Patients with chest trauma and multiple fractures are at high risk. It is unclear whether reamed nailing of long bone fractures causes it directly but may be implicated in the "second hit" phenomenon. Treatment is supportive (O_2, ventilator).
4. Fracture complications
   - Delayed union—defined as no progression of healing over serial radiographs. Treatment may include bone grafting and external bone stimulation.
   - Nonunion
     - □ Classification (Figure 11-1)
     - □ Biologic treatments—many new treatments, but scanty literature to support any one over the others
       - Calcium sulfate—short resorption time
       - Calcium phosphate—very long resorption time
       - Bone morphogenetic protein—expensive, indicated in some acute tibia fractures, and possibly useful in nonunions
       - Platelet-derived growth factors—seek to add osteoinductive factors to an osteoconductive matrix (cancellous bone, calcium)
     - □ Traditional treatment
       - Identify infection and treat appropriately.
       - Correct any deformity.

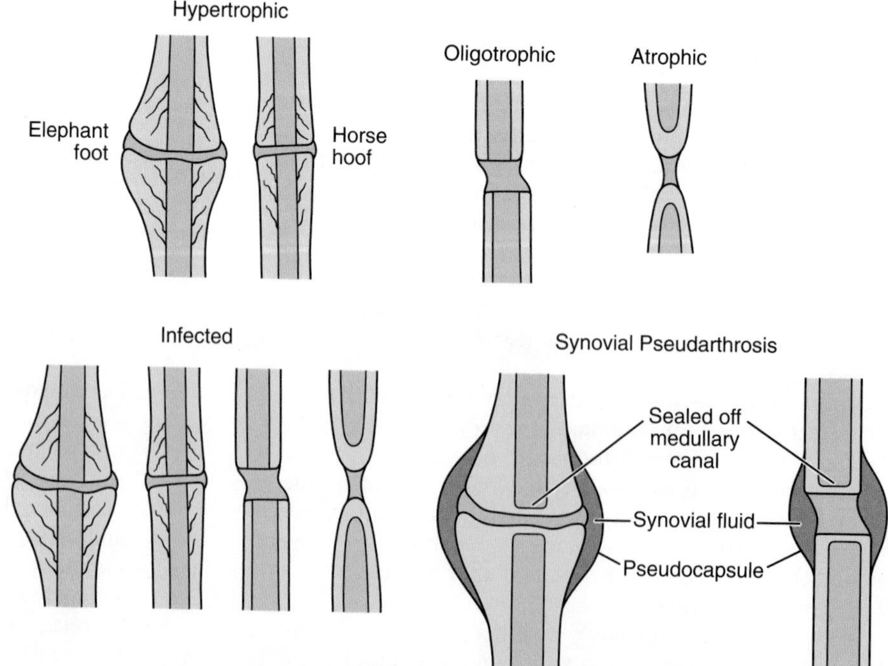

Figure 11-1 Classification of nonunions. (From Browner BD, et al, editors. *Skeletal trauma,* ed 4, Philadelphia, 2008, Elsevier.)

- Provide stability (for hypertrophic nonunions/infections).
- Preserve native biology.
  - Bone stimulator—no strong evidence for effectiveness of one method over the other
    - Ultrasound—delivers small, cumulative doses of ultrasound energy; thought to induce microfracture and healing response
    - Electromagnetic—attempts to promote healing by directing integral ion flow at cellular level of bone
- Segmental bone loss—Treatment includes treatment with bone graft, interposition free tissue transfer (free-fibula transfer), bone transport (Ilizarov or Taylor spatial frame), and amputation.
- Heterotopic ossification
  - Diagnosis—common in head-injured patients and in hip, elbow, and shoulder fractures. Any fracture associated with extensive muscle damage is at risk.
  - Prophylaxis—Indomethacin 25 mg orally three times a day or indomethacin (sustained release) 75 mg orally daily for 6 weeks may be effective in preventing heterotopic bone formation.
  - Radiation therapy (600-700 cGy) given 24 hours before or up to 72 hours after surgery; equal to indomethacin in effectiveness (but no issues with compliance with medication regimen)
  - Treatment—early, active range of motion (ROM) for the elbow and shoulder. Excision of problematic heterotopic ossification can be considered when no further growth (controversial how to assess—"quiet" bone scan, stable disease shown on radiographs, time >1 year)
- Osteomyelitis
  - Diagnosis
    - Definitive diagnosis—by bone biopsy
    - Other tests—may be used in combination with physical examination (draining wound, pain) to confirm the diagnosis
      - Magnetic resonance imaging (MRI)—95% sensitive and 90% specific
      - Technetium-99m (^{99m}Tc) study—85% sensitive and 80% specific
      - Indium study—95% sensitive and 85% to 90% specific
  - Treatment—based on grade and host type (Cierny/Mader)
    - Grade
      - Grade I—IM nail removal and reaming
      - Grade II—superficial; involves cortex; often seen in diabetic wounds; curettage
      - Grade III—localized; involves cortical lesion, with extension into medullary canal; requires wide excision, bone grafting, and perhaps stabilization
      - Grade IV—diffuse; indicates spread through cortex and along medullary canal; wide sequestrectomy, muscle flap, bone graft, and stabilization
    - Host
      - A—normal, healthy patient
      - B—locally compromised (vasculopathic)

Table 11-6 Classification of Closed Fractures with Soft Tissue Damage

Fracture Type	Description
0	Minimum soft tissue damage; indirect violence; simple fracture patterns *Example:* torsion fracture of the tibia in skiers
I	Superficial abrasion or contusion caused by pressure from within; mild to moderately severe fracture configuration *Example:* pronation fracture-dislocation of the ankle joint with soft tissue lesion over the medial malleolus
II	Deep, contaminated abrasion associated with localized skin or muscle contusion; impending compartment syndrome; severe fracture configuration *Example:* segmental "bumper" fracture of the tibia
III	Extensive skin contusion or crush injury; underlying muscle damage may be severe; subcutaneous avulsion; decompensated compartment syndrome; associated major vascular injury; severe or comminuted fracture configuration

From Tscherne H, Oestern HJ: Die Klassifizierung des Weichteilschadens bei offenen und geschlossenen Frakturen, *Unfallheilkunde* 85:111-115, 1982. © Springer-Verlag.

      - C—not considered a medical candidate for surgery; may require suppressive antibiotics
- Fractures caused by gunshot wounds
  - High-energy gunshot and shotgun wounds—These are considered grade III open fractures because they are often associated with considerable soft tissue injury (Table 11-6). They require extensive surgical débridement of necrotic tissue and require surgical stabilization of the fracture.
  - **Low-energy gunshot wounds—can be treated as a closed fracture but should get single-dose, first-generation cephalosporin and local wound care**
  - Bullets that pass through colon—may contaminate any fracture caused by the bullet after perforation (pelvis, spine). Bony fractures may be managed with antibiotics alone if extraarticular and the fracture pattern is stable.

III. BIOMECHANICS OF FRACTURE HEALING

Also see Chapter 1, Biomechanics

A. Stability and fracture healing

1. **Stability determines strain**
   - Absolute stability
   - Relative stability
2. Strain determines the type of healing.
   - Strain less than 2% results in primary bone healing (endosteal healing).
   - Strain 2% to 10% results in secondary bone healing (enchondral ossification).
   - Strain greater than 10% does not permit bone formation.
     - *Strain* is defined as change in fracture gap divided by the fracture gap (ΔL/L).

B. Relative stability
1. Micromotion at fracture site under physiologic load leads to callus formation.
2. **Strain** decreases as callus matures, leading to increased stability.
3. If there is too much motion, callus becomes hypertrophic as it tries to spread out force and **hypertrophic nonunion** can result.
4. Examples: casts, external fixators, IM nails, bridge plates

C. Absolute stability
1. No motion at fracture site under physiologic load
2. Bone heals through direct healing (no callus).
3. **Strain** is low or zero.
2. Healing times are longer and more difficult to confirm on by radiography.
5. Implants must have longer fatigue life.
6. **Examples: lag screws, compression plating, rigid locked plating (in nonbridging mode)**

D. Healing in different bone types
1. Diaphyseal (cortical)
   - Decreased blood supply leads to longer healing times.
   - Bone is more amenable to compression techniques (in short oblique/transverse fractures).
   - Strain is concentrated over a smaller surface area.
2. Cancellous (metaphyseal)
   - Larger surface area and better blood supply
   - Strain is lower as forces spread out over larger area.
   - Healing is more rapid.
   - However, joint surfaces tolerate very little malreduction (<2 mm) so there is often increased time to weight bear versus diaphyseal fractures.

IV. BIOMECHANICS OF ORIF

Also see Chapter 1, Biomechanics

A. Lag screws
1. Provide rigid interfragmentary compression (absolute stability)
2. Force is concentrated over a small area (around the screw) so typically a plate is needed to protect/neutralize the deforming forces.

B. Position screws
1. Compress plate to bone but will not provide interfragmentary compression
2. Friction between screw, plate, and bone resists pullout or bending.

C. Plating (Figure 11-2)
1. Plate length matters more for bending stability than number of screws in plate.
2. Torsional stability is more affected by position of screws (need end hole filled).
3. Longer plates spread the strain over more area (working length).
4. Plates are load bearing—will stress shield area covered by plate; important to protect area temporarily if plate removed after healing

D. Compression plating
1. Plate design (oval holes) or use of compression device allows plate to apply compressive forces across fracture.
2. Provides absolute stability when properly applied
3. Relies on friction between plate and bone (needs at least some nonlocking screws)

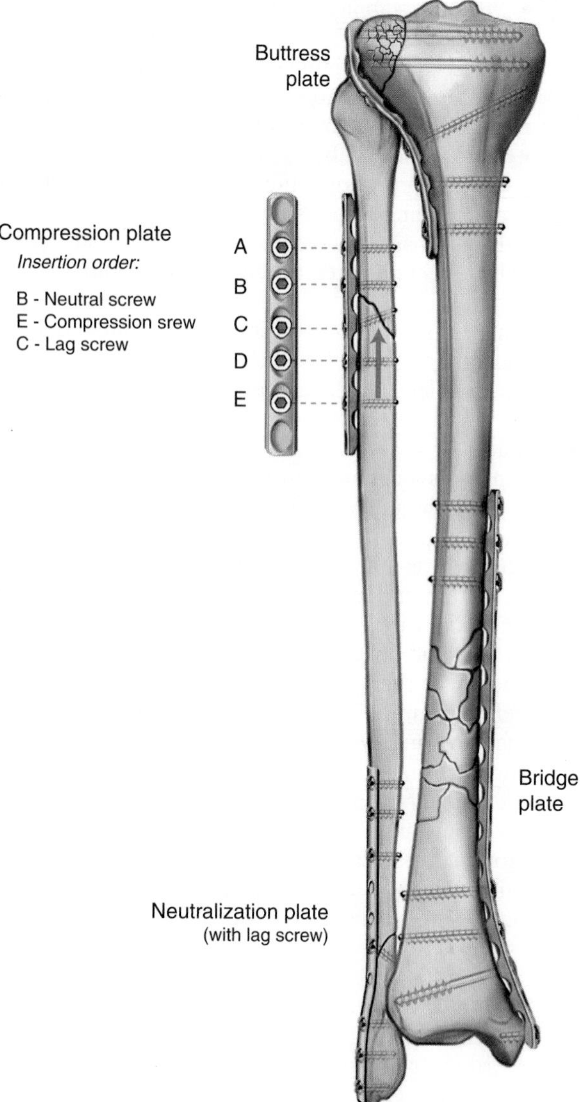

Figure 11-2 Plating modalities for various fracture patterns.

4. **May need pre-bend to eliminate gapping opposite plate**
5. **Insertion order is neutral position, then compression on opposite side of fracture, then lag screw (if placing through plate).**
6. **Tight contact of plate to bone when initially applied causes decreased periosteal blood flow and temporary osteopenia.**

E. Bridge plating
1. **Primarily for comminuted fracture patterns**
2. **Plate "bridges" area of comminution with fixation above and below fracture.**
3. **Allows some elastic deformation (relative stability)**
4. Avoid use of screws too close to fracture.
5. Number and types of screws to insert are fracture dependent—no clear, widely accepted guidelines.
6. Nonlocking screws compress plate to bone and can be used to lag in fragments; locking screws provide angular stability in short metaphyseal segments or in osteoporotic bone.

F. **Buttress plating**

1. Provides support at 90-degree angle to fracture—typically in depressed metaphyseal/articular fractures that have been reduced
2. Can provide absolute stability to metaphyseal fragments

G. **Submuscular/percutaneous plating**

1. To preserve biology at fracture site, plate may be placed in submuscular plane by sliding through small incisions proximal or distal to fracture and avoiding exposure of fracture site.
2. Typically used in bridge mode, although not exclusive
3. **Advantage is decreased soft tissue and biologic compromise.**
   - **Medullary and periosteal perfusion are better retained.**
4. Disadvantage: more prone to malreduction/malrotation

H. **Locked plating**

1. Screws have threads in head, which lock into corresponding holes in the plate.
   - Fail simultaneously, rather than sequentially
2. Does not depend on friction between plate and bone for stability
3. Provides fixed angle construct—similar to blade plate
4. **Most useful in unstable, short-segment metaphyseal fractures and osteoporotic bone**
5. **Fractures in which locking plate use is supported by data include**
   - **Periprosthetic fractures**
   - **Proximal humerus fracture**
   - **Intraarticular distal femur and proximal tibia**
   - **Humeral shaft nonunion in the elderly**
6. Unicortical locked screws
   - Typically for metaphyseal bone
   - Similar pullout strength to bicortical locked screws in good quality diaphyseal bone (but rare indications for use there)
   - **Weaker in torsion compared with bicortical screws**
7. Bicortical locked screws: biggest advantage is in osteoporotic, diaphyseal bone
8. **Multiaxial screws**
   - **May increase options for fixation in working around periprosthetic fractures**
   - **No advantage in strength or pullout**
9. **"Hybridization" describes the use of both locking and nonlocking screws in combination. This allows for both compression and fixed-angle support.**

I. **IM nails**

1. Load-sharing devices—relative stability
2. **Stiffness** depends on:
   - Material
     - □ Stainless is greater than titanium
   - Size
     - □ Increased diameter leads to increased stiffness: at a ratio of radius to the power of:
       - 3 in bending
       - 4 in torsion
   - Wall thickness
     - □ Larger = stiffer nail
3. **Radius of curvature of femoral nails is typically less than anatomic, improving frictional fixation.**
   - A large mismatch of curvature, however, results in difficult insertion, increased risk of intraoperative fracture, and malreduction in extension.
4. Nails resist bending very well and require interlocks to resist torsion or compression loads.
5. **Working length is the portion of the nail that is unsupported by bone when loaded.**
   - **Increased working length produces increased interfragmentary motion and may delay union.**
6. Advantage of intramedullary position is decreased lever arm for bending forces (especially useful in pertrochanteric fractures versus plate and screw construct).

SECTION 2 UPPER EXTREMITY

I. SHOULDER INJURIES (TABLES 11-7 AND 11-8)

A. **Sternoclavicular dislocation—"Serendipity" view or CT scan reveals dislocation of the sternoclavicular joint.**

1. **Anterior dislocation—more common, treated by closed reduction. The majority will remain unstable regardless of initial treatment modality, but these are typically asymptomatic.**
2. Posterior dislocation—more serious—30% associated with significant compression of posterior structures. May cause dysphagia or difficulty breathing and sensation of fullness in the throat. Treated by closed reduction with a towel clip in the operating room. A thoracic surgeon should be on standby.
3. Chronic dislocation—treated by resection of the medial clavicle, with preservation and reconstruction of costoclavicular ligaments
4. **Pseudodislocation—The medial clavicular epiphysis is the last to close at a mean age of 25 years. In patients younger than this, sternoclavicular dislocation is often a Salter-Harris type I or II fracture.**

B. **Clavicle fracture (Figure 11-3, *A* and *B*)**

1. Classification—classified by thirds
   - Middle—80%
   - Distal—15%
   - Medial—5%
2. Diagnosis—AP and 15-degree cephalad-oblique radiographic views
3. Associated injuries—**Open clavicle fractures are associated with high rates of pulmonary and closed-head injuries.**
4. Treatment
   - Nonoperative treatment—most mid-third fractures treated nonoperatively in a sling
     - □ **No difference in outcome between regular sling and figure-eight bandage**

Table 11-7 Adult Shoulder Dislocations/Ligamentous Injuries

Injury	Eponym/Other Name	Classification	Treatment	Complications
Anterior (GH) dislocation (most common)		Subcoracoid > subglenoid (also subclavicular and intrathoracic)	Must get axillary view of GH joint; reduce, immobilize (young patient, 4 wk; old patient, 2 wk); passive > active (Rockwood 7)	Axillary nerve neurapraxia, axillary artery injury, cuff injury (>40 yr old), recurrence (85% in <20 yr old), bone injury (head [Hill-Sachs], greater tuberosity, glenoid)
Recurrent/ multidirectional		Anterior dislocation/ subluxation atraumatic	Prolonged rehabilitation (rotator cuff strengthening); if failure, consider surgery (inferior capsular shift)	Look for generalized laxity; AMBRI
	Bankart repair: anterior capsule → anterior rim	Late instability		
	Staple capsulorrhaphy: capsule → glenoid	Late DJD, migration		
	Putti-Platt repair: subscapularis imbrication	Late DJD, ↓ ER		
	Magnuson-Stack repair: subscapularis → lesser tuberosity	Late DJD, ↓ ER		
	Bone block: crest graft, anterior	↓ Range of motion, migration		
	Bristow repair: coracoid transfer	Nonunion, ↓ ER, migration		
	Capsular shift: redundant capsule, advanced	Minimum procedure of choice with multidirectional instability		
Posterior dislocation	Subacromial (seizures and shocks) (most common)	Reduce, immobilize for 3-6 wk; rotator cuff strengthening; operate if recurrent (glenoid osteotomy, bone block, posterior capsular shift)	Lesser tuberosity fracture, late recognition (may require advancement of lesser tuberosity into defect or total shoulder arthroplasty [place in less retroversion]); avoid by checking axial view	
Inferior GH	Luxatio erecta		Reduce and immobilize; rotator cuff strengthening, rehabilitation	Neurovascular injury can resolve after reduction; axillary artery thrombosis; watch for rotator cuff tear
AC injury		I—AC sprain	7-10 days rest/ immobilization, sling	Joint stiffness, deformity, CC ligament and soft tissue calcification, AC DJD, associated fractures, distal clavicle osteolysis
		II—AC tear, CC sprain	Sling for 2 wk, rehabilitation, late-excision arthroplasty if required	
		III—AC tear, CC tear	Conservative vs. repair (athletes, laborers); Weaver-Dunn	
		IV—clavicle through trapezius posteriorly	Reduce and repair	
		V—clavicle 100%-300% elevated; trapezius, deltoid detached	Reduce and repair (Weaver-Dunn)	
		VI—clavicle inferior to coracoid	Reduce and repair	

Table 11-7 Adult Shoulder Dislocations/Ligamentous Injuries—cont'd

Injury	Eponym/Other Name	Classification	Treatment	Complications
Sternoclavicular injury		Anterior dislocation	Evaluate with "serendipity" view or computed tomography closed reduction with traction	Bump (cosmetic), DJD, mediastinal impingement (dysphagia, throat fullness), hardware migration (with operative treatment)
		Posterior dislocation	Closed reduction with towel clip or open; thoracic surgeon on standby	
		Chronic dislocation	Medial clavicle resection or ligament reconstruction (thoracic surgeon on standby)	
		Spontaneous atraumatic subluxation	Nonoperative	

AC, acromioclavicular; AMBRI, *a*traumatic, *m*ultidirectional, *b*ilateral, treated by *r*ehabilitation *i*nstability; CC, coracoclavicular; DJD, degenerative joint disease; ER, external rotation; GH, glenohumeral.

- **Risk of nonunion after midshaft fractures is higher in females and elderly and those fractures that are displaced, shortened more than 2 cm, or comminuted.**
- **Lateral fractures have higher rates of nonunion compared with midshaft fractures.**
- Operative treatment
  - **Middle third**
    - If shortened more than 2 cm or comminuted
      - Have higher rates of nonunion and decreased shoulder strength and endurance (~15%)
  - Lateral third

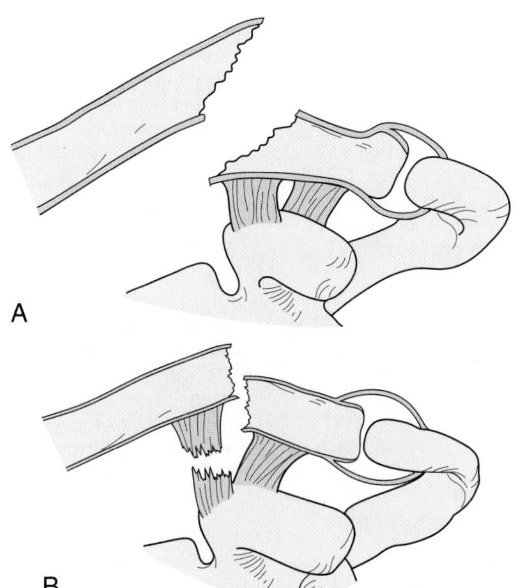

Figure 11-3 When the distal end of the clavicle is fractured, the ligaments may either remain intact and maintain apposition of the fracture fragments (type I) or rupture, allowing wide displacement of the fragments (type II). (Redrawn from Rockwood CA, Green DP, editors: *Fractures,* ed 4, vol 1, Philadelphia, 1996, JB Lippincott.)

    - Some authors recommend operative treatment of distal fractures that extend into the acromioclavicular joint, whereas others recommend a late Mumford procedure.
- Fixation options
  - Plate—typically dynamic compression plate; apply to superior aspect (better biomechanical strength but more prominent = hardware removal) or to anterior-inferior aspect (less hardware removal).
  - IM rod and screw—may be inserted percutaneously; higher rates of hardware irritation and complication
  - Avoid Steinmann pins, especially nonthreaded—can migrate.

C. **Acromioclavicular dislocation**

1. Classification—classified by extent of involvement of the ligamentous support and direction and magnitude of displacement (Figure 11-4). Coracoclavicular (CC) and acromioclavicular (AC) ligaments may be ruptured.
   - Type I—sprain of AC joint
   - Type II—rupture of AC ligaments and sprain of CC ligaments
   - Type III—rupture of both AC and CC ligaments
   - Type IV—The clavicle is buttonholed through the trapezius posteriorly.
   - Type V—The trapezius and deltoid are detached.
   - Type VI—The clavicle is translocated beneath the coracoid.
2. Treatment
   - Types I and II—always treated with brief immobilization in a sling
   - Type III—may be treated nonoperatively, but many would advocate early operative treatment in patients who are heavy laborers and throwers. The Weaver-Dunn procedure is the treatment of choice.
   - Types IV to VI—usually treated operatively

D. **Scapula fracture—associated with pulmonary contusion, pneumothorax, clavicle fracture (i.e., floating shoulder), rib fracture, head injury, brachial plexus injury, upper extremity vascular injury, pelvic or**

Table 11-8 Adult Shoulder Fractures

Injury	Eponym	Classification	Treatment	Complications
Proximal humerus fracture		Neer (parts > 1 cm or 45-degree displacement)		Missed dislocation, adhesive capsulitis (moist heat, gentle range of motion), malunion (reconstruction or TSA required), avascular necrosis (TSA required), nonunion (surgical neck, tuberosity fractures: ORIF), disrupted rotator cuff
		One-part (most common); impaction of the humeral neck	Sling for comfort, early motion; isometrics initially, advancing to progressive resistance	
		Two-part; displacement of the greater tuberosity >1 cm	Closed reduction unless articular segment (ORIF), shaft (impacted and angulated: traction, Velpeau; unimpacted: closed reduction, CRPP or ORIF), greater tuberosity (repair cuff), tuberosity with block to internal rotation (ORIF)	
		Three-part; displacement of the greater or lesser tuberosities >1 cm	ORIF in younger, ORIF/prosthesis in older; repair of rotator cuff	
		Four-part; displacement of lesser and greater tuberosities >1 cm head splitting is variant	Same as three-part; nonoperative in elderly/ diabetic/impacted four-part valgus pattern	
Proximal humerus		Anterior (greater tuberosity displacement)	Closed reduction; if >1 cm after reduction, open repair	As above, with the addition of axillary nerve or plexus injury, myositis ossificans (wait >1 yr to excise heterotopic bone)
Fracture-dislocation		Posterior (lesser tuberosity displacement)	Closed reduction, ORIF if three-part; treatment for fracture as above	
Impression/impaction of humeral head	Hill-Sachs	Stable (<20% articular surface)	Closed treatment	Avascular necrosis, DJD (TSA)
		Unstable (20%-50%)	Transfer of lesser tuberosity → defect (McLaughlin)	
		Unstable (>45%)	Prosthesis vs. rotational osteotomy	
Scapula fracture		Zdravkovic and Damholt		Associated injuries (clavicle, rib, pulmonary contusion, pneumothorax), axillary artery injury, plexus palsy, pressure symptoms, vascular and plexus injuries
		I—body	Most treated nonoperatively	
		II—coracoid and acromion	Associated injury common; ORIF of large, displaced fragments	
		III—neck and glenoid	ORIF of large, unstable fractures (glenoid with displaced clavicle fracture)	
Clavicle fracture		Middle one third (most common)	Nonoperative: sling, figure-eight brace ORIF: displacement, ipsilateral displaced glenoid neck fracture	Vascular injury/pneumothorax, ligament injury (CC or AC), skin necrosis, malunion (osteotomy for young, active patient); nonunion (ORIF and bone graft), nerve injury (rare); muscle fatigue/ weakness, DJD (if articular)
		Distal one third (Neer)	TSA if symptomatic	
		I—minimum interligamentous displacement (CC, AC)	Nonoperative; sling for comfort	
		II—fracture medial to CC ligaments	Nonoperative if nondisplaced; consider ORIF for displaced fracture	

Table 11-8 Adult Shoulder Fractures—cont'd

Injury	Eponym	Classification	Treatment	Complications
Clavicle fracture, cont'd		IIA—both ligaments attached to distal fragment	ORIF	
		IIB—conoid torn, trapezoid attached to distal fragment	ORIF	
		III—AC joint	Closed treatment; late-excision arthroplasty if required	
		Proximal one third	Closed treatment	
Glenoid fracture		Ideberg I—anterior avulsion fracture II—transverse/oblique fracture, inferior glenoid free III—upper one third of glenoid and coracoid IV—horizontal glenoid through body V—combination of II-IV	Nonoperative treatment if nondisplaced >25% of surface: ORIF if head is subluxated with major fragment; posterior approach	
Scapulothoracic dissociation (seen on scapular lateral or chest radiograph)			Closed reduction, sling immobilization	Vascular and brachial plexus injuries, associated clavicle fracture

AC, acromioclavicular; CC, coracoclavicular; CRPP, closed reduction with percutaneous pinning; DJD, degenerative joint disease; ORIF, open reduction with internal fixation; TSA, total shoulder arthroplasty.

acetabular fracture and spine fracture. Scapula body fractures are generally treated in a sling for 7 to 10 days and then with early ROM.

E. Glenoid fracture

1. Nonoperative treatment—used for nondisplaced fractures
2. Operative treatment—indicated for intraarticular fractures that are displaced more than 2 mm or widely displaced extraarticular fractures. The approach is usually through a posterior portal, although the Neviaser portal may be used to place a superoinferior screw in the glenoid.

F. Glenoid neck fracture

1. Nonoperative treatment—Many authors advocate nonoperative treatment in almost all cases.
2. Operative treatment—**indicated when glenoid neck and humeral head are translocated anterior to the proximal fragment or are medially displaced. Reduction and plating is through a posterior approach between infraspinatus (suprascapular nerve) and teres minor (axillary nerve). The suprascapular nerve and artery are at risk from excessive superior retraction, whereas the circumflex scapular artery is at risk during the approach.**

G. Scapulothoracic dissociation—the result of significant trauma to the chest wall, lung, and heart. Severe cases are treated essentially with a closed forequarter amputation.

1. Associated with:
   - Brachial plexus avulsion
   - Subclavian or axillary artery injury
   - AC dislocation, clavicle fracture, and sternoclavicular dislocation
   - **Mortality rate of 10%**
2. **Diagnosis should be suspected when there is a neurologic and/or vascular deficit. Lateral displacement of the scapula more than 1 cm on a chest radiograph is also suggestive.**
3. Management
   - Hemodynamically stable—angiography before surgery. Vascular injury may potentially be treated nonoperatively owing to the extensive collateral network around the shoulder.
   - Hemodynamically unstable—high lateral thoracotomy or median sternotomy to control bleeding
   - Musculoskeletal injury treatment is controversial but is often nonoperative if vascular repair is not undertaken.
4. **Functional outcome is based on severity of associated neurologic injury.**

H. Floating shoulder—fracture of the glenoid neck and clavicle

1. Some authors recommend fixation when a clavicle fracture is associated with a displaced glenoid neck fracture, whereas others do not consider it necessary (depends on stability of superior shoulder suspensory complex [SSSC]).

I. Proximal humerus fracture (Figure 11-5)

1. Neer classification ("part" is defined as displacement of more than 1 cm or angulation of more than 45 degrees). Parts are articular surface, greater tuberosity, lesser tuberosity and shaft
   - One-part—nondisplaced or minimally displaced fracture (often of the humeral neck)
   - Two-part—displacement of tuberosity of more than 1 cm; or surgical neck with head/shaft angled or displaced

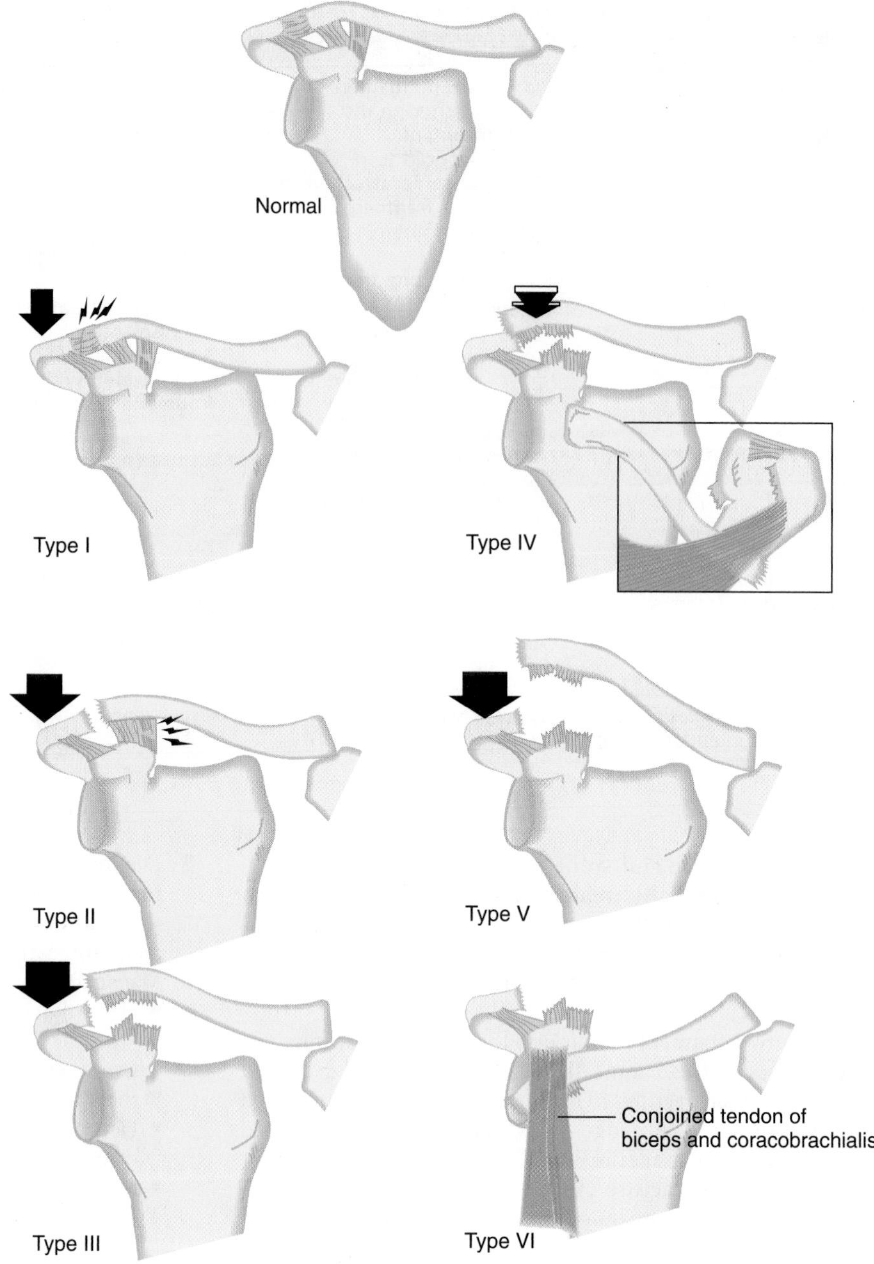

Figure 11-4 The classification of the ligamentous injuries that can occur to the acromioclavicular (AC) joint. In a type I injury, a mild force applied to the point of the shoulder does not disrupt either the AC or coracoclavicular (CC) ligament. In a type II injury, a moderate to heavy force applied to the point of the shoulder disrupts the AC ligaments but the CC ligaments remain intact. In a type III injury, when a severe force is applied to the point of the shoulder, both the AC and the CC ligaments are disrupted. In a type IV injury, not only are the ligaments disrupted but the distal end of the clavicle is also displaced posteriorly into or through the trapezius muscle. In a type V injury, a violent force applied to the point of the shoulder not only ruptures the AC and CC ligaments but also disrupts the muscle attachments and creates a major separation between the clavicle and the acromion. A type VI injury is an inferior dislocation of the distal clavicle in which the clavicle is inferior to the coracoid process and posterior to the biceps and coracobrachialis tendons. The AC and CC ligaments have also been disrupted. (From Rockwood CA Jr, Williams GR Jr, Young DC: Disorders of the acromioclavicular joint, In Rockwood CA Jr, et al, editors: *The shoulder,* ed 3, Philadelphia, Saunders, 2004.)

- Three-part—displacement of the greater or lesser tuberosities and articular surface
- Four-part—displacement of shaft, articular surface and both tuberosities. "Head splitting" is a variant, with split through the articular surface (usually requires replacement for treatment).

2. Treatment
   - One-part—sling for comfort and early mobilization
   - Two-part—repair of the displaced tuberosity with sutures or tension band wiring; surgical neck fractures can normally be managed nonoperatively. Unstable, unimpacted fractures may be treated with closed reduction with percutaneous pinning (CRPP).
     - Immediate physical therapy during nonoperative management results in faster recovery.
   - Three-part
     - **Open reduction with internal fixation (ORIF) for young patients, with repair of the tuberosities or rotator cuff**
     - **Hemiarthroplasty for older patients, with repair of the rotator cuff/tuberosities**
   - Four-part—same as for three-part
     - Humeral height can be judged most reliably using the superior border of the pectoralis major insertion.
       - Nonanatomic placement of the tuberosities leads to significant impairment in external rotation kinematics and an eightfold increase in torque requirements.
3. **Complications**
   - **Avascular necrosis**

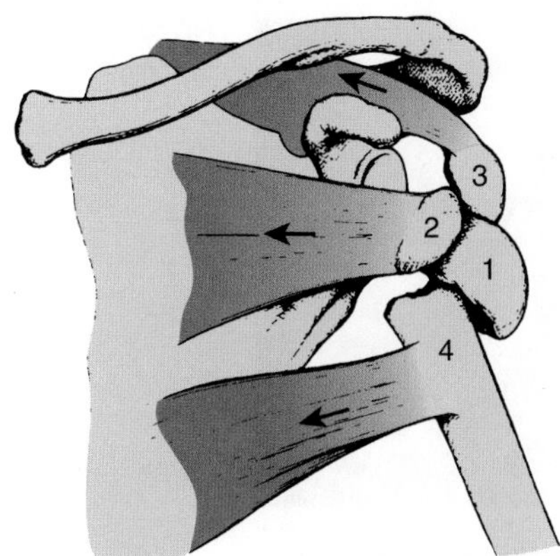

Figure 11-5 Proximal humeral fracture. There are four parts: *1,* head; *2,* lesser tuberosity; *3,* greater tuberosity; and *4,* humeral shaft. (From Neer CS, Rockwood CA: Fractures and dislocations of the shoulder. In Rockwood CA, Green DP, editors: *Fractures in adults,* ed 2, Philadelphia, 1984, JB Lippincott, p 696.)

- ▫ Factors associated with humeral head ischemia:
  - Disruption of the medial periosteal hinge
  - Medial metadiaphyseal extension less than 8 mm
  - Increasing fracture complexity
  - Displacement greater than 10 mm
  - Angulation greater than 45 degrees
- Neurovascular injury
  - ▫ Axillary nerve injury
    - Lateral pins placed during CRPP place the nerve most at risk.
  - ▫ **Anterior pins placed during CRPP risk the biceps tendon, cephalic vein, and musculocutaneous nerve.**
- **Hardware failure**
  - ▫ **The most common complication after locking plate fixation is screw cut out.**
- Nonunion
  - ▫ Most common after two-part fracture of surgical neck
  - ▫ **Nonunion of greater tuberosity following arthroplasty—loss of active shoulder elevation**

J. Shoulder dislocation

1. Anterior or anteroinferior (Figure 11-6) *most common*
   - Diagnosis
     - ▫ Apprehension sign
     - ▫ **The axillary view is diagnostic.**
     - ▫ Usually traumatic and unilateral
     - ▫ Usually painful
   - Treatment—reduction (multiple maneuvers available)
     - ▫ Sling for 2 weeks in the elderly and 4 weeks in the young, followed by rotator cuff strengthening
     - ▫ Consider operative treatment in cases of recurrence or rotator cuff tear.
       - The most common associated injury at arthroscopy after acute dislocation is anterior labral tear, followed by anterior capsular insufficiency and Hill-Sachs lesion.
     - ▫ High recurrence rate in young patients (owing to unstable labral tear)
     - ▫ **High incidence of rotator cuff injury in older patients (>45 years)**
2. Multidirectional
   - Diagnosis
     - ▫ Often bilateral
     - ▫ Often atraumatic, not painful
     - ▫ Examination of the shoulder reveals subluxation posteriorly as well as anteriorly and inferiorly.
     - ▫ Generalized ligamentous laxity
   - Treatment
     - ▫ Rotator cuff strengthening
     - ▫ Inferior capsular shift is indicated if instability is refractory to nonoperative treatment.
3. Posterior (Figure 11-7)
   - Diagnosis
     - ▫ Associated with seizures and electrical shock
     - ▫ Often missed but easily seen on axillary view
     - ▫ May have fracture of lesser tuberosity or reverse Hill-Sachs lesion
   - Treatment
     - ▫ Immobilization for 3 to 6 weeks
     - ▫ Rotator cuff strengthening
     - ▫ Possible open bone grafting of humeral head defect and repair of posterior labral tear
     - ▫ Allograft, coracoid transfer, or resurfacing for large defects
4. Inferior (luxatio erecta)
   - Diagnosis
     - ▫ Associated with motor vehicle collision or sporting injury
     - ▫ **Arm is typically abducted between 100 and 160 degrees.**
     - ▫ Diminished or absent pulses
   - Treatment
     - ▫ Closed reduction successful in 50%
     - ▫ Capsular reconstruction if unstable

II. HUMERAL INJURIES

A. Shaft fracture (Table 11-9)

1. Classification—by location and fracture pattern
2. Treatment
   - Nonoperative treatment—functional brace if there is less than 20 degrees of anterior angulation, less than 30 degrees of valgus/varus angulation, or less than 3 cm of shortening
   - **Operative treatment—open fracture, floating elbow, polytrauma, pathologic fracture, associated brachial plexus injury**
     - ▫ ORIF
       - Probably the gold standard
         - ▫ Anterolateral approach—proximal two thirds
         - ▫ Distal half—posterior approach
         - ▫ Need for radial nerve exploration—lateral approach
       - Higher union rates and decreased secondary operations
       - Weight bearing to tolerance is safe after plate fixation.
     - ▫ IM nail
       - Possibly better for segmental or shaft/proximal humerus combination as well as pathologic fracture

AP in scapular plane.

Arm supported in sling.

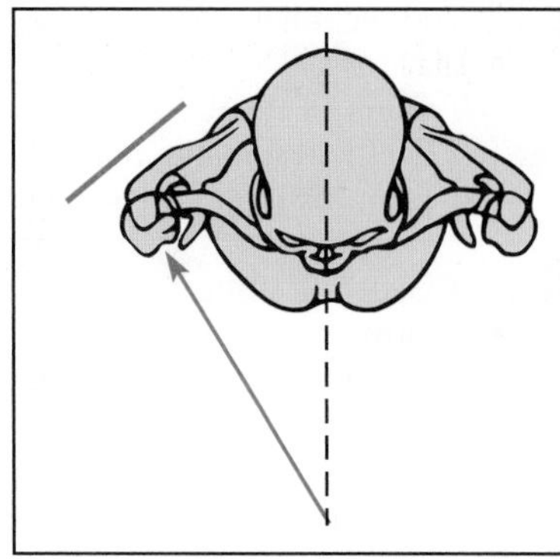

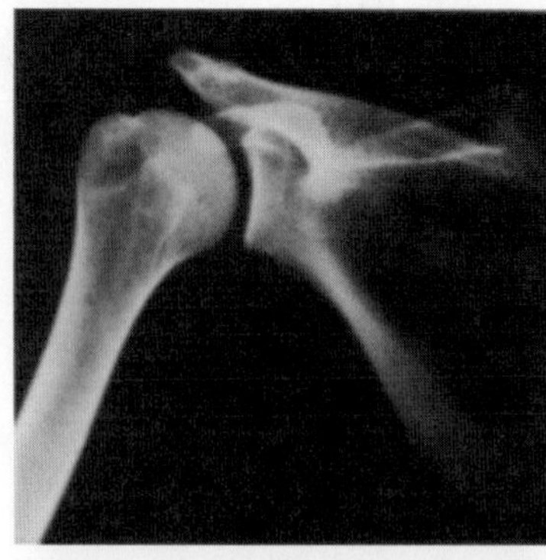

No overlap of head and glenoid.

Lateral in scapular plane.

Arm supported in sling.

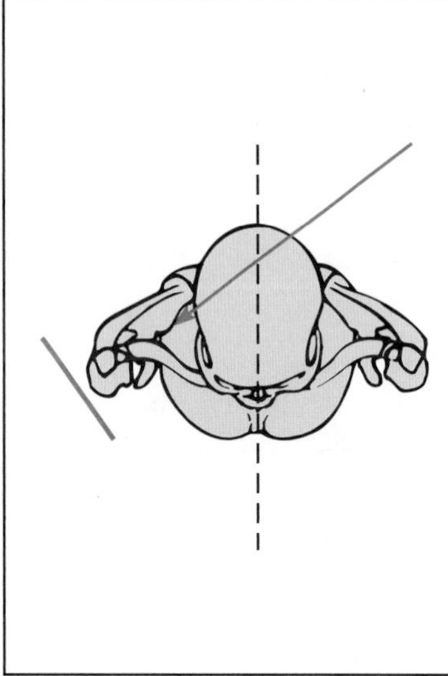

90 to AP.

Head in center of glenoid.

Identify anterior and posterior displacement.

Identify greater tuberosity displacement.

Evaluate shape of acromion for cause of impingement or cuff tears.

Emergency axillary.

Arm is gently abducted.

Tube at the hip.

Involved shoulder supported on pad.

Arm holds IV pole or is supported by assistant.

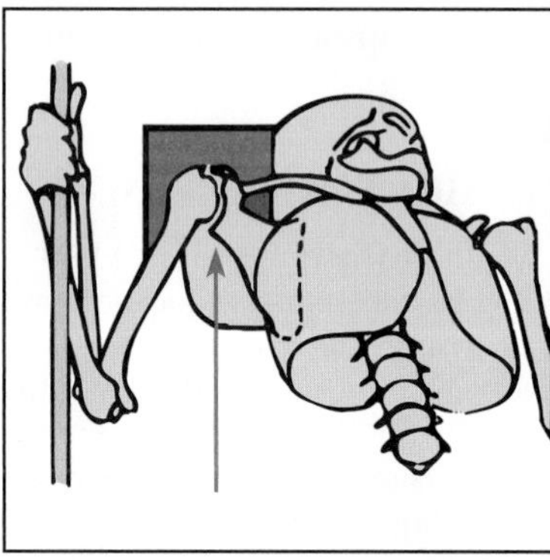

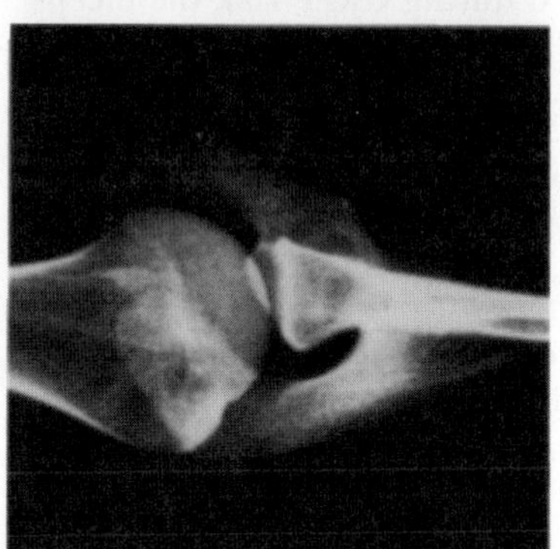

Evaluate glenoid for uneven wear or rim fractures.

Identify anterior and posterior dislocation.

Identify displaced tuberosities.

Identify unfused acromial epiphysis.

Figure 11-6 Trauma series views. (From Norris TR: In Chapman MW, Madison M, editors: *Operative orthopaedics,* Philadelphia, 1988, JB Lippincott, pp 203-220.)

- **Complication rate may be higher and associated with higher rates of reoperation compared with plate fixation.**
- **Distal locking screw risks:**
  - **Radial nerve with lateral to medial screw**
  - **Musculocutaneous nerve with anteroposterior screw**

3. Complications
   - **Radial nerve palsy (5%-10%)**
     - When to observe:
       - The vast majority (up to 92%) resolve with observation for 3 to 4 months.
       - Brachioradialis followed by extensor carpi radialis longus are the first to return, whereas extensor pollicis longus and extensor indicis proprius are last to return.
     - When to explore:
       - Open fracture
         - A higher likelihood of transection
         - Perform ORIF of fracture at time of exploration.
     - Controversial whether to observe or explore:
       - Secondary nerve palsy (i.e., after fracture manipulation)

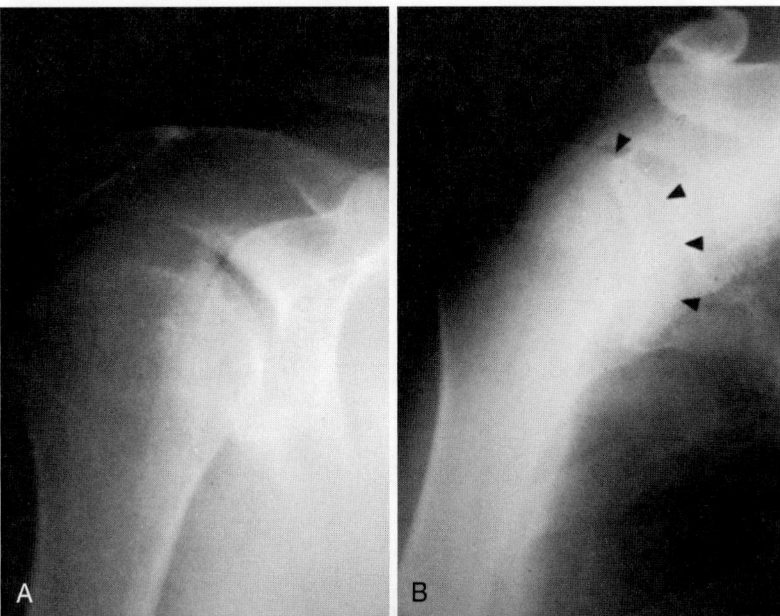

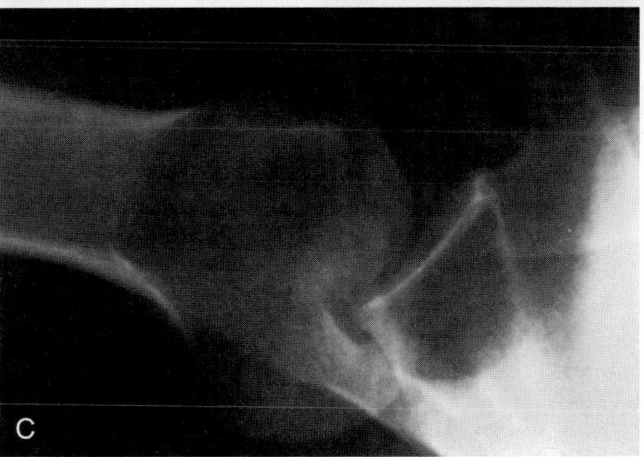

Figure 11-7 Anteroposterior radiographs. **A,** In the sagittal plane of the body (missed posterior dislocation). **B,** In the sagittal plane of the scapula, overlap of the head and glenoid *(arrowheads)* indicates a dislocation. **C,** Axillary or CT scans are the best views for diagnosing posterior dislocation or fracture-dislocation. (From Browner BD, et al, editors: *Skeletal trauma,* ed 4, Philadelphia, 2008, Elsevier.)

- Spiral or oblique fracture of distal third (Holstein-Lewis fracture)
  - Management of palsy that does not recover is also controversial as to timing of electromyography, nerve exploration, and tendon transfers.
- **Nonunion—Treat with compression plate with bone graft if atrophic.**
- Shoulder pain—Some papers report a high incidence of shoulder pain, whereas others do not. **Overall incidence is higher with IM nails.**

B. Supracondylar fracture—rare injury in adults

1. Classification
   - Anatomic location—high, low, abduction, and adduction (Figure 11-8)
   - AO/OTA distal humerus classification
     - Type A—extraarticular
     - Type B—intraarticular, single column
     - Type C—intraarticular, with both columns fractured and no portion of the joint contiguous with the shaft

Table 11-9 Adult Humeral Shaft Fractures

Indications	Eponym	Classification	Treatment	Complications
Pathologic fracture, open fracture, floating elbow Relative indications: segmental fracture, distal spiral with nerve injury (Holstein-Lewis), obesity, thoracic trauma, polytrauma	Holstein-Lewis (distal one third)	Based on location/ fracture pattern	*Nonoperative:* coaptation splint or cast brace if <20-degree anterior angulation, <30-degree varus/valgus, <3-cm shortening *Operative:* consider open reduction with internal fixation (compression plate) vs. IM nail	Nonunion (treat with compression plate and bone graft), malunion, radial nerve injury (5%-10% incidence; observe unless open fracture or persisting for 3-4 months), vascular injury; shoulder pain (IM nail)

IM, intramedullary.

Figure 11-8 **A** to **F**, Transcolumn fractures. These fractures occur in four basic patterns: high, low, abduction, and adduction. The high and low fractures can be further subdivided into extension and flexion patterns. When compared with other fractures of the distal end of the humerus, transcolumn fractures are uncommon. (From Browner BD, et al, editors: *Skeletal trauma,* ed 4, Philadelphia, 2008, Elsevier.)

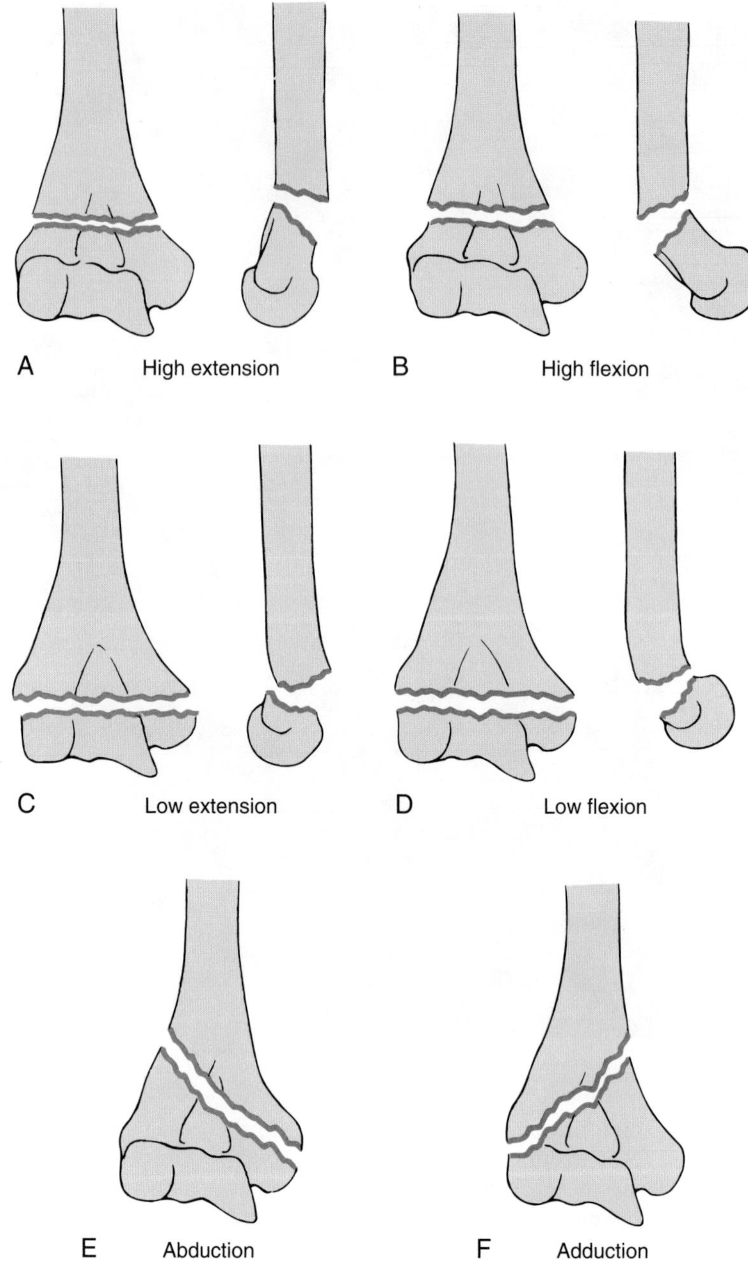

2. Treatment—ORIF
3. Complications—neurovascular injury, nonunion, malunion, and loss of motion (contracture, fibrosis, bony block)

C. Distal single-column (condyle) fracture

1. Classification
   - Classified as Milch types I and II lateral condyle fractures (more common) and types I and II medial condyle fractures. In type I lateral condyle fractures the lateral trochlear ridge is intact, and in type II lateral condyle fractures there is a fracture through lateral trochlear ridge (Figure 11-9).
   - AO/OTA distal humerus classification (see earlier)
2. Treatment—type I nondisplaced: immobilize in supination (lateral condyle fracture) or pronation (medial condyle fracture); otherwise, CRPP or ORIF

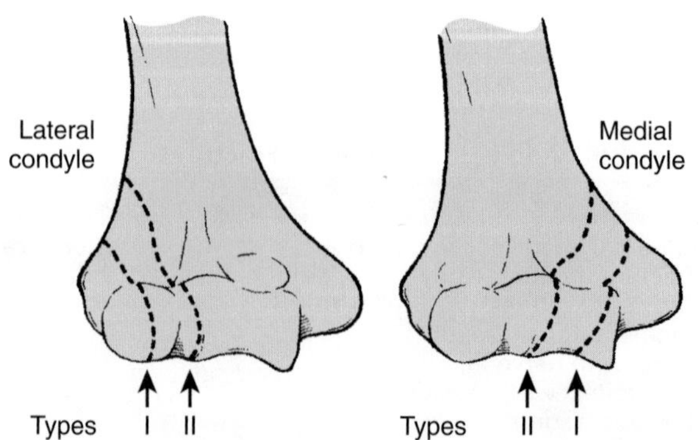

Figure 11-9 Humeral condyle fractures. (From Gelman MI: *Radiology of orthopedic procedures: problems and complications,* vol 24, Philadelphia, 1984, WB Saunders, p 56, reprinted by permission.)

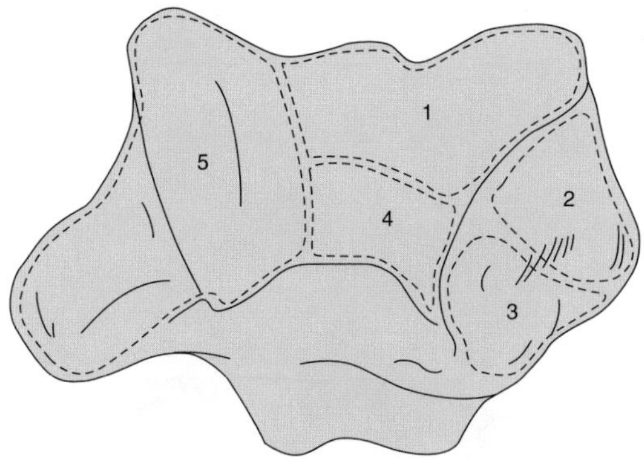

Figure 11-10 Schematic representation of the articular surface of the distal humerus showing the constituent parts of the articular fracture. *1,* Capitellum and lateral portion of the trochlea. *2,* Lateral epicondyle. *3,* Lateral epicondyle, posterior metaphyseal portion. *4,* Posterior aspect of the trochlea. *5,* Medial aspect of the trochlea and medial epicondyle. (From Tornetta P III, Baumgaertner M: *Orthopaedic knowledge update: trauma 3*, Rosemont, Ill, American Academy of Orthopaedic Surgeons, 2005, p 183.)

3. Complications—cubitus valgus (lateral) or cubitus varus (medial), ulnar nerve injury, and degenerative joint disease (DJD)

D. Distal two-column fracture

1. Presentation—Five major articular fragments are identified: capitellum/lateral trochlea, lateral epicondyle, posterolateral epicondyle, posterior trochlea, and medial trochlea/epicondyle (Figure 11-10)
2. Classification
   - Jupiter classification (Figure 11-11)
     - High T—proximal or at level of olecranon fossa
     - Low T (common)—transverse component just proximal to the trochlea
     - Y—oblique portion through both columns with distal vertical fracture
     - H—trochlea is free fragment (**avascular necrosis [AVN]**)
     - Medial lambda—proximal fracture exits medially
     - Lateral lambda—proximal fracture exits laterally
     - Multiplane—T type with additional fracture in coronal plane
   - AO/OTA distal humerus classification (see earlier)
3. Treatment (goal is early ROM with less than 3 weeks of immobilization)
   - **ORIF using a posterior approach with two plates applied to either column**
     - Biomechanical studies support both parallel placement (one plate medial, one plate lateral) and perpendicular placement (one plate medial, one plate posterolateral) configurations
     - Used with olecranon osteotomy or triceps split/peel (final muscle strength similar with both)
     - In an open fracture, use ORIF by means of a triceps split through the defect, producing better results than osteotomy.
     - Low-T fractures are more difficult and frequently require reoperation (almost 50%) for stiffness, but they can have good results.
   - "Bag-of-bones" technique—reasonable for demented patients and those who have severe medical comorbidities that prevent surgical treatment
   - **Total elbow arthroplasty—useful for patients older than age 65 years, particularly with osteoporosis or rheumatoid arthritis**
4. Complications
   - **Stiffness**
     - **Most common complication**
     - **Initially treat with static-progressive splinting**
   - **Loss of elbow muscle strength of 25%**
   - Ulnar nerve injury
     - Treat with anterior transposition
   - Heterotopic ossification (4%)
   - Infection

E. Capitellum fracture

1. Classification
   - Bryan-Morrey (Figure 11-12)
     - Type I—Hahn-Steinthal; complete fracture of capitellum
     - Type II—Kocher-Lorenz; shear fracture of articular cartilage
     - Type III—comminuted
   - **McKee modification**
     - **Type IV—coronal shear fracture including capitellum and trochlea** (Figure 11-13)
2. Treatment
   - Type I—If nondisplaced, splint for 2 to 3 weeks and then allow motion; if displaced more than 2 mm, use ORIF.
   - Type II—If nondisplaced, splint for 2 to 3 weeks and then allow motion; if displaced, excise fragments.
   - Type III—If displaced, excise fragments.
   - **Type IV—ORIF; lateral approach recommended**
3. Complications—nonunion (1%-11% with ORIF), olecranon osteotomy nonunion, ulnar nerve injury, heterotopic ossification (4% with ORIF), and AVN of capitellum

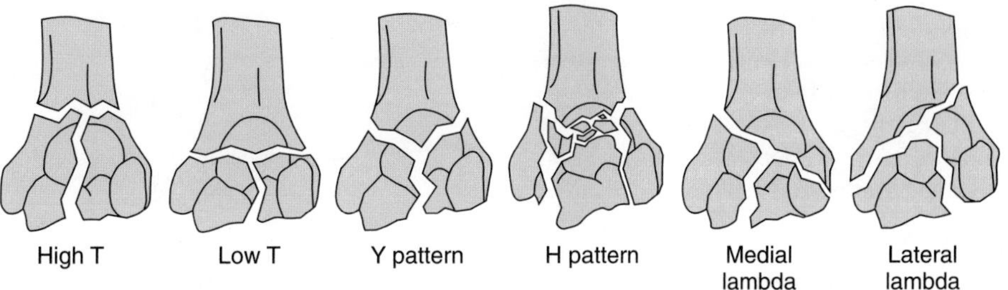

Figure 11-11 Jupiter classification of two-column distal humerus fractures. (From Jupiter J: *Skeletal trauma,* vol 2, Philadelphia, 1992, WB Saunders, pp 1159-1163, reprinted by permission.)

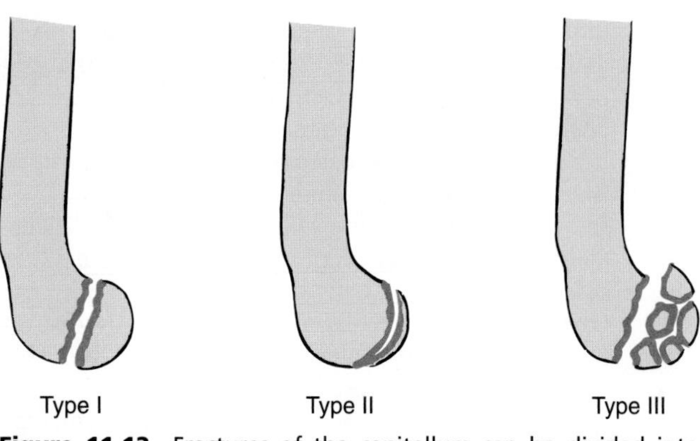

Figure 11-12 Fractures of the capitellum can be divided into type I, a complete capitellar fracture; type II, the more superficial lesion of Kocher-Lorenz; and type III, a comminuted capitellar fracture. (From Browner BD, et al, editors: *Skeletal trauma,* ed 2, Philadelphia, 1998, WB Saunders, p 1511.)

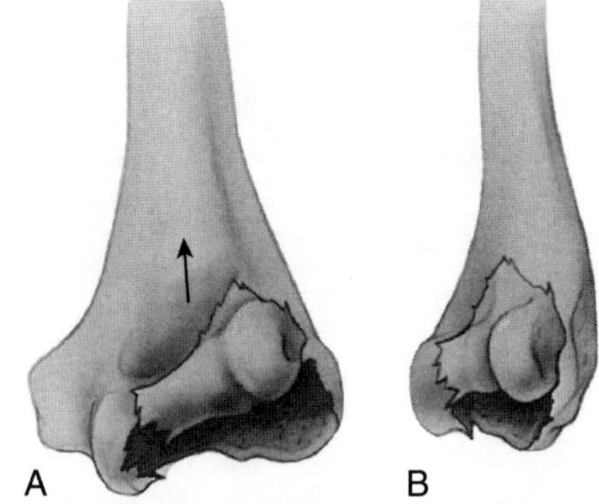

Figure 11-13 Coronal shear fracture of the distal humerus. **A,** Diagram showing separation and proximal migration rotation *(arrow)* of the distal fragment, which includes most of the anterior joint surface. **B,** Oblique view. (From Browner BD, et al, editors: *Skeletal trauma,* ed 2, Philadelphia, 1998, WB Saunders, p 1512.)

III. ELBOW INJURIES (TABLE 11-10)

A. Olecranon fracture

1. Classification—Colton (Figure 11-14)
   - Type I—avulsion
   - Types IIA to IID—oblique fractures with increasing complexity
   - Type III—fracture-dislocation
   - Type IV—atypical, high-energy, comminuted fractures
2. Treatment
   - Less than 1 to 2 mm displaced—Splint at 60 to 90 degrees for 7 to 10 days, followed by gentle active ROM exercises.
   - Tension band—Use stainless steel wire or braided cable, not braided suture material.
     - **The wire loop should be dorsal to the midaxis of the ulna, thus transforming tensile forces at the fracture site into compressive forces.**
     - **Bury Kirschner wires in anterior cortex for increased stability. Protrusion through the anterior cortex, however, is associated with reduced forearm rotation.**
     - Migration of Kirschner wires and prominent or painful hardware occurs in 71%.
   - IM screw fixation—It is inadequate by itself, but a properly placed 7.3-mm partially threaded screw with tension band wiring works well.
   - **Plate fixation (dorsal or tension side)—preferred technique for oblique fractures that extend distal to**

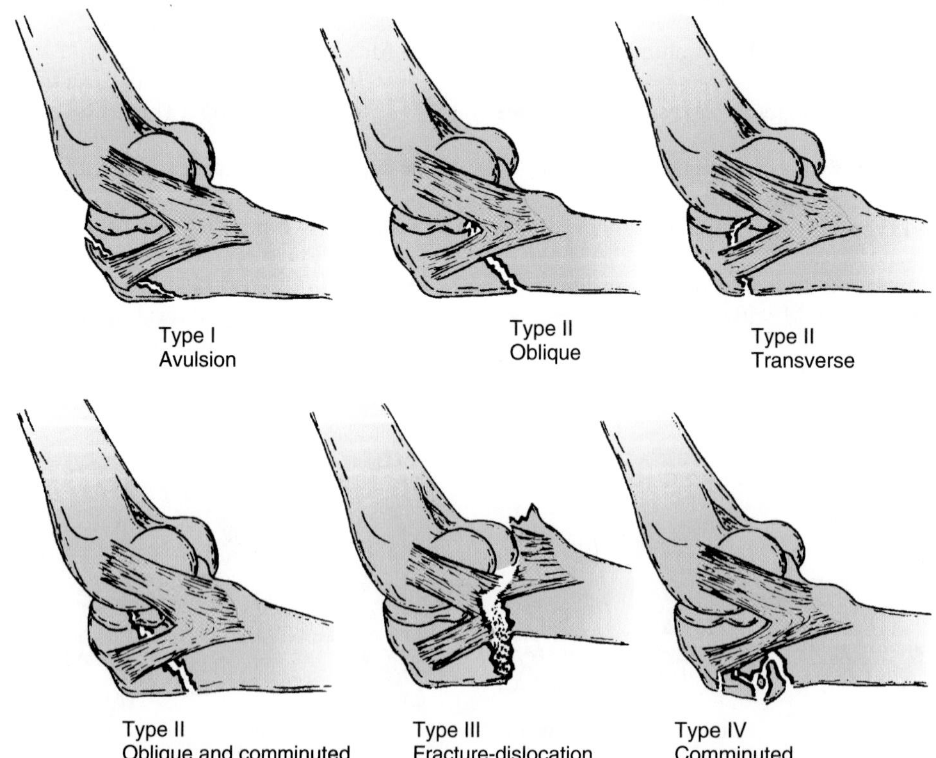

Figure 11-14 Colton classification of olecranon fractures. (From Browner BD, et al, editors: *Skeletal trauma,* ed 2, Philadelphia, 1998, WB Saunders, p 1469.)

Table 11-10 Adult Elbow Fracture-Dislocations

Injury	Eponym	Classification	Treatment	Complications
Supracondylar fracture		AO/OTA classification of distal humerus Type A—extraarticular Type B—intraarticular single column Type C—intraarticular with both columns fractured and no portion of the joint contiguous with the shaft	Displaced: ORIF (double plating)	Neurovascular injury, nonunion, malunion, contracture, pain, decreased ROM (fibrosis, bony block)
Bicolumn fracture		Jupiter I—high T pattern (at level of olecranon fossa) II—low T pattern (proximal to trochlea) III—Y pattern (through both columns, distal vertical fracture) IV—H pattern (trochlea is free fragment) V—medial lambda pattern (proximal fracture exits medially) VI—lateral lambda pattern (proximal fracture exits laterally) VII—multiplane: T type with additional fracture in coronal plane	Nondisplaced: immobilize for 2 wk, then gentle motion Displaced: ORIF (posterior approach, olecranon osteotomy or triceps split/peel): fix condyles first, then epitrochlear ridge to humeral metaphysis Arthroplasty (total elbow arthroplasty) in elderly (consider >6 "Bag of bones" technique for demented patients or those medically unfit for surgery)	Stiffness, heterotopic ossification, infection, ulnar neuropathy (treat with anterior transposition), AVN
Transcondylar fracture	Kocher	Intraarticular (fragment posterior to humerus)	ORIF	↓ROM
	Posadas	Intraarticular (fragment anterior to humerus)	ORIF	
Capitellar fracture		Bryan-Morrey		Nonunion (1%-11% with ORIF), olecranon osteotomy nonunion, ulnar nerve injury, heterotopic ossification (4% with ORIF), AVN of capitellum
	Hahn-Steinthal	I—complete fracture of capitellum, large trochlear piece	Nondisplaced: splint for 2-3 wk, then motion; displaced >2 mm: ORIF	
	Kocher-Lorenz	II—minimum subchondral bone (shear fracture of articular cartilage)	Nondisplaced: splint for 2-3 wk, then motion; displaced: excise displaced fragment	
		III—comminuted fracture	Excise if displaced and unsalvageable	
		IV (McKee modification)—coronal shear fracture, including capitellum and trochlea	ORIF	
Condylar fracture		Milch (lateral >> medial) I—lateral trochlear ridge intact II—fracture through lateral trochlear ridge	*Nondisplaced:* immobilize in supination (lateral condyle), pronation (medial condyle) *Displaced:* CRPP vs. ORIF	Cubitus valgus (lateral), cubitus varus (medial), ulnar nerve neurapraxia, DJD
Trochlear fracture	Laugier	Rare	*Nondisplaced:* splint for 3 wk *Displaced:* ORIF	
Epicondylar fracture	Granger	Medial >> lateral	Manipulation, immobilization for 10-14 days	Painful, unsightly fragment or ulnar nerve symptoms—late excision
Coronoid fracture	Regan and Morrey	Type I—fracture of the tip	Early motion if stable; ORIF with cerclage wire or suture if unstable	Instability (medial) and DJD
		Type II—fracture of <50% of coronoid	ORIF	
		Type III—fracture of >50% of coronoid	ORIF	

Continued

Table 11-10 Adult Elbow Fracture-Dislocations—cont'd

Injury	Eponym	Classification	Treatment	Complications
Olecranon fracture	Colton (modified)	Type I—avulsion Type II (A-D)—oblique fractures with increasing complexity Type III—fracture-dislocations Type IV—atypical high-energy, multifragmented fractures	Minimally displaced (<1-2 mm): splint at 60-90 degrees for 7-10 days, then motion Displaced: ORIF Tension band: use stainless steel wire or braided cable; migration of wire/ prominent hardware in 71% Intramedullary 7.3-mm screw and tension band Plate fixation for oblique and comminuted fractures Excision for unreconstructible proximal olecranon fractures; reattach close to articular surface; avoid >50% resection	↓ROM, DJD, nonunion, ulnar nerve neurapraxia, instability (with removal of >80% of olecranon), symptomatic hardware/need for hardware removal
Radial head fracture	Mason (and Johnston)	I—nondisplaced	Nonoperative; splint for 7 days, then early motion with or without aspiration	Loss of motion, posterior interosseous nerve injury; intraosseous membrane rupture; distal radioulnar joint disruption; Essex-Lopresti (distal radioulnar joint disruption); synovitis if Silastic radial head implant
		II—partially articular with displacement	If elbow stable and no block to motion: splint and early motion; otherwise, ORIF vs. arthroplasty	
		III—comminuted fractures involving the entire head of the radius	Arthroplasty; ORIF if <three pieces, good bone quality; excise in elderly, low functional demands	
		IV—fractures associated with ligamentous injury (elbow dislocation) or other associated fractures	Reduce dislocation and then address fracture surgically (arthroplasty for stability)	
Dislocation (pure ligamentous)		Posterolateral (most common), posterior, anterior, medial, lateral, divergent; simple (no fracture) or complex (fracture)	Closed reduction; check ROM/stability; splint for 2-7 days and then gentle, active ROM; open reduction unstable/ interposed soft tissue ORIF complex (fracture) dislocations	Irreducibility, median and ulnar nerve injury, brachial artery injury, flexion contracture, heterotopic ossification, fractures (medial epicondyle, radial head, coronoid)

AVN, avascular necrosis; CRPP, closed reduction with percutaneous pinning; DJD, degenerative joint disease; ORIF, open reduction and internal fixation; ROM, range of motion.

the coronoid process; more stable than tension band wiring

- **Excision with triceps advancement—used for nonreconstructible proximal olecranon fractures in low-demand patients**. Reattach close to the articular surface. Avoid resecting more than 50% of the olecranon.

3. Complications—decreased ROM, DJD, nonunion, ulnar nerve neurapraxia, and instability

B. Coronoid fracture

1. Classification—Regan and Morrey (Figure 11-15)
   - Type I—fracture of the tip of the coronoid process
   - Type II—fracture of 50% or less of coronoid
   - Type III—fracture of more than 50%

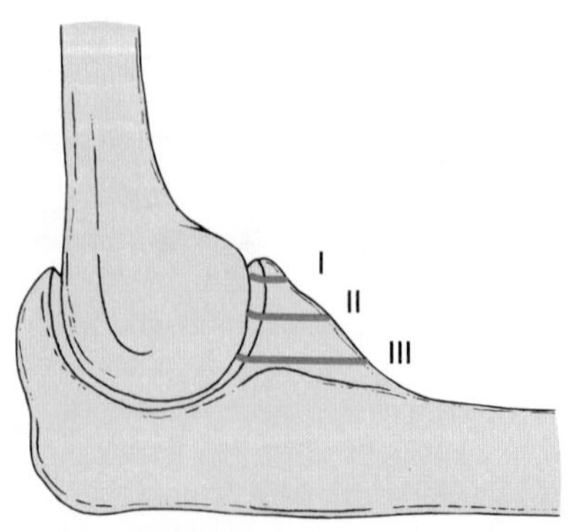

Figure 11-15 The coronoid fracture has been classified into three types by Regan and Morrey. (From Browner BD, et al, editors: *Skeletal trauma,* ed 4, Philadelphia, 2008, Elsevier.)

2. Treatment
   - Type I—associated with episodes of elbow instability. If instability persists, apply cerclage wire or No. 5 suture through drill holes; if instability does not persist, no operation.
   - Types II and III—ORIF helps restore elbow stability; must confirm stability before nonoperative treatment begins
3. Complications—instability (particularly medial) and DJD

C. Radial head fracture

1. Classification (Figure 11-16)
   - Type I—nondisplaced
   - Type II—partial articulation with displacement
   - Type III—comminuted fractures involving the entire head of the radius
   - Type IV—fractures associated with ligamentous injury or other associated fractures
2. Treatment
   - **Type I—Splint for no more than 7 days, and then allow motion.**

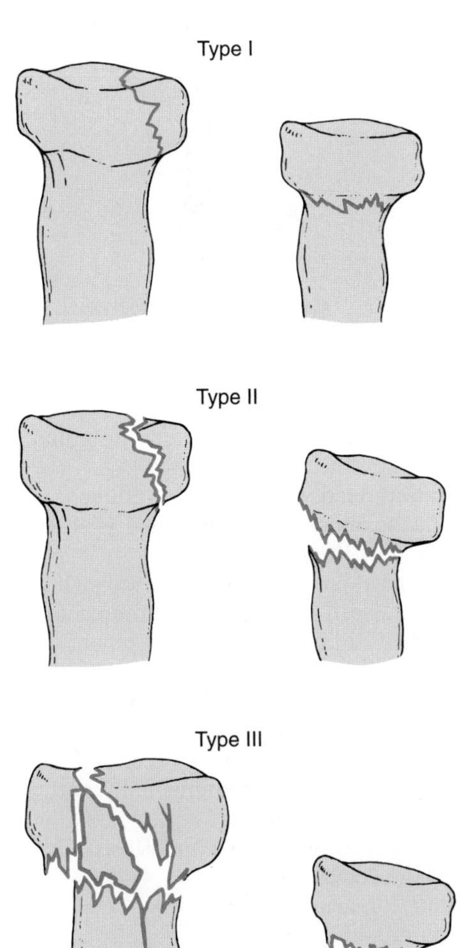

Figure 11-16 Modified Mason classification system for radial head fractures. (From Browner BD, et al, editors: *Skeletal trauma*, ed 4, Philadelphia, 2008, Elsevier.)

   - Type II—Treatment is nonsurgical, with analgesics and active ROM as symptoms resolve, if the elbow is stable and there is no block to motion with good reduction. Otherwise, use ORIF. Surgery provides better results (90%-100% good or excellent).
   - **Type III—Replace the radial head, usually with a metal implant. Use ORIF if fewer than three pieces. Excise only in elderly patients with low functional demands.**
   - Type IV—requires surgical repair: must use either ORIF or metallic radial head replacement. Do not excise without adding radial head implant.
     - **Safe zone for ORIF of radial head/neck is 110-degree arc (i.e., 25%) along lateral side, defined by radial styloid and Lister tubercle.**
3. Complications
   - Loss of motion
   - **Posterior interosseous nerve injury**
     - **Pronate arm to avoid injury.**
   - Radial shortening if Essex-Lopresti injury
   - Synovitis if a Silastic radial head implant is used

D. Dislocation

1. Classification (Figure 11-17)
   - Eighty percent are posterolateral; the rest are posterior, anterior, medial, lateral, or divergent.
   - Simple (no associated fracture) or complex (fracture)
     - Associated injuries
       - Avulsion fracture of medial or lateral epicondyle
       - Radial head and neck fractures
       - Coronoid fractures
       - Osteochondral injury
2. Treatment
   - **Simple—brief immobilization (1 week) for most and then allow motion. Long-term results are good.**
   - Complex—Surgical treatment is indicated. Anterior or divergent dislocations are usually high-energy injuries with a much higher incidence of open wounds, neurovascular injury, fracture, and recurrent instability.
3. Complications
   - Stiffness and flexion contracture
     - Directly correlated with period of immobilization greater than 3 weeks
   - Heterotopic ossification (collateral ligaments)
   - Ulnar or median nerve injury
   - Brachial artery injury

E. Terrible triad of the elbow

1. Elbow dislocation with lateral collateral ligament injury, radial head fracture, and coronoid fracture
   - **The lateral collateral ligament injury is typically a ligamentous avulsion from the origin on the distal humerus.**
2. **Always unstable and requires treatment**
3. **Treatment**
   - **Coronoid ORIF**
   - **Radial head ORIF or replacement**
   - **Lateral collateral ligament repair (typically to distal humerus)**
   - **Possible medial collateral ligament repair depending on stability**

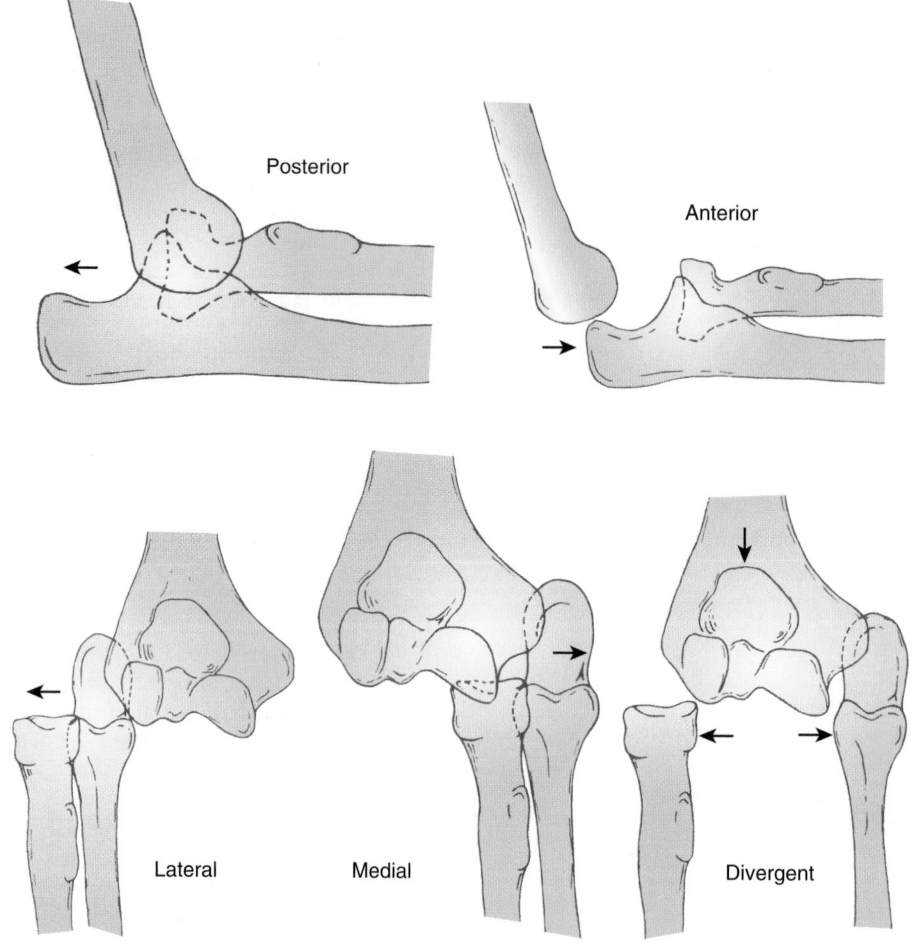

Figure 11-17 Classification of simple elbow dislocations. (Courtesy of Jupiter JB, Mehne DK: Fractures of the adult elbow. In Skirven T, et al, editors: *Rehabilitation of the hand and upper extremity,* ed 6, Philadelphia, 2011, Elsevier.)

IV. FOREARM FRACTURES (TABLE 11-11)

A. Monteggia fractures

1. Diagnosis/classification
   - Bado classification (Figure 11-18)
     - Type 1 (60%)—anterior radial head dislocation and apex anterior proximal third ulna fracture
     - Type 2 (15%)—posterior radial head dislocation and apex posterior proximal third ulna fracture
     - Type 3—lateral radial head dislocation and proximal ulnar metaphyseal fracture
     - Type 4—anterior radial head dislocation and proximal third radius and ulna fractures
     - "Monteggia-equivalent or variant"—radial head fracture instead of dislocation
   - Interosseous membrane evaluation is important with Monteggia and Monteggia-equivalent injuries.
     - Physical examination—considered abnormal if greater than 3-mm instability is noted when the radius pulled proximally, indicating injury. If injury is greater than 6 mm, both the interosseous membrane and the triangular fibrocartilage complex are injured.
     - Confirm diagnosis with findings on MRI or ultrasonography.
     - Middle third is strongest and most important for stability.
2. Treatment—All Monteggia fractures in adults should be treated with ORIF.
   - **The radial head will normally reduce and be stable. If not, the most common cause is a nonanatomic reduction of the ulna.**
   - If the ulna is anatomic and the radial head does not reduce, an open reduction with a separate approach is required to address the annular ligament.
3. Complications
   - **The complication rate is higher for Monteggia-equivalent and Bado type II injuries.**
   - **PIN injury**
     - **Usually resolves spontaneously and should be observed for 3 months**
   - Redislocation/subluxation, synostosis, and loss of motion

B. Both-bone forearm fractures

1. Classification—displaced versus nondisplaced
2. Treatment
   - ORIF in adults
   - **ORIF with cancellous bone graft**
     - **Significant segmental bone loss**
     - **Bone loss associated with open injury**
     - **Routine use of bone graft for closed, comminuted fractures is no longer indicated.**

Table 11-11 Adult Radial and Ulnar Shaft Fractures and Dislocations

Injury	Eponym/Other Name	Classification	Treatment	Complications
Radius and ulna fractures	"Both-bone"	Degree of displacement	ORIF with six-hole DCP; external fixation for type III open fracture, bone graft if >one-third (shaft) comminution	Malunion/nonunion, vascular injury, posterior interosseous nerve (PIN) injury, compartment syndrome, synostosis, infection, refracture (after plate removal)
Ulna fracture	Nightstick	Nondisplaced	Distal two thirds, <50% displaced, <10-degree angulation: long arm cast to functional brace with good interosseous mold	Malunion, nonunion
		Displaced	Proximal one third, >50% displaced, >10-degree angulation: ORIF; look for wrist/elbow injury	
Proximal ulna and radial head fracture	Monteggia	Bado		Posterior intraosseous nerve injury (usually spontaneously resolves), redislocation/ subluxation (inadequate reduction), synostosis, loss of motion
		Type I (60%)—radial head dislocation, anterior and apex anterior proximal one-third ulna fracture	ORIF of ulna (DCP), closed-reduction head, immobilize; if radial head irreducible, ulna fracture reduction may be nonanatomic	
		Type II (15%)—radial head dislocation, posterior and apex posterior proximal one-third ulna shaft fracture	ORIF of ulna (DCP), closed reduction head, immobilize at 70 degrees	
		Type III—radial head dislocation, lateral and proximal ulnar metaphyseal fracture	ORIF of ulna (DCP), closed reduction head, immobilize	
		Type IV—radial head dislocation, anterior fracture and forearm fracture of both bones	ORIF of radius and ulna, closed reduction head, immobilize	
Proximal radius fracture		Nondisplaced	Long-arm cast in supination, close follow-up	
		Displaced	Proximal one fifth: closed; one fifth–two thirds: ORIF	
Distal radius (distal one third) and radioulnar dislocation	Galeazzi/Piedmont	Supination/pronation (signs of instability: ulnar styloid fracture, widened distal radioulnar joint on posteroanterior view, dislocation on lateral view, ≥5-mm radial shortening)	ORIF of radius (volar), closed reduction with or without percutaneous pinning to radioulnar joint (in supination) if unstable	Angulation, distal subluxation, malunion, nonunion; displaced by gravity, pronator quadratus, brachioradialis

DCP, dynamic compression plate; ORIF, open reduction and internal fixation.

3. Complications
   - **Malunion (stiffness/deformity)**
     - **Restoration of the radial bow is directly related to functional outcome.**
   - Nonunion
     - Typically due to technical error or use of IM fixation
     - **Treat with ORIF and bone grafting.**
   - **Refracture after plate removal**
     - **Associated with premature plate removal at less than 12 to 18 months**
     - After plate removal, a functional forearm brace should be worn for 6 weeks and activity protected for 3 months.
   - **Synostosis**
     - **Associated with single incision approach to ORIF**
     - **Treated with early excision, irradiation, and indomethacin**

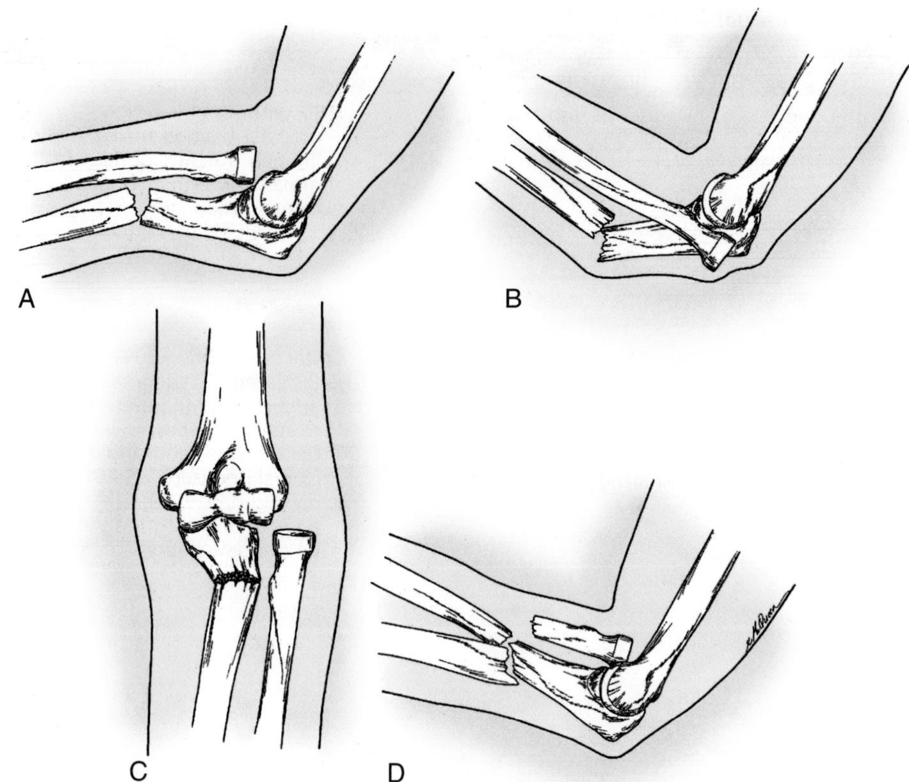

Figure 11-18 Monteggia fracture-dislocations. **A,** Type 1. **B,** Type 2. **C,** Type 3. **D,** Type 4. (From Crenshaw AH: Adult fractures and complex joint injuries of the elbow. In Stanley D, Kay NRM, editors: *Surgery of the elbow: practical and scientific aspects,* London, 1998, Arnold.)

- **Posterior interosseous nerve injury**
  - **Henry (volar) approach to the middle and upper third of radial diaphysis**
- Vascular injury

C. Ulna "nightstick" fractures

1. Classification—stable (traditional definition is <50% displacement) versus unstable (newer literature suggests that 25%-50% displacement or 10-15 degrees angulation is unstable)
2. Treatment
   - **Distal two thirds, less than 50% displaced, and less than 10 degrees angulation—short arm cast to functional fracture brace with good interosseous mold**
   - Proximal third, very distal shaft/head, over 50% displaced, or over 10 degrees angulation—ORIF
3. Complications—malunion/nonunion

D. Distal third radius fracture with radioulnar dislocation (Galeazzi)

1. Diagnosis/classification—fracture of the radius (usually at the junction of the middle and distal thirds), with distal radioulnar joint (DRUJ) instability
   - DRUJ instability
     - DRUJ is unstable in 55% of patients when the radial fracture is less than 7.5 cm from the articular surface.
     - DRUJ is unstable in 6% of patients when the radial fracture is more than 7.5 cm away from the articular surface.
     - Signs of DRUJ instability include ulnar styloid fracture, widened DRUJ on posteroanterior view, dislocation on lateral view, and greater than or equal to 5 mm of radial shortening.
2. Treatment
   - **Perform ORIF of the radius and then supinate the forearm and assess DRUJ.**
     - Reduced and stable—protective splint and early motion
     - Reduced and unstable
       - Large ulnar styloid fragment—Perform ORIF of styloid and immobilize in supination.
       - No fragment—Pin ulna to radius and immobilize in supination.
     - **Irreducible**
       - **Most commonly due to interposition of extensor carpi ulnaris tendon**
       - **Approach DRUJ via dorsal incision and remove block.**
3. Complications—malunion/nonunion and DRUJ subluxation

V. WRIST FRACTURES (TABLE 11-12)

A. Distal radius fractures

1. Classification
   - Frykman classification—types I to VIII (Figure 11-19)
     - Types II, IV, VI, and VIII—include the ulnar styloid
     - Type I—extraarticular
     - Type III—enters radiocarpal joint
     - Type V—enters radioulnar joint
     - Type VII—enters both joints
   - Melone classification (Figure 11-20—describes radiocarpal joint as four fragments:
     - Radial styloid

Table 11-12 Adult Wrist and Carpal Fractures

Injury	Eponym	Classification	Treatment	Complications
Distal radius fracture	Colles (dorsal displacement)	Frykman (I-VIII; even number = ulnar styloid fracture) I—extraarticular III—intraarticular radiocarpal joint fracture V—intraarticular radioulnar joint fracture VII—displaced intraarticular radiocarpal and radioulnar joint fractures	Distract, manipulate, splint 15 degrees palmar flexion and ulnar deviation, external fixation, and/or ORIF if comminuted/unstable; external fixation for severe comminution, ORIF for large fragments with a >15-degree dorsal tilt; >1-2–mm articular displacement; bone graft comminuted fractures	Loss of reduction, nonunion, malunion, median neuropathy/carpal tunnel syndrome, weakness, tendon adhesion/rupture, instability, extensor pollicis longus rupture, DISI >15 degrees (extension), ulnar side pain (shortening), CRPS, Volkmann ischemic contracture
Smith (volar displacement)	Intraarticular vs. extraarticular	Distract, manipulate, splint in supination, flexion; CRPP vs. ORIF (volar approach)	Missed diagnosis, similar to Colles fracture	
Dorsal rim of radius fracture	Dorsal Barton	Fernandez type II	Majority: ORIF with dorsal approach	Similar to Colles fracture
Radial styloid fracture	Chauffeur	Fernandez type II	Reduction, CRPP, cannulated screw or plate; immobilize in ulnar deviation	Similar to Colles fracture; rule out associated perilunate injury (ORIF)
Volar rim of radius fracture	Volar Barton	Fernandez type II	Majority: ORIF with volar buttress plate	Similar to Colles fracture
Distal radioulnar joint dissociation		Based on ulna displacement; fracture of base of ulnar styloid associated with TFCC tear	Dorsal—reduction, full supination, long arm cast for 6 wk Volar—reduction (may require open reduction), long-arm cast for 6 wk in pronation	Osteochondral fracture, TFCC injury, ulnar nerve compression, instability, arthrosis, weak grip, decreased forearm rotation
Scaphoid fracture		Based on anatomic location (neck, waist, body, proximal pole)	Evaluate with anteroposterior, lateral, navicular, and clenched-fist views; plain radiographs; MRI for occult fracture; CT to characterize fracture, evaluate nonunion Nondisplaced: thumb spica (long-arm cast for proximal and mid-body, short arm cast for distal pole) ORIF if displaced, unstable, proximal pole, nonunion	Nonunion (CT evaluation; bone graft), instability, refracture, nerve injury, CRPS, DJD, pain, missed fracture (MRI best for diagnosis of occult injury)
Triquetrum fracture		Dorsal shear (most common) vs. body (rare)	Short-arm cast for 4 wk; ORIF if displaced body fracture	
Pisiform fracture		Uncommon (1%-3% of all carpal fractures)	Short-arm cast in flexion/ulnar deviation for 6 wk	Nonunion (treat with excision); associated with distal radius, hamate, triquetrum fractures
Trapezium fracture		Body, trapezial ridge	Nonoperative: short-arm cast with molded abduction of first ray; ORIF of intraarticular displaced-body fractures	Body: associated CMC dislocation or Bennett fracture; trapezial ridge fracture: chronic pain (treat with excision)
Capitate fracture		Rare	Closed treatment if nondisplaced, ORIF if displaced	Associated with perilunate dislocations, scaphoid fractures, and CMC fracture-dislocations; osteonecrosis; nonunion (treat with fusion of capitate, scaphoid, and lunate)
Perilunate instability/dislocation (with or without scaphoid fracture)		Mayfield I—scapholunate dissociation II—lunocapitate disruption III—lunotriquetral disruption IV—lunate dislocation	Early (6-8 wk): open (dorsal) ligament repair and ORIF scaphoid fracture (if present) Late: triscaphoid fusion, proximal row carpectomy, or wrist fusion	Rotatory instability of scaphoid, median nerve palsy, late flexor rupture

Continued

Table 11-12 Adult Wrist and Carpal Fractures—cont'd

Injury	Eponym	Classification	Treatment	Complications
Rotatory scapholunate dissociation	Terry Thomas sign	>3-mm scapholunate interval on anteroposterior vs. contralateral wrist view; scapholunate angle > 60 degrees, scaphoid ring sign	Closed reduction, immobilization; ORIF if scaphoid fracture displaced; open repair of ligaments (volar and dorsal, capsulodesis)	Late DJD (advanced collapse of scapholunate)
Lunate fracture		Based on fracture location (volar pole most common)	ORIF for displaced fracture; nonoperative for nondisplaced injury	Disorganization, disintegration; distinguish from Kienböck
Hamate fracture		Based on location and size of fragment—body or hook	Body: closed treatment if nondisplaced; CRPP or ORIF if displaced or unstable Hook: closed treatment if acute, excise if chronic and symptomatic	Missed on plain films (CT view required); body: associated with fourth and fifth CMC fracture-dislocation; hook: ulnar nerve symptoms, flexor tendon problems
Carpal instability		DISI (most common), scapholunate angle > 70 degrees VISI, scapholunate angle < 35 degrees Axial injury	Closed reduction of acute injuries followed by early repair; open scapholunate reconstruction for failed/late reduction/ SLAC for wrist; ORIF axial injuries	DISI, VISI: DJD, stiffness, treatment for chronic instability controversial; axial: usually high energy with soft tissue injury, nerve/vascular/ muscle injury

CMC, carpometacarpal; CRPP, closed reduction with percutaneous pinning; CRPS, complex regional pain syndrome; CT, computed tomography; DISI, dorsal intercalated segment instability; DJD, degenerative joint disease; MRI, magnetic resonance imaging; ORIF, open reduction and internal fixation; SLAC, scapholunate advanced collapse; TFCC, triangular fibrocartilage complex; VISI, volar intercalated segment instability.

    - Shaft
    - Volar medial
    - Dorsal medial
    - Types I to IV represent increasingly comminuted fractures of the aforementioned four anatomic regions and their parts.
    - Type V is an extremely comminuted, unstable fracture without large, identifiable facet fragments).
  - Fernandez classification (Figure 11-21)—based on the mechanism of injury and designed to guide treatment decision making
    - Type I—bending fractures
    - Type II—articular shear fractures
    - Type III—compression fractures
    - Type IV—fracture-dislocations (associated with ligamentous injury)
    - Type V—combined mechanisms
2. Treatment—based on the Fernandez classification
  - Type I—usually an extra-articular metaphyseal fracture. Comminution determines stability. The volarly displaced radial fracture is much more unstable. Use conservative treatment with reduction and casting if stable and CRPP versus internal/external fixation if unstable.
  - Type II—shearing injury of the joint surface (volar or dorsal lip or radial styloid). This type is usually unstable, and carpal subluxation frequently occurs. Treatment is with ORIF.
  - Type III—Articular compression (die-punch) injuries follow the patterns described by Melone.
    - Conservative treatment if nondisplaced
    - ORIF with disimpaction of the articular surface if displaced. Arthroscopy may be adjunct.
  - Type IV—rare and follows high-energy trauma
    - These are avulsion fractures with radiocarpal fracture dislocations.
    - Surgical repair of the avulsed styloid usually restores stability. Treat with closed or, more frequently, open reduction, pin or screw fixation, or tension wiring.
  - Type V—combination fractures of types I to IV after high-energy trauma. These are very severe and unstable fractures. There are always associated injuries. Treatment is open, with combined methods.
3. Outcomes—Restoration of anatomic alignment is the best predictor of a good outcome.
  - The loss of radial length and volar tilt is the most important, and radial inclination is less important.
  - Articular step-offs of more than 1 to 2 mm also predict poor outcome.
4. Complications—loss of reduction, malunion/nonunion, median nerve neuropathy, weakness, tendon adhesion, instability, extensor pollicis longus rupture, dorsal intercalated segment instability (DISI), and Volkmann ischemic contracture

B. Other variants and eponyms

1. Dorsal rim radius fractures—dorsal Barton (Figure 11-22)
  - Classification—Fernandez type II
  - Treatment—ORIF with dorsal approach in the vast majority
  - Complications—same as for distal radius fracture
2. Radial styloid fractures—chauffeur fracture (Figure 11-23)
  - Diagnosis/classification—frequently high-energy trauma in young adults. Fernandez type II is associated with perilunate injuries.
  - Treatment—CRPP or ORIF with screws; immobilize in ulnar deviation.
  - Complications—same as for distal radius fracture

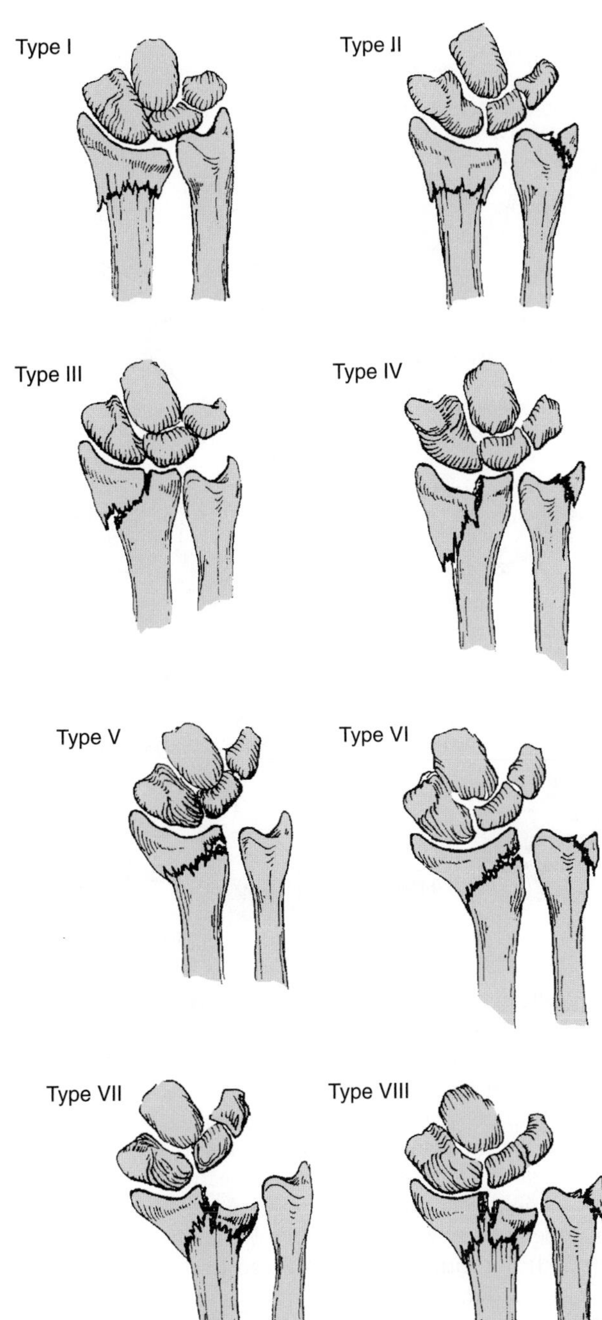

Figure 11-19 **The Frykman classification of distal radius fractures. Note even numbers with ulnar styloid involvement.** (From Kozin SH, Berlet AC: *Handbook of common orthopaedic fractures,* West Chester, Penn, 1989, Medical Surveillance, pp 17, 19.)

3. Volar rim radius fractures—volar Barton fracture (Figure 11-24)
   - Classification—Fernandez type II
   - Treatment—usually with ORIF by means of the volar approach; closed reduction (rarely)
   - Complications—same as for distal radius fracture
4. DRUJ injuries
   - Diagnosis/classification—fracture of the base of the ulnar styloid, associated with triangular fibrocartilage complex tear
   - Treatment—closed or open reduction to achieve anatomic ulnar styloid reduction; immobilize in supination
   - Complications—osteochondral fracture, ulnar nerve compression, instability, arthrosis, weak grip, and decreased forearm rotation

VI. CARPAL INJURIES

See Table 11-12.

A. Scaphoid fracture

1. Classification—based on anatomic location (Figure 11-25)
   - Neck
   - Waist
   - Body
   - Proximal pole
2. Diagnosis
   - Radiographs—anteroposterior, lateral, navicular, and clenched-fist views
   - MRI—to rule out occult fracture
   - CT with sagittal and coronal reconstructions—characterizes fracture and evaluates union
3. Treatment
   - General principles
     - Short-arm–thumb spica immobilization until definitive diagnosis and treatment plan are made.
     - Rule out occult fracture in those with a high index of suspicion and negative plain radiographs.
     - Stable fixation and immobilization
   - Nonoperative treatment
     - Nondisplaced distal fracture—short arm–thumb spica cast for 8 to 12 weeks
     - Nondisplaced proximal and midbody fractures—long arm–thumb spica cast for 6 weeks, followed by short-arm–thumb spica cast until union
   - Operative treatment
     - Indications—Operative treatment is used for displaced fractures, unstable fractures, proximal pole fractures, and delayed diagnosis.
     - ORIF—percutaneous screw fixation under arthroscopic assistance using headless variable-pitch screws
4. Complications
   - Nonunion (treat with Russe bone graft)
   - Instability
   - Refracture
   - Nerve injury
   - DJD
   - Pain
   - Missed fracture (bone scan or MRI helpful)

B. Lunate fracture

1. Diagnosis/classification—The mechanism of injury is direct trauma. The classification is based on fracture location, with fracture of the volar pole being most common. Lunate fracture must be distinguished from Kienböck disease.
2. Treatment
   - Nonoperative treatment—used for nondisplaced fractures
   - Operative treatment—ORIF used for displaced fractures
3. Complications—disorganization and disintegration of the lunate

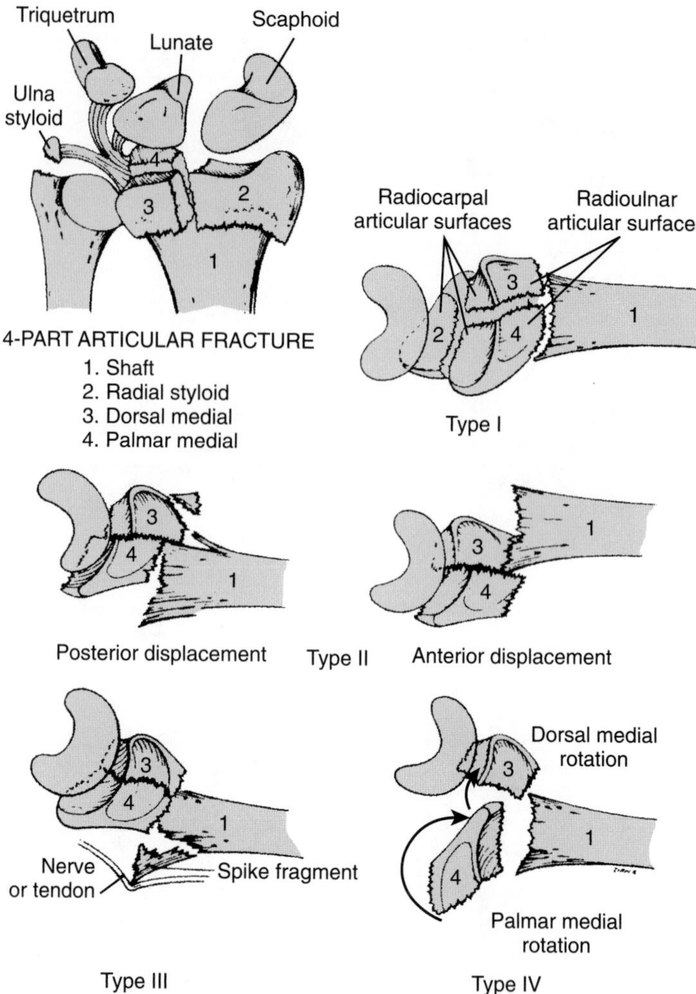

Figure 11-20 The Melone classification of distal radius fractures. (From Melone CP Jr: Open treatment for displaced articular fractures of the distal radius, *Clin Orthop Relat Res* 202:104, 1986, reprinted by permission.)

C. Triquetrum fracture
1. Diagnosis/classification
   - Dorsal shear injury—very common; the third most common carpal fracture after scaphoid and lunate
   - Body fracture (rare)
2. Treatment
   - Nonoperative treatment
     - Dorsal shear injury—closed treatment for 4 to 6 weeks; excision of fragment if symptoms continue
     - Body fracture—closed treatment if nondisplaced
   - Operative treatment—ORIF for displaced body fracture
3. Complications—usually asymptomatic

D. Pisiform fracture
1. Diagnosis/classification
   - Uncommon—1% to 3% of all carpal fractures
   - Fifty percent with distal radius, hamate, or triquetrum fracture
2. Treatment—short arm cast with 30 degrees of wrist flexion and ulnar deviation for 6 weeks
3. Complications—nonunion (treat with excision)

E. Trapezium fracture
1. Classification
   - Body fracture
   - Trapezial ridge fracture
     - Base of ridge
     - Tip of ridge
2. Treatment
   - Nonoperative treatment
     - Trapezial ridge I—attempted closed treatment and early excision for nonunion common
     - Trapezial ridge II—closed treatment for 6 weeks (molded abduction of first ray)
   - Operative treatment—For body fractures, treatment is ORIF for intraarticular displaced fracture.
3. Complications
   - Body—associated carpometacarpal dislocation or Bennett fracture
   - Trapezial ridge I fracture—chronic pain (requires excision)

F. Capitate fracture
1. Evaluation—rarely occurs in isolation
2. Treatment—ORIF
3. Complications
   - Associated with perilunate dislocations, scaphoid fracture, and carpometacarpal fracture-dislocation
   - Osteonecrosis
   - Nonunion (may be treated by fusion of the capitate, scaphoid, and lunate)

G. Hamate fracture
1. Diagnosis/classification
   - Body fracture—uncommon
   - Hook-of-hamate fracture—common in golf, baseball, and racquet sports

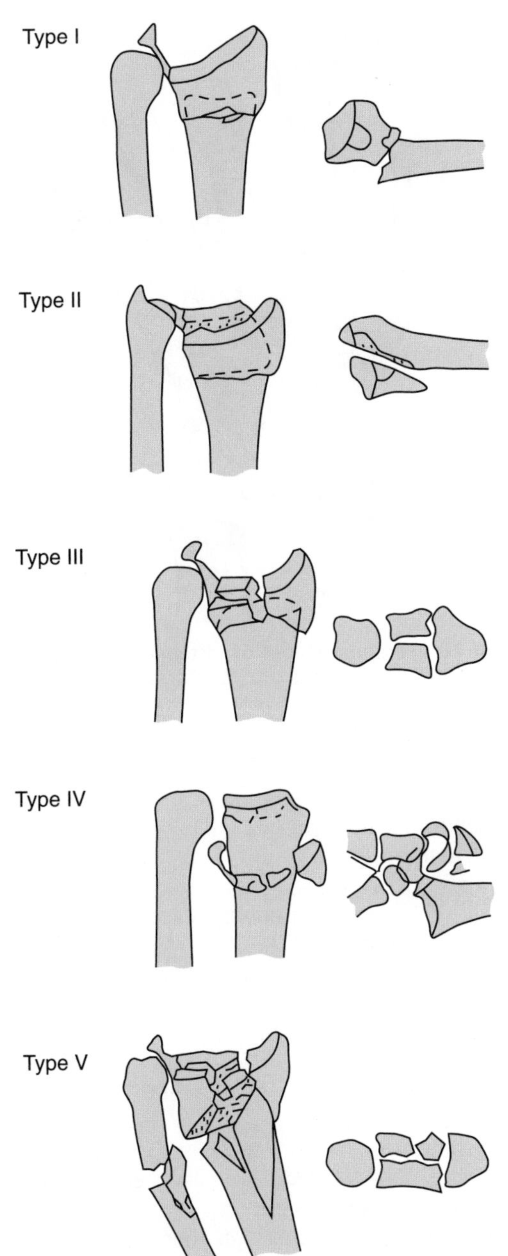

Figure 11-21 The Fernandez classification of distal radius fractures (fracture types in adults based on the mechanism of injury). (From Tornetta P III, Baumgaertner M: *Orthopaedic knowledge update: trauma 3,* Rosemont, Ill, 2005, American Academy of Orthopaedic Surgeons, p 206.)

2. Treatment
   - Nonoperative treatment
     - Body fracture—closed treatment for nondisplaced fracture
     - Hook-of-hamate fracture—closed treatment for 6 weeks if acute
   - Operative treatment
     - Body fracture—CRPP or ORIF if displaced or unstable
     - Hook-of-hamate fracture—excision or (rarely) ORIF
3. Complications
   - Body fracture—associated with fourth and fifth carpometacarpal fracture-dislocation

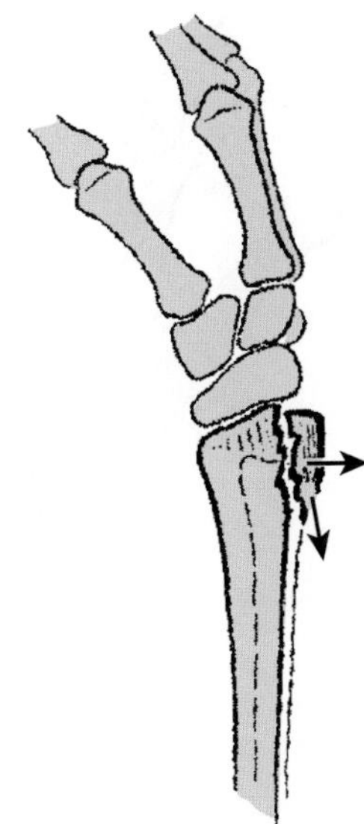

Figure 11-22 The Barton fracture (dorsal). (From Connolly JF, editor: *DePalma's the management of fractures and dislocations: an atlas,* ed 3, Philadelphia, 1981, WB Saunders, p 1032, reprinted by permission.)

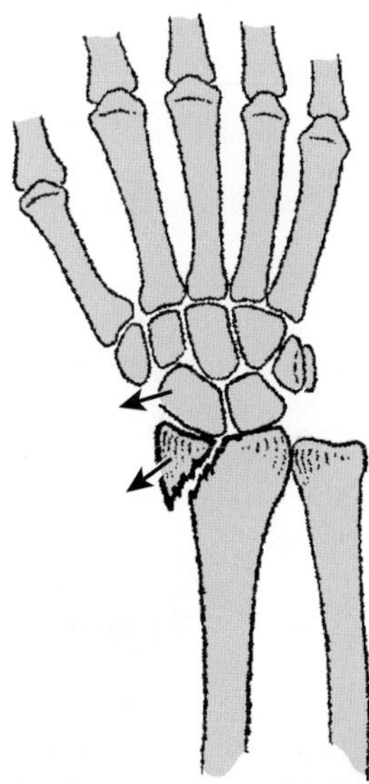

Figure 11-23 Radial styloid fractures. (From Connolly JF, editor: *DePalma's the management of fractures and dislocations: an atlas,* ed 3, Philadelphia, 1981, WB Saunders, p 1033, reprinted by permission.)

   - Hook-of-hamate fracture—ulnar nerve and flexor tendon symptoms or attritional rupture

H. Perilunate instability

1. Mayfield classification (Figure 11-26)
   - Scapholunate dissociation
   - Lunocapitate disruption
   - Lunotriquetral disruption
   - Lunate dislocation
2. Operative treatment
   - Early (6 to 8 weeks)—open (dorsally); ligament repair and ORIF scaphoid fracture (if present)
   - Late—triscaphoid fusion, proximal row carpectomy, or wrist fusion
3. Complications—rotatory instability of the scaphoid, median nerve palsy, and late flexor rupture

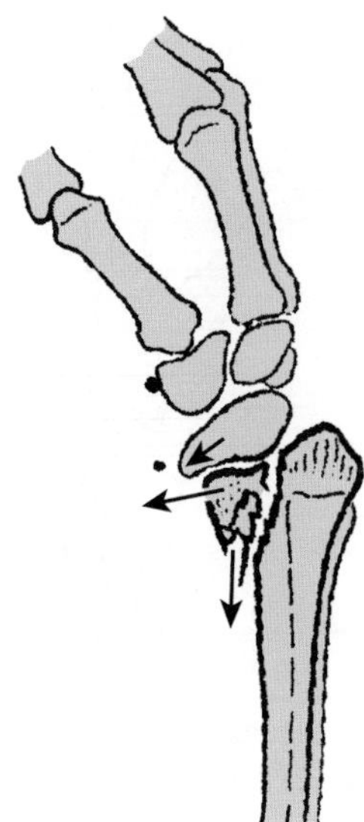

Figure 11-24 The Barton fracture (volar). (From Connolly JF, editor: *DePalma's the management of fractures and dislocations: an atlas,* ed 3, Philadelphia, 1981, WB Saunders, p 1028, reprinted by permission.)

I. Scapholunate dissociation

1. Diagnosis
   - Terry Thomas sign
     - Scapholunate angle greater than 60 degrees
     - Scaphoid ring sign
   - A 3-mm or larger scapholunate gap versus the opposite side
2. Treatment
   - Nonoperative treatment—closed treatment if minor
   - Operative treatment—for early treatment (<3 weeks), open reduction of scaphoid and lunate, with ligament repair and pinning

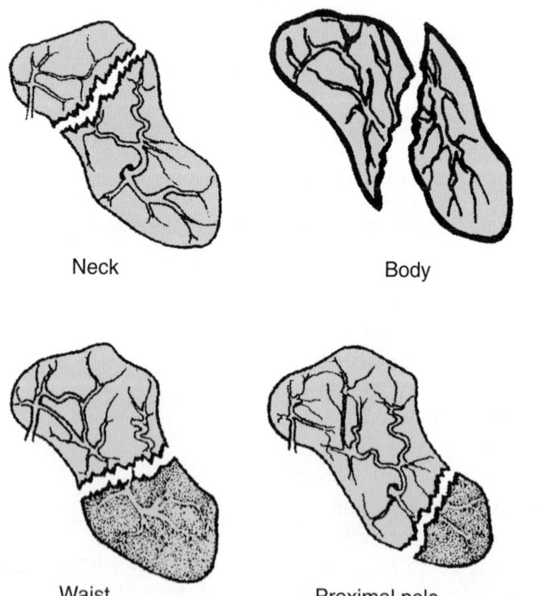

Figure 11-25 Classification of scaphoid fractures. Note progressive risk of avascular necrosis with proximal transverse fractures. (From Weissman BN, Sledge CB: *Orthopedic radiology,* Philadelphia, 1986, WB Saunders, 1986, p 1060, reprinted by permission.)

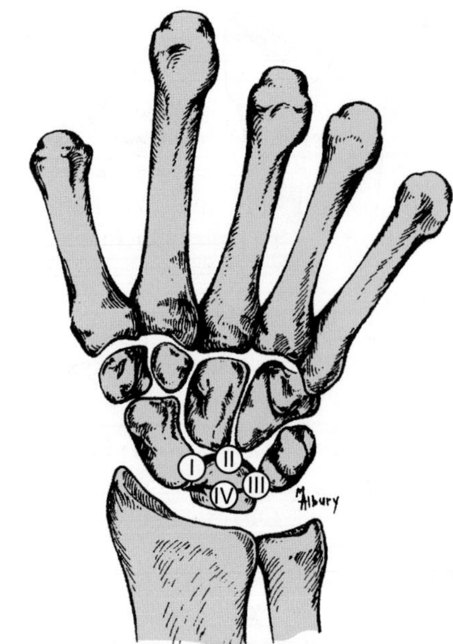

Figure 11-26 Perilunar stages of instability. *I,* Scapholunate. *II,* Capitolunate. *III,* Triquetrolunate. *IV,* Dorsal radiocarpal (leading to lunate dislocation). (From Mayfield JK: Mechanism of carpal injuries, *Clin Orthop Relat Res* 149:50, 1980, reprinted by permission.)

3. Complications—Widening of scapholunate is common. Another complication is late DJD.

J. Carpal instability

1. Diagnosis
   - DISI—The most common (scapholunate angle >70 degrees) (Figure 11-27)
   - Volar intercalated segmental instability (VISI) (volar scapholunate angle <35 degrees)
   - Axial injury
2. Treatment—operative
   - DISI and VISI—open reduction and ligament repair
   - Axial injury—ORIF
3. Complications
   - DISI and VISI—DJD and stiffness; treatment for chronic instability is controversial.
   - Axial injury—usually of high energy, with skin and soft tissue, neurovascular (ulnar nerve the most common), and intrinsic muscle injuries

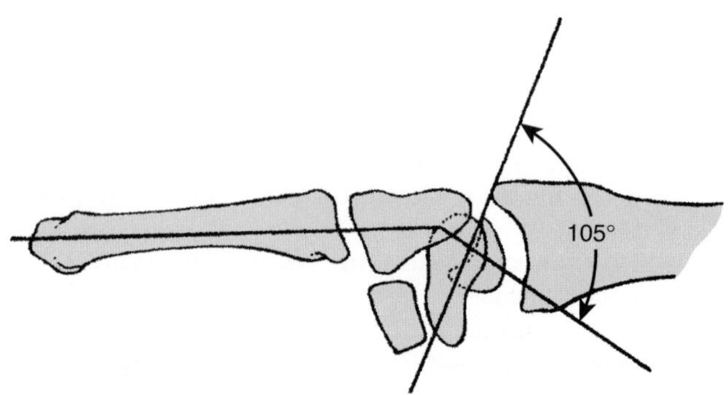

Figure 11-27 Dorsal intercalary segmental instability (DISI). Note scapholunate angle greater than 70 degrees, consistent with a DISI pattern. (From Connolly JF, ed: *DePalma's the management of fractures and dislocations: an atlas,* ed 3, Philadelphia, 1981, WB Saunders, p 1085, reprinted by permission.)

VII. HAND INJURIES (TABLES 11-13 AND 11-14)

A. Hamatometacarpal fracture-dislocation

1. Cain classification
   - IA—ligamentous injury
   - IB—dorsal hamate fracture (most common)
   - II—comminuted dorsal hamate fracture
   - III—coronal hamate fracture
2. Treatment
   - IA—stable, cast; unstable, CRPP
   - IB—stable, cast; unstable, ORIF
   - II—ORIF to restore dorsal buttress
   - III—ORIF to restore congruent joint surface

B. First carpometacarpal dislocation (Figure 11-28)

1. Evaluation—rare injury without associated fracture
2. Treatment—CRPP with traction/pronation
3. Complication—chronic instability

C. First metacarpal fracture

1. Classification
   - Bennett fracture—volar ulnar lip fracture
   - Rolando fracture—comminuted intraarticular fracture
   - Extraarticular fracture—can be transverse or oblique
2. Treatment
   - Bennett fracture
     - CRPP if the volar-ulnar fragment is too small for screw fixation and anatomic reduction is achieved
     - ORIF if there is a large fragment and/or the fracture is irreducible
   - Rolando fracture—ORIF with 2-mm T-plate or blade plate if there are larger fragments, Kirschner wires for smaller fragments, and spanning external fixator for very severe comminution
   - Extraarticular—spica cast for 4 weeks and CRPP if there is greater than 30 degrees angulation

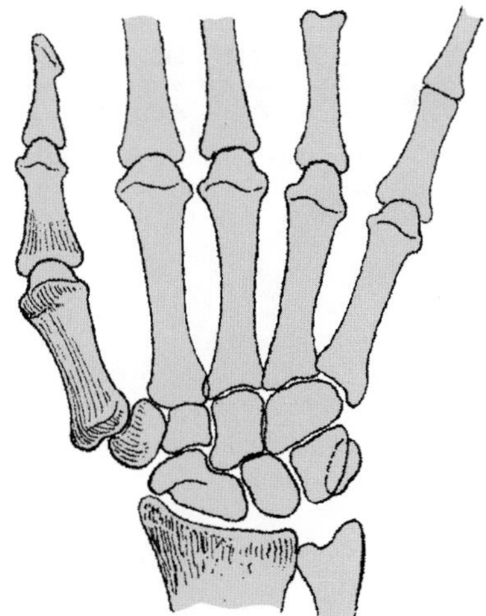

Figure 11-28 Subluxation/dislocation of the thumb carpometacarpal joint. (From Connolly JF, ed: *DePalma's the management of fractures and dislocations: an atlas,* ed 3, Philadelphia, 1981, WB Saunders, p 1165, reprinted by permission.)

D. First metacarpophalangeal joint injury/dislocation

1. Diagnosis/classification
   - Ulnar collateral ligament injury (gamekeeper's thumb)—the most common injury (Figure 11-29)
     - Sprain (joint opens <35-45 degrees) or complete tear
     - Stener lesion—interposition of adductor aponeurosis (prevents ulnar collateral ligament from healing back to bone)
   - Radial collateral ligament injury (rare)
   - Dorsal—simple or complex (interposition of the volar plate)

Table 11-13 Adult Hand Dislocations

Injury	Eponym/Other Name	Classification	Treatment	Complications
Distal interphalangeal dislocation		Dorsal dislocation (most common)	Closed reduction; immobilize for 2 wk, then range of motion; late diagnosis or irreducible: ORIF	Extensor lag—treated with 8-wk course of splinting, similar to a mallet finger
Collateral ligament injury			Sprain: buddy tape for 3-6 wk Tear: repair radial collateral of index, ring, middle finger; ulnar collateral of small (dominant hand)	
Proximal interphalangeal dislocation		Dorsal dislocation (most common) (volar plate disruption)		
		I—hyperextension, volar plate avulsion	Buddy tape or extension block splint for 4 days, then motion	Stiffness, contractures (treat with volar plate arthroplasty)
		II—dislocation, major ligamentous injury	Extension block splint	
		III—proximal dislocation (middle phalanx fracture)	If >4-mm displacement, reduce; ORIF if irreducible	

Continued

Table 11-13 Adult Hand Dislocations—cont'd

Injury	Eponym/Other Name	Classification	Treatment	Complications
Boutonniere		Volar dislocation (central slip injury)	Closed reduction; splint in full extension for 6 wk if congruous	Late recognition: therapy to restore motion, ORIF or volar plate arthroplasty
Rotatory			ORIF if irreducible or incongruous	
Dorsal fracture-dislocation			Extension block splint if congruous; if unstable, ORIF or volar plate arthroplasty	
Thumb MCP dislocation	Gamekeeper/skier thumb	Ulnar collateral ligament injury (most common)	Sprain: does not open >35 degrees with stress; treat with thumb spica cast for 4 wk	Unrecognized Stener lesion, chronic pain, instability, degenerative joint disease
			Complete rupture: open repair (interposition of adductor aponeurosis—Stener lesion)	
Radial collateral ligament injury (rare)			Splint vs. repair if complete rupture and symptomatic	
Dorsal (simple or complex [interposition of volar plate])			Simple: splint; complex: open	
MCP dislocation		Collateral ligament injury (index finger most common)	Reduce with traction/volar–directed force to proximal phalanx; splint in 50-degree MCP flexion for 3 wk, then buddy tape for 3 additional wk	Late recognition—injection, splinting, operation (rare)
		Dorsal dislocation (most common)	Open if irreducible, >2-mm displacement of associated fracture fragments, or 20% of joint	
		Simple	Closed reduction, immobilization for 7-10 days	Failure to recognize complex dislocation
		Complex	Soft tissue volar plate interposition (pucker, sesamoid in joint, and parallelism of metacarpal and P1 [phalanx] require ORIF and volar plate arthroplasty)	Stiffness, contractures, neurovascular injury (open)
		Volar dislocation	Rare, requires ORIF	
CMC dislocation			CRPP; ORIF—fourth CMC dislocations and open dislocations	
Thumb CMC dislocation		Rare injury without associated fracture	CRPP with traction/pronation; immobilize for 6-10 wk	Chronic instability
Hamate/metacarpal fracture-dislocation		Cain IA—ligamentous injury IB—dorsal hamate fracture (most common) II—comminuted dorsal hamate fracture III—coronal hamate fracture	Reduce—if stable, cast; if unstable, CRPP reduce—if stable, cast; if unstable, ORIF ORIF, restore dorsal buttress ORIF, restore congruent joint	Delay in diagnosis (pronation oblique films required)

CMC, carpometacarpal; CRPP, closed reduction with percutaneous pinning; MCP, metacarpophalangeal; ORIF, open reduction and internal fixation.

Table 11-14 Adult Hand Fractures

Injury	Eponym	Classification	Treatment	Complications
Distal phalanx (P3) fracture		Longitudinal, comminuted, transverse, crush (frequent)	Splint DIP joint for 3-4 wk; evacuate hematoma and repair nail bed with fine absorbable suture	Nail bed injury
Extensor digitorum communis avulsion	Mallet finger	Watson-Jones	Volar/stack splint for 6-8 wk full time, then 4 wk at night only; CRPP/ORIF if >50% of articular surface; volar subluxation of P3 or occupation prevents splinting	Dorsal skin necrosis, deformity, nail bed injury (with ORIF), subluxation, extensor lag, nail bed deformity, pin tract infections, osteomyelitis, hot-cold intolerance, hypersensitivity
Extensor tendon stretch: >15- to 30-degree extensor lag				
Extensor tendon rupture: 30- to 60-degree extensor lag				
Bony mallet				
Flexor digitorum profundus avulsion	Jersey finger	Leddy and Packer		Can lead to lumbrical and finger (late), missed diagnosis (therapy or fuse DIP late); quadregia if flexor digitorum profundus advanced >1 cm during repair
		I—tendon in palm	Repair within 7-10 days (vincula disruption)	
I		I—tendon at level of PIP joint (held by A3 pulley)	Repair within 6 wk	
		III—tendon at level of A4 pulley	ORIF of large, bony fragment with Kirschner wires; keep A4 pulley intact with repair	
		IV—bony fragment at P3 base	Early fixation of bony fragments and tendon	
Proximal (P1) and middle (P2) phalanges fracture		Extraarticular base (stable)	Buddy tape	Decreased ROM (flexor tendon adhesions), contractures, malunion/malrotation (may require osteotomy), lateral deviation, volar angulation (osteotomy), nonunion, tendon adherence
		Extraarticular base (unstable)	Reduce and immobilize (CRPP/ORIF if irreducible; external fixation for comminuted fractures, soft tissue injuries)	
		Intraarticular nondisplaced	Buddy tape, early ROM, close follow-up	
		Intraarticular condylar	Reduction, CRPP, or ORIF; restore articular surface if >1-mm displacement	
		Intraarticular P1 base	Small/nondisplaced—buddy tape Large/displaced—ORIF	
	Boutonniere	Intraarticular P2 base	Splint PIP (extension) for 6 wk; ORIF if large, bony fragment	

Continued

Table 11-14 Adult Hand Fractures—cont'd

Injury	Eponym	Classification	Treatment	Complications
Metacarpal (MC) fracture		Head (transverse, oblique, spiral, comminuted)	ORIF for large piece, external fixation with early motion of comminuted fractures	Soft tissue injury (look for fight bite!), malunion (rotation); prominent MC head in palm (affects grip); loss of reduction (no volar buttress); nonunion, contracture of intrinsic muscles; claw deformity with extrinsic tendon imbalance
	Boxer	Neck—fourth and fifth MCs	40- to 70-degree angulation; reduce with Jahss maneuver, splint; operative if rotational deformity, extensor lag, multiple fracture, irreducible	
		Neck—second and third MCs	Usually requires CRPP to adjacent MC or ORIF	
		Shaft—transverse	Closed reduction, immobilize, or CRPP; accept 20-30–degree angulation in IV and V, 10-degree angulation in II and III; ORIF if irreducible	
		Shaft—oblique	ORIF if >5-mm shortening or rotated	
		Shaft—comminuted	Nondisplaced: splint; displaced: CRPP to adjacent MC or ORIF	
Thumb (first) MC base fracture	Bennett	I—intraarticular volar ulnar lip	Attempt CRPP to trapezium; ORIF if irreducible	Displaced by abductor pollicis longus
	Rolando	II—intraarticular "Y" (volar and dorsal)	Large fragments: ORIF; comminuted: external fixation or early motion	Degenerative joint disease
		III—extraarticular (transverse or oblique)	Closed reduction, splint for 4 wk; CRPP if angulation >30 degrees	
Small (fifth) MC base fracture	"Baby Bennett"	Base fracture (epibasal, two-part, three-part, comminuted)	Evaluate with semipronated, semisupinated, distraction views; CRPP to adjacent MC or ORIF	Watch carpometacarpal fracture-dislocation, painful arthritis, fragment displaced by extensor carpi ulnaris

CRPP, closed reduction with percutaneous pinning; DIP, distal interphalangeal; MC, metacarpal; ORIF, open reduction and internal fixation; PIP, proximal interphalangeal; ROM, range of motion.

2. Treatment
   - Gamekeeper's thumb
     - Sprain—thumb spica cast for 4 to 6 weeks
     - Stener lesion—open-repair aponeurosis
   - Radial collateral ligament injury—splint; late reconstruction only if necessary
   - Dorsal—For a simple dislocation, splint for 3 weeks; for a complex dislocation, perform open repair.
3. Complications—unrecognized injury or Stener lesion, leading to chronic instability and pain

E. Finger metacarpophalangeal dislocation

1. Diagnosis/classification—index finger most often affected; characteristic skin puckering in the palm at the level of injury
   - Collateral ligament injury—uncommon aponeurosis
   - Dorsal—by far the most common (simple or complex)
   - Volar—rare
2. Treatment—Reduce with volar force to the dorsal base of the proximal phalanx. May be irreducible; do not make multiple forceful attempts at reduction.
   - Collateral ligament injury—Splint in 50 degrees metacarpophalangeal flexion for 3 weeks and then buddy tape for 3 more weeks. Use ORIF if there is an avulsion fragment with greater than 2-mm displacement or greater than 20% articular involvement.
   - Dorsal—For a simple dislocation, splint for 7 to 10 days and then buddy tape. For a complex dislocation, perform open reduction (irreducible).
   - Volar—open reduction
3. Complications—loss of motion (can be severely disabling)

F. Proximal interphalangeal dislocation

1. Diagnosis/classification
   - Dorsal—the most common dislocation

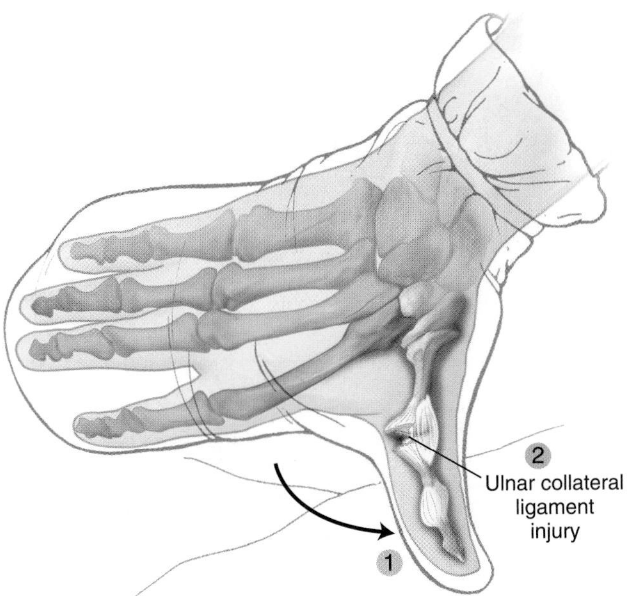

Figure 11-29 Gamekeeper's thumb.

- Avulsion of the volar plate occurs first, followed by a rent between the accessory and proper collateral ligaments.
- It can be further classified as stable or unstable as determined by maintenance of reduction.
- A fracture-dislocation of greater than 40% of the middle phalangeal joint surface will yield an unstable fracture-dislocation.

- Lateral
- Volar

2. Treatment—Reduce with volar force to the dorsal base of the proximal phalanx. May be irreducible; do not make multiple forceful attempts at reduction.
   - Dorsal dislocation—Reduce with digital block anesthesia, longitudinal traction, and dorsal pressure applied to the proximal phalangeal head. Confirm concentric reduction and then apply dorsal block (about 30 degrees) splinting for 4 days, followed by vigorous joint motion to avoid stiffness.
   - Dorsal fracture-dislocation—similar reduction and stability test in extension. If stable, apply dorsal block splinting, excluding the last 45 degrees of extension; apply 30-degree block after 5-7 days; and buddy tape a week later. Unstable fracture-dislocation requires surgical fixation.
   - Volar or lateral dislocation—closed reduction; ORIF if irreducible or incongruous. Try to reduce volar dislocation with metacarpophalangeal and proximal interphalangeal joints in flexion to avoid irreducible dislocation. Open treatment can be with pinning, external fixation, or open screw fixation.
3. Complications—Loss of motion (can be severely disabling)
   - Dorsal dislocations are at significant risk for permanent stiffness and contractures (treat with volar plate arthroplasty).
   - Central slip avulsion or marginal fracture avulsion—Look for these conditions with volar dislocations, leading to boutonniere deformity. Treat with acute ORIF repair of central slip.

G. Distal interphalangeal dislocation

1. Diagnosis/classification
   - Dorsal—most common dislocation
   - Collateral ligament injury
2. Treatment—Reduce with volar force to the dorsal base of the distal phalanx. May be irreducible; do not make multiple forceful attempts at reduction.
   - Dorsal—If the dislocation is acute, use closed reduction and splint for 1 to 2 weeks. If it is chronic or irreducible, use open reduction.
   - Collateral ligament injury—For a sprain, buddy tape for 3 to 6 weeks. For a tear, perform open repair.
3. Complications—extensor lag, which is treated with 8-week course of splinting, similar to a mallet finger

H. Small metacarpal base fractures

1. Diagnosis—reverse or baby Bennett fracture. Radiographic diagnosis can be difficult. Confirm the diagnosis with direct examination and special radiographs (semi-pronated, semi-supinated, or distraction films).
2. Classification
   - Epibasal
   - Two-part
   - Three-part
   - Comminuted
3. Treatment—controversial whether to use nonsurgical management or ORIF. If surgical treatment is elected, use CRPP and cast for 6 weeks or ORIF.
4. Complications—painful arthritis and displacement by extensor carpi ulnaris.

I. Metacarpal shaft fracture

1. Classification (descriptive)
   - Transverse
   - Oblique
   - Spiral
   - Comminuted
2. Treatment
   - Transverse—Reduce and immobilize or use percutaneous pinning (PCP).
     - Accept 10 degrees angulation for the index and long fingers and 20 to 30 degrees for the ring and small fingers.
     - Use ORIF if fracture is irreducible. No rotational deformity acceptable.
   - Oblique and spiral—CRPP or ORIF if fracture is unstable and/or displaced
   - Comminuted—For a nondisplaced fracture, splint. For a displaced fracture, pin to adjacent metacarpal (preferred) or ORIF.

J. Metacarpal neck fracture

1. Diagnosis/classification—common injury from flexed metacarpal head striking an unyielding object. A fracture of the fifth metacarpal neck is called a boxer fracture.
2. Treatment
   - Nonoperative treatment—Reduce with the Jahss maneuver (flexed metacarpophalangeal joint with dorsally directed force through metacarpal head and proximal phalanx). It is critical to assess rotational deformity. Splint in metacarpophalangeal and PIP extension for 2

to 3 weeks, and then free the PIP joint and start motion. Metacarpal motion begins after 4 to 5 weeks.
- Operative treatment—usually percutaneous pinning. Indications are rotational deformity despite closed reduction, extension lag due to excessive metacarpal head flexion, multiple fractures, or excessive displacement (>50 to 60 degrees for the ring and small fingers and >15 to 20 degrees for the index and long fingers).

3. Complications—claw deformity with extrinsic tendon imbalance, prominent metacarpal head in palm (may impair grip), loss of reduction, nonunion, and intrinsic contracture

K. Metacarpal head fracture

1. Diagnosis—Check carefully; these are frequently open fractures (look for "fight bite").
2. Classification (descriptive)
   - Vertical
   - Horizontal
   - Oblique
   - Comminuted
3. Treatment—ORIF for large fragments and external fixation with early motion if fracture is comminuted

L. Proximal and middle phalanx fracture

1. Diagnosis/classification
   - Transverse, oblique, spiral, or comminuted for diaphyseal fracture
   - Other anatomic locations—extraarticular base, neck, and condylar region
   - Intraarticular base—three types of fractures
     - Collateral ligament avulsion
     - Compression
     - Vertical shear
   - Diaphyseal
   - Neck
   - Condylar
2. Treatment
   - Extraarticular base fracture—Eaton-Belsky technique of transarticular pinning is popular for the proximal phalanx (Figure 11-30).
   - Collateral ligament avulsion—tension band or ORIF if it is displaced or unstable and buddy tape if nondisplaced
   - Compression fracture of intraarticular base—ORIF with bone graft if needed
   - Vertical shear—ORIF or CRPP
   - Diaphyseal fracture—Buddy tape if fracture is stable and CRPP or ORIF if unstable. There is no difference in recovery rate, pain score, alignment, motion, or grip strength in a trial between ORIF with screws and CRPP.
   - Neck—CRPP
   - Condylar
     - Nondisplaced: digital splint for 7 to 10 days
     - Displaced: ORIF
3. Complications—flexor tendon adhesions, flexion contracture, malunion or nonunion, malrotation, volar angulation (watch with proximal phalanx fractures; the middle phalanx may angulate toward either the volar or dorsal apex), and lateral deviation

M. Distal phalanx fracture

1. Diagnosis/classification
   - Descriptive—longitudinal, comminuted, and transverse
   - Frequently crush injuries

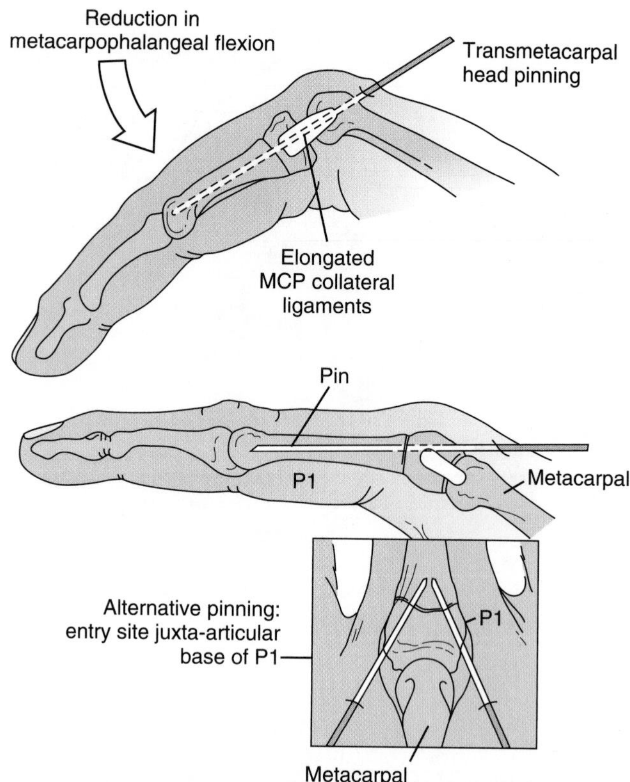

Figure 11-30 Intramedullary (Eaton-Belsky) pinning of proximal phalangeal base fractures. MCP, metacarpophalangeal. (From Stannard J, Schmidt A, Kregor P: *Surgical treatment of orthopaedic trauma,* New York, 2007, Thieme.)

2. Treatment
   - Associated nail bed injuries may require surgery and are open fractures. Irrigate/débride, reduce, and splint with a digital splint and with the distal interphalangeal joint extended and proximal interphalangeal joint free.
   - Repair nail bed sterile matrix

N. Extensor digitorum communis avulsion (mallet finger)

1. Classification—Watson-Jones classification
   - Extensor tendon stretch—15-30 degrees extensor lag
   - Extensor tendon torn—30-60 degrees extensor lag
   - Extensor tendon avulsion with bone flaking
   - Extensor tendon avulsion fragment—bony mallet
2. Treatment
   - Vast majority are treated closed with splinting. The first three classifications are treated with extensor splint for 6 to 8 weeks, followed by 3 to 4 weeks of night splinting.
   - CRPP if occupation prevents splinting
   - Volar subluxation of distal phalanx (absolute indication) or greater than 50% of the articular surface involved (relative indication at best): CRPP with extension block pinning (Figure 11-31) or ORIF
3. Complications—dorsal skin necrosis, extensor lag, permanent nail deformities, pin tract infections, and osteomyelitis (reported in up to 41% of surgically treated patients)

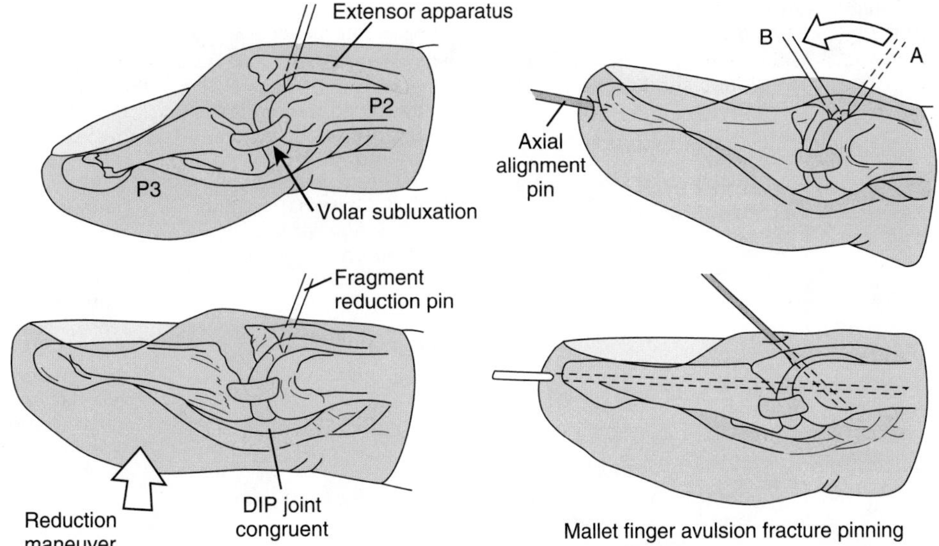

Figure 11-31 Technique of reduction and stabilization of a displaced mallet fracture with volar subluxation. The dorsal pin "levers" the avulsion fragment attached to the terminal tendon into place. The body of the phalanx is reduced and secured with a transarticular pin. DIP, distal interphalangeal joint. (From Stannard J, Schmidt A, Kregor P: *Surgical treatment of orthopaedic trauma,* New York, 2007, Thieme.)

O. Flexor digitorum profundus avulsion (jersey finger)—Typical mechanism is sports related: fingertip grabs jersey or pants and is forcibly extended while maximally contracting the flexor digitorum profundus muscle belly.

1. Classification—Leddy and Packer
   - Type I—nonbony avulsion retracting into the palm
   - Type II—avulsion, with small fragment retracting to proximal interphalangeal joint (held by A3 pulley)
   - Type III—large-fragment avulsion to A4 pulley (just proximal to the DIP joint) (less common)
2. Treatment—All three types should be treated surgically.
   - Type I—Repair as acutely as possible (7-10 days maximum) owing to complete disruption of vincula/blood supply
   - Type II—Repair by 6 weeks at the latest (easiest in first 7-10 days)
   - Type III—ORIF on large, bony fragment with Kirschner wires
3. Complications—Missed diagnosis leads to lumbrical-plus finger requiring therapy or distal interphalangeal arthrodesis (late); bony avulsion can have tendon avulsion separate from fragment, requiring fixation within 7 to 10 days.

SECTION 3 LOWER EXTREMITY AND PELVIS

I. PELVIC AND ACETABULAR INJURIES

A. Pelvic ring injuries (Table 11-15)

1. Diagnosis
   - Mechanism of injury
     - Often high energy
     - Associated injuries common (chest, head, other orthopaedic)
     - Nonpelvic sources of bleeding must be ruled out.
     - Mortality usually related to nonpelvic injuries
   - Radiographs
     - Anteroposterior pelvis
     - Inlet—Evaluate anteroposterior displacement of sacroiliac joint and internal/external rotational deformity.
     - Outlet—Evaluate vertical displacement of sacroiliac joint and flexion of hemipelvis.
   - CT—particularly useful to evaluate posterior pelvic injury patterns
2. Classification
   - Young-Burgess (Figure 11-32)—based on injury mechanism
     - Lateral compression (LC)—All have anterior transverse pubic ramus fracture.
       - I—sacral compression fracture
       - II—posterior iliac wing fracture
       - III—contralateral anteroposterior compression injury ("windswept pelvis")
         - Thought to be due to a rollover mechanism
     - Anteroposterior compression (APC)—All have symphyseal diastasis.
       - I—symphyseal diastasis less than 2.5 cm
         - Stretching of anterior sacroiliac ligaments
       - II—symphyseal diastasis greater than 2.5 cm with widening of sacroiliac joint anteriorly
         - **Rupture of sacrotuberous, sacrospinous, and anterior sacroiliac ligaments**

Table 11-15 Adult Pelvic Fractures

Injury	Eponym	Classification	Treatment	Complications
Pelvic fracture		Young and Burgess	Emergent management (advanced trauma life support, resuscitation, embolization of bleeding arteries if necessary, binder/external fixation/traction/pelvic C-clamp based on injury pattern)	Posterior skin slough, life-threatening hemorrhage, gastrointestinal injury, genitourinary injury (bladder, urethra, impotency), neurologic injury, nonunion, post-traumatic degenerative joint disease, pain, deep venous thrombosis, pulmonary embolism, loss of reduction, sepsis, thrombophlebitis, malunion (leg-length discrepancy, sitting problems), vascular injuries (including aortic rupture), SI pain; APC type III highest rate of associated injury
Lateral compression		I (most common)—transverse rami fracture and sacral compression fracture	Protected weight bearing, pain control	
		II—rami fracture and posterior iliac wing fracture	Protected weight bearing or delayed ORIF	
		III—symphysis or rami and anterior and posterior SI ligament torn	Based on contralateral injury (ORIF of unstable injuries)	
Anteroposterior compression		I—symphysis (<2.5 cm) or rami (vertical) and anterior SI ligament stretched	Bed rest, early mobilization, pain control	
		II—symphysis or rami and anterior SI ligament torn	Acute external fixation/anterior ORIF if concurrent laparotomy	
		III—symphysis or rami and anterior and posterior SI ligament torn	Acute external fixation/anterior ORIF if concurrent laparotomy; posterior SI ORIF	
	Malgaigne	Vertical shear—anterior and posterior vertical displacement	Acute external fixation/anterior ORIF if concurrent laparotomy; posterior SI ORIF (SI screws, anterior SI plate, posterior transiliac sacral bars, spinal-pelvic fixation)	
		Combined mechanical—combination of other injuries	Based on injuries; ORIF if posterior SI displaced	
Sacral fracture	Denis—fracture location relative to foramen	Stable, nondisplaced	Nonoperative (weight bearing as tolerated if fracture incomplete, toe-touch weight bearing for complete fracture)	Neurologic (highest with zone II fractures), chronic low-back pain, malunion
		Unstable, displaced (>1 cm)	Percutaneous SI screws, posterior ORIF, transiliac sacral bars, open foraminal decompression for nerve root injury with zone II fractures	

APC, Anteroposterior compression; ORIF, open reduction and internal fixation; SI, sacroiliac.

- III—symphyseal diastasis greater than 2.5 cm with complete disruption of sacroiliac joint, both anteriorly and posteriorly
  - Rupture of sacrotuberous, sacrospinous, and anterior and posterior sacroiliac ligaments
  - Complete separation of hemipelvis from pelvic ring
  - Vertical shear
  - Combined mechanism
    - Stable types are lateral compression type I and anteroposterior compression type I
- Tile—Based on fracture stability
  - Stable (posterior arch intact)
    - Avulsion fractures

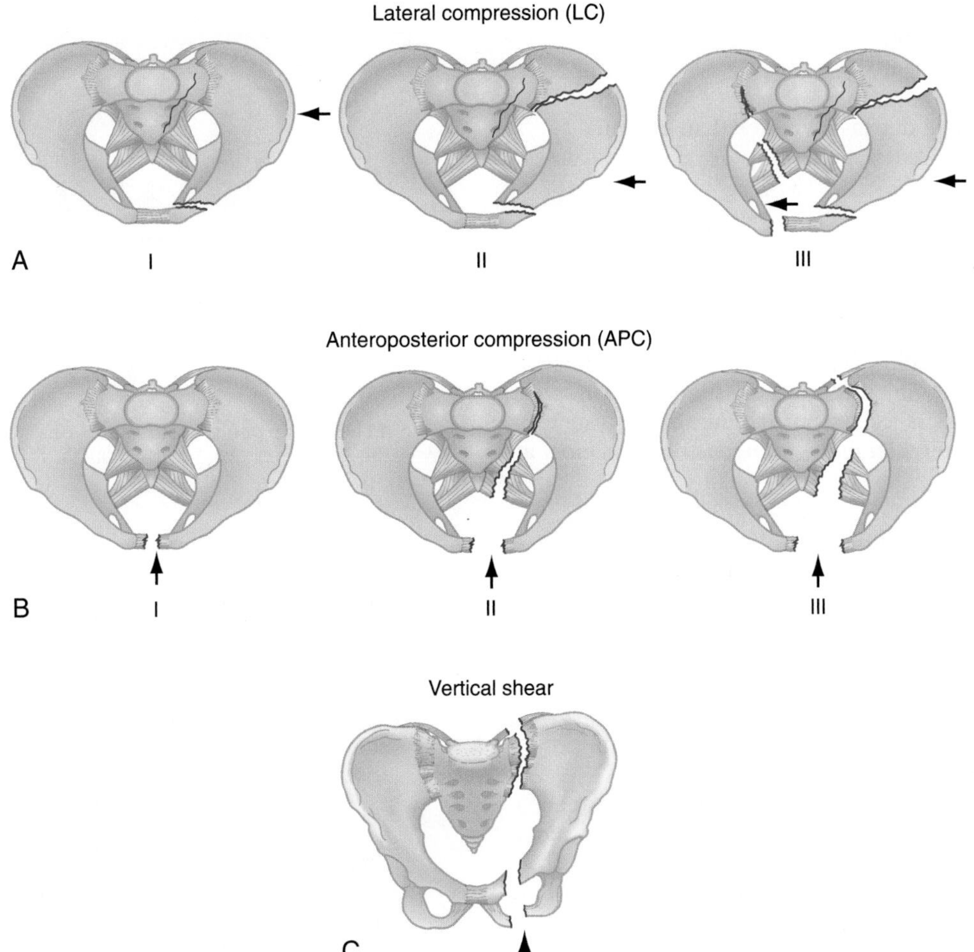

Figure 11-32 Young-Burgess classification. **A,** Lateral compression. Type I: a posteriorly directed force causing a sacral crushing injury and horizontal pubic ramus fractures ipsilaterally. Type II: a more anteriorly directed force causing horizontal pubic ramus fractures with an anterior sacral crushing injury and either disruption of the posterior sacroiliac joints or fractures through the iliac wing. Type III: an anteriorly directed force that is continued, causing external rotation of the contralateral side; the sacroiliac joint is opened posteriorly, and the sacrotuberous and spinous ligaments are disrupted. **B,** Anteroposterior compression. Type I: symphysis disrupted but with intact posterior ligamentous structures. Type II: continuation of a type I fracture with disruption of the sacrospinous and potentially the sacrotuberous ligaments and an anterior sacroiliac joint opening. Type III: continuation force disrupts the sacroiliac ligaments. **C,** Vertical shear: vertical fractures in the rami and disruption of all posterior ligaments. This injury is equivalent to an anteroposterior type III or a completely unstable and rotationally unstable fracture. *Arrow* indicates the direction of force. (Redrawn from Young JWR, Burgess AR: *Radiologic management of pelvic ring fractures,* Baltimore, 1987, Urban & Schwarzenberg.)

- Iliac wing fractures
- Transverse sacral fractures
- Partially stable—rotationally unstable and vertically stable
  - External rotation
    - Anterior pelvic disruption alone
    - Anterior sacroiliac ligaments too
    - Anterior and posterior sacroilliac ligaments
  - Lateral compression
    - Ipsilateral
    - Contralateral (bucket handle)
    - Bilateral
- Unstable (complete disruption of posterior arch)
  - Unilateral
  - Bilateral but one side B type and one side C type
  - Bilateral C type

3. Treatment
   - **General principles**
     - **Emergent treatment—to control hemorrhage and provisionally stabilize the pelvic ring:**
       - **Volume resuscitation**
       - **Pelvic binder**
       - **Angiographic embolization**
       - **External fixation**
         - **Place before emergent laparotomy**
       - **Skeletal traction—for vertically unstable patterns**
       - **Pelvic C clamp (rarely used)**
   - Nonoperative treatment
     - **Indicated for stable fracture patterns**
     - **Weight bearing as tolerated for isolated anterior injuries**

- Protected weight bearing for ipsilateral anterior and posterior ring injuries
- Operative treatment
  - Indications
    - **Symphysis diastasis greater than 2.5 cm**
    - Anterior and posterior sacroiliac ligament disruption
    - Vertical instability of posterior hemipelvis
    - Sacral fracture, with displacement greater than 1 cm
  - Anterior injuries
    - ORIF with plate fixation
    - External fixation via pins through anterior-inferior iliac spine (biomechanically stronger than illiac wing but less well tolerated clinically) or iliac wing
      - **The lateral femoral cutaneous nerve is most at risk.**
  - Posterior injuries
    - Percutaneous iliosacral screw fixation
      - **Vertical sacral fractures are a higher risk for loss of fixation.**
    - Anterior plate fixation across the sacroiliac joint
    - Posterior transiliac sacral bars or sacral plating
    - Spinal-pelvic fixation considered for bilateral sacral fractures
  - Vertically unstable patterns with anterior and posterior dislocations
    - **Anterior ring internal fixation and percutaneous sacroiliac screw has been shown to be most stable fixation construct.**
    - Spinal-pelvic fixation may also be considered.

4. Complications
   - Severe, life-threatening hemorrhage
     - **Highest risk with APC II, APC III, and LC III patterns**
   - Neurologic injury
   - Urogenital injury/dysfunction
     - **Urethral stricture most common in men**
     - **Dyspareunia and need for cesarean section childbirth common in women**
   - Malunion
   - Nonunion
   - DVT and/or pulmonary embolus
     - **DVT is the most common complication if thromboprophylaxis is not used.**
   - Infection—open fracture and associated contaminated laparotomy
   - Death
     - Risk factors for death identified during initial treatment:
       - **Blood transfusion requirement in first 24 hours**
       - **Unstable fracture type (APC II, APC III, LC II, LC III, vertical shear, combined mechanism)**
         - Young-Burgess fracture type does not predict mortality well.
       - Open fracture

B. Sacral fractures

1. Diagnosis
   - Mechanism of injury—high energy
   - Radiographs—anteroposterior pelvis, inlet, outlet, and lateral views
   - CT (usually required)

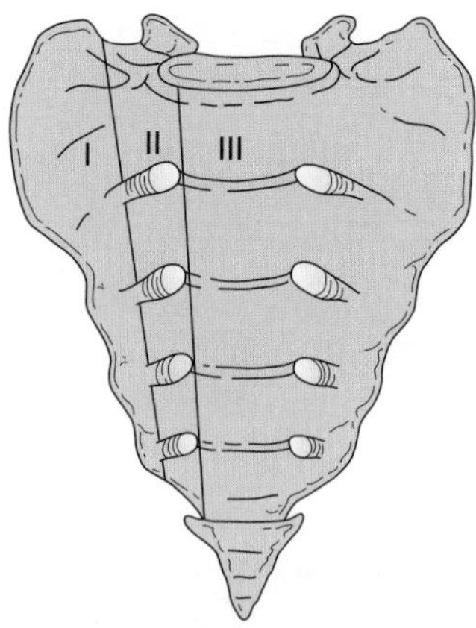

Figure 11-33 The Denis classification of sacral fractures. (From Browner BD, et al, editors: *Skeletal trauma,* Philadelphia, 1992, WB Saunders, p 820.)

2. Classification—Denis classification (Figure 11-33) based on fracture location relative to foramen (zones I, II, and III)
3. Treatment
   - Nonoperative treatment
     - Indicated for stable and minimally displaced fractures
     - Weight bearing as tolerated for incomplete fractures in which the ilium is contiguous with the intact sacrum (e.g., anterior impaction fractures from lateral compression mechanism or isolated sacral ala fractures)
     - Touch-toe weight bearing for complete fractures
   - Operative treatment
     - Indicated for displaced fractures (>1 cm)
     - Percutaneous iliosacral screws
       - Appropriate fluoroscopic visualization of anatomic landmarks is mandatory before surgery.
       - **The pelvic outlet radiograph allows optimal visualization of the S1 neural foramina to avoid injury.**
       - **The lateral sacral view identifies the sacral alar slope and minimizes risk to the L5 nerve root.**
     - Posterior plating
     - Transiliac sacral bars
     - Open foraminal decompression considered for neurologic injury associated with zone II fracture
4. Complications
   - Neurologic injury
     - Highest incidence with displaced zone II fractures
     - L5 nerve root usually involved with zone II fractures
     - Cauda equina syndrome can be associated with zone III injuries
   - Chronic low back pain
   - Malunion

C. Acetabular fractures (Figure 11-34 and Table 11-16)

1. Diagnosis
   - Mechanism of injury
     - Pattern of injury dependent on position of hip and direction of impact
     - Flexed hip with axial load (dashboard injury mechanism) most common

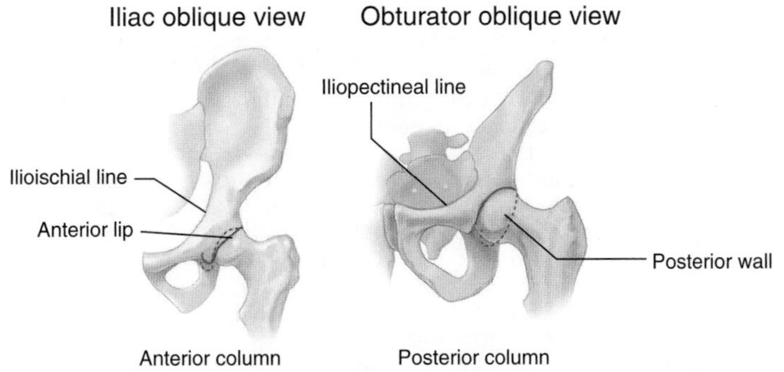

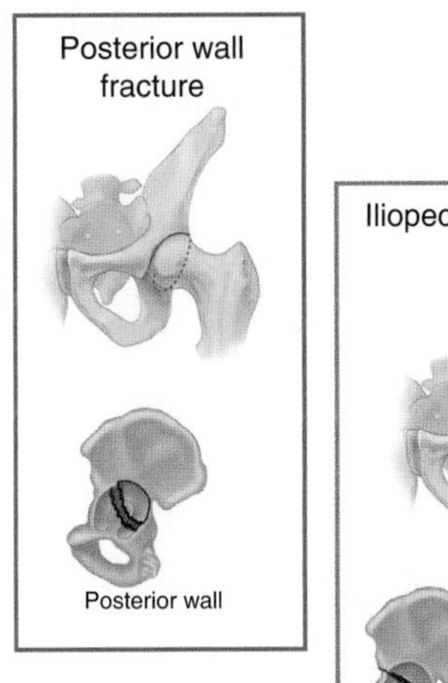

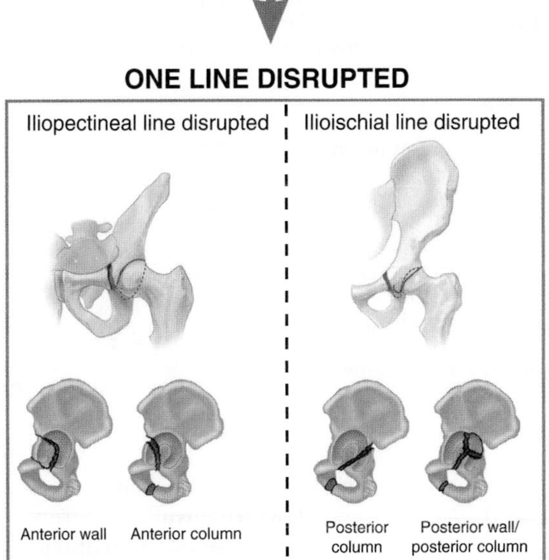

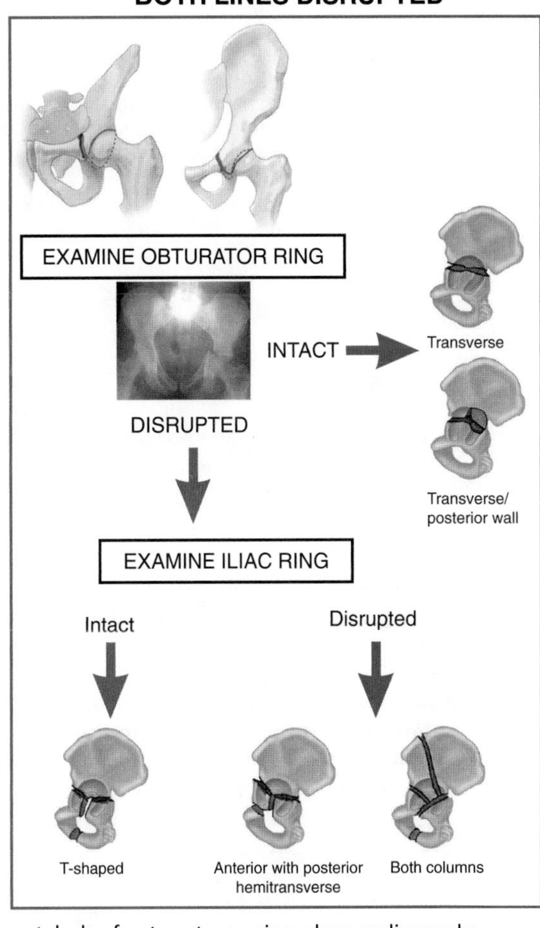

Figure 11-34 Acetabulum. Systematic evaluation for determining acetabular fracture type using plane radiographs.

- Plain radiographs
  - Anteroposterior pelvis—six cardinal lines (Figure 11-35)
  - **Obturator oblique—profiles anterior column and posterior wall** (Figure 11-36)
  - **Iliac oblique—profiles posterior column and anterior wall** (Figure 11-37)
- CT
  - Thin-cut (1-2 mm) axial
  - Three-dimensional reconstruction, with femur subtracted

2. Classification—Letournel classification (Figure 11-38) based on involvement of acetabular columns and walls
   - Simple types
     - Posterior wall (PW)
       - The most common simple type
     - Posterior column (PC)
     - Anterior wall (AW)
     - Anterior column (AC)
     - Transverse
       - Involves both the anterior and posterior columns
   - Associated types
     - Posterior column/posterior wall (PC/PW)
     - Transverse/posterior wall (TPW)
     - T-type
       - Transverse with vertical limbs through ischium
     - Anterior column/posterior hemitransverse (ACPHT)
       - Least common type
     - Associated both column (ABC)
       - Most common associated type
       - **Dissociation of acetabular dome from intact ilium**

Table 11-16 Adult Acetabular Fractures

Classification	Treatment	Complications
Letournel—based on involvement of acetabular columns and wall *Simple types:* Anterior wall (AW) Anterior column (AC) Posterior wall (PW)—most common simple type Posterior column (PC) Transverse—involves both AC and PC *Associated types:* PC/PW Transverse/PW—AC/posterior hemitransverse (ACPHT)—least common type T-type—transverse with vertical limb through ischium Associated both column (ABC)—dissociation of acetabular dome from axial skeleton. "Spur sign" seen on obturator oblique view (most common associated type)	Nonoperative: <1-mm step-off and <2-mm gap; roof arc angle > 45 degrees on anteroposterior, inlet, and outlet views—computed tomographic correlate is fracture >10 mm from dome apex; PW fractures without instability (<20% of PW); associated fractures of both columns (BCs) with secondary congruence; severe comminution in elderly in whom total hip arthroplasty is planned after fracture healing Relative contraindications to surgery: morbid obesity, physiologically elderly/nonambulatory, contaminated wound, delay to operation >4 wk, presence of deep venous thrombosis with contraindication for filter Operative: displaced fracture, incongruous or unstable joint, intraarticular bone fragments, irreducible fracture-dislocation ***Surgical approaches:*** Kocher-Langenbeck (posterior approach) indicated for PW, PC, transverse, transverse/PW (when PW requires fixation), PC/PW, T-type Ilioinguinal (anterior approach) indicated for AW, AC, ACPHT, BCs Extensile approaches considered for fractures >3 wk old and complex associated fractures Combined anterior and posterior approaches Extended iliofemoral Triradiate Posterior with trochanteric osteotomy	Nerve injury (sciatic 16%-33%, femoral, superior gluteal), vascular injury (inferior gluteal artery), heterotopic ossification (3%-69%—consider radiation therapy or indomethacin), avascular necrosis (with posterior injury), chondrolysis, post-traumatic degenerative joint disease, soft tissue degloving (Morel-Lavalle lesion), osteonecrosis (damage to medial femoral circumflex artery), malreduction (delay to surgery), bleeding (shorter time to surgery)

- "Spur sign" seen on obturator oblique view
  - Represents the posterior ilium that is undisplaced (Figure 11-39)

3. Radiographs
   - A systematic evaluation can be used to classify most acetabular fractures using plain radiographs (see Figure 11-34):
     - Examine the iliopectineal and ilioischial lines.

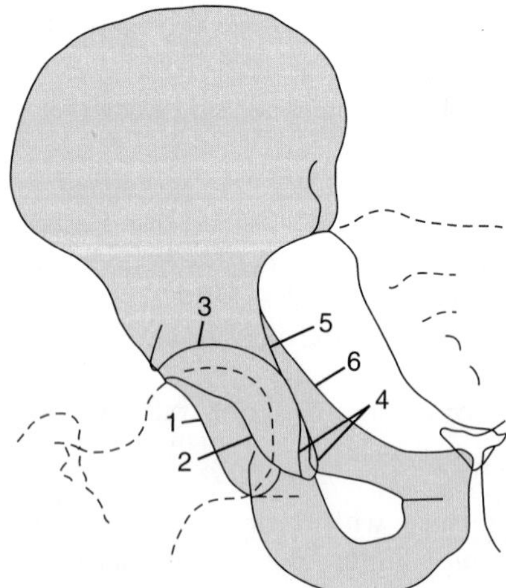

Figure 11-35 Six cardinal radiographic lines of the acetabulum. *1,* Posterior wall. *2,* Anterior wall. *3,* Roof. *4,* Teardrop. *5,* Ilioischial line. *6,* Iliopectineal line. (From Tornetta P III, Baumgaertner M: *Orthopaedic knowledge update: trauma 3,* Rosemont, Ill, 2005, American Academy of Orthopaedic Surgeons, p 264.)

     - If both lines are intact:
       - Posterior wall fracture
     - If only one line disrupted:
       - Iliopectineal line
         - Anterior wall fracture
         - Anterior column fracture
       - Ilioischial line
         - Posterior column fracture
         - Posterior column and posterior wall fracture
     - If both lines disrupted:
       - Look at the obturator ring and determine if it is intact.
         - Obturator ring intact
           - Transverse fracture
           - Transverse/posterior wall
         - Obturator ring disrupted
           - Look at iliac wing.
           - Iliac wing intact
             - T-type
           - Iliac wing disrupted
             - Anterior column–posterior hemitransverse
             - Associated both column fracture
   - CT
     - Typically used to evaluate posterior injuries, articular fragments, marginal impaction, and congruency of the hip joint
     - Axial CT may be useful to aid in fracture classification.

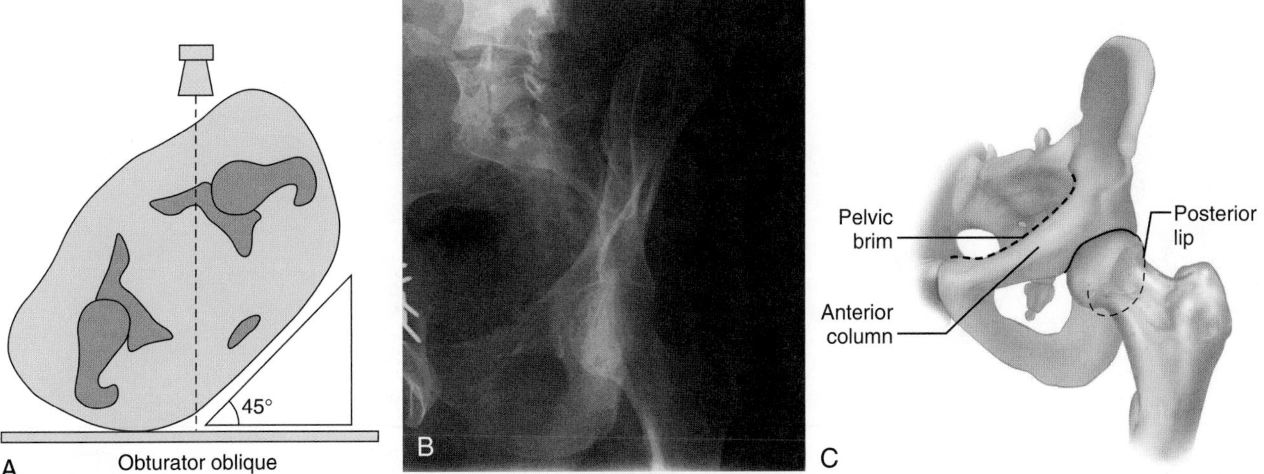

Figure 11-36 **A,** Obturator oblique view of the pelvis obtained with the patient tilted 45 degrees, with the unaffected hip down and adjacent to the x-ray cassette. The x-ray beam was centered over the affected hip. **B,** Obturator oblique radiograph profiles the anterior column and the posterior wall of the acetabulum. **C,** Obturator oblique–related landmarks. (**A** and **B** from Tornetta P III, Baumgaertner M: *Orthopaedic knowledge update: trauma 3,* Rosemont, Ill, 2005, American Academy of Orthopaedic Surgeons, p 263; **C** from Schemitsch E: *Operative techniques: orthopaedic trauma surgery,* Philadelphia, 2010, Elsevier.)

- **Vertical fracture line**
  - **Transverse or T-shaped fracture**
  - **If the wall can clearly be visualized, then anterior or posterior wall fracture**
    - **Horizontal fracture line**
      - **Column fracture**
- **Sequential axial CT cuts that demonstrate no intact support between the acetabular articular surface and axial skeleton through the sacroiliac joint are associated both-column fractures**

4. Treatment
   - General principles
     - Restore articular congruity and hip stability.
     - Avoid injury to blood supply to femoral head.
     - DVT screening and prophylaxis
   - Nonoperative treatment
     - Indications
       - Nondisplaced or minimally displaced fracture (<1-mm step and <2-mm gap)

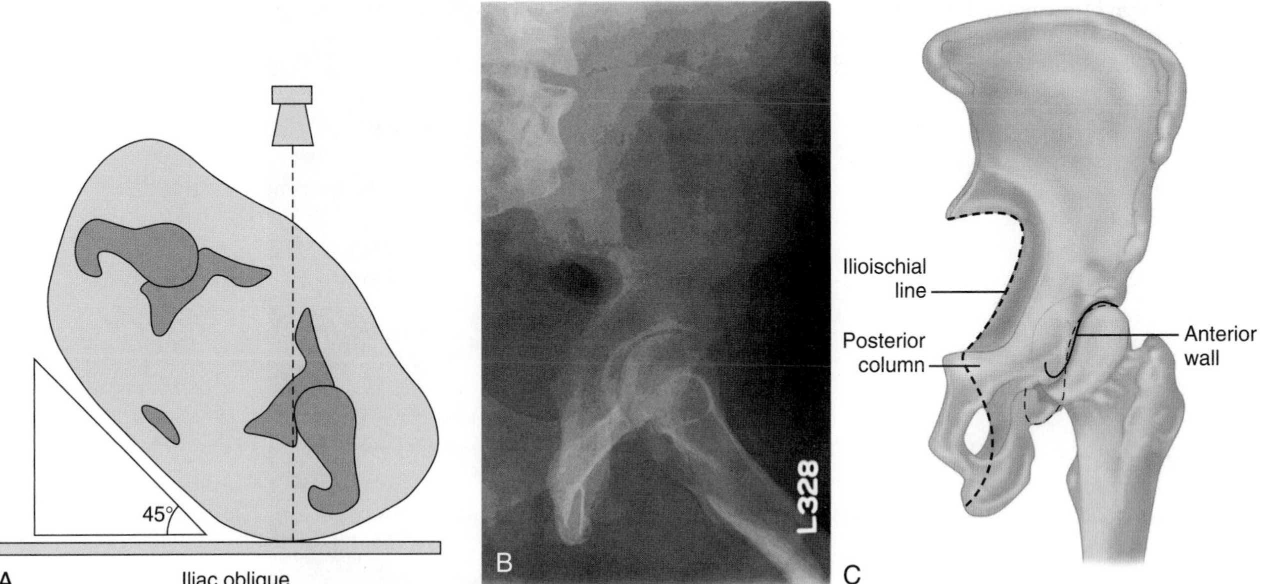

Figure 11-37 **A,** Iliac oblique view of the pelvis obtained with the patient tilted 45 degrees, with the affected hip down and adjacent to the x-ray cassette. The x-ray beam was centered over the affected hip. **B,** Iliac oblique radiograph profiles the posterior column and the anterior wall of the acetabulum. **C,** Iliac oblique–related landmarks. (**A** and **B** from Tornetta P III, Baumgaertner M: *Orthopaedic knowledge update: trauma 3,* Rosemont, Ill, 2005, American Academy of Orthopaedic Surgeons, p 263; **C** from Schemitsch E: *Operative techniques: orthopaedic trauma surgery,* Philadelphia, 2010, Elsevier.)

Simple

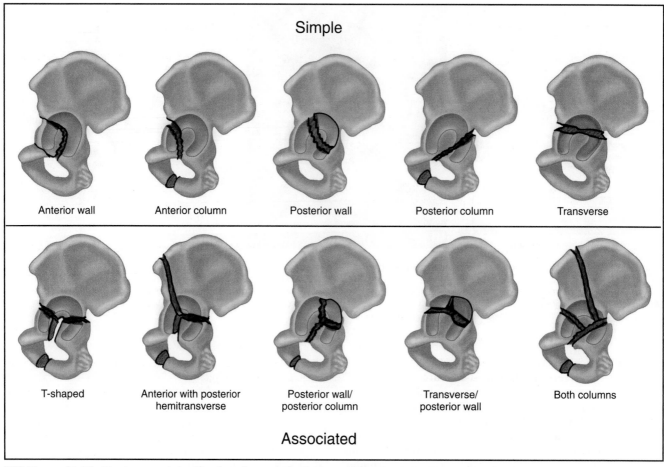

Anterior wall | Anterior column | Posterior wall | Posterior column | Transverse

T-shaped | Anterior with posterior hemitransverse | Posterior wall/ posterior column | Transverse/ posterior wall | Both columns

Associated

Figure 11-38 The Letournel classification of acetabular fractures. (From Tornetta P III, Baumgaertner M: *Orthopaedic knowledge update: trauma 3,* Rosemont, Ill, 2005, American Academy of Orthopaedic Surgeons, p 370.)

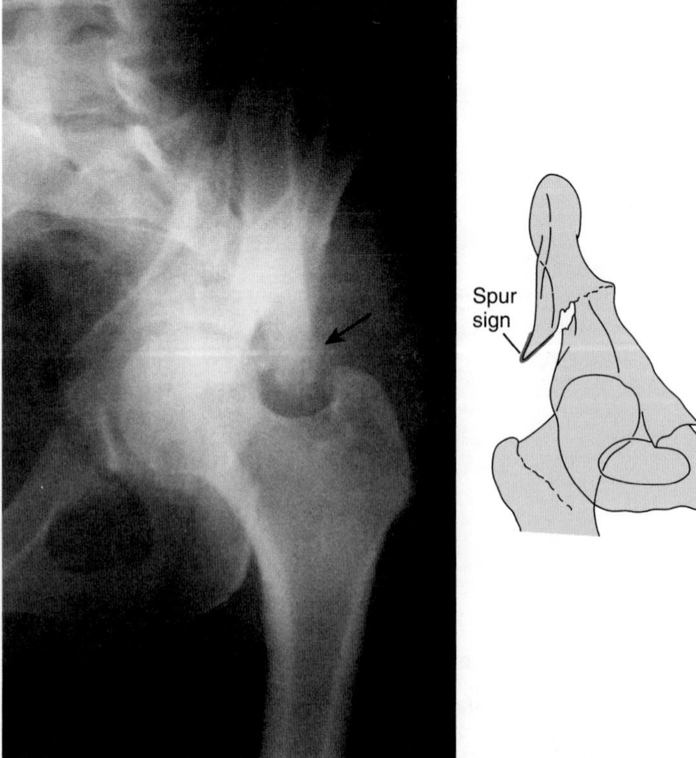

Figure 11-39 Spur sign. Obturator oblique radiograph and drawing of a both-column fracture. Note the medial translation of the dome of the acetabulum and the femoral head. The spur sign represents the intact portion of the iliac wing that remains in its anatomic position.

- Roof arc angle greater than 45 degrees on anteroposterior, iliac oblique, and obturator oblique—CT correlate is a fracture greater than 10 mm from the dome apex.
- Posterior wall fracture without instability (<20%-30% of posterior wall—exact number controversial)
- Fracture of both columns, with secondary congruence
- **Severe comminution in the elderly in whom total hip replacement is planned after fracture healing**
  - Protected weight bearing for approximately 6 weeks
  - For unstable injuries that cannot be operated on—femoral traction for 2 to 3 weeks, followed by toe-touch weight bearing for 3 to 4 weeks
- Operative treatment
  - Indications
    - Displacement with a greater than 1-mm step or greater than 2-mm gap associated with the roof is an angle less than 45 degrees on any view or documented instability with stress examination.
    - Posterior wall fracture of greater than 20% to 30% or hip instability
    - Intraarticular bone fragments
    - Irreducible fracture-dislocation
  - Relative contraindications to surgery
    - Morbid obesity
    - Physiologically elderly and nonambulatory
    - Presence of DVT, with contraindication to inferior vena cava filter
    - Contaminated wound compromising surgical approach
    - Delay to operation more than 3 weeks
  - Surgical approaches
    - Kocher-Langenbeck
      - Posterior approach
      - **Indicated for PW, PC, transverse, transverse/PW (when PW requires fixation), PC/PW, and some T-type**
    - Ilioinguinal
      - Anterior approach procedure
      - **Indicated for AW, AC, ACPHT, associated both column, and some T types (if limited posterior wall involved)**
      - **Can be divided into three "windows": lateral (iliac), middle (vascular), and medial (Stoppa)**
        - **The modified Stoppa exposes the internal pelvis and quadrilateral surface.**
    - **Extensile approaches considered for fractures more than 3 weeks old, complex associated fractures, and need for posterior column reduction**
      - Combined anterior and posterior approaches
      - Extended iliofemoral procedure
      - Triradiate
      - Posterior with trochanteric osteotomy
  - **Treatment with ORIF and acute total hip arthroplasty**
    - **Relative indications:**
      - **Age older than 60 with presence of superomedial dome impaction on radiograph ("gull sign")**
      - Displaced femoral neck fracture
      - Significant preexisting arthrosis

5. Complications
   - Soft tissue degloving (Morel-Lavallée lesion) associated with higher infection rates
   - DVT
     - Preoperative screening and inferior vena cava filter when DVT present. Postoperative screening and anticoagulation if DVT is present
   - Pulmonary embolism—treatment similar to that for DVT
   - Heterotopic ossification
     - Associated with extended approaches (20%-50%) greater than Kocher-Langenbeck (8%-25%) greater than anterior approach (2%-10%)
     - Prophylaxis with indomethacin or external-beam radiation therapy of 600 cGy within 48 hours of surgery
   - Neurologic injury
     - Sciatic nerve injury associated with posterior dislocations, especially peroneal division (<50% with full recovery)
     - Intraoperative monitoring is not associated with reduced iatrogenic nerve injury.
     - **Hip extension and knee flexion reduce tension on sciatic nerve.**
     - Iatrogenic injury to lateral femoral cutaneous nerve with anterior approach
   - Osteonecrosis—the highest incidence with posterior fractures, especially fracture-dislocations; iatrogenic damage to medial femoral circumflex artery
   - **Post-traumatic DJD**
     - Highest in patterns with posterior wall involvement
     - **Quality of reduction is most important predictor.**
   - **Malreduction**
     - **Associated with greater delay to surgery**
   - Bleeding—associated with shorter time to surgery
   - Functional deficit—especially abductor weakness (posterior more than anterior approach)

II. FEMORAL AND HIP INJURIES (TABLES 11-17 AND 11-18)

A. Hip dislocations

1. Diagnosis
   - Mechanism of injury—axial load. The position of the hip determines the direction of dislocation.
   - Plain radiographs—anteroposterior and lateral views of the hip; anteroposterior pelvis and Judet views after reduction to evaluate associated acetabular fractures
   - CT—performed after reduction to evaluate associated acetabular and/or femoral head fracture and loose bodies in joint
2. Classification—based on direction of dislocation and presence or absence of associated acetabular or femoral head fracture
   - Posterior dislocation—most common; associated with posterior wall acetabular fracture and anterior femoral head fracture—leg flexed, adducted, and internally rotated at hip
     - **Ipsilateral associated knee injury; 30% rate of meniscal tear**

Table 11-17 Adult Hip Dislocations

Injury	Classification	Treatment	Complications
Hip dislocation	Direction: posterior (most common), anterior, obturator; associated fractures (acetabular, femoral head)	Emergent, closed reduction (open if irreducible); computed tomography/plain films (Judet views) after reduction; traction/abduction pillow (depends on stability); weight bearing as tolerated if hip stable	Associated with increased-energy trauma and often associated with other injuries; femoral artery/nerve injuries (anterior dislocation), sciatic nerve injury (up to 20%; peroneal division most common), osteonecrosis (up to 15%), post-traumatic arthritis, recurrent dislocation (rare), post-traumatic degenerative joint disease (especially with retained fragments); instability (with >30%-40% fracture of posterior wall); unrecognized femoral neck fracture

- Anterior dislocation—uncommon; leg extended, abducted, and externally rotated at hip

3. Treatment
   - **Emergent, closed reduction**
   - Emergent, open reduction if irreducible after closed reduction
   - Evaluate stability after reduction.
   - Traction and/or hip abduction pillow for unstable injuries pending definitive management of associated injuries (e.g., acetabular fracture)
   - Postreduction radiographs (anteroposterior pelvis and Judet views) and CT to rule out associated acetabular fracture, femoral head fracture, and intraarticular loose bodies
   - Weight-bearing as tolerated (if hip is stable and without associated injuries)
4. Complications
   - **Osteonecrosis (up to 15%)**
   - Post-traumatic arthritis—Less common when associated with PW acetabular fracture
   - Sciatic nerve injury (up to 20%)—peroneal nerve division usually most affected
   - Recurrent dislocation (rare)

B. Femoral head fractures

1. Diagnosis
   - Plain radiographs—anteroposterior and lateral views of hip
   - CT—to evaluate location and size of fragment and rule out associated acetabular fracture.
2. Classification—Pipkin classification (Figure 11-40) based on location of fracture relative to fovea and presence or absence of associated fractures of the acetabulum or femoral neck
   - Type I—fracture below fovea
   - Type II—fracture above fovea
   - Type III—associated femoral neck fracture
   - Type IV—associated acetabular fracture
3. Treatment
   - General principles
     - **Restore articular congruity of weight-bearing portion of head and hip stability.**
     - **Remove associated loose bodies.**
     - Treat associated acetabular fracture if unstable.
     - Avoid injury to structures involved in blood supply to femoral head.
   - Nonoperative treatment
     - Indications
       - Pipkin type I—small fragment and congruent joint or nondisplaced larger fragment
       - Pipkin type II—nondisplaced; frequent (weekly) radiographs for 3 to 4 weeks to rule out secondary displacement
     - Protected weight bearing for 4 to 6 weeks
   - Operative treatment
     - Indications
       - Greater than 1-mm step-off (except small Pipkin type I)
       - Associated loose bodies in joint
       - Associated neck or acetabular fracture requiring surgical management
     - **Fixation with headless countersunk lag screws**
       - **Anterior approach via Smith-Petersen approach for Pipkin types I and II without associated operative posterior wall fracture**
       - **Posterior approach for Pipkin type IV**
     - Hip arthroplasty for older patient

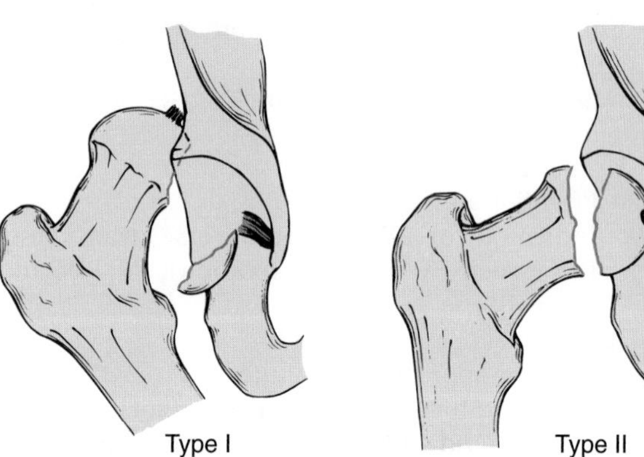

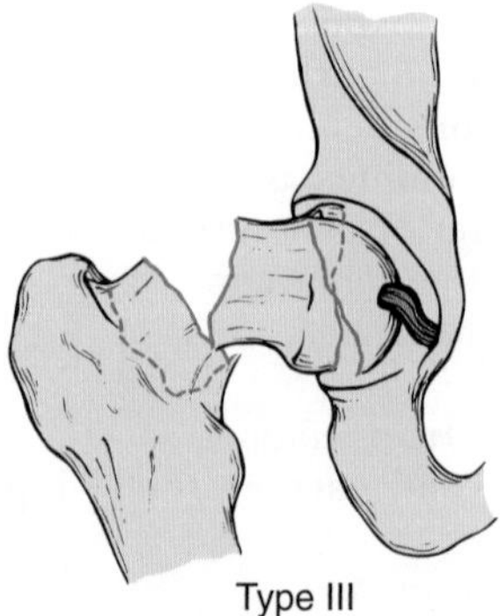

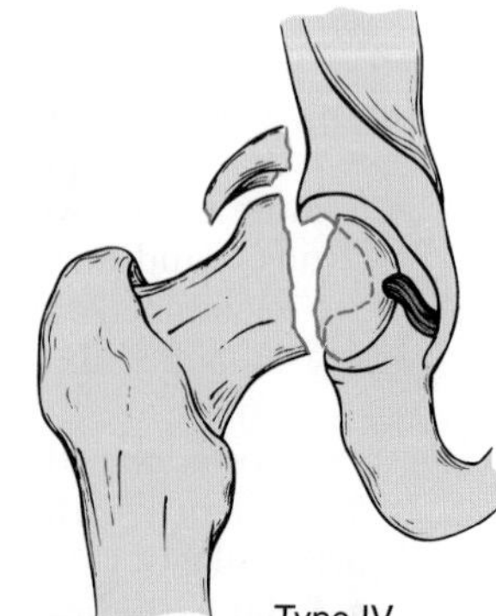

Figure 11-40 Pipkin classification system of posterior hip dislocations associated with femoral head fractures. (From Browner BD, et al, editors: *Skeletal trauma*, ed 4, Philadelphia, 2008, Elsevier.)

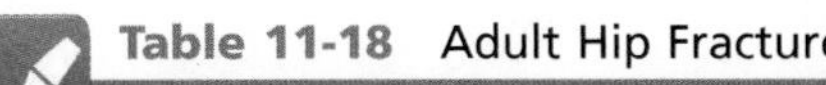

Table 11-18 Adult Hip Fractures

Injury	Classification	Treatment	Complications
Femoral head fracture	Pipkin—based on location of fracture relative to fovea and associated fractures of acetabulum or femoral neck	Restore articular congruity (ORIF when >1-mm step-off), restore hip stability, remove loose bodies, treat associated fractures, avoid injury to femoral head blood supply	Osteonecrosis (up to 15%), post-traumatic arthritis, sciatic nerve injury (up to 20%), recurrent dislocation (rare); Pipkin III highest rate of avascular necrosis
	Type I—fracture below fovea	Nonoperative if small fragment, congruent joint, protected weight bearing; ORIF with anterior approach (headless countersunk screws)	
	Type II—fracture above fovea	Nonoperative if stable, nondisplaced fragment, protected weight bearing; ORIF with anterior approach (headless countersunk screws)	
	Type III—associated femoral neck fracture	ORIF of femoral neck and head; arthroplasty if older patient	
	Type IV—associated acetabular fracture	ORIF of acetabulum and head via posterior approach; arthroplasty if older patient	
Femoral neck fracture	Garden (low energy in elderly)	Based on orientation of trabecular lines and displacement	Osteonecrosis (10%-40%; injury to medial femoral circumflex), nonunion (10%-30% of displaced fractures), infection, malunion (accept <15 degrees valgus and 10 degrees anteroposterior displacement); infection, pulmonary embolism, mortality (≈30% at 1 year; increases with advancing age, medical problems, males); cardiopulmonary decompensation with cemented stems
	I—incomplete/valgus impaction (stable) II—complete, nondisplaced (stable) III—complete, partially displaced (unstable) IV—complete, totally displaced (unstable)	Medical optimization; CRPP with 3 screws or sliding compression hip screw with derotation screw; prosthesis for elderly (>70-yr old physiologically), sick, pathologic fracture, Parkinson, rheumatoid arthritis, phenytoin (Dilantin) therapy with displaced fractures (Garden III or IV); results of unipolar vs. bipolar prosthesis similar; consider total hip arthroplasty for more active patients, acetabular degenerative joint disease (higher dislocation rate than hemiarthroplasty)	
	Pauwels (high energy in the young)	Based on orientation of fracture line; increased vertical orientation associated with less stability; ORIF with sliding hip screw (fixed-angle device) for vertically oriented fracture lines	
Intertrochanteric fracture	Number of fracture fragments, ability to resist compressive loads when fixed	Nonoperative treatment with nondisplaced fractures in compliant patients, those with high operative risk	Excessive collapse (limb shortening, medialization of shaft, sliding hip screw >> IM device), prominent hardware; nail cutout (TAD > 25 mm); loss of fixation (increased with superolateral screws); joint penetration (screw ideally placed center-center and deep); mortality, infection
	Two-part: stable with little risk of collapse Three-part: intermediate stability Four-part and comminuted: least stable	ORIF with sliding compression hip screw and side plate most reliable; lag screw in center-center position (TAD <25 mm); IM nail for unstable, reverse oblique, subtrochanteric fractures; calcar-replacing arthroplasty for patients with severe osteopenia, comminution	
Greater trochanteric fracture	Amount of displacement	ORIF if >1 cm displacement in young patient	
Lesser trochanteric fracture	Amount of displacement	ORIF if >2 cm displacement in young athlete	Consider pathologic fracture
Subtrochanteric fracture	Russell-Taylor—based on involvement of lesser trochanter and piriformis fossa	Restore limb length, alignment, rotation; indirect reduction (open or percutaneous if necessary); avoid piriformis entry when fossa involved; fixed-angle device (95-degree blade plate) for proximal comminution	Apex anterior and varus most common deformity; nonunion (minimized with IM nail), infection (increased with soft tissue dissection)
	IA—fracture below lesser trochanter	IM nail, standard proximal interlock	

Continued

Table 11-18 Adult Hip Fractures—cont'd

Injury	Classification	Treatment	Complications
	IB—fracture involves lesser trochanter; greater trochanter intact	IM nail, reconstructed interlock	
	IIA—greater trochanter involved, lesser trochanter intact	IM nail, standard proximal interlock	
	IIB—greater and lesser trochanters involved	ORIF with fixed-angle device (95-degree blade plate) vs. IM nail, reconstructed interlock	

CRPP, closed reduction with percutaneous pinning; IM, intramedullary; ORIF, open reduction and internal fixation; TAD, tip to apex distance.

4. Complications
   - Same as those for hip dislocation
   - AVN rate highest for Pipkin type III injuries. Rate of AVN is related to degree of displacement of femoral neck fracture.

C. **Femoral neck fractures**

1. Diagnosis
   - Mechanism of injury
     - Low energy (fall from standing height) in elderly—associated with osteoporosis
     - **High energy in young patients—associated with vertical fracture orientation and femoral shaft fractures**
   - Plain radiographs
     - Anteroposterior and lateral views of hip
       - **Legs should be in internal rotation to compensate for femoral anteversion.**
     - Anteroposterior and lateral views of femur
     - Anteroposterior pelvis
   - MRI or bone scan to rule out occult fracture—MRI more sensitive if less than 24 hours from injury
2. Classification
   - Garden classification (Figure 11-41) based on orientation of trabecular lines and displacement
     - Garden types I and II considered stable
     - Garden types III and IV considered unstable
   - Pauwels classification (Figure 11-42) based on orientation of fracture line
     - Increased vertical orientation associated with more shear force and reduced inherent stability
     - Nonunion and AVN associated with vertical patterns (Pauwels type III)
3. Treatment
   - General principles
     - **Rapid preoperative medical optimization**
       - Mortality reduced if surgery within 48 hours
     - Stable fixation and early mobilization
   - Nonoperative treatment
     - Indications
       - Nondisplaced fractures in patients able to comply with weight-bearing restrictions
       - Displaced fractures in patients with extremely limited functional demands and/or those with high risk for surgery
         - Toe-touch weight bearing for 6 to 8 weeks
   - Operative treatment
     - Indications
       - Displaced fractures
       - Most nondisplaced fractures
     - Internal fixation
       - Indicated for Garden types I, II, and III fractures in young patients, occult fractures, and displaced fractures in young patients

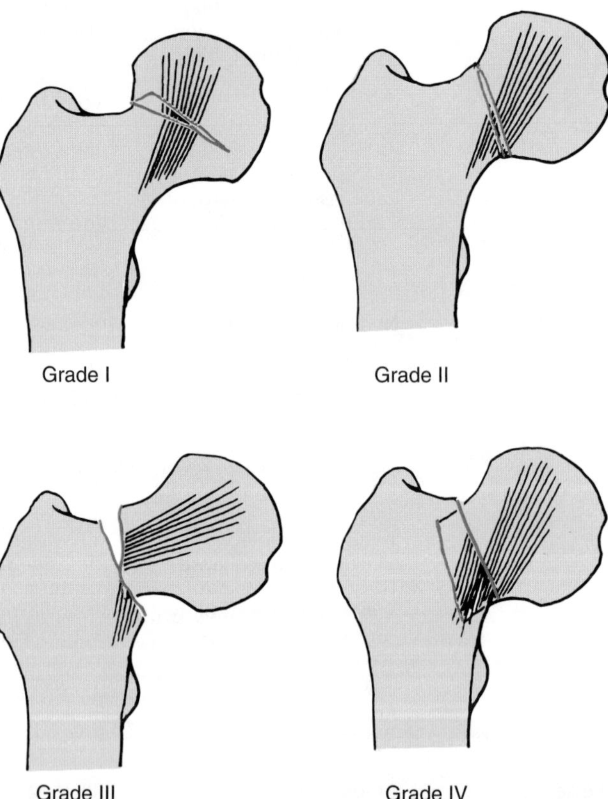

Figure 11-41 The Garden classification of femoral neck fractures. Grade I is an incomplete, impacted fracture in valgus malalignment (generally stable). Grade II is a nondisplaced fracture. Grade III is an incompletely displaced fracture in varus malalignment. Grade IV is a completely displaced fracture with no engagement of the two fragments. The compression trabeculae in the femoral head line up with the trabeculae on the acetabular side. Displacement is generally more evident on the lateral view in grade IV. For prognostic purposes, these groupings can be lumped into nondisplaced/impacted (grades I and II) and displaced (grades III and IV) because the risk of nonunion and aseptic necrosis is similar within these grouped stages. (From Browner BD, et al, editors: *Skeletal trauma,* ed 4, Philadelphia, 2008, Elsevier.)

30°

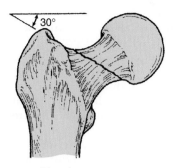

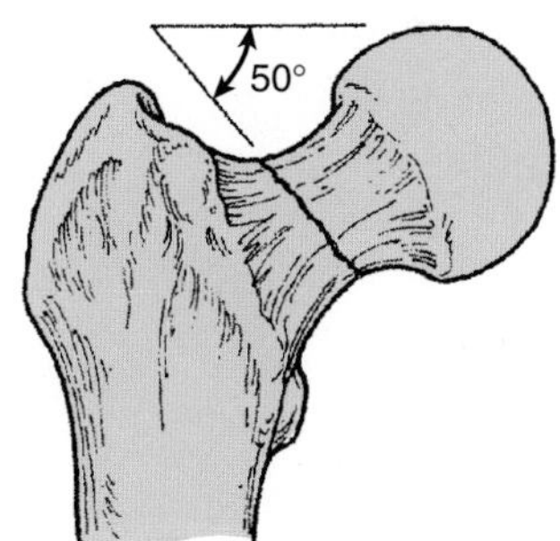

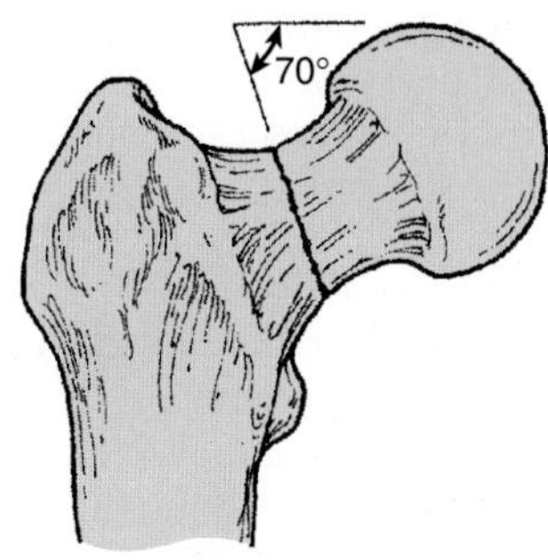

Type I Type II Type III

Figure 11-42 **The Pauwels classification of femoral neck fractures. With progression from type I to type III, there are increasing shear forces placed across the fracture site.** (From Evarts CM, editor: *Surgery of the musculoskeletal system,* ed 2, New York, 1990, Churchill Livingstone, p 2556.)

    - Three parallel screws for Garden types I and II and occult fractures
        - Inverted-V pattern
        - **Avoid start point distal to lesser trochanter (associated with increased risk of peri-implant subtrochanteric fracture).**
        - Consider fourth screw when posterior comminution exists.
    - Sliding hip screw (fixed-angle device) plus derotation screw indicated for basal cervical fractures and vertically oriented fractures
    - Anatomic reduction associated with the best results for displaced fractures in young patients
        - Open reduction often required
        - Anatomic reduction more critical than reduced time to fixation
    - Decompression of intracapsular hematoma thought to reduce risk of AVN (not proven and controversial)
    - Internal fixation associated with decreased perioperative morbidity (vs. hemiarthroplasty)
    - Failure rate for internal fixation up to 30% requiring secondary procedure (typically arthroplasty)
- Hemiarthroplasty
    - Indicated for elderly patients with displaced fractures
    - **Lower risk of dislocation than in total hip arthroplasty, especially in patients unable to comply with dislocation precautions (e.g., dementia, Parkinson disease)**
    - Cemented femoral component better than uncemented component in patients with "stove pipe"–type canals (but higher cardiopulmonary complications if preexisting disease)
    - The functional results of unipolar and bipolar prostheses are similar.
- Total hip arthroplasty
    - **Indicated for "active" elderly patients with displaced fractures**
    - Preferred to hemiarthroplasty for patients with preexisting hip arthropathy (osteoarthritis and rheumatoid arthritis)
    - **Better functional results than those associated with hemiarthroplasty in active patients**
    - Higher dislocation rate than hemiarthroplasty

4. Complications
    - Osteonecrosis—10% to 40%; associated with injury to femoral head blood supply (terminal branch of the medial femoral circumflex artery)
        - Higher risk with greater initial displacement
        - Higher risk with poor or deficient reduction
        - Decompression of intracapsular hematoma may reduce risk (controversial).
        - Reduced time to reduction may reduce risk (controversial).
    - Nonunion—occurs in 10% to 30% of displaced fractures
        - **Higher risk with malreduction (particularly varus)**
        - **Treatment options include conversion to hip arthroplasty (worse results than those associated with primary arthroplasty) and valgus osteotomy.**
    - Infection
    - **Decreased functional status**
        - **Preinjury cognitive function and mobility predict postoperative functional outcome.**
    - Mortality—1-year mortality in elderly patients approximately 30%

D. Intertrochanteric fractures

1. Diagnosis
    - Mechanism of injury—fall from standing height
    - Risk factors—osteoporosis, prior hip fracture, and risk of falls
    - More common than femoral neck fracture in patients with preexisting hip arthritis
    - Plain radiographs
        - Anteroposterior and lateral views of hip
        - Anteroposterior and lateral views of femur
        - Anteroposterior pelvis
    - MRI or bone scan to rule out occult fracture
        - MRI more sensitive if less than 24 hours from injury
2. Classification—based on the number of fracture fragments and ability to resist compression loads once they are reduced and fixed.
    - Two-part fractures—usually stable, with little risk of excessive collapse
    - Three-part fractures—intermediate stability
        - **Size and location of lesser trochanteric fragment determine stability.**
        - Large posterior medial fragments are less stable.

- Four-part and severely comminuted fractures are the least stable. They have the highest risk for excessive shortening, varus collapse, and nonunion.

3. Treatment
   - General principles
     - Stable fixation to allow early weight bearing
     - Minimize potential for implant failure
   - Nonoperative treatment
     - Indications
       - Nondisplaced fractures in patients able to comply with non–weight-bearing restrictions
       - Displaced fractures in nonambulatory individuals or those with prohibitive operative risk
     - Management with toe-touch weight bearing for 6 to 8 weeks
   - Operative treatment
     - Indications
       - Displaced fractures
       - Most nondisplaced fractures
     - Internal fixation indicated for the vast majority of intertrochanteric fractures
       - Sliding hip screw device
         - **Indicated for most intertrochanteric fractures except reverse oblique fractures, subtrochanteric fractures, and fractures without an intact lateral femoral wall**
         - High union rate
         - **Associated with moderate amount of collapse, resulting limb shortening, and medialization when used for unstable fractures; more collapse than that seen with IM implants.**
         - Lower peri-implant fracture rate than that seen with IM implants
         - **Lag screw placed in center—Center position with tip-apex distance of less than 25 mm is associated with the lowest screw failure rate** (Figure 11-43).
         - Two-hole side place sufficient for stable fractures

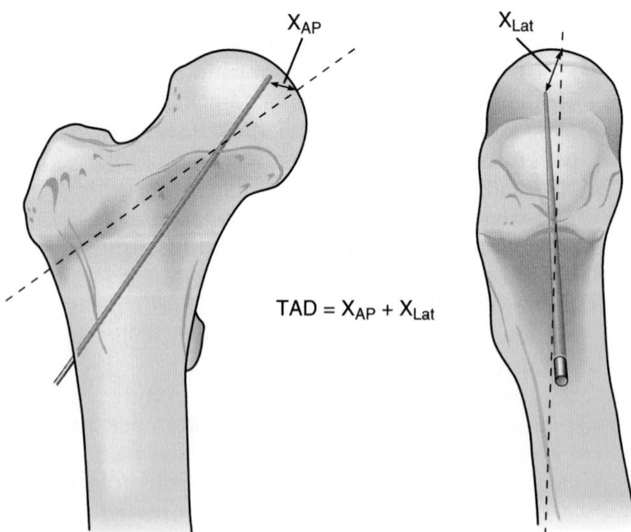

Figure 11-43 Tip-apex distance (TAD) should be less than 25 mm. (Redrawn from *Orthopaedic knowledge update: trauma* 2, Rosemont, Ill, 2000, American Academy of Orthopaedic Surgeons, p 127.)

       - IM nail
         - Indicated for most intertrochanteric fractures
         - Reduced collapse relative to sliding hip screw plate devices due to IM buttress effect of nail
         - Short nails indicated for standard obliquity fractures, with distal interlocking optional
         - **Long nails indicated for standard obliquity, reverse obliquity, and subtrochanteric fractures.**
           - **Risk of distal anterior perforation due to mismatch of anterior bow between femur and nail.**
         - Higher peri-implant fracture rate than that associated with sliding hip screw plate devices
         - Multiple screws into head fragment may provide improved rotational control (advantage controversial)
         - Single lag screw design should aim for center—Center in head with less than 25 mm tip-apex distance.
       - Ninety-five-degree fixed-angle plate device or locking proximal femoral plate—indicated for reverse obliquity, comminuted fracture, and nonunion repair
     - Arthroplasty
       - Indicated for severely comminuted fractures
       - Still requires union of greater trochanter to shaft
       - Calcar-replacing design often required

4. Complications
   - Excessive collapse—stable fixation to allow early weight bearing
     - Results in limb shortening and medialization of shaft
     - Reduced abductor moment arm may cause functional deficit.
     - Associated with displacement of lesser trochanter
     - More collapse associated with sliding hip screw device than with IM implant
     - May result in painful, prominent hardware
   - Implant failure/cutout—associated with tip-apex distance (see Figure 11-43) greater than 25 mm
   - Peri-implant fracture
     - **More common with nails than plates**
     - Low risk with current nail designs
       - Smaller distal interlocking screws further from tip of nail than earlier designs
       - Reduced trochanteric bend compared with earlier designs
   - Infection
   - Mortality (often due to medical comorbidities)
     - American Surgical Association classification predicts mortality.

E. Subtrochanteric fractures

1. Diagnosis
   - Mechanism of injury—higher energy than intertrochanteric fractures
   - Plain radiographs
     - Anteroposterior and lateral views of hip
     - Anteroposterior and lateral views of femur
2. Classification—Russell-Taylor classification (Figure 11-44) based on involvement of lesser trochanter and piriformis fossa

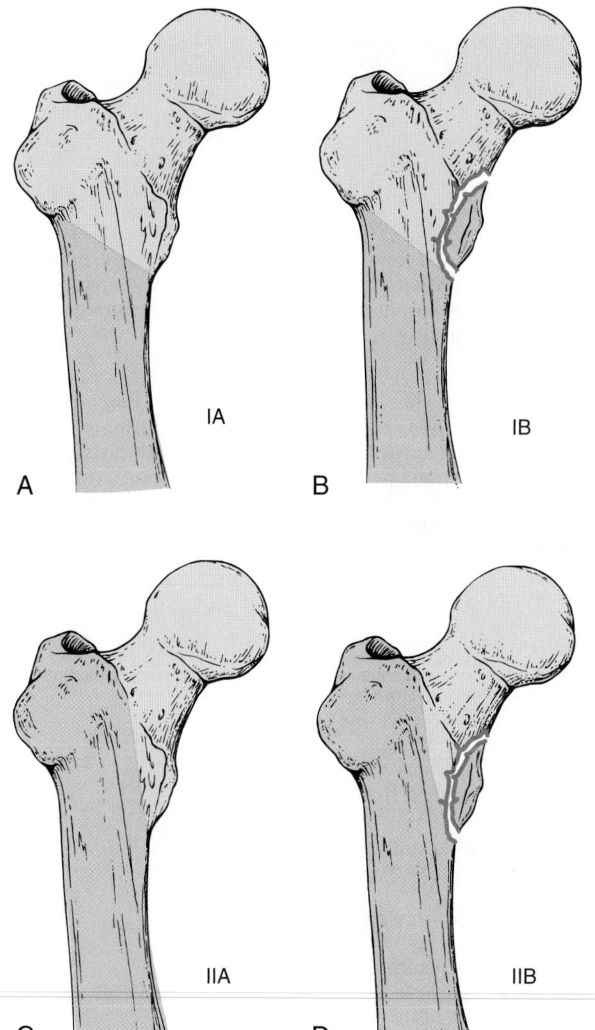

Figure 11-44 Russell-Taylor classification of subtrochanteric fractures. Fracture lines within red zones determine the type. In type I fractures, the piriformis fossa remains intact. Involvement of the piriformis fossa intramedullary nail entry site is the hallmark of type II fractures. Subtype A fractures do not involve the lesser trochanter, but in subtype B the lesser trochanter is a separate fragment. **A,** Type IA subtrochanteric fracture, suitable for first-generation locking nail. **B,** Type IB subtrochanteric fracture, which requires a cephalomedullary nail. **C,** Type IIA subtrochanteric fracture. The piriformis entry site is involved, but the lesser trochanter is intact. **D,** Type IIB subtrochanteric fracture. The nail entry site is involved, and lesser trochanteric comminution increases instability. (Modified from Tencer AF, et al: *Orthop Biomech Lab Report #002,* Memphis, Tenn, 1985, Richards Medical Co.)

- □ Type IA—fracture below lesser trochanter
- □ Type IB—fracture involves lesser trochanter; greater trochanter intact
- □ Type IIA—greater trochanter involved; lesser trochanter intact
- □ Type IIB—greater and lesser trochanter involved

3. Treatment
   - ▪ General principles
     - □ Restore limb length alignment and rotation.
     - □ Indirect reduction techniques obviate the need for bone grafting in acute fractures.
     - □ Nonoperative treatment is rarely indicated.
     - □ Operative treatment—Implant must withstand high medial compressive loads and high lateral tensile loads.
       - ▪ Indications—most subtrochanteric fractures
       - ▪ IM fixation
         - □ Indirect reduction preserves biologic environment.
         - □ Standard proximal interlocking for fractures with intact lesser trochanter
         - □ Reconstruction interlocking for fractures with involvement of lesser trochanter
         - □ Piriformis entry nail is a contraindication for fractures involving piriformis fossa.
           - ▪ **Apex anterior and varus angulation are the most common deformities.**
       - ▪ The psoas and abductors lead to flexion, abduction, and external rotation of the proximal fragment.
         - □ Open or percutaneous reduction indicated when closed reduction inadequate (frequent)—Union rates are same as with closed reduction.
         - □ **Lateral positioning allows easier alignment of the distal segment to the flexed proximal segment.**
       - ▪ Fixed-angle plate fixation/proximal femoral locking plates
         - □ Indicated for fractures with proximal comminution and nonunion
         - □ 95-degree devices
         - □ Devices of 135 degrees contraindicated
         - □ Must avoid soft tissue stripping
         - □ Acute bone grafting usually not required when biologic plating techniques are used
4. Complications
   - ▪ Nonunion—minimized with IM nailing and biologic plating
   - ▪ Malalignment—varus and apex anterior angulation with IM nailing. Consider adjunctive reduction aids and percutaneous reduction.
   - ▪ Infection—associated with increased soft tissue dissection

F. Femoral shaft fractures (Table 11-19)

1. Diagnosis
   - ▪ Mechanism of injury—Often associated with high-energy mechanisms
   - ▪ Associated fractures and other injuries are common.
   - ▪ **Associated neck fractures are uncommon (<10%); but when present, they are often missed (up to 50%).**
   - ▪ Plain radiographs
     - □ Anteroposterior and lateral views of femur
     - □ Anteroposterior and cross-table lateral hip to rule out femoral neck fracture
   - ▪ CT scan to rule out occult femoral neck fracture
     - □ If the scan is obtained for abdominal or pelvic evaluation, it should be reviewed.
     - □ Consider dedicated, thin-cut CT.
2. Classification—Winquist-Hansen classification (Figure 11-45) based on degree of comminution and amount of cortical continuity
   - ▪ Type 0—no comminution
   - ▪ Type I—comminution less than 25%
   - ▪ Type II—comminution 25%-50%
   - ▪ Type III—comminution greater than 50%
   - ▪ Type IV—comminution 100%

Table 11-19 Adult Femoral Shaft Fractures

Injury	Eponym/Other Name	Classification	Treatment	Complications
Femoral fracture (2.0 cm below lesser trochanter to 8 cm from knee joint)		Winquist—based on degree of comminution and amount of cortical continuity I—transverse, comminution <25% of circumference (e.g., butterfly fragment) II—comminution 25%-50% of circumference III—>50% comminution (unstable) IV—extensive (100%) comminution, no cortical contact, unstable V—segmental bone loss (unstable)	Most often high-energy mechanism; early stabilization as patient status permits; most fractures are treated by closed IM nail; statically locked, reamed nail for most fractures; antegrade (piriformis or trochanter) or retrograde; obesity a relative indication for trochanteric entry nail; multitrauma patients temporized with external fixation (damage control), converted to IM nail later; plate fixation for neck/shaft fractures, periprosthetic treatment (lower union, higher infection, longer time to weight bearing)	Infection (<5% closed fractures), nonunion (<5% closed fractures; treat with exchange nail vs. ORIF/ICBG), delayed union (exchange nail vs. dynamization), malalignment (malrotation, limb length discrepancy), hip pain/weakness (antegrade nail), knee pain (retrograde nail), pudendal nerve injury (excessive traction through post), missed knee ligament injury, knee stiffness (especially with distal external fixation), refracture, failure of fixation, deep venous thrombosis, pulmonary embolism, ARDS
Femoral neck and shaft fractures		Garden or Pauwels/ Winquist (2.5%-5.0% of femoral shaft fractures, *but* ≈30% are missed)	Neck takes priority; 135-degree fixed-angle device vs. parallel screws for neck, retrograde nail vs. plate for shaft; reconstruction nail for nondisplaced neck or intertrochanteric and shaft fractures	Infection, delayed union, nonunion, loss of fixation, avascular necrosis
Periprosthetic femur fracture		Vancouver	Stable prosthesis—lateral plate vs. lateral plate and allograft strut Unstable prosthesis—revision arthroplasty with uncemented long stem and lateral plate Allograft struts for bone loss	
Femoral and tibial shaft fractures	"Floating knee"		Retrograde nail for femur, antegrade nail for tibia	Multiple other injuries, fat emboli syndrome, ARDS

ARDS, acute respiratory distress syndrome; ICBG, iliac crest bone graft; IM, intramedullary; ORIF, open reduction and internal fixation.

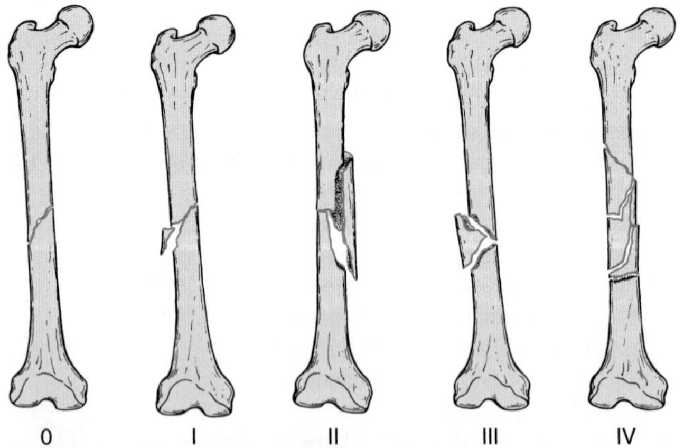

Figure 11-45 Winquist-Hansen classification of femoral shaft comminution. *0,* Non-comminuted; *I,* single small wedge ("butterfly") fragment; *II,* wedge fragment, greater than 50% shaft cortical contact; *III,* wedge fragment, less than 50% shaft cortical contact; *IV,* segmental comminution, no shaft cortex contact between proximal and distal main fragments. (From Browner BD, et al, editors: *Skeletal trauma,* ed 4, Philadelphia, 2008, Elsevier.)

3. Treatment
   - General principles
     - Restore limb length, alignment, and rotation.
     - Early stabilization reduces systemic complications associated with multiply injured patients.
   - Nonoperative treatment (rarely indicated)
     - Long leg cast or brace for nondisplaced distal shaft fracture
     - Pillow splint for nonambulatory individuals
   - Operative treatment—indicated for most fractures
     - IM nail
       - Indicated for most femoral shaft fractures
       - High union rates (>95%)
       - More hip problems with antegrade than retrograde insertion (pain/weakness)
       - More knee problems retrograde than antegrade insertion (pain and chondral injury to patella if nail left proud)
       - **Piriformis and trochanteric starting points indicated when they are used with appropriately designed nails**

- **Piriformis entry contraindicated when fracture extends to piriformis fossa**
- **Anterior starting point in piriformis fossa associated with increased hoop stress and risk of iatrogenic comminution**
- **Anterior trochanteric starting point with minimal hoop stress**
- **Trochanteric starting point risks medial comminution of shaft due to off-axis starting point and varus if straight (no trochanteric bend) nail used**

- **Static interlocking for most fractures**
- **Reamed nailing for most fractures**
  - **Higher union rates than unreamed nails**
  - Unreamed nails associated with decreased fat embolization; clinical relevance unclear
  - Appropriate reaming technique includes sharp reamers, slow advancement, less heat generation, and less embolization.
  - Minimum cortical reaming preferred
  - Nail diameter 1 to 2 mm smaller than largest reamer
- **Multiply injured patients may benefit from delayed nailing with immediate provisional external fixation (damage control principles).**
- **Benefits include reduced blood loss, reduced hypothermia, and reduced inflammatory mediator release.**

- **External fixation**
  - **Indicated for provisional fixation**
    - **Application of damage control principles**
    - Severe contamination requiring repeated access to medullary canal
    - Vascular injury
  - **Safely converted to IM nail in absence of pin tract infection up to at least 3 weeks with equal union and infection rates**
- Plate fixation
  - Indicated for periprosthetic fractures
  - Indicated for neck component of neck-shaft fractures
  - Reduced union rate, higher infection and implant failure rates, and longer time to weight bearing than with use of IM nail

4. Complications
   - Infection—less than 5% of closed fractures
   - Nonunion—less than 5% of closed fractures
     - Exchange nailing less successful than repair with plate and screws and bone grafting.
   - Delayed union—less than 5% of closed fractures
     - **Dynamization is less successful than exchange nailing.**
   - **Malalignment**
     - Proximal fracture more often malaligned with retrograde than antegrade nailing
     - Distal fractures more often malaligned with antegrade than retrograde nailing
     - Malrotation difficult to diagnose, especially with comminuted fractures
       - **Compare with the contralateral limb before leaving operating room**
       - Supine nailing has a higher incidence of internal rotation.
       - Lateral nailing has a higher incidence of external rotation.
       - **Fracture table use has a higher incidence of internal rotation compared with manual traction.**
   - Length discrepancy is associated with comminuted fractures.
   - **Hip pain/weakness is associated with antegrade nailing.**
   - **Knee pain is associated with retrograde nailing.**
   - Patellar chondral injury is associated with retrograde nailing, with nail left protruding into the knee joint.
   - Pudendal nerve injury is associated with excessive traction.
   - HO is associated with antegrade nailing (rarely clinically relevant).
   - **Osteonecrosis in adolescents with open physes treated with a piriformis-starting IM nail**
5. Special circumstances
   - Obese patients
     - Higher complication rates with piriformis nailing
     - Relative indication for retrograde nailing
   - **Ipsilateral femoral neck and shaft fractures**
     - Uncommon (<10%) but, when present, missed in up to 50% of cases
     - **Neck component the highest priority**
       - **Neck fracture often nondisplaced, vertical and basicervical**
       - **Use of 135-degree sliding hip screw or parallel screws preferred for femoral neck**
       - **Retrograde nail or plate fixation for shaft**
       - Reconstruction nail for nondisplaced neck fractures or associated intertrochanteric and shaft fractures
         - Use of a single device is associated with increased risk of malreduction of either shaft or neck.
   - Multiply injured patient—Consider damage control principles.
     - **Provisional external fixator with conversion to IM nail when stable (within 3 weeks)**
     - May be more applicable with associated lung/chest injury
   - Periprosthetic fracture
     - Stable prosthesis—A lateral plate with the use of biologic plating techniques yields results similar to those obtained with a lateral plate and an allograft strut. Newer techniques use lateral locking plate.
     - Unstable prosthesis—revision arthroplasty with uncemented long stem + lateral plate
     - **Allograft struts indicated for bone loss**
     - Longer plates are better than shorter plates if in doubt on overlap of prosthesis.

G. Supracondylar and intracondylar fractures

1. Diagnosis
   - Mechanism of injury—high energy in young patients and low energy in older patients
   - Plain radiographs
     - Anteroposterior and lateral views of femur
     - Anteroposterior and lateral views of knee
   - **CT**
     - **If intracondylar extension**

- **Coronal fracture (Hoffa fracture) incidence—40%**
  - **Lateral femoral condyle fracture incidence—80%**
  - **Plain radiographs frequently miss this injury.**

2. Classification—OTA classification (Figure 11-46) based on the degree of comminution and articular involvement
   - 33-A—Extraarticular
   - 33-B—Simple articular (unicondylar)
   - 33-C—Complex articular
3. Treatment
   - General principles
     - Restore articular congruity.
     - Rigid stabilization of articular fracture
     - Indirect reduction of metaphyseal component to preserve vascularity to fracture fragments
     - Stable (not necessarily rigid) fixation of articular block to shaft
     - Early knee ROM
   - Nonoperative treatment—indicated for nondisplaced fractures
     - Brace or knee immobilized
     - Full-time bracing for 6 to 8 weeks
     - Closed-chain ROM at 3 to 4 weeks
   - Operative treatment—indicated for most displaced fractures
     - Plate fixation—indicated for most fractures

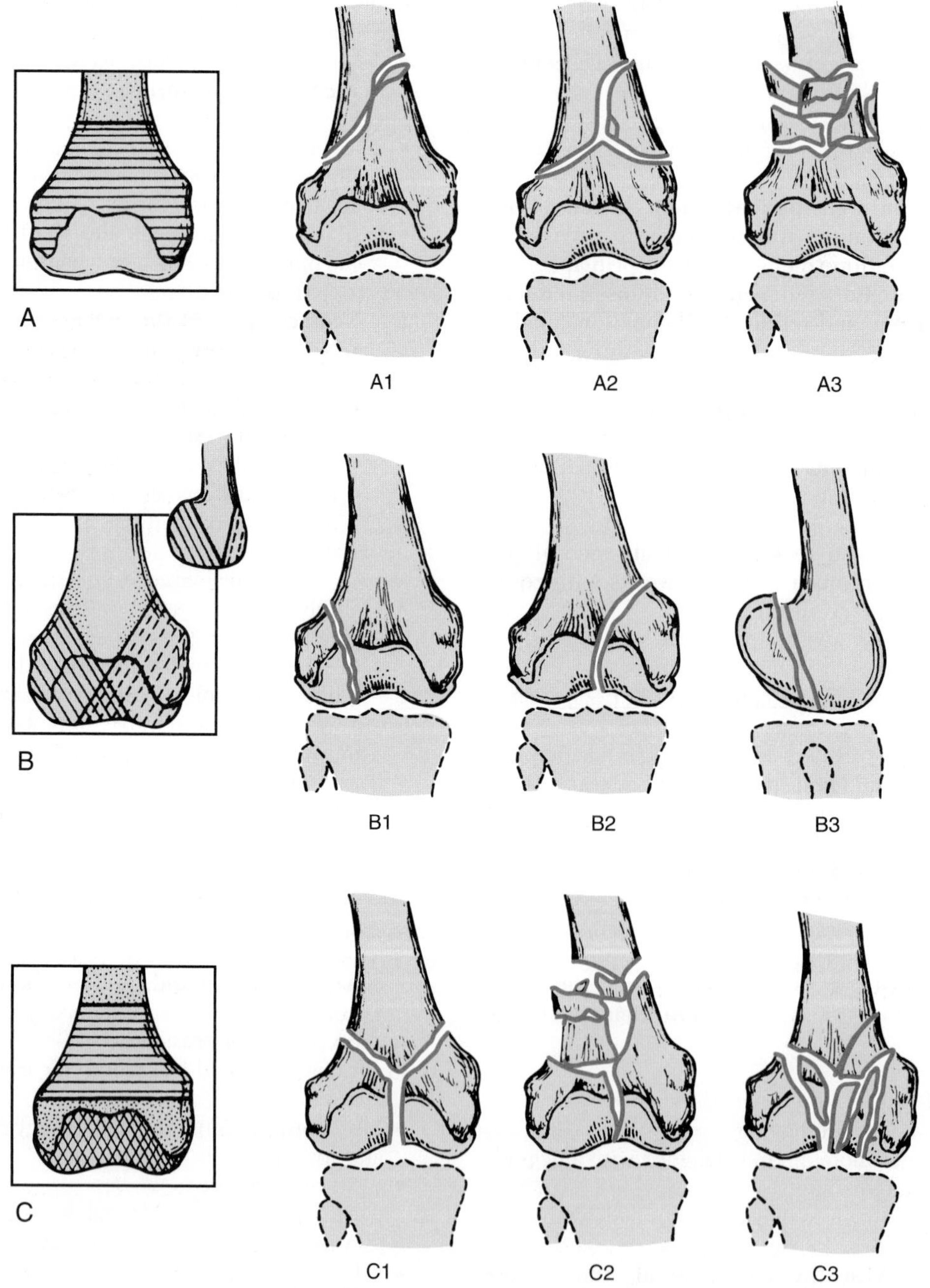

Figure 11-46 The AO/OTA classification of distal femoral fractures. (From Browner BD, et al, editors: *Skeletal trauma,* ed 4, Philadelphia, 2008, Elsevier.)

- Fixed-angle plates required when metaphyseal comminution exists
  - Traditional 95-degree devices limited by number and location of distal fixation
  - Locked plates offer multiple fixed-angle points of fixation in distal fragment in multiple planes.
  - Non–fixed-angle plates prone to varus collapse, especially in metaphyseal comminution
- High union rates (>80%) with indirect reduction technique without bone graft
- Lateral approach—indirect reduction of metaphyseal fracture and arthrotomy with direct reduction of articular component
  - Sagittal intraarticular split most common
  - Condyles are malrotated in sagittal plane with respect to each other.
  - Coronal (Hoffa) fractures require interfragmentary lag screws.
  - Laterally applied condylar plate spans fracture (locked plate preferred).

- Retrograde IM nail
  - Indicated for extraarticular fractures and simple intraarticular fractures
  - Reduced stability compared with plate fixation for osteoporotic fractures, especially those with wide metaphyseal flares
    - Blocking screws can help provide reduction and improved stability.
    - Fixed-angle, distal interlocking screws may provide improved stability.
  - Long nails that cross the femoral isthmus are preferred to short "supracondylar" nails.
- Arthroplasty
  - Indicated when associated with preexisting joint arthropathy and select cases when stable internal fixation not achievable
  - Usually requires distal femoral replacement prosthesis
  - Reduced longevity compared with internal fixation
  - Allows immediate weight bearing

4. Complications
   - Nonunion—associated with soft tissue stripping in metaphyseal region
   - Malalignment
     - Valgus malreduction most common (plate fixation)
     - Malalignment more common with IM nails
   - Loss of fixation
     - Varus collapse most common
       - Plate fixation associated with toggle of distal non–fixed-angle screws used for comminuted metaphyseal fractures
       - IM nail fixation
     - Proximal (diaphyseal) screw failure associated with short plates and nonlocked diaphyseal fixation—Plate fixation is associated with toggle of distal non–fixed-angle screws used for comminuted metaphyseal fractures.
   - Infection—occurs in diabetic patients, especially those with active foot ulcers
   - Knee pain/stiffness
   - **Painful hardware—Avoid prominent medial screws.**

5. Special circumstances—periprosthetic fractures
   - Good results with locked plates
   - Retrograde nails require a sufficiently large intercondylar box.

III. KNEE INJURIES (TABLE 11-20)

A. Dislocation

1. Diagnosis/classification
   - Direction (Kennedy)—anterior (30%-40%), posterior (30%-40%), medial, lateral, and rotatory (posterolateral the most common) (Figure 11-47)
   - Schenck anatomic classification of knee dislocation (KD)
     - KD I—dislocation with either anterior cruciate ligament (ACL) or posterior cruciate ligament (PCL) still intact (variable collateral involvement)
     - KD II—torn ACL/PCL
     - KD III—**most common**
       - Torn ACL/PCL and either posterolateral corner (PLC-KD IIIL) or posteromedial corner (PMC-KD IIIM)
     - KD IV—torn ACL/PCL/PLC/PMC
     - KD V—fracture-dislocation
   - More than 50% present reduced (easily missed diagnosis)
   - Vascular injury—5% to 15% in recent studies.
     - **Selective arteriography with the use of a physical examination (including ankle-brachial index) rather than an immediate arteriogram is now the standard of care.**
     - The most common finding in patients with vascular injury is a diminished or absent pedal pulse.
   - Significant soft tissue injuries
2. Treatment
   - Emergent reduction if patient did not present with fracture reduced
   - Revascularize within 6 hours if there is significant arterial injury.
   - Care for soft-tissue injuries (open-knee dislocations).
   - Ligament repair or reconstruction
     - Reconstruction with allograft becoming the most common
     - Acute reconstruction may be better than chronic reconstruction.
     - Early motion rehabilitation
     - Possible role for hinged external fixator
3. Complications
   - **Vascular injury—the highest with KD IV; an ankle-brachial index of greater than 0.9 is associated with an intact artery**
   - Neurologic injury—Peroneal nerve injury is common (about 25%), but up to 50% recover at least partially; may benefit from neurolysis.
   - Stiffness/arthrofibrosis—most common complication (38%)
   - Ligamentous laxity also very common (37%)

B. Patella fractures

1. Diagnosis/classification
   - Descriptive—transverse, vertical (rarely requires surgical treatment), comminuted, proximal or distal (30%) pole, and nondisplaced (Figure 11-48)

Table 11-20 Adult Knee Fractures and Dislocations

Injury	Eponym	Classification	Treatment	Complications
Supracondylar fracture	"Hoffa" fracture (33-B3)	AO/OTA—degree of comminution and articular involvement 33-A—extraarticular 33-B—partially articular (unicondylar) 33-C—intraarticular	Restore articular congruity, rigid stabilization of articular fracture, preserve vascularity, stable fixation of joint to shaft, early ROM Nonoperative: brace or knee immobilizer, non–weight bearing for 6-8 wk, closed-chain ROM at 3-4 wk Plate fixation: most fractures; fixed-angle plate for metaphyseal comminution (nonfixed: varus collapse) Retrograde IM nail: extraarticular or simple intraarticular fractures, long nail preferred Arthroplasty when fixation not achievable, arthropathy present	Nonunion (soft tissue stripping of metaphyseal region), malalignment (valgus malreduction most common, nails >> plates), loss of fixation (varus collapse), infection, knee stiffness, DJD, unstable fixation, DVT, fracture fragments from missed coronal plane ("Hoffa fracture"), prominent hardware
Periprosthetic fracture			Locked plate vs. retrograde nail (need size of intercondylar box in total knee arthroplasty for nail to fit)	
Patella fracture		Nondisplaced, transverse, proximal or distal (30%) pole, comminuted, vertical (nonoperative)	Nonoperative: nondisplaced (<2 mm) with intact extensor mechanism; hinged knee brace in extension, progress in flexion after 2-3 wk ORIF (tension band wiring, screws) if patient cannot actively extend knee (extensor mechanism rupture) or there is a >2-mm separation or incongruent articular surface (>2-mm step-off); excise fragments that are extremely comminuted; avoid patellectomy	Symptomatic hardware, loss of reduction, nonunion (<5%), infection, arthrofibrosis/stiffness, quadriceps weakness, infection, DJD, extensor lag
Patella dislocation		Acute, recurrent, subluxation, habitual, usually lateral	Immobilize, controlled motion for 6 wk; arthroscopy for displaced or osteochondral fracture; recurrent: lateral release, medial plication (repair/reconstruct MPFL); bony transplant if abnormal Q angle. Avoid surgery in those with habitual dislocation.	Redislocation
Knee dislocation		Anterior (30%-40%), posterior (30%-40%), lateral, medial, rotatory (anteromedial, anterolateral, posteromedial, posterolateral) Schenck anatomic classification: KD I—dislocation with anterior cruciate ligament (ACL) or posterior cruciate ligament (PCL) intact KD II—torn ACL/PCL KD III—torn ACL/PCL and either posterolateral corner (PLC) or posteromedial corner (PMC) KD IV—torn ACL/PCL/PLC/PMC KD V—fracture-dislocation	May present spontaneously reduced—easily missed; reduce dislocations emergently; open reduction if needed (posterolateral rotation); arteriogram based on physical exam findings (absent/asymmetric pulses); repair vascular injuries (5%-15%); ligament repair (within 2-3 wk) or reconstruction, allograft vs. autograft, early motion	Vascular injury (5%-15%, highest with KD-IV; ankle-brachial index > 0.9 associated with intact artery); neurologic injury (tibial/peroneal nerve), stiffness/arthrofibrosis (most common complication), ligamentous laxity

Table 11-20 Adult Knee Fractures and Dislocations—cont'd

Injury	Eponym	Classification	Treatment	Complications
Quadriceps rupture		Generally older than 40 and metabolic disorders (chronic renal failure, rheumatoid arthritis, steroid use), M >> F	Incomplete rupture: nonoperative management	Strength deficit; stiffness, inability to resume preinjury athletic/recreational activity; bilateral ruptures (identify underlying medical problem, repair both); DVT; chronic ruptures (allograft reconstruction, quadriceps tendon lengthening)
			Complete: repair through osseous drill holes or suture anchors; repair acutely: >2 wk or ≤5-cm retraction	
Patella tendon rupture		Younger than 40, overload of extensor mechanism; increased risk with metabolic disorders (rheumatoid arthritis, diabetes mellitus, infection)	Direct repair with nonabsorbable suture and locking (Krackow) stitch through drill holes; can protect repair with cerclage	Missed diagnosis (high-riding patella seen on radiographs), stiffness, extensor weakness

DJD, degenerative joint disease; DVT, deep venous thrombosis; IM, intramedullary; MPFL, medial patellofemoral ligament; ORIF, open reduction and internal fixation; ROM, range of motion.

- An inability to extend the knee or do a straight-leg raise demonstrates an incompetent extensor mechanism.
- Displaced fracture is 3 mm fragment separation or 2 mm step-off.

2. Treatment—Preserve patella whenever possible (i.e., avoid patellectomy).
   - Nonoperative treatment—nondisplaced with intact extensor mechanism, hinged knee brace in extension, and progress in flexion after 2 to 3 weeks
   - Tension band wiring—simple fracture patterns; most common technique; can be done with K wires or cannulated screws (biomechanically stronger); may use wire or braided non-absorbable suture (less hardware irritation)
   - Cerclage and tension band wiring—minimally displaced stellate fractures with significant comminution
   - **Partial patellectomy—useful with extraarticular distal pole fractures and also used with severely comminuted fractures; preserve the largest pieces and reattach patella ligament** (Figure 11-49).
3. Complications—symptomatic hardware (very common), loss of reduction (22%), nonunion (<5%), infection, and arthrofibrosis/stiffness

C. **Patella dislocations**

1. Diagnosis—frequently involves young adults or adolescents, usually laterally, and involves injury to the medial patellofemoral ligament
2. Treatment—Reduce and immobilize with controlled motion for 6 weeks.
3. Complications—redislocation

D. **Patella ligament rupture**

1. Diagnosis/classification—occurs in patients younger than 40 with overload of extensor mechanism during athletic activity
   - Increased risk with metabolic disorders, rheumatologic disease, renal failure, corticosteroid injection, patellar tendinitis, and infection. Diagnosis is frequently missed.
2. Treatment—direct primary repair with a nonabsorbable suture and locking (Krackow) stitch through patellar drill holes; can supplement with semitendinosus graft and/or cerclage wire/suture to protect repair.
3. Complications—stiffness and extensor weakness

E. **Quadriceps tendon rupture**

1. Diagnosis—Patients may be younger than 40, but this condition most commonly occurs in older patients with medical problems.
   - Association with renal failure, diabetes, rheumatoid arthritis, hyperparathyroidism, connective tissue disorders, steroid use, and intraarticular injections in 20% to 33%
   - Males are affected more often (up to 8 : 1). The nondominant limb is affected two times more often than the dominant limb.
2. Treatment
   - Incomplete rupture—nonoperative management; warn of risk for future rupture.
   - Acute unilateral rupture—repair through osseous drill holes or suture anchors; repair acutely. Ruptures more than 2 weeks old may be retracted 5 cm.

Apparent Knee Dislocation

- Physical exam
- History
- X-rays

↔ Assess ASAP for
1. Other injuries
2. Arterial injury → Immediate evaluation and management
3. Neurologic injury → Delayed evaluation and management
   - EMG / NCV
   - Nerve repair / graft
   - Tendon transfers

Pedal Pulses

Absent | Present

Reduce dislocation
Closed, if possible
Open if not

↔ - Splint as needed to maintain reduction
- Repeat x-ray to confirm

Reassess Pulses

Still absent | Return after reduction | Still present

Still absent →
- Urgent vascular surgery consult
- Possible arterial imaging
  - Duplex ultrasonography
  - Percutaneous ED or OR arteriogram
  - Percutaneous digital subtraction (radiol)
  - CT arteriography
- ***Imaging contraindicated if it will delay revascularization***

→
- Vascular repair
- Fasciotomies

? External fixation

Return after reduction / Still present → **ABI**

<0.9 →
- Vascular consult
- Arterial imaging and repair if needed

≥0.9 →
- Observe in hospital
- Check pulses q4 h
- Reassess if ↓

→ **Knee MRI** (? from vascular repair)

→ **Delayed Ligament Repair** (? from vascular repair)

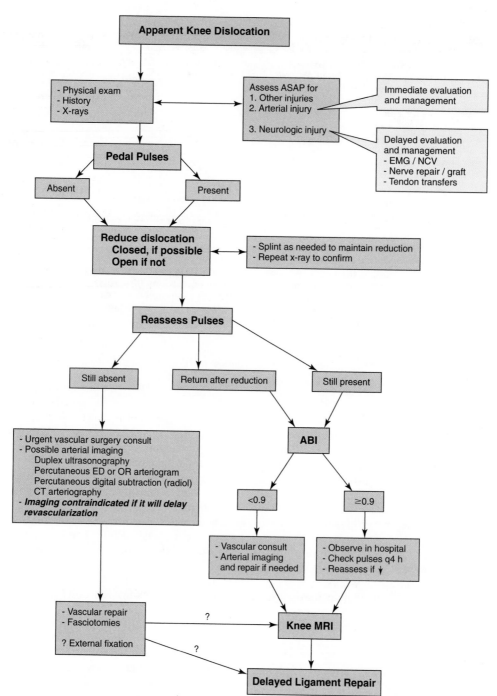

Figure 11-47 Treatment algorithm for dislocation of the knee. ABI, ankle-brachial index; CT, computed tomography; ED, emergency department; EMG/NCV, electromyelography/nerve conduction velocity; OR, operating room. (From Browner BD, et al, editors: *Skeletal trauma,* ed 4, Philadelphia, 2008, Elsevier.)

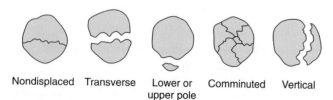

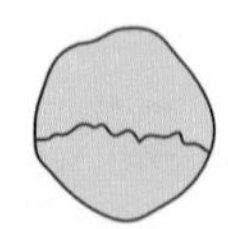

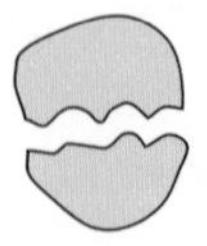

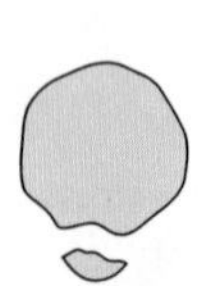

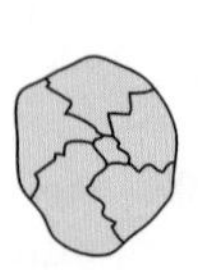

Figure 11-48 Types of patellar fractures. (From Weissman BN, Sledge CB: *Orthopedic radiology,*. Philadelphia, 1986, WB Saunders, p 553.)

- Bilateral ruptures—Identify the underlying medical problem; otherwise, treat the same as a unilateral rupture. Non–weight bearing and DVT prophylaxis are required.
- Chronic tendon ruptures—less successful than the acute ones; may require Codivilla procedure (V-Y lengthening) or quadriceps tendon lengthening.

3. Complications—strength deficit (33%-50% of patients), stiffness, and the inability to resume prior level of athletic/recreational activity (50%)

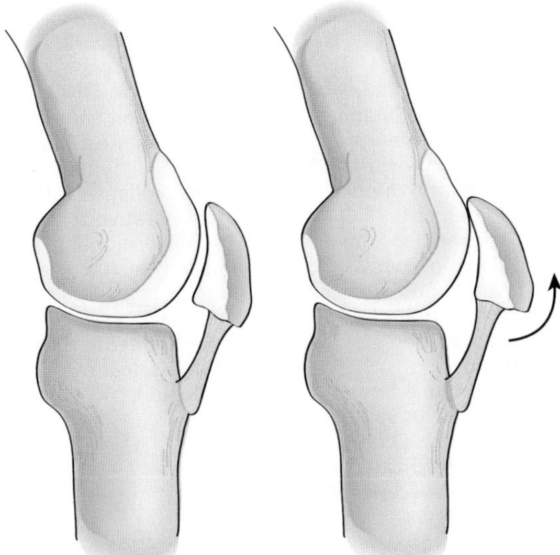

Figure 11-49 Anterior reattachment of the patellar ligament, which is recommended to prevent tilting of the patella superiorly. (Redrawn with permission from Marder RA, et al: Effects of partial patellectomy and reattachment of the patellar tendon on patellofemoral contact areas and pressures, *J Bone Joint Surg Am* 75:35-45, 1993.)

IV. TIBIAL INJURIES (TABLE 11-21)

A. Plateau fracture

1. Diagnosis/classification
   - Schatzker classification (Figure 11-50)
     - Type I—split
     - Type II—split depression
     - Type III—pure depression (rare)
     - Type IV—medial tibial plateau

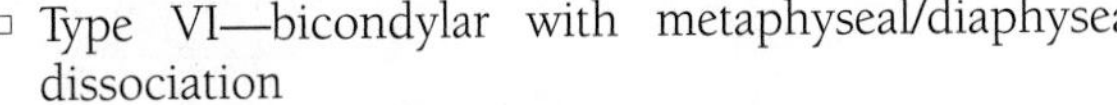

     - Type V—bicondylar with intact metaphysis
     - Type VI—bicondylar with metaphyseal/diaphyseal dissociation
   - AO/OTA classification (Figure 11-51)
     - 41-A—extraarticular fracture
     - 41-B—partial articular fracture (Schatzker I-IV)
     - 41-C—complete articular/bicondylar (Schatzker V and VI)
   - MRI changes treatment or classification in most cases.
     - Soft tissue injury is demonstrated (50%-90% incidence).
     - MCL and ACL injuries in 30% to 50%
     - **Meniscus tears in over 50% of cases**
       - **Lateral tears more common medial tears**
         - **Type II—lateral meniscal pathology**
         - **Type IV—medial meniscal pathology**
       - **Peripheral tears most common type**
   - Order of frequency—lateral greater than bicondylar greater than medial **(think *dislocation* with medial)**
2. Treatment
   - Nonoperative treatment—indicated in stable knees (<10 degrees coronal plane instability with the knee in full extension) with less than 3 mm articular step-off. Cast brace, early ROM, and delayed weight bearing for at least 4 to 6 weeks.
   - Operative treatment—indicated with articular step-off greater than 3 mm, condylar widening greater than 5 mm, **instability of the knee**, and all medial and bicondylar plateau fractures. **The goal of treatment is restoration of normal alignment. Development of arthritis does not correlate with articular step-off.**
     - ORIF
       - Plate fixation with early motion
       - **Percutaneous locked plating for poor-quality bone in bicondylar fractures; no stripping**

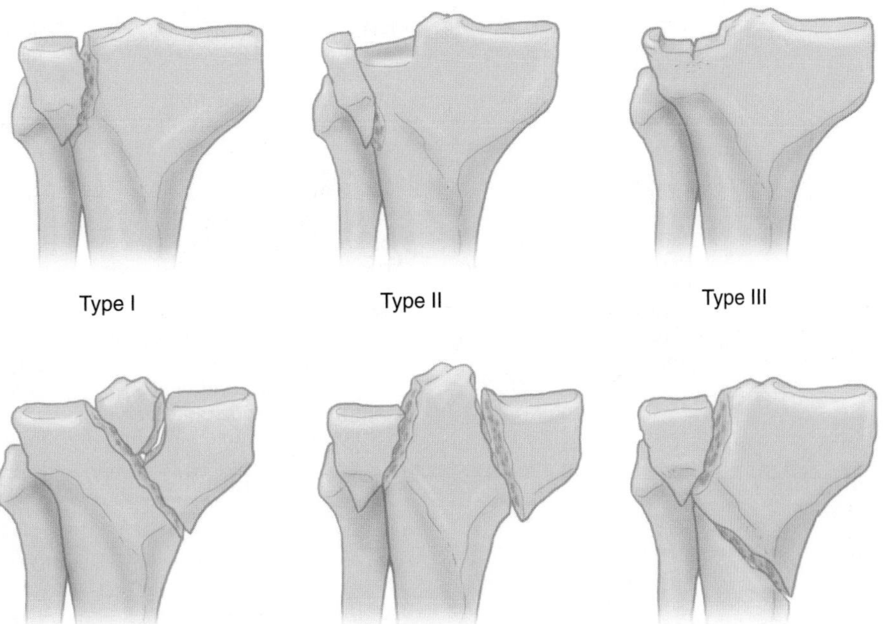

Figure 11-50 Schatzker classification of tibial plateau fractures. (Adapted from Lubowitz J, Elson W, Guttmann D: Part I: Arthroscopic management of tibial plateau fractures, *Arthroscopy* 20:1063-1070, 2004.)

Table 11-21 Adult Tibia Fractures and Dislocations

Injury	Eponym/Other Name	Classification	Treatment	Complications
Tibial plateau fracture		Schatzker classification I—split II—split depression III—pure depression IV—medial plateau split V—bicondylar with intact metaphysis VI—bicondylar with metaphyseal/diaphyseal dissociation AO/OTA classification 41-A—extraarticular fracture 41-B—partial articular fracture (Schatzker I–IV) 41-C—complete articular/ bicondylar (Schatzker V and VI)	Magnetic resonance imaging can change treatment or classification in most cases (soft tissue injury); medial collateral ligament > ACL; lateral > bicondylar > medial (think dislocation with medial); spanning external fixation for high-energy injuries (soft tissue stabilization) Nonoperative: stable knees (<10 degrees varus/valgus in full extension, <3 mm articular step-off); cast brace, early ROM, delayed weight bearing for 4-6 wk ORIF if articular step-off >3 mm, condylar widening >5 mm, knee unstable, medial and bicondylar; plate fixation (locked vs. nonlocked, single vs. dual [posteromedial] incision) vs. external fixation (bicondylar or severe soft tissue injury, wires >15 mm from joint)	DJD, infection (surgical approach most important factor), malunion (varus collapse with nonoperative treatment or conventional plates/ bicondylar fracture), ligament instability, peroneal nerve injury, compartment syndrome, stiffness, loss of reduction, avascular necrosis
Tibial spine fracture		I—anterior tilt II—complete anterior tilt III—no contact A—no rotation B—rotated	I/II/IIIA closed reduction, long-leg cast for 6 wk if knee can be brought into full extension; IIIB and all irreducible types require open reduction	Block to motion (arthroscopic loose-body removal), ACL laxity
Tibial tubercle fracture			ORIF with screw or staple	Loss of fixation, quadriceps weakness
Subchondral tibial fracture		Stable	Cast immobilization	Arterial injury, decreased ROM
		Displaced	ORIF with buttress plate	
Tibial stress fracture		Upper one third (recruits)	Modify activity for 6-10 wk	Progression to complete fracture
Tibial shaft fracture		Gustillo and Anderson—open fracture grade Grade I—no periosteal stripping, <1-cm wound Grade II—no periosteal stripping, >1-cm wound Grade IIIA—periosteal stripping, no flap required Grade IIIB—periosteal stripping, flap required Grade IIIC—periosteal stripping, flap required, vascular injury requiring repair	Most respond to closed reduction, LLC, wedge as needed, PTB at 6-8 wk; IM nail for transverse oblique fracture of mid–one third or segmental and also for vascular injury, bilateral injury, pathologic fractures, severe ligamentous injuries to knee (statically locked IM nail); open fractures: unreamed nail up to and including some IIIB injuries, early flap coverage, delayed bone grafting. Consider early amputation in grade IIIC injuries, posterior tibial nerve injury, warm ischemia >6 hr, and severe ipsilateral foot injury (unreconstructible limb).	Delayed union (>20 wk; increased with greater initial displacement and middle-third fractures; treatment includes fibulectomy and posterolateral bone graft), nonunion (posterolateral bone graft or reamed IM nail), infection (flap/graft or amputation), malunion (varus/valgus, shortening [accept <5 degrees varus/ valgus, <10 degrees anteroposterior angulation]), vascular injuries (upper one fourth of anterior tibial artery), compartment syndrome, peroneal nerve injury, CRPS
Tibial plafond fracture	Pilon	Ruedi and Allgöwer I—minimally displaced II—incongruous III—comminuted	Long-leg cast and non–weight bearing ORIF if displaced and ankle involved; consider minimally invasive small-pin external fixation techniques	DJD (may require late fusion), infection, varus/ valgus angulation, skin slough

Table 11-21 Adult Tibia Fractures and Dislocations—cont'd

Injury	Eponym/Other Name	Classification	Treatment	Complications
Fibular shaft fracture		Mid to lower one third (athletes)	Cast only if needed for pain relief	Missed syndesmotic injury
Proximal fibula fracture			Open if unstable	Injury to biceps, peroneal nerve
Proximal tibia-fibula dislocation		Anterior (most common), posterior, superior	Reduce (90 degrees flexion), ORIF fails with recurrence	
Chondral/ osteochondral fracture		Endogenous vs. exogenous	Arthroscopic evaluation of locked, acute condylar defects; remove small fragments (pin large fragments)	DJD

ACL, anterior cruciate ligament; CRPS, complex regional pain syndrome; DJD, degenerative joint disease; IM, intramedullary; ORIF, open reduction and internal fixation; PTB, patella tendon–bearing cast; ROM, range of motion.

- **Posteromedial fragments may not be captured via a lateral pate. Use a separate posteromedial incision if second plate is needed.**
- **Use of bone void fillers**
  - **Calcium phosphate cement has highest compressive strength.**
  - **Lower rate of subsidence compared with autogenous iliac bone graft**
- External fixation—hybrid or Ilizarov useful for bicondylar fractures with severe soft tissue injuries. Keep small wires at least 15 mm from the joint to avoid septic joint.

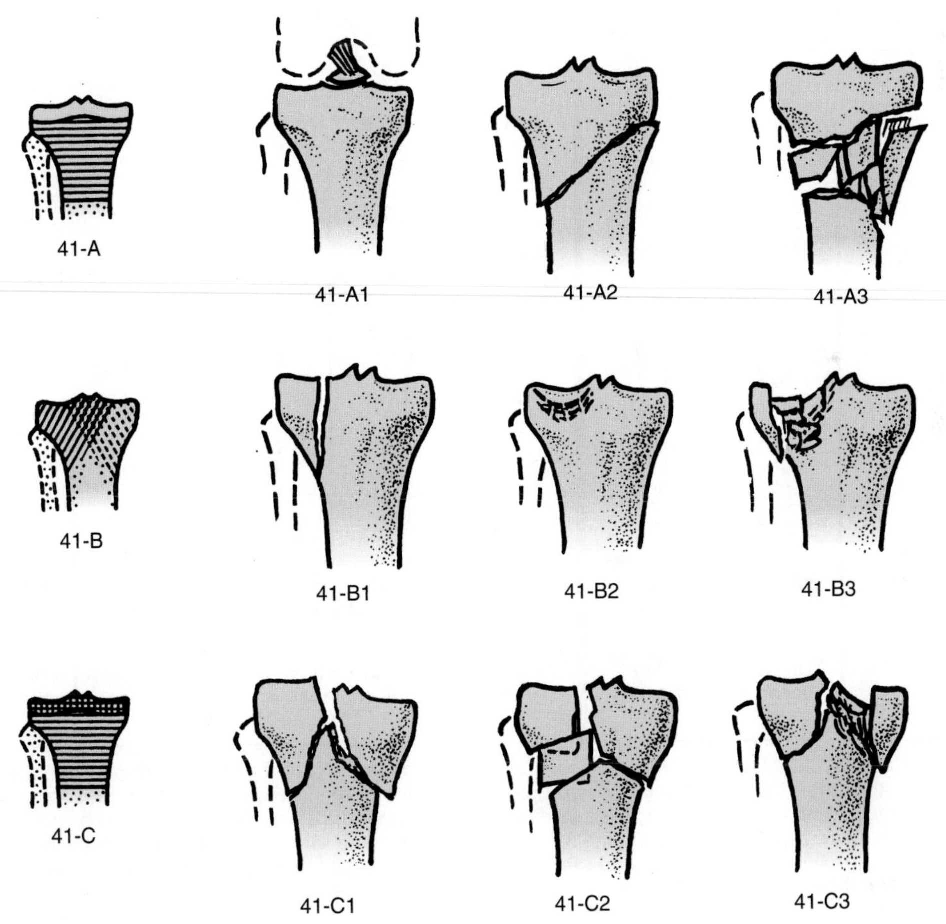

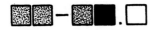

Figure 11-51 AO/OTA universal classification system for fractures of the tibial plateau (see text). (From Müller ME, et al, editors: *The comprehensive classification of fractures of long bones,* Berlin, 1990, Springer-Verlag.)

- **Spanning external fixators—used temporarily with selected high-energy injuries to allow for a reduction in soft tissue swelling before definitive fixation**

3. Complications—degenerative joint disease (DJD), infection (surgical approach the most important factor), malunion (varus collapse with nonoperative or conventional plates in severe bicondylar fractures), ligament instability (left untreated, has an adverse impact on outcome), peroneal nerve injury
   - Compartment syndrome—increased risk with more proximal fractures. Anterior and lateral compartments are at highest risk.

B. **Shaft fractures**

1. Diagnosis
   - Mechanism of injury
     - Low energy
       - Spiral oblique fracture
       - Tibia and fibula at different levels
       - Closed fracture with minor soft tissue trauma
     - High energy
       - Comminuted fracture
       - Tibia and fibula at same level
       - Transverse fracture pattern
       - Diastasis between tibia and fibula
       - Segmental fracture
       - Open fracture or closed with significant soft tissue trauma
   - The most common long bone fracture
   - Often associated with soft tissue injuries
     - Soft tissue management critical to outcome
     - Open fractures may require repeated incision and drainage.
       - Number of instances of débridement, type of irrigation, and pressure of irrigant controversial
       - Sharp débridement of nonviable soft tissue and bone the most important aspect of incision and drainage
   - Plain radiographs
     - Anteroposterior and lateral tibia views must include knee and ankle.
     - Dedicated knee and ankle radiographs for intraarticular extension
     - CT scan if significant intraarticular extension
2. Classification
   - OTA classification (Figure 11-52)—based on comminution
     - 42-A—simple (two parts)
     - 42-B—butterfly comminution
     - 42-C—comminuted; no direct contact between proximal and distal fragments

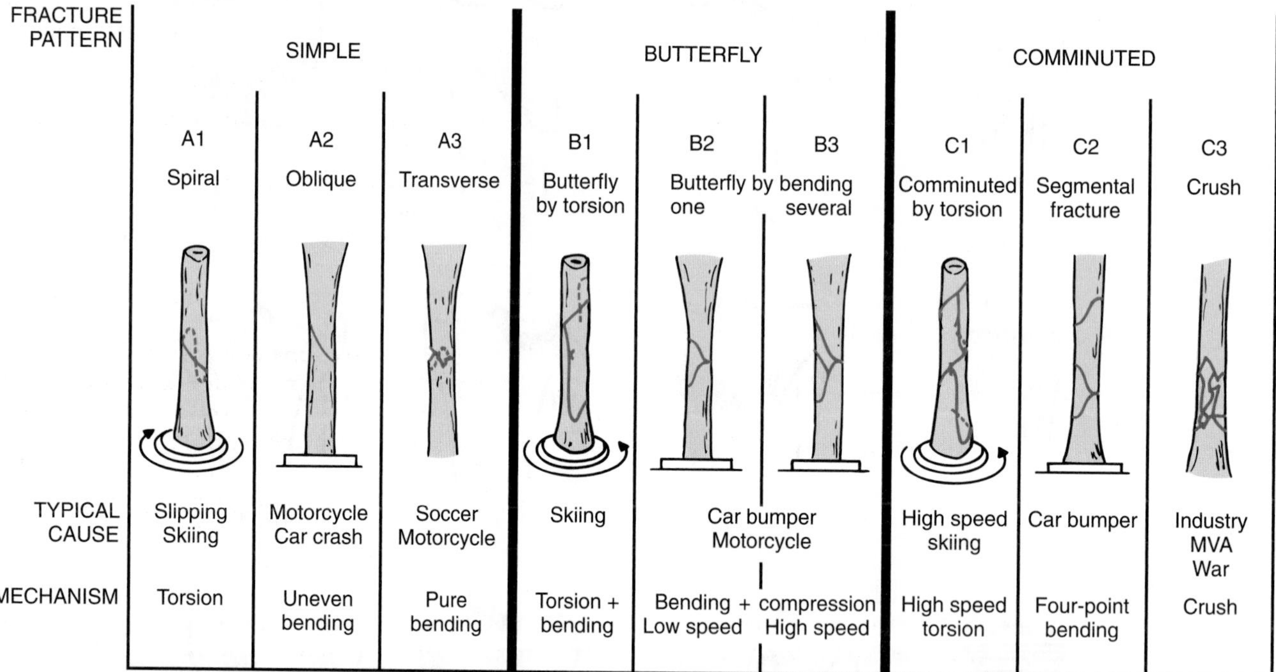

Figure 11-52 Johner and Wruhs' classification system for tibial shaft fractures. Note that neither displacement nor soft tissue wound severity is considered in this system. Nine alphanumeric groups (A to C, 1 to 3) are illustrated in this figure. Each group can be separated into three subgroups, each of which may have three qualifications. The subgroups are the same for each of the A and B groups: 1 = fibula intact, 2 = fibula fracture at a different level, and 3 = fibula fracture at the same level. The qualifications are also the same for all the A and B groups: (1) = proximal, (2) = middle, and (3) = distal. The subgroups within group C1 are .1, two intermediate fragments; .2, three intermediate fragments; and .3, more than three intermediate fragments. The C1 qualifications are (1) pure diaphyseal, (2) proximal metadiaphyseal, and (3) distal metadiaphyseal. The C2 subgroups are .1, single intermediate segmental fragment; .2, intermediate segmental and wedge fragments; and .3, two intermediate segmental fragments. For C2.1, the qualifications are (1) pure diaphyseal, (2) proximal metadiaphyseal, (3) distal metadiaphyseal, (4) oblique lines, and (5) transverse and oblique lines. For C2.2 the qualifications are (1) pure diaphyseal, (2) proximal metadiaphyseal, (3) distal metadiaphyseal, (4) distal wedge, and (5) three wedges, proximal and distal. For C2.3,the qualifications are (1) pure diaphyseal, (2) proximal metadiaphyseal, and (3) distal metadiaphyseal. For group C3 the subgroups are .1, two or three intermediate fragments; .2, limited shattering (<4 cm); and .3, extensive shattering (>4 cm). Qualifications for C3.1 are (1) two intermediate fragments and (2) three intermediate fragments. For C3.2 and C3.3, qualifications are (1) pure diaphyseal, (2) proximal metadiaphyseal, and (3) distal metadiaphyseal. MVA, motor vehicle accident. (Redrawn from Johner R, Wruhs O: Clin Orthop 178:7-25, 1983. In Browner N, Jupiter J, Trafton P, editors: *Skeletal trauma,* ed 3, Philadelphia, 2002, Elsevier.)

- Open fracture grade (Gustillo and Anderson)—based on degree of periosteal stripping and requirement for soft tissue coverage
  - Grade I—no periosteal stripping, less than 1-cm wound
  - Grade II—no or mild periosteal stripping or soft tissue injury, greater than 1-cm wound
  - Grade IIIA—periosteal stripping, contaminated wound, segmental fracture, no flap required
  - Grade IIIB—same as A but flap required to close soft tissue
  - Grade IIIC—same as A and vascular injury requiring repair
- Grade of closed-fracture soft tissue injury—Tscherne classification
  - Grade 0—injuries from indirect forces, with negligible soft tissue injury
  - Grade I—superficial contusion/abrasion, simple fracture
  - Grade II—deep abrasion, muscle/skin contusion; direct trauma, impending compartment syndrome
  - Grade III—excessive skin contusion; crushed skin or destruction of muscle, subcutaneous degloving, acute compartment syndrome, and rupture of a major blood vessel or nerve

3. Treatment
   - General principles
     - Degree of shortening and translation seen on injury radiographs can be expected to be present at union with nonoperative management.
     - Angular and rotational alignment well controlled with cast
     - Timely and thorough soft tissue management critical to outcome
     - Restore limb length, alignment, and rotation.
     - Stable fixation
     - Early ROM of knee and ankle
     - Prompt administration of antibiotics for open fractures
     - **BMP-2 is primarily used as an adjuvant for type III open tibia fractures treated with IM fixation, whereas BMP-7 is used in treatment of tibial nonunion.**
   - Nonoperative treatment
     - Indications
       - Low-energy fractures
       - Shortening less than 1 to 2 cm
       - Cortical apposition greater than 50%
       - Angulation maintained with cast
         - Varus—valgus less than 5 degrees
         - Flexion—extension less than 10 degrees
     - Long leg cast
       - Can control varus/valgus, flexion/extension, and rotation
       - **Shortening and cortical apposition seen on injury radiograph are equivalent to shortening at union.**
       - Convert to functional brace at 4 to 6 weeks
       - Non–weight bearing for 4 to 6 weeks
   - Operative treatment
     - Indications
       - Open fractures
       - Criteria for nonoperative management not met or failed nonoperative management
       - Soft tissue injury not amenable to cast
       - **Ipsilateral femoral fracture**
       - Polytrauma
       - Morbid obesity
     - IM nailing
       - **Reduced time of immobilization compared with cast management**
       - **Earlier weight bearing than that achieved with cast**
       - Union rate greater than 80% for closed injuries
       - Reamed nailing associated with higher union rates than those achieved with nonreamed nailing
         - Reamed nailing safe for open fractures
         - Severity of soft tissue injury more prognostic than reaming status
       - Static interlocking indicated for stable and unstable fractures
       - Dynamic interlocking indicated only for stable fracture (Winquist I or II)
       - Avoidance of malreduction of proximal third fractures associated with valgus and apex anterior angulation achieved by the following:
         - **Ensuring a laterally based starting point and anterior insertion angle**
         - **Blocking screws, placed posteriorly and laterally to the central axes of the proximal fragment (Figure 11-53)**
         - Provisional unicortical plates
         - Semiextended position for nailing
         - Femoral distractor
       - Gaps at fracture site associated with nonunion
     - External fixation
       - Temporary during application of damage control principles
       - Temporary or definitive for highly contaminated fractures
         - **Definitive fixation with external fixation for type III open tibia fractures have significantly longer time to union and poorer functional outcomes compared with IM nailing.**
       - Higher incidence of malalignment than IM nails
       - Circular frames indicated for very proximal and distal shaft fractures and when these fractures are associated with severe soft tissue injury
       - Can be safely converted to IM nail within 7 to 21 days (newer studies show longer then 7-day delay acceptable but exact safe timing unknown)
     - Plate fixation
       - For extreme proximal and distal shaft fractures
       - Higher infection risk than that for IM nailing in open fractures
       - **Use of a 13-hole percutaneous plate, such as a Less Invasive Stabilization System (LISS) plate, places the superficial peroneal nerve at risk for holes 11, 12, and 13. A larger incision with blunt dissection should be used for insertion of screws in this region.**
4. Complications
   - Nonunion
     - Rule out infection.

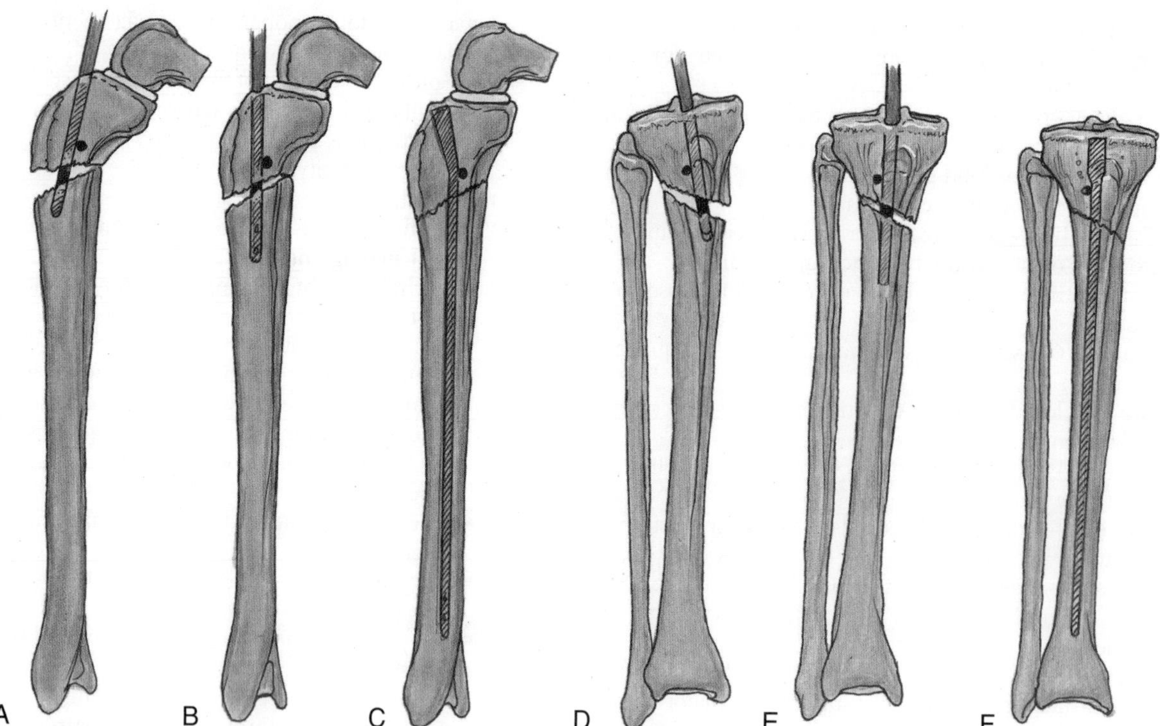

Figure 11-53 Shaft fractures. Blocking screws placed posteriorly and laterally to the central axes of the proximal fragment. (Reprinted with permission from Hiesterman TG, Shafiq BX, Cole PA: Intramedullary nailing of extra-articular proximal tibia fractures, *J Am Acad Ortho Surg* 19:11;690-700, 2011. © 2011 American Academy of Orthopaedic Surgeons.)

- Dynamization if axially stable
- **Reamed-exchange nailing**
- Bone graft for bone defects

- Malunion
  - Most common with proximal third fractures
    - Valgus and apex anterior
  - **May increase long-term risk of arthrosis, particularly in the ankle**
    - **More common with varus deformity**
    - **Rotational malalignment is common with distal third fractures.**
- **Delayed union**
  - **Risk factors for reoperation to achieve bony union within first postinjury year:**
    - **Transverse fracture pattern**
    - **Open fracture**
    - **Cortical contact less than 50%**
- Infection
  - Risk increases with increased severity of soft tissue injury and time to soft tissue coverage
  - **Use of vacuum-assisted closure for wound does not alter risk of infection.**
- Compartment syndrome
  - Diagnosed by compartment pressure within 30 mm Hg of diastolic blood pressure
  - Emergent fasciotomy indicated
  - Can occur even with open fractures
- **Anterior knee pain—occurs in more than 30% of IM nailing cases; resolves with removal of nail in 50% of cases**

5. Ipsilateral femoral shaft and tibial shaft fractures ("floating knee")—treated by retrograde femoral nailing and antegrade tibial nailing

C. **Tibial plafond fractures (pilon fractures)**

1. General principles—associated with motor vehicle collision, falls from height. Soft tissue handling is paramount.
2. Diagnosis
   - Radiographs—AP, lateral, mortise of ankle. tibia and foot films if extension
   - CT—will show location of comminution, fracture planes, etc. Obtain CT after temporary external fixation because fragment position will shift.
   - Three fragments typical because of intact ankle ligaments:
     - **Medial**
       - **Deltoid ligament**
     - **Posterolateral (Volkmann)**
       - **Anterior talofibular ligament**
     - **Anterolateral (Chaput)**
       - **Posterior tibiofibular ligament**
3. Classification
   - Ruëdi-Allgöwer (Figure 11-54)
     - Type I—a nondisplaced fracture
     - Type II—simple displacement of the articular surface
     - Type III—comminution of the articular surface
   - AO/OTA (Figure 11-55)
     - 43-A—extraarticular
     - 43-B—partial articular
     - 43-C—complete articular
4. Treatment
   - Nonoperative treatment—only if the patient is too ill or has significant risk of skin problems (diabetes and vascular disease)
   - Operative treatment
     - Limited internal fixation with external fixation
       - Proponents cite a decreased infection rate, soft tissue breakdown, and stiffness, even when ORIF is used.

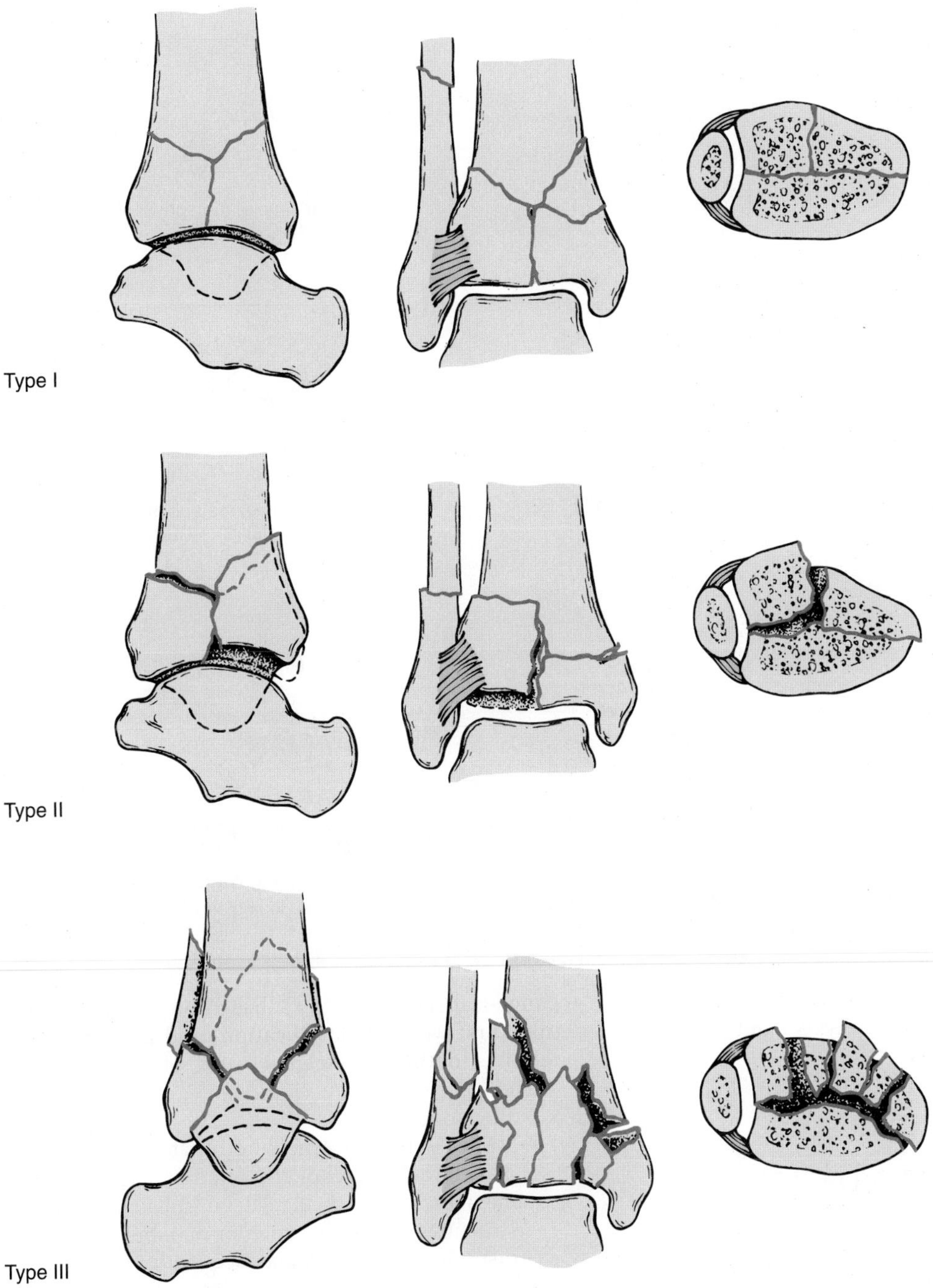

Type I

Type II

Type III

Figure 11-54 **Ruëdi and Allgöwer's classification of pilon fractures.** (Redrawn from Ruëdi TP, Allgöwer M: The operative treatment of intra-articular fractures of the lower end of the tibia, *Clin Orthop* 138:105-110, 1979.)

- With a hybrid fixator, thin wires may be placed within the joint capsule.
- Thin wires may often be placed within the zone of injury.
- Anatomic articular reconstruction may not be possible, especially when there is central depression.

□ **Primary temporizing external fixation with delayed ORIF**

- **Proponents advocate anatomic restoration of the joint despite a higher risk of wound problems and infection.**
- Typically ORIF of the fibula is done to maintain length and external fixation across the ankle; delay definitive ORIF of tibia until soft tissue swelling has subsided.
- Surgical approach depends on location of comminution or fracture lines.
- May be necessary for fractures with significant joint depression or displacement
- Four principles of ORIF:
  - □ Restoration of length
  - □ Reconstruction of the metaphyseal shell
  - □ Bone grafting
  - □ Reattachment of the metaphysis to the diaphysis
- Hardware may become prominent and require later removal.

- **Pilon fractures may continue to demonstrate clinical improvement for up to 2 years.**

5. Complications
   - Wound dehiscence: 9% to 30%—recommend waiting until soft tissue edema has subsided before ORIF (1-2 weeks)
   - Infection: 5% to 15%—may occur with either method of treatment

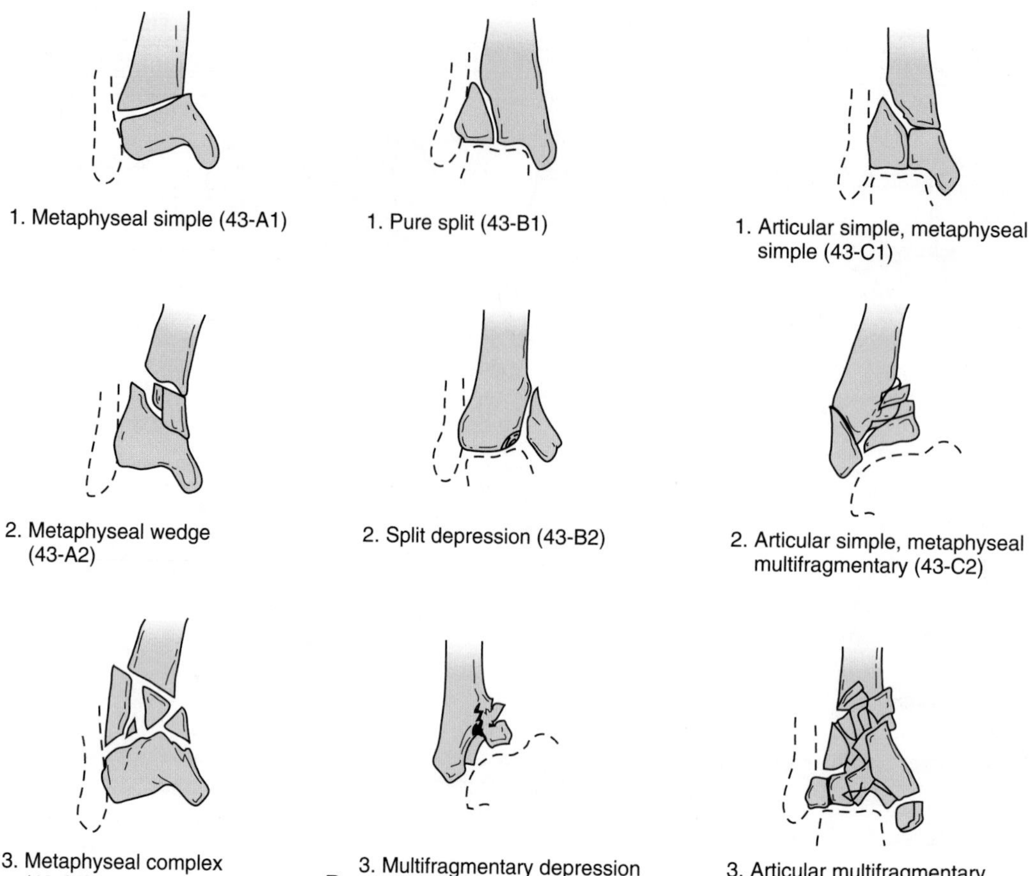

Figure 11-55 AO/OTA classification of tibial plafond fractures. **A,** Tibia/fibula, distal, extraarticular (43-A). **B,** Tibia/fibula, distal, partial articular (43-B). **C,** Tibia/fibula, distal, complete articular (43-C). (From the Orthopaedic Trauma Committee for Coding and Classification: Fracture and Dislocation Compendium, *J Orthop Trauma* 10[Suppl 1]:57, 1996.)

- Malunion
- **Nonunion—especially in metaphysis and more common with hybrid fixation**
- **Post-traumatic arthritis**
- Chondrolysis

V. ANKLE AND FOOT INJURIES (TABLES 11-22 AND 11-23)

A. Ankle fractures

1. Diagnosis
   - Mechanism of injury—rotation
   - Associated syndesmotic instability must be ruled out.
   - **Associated deltoid ligament incompetence must be ruled out.**
   - Systematic evaluation of ankle radiographs (Figure 11-56):
     - Medial clear space less than 4 mm
     - **Talocrural angle 83 ± 4 degrees**
     - Talar tilt less than 2 mm
     - **Syndesmotic tibial clear space less than 5 mm**
       - Medial border of fibula and incisura fibularis
     - **Tibiofibular overlap less than 10 mm or 42% of the width of the fibula**
     - Continuous curve between lateral talus and recessed tip of distal fibula
2. Classification
   - **Lauge-Hansen** (Box 11-1)**—based on the foot's position (first word of classification) and motion (talus) relative to the leg (second word of classification)** (Figure 11-57)
     - Supination-adduction
       - Stage I—transverse fracture of lateral malleolus at or below the level of the anterior talofibular ligament or a tear of the lateral collateral ligament structures, with the anterior talofibular ligament disrupted most often and frequently the calcaneofibular ligament also being torn
       - **Stage II—oblique or vertical fracture of the medial malleolus**
         - **Plafond impaction occurs in as many as 50% of cases and must be reduced.**
     - Supination—external (eversion) rotation (the most common)
       - Stage I—rupture of the anterior inferior tibiofibular ligament
       - Stage II—oblique fracture or spiral fracture of the lateral malleolus
       - Stage III—rupture of the post-tibiofibular ligament or fracture of the posterior malleolus of the tibia
       - **Stage IV—transverse (sometimes oblique) fracture of the medial malleolus *or* disruption of the deltoid ligament**

Table 11-22 Adult: Ankle Fractures and Dislocations

Classification	Treatment	Complications
Lauge-Hansen (position of foot—motion of foot relative to leg) *Supination-adduction* 1—transverse lateral malleolus fracture 2—oblique medial malleolus fracture *Supination–external rotation* 1—AITFL 2—spiral fracture of lateral malleolus 3—posteromedial fracture or PITFL injury 4—transverse/oblique medial malleolus fracture/ deltoid injury *Pronation-abduction* 1—transverse medial malleolus fracture/deltoid injury 2—anterior and posterior ITFL/posterior malleolus 3—oblique lateral malleolus (supramalleolar) fracture *Pronation–external rotation* 1—medial malleolus fracture/deltoid ligament injury 2—AITFL/intraosseous ligament 3—High fibular fracture 4—Posterior malleolus fracture *Pronation-dorsiflexion* 1—medial malleolus fracture 2—fracture of anterior lip of tibia 3—supramalleolar fibular fracture 4—posteromedial fracture or PITFL injury	Rotational injury; rule out syndesmotic injury and deltoid ligament incompetence Anatomic restoration of ankle mortise; 1-mm talar shift = 42% decrease in tibiotalar contact area; isolated lateral malleolus fractures with intact deltoid ligament can be treated with short-leg walking boot; isolated medial malleolus fractures ORIF: displaced bimalleolar/trimalleolar ankle fractures, displaced lateral malleolus with deltoid rupture, displaced medial malleolus, syndesmotic disruption, posterior malleolus > 25% ORIF fibula: lateral buttress plate with or without interfragment screw vs. posterolateral plate (peroneal irritation) ORIF medial malleolus: lag screws or tension band, buttress plate for vertical shear fractures ORIF posterior malleolus: anteroposterior/ posteroanterior lag screws, buttress plate	Wound complications (diabetics), deep infection (diabetics), stiffness, post-traumatic arthrosis, nonunion, malunion Diabetic complications: skin breakdown, loss of reduction, up to 30% amputation rate; augment fixation with transarticular screws/pins or syndesmotic fixation
Danis-Weber (AO/OTA; position of fibular fracture) 44-A—at or below the syndesmosis 44-B—obliquely up from joint 44-C—high fibula fracture	In general, treatment of AO/OTA type A fractures is closed; treatment of AO types B and C is ORIF. Assess syndesmosis stability.	

AITFL, anterior inferior talofibular ligament; ITFL, inferior talofibular ligament; ORIF, open reduction and internal fixation; PITFL, posterior inferior talofibular ligament.

- **Perform stress test to differentiate from supination–external rotation type II injury**
- Pronation-abduction
  - **Stage I—rupture of the deltoid ligament or transverse fracture of the medial malleolus**
  - **Stage II—rupture of the anterior and posterior inferior tibiotalofibular ligaments or bony avulsion**
  - Stage III—oblique fracture of the fibula at the level of the syndesmosis
- Pronation-eversion
  - Stage I—rupture of the deltoid ligament or transverse fracture of the medial malleolus
  - Stage II—rupture of the anterior inferior tibiotalofibular ligaments or bony avulsion
  - Stage III—spiral/oblique fracture of the fibula above the level of the syndesmosis
  - Stage IV—rupture of the posterior inferior tibiofibular ligament or fracture of the posterior malleolus
- Pronation-dorsiflexion
  - Stage I—fracture of the medial malleolus
  - Stage II—fracture of the anterior lip of the tibia
  - Stage III—fracture of the supramalleolar aspect of the fibula
  - Stage IV—rupture of the posterior inferior tibiofibular ligament or fracture of the posterior malleolus
- Danis-Weber and OTA classifications—based primarily on the location of the fibular fracture (see Figure 11-57)
  - 44-A—fibular fracture infrasyndesmotic
  - 44-B—fibular fracture trans-syndesmotic
  - 44-C—fibular fracture suprasyndesmotic
- Atypical malleolar fractures
  - Often caused by crushing or angulating forces
  - **Bosworth fracture-dislocation results when the distal portion of the fibula is entrapped behind the tibia. The posterolateral tibial ridge prevents reduction.**
  - Typically irreducible closed because of an intact interosseous membrane

3. Treatment
   - General principles
     - Anatomic reduction of ankle mortise required
     - One millimeter of lateral talar shift is equivalent to 42% decreased tibiotalar contact area
     - Confirm syndesmotic stability after operative fixation
   - Nonoperative treatment
     - Indications
       - Isolated lateral malleolus fractures with intact deltoid ligament
       - Isolated medial malleolus fractures—tip avulsion (nondisplaced or minimally displaced)
       - Nondisplaced bimalleolar fractures (need close follow-up)
     - Short leg weight-bearing cast or walker boot for 6 weeks
   - Operative treatment
     - Indications
       - Displaced bimalleolar and trimalleolar fractures
       - Displaced lateral malleolar fractures, with incompetent deltoid ligament

Table 11-23 Adult Trauma, Lower Extremity: Foot Fractures and Dislocations

Injury	Eponym/Other Name	Classification	Treatment	Complications
Talar neck fracture	Aviator astragalus	Hawkins and Canale I—nondisplaced II—displaced and subtalar dislocation/subluxation III—displaced and talar body dislocation IV—with talar body and head dislocation (pantalar dislocation)	Nonoperative: nondisplaced fracture, poor soft tissue; short leg cast, non–weight bearing for 8-12 wk (high shear stresses) ORIF: obtain and maintain anatomic reduction	AVN (especially types III/IV [Hawkins sign indicates a good prognosis]); delayed/nonunion, malunion, post-traumatic arthrosis, skin necrosis
Talar body fracture		Rare	Usually requires ORIF with or without medial malleolus osteotomy for exposure	AVN, malunion, DJD
Talar head fracture		Rare	Nondisplaced—splint/ice/elevation	Talonavicular DJD
Talar process fracture		Lateral process >> medial	Short-leg cast for 6 wk; excise if comminuted, symptomatic ORIF if large and displaced	Medial malleolus fracture (26%); rule out os trigonum (50%)
	Shepherd	Posterior process	Short-leg cast for 3-6 wk, excise symptomatic nonunions	
Subtalar dislocation		Calcaneus medial displacement (most common)	Reduce, immobilize for 4 wk, open reduction if irreducibly closed	Posterior tibial tendon entrapment
Total talar dislocation		Talar and Chopart injury	Open reduction, late fusion	AVN
Calcaneal fracture (most common)		Extraarticular (anterior process, tuberosity, medial process, sustentaculum talus, body)	Principles of treatment: avoid wound complications, restore articular congruity, restore height and width; computed tomographic scan helpful	Wound complications in up to 20% of cases; diabetics and smokers at increased risk; subtalar arthritis (need for fusion), peroneal tendon subluxation, neuroma, chronic pain (heel widening, nerve entrapment), DJD, malunion, associated fractures (spine, lower extremity), heel skin slough, compartment syndrome
		Intraarticular (nondisplaced, tongue, joint depression, comminuted), (Böhler angle and crucial angle of Gissane)	Nonoperative for nondisplaced and extraarticular fractures and high-risk patients (smokers, diabetics); walking boot/cast, non–weight bearing for 8-10 wk, early range of motion, edema control	
		Sanders classification Type I—nondisplaced fracture Type II—two-part fracture Type III—three-part fracture with central depression Type IV—comminuted fracture of four or more parts A, B, or C, depending on location of primary fracture line(s) from lateral to medial (see Figure 11-60)	ORIF: lateral approach after soft tissue subsides, articular reduction, internal fixation with or without bone graft (controversial)	
Navicular fracture		Anatomic location (body, tuberosity, avulsion), mechanism of energy (high vs. low energy) Compressed medial column	ORIF: displaced intraarticular and tuberosity fractures; stress fractures—short-leg cast, non–weight bearing for 6 wk; avulsion fracture: treat as symptomatic sprain	Osteonecrosis (ORIF nonunion), associated with midfoot fractures

Table 11-23 Adult Trauma, Lower Extremity: Foot Fractures and Dislocations—cont'd

Injury	Eponym/Other Name	Classification	Treatment	Complications
Cuboid fracture	Nutcracker	Compressed calcaneus and metatarsals (lateral column)	ORIF with bone graft or external fixation to 5th metatarsal to maintain length of lateral column short-leg cast, non–weight bearing for 6-8 wk	Nonunion, malunion, chronic pain, stiffness
Tarsometatarsal fracture-dislocation	Lisfranc (Lisfranc ligament from base of second metatarsal to medial cuneiform)	High (forced dorsiflexion) vs. low (dorsiflexion/twisting) energy	Anatomic reduction of all affected joints; avoid soft tissue complications	Chronic pain or disability (arthrodesis preferred); post-traumatic arthritis; delay in diagnosis (medial border of second metatarsal base must align with medial border of middle cuneiform); compartment syndrome; broken implants—removal not required
		Homolateral—all five digits in same direction	Nonoperative management for low-grade sprains, no subluxation	
		Partial (isolated)—first or second metatarsal displaced	ORIF for displaced fracture-dislocation vs. closed reduction with or without percutaneous pinning; ORIF of metatarsal disruptions with screws is successful; consider primary arthrodesis for pure ligamentous disruptions	
		Divergent—displacement in sagittal and coronal planes		
Metatarsal fracture		Shaft	Majority treated nonoperatively; CRPP if needed; short leg walking cast for 4 wk	Post-traumatic DJD, nonunion (most common with Jones fracture; ORIF, bone graft)
	March	Second metatarsal stress fracture (most common)	Symptomatic; short-leg walking cast if late	
		Head	Reduction (traction and manipulation), cast; CRPP vs. ORIF if needed (avoid plantar prominent metatarsal head)	
	Pseudo-Jones	Base avulsion (fifth metatarsal)	Short-leg walking cast for 2-3 wk, late removal of fragments if needed	
	Jones	Fifth metatarsal base transverse fracture (differentiate from metadiaphyseal stress fracture)	6-8 wk NWB, short-leg cast vs. percutaneous screw for faster recovery (return to play)	
Metatarsophalangeal dislocation		Direction of dislocation (dorsal, first metatarsophalangeal joint most common)	Reduce promptly, immobilize (consider CRPP)	Post-traumatic arthrosis
Phalangeal fractures		Crush, associated nail bed injury	Majority treated nonoperatively; buddy tape for comfort, weight bearing as tolerated; ORIF of intraarticular fracture of hallux (great toe)	Post-traumatic arthrosis

AVN, avascular necrosis; CRPP, closed reduction with percutaneous pinning; DJD, degeneration joint disease; ORIF, open reduction and internal fixation.

Figure 11-56 Restoration of the ankle mortise requires anatomic reduction of the lateral malleolus so that its articular surface is congruous with the reduced talus. **A,** On a mortise view radiograph, the condensed subchondral bone should form a continuous line around the talus and there should be no proximal displacement, malrotation, or angulation of the lateral malleolus. **B** and **C,** A proper talocrural angle and normal joint space width also indicate normality. The medial joint space should be less than 4 mm and the superior joint space within 2 mm medially of its width laterally. **D,** Adequate tibiofibular overlap on the anteroposterior view indicates a proper syndesmotic relationship. The space between the medial wall of the fibula and the incisural surface of the tibia should be less than 5 mm. The anterior tubercle of the tibia should overlap the fibula by at least 10 mm. **E** and **F,** Talar malalignment is indicated by its lateral displacement or tilt into valgus. **G,** Although the talus may be reduced by external pressure, its alignment is not maintained by a shortened, malrotated lateral malleolus, as shown. (From Browner BD, et al, editors: *Skeletal trauma,* ed 3, Philadelphia, 2002, Elsevier.)

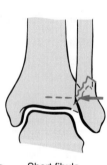

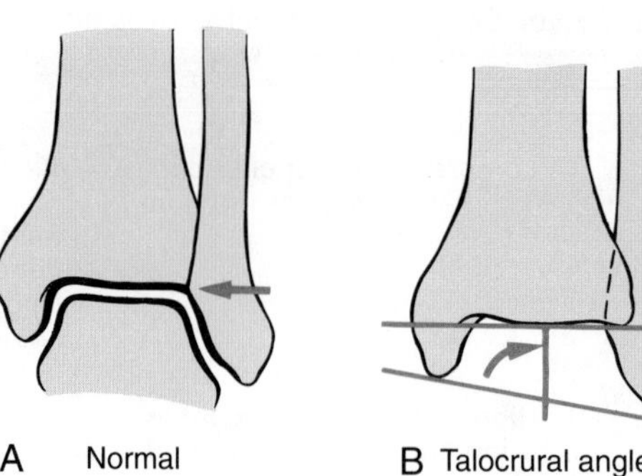

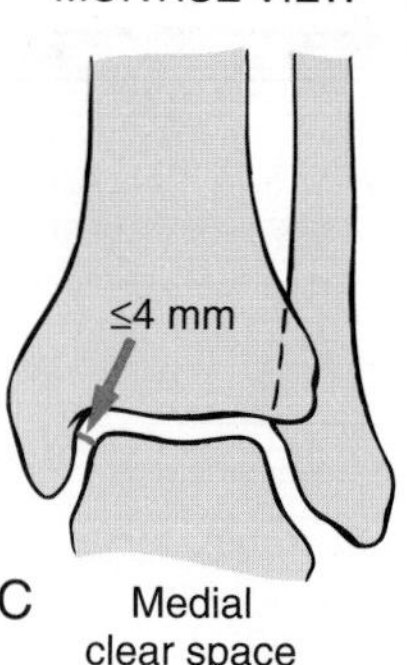

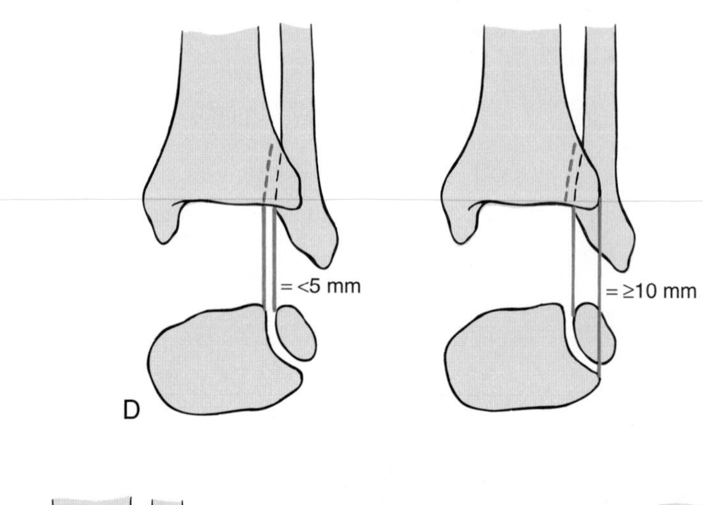

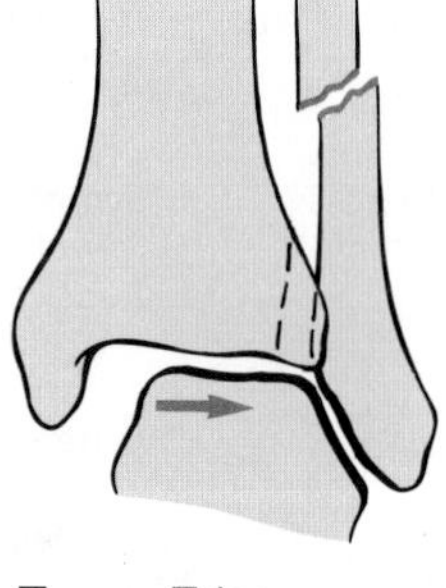

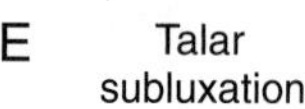

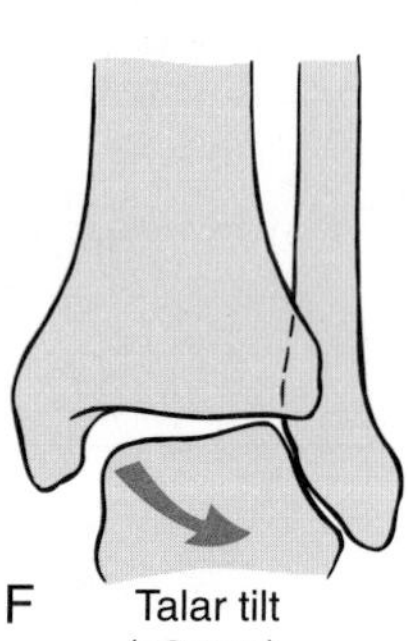

- Displaced medial malleolus fractures
- Syndesmotic disruption
- Posterior malleolar fractures greater than 25%
  - ORIF
    - Fibular fixation
      - Lateral plate with anteroposterior lag screw (for spiral/oblique patterns)
      - **Posterior lateral plate—more stable than the lateral plate but more soft tissue irritation (peroneal tendon)**
    - Medial malleolar fixation
      - Medial lag screws or tension band for transverse fractures
      - **Medial buttress plate for vertical fractures**
    - Posterior malleolus
      - Anteroposterior lag screws
      - Posterior buttress plate
    - Cast or walker boot for 6 weeks

4. Complications
   - Wound complications, especially with diabetics
   - Deep infection, especially in diabetics
   - Stiffness (common)
   - Post-traumatic arthrosis—associated with persistent mortise instability or malreduction
5. Special circumstances
   - Diabetic patients
     - High rate of complications with both nonoperative and operative management

Box 11-1

The Lauge-Hansen Classification

SUPINATION-ADDUCTION

- Stage 1: Transverse fracture of the lateral malleolus at or below the level of the anterior talofibular ligament or a tear of the structures of the lateral collateral ligament, with the anterior talofibular ligament most often disrupted. The calcaneofibular ligament is also frequently torn.
- Stage 2: Oblique fracture of the medial malleolus

SUPINATION–EXTERNAL (EVERSION) ROTATION*

- Stage 1: Rupture of the anterior inferior tibiofibular ligament
- Stage 2: Oblique fracture or spiral fracture of the lateral malleolus
- Stage 3: Rupture of the post–tibiofibular ligament or fracture of the posterior malleolus of the tibia
- Stage 4: Transverse (sometimes oblique) fracture of the tibial malleolus

PRONATION-ABDUCTION†

- Stage 1: Rupture of the deltoid ligament or transverse fracture of the medial malleolus
- Stage 2: Rupture of the anterior and posterior inferior tibiotalofibular ligaments or bony avulsion
- Stage 3: Oblique fracture of the fibula at the level of the syndesmosis

PRONATION-EVERSION

- Stage 1: Rupture of the deltoid ligament or transverse fracture of the medial malleolus
- Stage 2: Rupture of the anterior inferior tibiotalofibular ligaments or bony avulsion
- Stage 3: Spiral/oblique fracture of the fibula above the level of the syndesmosis
- Stage 4: Rupture of the posterior inferior tibiofibular ligament or fracture of the posterior malleolus

PRONATION-DORSIFLEXION

- Stage 1: Fracture of the medial malleolus
- Stage 2: Fracture of the anterior lip of the tibia
- Stage 3: Fracture of the supramalleolar aspect of the fibula
- Stage 4: Rupture of the posterior inferior tibiofibular ligament or fracture of the posterior malleolus

*40% to 70% of all ankle fractures.
†Less than 5% of ankle fractures.

            - Worse in patients with neuropathy
            - Skin breakdown, loss of reduction, and nonunion with cast treatment
            - Wound complications, deep infection, loss of reduction, and hardware failure with operative management
            - Up to 30% amputation rate
        - Augment fixation with transarticular screws or pins or with syndesmotic fixation.
        - Double immobilization time and expected healing time
    - Open fractures
        - Emergent incision and drainage
        - Immediate ORIF if clean, otherwise external fixation
        - Results similar to those of closed fractures
    - Syndesmotic instability
        - **Common with fibula fractures more than 6 cm above the ankle joint**
        - **Uncommon after fixation of low fibula fractures—Test stability after fixation.**
            - **Cotton test with clamp on fibula pulling laterally or external rotation of foot**
        - The reduction of joints of the tibia-fibula should be compared with uninjured side on true lateral view.
        - Malreduction associated with poor functional results
        - Fixation with two 3.5-mm position screws (not lag screws)
        - No weight bearing for 6 to 8 weeks
        - Screw removal after 3 months (optional)

B. Talus fractures

1. Diagnosis
    - Mechanism of injury—usually high-energy injuries; forced dorsiflexion with axial load
    - Neck fractures most common
    - Associated dislocation surgical emergency due to skin tenting and neurovascular stretch injury
2. Classification—Hawkins classification (Figure 11-58) based on displacement and associated dislocation
    - Type I—nondisplaced
    - Type II—displaced, with subtalar dislocation
    - Type III—displaced, with talar body dislocation (subtalar and tibiotalar dislocations)
    - Type IV—displaced, with talar body and head dislocation (plantar dislocation)
3. Treatment
    - General principles—Avoid secondary displacement, provide proper foot alignment, and avoid AVN.
    - Nonoperative treatment—Indicated for nondisplaced fractures is use of a short leg cast with non–weight bearing for 10 to 12 weeks; high shear stress requires prolonged immobilization and no weight bearing.
    - Operative treatment
        - Indicated for displaced fractures
        - Associated dislocations often require open reduction.
        - **Dual-incision approach recommended to ensure anatomic reduction**
            - Medial and anterolateral
            - Medial has greatest risk to vascular supply. Preserve dorsal and plantar capsular attachments.
        - Posterior-to-anterior or anterior-to-posterior screws
        - No weight bearing for 10 to 12 weeks
4. Complications
    - AVN—increased risk with increased initial displacement and associated dislocation; appears as relative sclerosis of talar body and associated with subchondral fracture or collapse
        - **Hawkins sign is classic early indicator of vascularity and appears at between 6 and 8 weeks. It represents patchy subchondral osteoporosis and relative radiolucency and is a reliable sign of vascular integrity** (Figure 11-59).
    - Nonunion
    - Post-traumatic arthritis of tibiotalar and subtalar joints
    - **Malunion (varus more common due to medial comminution)**
5. Special circumstances
    - Talar body fractures—unusual; treated with ORIF with or without medial malleolar osteotomy for exposure

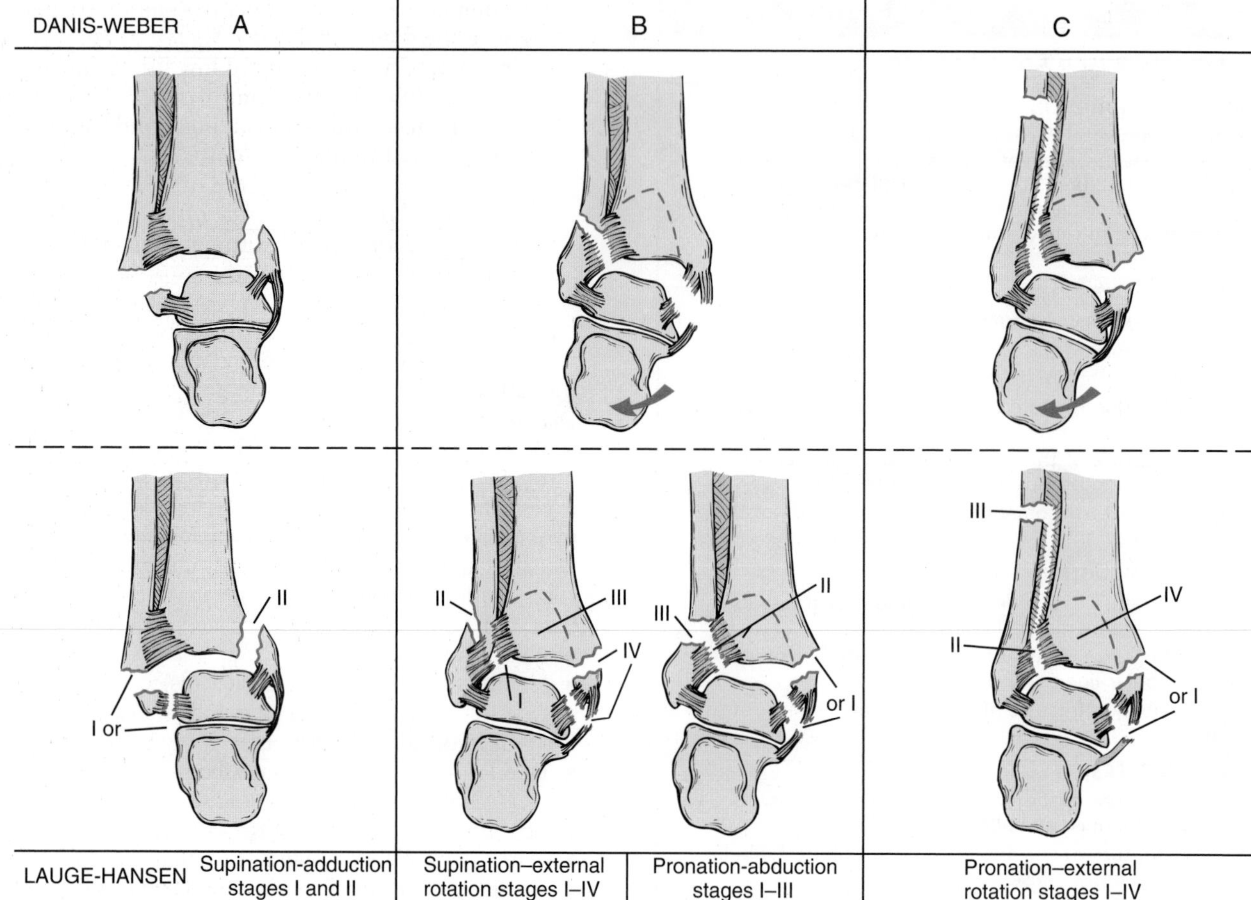

Figure 11-57 Correlation of the Danis-Weber (AO/ASIF) and the Lauge-Hansen classification systems for malleolar fractures. The Danis-Weber system is based on the level of the fibular fracture, and the Lauge-Hansen system is based on experimentally verified injury mechanisms. Type B injuries can be produced by two mechanisms: supination-external rotation and pronation-abduction. (From Browner BD, et al, editors: *Skeletal trauma,* ed 3, Philadelphia, 2002, Elsevier.)

- Talar process fractures
  - Lateral more common than medial
  - Often misdiagnosed as ankle sprain
  - Treat with short-leg cast and subsequent protected weight bearing for 6 weeks
- **Open fracture with extruded fragment—Preserve extruded fragment when it is articular and large.**
- Subtalar dislocations
  - Described by direction of foot relative to talus—medial (85%) or lateral (15%)
    - Lateral dislocation requires more energy and has a higher rate of associated injuries and typically has a worse outcome when there is an associated injury.
    - Direction of dislocation does not impact outcome in isolated subtalar dislocations.
  - Lack of associated bony injuries associated with best long-term outcomes
  - Associated injuries:
    - **Tarsal fracture—90%**
      - Medial—dorsomedial talar head, posterior tubercles of talus, lateral navicular
      - Lateral—cuboid, anterior process of calcaneus, lateral process of talus and lateral malleolus
    - Approximately 40% open injuries
  - Closed reduction in emergency department versus general anesthetic
  - **If irreducible—typically entrapped soft tissue or articular impaction**
    - **Medial—extensor digitorum brevis/capsule**
    - **Lateral—posterior tibial tendon**

C. **Calcaneus fractures**

1. Diagnosis
   - Mechanism of injury—forced dorsiflexion with axial load typically with fall from height or from motor vehicle collision
   - Significant soft tissue injury often associated with fracture
   - Typical deformity—heel shortened, widened, and in varus
2. Classification—Sanders classification (Figure 11-60) based on location and comminution of posterior facet on coronal CT scan
3. Treatment
   - General principles
     - Avoid wound complications
     - Restore articular congruity
     - Restore normal calcaneal width and height
     - Maximum functional recovery may take longer than 12 months.
   - Nonoperative treatment
     - Indicated for nondisplaced fractures, extraarticular fractures, and those at high risk for operative complications (diabetics and smokers)

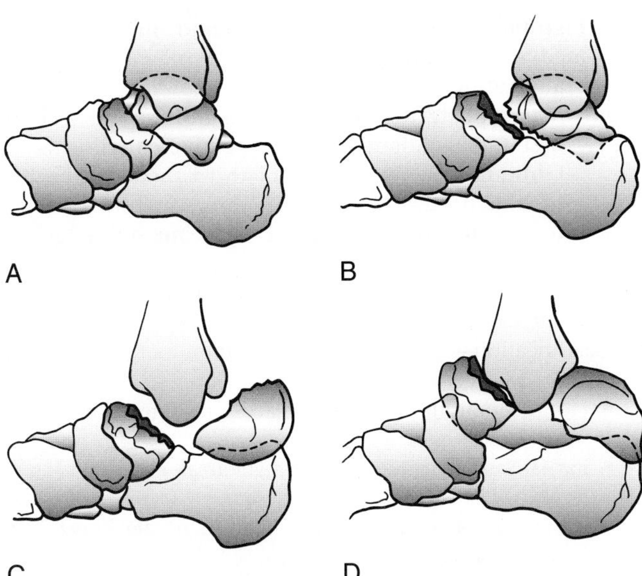

Figure 11-58 Hawkins classification. **A,** Group I: nondisplaced talar neck fractures. **B,** Group II: displaced talar neck fractures with subluxation or dislocation of the subtalar joint. **C,** Group III: displaced talar neck fractures with associated dislocation of the talar body from both subtalar and tibiotalar joints. **D,** Canale and Kelly group IV: displaced talar neck fracture with associated dislocation of the talar body from the subtalar and tibiotalar joints and dislocation of the head-and-neck fragment from the talonavicular joint. (From Sangeorzan BJ: Foot and ankle joint. In Hansen ST Jr, Swiontkowski MF, editors: *Orthopaedic trauma protocols,* New York, 1993, Raven, p 350.)

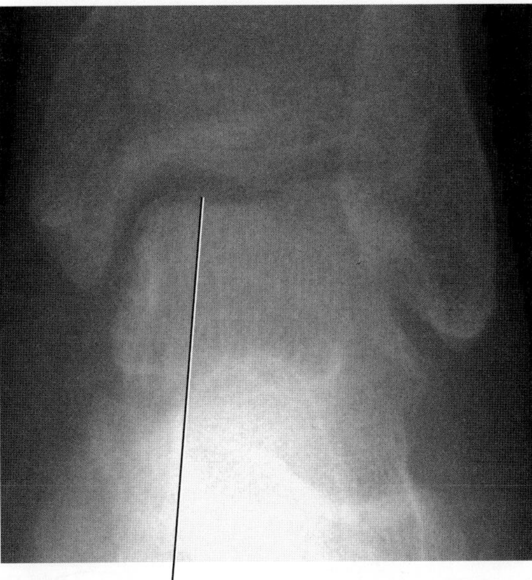

Figure 11-59 Hawkins sign. Anteroposterior radiograph shows a subchondral linear lucency involving the talar dome within the first 6 weeks after injury. This indicates hyperemia and is a sign that avascular necrosis is unlikely to occur. (From Morrison WB, Sanders TG: *Problem solving in musculoskeletal imaging,* Philadelphia, 2008, Elsevier.)

- Cast or walker boot, non–weight bearing for 8 to 10 weeks, early ROM, and compression stocking to control swelling
- Operative treatment
  - Indicated for displaced intraarticular fractures
  - Extensile lateral approach associated with up to 20% wound complications
  - Low-profile implants
    - **Care must be taken when drilling through the medial cortex due to the flexor hallucis longus tendon and medial neurovascular bundle**
  - Percutaneous reduction and screw fixation (if indicated) can decrease risk of extensile exposure.
  - Delay surgery until soft tissue envelope shows wrinkling (7-14 days).
  - Primary subtalar fusion (controversial) may be indicated for Sanders type 4 fracture or if surgery is delayed.

4. Complications
   - **Wound complications in up to 20% of cases (increased in diabetics and smokers)**
     - Local wound care and oral antibiotics usually sufficient
     - Implant removal usually not required
   - Subtalar arthritis
   - Peroneal impingement with nonoperative treatment from lateral wall blowout
   - **Poor functional outcome in patients older than age 50, obese patients, manual laborers, and those receiving workers' compensation**
   - **Best surgical results in young females with nonlabor jobs**
   - Compartment syndrome
5. Special circumstances—open fractures
   - Usually a medial open wound
   - **Poorer results than those associated with closed fractures**
   - Associated with severe comminution

D. Navicular fractures

1. Diagnosis/classification
   - High-energy fractures usually via compression of medial column (nutcracker)
   - Low-energy injuries—avulsions
     - Dorsal avulsion of joint capsule
     - Tuberosity fracture—avulsion of posterior tibial tendon
   - Stress fracture
2. Treatment
   - Displaced intraarticular fractures—ORIF
   - Avulsion fractures—protocol for symptomatic sprains
   - Stress fracture—short-leg cast with no weight bearing for 6 weeks

E. Cuboid fractures

1. Diagnosis—compression of lateral column
2. Treatment
   - Restore column length—ORIF or external fixation spanning from the calcaneus to the fifth metatarsal
   - Short-leg cast with no weight bearing for 6 to 8 weeks

F. Tarsometatarsal fracture-dislocations (Lisfranc injury)

1. Diagnosis
   - Mechanism of injury
     - High energy—forced dorsiflexion
     - Low energy—dorsiflexion/twisting
   - **High index of suspicion for subtle injury when it is associated with midfoot swelling and/or tenderness**
     - **Stress view (standing)**
     - **Comparison view of noninjured foot**

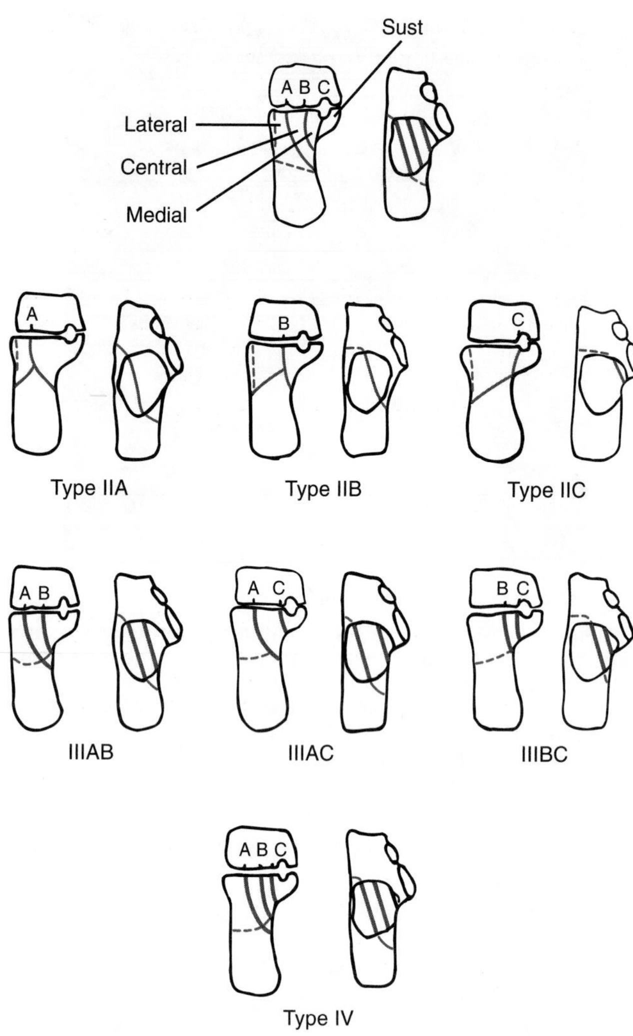

Figure 11-60 Sanders computed tomography classification of calcaneal fractures. *Sust,* Sustentaculum tali. (Redrawn from Sanders R: Intraarticular fractures of the calcaneus: present state of the art, *J Orthop Trauma* 6:252-265, 1992.)

- **Lisfranc ligament—base of second metatarsal to medial cuneiform**
- **Plain radiographs**
  - **Anteroposterior—medial bases of first and second metatarsals aligned with respective cuneiforms**
  - **Oblique—medial border of third metatarsal with medial border lateral cuneiform; medial base of fourth metatarsal aligned with medial edge of cuboid**
  - Lateral—dorsal surfaces of tarsal and metatarsals aligned

2. Classification—based on the direction of dislocation (Figure 11-61)
   - Homolateral (all joints displace in same direction—medial or lateral)
   - Partial (isolated)—first tarsometatarsal joint or rays 2 to 5
   - Divergent—first tarsometatarsal joint medial, rays 2 to 5 lateral
3. Treatment
   - General principles
     - Anatomic reduction of all affected joints
     - Avoid soft tissue complications.
     - Immediate reduction of widely dislocated joints—minor subluxation acceptable
     - Definitive management after recovery of soft tissues
     - Provisional Kirschner wire fixation for grossly unstable joints
   - Nonoperative treatment—indicated for low-grade sprains with no subluxation
   - **Operative treatment**
     - **Indicated for displacement**
     - Screw fixation of affected medial joints (minimal motion so hardware can remain)
     - Screw or Kirschner wire fixation of lateral joints (maximal motion so need implant removal)
     - No weight bearing for 6 to 8 weeks; no removal of implants before 12 weeks (except Kirschner wires laterally)

Figure 11-61 Classification of midfoot tarsometatarsal injuries.

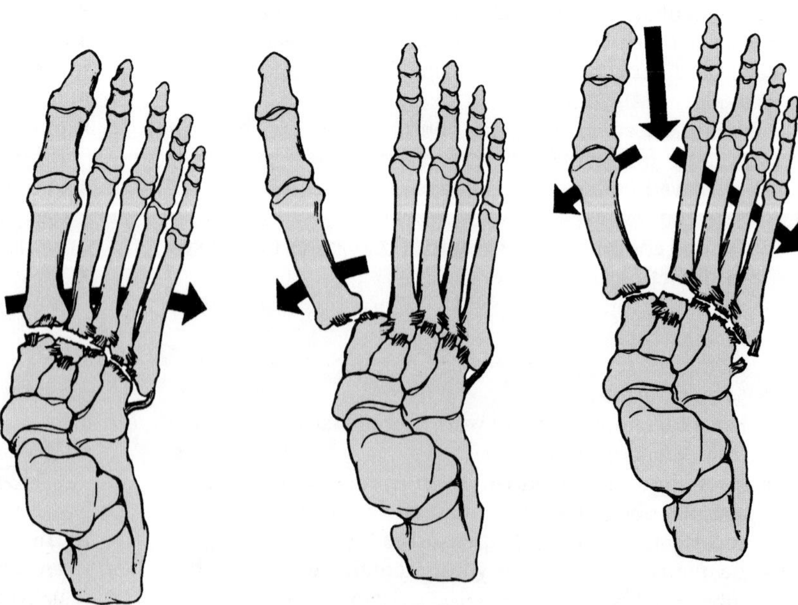

- Primary fusion may be indicated for purely ligamentous displaced injuries (controversial)

4. Complications
   - Long-term pain and/or disability—maximum recovery longer than 12 months
   - **Post-traumatic arthritis**
     - **Missed Lisfranc injury treated with tarsometatarsal arthrodesis**
   - Fractured implants—removal not required unless symptomatic

G. Metatarsal fractures

1. Diagnosis/classification
   - Rule out associated Lisfranc injury especially if base of first to fifth metatarsals
   - Distinguish midshaft, distal (neck), and base fifth metatarsal fractures
   - Jones fracture at metaphyseal diaphyseal junction of fifth metatarsal
     - Vascular watershed area
     - Relatively high healing complication rate with weight-bearing protocols
     - Requires prolonged no weight bearing
   - Pseudo-Jones fracture—more proximal than Jones; avulsion of peroneus brevis tendon or plantar ligaments
     - Healing much more reliable than true Jones fracture
     - Weight-bearing protocol acceptable
2. Treatment
   - Shaft fractures usually treated nonoperatively
   - Avoid prominent metatarsal heads—need reduction and pinning versus ORIF
   - Jones fracture—short-leg cast with no weight bearing for 6 to 8 weeks or percutaneous screw fixation for faster recovery (athletes)
   - Pinning for widely displaced shaft fractures or distal fractures
3. Complications
   - Nonunion—most common complication with Jones fracture; treated by screw fixation with or without bone grafting
   - Malunion—leads to pain and prominence on plantar or dorsal surface causing shoe wear difficulties

H. Metatarsophalangeal joint dislocation

1. Classification
   - First metatarsophalangeal (the most common dislocation)
   - Dorsal
2. Treatment—closed reduction, a hard shoe, and weight bearing as tolerated

I. Phalangeal fractures

1. Diagnosis
   - Result from dropping object (comminuted or transverse fracture) or stubbing toe—axial load (spiral/oblique fracture)
   - Watch for associated nail bed injury in distal phalanx.
2. Treatment
   - Nonoperative for most
   - Buddy taping for comfort
   - Weight bearing as tolerated
   - Consider operative for intraarticular fractures of the great toe.

SECTION 4 SPINE

I. UPPER CERVICAL SPINE INJURIES (TABLE 11-24)

A. General concepts—The first goal of treatment is stabilization.

1. Traction should not be used in distraction injuries.
   - Distraction injuries tend to be more unstable than compression injuries.
2. Neurogenic shock is rare, characterized by massive vasodilation causing the loss of autonomic tone. Treatment is with vasopressors.
3. The role of steroids is unclear and still controversial.
   - If they are given within 3 hours, administer for 24 hours.
   - If they are given within 3-8 hours, administer for 48 hours.
   - A bolus of 30 mg/kg over 15 minutes, with a maintenance infusion of 5.4 mg/kg per hour

B. American Spinal Injury Association (ASIA) classification

- A—0/5 motor score, complete sensory deficit
- B—0/5 motor score, incomplete sensory deficit
- C—**less than 3/5 motor score, incomplete sensory deficit**
- D—greater than 3/5 motor score, incomplete sensory deficit
- E—5/5 Motor score, no sensory deficit

C. Clinical syndromes

- Brown-Séquard syndrome (spinal cord hemisection)
- Motor function is disrupted on the side of injury, while pain and temperature are affected on the contralateral side.
- 90% of patients will recover the ability to walk.
- Typical cause is penetrating trauma.

2. **Central cord syndrome**
   - **The upper extremity is affected more than the lower extremity and distal muscles more than proximal.**
   - **The prognosis is good for the recovery of ambulation, but the patient is less likely to recover upper extremity function.**
   - Typical mechanism is hyperextension with preexisting canal stenosis.
3. Anterior cord syndrome (spinothalamic tract injury)
   - Motor response, pain reception, and temperature reception are not functioning; vibration sensation, proprioception, and deep pressure sensation are intact.
   - The prognosis for motor recovery is poor.

D. Occipitocervical dissociation

1. Head is disconnected from C1.
2. Frequently fatal
3. Diagnosis challenging on plain films (CT/MRI about 85% sensitive)

Table 11-24 Adult Spine Trauma

Level	Injury Type	Classification	Common Name	Mechanism of Injury	Risk of Neurologic Injury	Treatment	Indication for Surgery	Important Points
Occipitocervical dislocation	I	Traynelis et al	Anterior	Anterior translation	Very high	Occipitocervical fusion	Surgery indicated	Very unstable; rarely survive injury
	II		Distraction	Pure distraction	Very high	Occipitocervical fusion	Surgery indicated	Very unstable; rarely survive injury
	III		Posterior	Posterior translation	Very high	Occipitocervical fusion	Surgery indicated	Very unstable; rarely survive injury
Occipital condyle fracture	I	Anderson-Montesano	Impacted condyle fracture	Compression of skull	Low	Collar	Usually not required	Alar ligament and tectorial membrane usually intact
	II		Occipital condyle and basilar skull fracture	Compression of skull	Low	Collar	Usually not required	Alar ligament and tectorial membrane usually intact
	III		Avulsion fracture of alar ligament	Distraction of skull	Moderate to high	Collar, halo, or surgery, depending on stability	More than 1 mm of displacement	Potential for ligament disruption
C1 ring fracture	Posterior arch fracture		Lamina fracture	Hyperextension	Low	Immobilization	Not indicated	Hyperextension
	Two- and three-part fractures		Lateral mass fracture	Lateral compression	Low	Immobilization	Not indicated	
	Four-part fracture		Jefferson fracture	Axial compression	Low	Immobilization, sometimes traction	Optional for widely displaced lateral masses	>7-mm offset of lateral mass indicates transverse ligament rupture
C2 fracture	Traumatic spondylolisthesis	Levine	Hangman fracture					
	I or IA		IA called atypical hangman	Hyperextension	Low	Collar		Prove stable with supervised flexion–extension radiographs
	II or IIA			Hyperextension with secondary flexion	Low to moderate	Immobilization; avoid traction with IIA	Osteosynthesis optional	Type II, use traction; type IIA, avoid traction
	III		Bilateral facet dislocation	Hyperextension with secondary flexion/distraction	High	Surgical reduction of facet dislocation and C2-C3 fusion	Surgery required to reduce facets	Open reduction of facets required
	Odontoid fracture							
	I	Anderson-D'Alonso	Avulsion fracture	Hyperextension of distraction	Low	Collar	None	Watch for associated occipitocervical instability
	II		Fracture at junction of odontoid and body	Multiple mechanisms	Moderate	Halo vs. internal fixation	Unstable fracture or nonunion	Most common; high rate of nonunion
	III		Fracture into C2 body	Multiple mechanisms	Moderate	Halo vest immobilization	Displacement, instability	Usually stable
C2 body fracture				Similar to subaxial cervical spine	Low			
Transverse ligament disruption			C1-C2 instability	Severe flexion	Moderate to high	C1-C2 fusion	ADI > 3-5 mm	Often associated with dizziness, syncope, respiratory problems, and blurred vision

C1-C2 rotatory subluxation	I	Fielding-Hawkins	Rotatory fixation	Rotational trauma	Low	Immobilization/traction/surgery	Indicated for chronic cases with fixed deformity and spasm or instability	Many causes; infection and trauma most common
	II		Rotatory fixation with 3-5 mm of anterior displacement	Rotational trauma	Moderate	Immobilization/traction/surgery	Indicated for chronic cases with fixed deformity and spasm or instability	
	III		Rotatory fixation with >5 mm anterior displacement	Rotational trauma	Moderate	Immobilization/traction/surgery	Indicated for chronic cases with fixed deformity and spasm or instability	
	IV		Rotatory fixation with posterior displacement	Rotational trauma	Moderate to high	Immobilization/traction/surgery	Indicated for chronic cases with fixed deformity and spasm or instability	
Subaxial cervical spine		Allen-Ferguson		Mechanisms implied by name	Depends on stage of injury	Depends on stage of injury		
	Compressive flexion			Compression and flexion	Low to high		Instability or neurologic deficit with cord compression	
	Distractive flexion			Distraction and flexion	Low to high		Instability or neurologic deficit with cord compression	
	Axial compression			Axial compression	Low to high		Instability or neurologic deficit with cord compression	
	Compressive extension			Compression and extension	Low to high		Instability or neurologic deficit with cord compression	
	Distractive extension			Distraction and extension	Low to high		Instability or neurologic deficit with cord compression	
	Lateral flexion			Lateral bending	Low to moderate		Instability or neurologic deficit with cord compression	
	Compression		Compression	Flexion	Low	Collar		Watch for signs of posterior ligament disruption

Continued

Table 11-24 Adult Spine Trauma—cont'd

Level	Injury Type	Classification	Common Name	Mechanism of Injury	Risk of Neurologic Injury	Treatment	Indication for Surgery	Important Points
Subaxial cervical spine (cont'd)	Burst		Burst	Axial compression	Moderate to high	Halo vs. anterior decompression/fusion	Cord compression	Anterior decompression specifically indicated in cases of incomplete cord injury
			Flexion teardrop	Compression and flexion	High	Halo vs. anterior decompression/fusion	Cord compression	Very unstable
			Facet dislocation	Flexion and distraction	High	Reduction of facet, fusion	Bilateral facet dislocation	Possible disc herniation; consider MRI before reduction
	Posterior element fracture		Spinous process	Extension (sometimes flexion or rotation)	Low	Collar	Floating lateral mass	Most are stable
Thoracolumbar spine	Compression	Denis		Flexion and axial loading		Bracing	>50% anterior collapse or widening of spinous process	Osteoporotic compression fracture requires workup and treatment of underlying condition; watch for ileus
	Burst			Axial loading				
	Stable					Bracing	Progressive deformity or neurologic compromise	Watch for any signs of posterior ligament rupture vs. MRI; watch for ileus
	Unstable					Surgery	>30 degrees kyphosis; incomplete cord injury with cord compromise	Cord decompression required if neurologic deficit present
	Seatbelt injury		Chance fracture (bony injury)	Distraction and flexion		Surgery for posterior ligament ruptures, bracing for postoperative treatment	>17% kyphosis with bony injury, posterior ligament injury	High rate of associated intraabdominal injury
	Fracture-dislocation			Rotation and shear		Surgical alignment, fusion, instrumentation	All require surgery	Long segmental posterior construct

ADI, atlanto-dens interval; MRI, magnetic resonance imaging.

4. Radiologic measurements
   - The Powers ratio (Figure 11-62)
     - Measure distance from basion to posterior arch; divide by distance of anterior arch to opisthion.
     - Greater than 1.0 indicates instability of the atlanto-axial junction (from possible dislocation)
   - Harris method
     - Basion-axial interval—distance from basion to line drawn tangential to posterior border of C2 (normal: 4-12 mm)
     - Basion dental interval—distance from basion to odontoid
       - The distance between the odontoid and basion is 4 to 5 mm in adults and up to 10 mm in children. More than 12 is abnormal.
5. Classification—Harborview classification
   - Stage I—MRI evidence of injury to ligamentous stabilizers, alignment within 2 mm of normal, and distraction of 2 mm or less on manual traction radiograph
   - Stage II—same as stage I, except distraction of less than 2 mm on a manual-traction radiograph
   - Stage III—distraction of more than 2 mm on static radiographs
6. Treatment
   - Operative treatment indications—stage II or III injuries or any injury with associated neurologic deficit
7. Operative procedure—occipitocervical fusion

E. Occipital fracture

1. Classification—Anderson-Montesano classification
   - Type I—comminuted impaction fracture of occiput; generally stable
   - Type II—shear or compression fracture extending into the base of the skull; variably stable
   - Type III—avulsion injuries that have a transverse fracture component; generally unstable—may be associated with occipitocervical dissociation
2. Treatment
   - Operative treatment—indicated with evidence of instability or neurologic deficit
   - Stable vs. unstable injuries—a cervical collar for stable injuries and surgical stabilization for unstable injuries

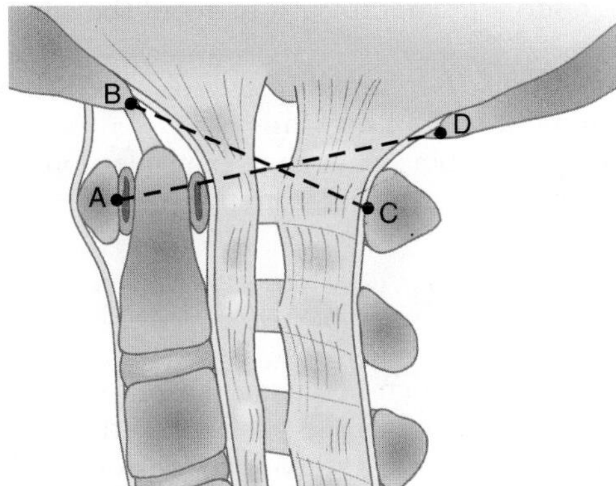

Figure 11-62 Powers ratio. The ratio of BC/OA should always equal 1 or less. If it is greater than 1, the patient most likely has an anterior occipitocervical subluxation or dislocation. *B,* basion; *D,* opisthion; *A,* anterior arch of the atlas; *C,* posterior arch of the atlas.

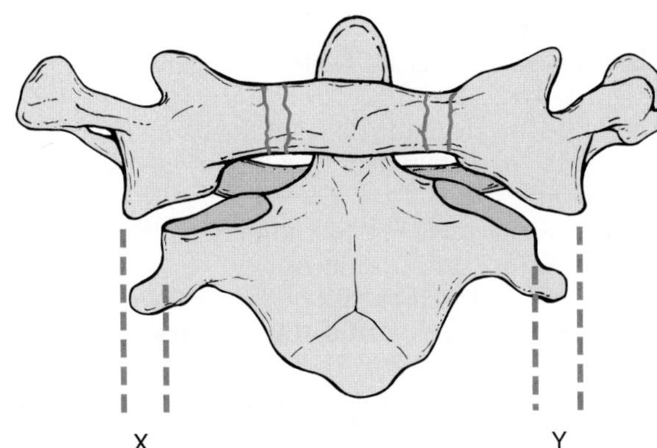

Figure 11-63 Atlantoaxial offset. If X + Y is greater than 6.9 mm, transverse atlantal ligament rupture is implied.

F. C1 fracture

1. Classification—Levine and Edwards
   - Posterior arch fractures—hyperextension
   - Lateral mass fractures—axial load with lateral bend
   - Isolated anterior arch fractures—hyperextension
   - **Burst fractures (Jefferson)—axial load**
2. Treatment—operative treatment
   - Indications
     - **Combined lateral mass displacement of 7 mm (8.1 mm with standard radiographic magnification) indicates transverse ligament rupture** (Figure 11-63).
     - Atlanto–dens interval
       - If greater than 3 mm, indicates that the transverse ligament is damaged
       - If greater than 5 mm, indicates that both the transverse and alar ligaments are damaged
     - Residual displacement after halo of more than 7 mm or atlanto–dens interval of more than 3 mm
   - A halo for 6 to 12 weeks for fractures with an intact transverse ligament
   - **Posterior spinal fusion (C1-C2 or occiput-C2) if the transverse ligament is incompetent**

G. Atlantoaxial instability

1. Classification—Fielding and Hawkins
   - Type I—rotationally unstable but transverse alar ligament intact. The odontoid is the pivot point.
   - Type II—rotationally unstable, with transverse alar ligament incompetence; one facet acts as the pivot.
   - Type III—both facets subluxed anteriorly, more than 5 mm atlanto–dens interval
   - Type IV—both facets subluxed posteriorly
   - Type V—frank dislocation
2. Treatment—operative treatment
   - Indications
     - Chronic deformity
     - Less than 2-mm distraction
     - Types IB and IC
     - Failure of immobilization
   - A halo for 3 months—types IIA and IIB
   - C1-C2 posterior fusion—Include the occiput if the instability is associated with occipitocervical dislocation.

H. Odontoid fracture

1. Classification—Anderson-D'Alonso (Figure 11-64)
   - Type I—avulsion of the alar ligaments from the tip
   - Type II—fracture at the base of the odontoid
   - Type IIA—comminuted fracture of the base of the odontoid
   - Type III—fractures that extend into the body of C2
2. Treatment—operative treatment
   - Indications—based on risk of developing nonunion
     - **Displaced types II and IIA fractures are generally considered operative because of the high rate of nonunion with nonoperative treatment, particularly in those older than age 50 years.**
     - **Risk factors for nonunion in type II:**
       - **Displacement greater than 5 mm**
       - **Angulation greater than 10 degrees**
       - **Posterior displacement**
       - **Age older than 40 years**
       - **Delayed treatment**
   - **Immobilization in rigid cervical orthosis for type I and nondisplaced type II (controversial)**
   - **Posterior C1-C2 fusion for type II**
   - **An anterior screw may be used in type II fractures unless body habitus, fracture geometry ("anterior oblique")**, or other injuries preclude it. This procedure is associated with a higher failure rate than posterior fusion, but it does preserve atlantoaxial motion.

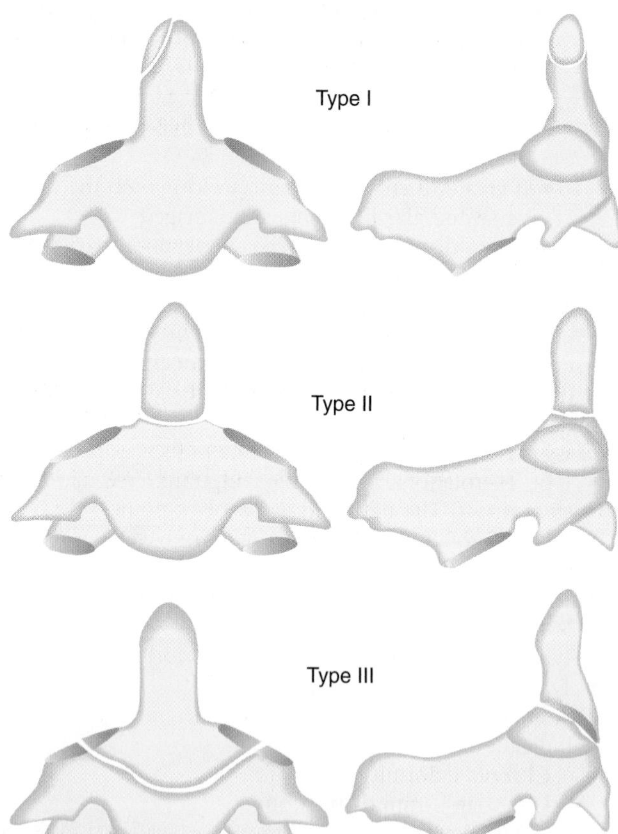

Figure 11-64 Anderson-D'Alonso classification of odontoid fractures. Type I is an oblique avulsion fracture from the upper portion of the odontoid. Type II is a fracture of the odontoid process at its base. Type III is an odontoid fracture through the body of C2.

   - **Halo vest for type III—Consider operative treatment if initial displacement is greater than 5 mm.**
3. **Complications**
   - Overall nonunion rate for type II is approximately 32%.
   - **Patients older than age 80 do poorly, regardless of operative or nonoperative management.**
     - **Airway problems postoperatively or with halo vest immobilization**

I. C2 fracture (traumatic spondylolisthesis of the axis or hangman fracture)

1. Classification—Levine
   - Type I—minimally displaced fracture of the pars secondary to hyperextension and axial loading (<3 mm displacement, no angulation)
   - Type IA—same as type I except fracture lines are asymmetric
   - Type II—displaced fractures (>3 mm) of the pars, with subsequent flexion after hyperextension and axial loading
   - Type IIa—flexion without displacement; *be careful* not to mistake this for a type I fracture, which represents total disc avulsion because traction may worsen fracture.
   - Type III—bilateral pars fracture with bilateral facet dislocations (rare)—has flexion-distraction then hyperextension mechanism
2. Treatment
   - Indications
     - Operative treatment for type II fractures with more than 3- to 5-mm displacement
     - Operative treatment for other type fractures
   - Type I—rigid cervical orthosis
   - Type IIA—halo vest or surgery (no traction!)
   - Type III—generally operative, usually C2-C3 fusion
3. Complications—vascular injury; vertebral artery injury is rare but increasingly diagnosed by magnetic resonance angiogram (MRA)

J. Halo vest immobilization

1. Indicated in Jefferson fracture, odontoid fracture (type III and nondisplaced type II), hangman fracture (type II), fracture associated with ankylosing spondylitis
2. **Effective in controlling most spinal motions, except axial distraction**
3. **Safe zone for anterior pin placement: above the eyebrow in the middle to lateral third to avoid the supraorbital nerve**
4. **Adults: 4 pins (6-8 inch-lb pressure pins), children: 8 to 10 pins (2 inch-lb pressure pins)**
5. Complications—pin loosening, pin infection, pressure sores, nerve injury, dural penetration

II. LOWER CERVICAL SPINE INJURIES

See Table 11-24.

A. Classification—Allen-Ferguson (based on mechanism); described as the position of the head and neck at the time of injury (flexion/extension) and the mode of failure (distraction/compression). First three are most common, last two are least common:

1. Compressive flexion
2. Distractive flexion
3. Compressive extension

4. Vertical compression
5. Distractive extension
6. Lateral flexion

B. Stability

1. White and Punjabi—point system based on anatomic, radiographic, and neurologic criteria; less than 5 points is equivalent to instability.
2. Several patterns are inherently unstable:
   - "Teardrop" fractures, which result from compressive flexion injury, contrast to the small avulsion-type teardrop injury, which may be treated with immobilization.
   - Flexion-type injuries tend to be more unstable than extension injuries.
   - Any fracture associated with neurologic injury is assumed to be unstable.
   - Facet dislocations
   - Fractures with significant initial displacement

C. Treatment

1. Fractures that are primarily bony without ligamentous injury are usually treated with immobilization.
2. Posterior ligamentous injury is usually treated with surgical stabilization.
3. Facet fracture-dislocations (jumped facets)
   - The role of MRI to evaluate the disc before or after closed reduction is controversial, particularly as it relates to neurologic status.
   - The purpose is to identify potential anterior causes of impingement to the spinal cord during the reduction maneuver.
     - Closed reduction before MRI
       - Patient must be awake, alert, and cooperative.
     - MRI before closed reduction
       - Obtunded patient
   - Closed reduction is with Gardner-Wells tongs or halo and slow progressive application of traction.
   - MRI is generally required before open reduction.
   - If patient is obtunded, develops neurologic symptoms, or fails closed reduction, obtain MRI to evaluate disc.

III. THORACIC SPINE INJURIES

See Table 11-24.

A. Classification—Magerl

1. Type A—compression fractures caused by axial loading
2. Type B—distraction injuries with ligamentous (B1) or osseoligamentous (B2) injury posteriorly
3. Type C—multidirectional injuries, often fracture-dislocations; very unstable with very high likelihood of neurologic injury

B. Treatment

1. Most burst fractures and compression fractures can be treated with an orthosis for 12 weeks and a shorter period of time for less severe fractures.
2. Flexion-distraction injuries with a bony avulsion posteriorly (type B2) can be treated with an orthosis.
3. Types B1 and C injuries usually require surgical stabilization.
4. Some compression fractures with more than 50% anterior collapse may also require stabilization.

IV. THORACOLUMBAR AND LUMBAR SPINE INJURIES

See Table 11-24.

A. Classification—Denis

1. Columns
   - The anterior column is equivalent to the anterior one third of the body and annulus and the anterior longitudinal ligament.
   - The middle column is equivalent to the posterior two thirds of the body and annulus and the posterior longitudinal ligament.
   - The posterior column is equivalent to the spinous process, lamina, pedicles, transverse process, and ligamentum flavum; interspinous ligament; supraspinous ligament; and facets.
2. Compression fractures involve only the anterior column.
3. Burst fractures involve the middle and anterior and often the posterior columns.
4. **Flexion-distraction injuries involve failure of the posterior and middle columns in tension.**
5. Fracture-dislocations involve the failure of all three columns.
6. Fractures in T11-L2 are the most common (more than 50% of thoracic and lumbar spine fractures)

B. Associated injuries

1. Adynamic ileus is common.
2. Calcaneus fractures are associated in approximately 10% of cases.

C. Treatment

1. Most compression fractures can be managed in an orthosis unless kyphosis is greater than 30 degrees.
2. **Burst fractures may be treated in an orthosis if kyphosis is less than 30 degrees, there is no neurologic deficit, canal compromise is less than 50%, and there is less than a 50% loss of anterior body height; otherwise, they are operative.**
3. **Flexion-distraction and fracture-dislocations are routinely treated with surgical stabilization via posterior approach with some requiring additional anterior decompression and stabilization.**

SECTION 5 PEDIATRIC TRAUMA

I. INTRODUCTION

A. Several features of fractures and dislocations in children are not found in adults (Tables 11-25 through 11-36; see Figures 11-65 through 11-83).

1. Children's bones are more ductile than adults' bones, and bowing is thus unique to children.
2. The terms ***greenstick*** and ***torus*** imply a partial fracture with some part of the bone intact.
3. The periosteum in children is much thicker and often remains intact on the concave (compression) side, allowing for less displacement and better reduction of fractures.

Table 11-25 Salter-Harris Classification of Physeal Injuries

Type	Description	Prognosis
I	Transverse fractures through the physis	Excellent
II	Fractures through the physis, with metaphyseal fragment	Excellent
III	Fractures through the physis and epiphysis	Good but with the potential for intraarticular deformity; may require ORIF
IV	Fractures through the epiphysis, physis, and metaphysis	Good but unstable; fragment requires ORIF
V	Crush injury to the physis	Poor, with growth arrest
VI	Injury to the perichondrial ring	Good; may cause angular deformities

ORIF, open reduction with internal fixation.

4. Children's fractures heal more quickly and with less immobilization than adults' fractures. Contractures are also less likely.
5. Because bones are actively growing in pediatric fractures, malunion and growth plate injuries are important concerns. Remodeling is more thorough; thus, displacement and angulation that would not be acceptable in an adult are often acceptable in children.
6. The exception to this rule is an intraarticular fracture, in which the same axioms apply. However, the presence of nearby physeal structures can affect fixation options.

II. CHILD ABUSE

A. Introduction

1. One must always be alert for the "battered child."
2. **All states now require physicians to report suspected child abuse.**
3. **Suspicion should be raised when fractures are seen in children younger than 3 years old (the most common age group for sustaining abuse), with multiple healing bruises, skin marks, burns, unreasonable histories, and signs of neglect, among other indications.**
4. Osteogenesis imperfecta is often in the differential diagnosis in a child with multiple fractures.

B. Fracture location

1. The most common locations of fractures in children of abuse are the humerus, tibia, and femur, in that order.
   - **Spiral humerus fractures and distal humeral physeal separations are highly suggestive.**
   - **Spiral femur fractures in nonambulatory children are also highly suspicious.**

Table 11-26 Pediatric Hand and Wrist Trauma

Injury	Eponym/Other Name	Classification	Treatment	Complications
Phalanx fracture (watch for mallet equivalent)		Based on phalanx and SH classification	Closed reduction for most; ORIF if condylar, SH III/IV >25 degrees if <10 yr old, >10 degrees if >10 yr old; dynamic traction for pilon equivalents	Residual deformities, tendon imbalance, nail deformities
MC fracture		Based on location	Reduce; ORIF if irreducible	Avascular necrosis of metacarpal head
Thumb MC fracture	Type D = Bennett equivalent	Type A—metaphyseal Type B—SH II (medial) Type C—SH II (lateral) Type D—SH III	Closed reduction except for type D, which requires ORIF	
Interphalangeal dislocation			Closed reduction and splint; ORIF if unable to obtain or maintain a congruous reduction	
MCP dislocation			Attempt closed reduction; ORIF if irreducible	
CMC dislocation			Reduce with finger traps; CRPP with Kirschner wire to carpus and adjacent MC	
Distal radius fracture		SH fractures I-V	CRPP types III and IV	Deformity, loss of reduction, infection with open fracture, Volkmann contracture, growth arrest, malunion, refracture, TFCC tears, carpal tunnel syndrome
Torus	Tension side intact	Short-arm cast for 3 wk		
Greenstick	Tension side with plastic deformation	Reduce if angulation >10 degrees		
Complete	Both cortices disrupted	Reduce and place in long-arm cast		

CMC, carpometacarpal; CRPP, closed reduction with percutaneous pinning; MC, metacarpal; MCP, metacarpophalangeal joint; ORIF, open reduction with internal fixation; SH, Salter-Harris; TFCC, triangular fibrocartilage complex.

Table 11-27 Pediatric Radial and Ulnar Shaft Trauma

Injury	Eponym/Other Name	Classification	Treatment	Complications
Radius and ulna fractures	"Both-bone"	Greenstick, compression, complete	Correct rotation, with pronation/supination and <10 degrees angulation: long-arm cast 3-4 wk if <10 yr old; bayonet apposition OK if growth remains	Refracture, limb ischemia, malunion (especially in <10 yr old with inadequate reduction), nerve injury, synostosis
Plastic deformation		Based on bones involved (ulna > radius)	Reduction with pressure as a fulcrum, the most deformed bone first; must reduce >20 degrees in 4 yr old, less in older children	Persistence of deformity
Ulna fracture and radial head dislocation (see Figure 11-18)	Monteggia	Type I—ulna angulation and radial head anterior (extension)	Reduce (traction flexion); long-arm cast, 100 degrees flexion in supination	Late diagnosis (reconstruct annular ligament), decreased ROM Missed wrist injury, nonunion, persistent radial head dislocation, periarticular ossification
		Type II—ulna angulation and radial head posterior (flexion)	Reduce (traction extension); long-arm cast in some extension	
		Type III—ulna anterior angulation, radial head lateral (adduction)	Reduce (extension); long-arm cast, 90 degrees flexion in supination	
		Type IV—ulna and proximal (one third) radius fracture (both anterior angulation)	Reduce (supinate); may require ORIF	
Radial head dislocation (anterior)	Monteggia equivalent		Supination and pressure on radial head; long-arm cast, 100 degrees flexion in supination	Synostosis, PIN injury, loss of reduction
Ulna and radial neck fractures	Check for Monteggia equivalent		Reduce (traction, pressure on radial head, varus stress); long-arm cast, 90 degrees flexion	
Ulna and proximal radius fractures	Check for Monteggia equivalent		Reduce (traction supination); long-arm cast, 90 degrees in supination	
Radius fracture and distal radioulnar dislocation	Galeazzi		Reduce (traction supination if ulna dorsal, pronation if ulna volar); ORIF if >12 yr old or reduction fails	Malunion, nerve injury (AIN), radioulnar subluxation, loss of radial bow

AIN, anterior interosseous nerve; ORIF, open reduction with internal fixation; PIN, posterior interosseous nerve; ROM, range of motion.

2. **If suspicion is high, skeletal surveys are appropriate in children with delayed development and in some metaphyseal and spiral fractures.**
3. **Corner fractures (at junction of metaphysis and physis) and posterior rib fractures are described as pathognomonic for abuse** (Figure 11-65).
4. However, diaphyseal fractures are more common in abuse cases (four times as likely as metaphyseal fractures).
5. Skeletal surveys are not as helpful in children older than 5 years old. Instead, a bone scan may be done as an alternative or adjunctive study.
6. **Nonorthopaedic injuries found in abuse include skin injuries, head injuries, burns, and blunt abdominal visceral injuries.**

C. Treatment—In addition to normal fracture care, early involvement of social workers and pediatricians is essential. If the abuse is missed, there is a greater than 33% chance of further abuse and a 5% to 10% chance of death in affected children.

III. PHYSEAL FRACTURES

A. Introduction—Fracture of the physis, or growth plate, is more likely than injury to attached ligaments; thus, assume that there is a fracture of the physis until evidence proves otherwise (young children rarely get sprains).

B. Characteristics

1. Although physeal fractures are classically thought to be through the zone of provisional calcification (within the zone of hypertrophy) of the growth plate, the fracture can be through many different layers.

Table 11-28 Pediatric Elbow Trauma

Injury	Eponym/Other Name	Classification	Treatment	Complications
Supracondylar fracture (6-8 yr old) (see Figure 11-71)		I—extension (98%), nondisplaced	Immobilize 3 wk Minimally displaced (<2 mm), splint	Nerve injury (AIN and radial), vascular injury (1%), decreased ROM; if pulse present but then lost, explore; if pulse present but then lost, explore; if no pulse present but pink hand, watch; if no pulse present and cold, explore HO, cubitus varus (5%-10%), ipsilateral fractures Nerve injury (ulnar), malunion (decreased extension)
		II—displaced (posterior cortex intact)	Reduce; cast vs. CRPP (must re-create Baumann angle) (see Figure 11-69)	
		III—displaced (posterior periosteal hinge intact)	Reduce; CRPP vs. open pinning	
		IV—displaced (posterior periosteal hinge disrupted)	Reduce; CRPP vs. open pinning	
		Flexion (distal fragment anterior)	Reduce; CRPP vs. ORIF	
Lateral condyle fracture (6 yr old) (see Figure 11-72)		Milch I—SH IV Milch II—SH II into trochlea	Minimally displaced (<2 mm), splint; displaced, ORIF with pins or cannulated screws	Overgrowth/spur "fish tail" deformity, nonunion, cubitus valgus, AVN, ulnar nerve palsy
Medial condyle fracture (9-14 yr old)		Nondisplaced— <10 mm displacement		Cubitus varus, AVN
Displaced— >10 mm displacement			Minimally displaced, splint Displaced, ORIF	
Entire distal humeral physis fracture (<7 yr old) (see Figure 11-74)		A—infant (SH I) B—7 mo-3 yr old (SH I) C—3-7 yr old (SH II)	Closed reduction, long-arm cast; displaced, CRPP	Child abuse, common late diagnosis, cubitus varus
Medial epicondylar apophysis fracture (11 yr old) (see Figure 11-73)	Little Leaguer's elbow	I—acute injuries		Highly associated with elbow dislocation (50%), valgus instability, loss of extension
		A—nondisplaced	Immobilize 1 wk	
		B—minimally displaced	Immobilize 1 wk	
		C—significantly displaced (may be dislocated)	ORIF for valgus instability; otherwise, early ROM	
		D—entrapment of fragment in joint	Manipulative extraction, ORIF (especially with ulnar nerve entrapment)	
		E—fracture through epicondylar apophysis	Immobilization vs. ORIF	
		II—chronic tension stress injury	Change in throwing activities	
T condylar fracture		Based on fracture	ORIF with cannulated screws	Decreased ROM
Radial head and neck fractures (<4 yr old)		A—SH I or II physeal fracture B—SH IV fracture C—transmetaphyseal fracture D and E—with elbow dislocation	Immobilize if <60 degrees in pronation/supination; ORIF if markedly displaced or >60 degrees primarily	Decreased ROM, radial head overgrowth, neck notching, AVN, synostosis, nonunion
Proximal olecranon physis fracture (rare)		I—physeal-metaphyseal border (younger children) II—physis with large metaphyseal fragment (older children)		

Table 11-28 Pediatric Elbow Trauma—cont'd

Injury	Eponym/Other Name	Classification	Treatment	Complications
Olecranon metaphysis fracture		A—flexion	If undisplaced (<3 mm), immobilize 3 wk; ORIF if defect	Rare: delay/nonunion
		B—extension	Reduction in extension	
		C—shear	Immobilize in hyperflexion ORIF if periosteal tear	
Elbow dislocation (11-20 yr old)		Based on direction of dislocation	Reduction and cast for <2 wk	Watch for associated fractures and nerve injuries (ulnar > median), HO, recurrent dislocation
Radial head subluxation (15 mo-3 yr old)	Nursemaid's elbow		Stretching of annular ligaments Reduce (supination/flexion)	

AIN, anterior interosseous nerve; AVN, avascular necrosis; CRPP, closed reduction with percutaneous pinning; HO, heterotopic ossification; ORIF, open reduction with internal fixation; ROM, range of motion; SH, Salter-Harris.

Table 11-29 Pediatric Shoulder Trauma

Injury	Classification	Treatment	Complications
Humeral shaft fracture	Neonate	Small splint or splint to side	Compartment syndrome, radial nerve palsy, rotational palsy
	<3 yr old	Collar and cuff OK	
	3-12 yr old	Sarmiento brace	
	>12 yr old	Sarmiento brace	
Proximal humeral physis fracture	SH (I most common in <5 yr old)	Sling if minimally displaced, gentle manipulation for displaced fractures, CRPP vs. ORIF for <50% apposition, >45 degrees angulation	
Proximal humeral metaphysis fracture (common)	Based on location	Sling	
Midshaft clavicle fracture	≤2 yr old	Supportive sling if symptomatic	Rare: malunion or nonunion, neurovascular compromise
	>2 yr old	Figure-eight brace vs. sling	
Medial clavicle fracture	Usually SH I or II physeal separations	Sling for 1 wk	
Lateral clavicle fracture	I—nondisplaced; intact AC and CC ligaments IIA—clavicle displaced superiorly; fracture medial to CC ligament IIB—clavicle displaced superiorly; conoid ligaments tear	Sling vs. figure-eight brace Type II may need ORIF	
AC joint injury	Same as adult	Same as adult	Watch for coracoid fracture
SC joint injury	Anterior and posterior	Same as adult	
Clavicle dislocation (rare)	Anterior and posterior	ORIF with repair of periosteal tube	
Scapula fracture	Anterior and posterior	Same as adult	
Glenohumeral dislocation	Anterior and posterior	Initial immobilization followed by rehabilitation; reconstruction for recurrent instability	Recent research shows >60% chance of redislocation when patient is <21 yr old

AC, acromioclavicular; CC, coracoclavicular; ORIF, open reduction with internal fixation; CRPP, closed reduction with percutaneous pinning; SC, sternoclavicular; SH, Salter-Harris.

Table 11-30 Pediatric Spine Trauma

Injury	Eponym/Other Name	Classification	Treatment	Complications
Occiput-C1 dissociations			Reduced with traction; craniovertebral fusion later	Often fatal
C1-C2 dissociations		Traumatic ligament disruption	Reduce in extension, immobilize with halo for 8-12 wk	Vertebral artery is at risk with surgery
Grisel syndrome		Ligament laxity from local inflammation	Traction; immobilize for 6-8 wk	
Rotatory subluxation		I—without C1 shift II—<5 mm C1 anterior shift III—>5 mm C1 anterior shift IV—posterior shift Odontoid physeal or os odontoideum	Traction; if no improvement, then open reduction and fusion	
C2-C3 dislocation		True vs. pseudo (more likely)		
Cervical facet dislocation			Same as in adults	
Thoracic and lumbar fractures		Same as in adults	Same as in adults	
Spondylosis		Stress fracture of pars (likely at L5-S1)	Acute: immobilize in brace; otherwise, surgical treatment; fusion for refractory cases	
Spinal cord injury without radiographic abnormality		Spinal cord injury without radiographic abnormality	Evaluation with magnetic resonance imaging and supportive treatment	Scoliosis (especially <8 yr old)

Table 11-31 Pediatric Pelvic Fracture*

Classification (Key and Cornwell)	Eponym	Treatment	Complications
I—Ring Intact			
Avulsions (ASIS, AIIS, IT)		BR flexed hip for 2 wk; guarded WB for 4 wk	Loss of reduction, delayed union
Pubis/ischium	Duverney	BR 3-7 days; limited WB for 4 wk	DJD, malunion, organ injury
Iliac wing		BR with leg abducted; progress to full WB	Sacral nerve injury
Sacrum/coccyx		BR 3-6 wk, conservative management if <1 cm displaced, otherwise ORIF	
II—Single Break in Ring			
Ipsilateral rami		BR 2-4 wk; non-WB	
Symphysis pubis		BR with sling or spica; ORIF if undergoing laparotomy or widely displaced	
SI joint (rare)		BR with progressive WB	
III—Double Break in Ring	Straddle		
Bilateral pubic rami	Malgaigne	BR with flexed hip 2-4 wk	Often unstable, with associated injuries
Anterior and posterior ring with migration		Skeletal traction; external fixator for 3-6 wk	
IV—Acetabular Fractures			
Small fragment with dislocation		BR followed by progressive ambulation	
Linear: nondisplaced		Treat associated pelvic fracture	
Linear: hip unstable		Skeletal traction; ORIF if incongruous	
Central		Lateral traction for reduction; ORIF if severe	HO, especially if severe

AIIS, anterior inferior iliac spine; ASIS, anterior superior iliac spine; BR, bed rest; DJD, degenerative joint disease; HO, heterotopic ossification; IT, ischial tuberosity; ORIF, open reduction with internal fixation; SI, sacroiliac; WB, weight bearing.

*In general, less than adults because of remodeling.

Table 11-32 Pediatric Hip Trauma

Injury	Classification	Treatment	Complications
Hip fracture (see Figure 11-75)	Delbet	Closed reduction or ORIF with pin	AVN close to 100%
	IA—transepiphyseal with dislocation		
	IB—transepiphyseal without dislocation	CRPP with spica	AVN in up to 60%
	II—transcervical	CRPP with spica	Coxa vara (25%): treat with subtrochanteric valgus osteotomy
	IIIA—cervical trochanteric (displaced)	CRPP with spica	Nonunion (6%)
	IIIB—cervical trochanteric (nondisplaced)	Spica cast in abduction	Growth arrest
	IV—intertrochanteric	Spica cast; ORIF if unstable	May cross physis if it creates greater fracture stability
Femoral neck stress fracture	Devas Superior transverse Inferior (compressive)	CRPP (otherwise is displaced) NWB	Displacement causes more problems; varus deformities
Traumatic dislocation	Posterior or anterior	Closed reduction; open if joint incongruous	AVN (10%), recurrent dislocation, HO, DJD

AVN, avascular necrosis; CRPP, closed reduction with percutaneous pinning; DJD, degenerative joint disease; HO, heterotopic ossification; NWB, non–weight bearing; ORIF, open reduction with internal fixation.

2. The blood supply of the epiphysis is tenuous, and injuries can disrupt small physeal vessels supplying the growth center. This can lead to many complications associated with these injuries (e.g., limb-length discrepancies, malunion, bony bars).
3. The most common physeal injuries occur in the distal radius, followed by the distal tibia.

C. **Classification**

1. The **Salter-Harris** (SH) classification modified by Rang is the gold standard for physeal injuries (Figure 11-66; see Table 11-25).
   - It can be recalled using the mnemonic SALTR
     - I—**S**lipped—separation physis
     - II—**A**bove—metaphysis and physis
     - III—**L**ower—epiphysis and physis
     - IV—**T**hrough—metaphysis, physis, epiphysis
     - V—**R**uined—crushed physis
   - SH type I fracture is through the zone of hypertrophic cells of the physis.

D. **Treatment and results**

1. Gentle reduction should be attempted initially for SH I and II fractures, sometimes using conscious sedation protocols. With reduction and immobilization, these fractures will do well without a significant amount of growth arrest (except in the distal femur).
2. SH III and IV fractures are intraarticular by definition and usually require ORIF. Follow-up radiographs are required for all physeal injuries.
3. Remodeling is also common in pediatric fractures (up to 20 degrees). This depends on the location and age of the patient.
4. Harris-Park growth arrest lines (transverse radiodense lines) may be the only evidence of a physeal injury on follow-up radiographs.

E. **Partial growth arrest**

1. Physeal bars or bridges result from growth plate injuries that arrest a part of the physis and leave the uninjured physis to grow normally. This results in angular growth and deformity.
2. Physeal bridge resection with interposition of a fat graft or artificial material is reserved for patients with over 2 cm of growth remaining and less than 50% physeal involvement.
3. Treatment of smaller peripheral bars in young patients have the highest success rate.
4. MRI and CT can help define the location and amount of physeal closure.
5. Arrest involving more than 50% of the physis should be treated with ipsilateral completion of the arrest and contralateral epiphysiodesis or ipsilateral limb lengthening.

IV. PEDIATRIC POLYTRAUMA

A. **Introduction**

1. Trauma is the most common cause of death in children older than 1 year old.

Table 11-33 Pediatric Femoral Shaft Trauma

Injury	Classification	Treatment	Complications
Femur fracture (including subtrochanteric fractures)	≤6 yr old	Spica cast; may need short period of traction if shortened >2 cm and followed by spica casting	LLD: Angular deformity (avoid >10 degrees frontal and >10 degrees sagittal malalignment)
	6-13 yr old	Current trend to use flexible titanium nails, with possible additional immobilization, but may also use external fixation (higher refracture rate), plate (need to remove, causes large scar formation), or traction (rare)	Rotational deformity (>10 degrees); expect 0.9 cm overgrowth in <10 yr old
	≥14 yr old	IM nail (trochanteric entry)	AVN reported with IM nails in children with growth remaining

AVN, avascular necrosis; IM, intramedullary; LLD, leg-length discrepancy.

Table 11-34 Pediatric Knee Trauma

Injury	Eponym/Other Name	Classification	Treatment	Complications
Distal femoral epiphysis fracture (see Figure 11-77)	"Wagon wheel"	SH I-IV (II most common)	Closed reduction: LLC; CRPP in SH III or IV; open if soft tissue interposition or displaced III and IV	Popliteal artery or peroneal nerve injury, recurrent displacement; growth plate injuries because of undulating physis
Proximal tibial epiphysis fracture		SH I-IV (II most common)	*Nondisplaced:* long-leg cast in 30 degrees of flexion *Displaced:* CRPP	Popliteal artery injury, growth plate injury
Floating knee		Letts		Infection, nonunion, malunion, injuries
		A—both fractures diaphyseal	ORIF in one, closed reduction in the other	
		B—one fracture diaphyseal and one metaphyseal	ORIF of diaphyseal and closed reduction of metaphyseal	
		C—one fracture diaphyseal and one epiphyseal	CRPP of epiphyseal and ORIF of diaphyseal	
		D—one fracture open and one closed	Débride/external fixation, open and closed reductions of closed fracture	
		E—both fractures open	Débride/external fixation of both	
Tibial tubercle avulsion fracture (14-16 yr old in jumping sport) (see Figure 11-80)		Ogden		
		1—small distal piece fractured	If minimally displaced with extension, then cast; otherwise, ORIF	Genu recurvatum, decreased ROM, laxity
		2—fracture at junction of primary and secondary ossification centers		
		3—fracture through one epiphysis (SH III)		
Tibial spine fracture (most common hemarthrosis in preadolescent) (see Figure 11-79)		Meyers and McKeever		
		I—incomplete/ nondisplaced	Attempt closed reduction in extension for all; if it remains displaced, then may use arthroscope and ACL guide to fix with suture	Meniscal entrapment
		II—hinged (posterior rim intact)		
		III—completely displaced		
Patella fracture		Nondisplaced	Aspiration and cast vs. brace in 5 degrees of flexion	Patella alta, extensor lag, infection
		Displaced (>2 mm)	ORIF with tension band	
Sleeve fracture (see Figure 11-78)		Avulsion of the distal pole and articular cartilage	ORIF with tension band	
Femorotibial dislocation		Same as in adults	Same as in adults: arteriogram	Popliteal artery injury
Patella dislocation		Same as in adults	Closed-reduction cast for 3 wk; consider fixing MPFL; open if fragment	Predisposition: Down syndrome, arthrogryposis

ACL, anterior cruciate ligament; CRPP, closed reduction with percutaneous pinning; LLC, long-leg cast; MPFL, medial patellofemoral ligament; ORIF, open reduction with internal fixation; ROM, range of motion; SH, Salter-Harris.

Table 11-35 Pediatric Tibial Shaft Trauma

Injury	Eponym/Other Name	Classification	Treatment	Complications
Tibia-fibula fracture	Greenstick	Incomplete	Long-leg cast in slight flexion for 6-8 wk unless >10 degrees AP or >5 degrees varus/valgus; then must do manipulation	Angular deformity (valgus)
Complete			Closed reduction and cast	LLD (may see overgrowth with <10 yr old), malrotation, vascular injury
Tibial spiral fracture		Spiral fracture in <6 yr old	Long-leg cast for 3-4 wk	
Bike spoke injury		Soft tissue disruption	Admit and observe	Compartment syndrome; need for soft tissue coverage
Proximal tibial metaphysis fracture (see Figure 11-81)	Cozen	Greenstick in 3-6 yr old (complete in older children)	Long-leg cast in varus for 6 wk	Genu valgum, arterial injury, physeal injury

AP, anteroposterior; LLD, leg length discrepancy.

- Death is most closely associated with the severity of traumatic brain injury.

2. The most common cause of polytrauma is fall from height and motor vehicle collision.

B. Treatment

1. Cervical spine immobilization for children younger than age 6 years requires use of a backboard with occipital cut out because of the large head size of children.
   - Adult backboard use can result in neck flexion.
2. Timing of orthopaedic management
   - Early operative fixation (within 2-3 days) decreases intensive care unit and overall hospital stay.

V. SHOULDER AND ARM INJURIES

A. Clavicle fractures

1. Principles and presentation
   - Most frequent fracture in children
   - 90% of obstetric fractures; often associated with brachial plexus palsies
   - Birth injury mechanism—direct pressure from the symphysis pubis
   - Older children mechanism—fall on an outstretched hand; direct trauma to the clavicle or acromion
2. Diagnosis and radiographs

Table 11-36 Pediatric Ankle and Foot Trauma

Injury	Eponym/Other Name	Classification	Treatment	Complications
Ankle fracture		SH and Dias-Tachdjian (see Figure 11-66)	If SH I or II injury, treat with short-leg walking cast; if SH III or IV injury, treat with CRPP vs. ORIF	Angular deformity, bony bridge (poor prognosis with distal tibia), LLD, DJD, rotational deformity, AVN
	Juvenile Tillaux (see Figure 11-82)	SH III of lateral tibial physis (because distal-medial tibial physis is closed in this age group)	May use long-leg cast if <2 mm displacement; if greater, treat with ORIF and visualization of joint line	
	Wagstaff	SH III of distal fibular physis	Closed reduction and cast; ORIF if necessary	
	Triplane (see Figure 11-83)	Complex SH IV, with components in all three planes	ORIF if >2 mm articular step-off (fixation achieved parallel to physis in metaphysis and epiphysis)	Must use CT to delineate fracture
Talus fracture		Same as in adults	Closed reduction and cast unless >5 mm or 5 degrees of displacement	AVN
Calcaneus fracture	Essex-Lopresti	Same as in adults	Same as in adults	
Tarsometatarsal fracture		Fracture of base of second metatarsal and cuboid fracture	Closed reduction vs. CRPP if unstable	
Base of the fifth metatarsal fracture	Jones/pseudo-Jones	Same as in adults	Same as in adults	Nonunion

AVN, avascular necrosis; CRPP, closed reduction/percutaneous pinning; CT, computed tomography; DJD, degenerative joint disease; LLC, long-leg cast; LLD, leg-length discrepancy; ORIF, open reduction with internal fixation; SH, Salter-Harris.

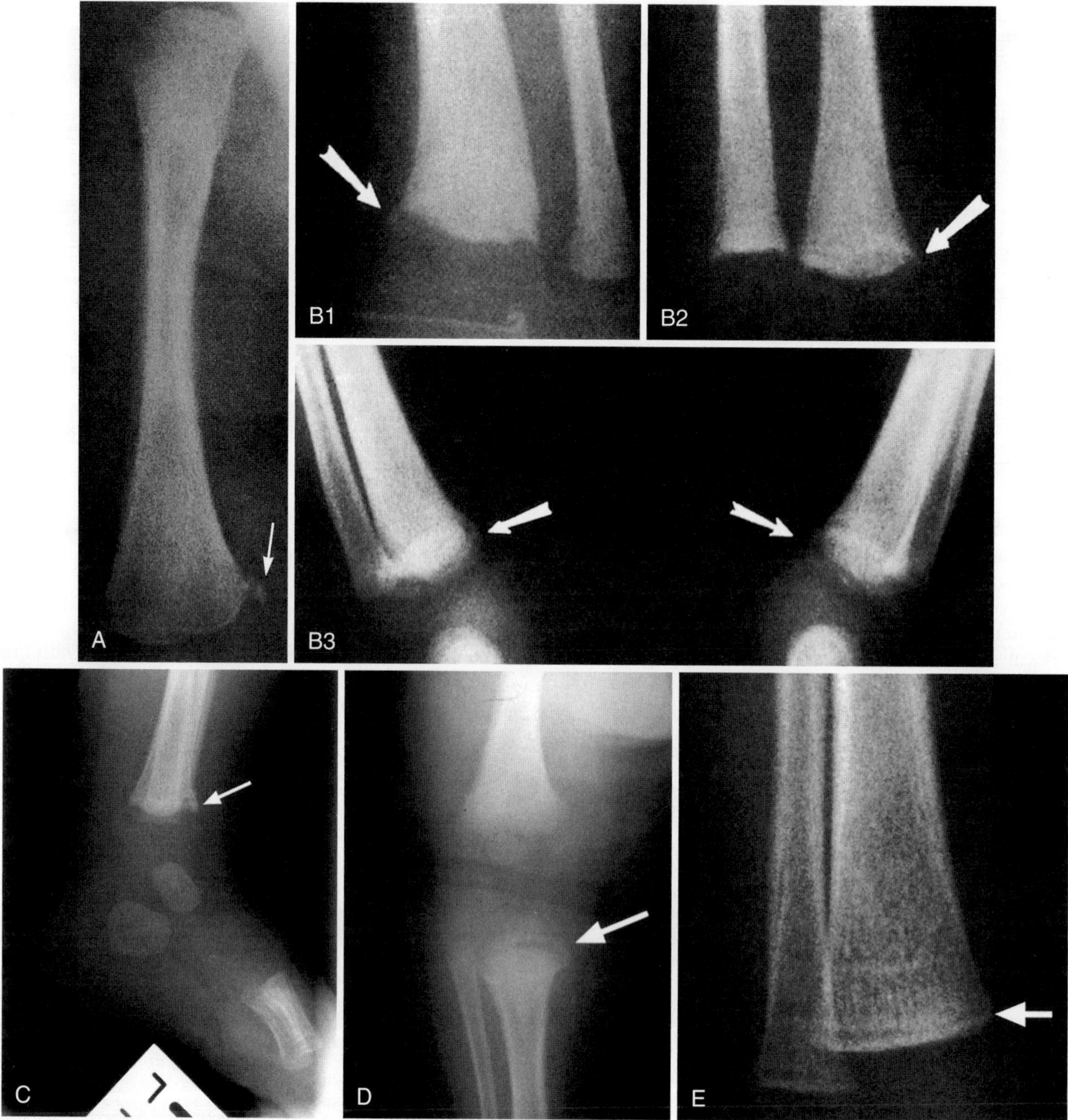

Figure 11-65 Metaphyseal fractures. Radiographs of the right femur **(A)** and both ankles **(B)** of a 2-month-old abused infant demonstrating metaphyseal corner fractures of the distal femur and both distal tibia *(arrows).* Angled tangential view reveals the "bucket handle" appearance of the fracture. **C,** Radiograph of the left ankle of an infant demonstrates a metaphyseal corner fracture of the distal tibia *(arrow).* **D,** Angled tangential view of the right lower limb of an abused infant demonstrates the "bucket handle" appearance *(arrow).* **E,** Radiograph of the right ankle of a 6-week-old abused neonate with subtle metaphyseal fractures evident as a metaphyseal lucent line *(arrow).* (From Adam A, Dixon A, editors: *Grainger & Allison's diagnostic radiology,* ed 5, Edinburgh, UK, 2007, Elsevier.)

- Ultrasound for obstetric fractures
- Cephalic tilt views (cephalic tilt of 35-40 degrees)
- Apical oblique view (ipsilateral side rotated 45 degrees and cephalic tilt of 20 degrees toward beam)
- CT axial imaging for medial clavicle fractures and physeal separation evaluations

3. Classification—Allman
   - Middle third (80%)
   - Lateral third (10%-15%)
     - Distal to coracoclavicular ligaments
   - Medial third (5%-10%)
4. **Treatment**
   - **Newborn—nonoperative treatment**
   - **Adolescents—Nonoperative treatment is standard of care.**
   - **Sternoclavicular physeal fracture-dislocations**
     - **Anterior—closed reduction, often unstable but can remodel**
     - Posterior—reduction with CT surgery backup after CT scan to evaluate for mediastinal impingement
   - Operative treatment controversial for middle third clavicle fractures

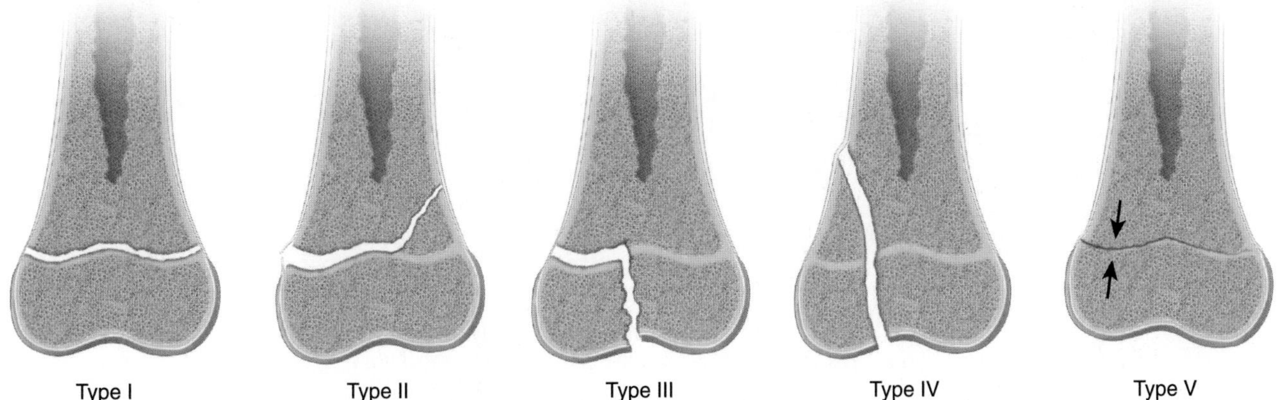

Figure 11-66 **Salter-Harris classification of physeal fractures.** (From Herring J: *Tachdjian's pediatric orthopaedics,* ed 4, Philadelphia, 2007, Elsevier.)

- Absolute indications—open fractures, neurovascular compromise
- Relative indications—nonunion, malunion, displacement greater than 2.0 cm
- Pin fixation should be avoided.
- Plate fixation or intramedullary nailing acceptable operative options

5. Complications
   - Nonunion (1%-3%)—rare in children; beware of congenital pseudarthrosis
   - Malunion—rare in younger populations; rates increase as age increases.
   - Neurovascular compromise
   - Pneumothorax

B. Proximal humerus fractures

1. Principles and presentation
   - In 80% to 90% humeral growth occurs at proximal physis; increased remodeling potential (Figure 11-67)
   - **Less than 5% of pediatric fractures**
   - Three ossification centers (humeral head, greater and lesser tuberosities) coalesce at ages 6 to 7.
   - Proximal fragments rotated into abduction and external rotation by rotator cuff muscles
   - **Distal fragments pulled into adduction and shortened by the pectoralis major and deltoid**
     - **Accordingly, gravity can be a useful reduction aid.**
2. Diagnosis and radiographs
   - AP, scapular Y, and axillary views
3. Classification
   - SH classification commonly applied to these fractures
   - SH I fractures most common in children younger than 5 years old
   - SH II fractures most common in children older than 12 years old
   - Metaphyseal fractures common in children between 5 and 12 years old
   - "Little Leaguer's shoulder" represents an SH I fracture.
4. Treatment
   - **Nonoperative treatment with temporary immobilization is usual treatment due to remodeling potential** (see Figure 11-67).
   - Operative indications
     - Absolute—open fractures, neurovascular injuries, intraarticular extension
     - Relative—young children younger than 12 years old; 70 degrees and 100% displacement acceptable
     - Age older than 12 years, controversial, 30 to 40 degrees, and 50% displacement
5. Complications
   - Malunion—varus deformity well tolerated due to shoulder motion

C. Diaphyseal humerus fractures

1. Principles and presentation
   - Uncommon in children
   - Radial nerve palsy can accompany middle or distal third fractures; usually neurapraxia and transient
2. Diagnosis and radiographs
   - AP and lateral radiographs of the humerus
   - Always evaluate elbow and shoulder appropriately.
3. Treatment
   - Nonoperative treatment with sling or clam-shell type splint immobilization
   - Operative indications—open fractures, vascular compromise after reduction
4. Complications
   - Radial nerve palsy—usually transient; exploration rarely indicated

VI. ELBOW INJURIES

A. Principles of elbow fractures

1. Skeletal anatomy (Figure 11-68)
   - Secondary ossification centers in order of ossification can be recalled using the mnemonic CRITOE and age at ossification can be roughly estimated based on odd numbers 1, 3, 5, 7, 9, 11:
     - Capitellum
     - Radial head
     - Internal (medial) epicondyle
     - Trochlea
     - Olecranon
     - External (lateral) epicondyle
   - Radial head, trochlea, and olecranon may appear as multiple ossification sites.

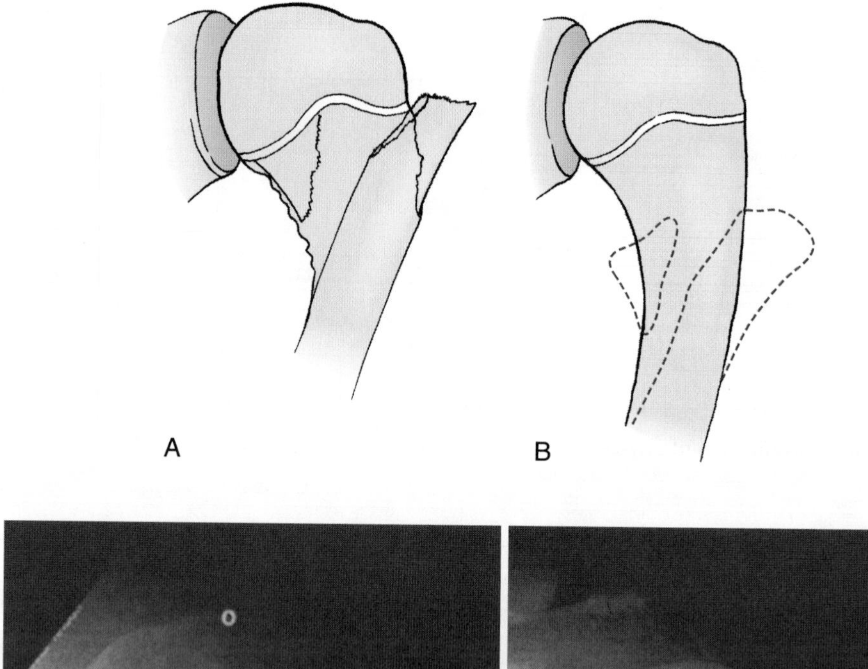

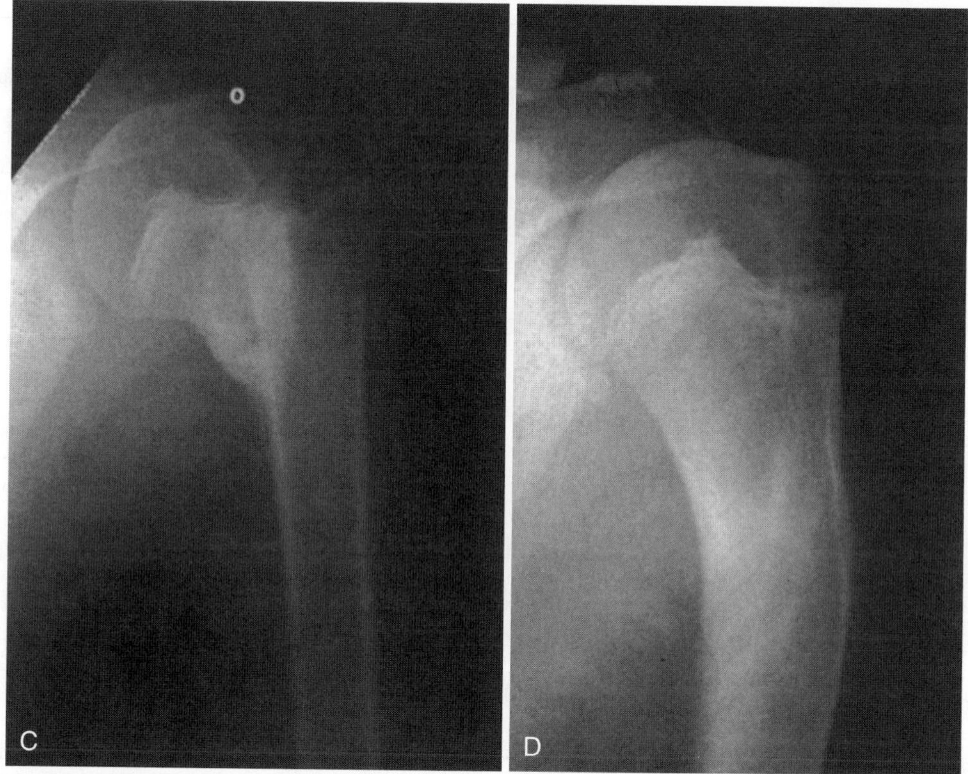

Figure 11-67 The remodeling potential of the proximal end of the humerus is great because of the amount of growth (80% of the entire humerus) coming from the proximal physis, as well as the universal motion of the shoulder joint. **A** and **C,** Early remodeling. **B** and **D,** Late remodeling. (From Herring J: *Tachdjian's pediatric orthopaedics,* ed 4, Philadelphia, 2007, Elsevier.)

2. Radiographic anatomy
   - A five-part systematic approach is key to avoiding missing injury (Figure 11-69):
     - Proximal radius should align with capitellum in all views.
     - Long axis of ulna should align and be slightly medial to humerus on AP radiograph.
     - Anterior humeral line should bisect capitellum on true lateral radiograph.
     - Humeral-capitellar (Baumann) angle should be in valgus and fall between 9 and 26 degrees.
     - The soft tissue shadows may demonstrate an anatomic anterior fat pad.
   - Abnormalities in radiographic anatomy (Box 11-2)

B. Distal humerus fractures

1. Distal humeral physeal separation (Figure 11-70)
   - Principles and presentation
     - Usually occur in pediatric patients younger than 6 to 7 years old
     - **Consider evaluation for child abuse in young patients with questionable presentation.**
     - Young patients may present with pseudoparalysis.
     - Often confused for elbow dislocations (which are rare in young children)
   - Diagnosis and radiographs
     - Radiographs demonstrate intact relationship between radius and capitellum. Radius and ulna lose normal relationship with distal end of humerus.

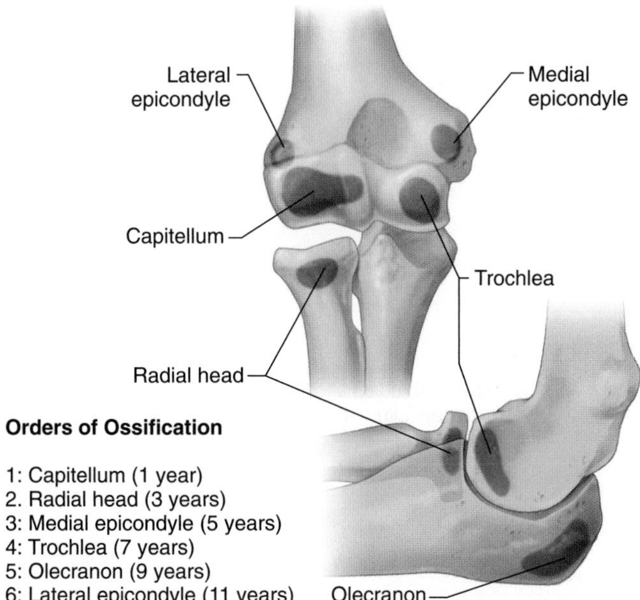

Figure 11-68 Ossification centers of the elbow in order of appearance and approximate age of ossification.

- Ultrasound or MRI evaluation may be necessary for young children.
- Arthrography can be used to evaluate for intraarticular extension.
- Treatment
  - Closed reduction and percutaneous pinning
  - Avoid closed reduction if diagnosis is made late to avoid iatrogenic injury to the physis.
- Complications
  - Misdiagnosis is most common, and these injuries can be mistaken for elbow dislocations or soft tissue injuries.
    - Physeal separations are typically medial whereas elbow dislocations are typically lateral.

2. Supracondylar humerus fractures
   - Principles and presentation
     - 50% to 60% of pediatric elbow fractures
     - 95% to 98% extension type; typically occur from a fall on outstretched hand with elbow in extension or hyperextension
     - 2% to 5% flexion type; typically occur from a fall onto the flexed elbow
     - Peak incidence in children between 5 and 8 years old
     - 1% associated with vascular injuries
     - **Anterior interosseous nerve injury most common for extension type; usually neurapraxia**
     - **Ulnar nerve injury usually iatrogenic from medial pinning and also the most common nerve injury from flexion type**
   - Diagnosis and radiographs
     - AP and lateral radiographs essential
       - AP view should be examined for Baumann angle; may need to compare with contralateral arm
       - Lateral radiograph should be examined to see if the anterior humeral line intersects the middle third of the capitellar ossification center.
       - Anterior and posterior fat pad signs should be examined.
         - Anterior fat pad displacement has low specificity and can be normal.
         - Posterior fat pad displacement is always pathologic and can indicate a nondisplaced fracture.
   - Classification and treatment—Gartland classification (Figure 11-71)
     - Type I—nondisplaced
       - Treated closed in a long-arm cast for 2 to 3 weeks
     - Type II—displaced with intact posterior cortex
       - Closed treatment for type II fractures is appropriate if all of the following criteria are met:
         - No significant swelling
         - Anterior humeral line intersects the capitellum
         - No medial distal humeral cortical impaction
       - Otherwise, closed reduction and percutaneous pinning is appropriate for type II fractures with postoperative long-arm immobilization at 90 degrees of flexion.
     - Type III—completely displaced; can be displaced posteromedially or posterolaterally
       - Treated with closed reduction and percutaneous pinning
       - Open reduction and internal fixation rarely needed
         - Rotationally unstable fractures, open fractures, or those associated with neurovascular injuries
         - Anterior approach preferred
       - **Crossed pin and lateral-entry pin configurations are often used.**
         - **Crossed pin considered more stable biomechanically.**
         - Medial pin can risk iatrogenic ulnar nerve (3%-8%).
         - Lateral-entry pin configuration has shown similar clinical results as crossed pin fixation when there is appropriate pin spread and engagement of both humeral columns.

Box 11-2

Abnormalities in Pediatric Radiographic Anatomy

Radiographic abnormality	Likely injury
Radius does not point to capitellum	Lateral condyle fracture Radial neck fracture Monteggia fracture or equivalent Elbow dislocation
Long axis of ulna not in line or not slightly medial to long axis of humerus	*Radial head and capitellum correctly aligned* → transphyseal injury or displaced supracondylar *Radius not pointing to capitellum* → elbow dislocation
Anterior humeral line does not bisect capitellum	*First, ensure true lateral radiograph* Center of capitellum posterior → extension-type supracondylar fracture Center of capitellum anterior → flexion-type supracondylar fracture
Baumann angle abnormal	Inadequate reduction of supracondylar fracture
Posterior fat pad present	76% rate of occult fracture when no other radiographic abnormality identified

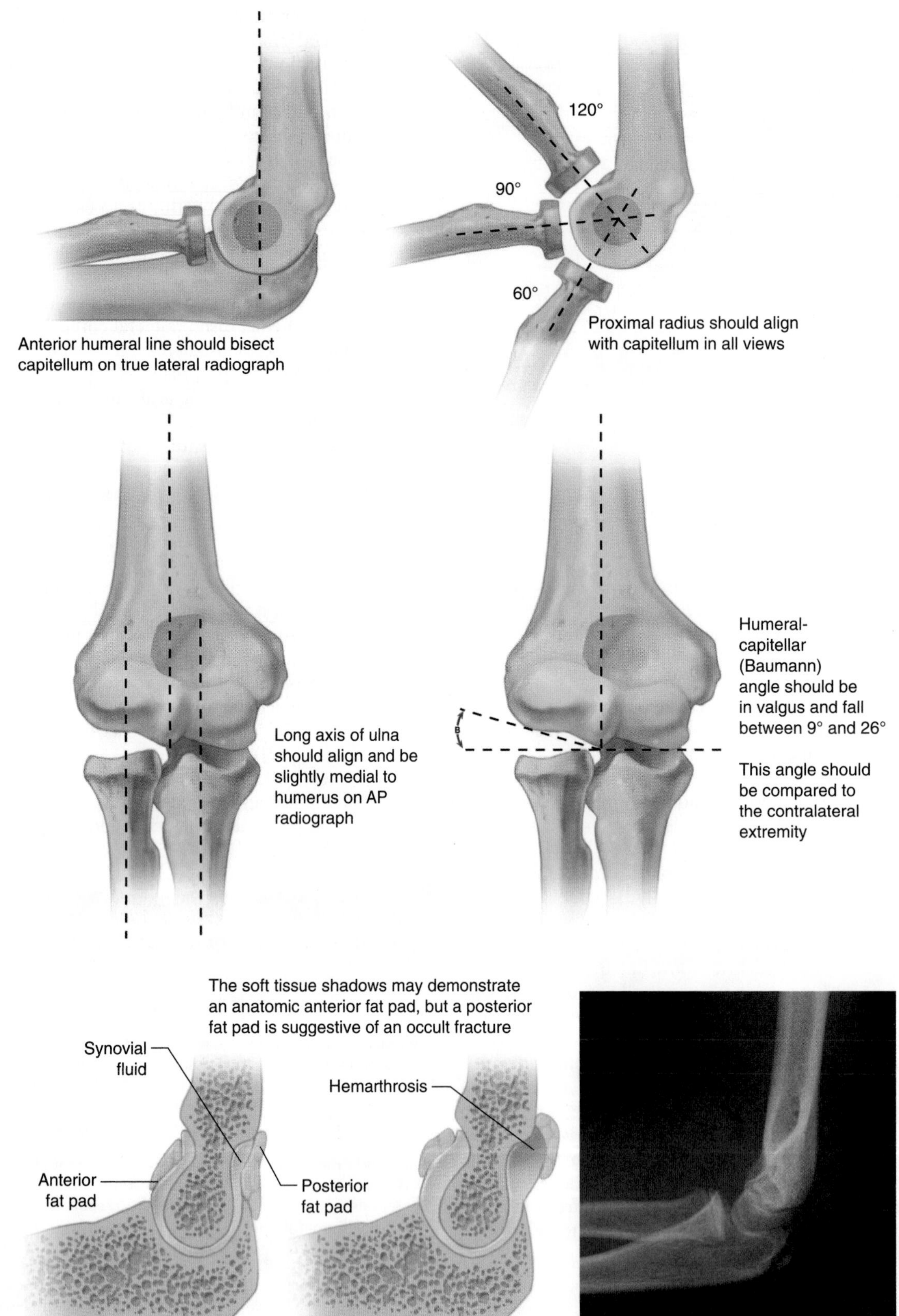
120°
90°
60°
Anterior humeral line should bisect capitellum on true lateral radiograph
Proximal radius should align with capitellum in all views
Long axis of ulna should align and be slightly medial to humerus on AP radiograph
Humeral-capitellar (Baumann) angle should be in valgus and fall between 9° and 26°
This angle should be compared to the contralateral extremity
The soft tissue shadows may demonstrate an anatomic anterior fat pad, but a posterior fat pad is suggestive of an occult fracture
Synovial fluid
Anterior fat pad
Posterior fat pad
Hemarthrosis

Figure 11-69 Radiographic anatomy of the pediatric elbow.

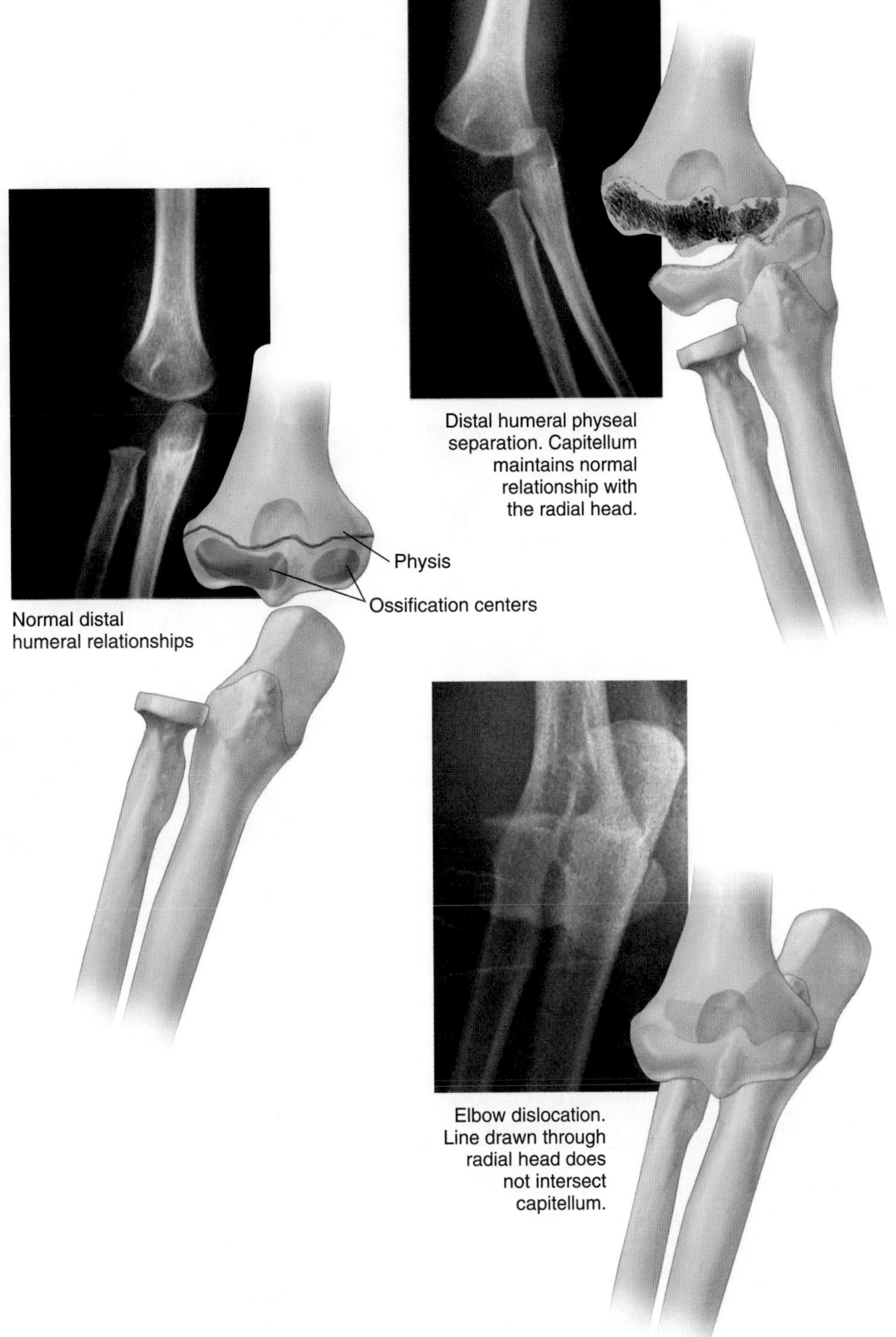
Distal humeral physeal separation. Capitellum maintains normal relationship with the radial head.
Physis
Ossification centers
Normal distal humeral relationships
Elbow dislocation. Line drawn through radial head does not intersect capitellum.

Figure 11-70 Injuries about the distal end of the humerus comparing distal humeral physeal separations and elbow dislocations.

- Flexion type
  - Similar management to extension type based on degree of displacement
  - Minimally displaced treated with immobilization in extension
  - Displaced treated with closed reduction and percutaneous pinning
- Supracondylar fracture with associated vascular injury
  - **Well-perfused hand, absent pulse ("pink, pulseless hand") (controversial)**
    - **Urgent closed reduction and percutaneous pinning**
    - Pulse returns in majority of cases. If not, observe as an inpatient and splint extremity.
    - If hand becomes poorly perfused, obtain vascular consultation and consider intervention.
  - **Poorly perfused hand, absent pulse**

Figure 11-71 Supracondylar fractures.

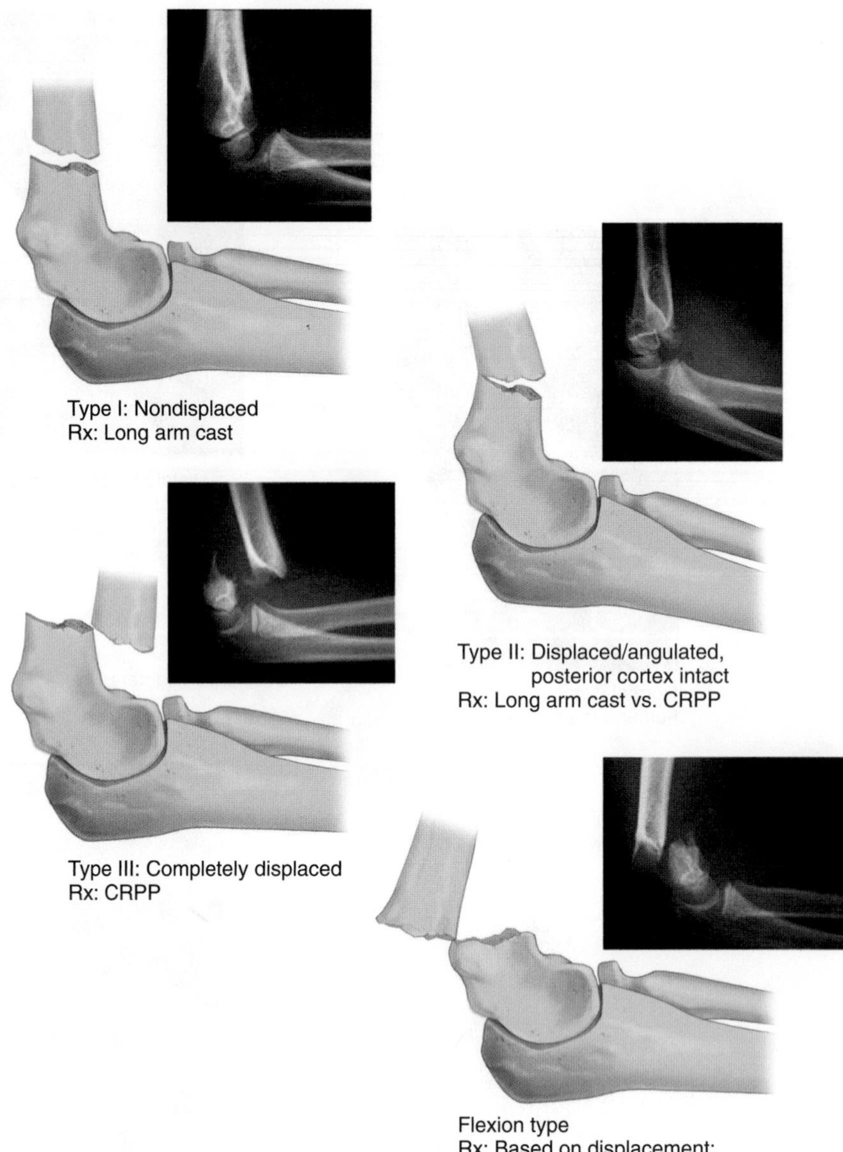

- **Urgent closed reduction and percutaneous pinning**
  - **Arteriography generally not warranted—the location of the injury is generally known.**
- If perfusion restored, observe as an inpatient.
- If hand remains poorly perfused, obtain vascular consultation.

- Complications
  - **Iatrogenic ulnar nerve injury with medial pin use (3%-8%)**
  - Compartment syndrome
    - Volkmann ischemic contracture is the most serious complication; beware of antecubital swelling and pressure from splint/cast.
  - Angular deformity
    - **Cubitus varus is typically the result of malunion, not growth arrest.** It results in a gunstock deformity associated with poor cosmesis but does not generally affect function
    - Recurvatum is poorly tolerated.
  - Stiffness
    - Rare if cast removal is done appropriately

3. Lateral condyle fractures
   - Principles and presentation
     - 17% of distal humeral fractures
     - Peak incidence around 6 years old
     - Loss of motion can be severe owing to intraarticular extension if the diagnosis is missed.
     - Increased incidence of growth disturbance
   - Diagnosis and radiographs
     - **AP, lateral, and oblique radiographs (especially internal oblique)**
     - Arthrogram can help distinguish transphyseal fractures from lateral condyle fractures.
   - Classification—Milch (historic, does not dictate treatment) (Figure 11-72)
     - Milch I—SH type IV fracture; fracture courses through the ossific center of the capitellum; less common
     - Milch II—SH type II fracture; fracture courses medial to the ossific center of the capitellum; more common

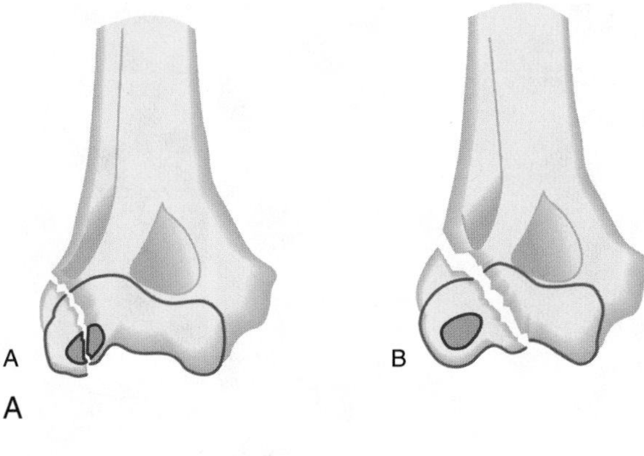

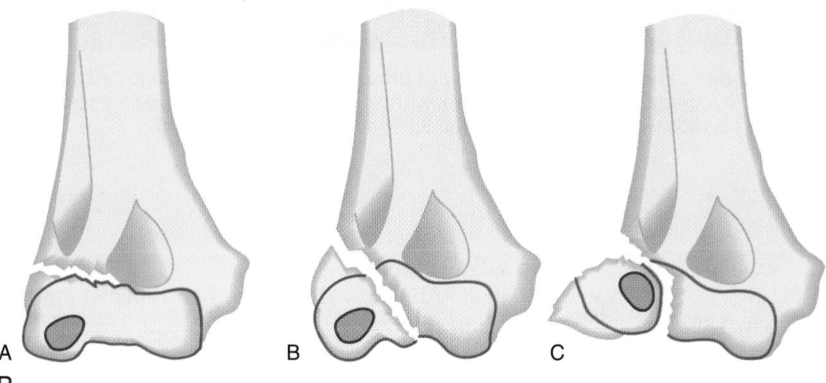

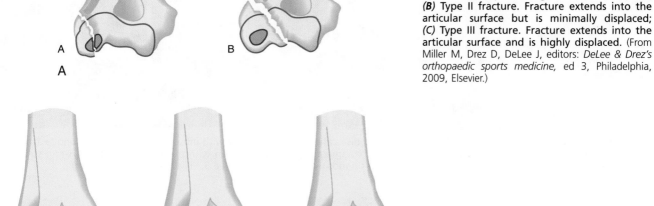

Figure 11-72 **A,** Lateral condyle drawing—Milch classification. *(A)* Milch type I fracture. The fracture line is through the ossific center of the capitellum; *(B)* Milch type II fracture. The fracture line is lateral to the ossific center of the capitellum. **B,** Lateral condyle drawing—Jakob classification. *(A)* Type I fracture. The fracture line does not enter the articular surface, permitting it to remain stable; ***(B)*** Type II fracture. Fracture extends into the articular surface but is minimally displaced; *(C)* Type III fracture. Fracture extends into the articular surface and is highly displaced. (From Miller M, Drez D, DeLee J, editors: *DeLee & Drez's orthopaedic sports medicine,* ed 3, Philadelphia, 2009, Elsevier.)

- Classification—Jakob (more clinically useful) (see Figure 11-61)
  - Type I—less than 2 mm displacement; intact intraarticular cartilage hinge
    - Can be treated with long-arm immobilization but can displace and need to be followed closely
  - Type II—2 to 4 mm displacement
    - Generally treated with closed reduction and percutaneous pinning
  - **Type III—greater than 4 mm displacement**
    - Closed reduction and percutaneous pinning if intraarticular reduction confirmed on arthrogram
    - **Open reduction can be necessary to ensure intraarticular reduction**
      - **Must preserve posterior blood supply**
- Complications
  - **Delayed union or nonunion**
    - Fracture fragment bathed in synovial fluid; relatively tenuous blood supply and primarily cartilage
  - Stiffness
    - Because of longer immobilization often needed and intraarticular extension
  - Angular deformity
    - Cubitus valgus more common due to lateral growth arrest
    - Tardy ulnar nerve palsy may result.
  - Osteonecrosis
    - **Iatrogenic—posterior blood supply must be preserved**

4. Medial condyle fractures
   - Principles and presentation
     - Rare injury less than 1% of elbow fractures
     - 8 to 12 years old
     - Can be mistaken for more common medial epicondylar fractures
   - Diagnosis and radiographs
     - AP, lateral, oblique views
     - In young children, arthrogram may help show intraarticular component.
   - Classification—Milch (same as lateral condyle)
     - Type I—through apex of trochlea (SH type II); very rare
     - Type II—through groove between capitellum and trochlea (SH type IV)
   - **Treatment**
     - **Similar treatment protocol as lateral condyle fractures**
   - Complications
     - Missed diagnosis; usually confused for a medial epicondylar fracture
5. Medial epicondyle fractures
   - Principles and presentation
     - **Traction injury resulting in an avulsion of the apophysis by the medial collateral ligament and flexor mass**
     - Last ossification center to fuse with metaphysis
     - **Associated with elbow dislocation approximately 50% of the time**

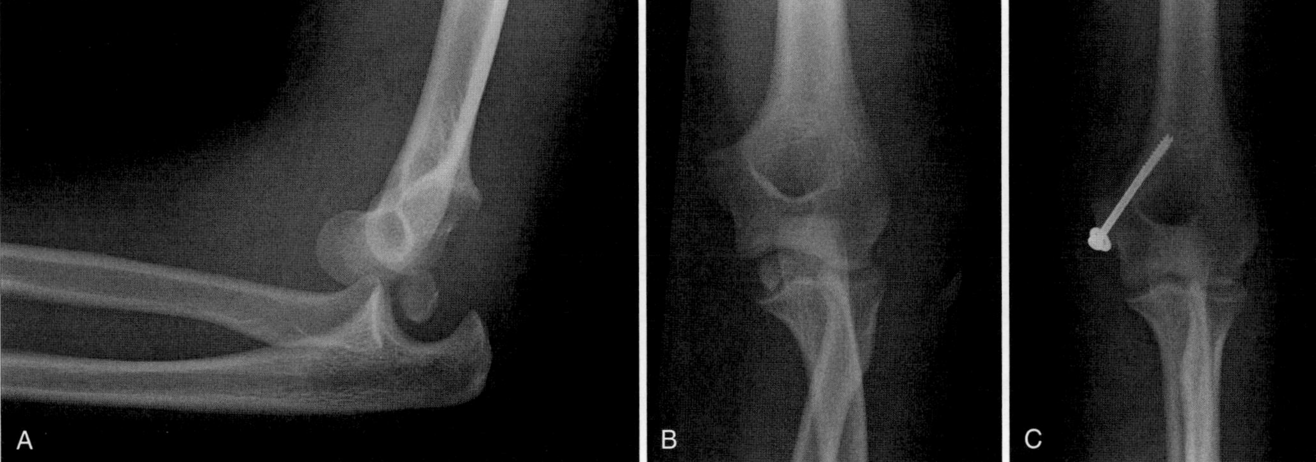

Figure 11-73 Medial epicondyle fracture following elbow dislocation. **A,** Lateral view with intraarticular medial epicondyle fragment. **B,** Anteroposterior view after reduction with incarcerated fragment. **C,** Internal fixation with a single cannulated 3.5-mm screw and washer. (From Miller M, Drez D, DeLee J, editors: *DeLee & Drez's orthopaedic sports medicine,* ed 3, Philadelphia, 2009, Elsevier.)

- Valgus force with contraction of flexor-supinator mass (same mechanism as in elbow dislocation)
  - **Can be incarcerated after reduction in 15% to 18% of cases** (Figure 11-73)
  - Also referred to as Little Leaguer's elbow
  - Ulnar nerve symptoms can accompany injury secondary to stretch during trauma or swelling.
- Diagnosis and radiographs
  - AP, lateral, oblique views
  - **If apophysis is missing from an AP view, carefully evaluate lateral and oblique views for possible incarceration.**
- Classification
  - Based on the amount of displacement whether it is incarcerated in the joint
- Treatment
  - Most can be treated nonoperatively with excellent functional results.
  - The amount of displacement that would necessitate surgical reduction and fixation in young athletic patients is controversial.
  - More than 5 mm was a traditional amount of acceptable displacement; however, has been shown to be difficult to assess the true displacement on standard radiographs.
  - **Incarceration of the fragment is an indication for surgical treatment.**
- Complications
  - Missed incarceration
  - Ulnar nerve symptoms (10% to 16%)
  - Nonunion—reported to occur in up to 60% of cases but good functional outcomes reported even with radiographic nonunion
  - Loss of extension—20%

C. **Radial head and neck fractures**

1. Principles and presentation
   - 5% of pediatric elbow fractures
   - 90% are physeal or metaphyseal; rarely involve the head
   - Often valgus injuries
   - Associated with elbow dislocations and medial epicondyle fractures
2. Diagnosis and radiographs
   - AP, lateral, oblique views
   - Radiocapitellar view (Greenspan)—oblique lateral directed 40 degrees proximally
3. Classification—Wilkins
   - Type A—SH I or II physeal fractures
   - Type B—SH III or IV intraarticular fractures (rare)
   - Type C—metaphyseal fractures
4. Treatment
   - **Multiple closed reduction maneuvers**
     - **Patterson maneuver**
     - **Israeli technique**
   - Indications for surgery
     - Less than 20 to 30 degrees of angulation and no translation acceptable; treated in long-arm immobilization
     - More than 30 degrees angulation, translation greater than 3 to 4 mm, and more than 45 degrees of rotation are indications for surgical intervention.
     - Surgical treatment using percutaneous wire correction or retrograde insertion of a wire with rotation of the wire accounting for reduction (Metaizeau)
     - Open reduction occasionally needed through a lateral approach
   - Complications
     - Decreased range of motion: usually loss of pronation and supination
     - Radial head overgrowth (20%-40%)
     - Physeal arrest—can lead to cubitus valgus deformity
     - AVN of the radial head—70% of AVN cases associated with open reduction
     - Neurologic injury—posterior interosseous nerve most commonly injured
     - Radioulnar synostosis—associated with open reduction

D. Radial head subluxation

1. Principles and presentation
   - Also known as nursemaid's elbow
   - Mechanism is usually traction on an extended elbow in children younger than 5 years old; peak age is 2 to 3 years old.
   - Arm usually held in slight flexion and pronation
   - Annular ligament subluxates over the radial head.
2. Diagnosis and radiographs
   - Usually normal and usually not necessary if clinical picture is appropriate
3. Treatment
   - **Closed reduction achieved by placing thumb over radial head and then progressively supinated and flexed.**
   - Immobilization is generally not needed.
4. Complications
   - Recurrence can be common in young patients but uncommon after age 5 as the distal attachment of the annular ligament strengthens.

E. Monteggia fractures

1. Principles and presentation
   - Proximal ulna fracture associated with a radial head dislocation
   - Radial head dislocation in children without an obvious fracture can often be secondary to plastic deformation of the ulna.
   - Peak incidence between 4 and 10 years old
2. Diagnosis and radiographs
   - All forearm fractures should be accompanied by elbow radiographs to evaluate for radial head dislocation; all radial head dislocations should be accompanied by forearm radiographs.
3. **Classification—Bado** (see Figure 11-18)
   - Anterior radial head dislocation and apex anterior proximal ulna fracture
   - Posterior radial head dislocation and apex posterior proximal ulna fracture
   - Lateral radial head dislocation and apex lateral proximal ulna fracture
   - Radial head fracture-dislocation and proximal ulna fracture
4. Treatment
   - Nonoperative treatment usually unsuccessful in adults
   - **If ulnar length restored either by closed reduction or intramedullary fixation, radial head reduction can be successfully maintained**
   - Chronic Montaggia fractures may require ulnar osteotomy and annular ligament reconstruction.
5. Complications
   - Neurovascular—posterior interosseous nerve neurapraxia (10%)

VII. FOREARM FRACTURES

A. Diaphyseal ulna and radius fractures

1. Principles and presentation
   - Forearm fractures make up 45% of all pediatric fractures; male predominance.
   - 80% occur after age 5 years.
   - Mechanism is usually a fall on an outstretched hand.
     - Pronation can lead to a flexion injury with dorsal angulation.
     - Supination can lead to an extension injury with volar angulation.
2. Diagnosis and radiographs
   - AP and lateral views of the forearm
   - Radiographic evaluation of the elbow and wrist also important
3. Classification
   - Can be described as incomplete (greenstick fractures) or complete fractures
   - Otherwise can be described by direction of apex angulation and amount of displacement
4. Treatment
   - **Nonoperative treatment with closed reduction and long-arm immobilization is usually successful in children.**
   - **In general, apex dorsal angulation should be accompanied by immobilization in supination.**
   - **In general, apex volar angulation should be accompanied by immobilization in pronation.**
   - Also, location of the fracture and associated deforming forces may dictate the proper arm rotation of immobilization: proximal third fractures in supination, middle third fractures in neutral, and distal third fractures in pronation.
   - Indications for surgery include open fractures, neurovascular compromise, compartment syndrome, more than 15 to 20 degrees of angulation in patients younger than 10 years old, more than 10 degrees of angulation in patients more than 10 years old, bayonet apposition in patients older than 10 years old, and greater than 30 degrees of malrotation.
5. Complications
   - Compartment syndrome
   - Malunion
     - Contributing factors include quality of initial reduction, quality of initial reduction in relation to initial displacement, and delay in diagnosis.
     - Mild loss of supination and/or pronation
     - Refracture
       - 5% to 12%

B. Distal ulna and radius fractures

1. Principles and presentation
   - Very common in pediatric patients
   - Important to evaluate forearm and elbow for associated injuries
2. Diagnosis and radiographs
   - AP and lateral views of the wrist
   - Radiographic evaluation of the forearm and elbow is also often necessary.
3. Classification
   - Generally classified by the Salter-Harris classification of physeal injuries
   - Metaphyseal fractures can be buckle or incomplete fractures or complete fractures.
4. Treatment
   - Generally treated with closed reduction and immobilization
   - **Acceptable sagittal angulation is up to 30 degrees in patients with greater than 5 years of growth**

remaining, with 5 degrees less accepted for each year less than 5 years of growth remaining.
- Acceptable coronal angulation is up to 10 to 15 degrees in patients with greater than 5 years of growth remaining.
- Surgical indications to pin these fractures include failure to maintain adequate closed reduction with casting alone, ipsilateral distal humerus fracture requiring operative intervention, and soft tissue concerns that would not allow for casting.

5. Complications
   - Similar to those of diaphyseal forearm fractures

VIII. LOWER EXTREMITY

A. Pelvis fractures

1. Principles and presentation
   - Less common in pediatric patients but associated (>50%) with multiple injuries and visceral injuries in the polytrauma patient
   - Avulsion fractures can be seen in adolescence, especially in athletes.
   - Ischial avulsions result from the pull of the hamstring or adductors (Figure 11-74).
   - Anterior superior iliac spine avulsions result from the pull of the sartorius.
   - Anterior inferior iliac spine avulsions result from the pull of the rectus femoris.
   - Iliac crest avulsions result from the pull of the abdominal muscles.
   - Lesser trochanter avulsions result from the pull of the iliopsoas.
2. Diagnosis and radiographs
   - AP, Judet views (acetabulum), inlet/outlet views (pelvic ring)
   - CT often necessary because 50% of all pelvic fractures may be missed on a plain AP pelvis view

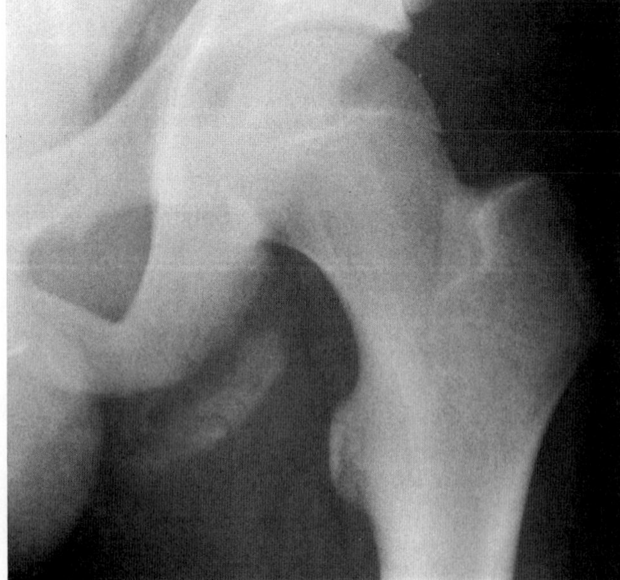

Figure 11-74 Ischial avulsion. (From Adam A, et al: Grainger & Allison's diagnostic radiology, ed 5, Philadelphia, 2008, Churchill Livingstone.)

3. Classification
   - Torode and Zieg
     - Type I—avulsions
     - Type II—iliac wing fractures
     - Type III—simple ring fractures without segmental instability
     - Type IV—ring disruptions with segmental instability
   - Tile
     - Type A—stable
     - Type B—rotationally unstable but vertically stable
     - Type C—rotationally and vertically unstable
4. Treatment
   - Pelvic ring fractures in the polytrauma patient who is hemodynamically unstable may necessitate placement of external fixation.
   - Vertically unstable and intraarticular displacement of acetabular fractures in pediatric patients are surgical indications.
   - **Nonoperative treatment is usually indicated for avulsion fractures with gradual return to athletics.**
   - Operative treatment of avulsion fractures may be necessary if these progress to symptomatic nonunions.
5. Complications
   - Premature closure of the triradiate cartilage
   - Leg-length discrepancies
   - Neurovascular injuries
   - Heterotopic ossification

B. Hip dislocations

1. Principles and presentation
   - More common than hip fractures in pediatric patients
   - New research may suggest an association with femoral acetabular impingement in athletes sustaining these injuries without high-energy trauma.
2. Diagnosis and radiographs
   - AP pelvis and cross-table lateral views
   - CT scans may be necessary post reduction to confirm the adequacy of the reduction and to rule out incarcerated fragments.
3. Classification
   - Generally described based on the direction of dislocation (anterior vs. posterior)
   - Posterior dislocations are 10 times more common than anterior dislocations.
4. Treatment
   - Closed reduction with sedation as soon as possible to reduce the risk of avascular necrosis
   - **Open reduction is indicated for failed closed reduction, nonconcentric reduction, or dislocation with associated femoral head, neck, or acetabular fracture.**
5. Complications
   - Avascular necrosis—8% to 10%
     - Decreased incidence in patients younger than age 5 years
     - Increased incidence a delay in reduction

C. Femoral neck fractures

1. Principles and presentation
   - Rare in pediatric patients
   - Usually the result of severe, high-energy trauma (75%-80%)
2. Diagnosis and radiographs
   - AP pelvis and cross-table lateral views

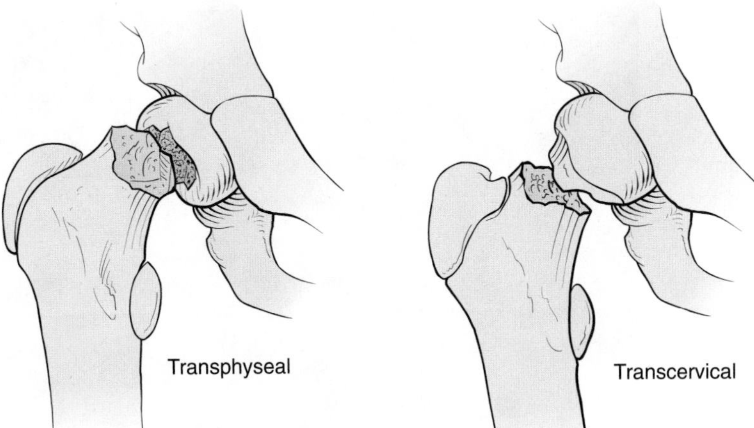

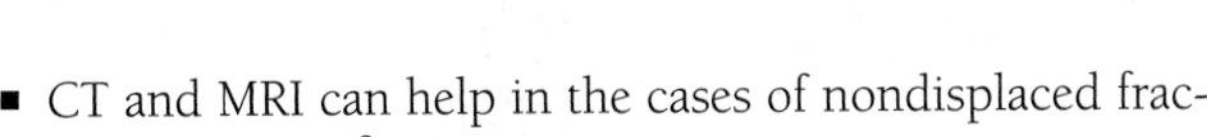

Figure 11-75 Delbet classification of children's hip fractures. (From Herring J: *Tachdjian's pediatric orthopaedics,* ed 4, Philadelphia, 2007, Elsevier.)

- CT and MRI can help in the cases of nondisplaced fractures or stress fractures.

3. Classification—Delbet (Figure 11-75)
   - Type I—transphyseal fractures
     - Very high risk of AVN (approaches 100%)
   - Type II—transcervical fractures
     - Moderate risk of AVN (50%)
   - Type III—basicervical or cervicothoracic fractures
     - **Low risk of AVN (20%-30%)**
   - Type IV—intertrochanteric fractures
     - Very low risk of AVN (10%-15%)
4. Treatment
   - **Types I to III represent a surgical emergency and should be treated with open reduction and internal fixation; smooth pins should be used for younger patients and threaded pins in adolescent patients.**
   - Postoperative spica casting may be necessary in some cases especially younger children and more severe injuries
5. Complications
   - AVN
   - Coxa vara
   - Nonunion
   - Physeal arrest

D. Diaphyseal femur fractures

1. Principles and presentation
   - Bimodal age distribution in pediatric patients with peaks between 2-4 years of age and later in adolescence
   - Consider child abuse in pediatric patients not yet walking.
2. Diagnosis and radiographs
   - AP and lateral views of the femur
   - Ipsilateral knee and hip views should be obtained to rule out associated injuries.
3. Treatment
   - **Based on fracture pattern and age of the patient**
   - Infants younger than 6 months old can be treated in Pavlik harness.
   - Patients younger than 5 to 6 years old can be treated with early spica casting or traction with delayed spica casting especially if minimal (<2 cm) shortening.
   - Patients between 5 and 11 years old can be treated with several approaches:
     - **Flexible intramedullary nailing is appropriate for more stable simple fracture patterns without significant shortening and is associated with poorer results in children older than 11 years old and in heavier obese children.**
     - Submuscular plate fixation is appropriate for more unstable fracture patterns especially with shortening and comminution.

- External fixation is appropriate for the poly trauma patient, open fractures, or those with soft tissue management concerns and is usually placed laterally to avoid the quadriceps.
- Patients over the age of 11 years old and those approaching skeletal maturity can be usually treated with antegrade intramedullary nailing.
  - **Trochanteric or lateral entry nailing required**
  - **Must avoid piriformis entry nailing because this risks the vascularity to the femoral head**
- External fixation is always an option in emergency setting in which the patient may be hemodynamically unstable, multiply injured, or has open fractures.

4. Complications
   - Malunion—rotational deformities do not remodel and need to be controlled at the time of reduction and fixation. Greater sagittal angulation is acceptable secondary to better remodeling capability than varus/valgus angulation.
   - Leg-length discrepancy
     - Overgrowth
       - Overgrowth of 0.7 to 2.0 cm is common in younger children (<10 years old). It is most common during the 2 years after injury.
     - Shortening
       - Up to 2.0 cm of shortening is acceptable in young children with the potential for overgrowth. Thus, older children and those with more than 2.0 cm of shortening need to have either traction applied to restore length or appropriate open reduction and internal fixation to address shortening.

E. Distal femur fractures

1. Principles and presentation
   - Most distal femoral physeal fractures occur in adolescence (two thirds).
   - Often the result of direct trauma with some degree of rotation or angulation
     - Physis often fails on the tension side while the metaphysis often fails on the compression side resulting in the Thurston-Holland fragment (in SH type II physeal fractures) (Figure 11-76)
   - Must be considered in adolescent patients possibly misdiagnosed with collateral ligament injuries
2. Diagnosis and radiographs (Figure 11-77)
   - AP, lateral, oblique views of the knee
   - **Stress views may help delineate subtle physeal injuries.**
   - CT may be necessary to evaluate for intraarticular extension
   - Angiograph is occasionally necessary to evaluate for a vascular injury especially those physeal fractures with wide displacement and posterior spiked fragments with a clinical presentation that warrants evaluation.
3. Classification (see Figure 11-66)
   - Salter-Harris physeal fracture classification is often used to describe these injuries.
4. Treatment
   - Nonoperative treatment with cast immobilization appropriate for nondisplaced fractures
   - Operative treatment indicated for open fractures, intraarticular fractures, or displacement through the physis

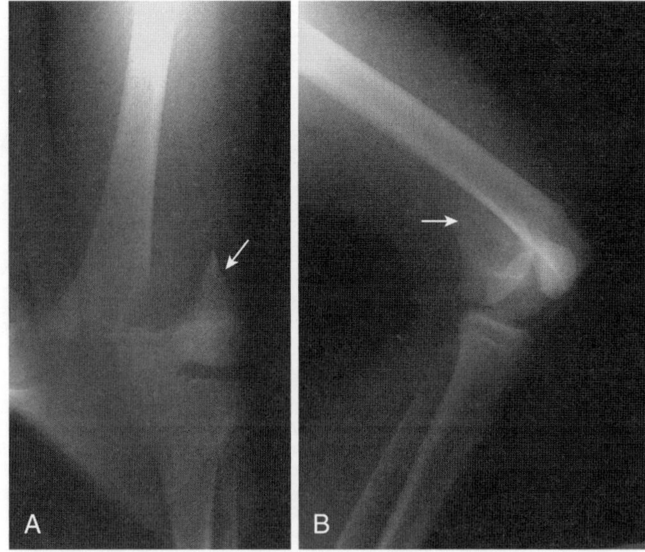

Figure 11-76 Anteroposterior **(A)** and lateral **(B)** images of a typical Salter-Harris type II fracture of the distal femur in a 15-year-old boy who sustained a valgus force to the knee while playing football. Note the significant displacement in the lateral Thurston-Holland fragment *(arrow)*. (From Herring J: *Tachdjian's pediatric orthopaedics,* ed 4, Philadelphia, 2007, Elsevier.)

   - **Smooth wires can be placed across the physis temporarily to hold the physeal reduction.**
   - Fixation across the Thurston-Holland fragment to the rest of the metaphysis may help the reduction but generally cannot hold the reduction of the physis alone.
5. Complications
   - **Growth arrest—very common (30%-50%); patients and families should be counseled about this at the time of initial evaluation; can also result in limb-length discrepancies and angular deformities**

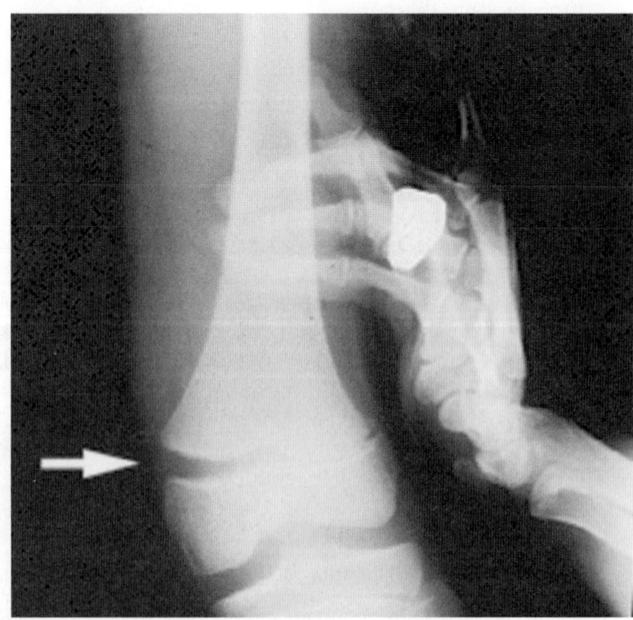

Figure 11-77 Stress radiograph of a physeal injury of the distal femur. An anteroposterior radiograph with valgus stress applied reveals unstable physeal disruption. (From Townsend C, et al: *Sabiston textbook of surgery,* ed 18, Philadelphia, 2007, Elsevier.)

depending on the amount of physis arrested and age of the patient

- Vascular injury (<2%)—especially with hyperextension injuries that have a posterior spike
- Peroneal nerve palsy (3%)—especially with varus injuries
- Knee instability (possibly up to 40%)—some degree of stretch of the cruciate ligaments is thought to occur during these injuries. Whether this stretch and instability causes functional deficits is unclear.

F. **Patella**

1. Principles and presentation
   - Presents similar to adult patellar fractures
   - Be aware of bipartite patella (5%)
   - **Can be missed secondary to difficult to visualize radiographically cartilaginous avulsion injury—"patellar sleeve" fracture**
     - Must look for patella alta and defect (Figure 11-78)
2. Diagnosis and radiographs
   - AP, lateral, and sunrise views
3. Treatment
   - Similar to adult patellar fractures
   - **Indications for surgery include extensor lag, inability to do a straight-leg raise, and intraarticular displacement.**
   - **Tension band constructs are often used if bone stock is sufficient.**
   - Soft tissue repair techniques with careful attention to repair of the retinacular structures if repair of the cartilaginous sleeve fracture is needed
4. Complications
   - Loss of range of motion—Fixation technique should allow for early motion.

G. **Proximal tibia**

1. Tibial spine fractures
   - Principles and presentation
     - **Similar to anterior cruciate ligament ruptures in terms of mechanism of injury; often while landing with a rotational component; hyperextension and valgus forces predominant**
     - Present with a hemarthosis
     - Often have an unstable Lachmans or pivot shift test
   - Diagnosis and radiographs
     - AP and lateral views
     - An AP view taken perpendicular to the tibial plateau accounting for the 5 to 10 degrees of posterior tibial slope can help visualize the often small osseous fragment.
   - Classification—Meyers and McKeever (Figure 11-79)
     - Type I—nondisplaced spine fragment
     - Type II—anterior angulation and displacement of the spine fragment hinging on the posterior cortex
     - Type III—completely displaced fragment
   - Treatment
     - **Type I and type II fractures that reduce with extension can be treated nonoperatively with initial immobilization in extension; range of motion can be progressed once bony union achieved usually at 4 to 6 weeks**
     - Type III are treated with operative fixation (both open and arthroscopic techniques can be utilized)
       - Often anterior horn of either meniscus can be found trapped in the fracture site.
         - Lateral meniscus was thought to be found most commonly trapped but Kocher et al found the medial meniscus to be trapped more commonly.
       - Fixation can be achieved with screw fixation if the fragment is big enough; otherwise, suture fixation is suggested
   - Complications
     - Knee stiffness and loss of extension—very common; loss of extension found in up to 60%
     - **Late anterior instability—up to 60%; possibly secondary to ligamentous stretch; unclear whether clinically significant**
     - Malunion can lead to impingement (similar to a Cyclops lesion after anterior cruciate ligament reconstruction)
2. Tibial tuberosity fractures
   - Principles and presentation
     - Most common between ages 14 to 16 years; often occurs in athletes
     - Tibial tubercle and tibial plateau physis closes from posterior to anterior.

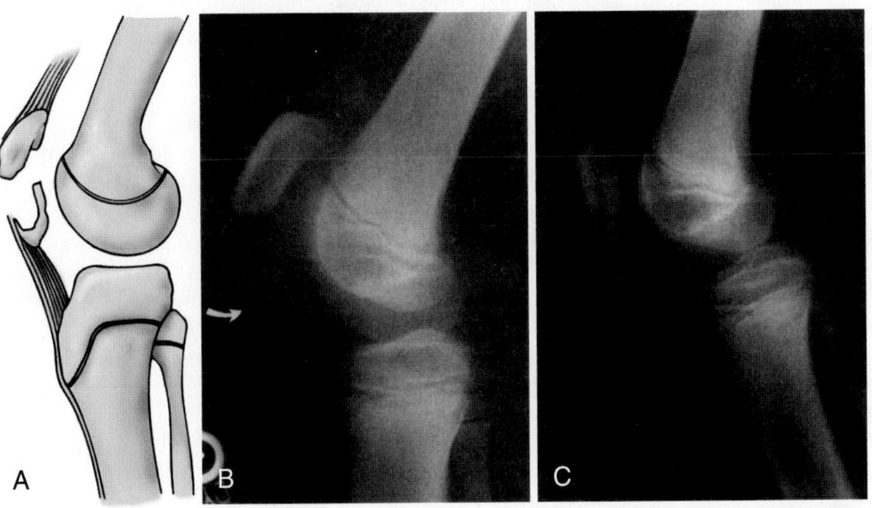

Figure 11-78 **A,** Sleeve fracture of the patella. **B,** The cartilage on the distal fragment is not seen in this projection, but the fracture fragment is evident. (From Scott WM, editor: *Insall & Scott surgery of the knee,* ed 4, Philadelphia, 2005, Elsevier.)

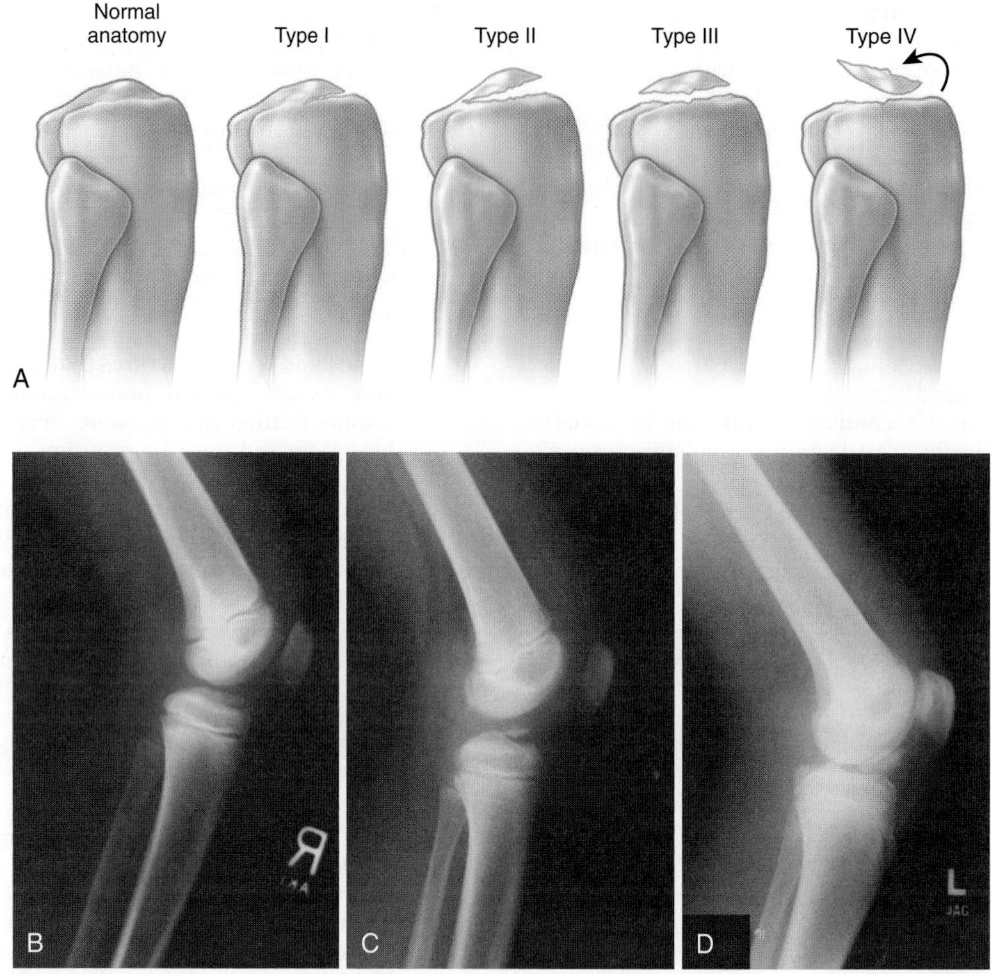

Figure 11-79 A, Meyers and McKeever classification of tibial spine injuries in children. **B,** Lateral radiograph demonstrating a nondisplaced type I tibial spine injury. **C,** Lateral radiograph demonstrating a type II tibial spine injury. **D,** Lateral radiograph demonstrating a type III tibial spine injury. (From Herring J: *Tachdjian's pediatric orthopaedics*, ed 4, Philadelphia, 2007, Elsevier.)

- Predisposing factors include patella baja, tight hamstrings, and history of Osgood-Schlatter disease.
- Diagnosis and radiographs
  - AP and lateral views
  - Patellar alta often observed on the lateral view
- Classification—Ogden modification of Watson-Jones (Figure 11-80)
  - Type I—small fragment displaced proximally
  - Type II—secondary ossification completely displaced proximally
  - Type III—fracture extends intraarticularly
  - A+B versions of each type denote increasing comminution and displacement.
- Treatment
  - Nondisplaced fractures can be treated with long-leg immobilization in a manner similar to tibial spine fractures.
  - Displaced fractures should be treated with open reduction and internal fixation.
    - Screws can be used in most of these patients because they are approaching skeletal maturity.
    - Intraarticular reduction must be confirmed for type III fractures (arthroscopically or through an arthrotomy).
- Complications
  - **Compartment syndrome—The anterior tibial recurrent artery can be tethered and torn as it enters the anterior compartment from the trifurcation posteriorly; increased risk of swelling.**
  - Growth arrest—most patients are approaching skeletal maturity; however, young patients may suffer from a recurvatum deformity if a growth arrest occurs.

3. Proximal tibial physeal fractures
   - Principles and presentation
     - More uncommon but often unstable
     - Vascular injury is most serious sequelae given the popliteal artery is tethered behind the knee.
   - Diagnosis and radiographs
     - AP and lateral views of the knee
     - Like the distal femur, stress views may help delineate a subtle injury but care must be taken to not stretch the neurovascular structures.
     - CT can help delineate an intraarticular extension or displacement.
   - Classification
     - Salter-Harris classification of physeal fractures often used
   - Treatment

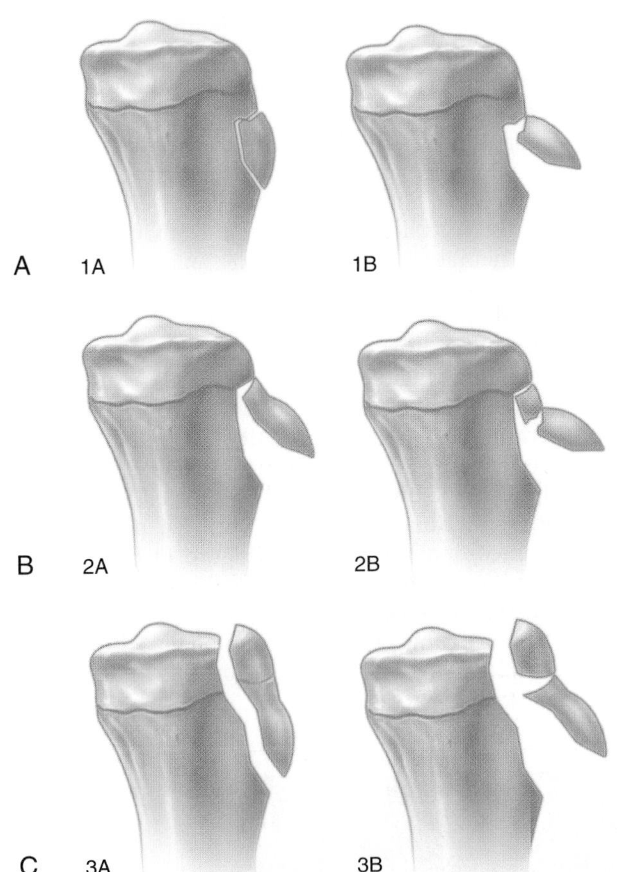

Figure 11-80 Ogden modification of the Watson-Jones classification of tibial tubercle fractures. **A,** Ogden classification. **B,** Lateral radiograph of a type II tibial tubercle fracture. **C,** Lateral radiograph of a type III tibial tubercle fracture. (From Herring J: *Tachdjian's pediatric orthopaedics*, ed 4, Philadelphia, 2007, Elsevier.)

- Nondisplaced fractures can be treated with immobilization but need to be followed closely because these injuries can be unstable.
- Displaced fractures can be treated with reduction, and smooth pin fixation that crosses the physis can be used when necessary.
- Intraarticular fractures (SH types III and IV) should be visualized by arthroscopy or arthrotomy to confirm reduction.

- Complications
  - Neurovascular injury—Popliteal injury is possible during the initial trauma; peroneal nerve is susceptible to stretch injuries from varus displacement.
  - Growth arrest—can result in leg-length discrepancies; partial arrests or bars can be associated with angular deformities.

4. Proximal tibia metaphyseal fractures
   - Principles and presentation
     - Common in 3- to 6-year-old children
     - **Heal rapidly but often present with late genu valgum (Cozen phenomenon) (Figure 11-81)**
       - **Unknown cause but resolve spontaneously over time.**
   - Diagnosis and radiographs
     - Standard AP, lateral views of the knee ± tibia
   - Treatment
     - Closed reduction and long-leg cast immobilization
   - Complications
     - Cozen phenomenon; resolves spontaneously

H. **Tibial shaft**

1. Principles and presentation
   - Common; accounts for 15% of all pediatric fractures
   - Average age: 8 years old
   - 30% associated with a fibular fracture
   - Most commonly secondary to pedestrian versus motor vehicle accidents (50%)
   - **"Toddler's fracture" is a nondisplaced oblique or spiral tibial shaft fracture with intact fibula.**
     - Typically occurs in child younger than 6 years old who sustained a twisting injury
     - **Occasionally mistaken for infection, because radiographs are often normal**
2. Diagnosis and radiographs
   - AP and lateral views of the tibia and fibula
   - Radiographic evaluation of the ipsilateral ankle and knee usually required
3. Treatment

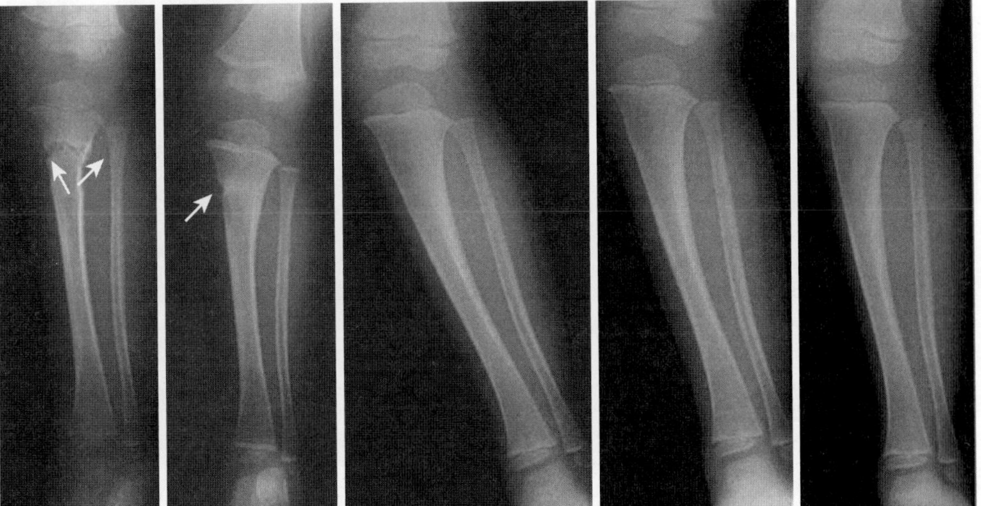

Figure 11-81 Posttraumatic tibial valgus with subsequent resolution. (Reprinted with permission from Macnicol MF: Paedatric knee problems, *Orthopaedics Trauma* 24[5]:369-380, 2010.)

- **Closed reduction and casting can be used for nondisplaced fractures and adequately reduced fractures.**
  - **Toddler's fractures should be placed into a long-leg cast for 2 weeks, and repeat radiographs obtained to demonstrate presence of callus, thus confirming diagnosis.**
- Indications for surgery include open fractures, neurovascular compromise, more than 5 degrees valgus angulation, more than 5 degrees posterior angulation, and more than 5 to 10 degrees varus or anterior angulation.
- Operative fixation techniques include percutaneous pinning (younger patients), screw and plate fixation, external fixation (especially in open fractures), and intramedullary nail fixation (especially in older patients).

4. Complications
   - Compartment syndrome
   - Leg-length discrepancy
   - Angular deformity
   - Unrecognized physeal injury proximally or distally

I. Distal tibia/ankle fractures

1. Principles and presentation
   - 25% to 38% of all physeal injuries
   - Second most common physeal injury (distal radius is most common)
   - Physeal injuries in the distal tibia and fibula are typically seen between ages 8 and 15 years.
   - Mechanism of injury is similar to that for adult ankle fractures; occasional direct trauma, usually rotation around a fixed foot and ankle
   - The distal tibial physis closes in a predictable pattern from central to medial, and the anterolateral portion closes last; this gives rise to unique "transitional" type physeal fractures.
   - **Tillaux fractures are SH type III fractures of the distal tibia (Figure 11-82).**
     - **External rotation force fractures off the anterolateral portion of the distal tibia.**
     - Usually in patients between 12 and 14 years old
   - **Triplane fracture are usually SH type IV fracture of the distal tibia that occurs in three planes: transverse, coronal, and sagittal (Figure 11-83).**
     - **Similar mechanism of external rotation through a partial closed physis**
     - **Intraarticular fracture component through the epiphysis is generally seen on the AP or mortise views.**

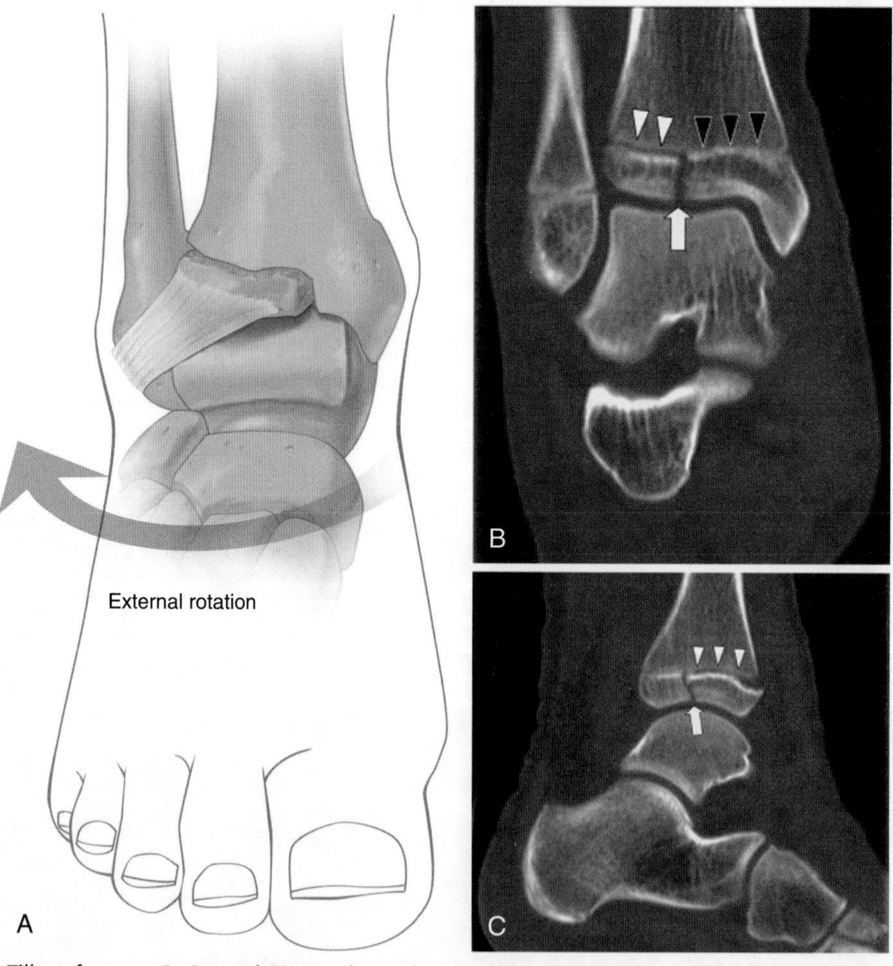

Figure 11-82 **A,** Tillaux fracture. **B,** Coronal CT scan shows the Salter-Harris type III fracture with a longitudinal component through the epiphysis *(arrow)* and a transverse component through the unfused lateral physis *(white arrowheads)*. The fused medial physis is indicated by the *black arrowheads*. **C,** Sagittal CT scan shows the Salter-Harris type III fracture with a longitudinal component through the epiphysis *(arrow)* and a transverse component through the unfused physis *(arrowheads)*.

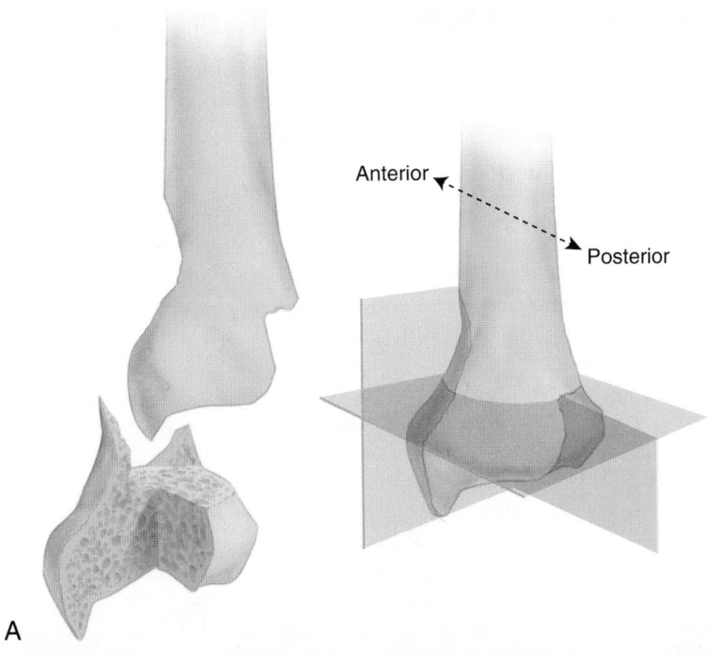

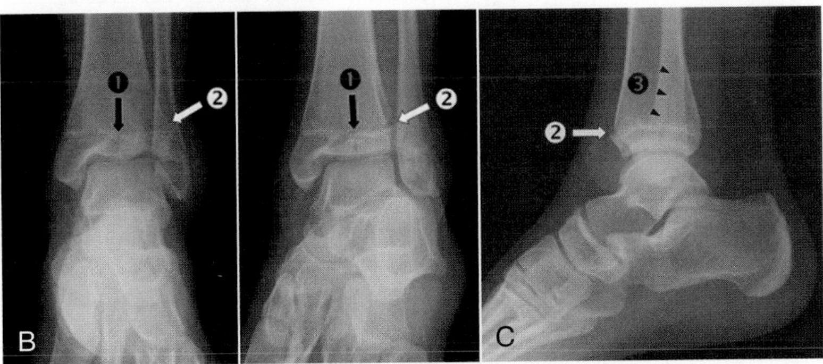

Figure 11-83 Triplane fractures are usually Salter-Harris type IV fractures. Non–weight-bearing anteroposterior **(A)** and mortise **(B)** radiographs. When minimally displaced, the fracture margins can be difficult to see on radiographs. The *black arrow* points to the epiphysis fracture, running vertically in the sagittal plane (plane 1). The *white arrow* points to the physis fracture, running horizontally in the axial plane (plane 2). **C,** Lateral non–weight-bearing radiograph. The *arrow* points to the physis fracture, running horizontally in the axial plane. The *arrowheads* point to the metaphysis fracture, running obliquely vertically in the coronal plane (plane 3).

  - **Thurston-Holland metaphyseal fragment is generally posterolateral and best seen on the lateral view.**
2. Diagnosis and radiographs
   - AP, mortise, and lateral views of the ankle
   - Proximal tibial views occasionally needed to rule out a Maisonneuve-type high fibular fracture
   - CT scan may be needed to examine the displacement of intraarticular extension of triplane or Tillaux type fractures.
3. Classification
   - Salter-Harris physeal fracture classification is generally used to describe these injuries.
   - Triplane can be described by the number of fracture fragments (two, three, or four parts) and their location.
4. Treatment
   - Nondisplaced fractures of the distal tibial and fibular physes can often be treated with immobilization and no weight bearing.
   - **Less than 2 mm of intraarticular displacement is generally considered the appropriate amount that can be tolerated; more displacement should be treated with open reduction and internal fixation or closed reduction and percutaneous pin or screw fixation.**
5. Complications
   - Growth arrest
     - Partial arrests can result in angular deformity; distal fibular arrests will result in a valgus deformity; medial tibial physeal arrests are associated with varus deformities.
     - Complete arrests can result in leg-length discrepancies; contralateral epiphysiodesis can address these issues if prompt diagnosis and remaining skeletal growth allows.
   - Post-traumatic arthrosis
     - Unrecognized intraarticular displacement or inadequate reduction can result in premature arthritic changes.

Acknowledgment

We would like to express our gratitude to David A. Volgas, William M. Ricci, Daniel J. Sucato, Todd A. Milbrandt, and Matthew R. Craig for their contributions to this chapter in the fifth edition.

TESTABLE CONCEPTS

SECTION 1 CARE OF THE MULTIPLY INJURED PATIENT

I. Principles of Trauma Care

- Failure to respond to a 2-L crystalloid bolus in a trauma patient should be considered to have an estimated blood loss greater than 30% of blood volume and require early blood product transfusion.
- Massive transfusion should be a 1 : 1 : 1 ratio of packed red blood cells, fresh frozen plasma, and platelets.
- The end points of adequate resuscitation are not clear. Hemodynamic parameter use is inadequate. Base deficit, as measured by lactate level, is a proxy for amount of anaerobic metabolism by the body.
  - Lactate levels are used to guide the adequacy of resuscitation.
- Hemorrhagic shock presents as increased heart rate and systemic vascular resistance. Central venous pressure and pulmonary capillary wedge pressure are low.
- Neurogenic shock presents as a low heart rate, low blood pressure, and failure to respond to crystalloids. Treatment is with dobutamine and dopamine.
- Damage-control orthopaedics should be employed in severely injured patients with elevated lactate levels. Acute stabilization is achieved primarily via external fixation.
- Pregnant patients should be placed into the left lateral decubitus position to alleviate potential vena cava compression by the uterus.

II. Care of Injuries to Specific Tissues

- Compartment syndrome is a clinical diagnosis with pain out of proportion to the injury and pain with passive stretch.
  - Intracompartmental pressure measurement is abnormal if pressure is within 30 mm of the diastolic pressure (ΔP) or greater than 30 mm of the absolute pressure (the criteria are debated).
  - Anesthesia may lower the diastolic blood pressure and give abnormally low ΔP values.
- Motor recovery potential after repair is poorest for the peroneal nerve. The best results are seen in the radial, musculocutaneous, and femoral nerves.
- Traumatic arthrotomies may be detected via a saline load test or reverse arthrocentesis. The knee may require more than 150 mL for correct diagnosis. However, small puncture wounds may be missed.
- Open segmental fractures and farm injuries are automatically Gustilo type III.
  - Types I and II → first-generation cephalosporin
  - Type III → cephalosporin and aminoglycoside
  - Farm → cephalosporin, aminoglycoside, and penicillin

III. Biomechanics of Fracture Healing

- Stability determines strain. Strain determines the type of healing. Fractures with less than 2% of strain result in primary bone healing, whereas strain between 2% and 10% results in secondary bone healing.
  - Examples of absolute stability include lag screws, compression plating, and rigid locked plating (in nonbridging mode).

IV. Biomechanics of ORIF

- Compression plating screw insertional order is neutral position, then compression on opposite side of fracture, then lag screw (if placing through plate).
  - May need pre-bend to eliminate gapping opposite plate
  - Tight contact of plate to bone when initially applied causes decreased periosteal blood flow and temporary osteopenia.
- Bridge plating spans an area of comminution with fixation above and below the fracture. It allows some elastic deformation.
- Submuscular plating advantages include retained medullary and periosteal bone perfusion.
- Locking plates are most useful in unstable, short segment, metaphyseal fractures, and osteoporotic bone.
  - Other indications: periprosthetic fractures, proximal humerus fractures, intraarticular distal femur and proximal tibia fractures, and humeral shaft nonunions in the elderly
  - Multiaxial locking screws increase options for fixation in working around periprosthetic fractures but do not offer strength or pullout advantages.
  - Locking plates with unicortical locked screws are weaker in torsion compared with bicortical screws.
  - Locked plating screws typically fail simultaneously rather than sequentially.
  - IM nail stiffness depends on material, size, and wall thickness.
  - Increased diameter results in increased stiffness at a ratio of radius to the power of 3 in bending and to the power of 4 in torsion.
  - The working length is the portion of the nail that is unsupported by bone when loaded.
  - Increased working length produces increased interfragmentary motion and may delay union.

SECTION 2 UPPER EXTREMITY

I. Shoulder Injuries

- Sternoclavicular dislocation is most commonly anterior. The majority will remain unstable, but these are typically asymptomatic.
  - The medial clavicular epiphysis is the last to close at a mean age of 25 years. In patients younger than this, sternoclavicular dislocation is often a Salter-Harris type I or II fracture.
- Clavicle fractures are most commonly middle third. Open clavicle fractures are associated with high rates of pulmonary and closed-head injuries
  - Treatment is controversial. Most middle third fractures are treated nonoperatively in a sling. There is no difference between sling and figure-eight bandage in outcomes.
  - Risk of nonunion after midshaft fractures is higher in females, elderly, and those fractures that are displaced, shortened more than 2 cm, or comminuted.

- Operative treatment is recommended for displaced and shortened clavicle fractures, owing to higher rates of nonunion and decreased shoulder strength and endurance.
- Scapula fractures are associated with pulmonary contusion, pneumothorax, clavicle fracture (i.e., floating shoulder), rib fracture, head injury, brachial plexus injury, upper extremity vascular injury, pelvic or acetabular fracture, and spine fracture. These fractures are generally treated nonoperatively.
- Glenoid neck fractures are almost always treated nonoperatively.
  - Operative treatment is indicated when the glenoid neck and humeral head are translocated anterior to the proximal fragment or are medially displaced. Preferred surgical approach is posterior between infraspinatus and teres minor.
- Scapulothoracic dislocation should be suspected when there is a neurologic and/or vascular deficit. Lateral displacement of the scapula more than 1 cm on a chest radiograph is also suggestive. Functional outcome is based on the severity of the associated neurologic injury.
- Proximal humerus fracture treatment can be divided based on the Neer classification. Two-part fractures treated nonoperatively should have immediate physical therapy to facilitate faster recovery.
  - Three- and four-part fractures may be treated with open reduction and internal fixation (ORIF) for young patients and hemiarthroplasty for elderly. During hemiarthroplasty, attention must be paid to humeral height, humeral version, and tuberosity reconstruction. The insertion of pectoralis major is a reliable landmark for determining height.
  - Avascular necrosis can be predicted by Hertel's criteria: disruption of the medial periosteal hinge, medial metadiaphyseal extension less than 8 mm, and increasing fracture complexity.
  - Locking plate constructs are associated with significant rates of screw cutout.
  - Nonunion of the greater tuberosity after arthroplasty results in a loss of active shoulder elevation.
- Shoulder dislocation must be evaluated with an axillary radiograph. The most common associated injury at arthroscopy is an anteroinferior labral tear. There is a high incidence of rotator cuff injury in patients older than age 45 years after a shoulder dislocation.
  - Inferior dislocation commonly presents with the arm abducted between 100 and 160 degrees.

II. Humeral Injuries

- Humeral shaft fractures may be treated nonoperatively if there is less than 20 degrees of anterior angulation, less than 30 degrees of valgus/varus angulation, or less than 3 cm of shortening.
- Indications for fixation include those fractures outside nonoperative parameters, open fracture, floating elbow, polytrauma, pathologic fracture, and associated brachial plexus injury.
  - ORIF (with plate/screws) has higher union rates and decreased secondary operations. Weight bearing to tolerance is safe after plate fixation
  - Intramedullary nails may be used for segmental or pathologic fractures. Complications include a higher rate of reoperation and shoulder pain. Distal locking options vary by nail design. Lateral to medial screws put radial nerve at risk, whereas anterior to posterior screws put musculocutaneous nerve at risk. Mini open incisions are recommended for interlocking screws.
- Radial nerve palsy occurs in 5% to 10% of cases.
  - *When to observe:*
    - The vast majority (up to 92%) resolve with observation for 3 to 4 months.
    - Brachioradialis followed by extensor carpi radialis longus are the first to return, whereas the extensor pollicis longus and extensor indicis proprius are last to return.
  - *When to explore:*
    - Open fracture: there is a higher likelihood of transection; perform ORIF of fracture at time of exploration.
  - *Controversial whether to observe or explore:*
    - Secondary nerve palsy (i.e., after fracture manipulation)
    - Spiral or oblique fracture of distal third (Holstein-Lewis fracture)
- Humeral shaft nonunion should be treated with compression plate and bone grafting if atrophic. Locking plates may be used in elderly patients.
- Distal humerus fractures involving both columns should be treated with ORIF using a posterior approach with two plates applied to either column.
  - Total elbow arthroplasty is a treatment option in severely comminuted fractures in patients older than age 65 years, particularly if they have rheumatoid arthritis.
  - The most frequent complication is stiffness, which is treated with static-progressive splinting.
  - Elbow muscle strength typically decreases 25%.
- Coronal shear fractures should be treated with ORIF via a lateral approach.

III. Elbow Injuries

- Olecranon fractures treated with a tension band construct should have the wire loop dorsal to the mid axis of the ulna, thus transforming tensile forces at the fracture site into compressive forces.
  - Kirschner wires should be buried in the anterior cortex of the ulna for increased stability. Protrusion through the anterior cortex, however, is associated with reduced forearm rotation.
  - Plate fixation is the preferred technique for oblique fractures that extend distal to the coronoid process, because this is more stable than tension band wiring.
  - Excision with triceps advancement is reserved for nonreconstructible proximal olecranon fractures in low-demand patients.
- Radial head fractures that are nondisplaced may be treated in a splint for no more than 7 days, followed by early motion.
  - Comminuted fractures less than three places may be treated with ORIF. Otherwise, treat with metallic radial head replacement.

Continued

- The safe zone for ORIF of a head fracture is a 110-degree arc between the radial styloid and the Lister tubercle.
- The posterior interosseous nerve is at risk, and the arm must be pronated to avoid injury.
- Simple elbow dislocations may be treated with brief immobilization.
- Terrible triad of the elbow is a complex dislocation with lateral collateral ligament injury, radial head fracture, and coronoid fracture. The lateral collateral ligament injury is most commonly a ligamentous avulsion from the origin on the distal humerus. This injury is always unstable and requires treatment.
  - Perform coronoid ORIF, radial head ORIF or replacement, lateral collateral ligament repair (typically to distal humerus), and possible medial collateral ligament repair, depending on stability.

IV. Forearm Fractures

- Monteggia fractures are ulnar fractures with associated radial head dislocation.
  - Treat with ORIF. The radial head will normally reduce and be stable.
  - Nonanatomic reduction of the ulna followed by interposition of the annular ligament are the most common causes for failure of radial head reduction.
  - Posterior radial head dislocation (Bado type II) or radial head fractures (Monteggia equivalent) are associated with higher complications. Posterior interosseous nerve injury is most frequent, typically resolves spontaneously, and should be observed for 3 months.
- Both-bone forearm fractures are almost universally treated with ORIF.
  - Restoration of the radial bow is directly related to functional outcome.
  - Refracture risk is elevated with removal of hardware in less than 12 to 18 months.
  - Synostosis is associated with single incision approach to ORIF and treated with early excision, irradiation, and indomethacin.
- Galeazzi fractures are radius fractures with distal radioulnar joint instability.
  - ORIF of the radius should be performed, followed by intraoperative assessment of the distal radioulnar joint.
  - Irreducible distal radioulnar joint is most commonly due to interposition of the extensor carpi ulnaris tendon. Recommended approach is dorsal to remove the block

SECTION 3 LOWER EXTREMITY AND PELVIS

I. Pelvic and Acetabular Injuries

Pelvic Fractures

- Pelvic ring injuries are commonly classified using the Young-Burgess system.
  - APC I → stretching of anterior sacroiliac ligaments
  - APC II → rupture of the anterior sacroiliac sacrotuberous and sacrospinous ligaments
  - APC III → rupture of sacrotuberous, sacrospinous, and anterior and posterior sacroiliac ligaments
- Emergent treatment of a hemodynamically unstable patient with a pelvic ring injury:
  - Volume resuscitation
  - Pelvic binder
  - Angiographic embolization
  - External fixation—place before emergent laparotomy
  - Skeletal traction—for vertically unstable patterns
  - Pelvic C clamp (rarely used)
- Nonoperative treatment is indicated for stable fracture patterns
  - Weight bearing as tolerated for isolated anterior injuries
- Anterior injuries are generally treated with plate fixation. External fixation with pins in the AIIS region is stronger than iliac wing pins but not stronger than internal fixation. The lateral femoral cutaneous nerve is most at risk "during ex fix pin placement."
- Posterior injuries with a vertically oriented sacral fracture are at higher risk for loss of fixation.
- Vertically unstable patterns with anterior and posterior dislocations can be treated with anterior ring internal fixation and percutaneous sacroiliac screw fixation. This is the most stable fixation construct.
- The risk of severe, life-threatening hemorrhage is highest in anteroposterior compression types II and III and lateral compression type III patterns and vertical shear.
- Urogenital injury is common.
  - Men: urethral stricture
  - Women: dyspareunia and need for cesarean section childbirth
- The most common complication of pelvic ring injury is deep venous thrombosis if thromboprophylaxis is not employed.
- Risk factors for death during initial treatment:
  - Blood transfusion requirement in first 24 hours
  - Unstable fracture type (anteroposterior compression types II and III, lateral compression types II and III, vertical shear, combined mechanism)
- Percutaneous sacroiliac screw insertion requires appropriate fluoroscopic visualization of anatomic landmarks. Use the pelvic outlet radiograph to visualize the S1 neural foramina. The lateral sacral view identifies the sacral alar slope and minimizes risk to the L5 nerve root.

Acetabular Fractures

- The obturator oblique view profiles the anterior column and posterior wall. The iliac oblique view profiles the posterior column and anterior wall.
- The Letournel classification divides acetabular fractures into five simple and five associated types.
- The associated both-column fracture represents a dissociation of the acetabular dome from the intact ilium. A "spur sign" is seen on the obturator oblique view and represents the intact portion of the iliac wing.
- Cardinal radiographic features of fracture types:
  - Posterior wall—iliopectineal and ilioischial lines intact
  - Posterior column or posterior column/posterior wall—ilioischial line disrupted
  - Anterior wall or anterior column—iliopectineal line disrupted

- Transverse or transverse/posterior wall—iliopectineal, ilioischial lines disrupted, obturator ring intact
- Both column or anterior column posterior hemitransverse—"T-type" iliopectineal, ilioischial, iliac wing and obturator foramen disrupted

- General guidelines for surgical approach based on fracture type:
  - Kocher-Langenbeck (posterior): posterior wall, posterior column, transverse, transverse/posterior wall (when posterior wall requires fixation), posterior column/posterior wall, and some T types
  - Ilioinguinal (anterior): anterior wall, anterior column, anterior column posterior hemitransverse, associated both column, and some T types (if limited posterior wall involved)
  - Extensile approaches: fractures more than 3 weeks old, complex associated fractures, and need for posterior column reduction
- Treatment with ORIF and acute total hip arthroplasty relative indications are age older than 60 years with presence of superomedial dome impaction on radiograph ("gull sign"), associated displaced femoral neck fracture, or significant preexisting arthrosis.
- The risk of neurologic injury can be reduced with hip extension and knee flexion.
- Quality of reduction is the most important predictor of post-traumatic osteoarthritis. Malreduction is associated with a greater delay to surgery.

II. Femoral and Hip Injuries

Hip Dislocations

- Hip dislocations require emergent closed reductions in an attempt to ameliorate the risk of osteonecrosis.
  - Posterior wall and anterior femoral head fractures are common associated injuries. There is a 30% rate of labral tear.

Femoral Head Fractures

- Treatment principles include restoration of articular congruity of the weight-bearing portion of the femoral head and to remove associated loose bodies.
- Smith-Petersen approach for ORIF recommended for Pipkin types I and II. Type IV fractures are typically fixed via a posterior approach.

Femoral Neck Fractures

- High-energy femoral neck fractures are typically vertical and associated femoral neck fractures.
- AP radiographs should be obtained with the legs in internal rotation to compensate for femoral anteversion.
- Treatment of femoral neck fractures is controversial and includes cannulated screws, sliding hip screws, hemiarthroplasty, and total hip arthroplasty.
  - Cannulated screw fixation start points should be above the lesser trochanter to decrease risk of peri-implant subtrochanteric fracture.
  - Hemiarthroplasty is associated with a lower risk of dislocation than in total hip arthroplasty, especially in patients unable to comply with dislocation precautions (e.g., dementia, Parkinson disease)
  - In "active" elderly patients, better functional results are seen with total hip arthroplasty.
- Osteonecrosis risk is increased with greater initial displacement and poor reduction.
- Nonunion risk is higher with varus malreduction. Treatment options include conversion to hip arthroplasty (worse results than those associated with primary arthroplasty) and valgus osteotomy.
- Pre-injury cognitive function and mobility predict postoperative functional outcome.

Intertrochanteric Hip Fractures

- The size and location of the lesser trochanteric fragment determine stability.
- A sliding hip screw device is indicated for most fractures.
  - *Exceptions:* reverse obliquity fractures, subtrochanteric fractures, and fractures without an intact lateral femoral wall
  - These fractures are associated with a moderate amount of collapse, resulting limb shortening, and medialization when used for unstable fractures. Collapse is more than that seen with intramedullary implants.
- Long intramedullary nails are indicated for standard and reverse obliquity and subtrochanteric fractures.
  - Risk of distal anterior perforation occurs owing to mismatch of anterior bow between femur and nail.
- Implant failure/cutout is associated with a tip-apex distance greater than 25 mm.
- Peri-implant fracture is more common with nails compared with plates.
- American Surgical Association classification predicts mortality in patients with intertrochanteric hip fractures.

Subtrochanteric Fractures

- Apex anterior and varus angulation are the most common deformities. The psoas and abductors lead to flexion, abduction, and external rotation of the proximal fragment.
- Lateral positioning allows easier alignment of the distal segment to the flexed proximal segment.

Femoral Shaft Fractures

- Piriformis and trochanteric starting points are indicated when they are used with appropriately designed nails.
  - Piriformis entry is contraindicated when fracture extends to piriformis fossa and in children with open physes (osteonecrosis).
  - Anterior starting point in piriformis fossa is associated with increased hoop stress and risk of iatrogenic comminution.
  - Anterior trochanteric starting point is associated with minimal hoop stress.
- Trochanteric starting point risks medial comminution of shaft owing to off-axis starting point and varus if straight (no trochanteric bend) nail used.
- Static interlocking for most fractures
- Reamed nailing for most fractures
  - Higher union rates than unreamed nails
- Multitrauma patients may benefit from delayed nailing with immediate provisional external fixation (damage control principles). Benefits include reduced blood loss,

Continued

reduced hypothermia, and reduced inflammatory mediator release.
  - External fixation can be safely converted to intramedullary nailing in absence of pin tract infection for up to at least 3 weeks with equal union and infection rates.
- Nonunion treatment is more successful with plate/screw/bone graft constructs compared with exchanged nailing. Dynamization is less successful than exchange nailing for treating delayed union.
- Malalignment is difficult to diagnose, but comparison must be made to the contralateral limb before leaving the operating room. Use of a fracture table is associated with increased risk of malalignment.
- Ipsilateral femoral neck and shaft fractures are uncommon (<10%), but when present they are missed in up to 50% of cases.
  - Neck component is typically vertical in orientation. It has the highest priority.
  - Preferred technique is to use parallel screws or sliding hip screw for the neck, followed by retrograde nail or plate fixation for the shaft.

Supracondylar Femur Fractures

- Intracondylar extension warrants CT evaluation for a coronal fracture (Hoffa fracture).
  - 40% incidence, with 80% affecting lateral femoral condyle
- Plate fixation is indicated for most fractures. Non–fixed-angle plates are prone to varus collapse, especially in metaphyseal comminution. Avoid prominent medial screws.

III. Knee Injuries

- Vascular injury is present in 5% to 15% of knee dislocations. Selective arteriography with the use of a physical examination (including ankle brachial index < 0.9) rather than an immediate arteriogram is now the standard of care.
- Patella fractures may be treated nonoperatively or with tension band wiring, cerclage, and tension band wiring and partial patellectomy.
  - Partial patellectomy is useful for extraarticular distal pole fractures. Preserve the patella wherever possible, however.

IV. Tibial Injuries

Tibial Plateau Fractures

- Meniscus tears occur in more than 50% of tibial plateau fractures. Lateral is more common than medial: Schatzker II—lateral; Schatzker IV—medial. Peripheral tears are the most common type.
- Medial fractures are uncommon. Think *knee dislocation* with spontaneous reduction.
- The goal of treatment is restoration of normal alignment. Post-traumatic arthrosis development does *not* correlate with articular step-off.
- Spanning external fixators are used temporarily with selected high-energy injuries to allow for a reduction in soft tissue swelling before definitive fixation.
- Use percutaneous locked plating for poor-quality bone in bicondylar fractures. Avoid stripping.
- Posteromedial fragments may not be captured via a lateral pate. Use a separate posteromedial incision if second plate is needed.
- Use of bone void fillers
  - Calcium phosphate cement has highest compressive strength.
  - There is a lower rate of subsidence compared with autogenous iliac bone graft

Tibial Shaft Fractures

- Indications for nonoperative management:
  - Shortening less than 1 to 2 cm
  - Cortical apposition greater than 50%
  - Varus-valgus less than 5 degrees
  - Flexion-extension less than 10 degrees
  - Shortening is the most difficult deformity to correct. Shortening and cortical apposition seen on injury radiograph are equivalent to shortening at union.
- Operative management in intramedullary nailing is associated with reduced time of immobilization compared with cast management and earlier weight bearing than that achieved with a cast.
- Avoidance of malreduction of proximal third fractures associated with valgus and apex anterior angulation is achieved by the following:
  - Ensuring a laterally based starting point and anterior insertion angle
  - Blocking screws, placed posteriorly and laterally to the central axes of the proximal fragment
- Definitive fixation with external fixation for type III open tibia fractures have significantly longer time to union and poorer functional outcomes compared with intramedullary nailing.
- Plate fixation for extreme proximal and distal shaft fractures is associated with a higher infection risk than that for intramedullary nailing in opening fractures.
  - Use of a 13-hole percutaneous plate, such as a Less Invasive Stabilization System (LISS) plate, places the superficial peroneal nerve at risk for holes 11, 12, and 13. A larger incision with blunt dissection should be used for insertion of screws in this region.
- Nonunion should be treated with reamed-exchange nailing after infection has been ruled out.
- Malunion is most common with proximal third fractures, resulting in valgus and apex anterior angulation.
  - This may increase long-term risk of arthrosis, particularly in the ankle (more common with varus deformity).
  - Rotational malalignment is common with distal one third fractures.
- Risk factors for reoperation to achieve bony union within the first year:
  - Transverse fracture pattern, open fracture, cortical contact less than 50%
- Infection risk increases with severity of soft tissue injury and time to soft tissue coverage. Use of wound vacuum-assisted closure does not alter the risk of infection.
- Anterior knee pain occurs in more than 30% of intramedullary nail cases and resolves with removal of the nail in 50% of cases.

Tibial Plafond (Pilon) Fractures

- Three fragments are typical because of intact ankle ligaments.
  - Medial → deltoid ligament
  - Posterolateral (Volkmann) → anterior talofibular ligament
  - Anterolateral (Chaput) → posterior tibiofibular ligament
- Treatment is generally staged with spanning external fixation followed by delayed ORIF.
- Pilon fractures may continue to demonstrate clinical improvement for up to 2 years
- Nonunion is most common in the metaphysis and more common with hybrid fixation. Post-traumatic arthritis is a common late complication.

V. Ankle and Foot Injuries

Ankle Fractures

- In patients with ankle injuries, both deltoid ligament and syndesmotic instability must be ruled out with stress testing.
- A systematic evaluation of ankle radiographs should be performed: talocrural angle 83 ± 4 degrees; medial tibial clear space less than or equal to 4 mm; tibiofibular overlap greater than 10 mm or 42% of the width of the fibula.
- Lauge-Hansen classification is based on the foot's position (first word) and motion of talus relative to the leg (second word). Simplified version:
  - Supination-adduction—transverse fibula and vertical medial malleolus
  - Supination-external rotation—spiral fibula (SER II) and either transverse medial malleolus (SER IV) or deltoid ligament disruption (SER IV equivalent; perform stress test)
  - Pronation-abduction—transverse medial malleolus and transverse fibula (with lateral wall comminution). stage II injury is syndesmosis failure.
  - Pronation-external rotation—spiral fracture of fibula above level of plafond with either transverse fracture of medial malleolus or rupture of deltoid ligament
- ORIF of the fibula with a posterior lateral plate is more stable than the lateral plate, but there is more peroneal tendon irritation.
- Medial malleolar ORIF should be with a medial buttress plate for vertical fractures and lag screws or a tension band for transverse fractures.
- Syndesmotic instability is common with fibula fractures more than 6 cm above the ankle joint. Intraoperative testing with the Cotton test is vital.

Talus Fractures

- A dual-incision approach is recommended to ensure anatomic reduction, particularly of the medial side.
- Hawkins sign is classic early indicator of vascularity and appears between 6 and 8 weeks. It represents patchy subchondral osteoporosis and relative radiolucency and is a reliable sign of vascular integrity.
- Medial comminution is common and can result in varus malunion.
- The extruded talus should be preserved when the portion is articular and large.
- Subtalar dislocations have a 90% rate of associated tarsal fractures.
  - Irreducible medial dislocations are typically the result of extensor digitorum brevis or the capsule, whereas lateral dislocations are due to interposed posterior tibial tendon.

Calcaneus Fractures

- Operative results are best in young patients, female patients, those without workers' compensation claims, and those with simple fracture types.
- Poor functional outcome in patients older than age 50, obese patients, manual laborers, and those receiving workers' compensation. Open fractures have poorer results compared with closed fractures.
- During ORIF, care must be taken when drilling through the medial cortex due to the flexor hallucis longus tendon and medial neurovascular bundle.
- Wound complications occur in 20% of patients and are increased in diabetics and smokers.

Lisfranc Injury

- The Lisfranc ligament is from the base of the second metatarsal to medial cuneiform.
- Plain radiographs
  - Anteroposterior—medial bases of first and second metatarsals aligned with respective cuneiforms
  - Oblique—medial base of forth metatarsal aligned with medial edge of cuboid
  - Standing views are mandatory if subacute or if diagnosis is in question.
- Operative treatment is recommended for any displaced Lisfranc injury.

SECTION 4 SPINE

I. Upper Cervical Spine Injuries

- ASIA classification of spinal cord injury is based on motor strength and complete versus incomplete sensory deficit. An ASIA C grade represents less than 3/5 motor score and incomplete sensory deficit.
- C1 burst fractures (Jefferson) may be stable or unstable, depending on the integrity of the transverse ligament. Combined lateral mass displacement greater than 7 mm indicates transverse ligament disruption. Posterior spinal fusion is recommended.
- Odontoid fracture treatment is based on the risk of developing nonunion.
  - Type I—rigid cervical orthosis
  - Generally, type II fractures are considered operative, particularly in those older than 50. For a posterior C1-C2 fusion an anterior screw may be used unless body habitus or anterior oblique fracture orientation prevents it.
  - Risk factors for type II nonunion: displacement greater than 5 mm; angulation greater than 10°; posterior displacement; age > 40 years; delayed treatment
  - Nondisplaced type II—rigid cervical orthosis versus halo
  - Type III—halo vest

Continued

- Hangman fracture acceptable reduction: less than 4 mm translation and less than 10-degrees angulation
- Halo vest orthosis is effective in controlling most spinal motions except axial distraction.
  - The safe zone for anterior pins is the middle to lateral third above the eyebrow to avoid the supraorbital nerve.
  - Adults require 4 pins at 6 to 8 inch-lb pressure. Children need 8 to 10 pins with 2 inch-lb pressure.

II. Lower Cervical Spine Injuries

- Bilateral facet joint dislocations demonstrate greater than 50% translation and are often associated with spinal cord injury.
- The role of MRI in reducing facet dislocations is controversial.
  - Most authors recommend obtaining an MRI before closed reduction in an obtunded patient. Closed reduction before MRI must be done in an awake, alert, and cooperative patient.

III. Thoracolumbar and Lumbar Spine Injuries

- Flexion-distraction injuries involve failure of the posterior and middle columns in tension.
  - These injuries are routinely treated with surgical stabilization via posterior approach. Occasionally they require additional anterior decompression and stabilization.
- Burst fractures may be treated in an orthosis if kyphosis is less than 30 degrees, there is no neurologic deficit, canal compromise is less than 50%, and there is less than a 50% loss of anterior body height; otherwise, they are operative.

SECTION 5 PEDIATRIC TRAUMA

I. Introduction

- Suspected child abuse must be reported. Suspicion should be raised in children younger than 3 years old who have inconsistent or developmentally incorrect histories.
- Skin injuries are most common, followed by fractures and head injuries.
  - Skeletal surveys are most helpful in children younger than age 5. If older than age 5, consider bone scan as alternative or adjunct.
  - The most common locations of fractures, in order of frequency, are the humerus, tibia, and femur.
  - Spiral femur fractures in nonambulatory children, as well as distal humeral physeal separations, are highly suggestive of abuse.
  - Corner fractures at the junction of the metaphysis and physis are said to be pathognomonic for abuse. They are four times less common than diaphyseal fractures, however.
- Salter-Harris type I fractures involve the zone of hypertrophy in the physis.
- Polytrauma outcomes are most closely linked with the severity of traumatic brain injury.

Upper Extremity Fractures

- Clavicle fractures represent 90% of obstetric fractures, frequently associated with brachial plexus palsies and almost universally treated nonoperatively.
- Proximal humerus fractures have increased remodeling potential, because 80% to 90% of humeral growth occurs at the proximal physis.
  - In children younger than age 12 years, 70-degree angulation and 100% displacement may be accepted.
  - The distal fragment is shortened and adducted by the deltoid and pectoralis major. Gravity can be a useful reduction aid.
- All pediatric elbow fractures should have a systematic evaluation of radiographic anatomy (see Figure 11-69).
- Distal humeral physeal separations occur in the young child and raise suspicion of child abuse. This injury is often confused with an elbow dislocation.
  - Radiographs demonstrate an intact relationship between the radius and capitellum with loss of relationship between the radius/ulna and distal humerus.
  - Treatment is with closed reduction and percutaneous pinning (CRPP).
- Supracondylar humerus fractures are 98% extension type and 2% flexion type.
  - Most common nerve injury:
    - Extension-type—anterior interosseous nerve
    - Flexion-type—ulnar nerve
  - Gartland classification guides treatment
    - I—nondisplaced—long-arm cast
    - II—displaced with intact posterior cortex—long-arm cast if no swelling, anterior humeral line intersects capitellum and no medial distal humeral cortical impaction; otherwise, CRPP
    - III—displaced—CRPP; crossed pins more stable biomechanically
  - Vascular abnormalities should be first treated with reduction, not angiography.
  - Complications of treatment include iatrogenic ulnar nerve injury and cubitus varus from malunion/malreduction.
- Lateral condyle fractures are historically classified using the Milch system, with a type I representing a Salter-Harris type IV fracture and a type II representing a Salter-Harris type II fracture. The Jakob classification, however, is more clinically useful.
  - Amount of displacement guides treatment
    - Less than 2 mm—Cast and closely observe.
    - 2 to 4 mm—CRPP
    - More than 4 mm—CRPP if arthrogram shows perfect reduction; otherwise, ORIF to ensure articular reduction
  - During ORIF, the blood supply arises posteriorly and should be protected.
  - This is one of the rare pediatric fractures that may proceed to nonunion
- Medial epicondyle fractures that occur in adolescents represent an apophyseal avulsion injury of the flexor mass and medial collateral ligament.

    - A 50% association occurs with elbow dislocation, which can result in an incarcerated fragment in 15% of cases.
        - Close attention must be given to identifying the apophysis on the AP view. If it is missing, look for an incarcerated fragment on a lateral or oblique view.
    - Most injuries are treated nonoperatively, but this is controversial.
    - Treatment of an incarcerated fragment is ORIF.
    - Never excise a medial epicondyle fracture.
- Radial neck fractures can be managed nonoperatively according to the "rule of 3s."
    - Less than 30-degree angulation, less than 3-mm translation, and less than one third of radial head involvement
    - There are multiple techniques for closed reduction.
- Radial head subluxation (nursemaid's elbow) occurs when the annular ligament subluxates over the radial head. Closed reduction is achieved by supination and flexion with a thumb placed over the radial head.
- Monteggia fractures can be classified as in adults. Plastic deformations and incomplete injuries may be treated with closed reduction and casting.
    - The key feature in treatment is based on ulnar length restoration. This will generally result in radial head reduction.
    - Diaphyseal "both bone" forearm fractures are generally treated nonoperatively with closed reduction and long-arm casting.
        - Apex dorsal angulation—supination
        - Apex volar angulation—pronation
- Distal radius fractures can be treated nonoperatively in the majority of cases.
    - Acceptable sagittal angulation is up to 30 degrees in patients with greater than 5 years of growth remaining, with 5 degrees less accepted for each year less than 5 years of growth remaining.

VII. Lower Extremity

- Avulsion fractures of the pelvis are relatively common in the pediatric population and generally treated nonoperatively.
- Femoral neck fractures resulting in avascular necrosis can be predicted using the Delbet classification, with type I transphyseal fractures approaching 100% risk.
    - Transphyseal, transcervical, and basicervical fractures represent a surgical emergency.
- Diaphyseal femur fracture management is based on fracture pattern and age of the patient.
    - Birth to 6 months—Pavlik
    - 6 months to 6 years—spica casting
    - 6 to 11 years—flexible nails for stable fractures and submuscular plating for unstable and external fixation for polytrauma
    - Older than 11 years—trochanteric-starting intramedullary nail
- Distal femur physeal fractures should be suspected in adolescent patients with "knee sprains" and can be diagnosed with stress views.
    - Nonoperative treatment is reserved for nondisplaced fractures.
    - Displaced fractures are treated with CRPP and casting versus ORIF.
    - Growth arrest occurs in approximately 50% of cases, resulting in either limb-length discrepancy (1 cm/yr) or angular deformity.
    - Up to 40% of patients sustain injury to the cruciate ligaments.
- Patellar sleeve fractures should be suspected when radiographs demonstrate patella alta. Indications for surgery include extensor lag, inability to straight-leg raise, and intraarticular displacement. A tension band construct can be used if bone-stock permits it.
- Tibial spine fractures are similar to anterior cruciate ligament ruptures in terms of mechanism.
    - Meyers and McKeever classification guides treatment:
        - I—nondisplaced—casting
        - II—anterior hinge—reduction in extension and casting
        - III—displaced—operative fixation
    - Both stiffness (arthrofibrosis) and late anterior instability are common complications occurring in up to 60% of cases. It is unclear whether late anterior instability is clinically significant.
- Tibial tuberosity fractures can be treated nonoperatively for nondisplaced fractures. The anterior tibial recurrent artery may be injured and increases the risk for compartment syndrome.
- Proximal tibial metaphyseal fractures may be termed *Cozen fractures* based on the phenomenon he described. These minimally displaced fractures present as late genu valgum that spontaneously resolves.
- Toddler's fracture is a nondisplaced oblique or spiral tibial shaft fracture with intact fibula. It may not be apparent on radiographs and can be confused with tibial osteomyelitis. Treatment is with a long-leg cast and repeat radiographs in 2 weeks looking for evidence of callus to confirm the diagnosis.
- Tillaux fractures are a Salter-Harris type III fracture due to external rotational force.
- Triplane fractures are a Salter-Harris type IV fracture due to external rotational force through a partially closed physis. It appears as a Salter-Harris type III on AP radiographs and type II on lateral radiographs. CT may be particularly helpful.
    - Less than 2 mm displacement may be treated nonoperatively.

SELECTED BIBLIOGRAPHY

The selected bibliography for this chapter can be found on www.expertconsult.com.

Chapter 12

PRINCIPLES OF PRACTICE

Marc M. DeHart

CONTENTS

SECTION 1 PRINCIPLES OF PRACTICE

I. INTRODUCTION

A. Orthopaedic practice involves managing relationships among the following:
1. Medical ethics of patient care
2. Business realities of medical practice
3. Legal environment that involves complex and changing laws

B. Conflicts of interest among ethical medical care, business goals, and legal considerations can arise. Wherever a conflict of interest arises, it must be resolved in the best interest of the patient.

C. The physician-patient relationship is the central focus of all ethical concerns.

D. Documents have been developed by the American Academy of Orthopaedic Surgeons (AAOS) with the help of other organizations to outline ethical principles of medicine and orthopaedic surgery (http://www.aaos.org/about/papers/ethics.asp):
1. *Medical Professionalism in the New Millennium: A Physician Charter* (2002)
2. *Principles of Medical Ethics and Professionalism in Orthopaedic Surgery* (2002)
3. *AAOS Standards of Professionalism* (http://www3.aaos.org/member/profcomp/sop.cfm)
4. *Guide to Professionalism and Ethics in the Practice of Orthopaedic Surgery* (2011)
5. *Code of Ethics and Professionalism for Orthopaedic Surgeons* (2009)

E. Most documents are aspirational.

F. AAOS Standards of Professionalism are unique in that they represent the minimal level of acceptable conduct.

G. Nonadherence to these principles can result in the loss of membership.

H. Violations of these standards:
1. May serve as grounds for formal complaints to AAOS
2. May be reviewed by the AAOS Professional Compliance Program
3. May result in action outlined in the AAOS Bylaws, including the following:
   - Reporting to the National Practitioner Data Bank
   - Reporting to State Medical Licensing Boards
   - Reporting to **American Board of Orthopaedic Surgery**
   - Censuring, suspension for a time, or expulsion from AAOS

II. PRINCIPLES OF ETHICS AND PROFESSIONALISM

A. *Ethics* is the discipline dealing with the principles or moral values that govern relationships between and among individuals and defines what the orthopaedic surgeon ought to do.

B. Key elements of the *AAOS Code of Ethics and Professionalism for Orthopaedic Surgeons* (2009):

1. The physician-patient relationship is the "central focus of all ethical concerns."
   - This relationship is based on trust but also has a contractual basis.
2. Conduct of the orthopaedic surgeon must have the following goals:
   - Emphasize the patient's best interests
   - Provide "competent and compassionate care"
   - Obey the law and maintain professional dignity and discipline
3. Conflicts of interest are common
   - They must be resolved in the best interest of the patient.
   - Relationships with industry and ownership of medical facilities are the most common areas of conflict and are best managed with full disclosure.
4. The other sections of the code address additional important issues.
   - Maintaining competence
   - Relationships with orthopaedic surgeons, nurses, and allied health professionals
   - Relationship to the public
   - General principles of care
   - Research and academic responsibilities
   - Responsibility to society as a whole

C. *Medical Professionalism in the New Millennium: A Physician Charter* (2002)

1. The AAOS adopted the charter crafted by physicians throughout the industrialized world who were concerned about changes in health care delivery systems that threaten the values of professionalism.
   - Three fundamental principles of professionalism define the basis of the contract between the field of medicine and society:
     - Primacy of patient welfare: serve the patient's interest
     - Autonomy: respect a patient's informed choices
     - Social justice: promote fair distribution of health care resources
2. The charter also defines a set of 10 professional responsibilities that apply to physicians.
   - Professional competence: Individual commitment and the profession must strive to ensure that its members are competent.
   - Honesty with patients: Good information must be provided before and after treatment, especially with unanticipated outcomes.
   - Patient confidentiality: Privacy reinforces trust in the profession, but it may have to be disregarded if the patient endangers other people.
   - Appropriate relations: Patients must never be exploited for sexual or financial advantage.
   - Improving the quality of care: Physicians must maintain knowledge, reduce errors, and create mechanisms to improve care.
   - Improving access to care: Physicians should reduce barriers to access that are based on laws, education, and finances.
   - Just distribution of finite resources: Physicians should promote the wise and cost effective use of limited resources.
   - Scientific knowledge: Physicians should promote research and create new knowledge and use it appropriately.
   - Managing conflicts of interest: Physicians must recognize and disclose to patients and to public when reporting results of clinical trials or guidelines.
   - Professional responsibilities: Physicians must work collaboratively and participate in self-regulating and self-disciplining other members of profession.

D. Standards of professionalism represent the mandatory *minimum* levels of acceptable conduct for orthopaedic surgeons (http://www3.aaos.org/member/profcomp/sop.cfm).

1. **Providing musculoskeletal services to patients** (2008):
   - Responsibility to the patient is paramount.
   - Provide equal treatment of patients regardless of race, color, ethnicity, gender, sexual orientation, religion, or national origin.
   - Provide needed and appropriate care or refer to a qualified alternative provider.
   - Present pertinent medical facts and obtain informed consent.
   - Advocate for the patient and provide the most appropriate care.
   - Safeguard patient confidentiality and privacy.
   - Maintain appropriate relations with patients.
   - Respect a patient's request for additional opinions.
   - Pursue lifelong scientific and medical learning.
   - Provide services and use techniques only for which he or she is qualified by personal education, training, or experience.
   - If impaired by substance abuse, seek professional care and limit or cease practice as directed.
   - If impaired by mental or physical disability, seek professional care and limit or cease practice as directed.
   - Disclose to the patient any conflict of interest, financial or otherwise, that may influence care.
   - Do not enter into a relationship in which the surgeon pays for the right to care for patients with musculoskeletal disorders.
   - Make a reasonable effort to ensure that the academic institution, hospital, or employer does not pay for the right to care for patients.
   - Do not couple a marketing agreement or provision services, supplies, equipment, or personnel with required patient referrals.
2. **Professional relationships** (2005)
   - Responsibility to the patient is paramount.
   - Maintain fairness, respect, and confidentiality with colleagues and other professionals.
   - Act in a professional manner with colleagues and other professionals.
   - Work collaboratively to reduce medical errors, increase patient safety, and improve outcomes.
   - Facilitate and cooperate in transferring patient care.
3. **Orthopaedic expert witness testimony** (2010)
   - Do not testify falsely.
   - Provide fair and impartial opinions.
   - Evaluate care by standards of time, place, and context as delivered.
   - Do not condemn standard care or condone substandard care.
   - Explain the basis for any opinion that varies from standard.
   - Seek and review all pertinent records.

- Have knowledge and experience, and respond accurately to questions.
- Have current valid, unrestricted license to practice medicine.
- Have current board certification in orthopaedic surgery (i.e., American Board of Orthopaedic Surgery).
- Have an active practice or familiarity with current practices to warrant expert designation.
- Accurately represent credentials, qualifications, experience, or background.
- Fees should not be contingent on outcome.
- Expect reasonable compensation that is based on expertise, time, and effort needed to address issue.

4. **Research and academic responsibilities** (2006)
   - Responsibility to patient is paramount.
   - Informed consent is required.
   - Honor withdrawal requests.
   - Seek peer review, and follow regulations.
   - Be truthful with patients and colleagues.
   - Report fraudulent or deceptive research.
   - Claim credit only if substantial contributions made.
   - Give credit when presenting other's ideas, language, data, graphics, or scientific protocols.
   - Expose fraud and deception.
   - Make significant contributions when publishing manuscripts.
   - Disclose existence of duplicate publications.
   - Include and credit or acknowledge all substantial contributors.
   - Acknowledge funding sources or consulting agreements.
5. **Advertising by Orthopaedic Surgeons** (2007)
   - Advertising must not suggest any of the following:
     - A diagnosis can be made without consultation.
     - One treatment is appropriate for all patients.
     - A treatment is without risk.
   - Do not use false or misleading statements.
   - Use no misleading representation about ability to provide medical treatment.
   - Use no false or misleading images or photographs.
   - **Use no misrepresentations that communicate a false degree of relief, safety, effectiveness, or benefits of treatment.**
   - Surgeons will be held responsible for any violations of their office or public relations firms retained.
   - Surgeons will make efforts to ensure that advertisements by academic institutions, hospitals, and private practices are not false or misleading.
   - Advertisements shall abide by state and federal laws and regulations related to professional credentials.
   - Provide no false or misleading certification levels.
   - Provide no false or misleading representation of procedure volume or academic appointments orassociations.
   - Provide no false or misleading statements regarding development or study of surgical procedures.
6. **Orthopaedist-Industry Conflicts of Interest** (2007)
   - Surgeons shall regard their responsibility to the patient as paramount
   - Surgeons shall prescribe drugs, devices and treatments on the basis of medical considerations, regardless of benefit from industry.
   - Surgeons shall be subject to discipline by AAOS Professional Compliance Program if convicted of federal or state conflict-of-interest laws.
   - Surgeons shall resolve conflicts of interest in the best interest of the patient, respecting the patient's autonomy.
   - Surgeons shall notify the patient when withdrawing from a patient-physician relationship if a conflict cannot be resolved in the best interest of the patient.
   - Surgeons shall decline subsidies or support from industry except gifts of $100 or less, medical textbooks, or educational material for patients.
   - Surgeons shall disclose any relationship with an industry to colleagues, institution, and other entities.
   - Surgeons shall disclose to patients any financial arrangement, including royalties, stock options, and consulting arrangements with an industry.
   - Surgeons shall refuse any direct financial inducement to use a particular implant, device, or drug.
   - Surgeons shall enter into consulting agreements with industry only when agreements are made in advance in writing and have the following features:
     - They include documentation of an actual need for the service.
     - They include proof that the service was provided.
     - They include evidence that physician reimbursement for consulting services is consistent with fair market value.
     - They are not based on the volume or value of business that the physician generates.
   - Surgeons shall participate only in meetings that are conducted in clinical, educational, or conference settings conducive to the effective exchange of information.
   - Surgeons shall accept no financial support to attend social functions with no educational element.
   - **Surgeons shall accept no financial support to attend continuing medical education (CME) events except in the following situations:**
     - As residents and fellows when selected by and paid by their training institution or CME sponsor.
     - As faculty members of CME programs are allowed honoraria, travel and lodging expenses, and meals from sponsor.
   - Surgeons shall **accept only tuition, travel accommodations, and modest hospitality when attending industry-sponsored non-CME events.**
   - Surgeons shall accept no financial support for guests or other persons who have no professional interest in attending meetings.
   - Surgeons shall disclose any financial relationship with regard to procedure or device when reporting clinical research and experience.
   - Surgeons shall truthfully report research results with no bias from funding sources, regardless of positive or negative findings.

III. CHILD, ELDER, AND SPOUSAL ABUSE

A. Violence

1. Each year, intentional violence claims 20,000 lives, is responsible for more than 300,000 hospitalizations, and causes millions of injuries.

2. It is estimated that 1.4 million children in the United States suffer some form of maltreatment each year. As many as 2000 children die each year from abuse.

B. Child abuse

1. The U.S. Child Abuse Prevention and Treatment Act of 1974 requires orthopaedic surgeons to report all suspected cases of child abuse to local authorities.
2. Failure to report suspected child abuse might result in state disciplinary actions.
   - Child protective services and social workers should be alerted, and the events and home circumstances should be investigated.
   - These statutes provide legal immunity for physicians who report such cases, provided that they act in good faith, even if the information is protected by the physician-patient privilege.

C. Elder abuse

1. Elder abuse has been estimated to affect 2 million older Americans each year.
2. A 1989 Congressional study indicated that 1 of every 25 Americans older than 65 years suffers some serious form of abuse, neglect, or exploitation.
3. Many states have provided legislation to protect from liability the physicians who report elder abuse.
4. **Risk factors for elder abuse include increasing age, functional disability, cognitive impairment, and higher rates of child abuse within the regional population. Gender is not a risk factor.**

D. Spousal abuse

1. One in four women experience domestic violence. Women account for 85% of the victims of intimate partner violence (men only about 15%).
2. **The reporting of suspected spousal abuse is not required, and there is a corresponding absence of legal protection for physicians.**
3. A physician may encourage a patient to seek self-protection. If the physician believes that an individual is truly incapable of self-protection, a court order may be obtained to permit reporting.
4. **Risk factors for spousal abuse include pregnancy, women's age of 19 to 29 years in households earning less than $10,000/year, and African-American race with low socioeconomic status.**

IV. DIVERSITY IN ORTHOPAEDICS

A. Importance of diversity: The understanding of the value of diversity in race, gender, creed, and sexual orientation is increasing in all areas of life.

1. It is essential to be sensitive to diversity issues with regard to colleagues in orthopaedic surgery and medicine, professionals in fields of allied medicine, and patients.
2. Other important aspects of diversity and nondiscrimination include obesity, psychiatric disease, income class, physical disability, and the status of human immunodeficiency virus (HIV) infection.

B. Treatment decisions should not be made on any basis that would constitute illegal discrimination.

1. To include but not limited to race, color, gender, sexual orientation, religion, or national origin (AAOS Standards of Professionalism)

C. Sensitivity to diversity issues is an increasingly important aspect of professionalism.

1. Each practitioner must examine the attitudes, preconceptions, and emotions in this dimension that are exhibited in the workplace.
2. Practitioners must be aware of how speech and behaviors might be perceived by other people of different backgrounds.
3. It is possible for the actions of someone with good intentions to be interpreted as threatening or derogatory by other people of different backgrounds.

V. SEXUAL MISCONDUCT

A. Introduction

1. Avoiding sexual misconduct is an important aspect of professionalism in relationships with patients, coworkers, staff, and colleagues.
2. Sexual relationships, even if consensual, between individuals in a professional supervisor-trainee relationship create the potential for sexual exploitation and the loss of objectivity.

B. Sexual harassment in employment

1. Quid pro quo: Harassment is directly linked to employment or advancement.
2. Hostile environment harassment: Actual sexual advances are not necessary to create a hostile work environment.
   - Verbal or physical conduct (e.g., gestures, innuendo, humor, pictures) of a sexual nature may be interpreted as harassment.
   - General gender-based hostility that promotes a hostile environment in the workplace may be interpreted as harassment.
3. "Reasonable woman" test is the adopted standard for offensive behavior. If a "reasonable woman" would have found the behavior objectionable, then harassment may have occurred.
4. Individuals in medical training programs are considered employees of the school that is training them. This status allows them to pursue harassment claims under the Civil Rights Act.

C. Sexual misconduct in the patient care setting

1. Sexual misconduct with patients is a form of exploitation.
2. Such misconduct is unethical and may represent malpractice or even criminal acts of assault. Courts have maintained that a patient is unable to give meaningful consent to sexual or romantic advances by a physician. Physicians are encouraged to report instances of sexual misconduct by their colleagues.
3. Many states have laws prohibiting physicians from pursuing relationships with current or former patients.
4. The physician-patient relationship must be terminated before any romantic interest can be pursued between the two persons involved.
4. Even then, it may still be unethical if the physician exploits certain confidences, trust, or emotions learned while serving as the patient's physician.

VI. THE IMPAIRED PHYSICIAN

"Impairment" can include chemical impairment, dependence, misconduct, or incompetence.

A. A surgeon (resident, fellow, or attending physician) who discovers impairment in a colleague or supervisor has the responsibility to ensure that the problem is identified and treated.
B. Mechanisms exist for the proper identification and treatment of the impaired physician. Misconduct can be reported to state and local agencies.
C. When reporting such incidences, the practitioner must be sure to act in good faith with reasonable evidence.
D. When a patient is at risk for immediate harm, the practitioner should assert authority to relieve the impaired physician of the patient's care and address the problem with the senior hospital staff as soon as possible.

VII. ORTHOPAEDIC EDUCATION

A. Core competencies
The Accreditation Council for Graduate Medical Education has defined core competencies for all resident education:
1. Patient care skills—including the provision of "compassionate, appropriate, and effective" care—should be mastered.
2. Medical knowledge (biomedical, clinical, and cognate sciences) must be assimilated and applied to patient care.
3. Practice-based learning includes improving patient care with investigation and the appraisal of scientific evidence.
4. Interpersonal and communication skills facilitate effective and compassionate exchange of information with patients, families, and health professionals.
5. Professionalism consists of handling responsibilities while adhering to ethical principles and considering diversity issues in patient care and social services.
6. System-based practice is aided by an awareness of the larger context of medical decisions at the levels of the social, economic, and information systems.

B. Residency and Guidelines of the Accreditation Council for Graduate Medical Education
1. Work hour restrictions
   - Implemented by the Accreditation Council for Graduate Medical Education to address impaired performance with long duty hours
   - Failure to comply can result in probation or suspension of residency accreditation.
   - Effects on resident education are being monitored.
2. **Duty hours**
   - Defined as clinical (patient care), academic, and administrative work, including time on call.
   - Duty hours must be 80 hours or less per week averaged over a 4-week period. A 10% increase may be allowed by programs when the education value is justified by special circumstances.
   - One day in seven must be taken off, averaged over a 4-week period.
   - Time on call must be no more than 1 day per every 3 days in house; there must also be a 10-hour period off duty between daily clinical duties or after being on call.
   - **Results of early evaluations of "new" duty hours have raised concern about patient safety with regard to decreased continuity of care.**

C. Maintenance of certification
1. Practicing orthopaedic surgeons should strive to continually improve performance.
2. Formal education beyond a surgeon's practice is essential.
3. The American Board of Orthopaedic Surgery established a 10-year cycle:
   - Formal orthopaedic American Medical Association (AMA) Physician's Recognition Award (PRA) category 1 CME credits.
     - An average of 40 per year are needed, with at least 120 credits in each of two consecutive 3-year cycles.
     - Of these, at least 20 credits of scored and recorded self-assessment examinations are needed in each 3-year cycle.
   - Pass a formal computerized recertification examination.

VIII. RESEARCH

A. Research is considered "ethical" when the primary goal is to improve methods of detection or treatment of illness.
B. It should be designed to produce useful, reproducible information.
C. Studies should not be redundant or serve to further the interests of individuals or institutions, financially or professionally.
D. Results should be reported honestly, accurately, and in a timely manner. Misrepresentation or falsifying data is unethical.
E. Withholding critical information in order to protect financial interests may create an ethical conflict and jeopardize patient care.
F. Sponsorship by industry has represented a potential conflict of interest or bias:
1. Specific ethical problems arise with this type of research funding.
2. However, significant developments have been made possible by their involvement, and this form of cooperative effort is gaining acceptance.

G. Informed consent: Human research subjects must provide voluntary, informed consent before participating in any research protocol.
1. Their medical care must not be contingent on their participation, and they must be allowed to withdraw from the study at any time without penalty.
2. Each subject must be able to demonstrate understanding of the information and the ability to make a responsible decision.
3. The decision must be voluntary and not the result of undue pressure or influence. Consent can be voluntary and informed only when the following criteria are met:
   - The proposed procedure is explained.
   - The likely effects and risks of the procedure are detailed.
   - The possible side effects are explained in language easily understood by the patient.
   - Methods and conditions of participation are elucidated.

H. Animal use in research
1. According to the AAOS, the humane use of animals in research is justified in order to enhance the quality of life of both humans and animals.
2. The use of animals is ethical only when no suitable alternatives are available.

3. Experimental protocols should minimize the number of animals used, avoid abuse, and maintain all appropriate standards of animal care.
4. The approval of the Animal Care and Use Committee of the AAOS is mandatory.

I. Responsibilities of the principal investigator and coauthors

1. The principal investigator remains responsible for all aspects of the research project, even when duties have been delegated to other people.
2. The principal investigator is also responsible for accurately representing the efforts of individuals or agencies involved in the research and citing contributions from other researchers or publications.
3. The coauthors must have made a significant contribution to the design of, collection of data for, and formation of the research project.
4. Each coauthor should sign an affidavit stating that he or she has reviewed the manuscript of the research report and agrees with all the results and conclusions presented therein before its publication.
5. Resident research should be conducted under the supervision of an attending surgeon. However, the attending surgeon must contribute to the work in actual fact or in a consultative capacity.
6. Scientific publications convey information that affects other research and the direct care of patients.
7. If an error in scientific method or failure to replicate results is found, the principal investigator is responsible for accurately reporting it.

J. Ethical guidelines for human research are based on the duty of a physician to "promote and safeguard the health of the people."

1. *Declaration of Helsinki* (2000) by the World Medical Association
2. *Belmont Report* (1979) by National Commission for the Protection of Human Subjects in Biomedical and Behavioral Research

IX. IMPAIRMENT, DISABILITY, AND HANDICAP

A. Impairment

1. Loss of use or derangement of any body part, system, or function (e.g., muscle weakness, incontinence, pain, loss of joint motion, loss of body part)
2. Impairments are determined by the physician on the basis of the objective results of a physical examination.
3. In permanent impairment, the impairment has become static or well stabilized and is not likely to remit despite maximum medical treatment.
4. An impaired individual is not necessarily disabled.

B. Disability: loss of an individual's capacity to meet personal, social, or occupational demands because of impairment

1. The gap between what a person can do and what she or he needs or wants to do
2. A disability renders a person unable to perform any kind of substantial gainful work, in view of the individual's age, education, and work experience.
3. Permanent disability is disability that has become static or well established and is not likely to change despite medical or rehabilitative measures.
4. The provisions of the **Americans with Disabilities Act** apply to organizations in the private sector that employ 25 or more employees.
   - **Accommodation** refers to workplace modifications that enable a disabled employee to meet the job demands required of other workers.
   - Under the Americans with Disabilities Act, the identification of an individual as having a disability does not depend on the results of a medical examination.
   - An individual may be identified as having a disability if there is a record of an impairment that has substantially limited one or more major life activities.
5. Morbidity associated with disability:
   - Feelings of displacement, depression, and suicide increase as the disability becomes protracted.
   - There is a higher incidence of drug and alcohol abuse, family disruption, and divorce among disabled workers.
   - Return to employment must be the goal of treatment.

C. Handicap: related to, but different from, the concepts of disability and impairment

1. Under federal law, an individual is handicapped if impairment substantially limits one or more of the activities of daily living.
2. Example:
   - A surgeon who loses a hand has an impairment and will be disabled in terms of the ability to operate.
   - However, the surgeon may be fully capable of being the chief of a hospital medical staff and may not be at all disabled with regard to that occupation.
   - The surgeon has a handicap that impairs his ability to tie shoelaces or cut steak.

SECTION 2 ETHICS AND THE BUSINESS OF ORTHOPAEDICS

I. CONFLICT OF INTEREST

These issues best managed with **full disclosure.**

A. When a surgeon's financial or ownership interest in a durable medical goods provider, imaging center, surgery center, or other health care facility is not immediately obvious, the surgeon must disclose this information.

B. Disclosure is important with regard to intellectual property, royalties, and devices as well.

II. GLOBAL SERVICES

A. "Unbundling" is to bill individually for services that are properly considered a part of the "global service" package.

B. For example, a surgeon does not bill separately for office visits that are ordinarily scheduled for routine postsurgical follow-up for a period of 90 days.

III. REFERRALS AND OWNERSHIP OF MEDICAL SERVICES

A. The Stark laws* continue to be reinterpreted and modified but apply to physicians who serve Medicare and Medicaid patients.
B. Designated health services include most diagnostic and therapeutic services relevant to orthopaedic surgery.
C. The Stark laws prohibit the referral of patients to entities with which the referring physician or immediate family member has a financial relationship.
D. Exceptions exist for "in-house ancillary services" that are within a surgeon's own practice. These services play specific roles.

1. Provide convenience for the patient
2. Offer potential economic efficiency for the health care system
3. Constitute an important source of income for some groups
4. Raise a potential for abuse

IV. RELATIONSHIP WITH INDUSTRY[†]

A. Conflict of interest must be resolved in the best interest of the patient.

1. The surgeon's role is to select the best possible orthopaedic hardware, medication, or treatment for a particular patient's needs.
2. Decisions should be based on the following criteria:
   - Results of clinical trials in the published medical literature
   - The clinician's expertise
   - The clinician's perspective of the patient's preference
   - Monetary issues, which should enter into the decision process in the realm of cost effectiveness
     - Monetary considerations may include limitations of the patient's resources or needs.
     - In this decision, there is no role for factors that benefit the physician. This is particularly true for financial compensation.

B. Consulting and intellectual property and relationship with industry

1. This relationship has been described as being of four types:
   - Type I: A surgeon possesses intellectual property rights.
   - Type II: A consulting agreement is based on specific expertise.
   - Type III: A surgeon is compensated for product promotional activities—often an ethical violation.
   - Type IV: A surgeon is provided benefits in exchange for product use—always an ethical violation.

C. Procedure patents are unethical.

1. They deny all formal contributions from individuals, limit education, increase cost of delivered services, and may jeopardize ideal patient care.

V. SECOND OPINIONS

A. Consultation implies that the treating physician retains care for the patient; it is unethical for the consulting physician to solicit the care of a patient.
B. Referral implies that the treating physician desires to share the care of the patient with a specific service.
C. Transfer by the treating physician implies complete transfer of care to an accepting physician. All transfers must be made with the consent of the patient.
D. Second opinions secured by third-party payers before authorization of procedures are usually governed by contractual agreements.
E. Orthopaedic surgeons providing a second opinion are ethically responsible to inform the patient of all relevant facts, including instances in which surgeon error may have led to the current circumstances. However, there is no legal requirement to provide this information.

VI. INSURANCE AND REIMBURSEMENT

A. Centers for Medicare and Medicaid Services are federal agencies that administer public health programs in the United States.
B. Public health care programs were initiated as part of the Social Security Amendments of 1965 and have become some of the most important economic entities in modern health care.
C. Medicare is a federal health care insurance system for individuals 65 years of age and older.
D. Medicaid is a federally funded but state-administered health care insurance system for certain low-income and other individuals.
E. Insurance and reimbursement tools

1. **Relative value units** (RVUs): system through which physicians are reimbursed for patient care.
   - RVUs are assigned to patient care activities in the clinic, operating room, emergency room, or interventional suite.
   - The total RVU for patient care is based on the following:
     - Work (time, intensity, effort: about 50% of value)
     - Practice expense (overhead, staffing: about 45%)
     - Professional liability insurance (regional malpractice costs: about 5%)
   - The geographic practice cost index (GPCI) adjusts RVU payments by regional differences in cost of living, liability exposure, and political influences.
   - The RVU calculation for thousands of codes and procedures is complex.
   - Both government and physician groups throughout the AMA are represented in determining updates.
2. **Diagnosis-related groups** (DRGs): system by which hospitals are reimbursed for patient care.
   - For example, DRG 209 represents hospitalization that includes total knee and total hip arthroplasty.
3. **Gain-sharing:** an incentive plan in which both surgeon and hospital are encouraged to increase efficiency and lower costs
   - The high, and increasing, cost of implants is often the first target of these programs.
   - Ethical concerns and legality of gain-sharing are frequently discussed by the powerful stakeholders, including implant manufacturers and hospitals.
4. **Pay for performance (P4P):** a trend in reimbursement and quality assurance whose goal is to reimburse efforts to standardize patient care

---

*Federal laws that limit self-referrals by physicians to facilities that they own.
[†]See earlier discussion of Standards of Professionalism.

- Government, private insurers, or professional organizations define quality measures.
- The time when measures are met may entitle surgeons, hospitals, or both to increase payments or to avoid fines.
- *Quality measures* include either *process of care* goals (e.g., preoperative prophylactic antibiotic orders) or *outcome measurements* (e.g., decrease rates of infection).

VII. EMERGENCY ROOM CALL

Numerous factors have been cited as contributing to a decreasing desire among surgeons to cover an emergency room call:

A. Wide-ranging, unpredictable, and frequently difficult-to-treat pathologic processes in patients who display assorted levels of compliance

B. Economic components, including higher percentages of underinsured patients

C. Markedly smaller payer reimbursements in the presence of unrelenting increases in overhead costs

D. Night calls, which may interfere with a productive elective schedule during the day

E. Attitudes of younger surgeons toward work

F. Lifestyle issues and changing perception of parental duties in modern two-income families

G. Emergency Medical Treatment and Active Labor Act (EMTALA): places the responsibility to provide emergency services on the hospital

1. EMTALA laws govern how hospitals treat and transfer patients presenting with unstable medical conditions.
   - These laws are sometimes called "antidumping" laws.
   - In general, hospitals must evaluate any patient and "stabilize" an unstable medical condition, regardless of the patient's ability to pay.
2. EMTALA applies to hospitals that provide emergency services to Medicare and Medicaid patients and applies to nearly all hospitals.
   - The regulations apply to all patients at such hospitals, not just Medicare patients.
   - Any patient who comes to the emergency room requesting treatment must receive a screening examination to identify a possible emergency condition.
   - A patient in whom an emergency condition exists must receive treatment until the condition is "stabilized" or until transfer or discharge is unlikely to result in deterioration of the condition.
   - **Once the patient's condition is stabilized, the patient may be transferred if the benefits of transfer outweigh the risks (documented) and the receiving institution accepts the transfer.**
   - The patient's records must accompany the transfer.
3. EMTALA does not force orthopaedists to provide emergency services or to be on call.
   - Orthopaedists in every community have a responsibility to ensure that emergency patients receive appropriate and timely musculoskeletal care.
   - Local strategies must be employed by the orthopaedic surgeons and hospitals in each community.
   - Surgeons may be in violation of EMTALA in the following situations:
     - If a physician who is "on call" (by bylaw or contract) fails to respond to an emergency medical condition.
     - If a physician affirms that a patient in unstable condition is stable to authorize a transfer.
4. EMTALA does force hospitals to provide emergency care to patients.
   - Hospitals may fulfill their obligation by contracts with physicians or groups of physicians or by requirements in the hospital bylaws.
   - A growing trend exists for hospitals to hire surgeons directly, to pay for care that surgeons provide to uninsured patients, or to provide a stipend for covering the hospital's obligation.
   - According to the AAOS position, hospitals are obligated to assume a portion of the growing costs of providing emergency care.
5. The law is unclear in scenarios involving follow-up care.
   - An "on-call" orthopaedist who either sees the patient or formulates a plan of care without seeing the patient has established a relationship.
   - This does not constitute a clear obligation to provide follow-up care under EMTALA once the patient's condition has been stabilized.
   - However, the law may be interpreted in different ways, and the orthopaedist may have some obligation for ongoing care regardless of the patient's ability to pay.
   - It is in the best interests of the hospital, the orthopaedic surgeon, and the community to provide adequate compensation for unfunded care from the emergency room.

SECTION 3 ETHICS AND MEDICOLEGAL ISSUES

I. INFORMED CONSENT

This is a legal doctrine about obtaining permission for care in close association with the right to autonomy.

A. Informed consent is a process (not simply a document) representing an exchange of information that results in the selection of and agreement to undergo a specific form of treatment.

B. Without proper consent from a patient or a patient's family, the surgeon may be guilty of an assault, battery, or trespass against the patient.

C. Most litigation results from unexpected consequences of a procedure.

D. Properly informed patients are aware of, and have decided to accept, both the potential for benefits and the risks.

E. The attending surgeon should explain to patient (or legal representative) in layperson's terms the following information:

1. The patient's diagnosis and the nature of the condition or illness necessitating intervention

2. The nature and purpose of the proposed treatment or procedural plan
3. The risks and complications of the treatment or procedure
4. Options or alternatives (including no treatment), with their associated risks and complications
5. The probability of success (no guarantee of success should be expressed or implied)

F. In elective cases, informed consent should ideally be obtained by the physician in the office setting several days before surgery.

G. A patient (or legal representative) must have adequate decision-making capacity.

H. A professional translator should be present for patients who do not speak the same language as the physician. Avoid using a family member for translation whenever possible.

I. If a patient lacks the ability to make decisions, informed consent may be obtained by a legal guardian or, in situations deemed medically necessary, by a physician.

J. Special rules about informed consent apply in cases of emergencies and to minors.

1. **A medical emergency concerns an unconscious or incapacitated person with a life- or limb-threatening condition that necessitates immediate medical attention.**
   - **Treatment can proceed without informed consent; as soon as is practical, the reason for treatment should be documented.**
2. Consent rules for minors vary greatly from state to state. The surgeon must be aware of the rules that apply locally.
   - **In general, consent for treatment of minors is obtained from the parent or guardian for all conditions except emergencies.**

K. Documentation of consent is usually in the form of a hospital "permit" and a summary note in the patient's record (which constitute so-called double consent).

L. Standards of disclosure: The degree of disclosure varies among the states, and the courts have developed two standards that may be applied.

1. Professional or reasonable physician standard: used by most states, based on what is customary practice in a specific medical community for surgeons to divulge to their patients.
2. Patient viewpoint standard: based on the level of information that a "reasonable person" would want to know in a similar circumstance. (This viewpoint has received some preference in courts.)

II. PHYSICIAN-PATIENT CONTRACT

"Physician-patient relationship has a contractual basis and is based on confidentiality, trust, and honesty" (*AAOS Code of Medical Ethics*).

A. Both the patient and the orthopaedic surgeon are free to enter or discontinue the relationship within any existing constraints of a contract with a third party.

B. An orthopaedic surgeon has an obligation to render care only for the conditions that he or she is competent to treat.

1. The contract starts when a physician actually sees a patient in an office visit or hospital consultation.
2. Orthopaedic surgeons do have an obligation to adhere to the **"standard of care,"** although this concept is hard to define precisely:
   - What a "reasonable" orthopaedic surgeon might do under similar circumstances
   - Often considered to be regional or local in nature, but several legal cases have been decided on the notion of a national standard of care.
   - A complex concept that is often determined on a case-by-case basis
   - It is not ethical or legal to offer substandard care to a patient who is perceived as undesirable.
   - A physician is not required to provide therapy that is found to be ethically inappropriate or medically ineffective.
3. Terminating the physician-patient contract: Once a relationship has been established, it is expected that the relationship will continue except under certain circumstances:
   - Physicians must always provide emergency treatment to patients.
   - Physicians may terminate the relationship for patients who can no longer pay for services, as long as an alternative source of care can be identified.
     - When an alternative source cannot be identified, caution must be exercised in terminating the relationship.
     - Even for nonemergency care, there is debate over whether an orthopaedist may terminate care because of a patient's inability to pay.
   - Identifying an alternative source of care is best accomplished in writing and should provide the patient with ample time to establish care with the new provider.
     - This situation also applies if an orthopaedic surgeon withdraws from a managed care contract or no longer accepts an insurance plan.
   - Medical records should be forwarded to the accepting physician, including a medical history and a summary of the treatment rendered.
     - The dates of shipping and receipt of records should be documented.
4. **Abandonment**
   - Wrongful termination of the physician-patient relationship consists of four basic elements:
     - The physician-patient relationship must be established.
     - Patient must have a reasonable expectation that care will be provided.
     - Patient must have a medical need that necessitates medical attention, the absence of which will result in harm or injury.
     - Causation must be established. The failure to provide care must produce injury or harm.
   - Abandonment may take many forms.
     - Inadequate follow-up for common complications to be recognized
     - Failure to provide an appointment to an established patient, even if the patient has not paid previous bills, has missed other appointments, has been noncompliant, or has sought interim care from another provider
     - Premature discharge from an inpatient setting

- Failure to allow the patient the opportunity to seek care elsewhere when physician has illness, personal conflict, or vacation
- If a patient does not appear for important follow-up appointments, a certified letter should be sent instructing him or her to attend follow-up appointments.

5. **Scope of practice:** "An orthopaedic surgeon should practice only within the scope of his or her personal education, training, and experience" (*AAOS Code of Medical Ethics*).
   - The surgeon may decline to treat a patient with a pathologic condition that is outside the scope of the surgeon's practice.
   - Contractual obligations may also be important in the managed care setting or hospital contracts, in which an orthopaedic surgeon manages general musculoskeletal care.
     - "If an orthopaedic surgeon contracts to provide comprehensive musculoskeletal care, then he or she has the obligation to ensure that appropriate care is provided in areas outside of his or her personal expertise" (*AAOS Code of Medical Ethics*).

III. MEDICAL LIABILITY

A. Crisis and reform: It is commonly accepted that there is an ongoing crisis in medical liability that threatens the well-being of patients and physicians alike.

1. States whose politicians have reformed policies are rewarded with increasing numbers of physicians.

B. Malpractice: negligence by a health care provider that results in injury to a patient

1. **Malpractice suit:** a civil action filed by a patient alleging that a physician's negligence resulted in an injury for which the patient desires compensation
2. **Issues with physician-patient communication are frequently cited as the most common factor in the initiation of a malpractice lawsuit.**
3. **In general, if an error is discovered by the surgeon (such as use of an incorrect implant), it should be disclosed to the patient.**
4. **Femur fractures (particularly pediatric fractures), followed by tibia fractures, are the orthopaedic conditions that most commonly result in malpractice suits.** Displacement of an intervertebral disk is third most common, but it has the highest indemnity, both total and average.
5. The law requires proof of the allegation by a preponderance of the evidence.

C. Negligence: the result of failure to exercise the degree of diligence and care that a reasonable and prudent person would exercise under the same or similar conditions. Medical negligence comprises four elements: duty, breach of duty, causation, and damages.

1. **Duty** begins when the surgeon offers to treat the patient and the patient accepts the offer.
   - The duty of the physician is to provide care equal to the same standard of care ordinarily executed by surgeons in the same medical specialty.
     - There is no particular "institution" standard of care; the standard of care is usually established by **expert testimony.**
       - Validity of testimony: The testimony must be nonpartisan, scientifically correct, and clinically accurate.
       - Basis for testimony must be documented (personal experience, clinical references, and currently accepted orthopaedic opinion).
       - Ethics and requirements to testify (see earlier discussion of Standards of Professionalism, ***Orthopaedic Expert Witness Testimony*):**
       - Reasonable compensation commensurate with time and expertise is acceptable; *compensation based on the outcome of the litigation is unethical.*
     - ***Res ipsa loquitur*** ("the thing speaks for itself"): Certain cases do not require expert testimony.
       - When surgery is performed at the wrong site, when surgical equipment is inadvertently left inside the patient, and when a physician fails to attend to a patient in distress who complains persistently.
         - **The chance of wrong-site** surgery can be decreased by involving the patient in identifying the surgical site.
     - Residents and fellows are held to the same standard of care as that for board-certified orthopaedists.
2. **Breach of duty:** when action or failure to act deviates from the standard of care
   - Breach of duty takes the form of an **act of commission** (doing what should not have been done) or an **act of omission** (failing to do what should have been done).
3. **Causation:** when failure to meet the standard of care was the direct cause of the patient's injuries
4. **Damages:** monies awarded as compensation for injuries sustained as the result of medical negligence
   - **Special damages** are actual expenses, such as medical or rehabilitative expenses and lost wages.
   - **General damages**, or noneconomic losses, are awards for pain and suffering, disfigurement, and other adverse outcomes.
   - **Punitive or exemplary damages** serve as a penalty for blatant disregard or incompetence. (Seldom awarded in medical malpractice cases.)
   - ***Ad quod damnum* clause** specifies the amount of money sought for damages in a suit. (not allowed in some states)

D. Comparative negligence doctrine awards damages that are based on the percentage of responsibility for the result by each party.

E. Contributory negligence bars the recovery of damages if there was negligence on the part of the plaintiff.

F. Modified comparative fault bars the recovery of damages if the plaintiff's contributory negligence exceeds 50%.

G. Bad faith action: When a claim is filed and an action pursued regardless of the lack of reasonable grounds for filing the claim. In these circumstances, the physician may countersue for damages.

H. Statute of limitations: time limit for plaintiff to file a malpractice suit

1. In general, 2 years (the time limit varies by state)
2. For minors, generally 2 years from the time of the incident or until the individual's eighteenth birthday.

I. Discovery: the process by which both parties find out about each other's cases and is a period of information gathering

1. Techniques of gathering facts:
   - Interrogatories: written questions answered in writing under oath
   - Deposition: pretrial oral testimony given under oath
   - Production request: request to produce documents regarding a claim
   - Request for admission: request of one party that the other party admit or deny factual statements under oath

IV. MALPRACTICE INSURANCE

A. Two basic types

1. **Occurrence coverage** covers claims resulting from action that occurs during the coverage period of policy, regardless of when the claim is filed.
   - Very expensive; coverage extends even after physician stops work (i.e., so-called tail insurance is included).
2. **Claims-made coverage** covers claims resulting from action that occurs during the policy period that are reported during policy period.
   - Claims filed after the expiration of the policy are not covered even if the events occurred during the period of coverage (i.e., tail insurance is not included).

B. Other malpractice coverage

1. **Tail coverage** is a separate policy that covers the physician for all claims made for actions occurring during the period of coverage; this essentially constitutes an occurrence policy.
2. **Prior-act coverage** protects the insured physician from potential claims resulting from events for which claims have yet to be filed.
3. ***Locum tenens* coverage** provides extended insurance coverage to a physician who temporarily replaces the policyholder.
4. **Slot coverage** covers duties encountered during practice in a specific position through which several physicians may rotate.

C. Policies may have specific restrictions or exclusions

1. Some policies cover only direct patient care.
2. Activities such as peer review, quality assurance, and utilization review may be covered by the insurance policy or a health care contract.
3. Nearly all policies for residents and fellows have an exclusion for moonlighting.
   - Ensure that your employer provides such coverage, or purchase professional liability insurance in your own behalf.
4. **Hold harmless clause** is a contractual statement that attempts to shift liability from the employer to the physician. Insurance carriers do not generally cover this contractual obligation.

D. Surcharging or experience rating: Insurance plans may assess points against a physician on the basis of the number of claims filed and the dollar amounts awarded on behalf of the insured.

E. Good Samaritan Act: This act grants legal immunity for actions performed in good faith by persons at the scene of an emergency.

1. Legal immunity is not given if the action constitutes gross, willful, or wanton neglect.
2. It does not extend to care given in expectation of payment by persons who routinely render care in an emergency room or by the patient's admitting, attending, or treating physician.

F. The AAOS recommends that a resident or fellow make a point of obtaining evidence of insurance for each year of residency and saving this evidence in personal files.

V. LIABILITY STATUS OF RESIDENTS AND FELLOWS

A. Residents and fellows are licensed physicians who function as employees while in a training or educational program.

B. This creates a special relationship between them and their patients and supervisors.

C. Disclosure to patients: Failure to inform a patient of residency or fellow status may result in claims of fraud, deceit, misrepresentation, assault, battery, and lack of informed consent.

D. Levels of responsibility

1. Residents and fellows are responsible for their own actions.
2. Supervisors may be held accountable for the actions of the residents and fellows. This is known as **vicarious liability.**
3. ***Respondeat superior*** ("Let the master answer"): This doctrine is also known as "borrowed servant" or the "captain of the ship."
   - An agency relationship is established by the fact that the resident or fellow has been authorized to act for or represent the supervising physician.
   - While the resident or fellow is an agent for the supervisor, all acts of the relationship are considered to be under the direction of the supervisor.
   - This relationship is independent of the specific employer of the resident or fellow.
4. Residents and fellows are held to *the same standard of care as a fully trained, practicing orthopaedist*, regardless of their level of training.
   - Residents should not attempt to perform procedures that are beyond their level of training.
   - Appropriate consultation with their supervisors is imperative to avoid putting the resident or fellow at risk of acting independently of the supervisor.

E. The AAOS recommends that residents and fellows retain permanent documentation regarding the resolution of any adverse decision in which they may be named.

F. Adverse decisions are reported to the National Practitioner Data Bank, and the resulting information is made available to all health care facilities, as is information about any pending litigation.

G. Documentation regarding the individual cases and information on the resolution of adverse decisions is necessary when the resident or fellow seeks privileges at any health care facility.

VI. MEDICAL RECORDS

These are a systematic documentation of a patient's individual medical history and care.

A. Primary purpose: to allow continuity of care and communication between providers

B. Whether used in legal proceedings or not, the medical record is a legal document.

C. It is a business and administrative document justifying appropriate reimbursement when available.

D. The following statements cover several legal and practical aspects of the medical record:

1. The data in medical records belong to the patient (who may request copies at reasonable cost).
2. Medical records represent the best defense in a malpractice lawsuit.
   - Medical records must be maintained for 7 years after the last date of treatment.
   - Medical records are confidential and, without the patient's written approval, cannot be reproduced or discussed with parties not involved in treating the patient.
3. Accurate and complete medical records protect both the patient and physician from errors and misinterpretations. Records should be characterized as follows:
   - Well-documented, detailing the history, observations, reasons for the treatment provided, and patient noncompliance
   - Legible and clear
   - Accurate and should properly identify the patient
   - A logical sequence of the events and factors affecting treatment decisions
   - An outline of the treatment plan, including the risks, benefits, and alternatives
   - Free from editorial comments or casual criticism of the patient or other health care providers
4. **Medical records should never be altered.**
   - All corrections should be made by amendments. These amendments should accurately reflect the reason for correction and be placed after the last entry.
   - An errant entry should be lined through so that it remains legible. The reason for the correction, the date, the time, and the physician's initials must be included.
   - Removing or obscuring an entry shatters credibility and is indefensible.
   - Attempts to supplement or clarify entries after notification of a lawsuit constitute tampering.
5. On notification of a complaint or lawsuit, the medical records should be secured, inventoried, and copied.
   - Copies of the medical record must be made available to the patient or the attorney in a reasonable amount of time.
   - The medical record must not be withheld as ransom for outstanding bills.
6. **Health Insurance Portability and Accountability Act (HIPAA):** federal security and privacy laws that regulate the disclosure of a patient's personal medical records
   - Practices must develop specific policies on the use of private patient information.
   - In order for practices to release the private information, patients must sign notices that describe the policies.
   - Patients must authorize the release of their medical information before the information is released to a business for purposes not related to their health care (e.g., life insurer, bank, marketing firm).

TESTABLE CONCEPTS

SECTION 1 PRINCIPLES OF PRACTICE

- Advertising must not suggest that treatment is without risk or that one treatment is appropriate for all patients. Misrepresentations that that communicate a false degree of relief, safety, effectiveness, or benefits of treatment (e.g., "pain-free surgery") must not be made.
- Financial support to attend CME events is restricted to faculty members only. They are permitted to accept only tuition, travel accommodations, and modest hospitality when attending industry-sponsored non-CME events.
- The reporting of abuse varies by age and type.
  - Child abuse must be reported in all states, and failure to report may result in state disciplinary actions. Legal immunity is also provided for such reporting.
  - However, the reporting of suspected spousal abuse is not required, and there is a corresponding absence of legal protection for physicians who report it.
  - Requirements for reporting elder abuse are inconsistent; only some states mandate reporting. Provision of legal immunity is also inconsistent.
- A surgeon (resident, fellow, or attending physician) who discovers impairment in a colleague or supervisor has the responsibility to ensure that the problem is identified and treated. When a patient is at risk for immediate harm, the surgeon should assert authority to relieve the impaired physician of the patient care and address the problem with the senior hospital staff as soon as possible.

SECTION 2 ETHICS AND THE BUSINESS OF ORTHOPAEDICS

- When a surgeon's financial or ownership interest in a durable medical goods provider, imaging center, surgery center, or other health care facility is not immediately obvious, the surgeon must disclose this information.
- Disclosure is important with regard to intellectual property, royalties, and device.
- Orthopaedic surgeons providing a second opinion are ethically responsible to inform the patient of all relevant facts, including instances in which surgeon error may have led to the current circumstances. However, there is no legal requirement to provide this information.
- EMTALA places the responsibility to provide emergency services on the hospital. It does not force orthopaedists to provide emergency services.
  - A patient in whom an emergency condition exists must receive treatment until the condition is "stabilized" or until transfer or discharge is unlikely to result in deterioration of the condition.
  - Once the patient's condition is stabilized, the patient may be transferred if the benefits of transfer outweigh the risks (documented) and the receiving institution accepts the transfer.

SECTION 3 ETHICS AND MEDICOLEGAL ISSUES

- In elective cases, informed consent should ideally be obtained by the physician in the office setting several days before surgery.
- A professional translator should be present for patients who do not speak the same language as the physician. Avoid using a family member for translation whenever possible.
- In general, consent for treatment of minors is obtained from the parent or guardian for all conditions except emergencies.
- A medical emergency concerns an unconscious or incapacitated person with a life- or limb-threatening condition that necessitates immediate medical attention. Treatment can proceed without informed consent; as soon as is practical, the reason for treatment should be documented.
- Issues with physician-patient communication are frequently cited at the most common factor in the initiation of a malpractice lawsuit.
- In general, if an error is discovered by the surgeon (such as use of an incorrect implant), it should be disclosed to the patient.
- Femur fractures (particularly pediatric fractures), followed by tibia fractures, are the orthopaedic conditions that most commonly result in malpractice suits.
- Medical negligence comprises duty, breach of duty, causation, and damages. In proving breach of duty, it is not necessary to prove intent.
- The chance of wrong-site surgery can be decreased by involving the patient in identifying the surgical site.
- Medical records should never be altered. On notification of a complaint or lawsuit, the medical records should be secured, inventoried, and copied.

SELECTED BIBLIOGRAPHY

The selected bibliography for this chapter can be found on www.expertconsult.com.

Chapter 13

RESEARCH DESIGN AND BIOSTATISTICS

Joseph M. Hart

CONTENTS

SECTION 1 INTRODUCTION

Critical review of medical research is essential for orthopaedic surgeons. Experiments are conducted in both the clinical and basic sciences, and decisions are based on the results of these experiments and associated statistical analyses. The concepts that support or refute these decisions and generalizations must be understood by the astute consumer of medical literature.

Research starts with developing a question that is important to a particular area of investigation or clinical population; then the study population is defined, and the most appropriate outcome measures and variables are selected. It is important that the research team collaborate so that their combined expertise can contribute to the study aims.

This chapter describes some important concepts to consider in designing a research study and in analyzing and interpreting results.

SECTION 2 COMMON RESEARCH DESIGNS AND RESEARCH TERMINOLOGY

I. PROSPECTIVE STUDIES

A. Designed to assess outcomes occurring forward in time
B. Exposure has occurred or risk factor has developed; patients are monitored forward in time to determine the occurrence of an outcome of interest.

II. RETROSPECTIVE STUDIES

A. Designed to assess outcomes that have already occurred or data that has been collected in the past

III. LONGITUDINAL STUDIES

A. Designed to assess outcomes at multiple points (i.e., repeated measures) over time

IV. OBSERVATIONAL RESEARCH DESIGNS

These designs can be prospective, retrospective or longitudinal (Figures 13-1 and 13-2). Common observational designs are as follows:

A. Case reports

1. Descriptions of unique injures, disease occurrences, or outcomes in a single patient
2. No attempts at advanced data analysis are made.
3. Cause-effect relationships are not discussed, and generalizations are not made.

B. Case series

1. Outcomes are measured in patients with a particular disease or injury.
2. In orthopaedic research, these studies are typically retrospective and involve a thorough review of medical records.

C. Case-control studies

1. Outcomes measured in patients with a particular disease or injury are compared with outcomes in a control group (see subsection VII, Potential Problems with Research Designs, for more information about control groups).
2. Odds ratios (not relative risks) are appropriate measures of association from data collected in these study designs (see Section 4, Concepts of Epidemiology).

D. Cohort study

1. Groups of patients with a similar characteristic or similar exposure or risk factors are studied forward in time (prospective) or from existing data (retrospective).
2. Cohort studies are appropriate for estimating incidence of disease or injury and the relative risks.

E. Cross-sectional study designs

1. A specific patient population is studied at a given time.

Confidence that study conclusions and recommendations are valid ↑

	TYPE OF STUDY			
Level	**Therapeutic Studies** (Investigating the results of treatment)	**Prognostic Studies** (Investigating the outcome of disease)	**Diagnostic Studies** (Investigating a diagnostic test)	**Economic and Decision Analyses** (Developing an economic or decision model)
Level I	1. Randomized controlled trial a. Significant difference b. No significant difference but narrow confidence intervals 2. Systematic review[2] of level I randomized controlled trials (studies were homogeneous)	1. Prospective study[1] 2. Systematic review[2] of level I studies	1. Testing of previously developed diagnostic criteria in series of consecutive patients (with universally applied reference "gold" standard) 2. Systematic review[2] of level I studies	1. Clinically sensible costs and alternatives; values obtained from many studies; multiway sensitivity analyses 2. Systematic review[2] of level I studies
Level II	1. Prospective cohort study[3] 2. Poor-quality randomized controlled trial (e.g., <80% follow-up) 3. Systematic review[2] of level II studies or nonhomogeneous level I studies	1. Retrospective study[4] 2. Study of untreated controls from a previous randomized controlled trial 3. Systematic review[2] of level II studies	1. Development of diagnostic criteria on basis of consecutive patients (with universally applied reference "gold" standard) 2. Systematic review[2] of level II studies	1. Clinically sensible costs and alternatives; values obtained from limited studies; multiway sensitivity analyses 2. Systematic review[2] of level II studies
Level III	1. Case-control study[5] 2. Retrospective cohort study[4] 3. Systematic review[2] of level III studies	Case-control study[5]	1. Study of nonconsecutive patients (no consistently applied reference "gold" standard) 2. Systematic review[2] of level III studies	1. Limited alternatives and costs; poor estimates 2. Systematic review[2] of level III studies
Level IV	Case series	Case series	1. Case-control study 2. Poor reference standard	No sensitivity analysis
Level V	Expert opinion	Expert opinion	Expert opinion	Expert opinion

[1]All patients were enrolled at the same point in their disease course (inception cohort) with ≥80% follow-up of enrolled patients.
[2]A study of results from two or more previous studies.
[3]Patients were compared with a control group of patients treated at the same time and institution.
[4]The study was initiated after treatment was performed.
[5]Patients with a particular outcome ("cases" with, for example, a failed arthroplasty) were compared with those who did not have the outcome ("controls" with, for example, a total hip arthroplasty that did not fail).

Figure 13-1 Study design characteristics that are considered when various types of studies are assigned a "level of evidence." (Adapted from Wright JG, et al: Introducing levels of evidence to the journal, *J Bone Joint Surg Am* 85:1–3, 2003.)

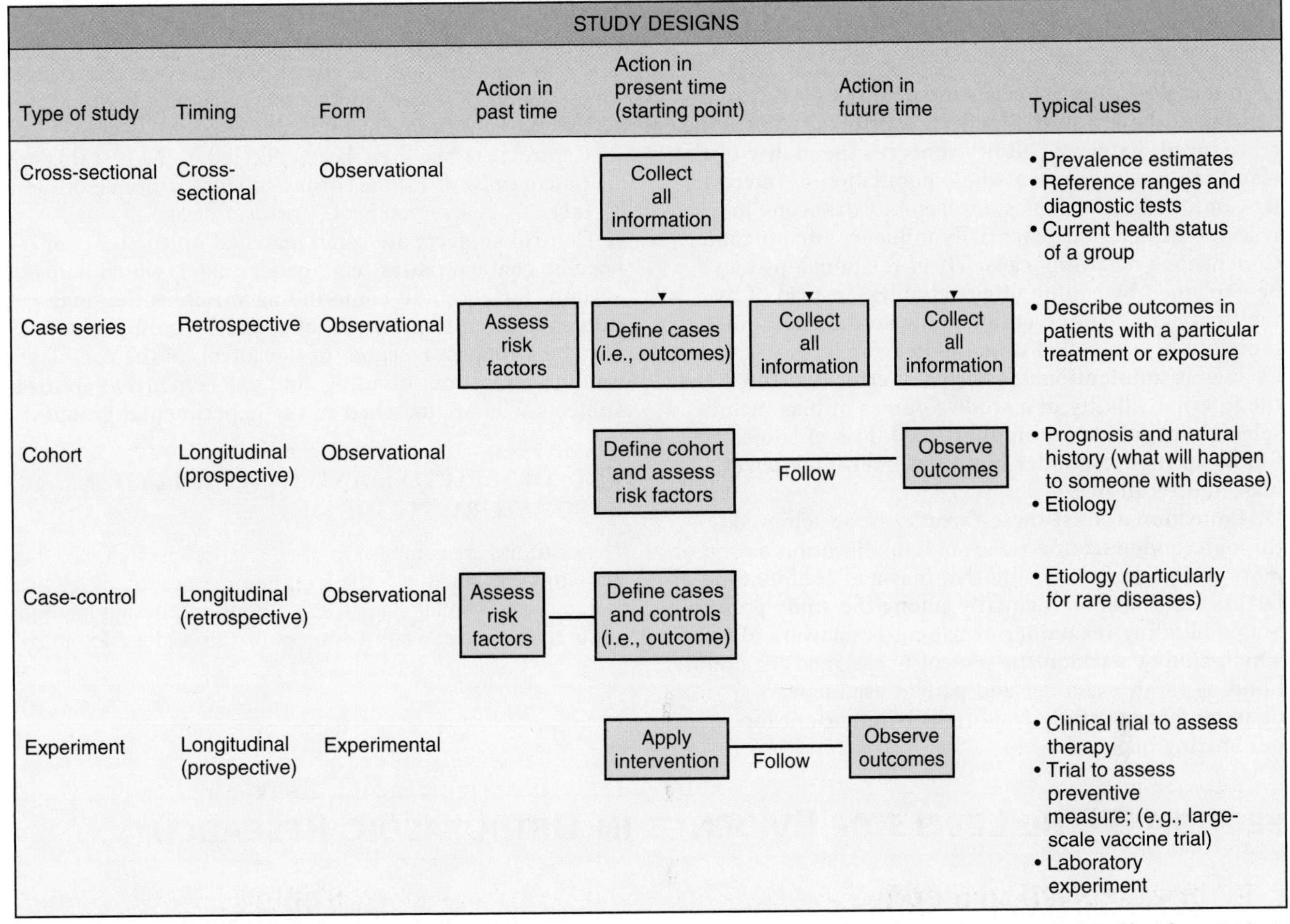

STUDY DESIGNS

Type of study	Timing	Form	Action in past time	Action in present time (starting point)	Action in future time	Typical uses
Cross-sectional	Cross-sectional	Observational		Collect all information		• Prevalence estimates • Reference ranges and diagnostic tests • Current health status of a group
Case series	Retrospective	Observational	Assess risk factors	Define cases (i.e., outcomes)	Collect all information; Collect all information	• Describe outcomes in patients with a particular treatment or exposure
Cohort	Longitudinal (prospective)	Observational		Define cohort and assess risk factors	Follow — Observe outcomes	• Prognosis and natural history (what will happen to someone with disease) • Etiology
Case-control	Longitudinal (retrospective)	Observational	Assess risk factors	Define cases and controls (i.e., outcome)		• Etiology (particularly for rare diseases)
Experiment	Longitudinal (prospective)	Experimental		Apply intervention	Follow — Observe outcomes	• Clinical trial to assess therapy • Trial to assess preventive measure; (e.g., large-scale vaccine trial) • Laboratory experiment

Figure 13-2 Characteristics and typical uses of various research design common in orthopaedic research. (Modified from Petrie A, Sabin C: *Medical statistics at a glance*, Oxford, UK, 2000, Blackwell Science.)

2. All measurements are made at once, with no follow-up period.
3. These studies are considered "snapshots" that are useful for describing the prevalence of a particular injury or disease of interest at a particular time.

C. Clinical studies can be designed to determine superiority of one treatment over another, whether one treatment is no worse than another (noninferiority), or whether both treatments are equally effective (equivalency).

D. Clinical research can be designed to assess outcomes data that are reported by the patient (subjective) or collected by an examiner (objective).

V. RESEARCH TERMINOLOGY

A. Instrument validity:

1. An instrument's ability to *accurately* describe truth or reality
2. In a validation study, measurements recorded by a particular instrument are tested against a "gold standard" measure.

B. Instrument reliability:

1. The ability to precisely describe a characteristic with repeated measurements
2. The precision of an instrument can be tested by different examiners on the same patient (interobserver reliability) or by the same examiner at consecutive times (intraobserver reliability).
3. The *intraclass correlation coefficient* is a common statistical method for testing the reliability or validity of an instrument. Values range from 0 to 1.0 (1.0 represents perfect accuracy or precision).

VI. EXPERIMENTAL RESEARCH DESIGNS

A. Clinical trials: allocate treatments and track outcomes in order to test a specific hypothesis

1. The clinical trial that is the "gold standard" and is based on the highest level of evidence is the randomized controlled trial.

B. Parallel designs: Treatments are allocated to different subjects or patients in a random or nonrandom manner.

C. Crossover designs: Each subject receives or undergoes a series of treatments of each treatment condition being studied.

1. Patients are monitored *longitudinally* for a period of time while receiving one treatment; then they start receiving a second treatment and are monitored for an additional period of time. One of the "treatment conditions" can be a control condition.

VII. POTENTIAL PROBLEMS WITH RESEARCH DESIGNS

A. Internal validity concerns the quality of a research design and how well the study is controlled and can be reproduced. External validity concerns the ability of the results to generalize to a whole population of interest.

B. Confounding variables are factors extraneous to a research design that potentially influence the outcome. Conclusions regarding cause-effect relationships may be explained by confounding variables, instead of by the treatment or intervention being studied and must therefore be controlled or accounted for.

C. Bias is unintentional, systematic error that threatens the internal validity of a study. Sources of bias include selection of subjects (sampling bias), loss of subjects to follow-up (nonresponder bias), observer/interviewer bias, and recall bias.

D. Protection against these threats can be achieved through randomization (i.e., random allocation of one or more treatments) to ensure that bias and confounding factors are distributed equally among the study groups. Single blinding (examiner or patient is unaware of to which study condition the patient is assigned) or double blinding (both examiner and patient are unaware of assignment of study condition) is important for minimizing bias.

E. Control groups can help account for the potential placebo effect of interventions.

1. Control groups may receive an intervention that reflects the standard of care, no intervention, a placebo (i.e., inactive substance), or a sham intervention.
2. Control data may have been collected in the past (historical controls) or may occur in sequence with one or more other study interventions (crossover design).

F. Control subjects are often matched on the basis of specific characteristics (e.g., gender, age), which helps account for potential confounding variables that may influence the interpretation of research findings.

G. The strongest research design involves the use of random allocation, blinding, and use concurrent control subjects who are matched to the experimental group(s).

VIII. DESCRIPTIVE AND CONTROLLED LABORATORY STUDIES

These studies are common in basic science research, but they may involve many of the common concepts of clinical research, and similar statistical methods and design methods are used to protect against sources of bias and confounding.

SECTION 3 THE LEVELS OF EVIDENCE IN ORTHOPAEDIC RESEARCH

I. EVIDENCE-BASED MEDICINE

A. Evidence-based medicine (or evidence-based practice) aims to apply evidence from the highest quality research studies to the practice of medicine.

B. Findings from the best designed and most rigorous studies have the greatest influence on decision making.

II. LEVELS OF EVIDENCE

A. The "levels of evidence" in medical research are listed in order from the most valid and what best describes cause-effect relationships (see Figure 13-1):

1. **Level I: high-quality clinical trials (randomized, controlled, blinded, and so forth)**
2. **Level II: cohort studies or lesser quality clinical trials**
3. **Level III: case-control studies**
4. **Level IV: case series studies**
5. **Level V: expert opinions**

SECTION 4 CONCEPTS OF EPIDEMIOLOGY

I. DEFINITIONS

Epidemiology is the study of the distribution and determinants of disease. The following measures are commonly used in this type of research.

A. Prevalence is the proportion of existing cases or conditions of injuries or disease within a particular population.

B. Incidence (absolute risk) is the proportion of *new* injuries or disease cases within a specified time interval (a follow-up period is required).

1. The incidence can be reported with regard to the number of exposures.
2. Example: Of 100 athletes on a sports team, 12 experience a sports-related injury during a 10-game season; the *incidence rate* would be reported as 12 injuries per 1000 athlete exposures.

D. Relative risk (RR) is a ratio between the incidences of an outcome in two cohorts. Typically, a treated or exposed cohort (in the numerator of the ratio) is compared with an untreated or unexposed (control) group (in the denominator of the ratio). Values can range from 0 to infinity and are interpreted as follows:

1. When RR = 1.0, the incidence of an outcome is equal between groups.
2. When RR > 1.0, the incidence of an outcome is greater in the treated/exposed group (higher incidence value in the numerator).

3. When RR < 1.0, the incidence of an outcome is greater in the untreated/unexposed group (higher incidence value in the denominator).

E. Odds ratios are calculated from the probabilities of an outcome in two cohorts.

1. Odds ratios are well suited for binary data or studies in which only prevalence can be calculated.

F. Interpreting relative risk and odds ratio:

1. Odds ratio and relative risk values are interpreted similarly.
2. When outcomes of two groups are compared, a relative risk or odds ratio of 0.5 would indicate that the likelihood that the treated/exposed patients will experience a particular outcome is half that of the untreated/control group.
3. A value of 2.5 would indicate that the likelihood that the treated/exposed group will experience the outcome is 2.5 times higher than that of the untreated/control group.

II. CLINICAL USEFULNESS OF DIAGNOSTIC TESTS

A. 2×2 contingency table (Figure 13-3) can be used to plot the occurrences of a disease or outcome of interest among patients whose diagnostic test results were positive or negative.

1. **"True positives"**: the number of individuals whose diagnostic test yielded positive results and who actually do have the disease or outcome of interest
2. **"True negatives"**: the number of individuals whose diagnostic test yielded negative results and who actually do *not* have the disease or outcome of interest
3. **"False positives"**: the number of individuals whose diagnostic test yielded positive results but who actually do *not* have the disease or outcome of interest
4. **"False negatives"**: the number of individuals whose diagnostic test yielded negative results but who actually do have the disease or outcome of interest

B. Analysis of diagnostic ability

1. **Sensitivity:**
   - The likelihood of a positive test result in patients who actually have the disease or condition of interest (i.e., ability to detect true positives among those with a disease)
   - Calculated as the proportion of patients with a disease or condition of interest who have a positive diagnostic test:

$$\text{Sensitivity} = \frac{\text{"True positives"}}{\text{Total patients with disease}}$$

   - □ Total number of patients with the disease of interest = "true positives" + "false negatives"
   - **Sensitive tests are used for screening** because they yield few false-negative results. They are unlikely to miss an affected individual.
   - When the result of a highly sensitive (Sn) test is negative (N), the condition can be ruled "OUT" (mnemonic: "SnNOUT").
2. **Specificity:**
   - The likelihood of a negative test result in patients who actually do *not* have the disease or condition of interest (i.e., ability to detect "true negatives" among those without a disease)
   - Calculated as the proportion of patients without a disease or condition of interest who have a negative test result:

$$\text{Specificity} = \frac{\text{"True negatives"}}{\text{Total patients without disease}}$$

   - □ Total number of patients without the disease or condition of interest = "true negatives" + "false positives"
   - **Specific tests are used for confirmation** because they yield few false-positive results and are therefore unlikely to result in unnecessary treatment of a healthy individual.
   - When the result of a highly specific (Sp) test is positive (P), the condition can be ruled "IN" (mnemonic: "SpPIN").
3. **Positive predictive value:**
   - The proportion of patients with a positive test result actually has the disease or condition of interest

	Disease present (+)	Disease absent (–)	
Diagnostic test (+)	True positives	False positives	Positive predictive value = True positives / Total patients with positive test result*
Diagnostic test (–)	False negatives	True negatives	Negative predictive value = True negatives / Total patients with negative test result†
	Sensitivity = True positives / Total patients with disease‡	Specificity = True negatives / Total patients without disease§	

Figure 13-3 Calculations of specificity, sensitivity, and positive and negative predictive values are presented in relation to a 2×2 contingency table. Data from all patients (*N*) can be calculated by summing the four boxes in the contingency table. *Total patients with positive diagnostic test results = number of patients with true-positive results + number of those with false-negative results. †Total patients with negative diagnostic test results = number of patients with false-negative results + number of those with true-negative results. ‡Total patients with disease = number of patients with true-positive results + number of those with false-negative results. §Total patients without disease = number of patients with false-positive results + number of those with true-negative results.

- Calculated as the proportion of patients who have a positive test result and actually do have the disease of interest (i.e., the disease is correctly diagnosed with a positive test result):

$$\text{Positive predictive value} = \frac{\text{“True positives”}}{\text{Total patients whose test results were positive}}$$

  - Total number of patients with positive test results = “true positives” + “false positives”

4. **Negative predictive value:**
   - The proportion of patients with a negative test result actually does NOT have the disease/condition of interest
   - Calculated as the proportion of patients with a negative test result who do not have the disease of interest (i.e., the absence of disease is correctly confirmed with a negative test result):

$$\text{Negative predictive value} = \frac{\text{“True negatives”}}{\text{Total patients whose test results were negative}}$$

     - Total number of patients with negative test results = “true negatives” + “false negatives”

5. **Likelihood ratio:**
   - Probability that a disease exists, according to a test result. Likelihood ratios account for both specificity and sensitivity of a given test.
     - Likelihood ratios close to 1.0 provide little confidence regarding the presence or absence of a disease.
   - **Positive likelihood ratios** (greater than 1.0) indicate a higher probability of disease when the diagnostic test result is positive.
     - Calculated as the ratio between the true-positive rate (sensitivity) and the false-positive rate (1 – specificity):

$$\text{Positive likelihood ratio} = \frac{\text{Sensitivity}}{(1 - \text{Specificity})}$$

   - **Negative likelihood ratios** (less than 1.0) indicate a higher probability that the disease is absent when the diagnostic test result is negative.

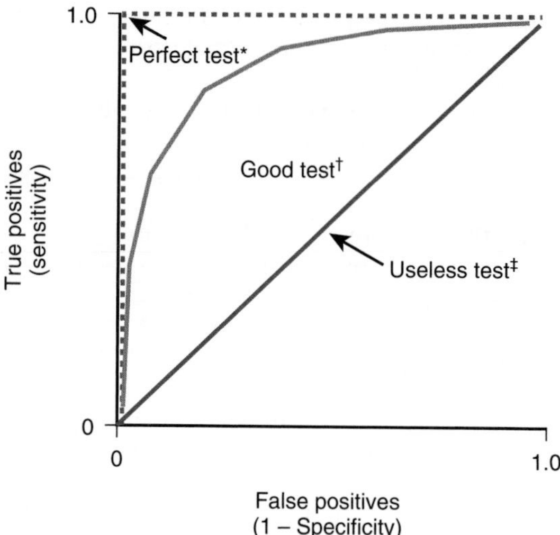

Figure 13-4 Graphic plot showing receiver operating characteristic (ROC) curves for perfect tests (*area under the curve value = 1.0), good tests (†area under the curve is less than 1.0 but greater than 0.5), and useless tests (‡area under curve = 0.5).

     - Calculated as the ratio between the false-negative rate (1 – sensitivity) and the true-negative rate (specificity):

$$\text{Negative likelihood ratio} = \frac{(1 - \text{Sensitivity})}{\text{Specificity}}$$

6. **Receiver operating characteristic (ROC)** curves are graphic representations of the overall clinical utility of a particular diagnostic test that can be used to compare accuracy of different tests in diagnosing a particular condition (Figure 13-4).
   - Tradeoffs between sensitivity and specificity must be considered in identifying the best diagnostic tests.
   - In ROC curves, the true-positive rate (sensitivity) and the false-positive rate (1 – specificity) are plotted on a graph.
   - The area under the ROC curve ranges from 0.5 (useless test, no better than a random guess) to 1.0 (test with perfect diagnostic ability).

SECTION 5 STATISTICAL METHODS FOR TESTING HYPOTHESES

Statistical tests match the purpose of a particular research study. Statistical analyses differ according to the goals of the researcher: for example, to compare groups to identify differences or establish relationships between groups (Table 13-1).

I. SAMPLING AND GENERAL TERMINOLOGY

A. A population consists of all individuals who share a specific characteristic of clinical or scientific interest. *Parameters* describe the characteristics of a population.

B. Study samples affords all members of a specific population equal chance of being studied or enrolled in a clinical study.

C. Sample populations are representative subsets of the whole population. Statistics describe the characteristics of a sample and are intended to be generalized to the whole population.

D. Populations are delimited on the basis of inclusion and exclusion criteria that are established before a study starts.

E. Types of data collected from samples:

1. **Discrete data have an infinite number of possible values (e.g., age, height, distance, percentages, time)**
2. **Categorical data have a limited or finite number of possible values or categories (e.g., excellent, good, fair, or poor; male or female; satisfied or unsatisfied).**

Table 13-1 Decision-Making Guide for Choosing Common Parametric and Nonparametric Statistical Tests According to the Desired Study Purpose

Desired Analysis	Parametric Statistics*	Nonparametric Statistics†
Comparison of two groups		
Paired	Dependent (paired)–samples *t*-test	Wilcoxon test
Unpaired	Independent-samples *t*-test*	Mann-Whitney *U* test
Comparison of three or more groups		
One outcome variable	Analysis of variance (ANOVA)	Kruskal-Wallis test
Repeated observations in same patient	Repeated-measures ANOVA	Friedman test
Multiple dependent variables	Multivariate analysis of variance (MANOVA)	
Analysis including a covariate	Analysis of covariance (ANCOVA)	
Establishing relationship or association	Pearson product-moment correlation coefficient	Spearman rho correlation coefficient
Prediction		
From one predictor variable	Simple regression	Logistic regression
From two or more predictor variables	Multiple regression	
Comparisons of categorical data		
Two or more variables	Chi-square	Chi-square
Better for low sample size	Fisher exact test	Fisher exact test

*Appropriate for normally distributed continuous data.
†Alternative tests appropriate for nonnormally distributed data, small sample sizes, or both.

- **Binary categorical data only have two options (e.g., "yes" or "no").**
- **Categorical data can be ordered (severity: mild, moderate, severe) or unordered (e.g., race).**

F. Data can be plotted in frequency distributions (histograms) to summarize basic characteristics of the study sample.

G. Cutoff points: Continuous data are often converted into categorical or binary data through the use of cutoff points. Cutoff points can be arbitrary or evidence based.

1. In evidence-based establishment of cutoff points, ROC curves are used, and a point that maximizes sensitivity, specificity, or both of a particular test is identified.
2. Example: A numerical value can be established as a cutoff point for white blood cell count to identify whether an infection exists.
3. Arrays of continuous data can be separated into **percentiles** to identify upper and lower halves, thirds, quartiles, and so forth.

II. DESCRIPTIVE STATISTICS

A. A *data distribution* histogram describes the frequency of occurrence of each data value. Distributions can be described in descriptive statistics such as the following:

1. **Mean** is calculated as the sum of all scores divided by the number of samples (n).
2. **Median** is the value that separates a dataset into equal halves; half of the values are higher and half are lower than the median.
3. **Mode** is the most frequently occurring data point.
4. **Range** is the difference between the highest value and the lowest value in a dataset.
5. **Standard deviation** is a value that describes the dispersion or variability of the data.
   - Standard deviation is higher when the variation in data points is wider.

B. Characteristics of a dataset (Figure 13-5):

1. **Normally distributed data** appear in a graph as a bell-shaped curve. The mean, median, and mode are the same value in a gaussian (normal) distribution.
2. **Skewed data** distributions are asymmetric and may be caused by outliers. Data distributions can be skewed to the left (negative skew) or skewed to the right (positive skew).
3. **Kurtosis** is a measure of the relative concentration of data points within a distribution. If data values cluster closely, the dataset is more kurtotic.
4. **Outliers** are data points that are considerably different from the rest of the dataset. Outliers can cause data distributions to be skewed.

C. Confidence intervals quantify the precision of the mean or of another statistic, such as an odds ratio or relative risk.

1. Confidence intervals are calculated to provide a range of values around a point estimate (such as a mean, proportion, relative risk, or odds ratio) that can be used to describe the level of *confidence* that the study data represent the truth.
2. Datasets that are highly variable (have large standard deviations) have larger confidence intervals and hence enable less accurate estimates of the characteristics of a population.
3. **A 95% confidence interval consists of a range of values within which researchers are 95% certain that the actual population parameter (e.g., mean, odds ratio, relative risk) is located.**
   - Example: "Mean = 40.5 (95% confidence interval: 35.5 to 45.5)" indicates that researchers are 95% confident that the population mean is somewhere between 35.5 and 45.5.

III. INFERENTIAL STATISTICS

A. Inferential statistics are used to test specific hypotheses about associations or differences among groups of subject or sample data.

B. The dependent variable is what is being measured as the outcome. There can be multiple dependent variables, depending on how many outcome measures are desired.

C. The independent variables include the conditions or groupings of the experiment that are systematically manipulated by the investigator.

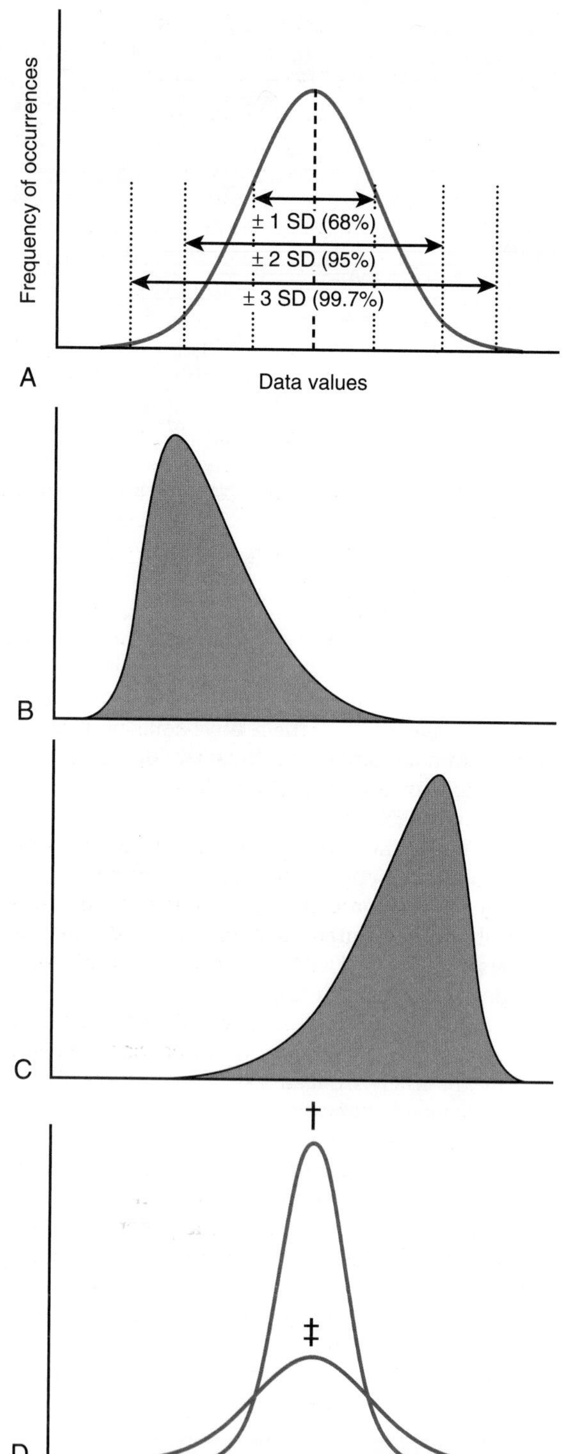

Figure 13-5 Data histograms. **A,** The dispersion of normally distributed data with regard to standard deviation. **B,** Data that are skewed to the right (positive skew). **C,** Data that are skewed to the left (negative skew). **D,** Data exhibiting excessively high (†) and low (‡) kurtosis.

1. For example, a researcher is measuring pain and prescription medication use in patients with shoulder pain who are receiving treatment A, B, or C. The dependent variables are pain and prescription medicine use. The independent variable is treatment condition, of which there are three (A, B, and C).

D. Inferential statistics can be generally divided into *parametric* and *nonparametric* statistics.

1. **Parametric inferential statistics** are appropriate for continuous data and rely on the assumption that data are normally distributed.
   - The mean and standard deviation are used when groups are compared or associations are identified.
   - The mean of a dataset is greatly influenced by outliers; thus, these tests may not be as robust for skewed datasets.
2. **Nonparametric inferential statistics** are appropriate for categorical and data that are not normally distributed.
   - The median and ranks are used in calculating these statistics, and the statistics are therefore more robust alternatives when data are not normally distributed.
3. The goal of inferential statistics is to estimate parameters.
   - Default tests should be parametric.
   - Nonparametric alternatives are justified if the basic underlying assumptions for using parametric statistics are violated, or if the sample sizes are very small.

IV. WHICH TEST TO USE

The decision on what statistical test to use is based on several factors inherent in research designs.

A. Some important distinctions:

1. How many groups are being studied
2. Whether the measures are being recorded in the same or different subjects
3. Whether the data are continuous or categorical
4. Whether the data are normally distributed

B. When two groups of data are compared, the *t*-test is used. There are two variations of the *t*-test:

1. **Dependent (paired)–samples *t*-test:**
   - Appropriate for comparing continuous, normally distributed data collected two times from the same subjects
   - Example: data from two time points measured in the same patient (e.g., before and after intervention)
   - This test is also appropriate for side-by-side comparison within the same subject or in matched pairs of subjects.
   - The nonparametric equivalent is the **Wilcoxon test.**
2. **Independent-samples *t*-test**
   - Appropriate for comparing continuous, normally distributed data from two separate groups
   - Example: data from two groups of patients who received different treatments
   - The nonparametric equivalent is the **Mann-Whitney *U* test.**

C. When three or more groups are compared, an analysis of variance is used. This is also known as the *F*-test.

1. **Analysis of variance (ANOVA)** is appropriate when three or more groups of continuous, normally distributed data are used.
   - The nonparametric equivalent is the Kruskal-Wallis test.
2. **Repeated-measures ANOVA** is a variation of the ANOVA that is appropriate for sequential measurements recorded from the same subjects.

- For example, this test would be used to compare a dependent variable (outcome measure) recorded at three or more time points (e.g., baseline, 1 month after intervention, 2 months after intervention).
- The nonparametric alternative is the Friedman test.

3. **Multivariate analysis of variance (MANOVA),** a variation of the ANOVA, is used when multiple dependent variables are compared among three or more groups.
4. **Analysis of covariance (ANCOVA)** is an appropriate test when confounding factors must be accounted for in the statistical analysis.
5. **Post hoc testing** is necessary after any ANOVA to determine the exact location of differences among groups.
   - ANOVAs describe whether a statistically significant difference exists in *some* way among the study groups.
   - For example, when three levels of the independent variable—treatment conditions A, B, and C—are compared, post hoc testing involves specific comparisons of conditions A and B, conditions B and C, and conditions A and C to determine the exact type of group differences. Post hoc testing is appropriate only if the ANOVA yields statistically significant findings (see Section 6, Important Concepts in Research and Statistics).
   - Common post hoc tests: Tukey Honestly Significant Difference, Sidak, Dunnet, and Scheffe
6. **Factorial designs** are used for multiple independent variables.
   - Hypotheses regarding an interaction among three different treatment groups from before to after intervention are tested in a 2×3 factorial design.
     - The expression "2×3" refers to the number of conditions of two independent variables: The first independent variable (time) has two levels (before and after intervention) and the second (treatment condition) has three levels (treatments A, B, and C).

D. Correlation and regression

1. **Correlation coefficients**
   - These describe the strength of a relationship between two variables.
   - The Pearson product correlation coefficient (r) used for continuous, normally distributed data.
     - The Spearman rho correlation coefficient (ρ) is the nonparametric equivalent.
   - Values range from −1.0 to 1.0: ranges between −0.33 and 0.33 are "weak"; those between −0.66 and −0.33 and between 0.33 and 0.66 are "moderate"; and those lower than −0.66 and higher than 0.66 are "strong."
   - Positive correlation coefficients are indicative of direct relationships: that is, patients who score high on one scale also score high on the other.
   - Negative correlation coefficients are indicative of inverse or indirect relationships: that is, patients who score high on one scale will score low on the other.
2. **Simple linear regression**
   - This statistic describes the ability of one independent (predictor) variable to predict a dependent (outcome) variable.
   - The coefficient of determination (R^2) is the square of r (Pearson product correlation coefficient) and indicates the proportion of variance explained in one variable by another.
   - R^2 ranges from 0 to 1.0, whereby higher values indicate more variance explained.
3. **Multivariate linear regression** describes the ability of several independent variables to predict a dependent variable.
4. **Logistic regression** is used when the outcome is categorical and the predictor variables can be either categorical or continuous data that are not normally distributed.

E. Statistical tests for categorical data

1. **Chi-square (χ^2) test**
   - **Used for two or more groups of categorical data**
   - **Example: to compare treatment A with treatment B when the outcome is either "satisfied" or "unsatisfied," the chi-square test can be used to identify relationships between treatment condition and outcome category**
     - If the result of the test is statistically significant, frequencies of each outcome can be visually compared between the two treatment groups to describe which treatment is superior.
2. **Fisher exact test**
   - Similar to the chi-square test but better for small sample sizes or when the number of occurrences in one of the categories is low (e.g., if only one patient who received treatment A had an unsatisfactory outcome, this test is preferred)

SECTION 6 IMPORTANT CONCEPTS IN RESEARCH AND STATISTICS

I. STATISTICAL ERROR

A. Type I error (α error, false-positive error)

1. **The probability that a statistical test result is *wrong* when the null hypothesis is rejected (e.g., the finding that groups are different when they actually are not).**
2. **It is accepted that this error may occur 5 times out of 100 tests; therefore, the probability value threshold for statistical significance is 0.05, or 5%.**

B. Type II error (β error. false-negative error)

1. **The probability that a statistical test result is *wrong* when the test fails to reject the null hypothesis (e.g., the finding that two groups are *not* different when they actually are different).**
2. **It is accepted that this may occur in up to 20% of tests.**

II. PROBABILITY (*P*) VALUES

A. Inferential test statistics (e.g., *t* statistic, *F* statistic, *r* coefficient) are accompanied by a probability (*P*) value. These values are on a scale from 0% to 100% and indicate the probability that the differences or relationships among study data occurred by chance.

B. P values less than 0.05 mean there is less than a 5% chance that the observed difference or relationship has occurred by chance alone and not because of the study intervention.

C. Typical threshold for "statistical significance": P value = 0.05 or less (type I error may occur in 5 of 100 tests)

1. The decision regarding the threshold for defining statistical significance is arbitrary, but this α level (type I error) is generally accepted.

D. Therefore, in accordance with the P value, the null hypothesis—which is that no differences or no association exists either is rejected (i.e., $P < 0.05$) or fails to be rejected ($P > 0.05$)

E. Bonferroni correction to the P value:

1. Adjusted threshold for statistical significance when multiple *t*-tests are performed for each of several dependent (outcome) variables. It is used to protect against type I error that may occur.
2. Calculated as $0.05/k$, where k is the number of comparisons being made
   - For example, when two groups are compared in a *t*-test for each of three outcome variables, the *t*-test result is statistically significant only if the P value is less than or equal to 0.05/3, or 0.017.

III. STATISTICAL POWER AND ESTIMATING SAMPLE SIZE

A. Research studies should have enough subjects or samples in order to obtain valid results that can be generalized to a population while minimizing unnecessary risk.

B. Sample size estimates are based on the desired statistical power (these estimates are often termed *power analyses*).

1. Statistical power is the probability of finding differences among groups when differences actually exist (i.e., avoiding type II error).
2. These differences are desirable in 80% or more of statistical tests.

C. Sample sizes are justified as the number of subjects needed for researchers to find a statistically significant difference or association (i.e., $P \leq 0.05$) while statistical power is maintained higher than 80%.

D. Higher sample sizes or highly precise measurements (lower variability) are necessary to find small differences between study groups.

E. Power analyses can be done before the study starts (a priori) or after the study has been completed (post hoc).

1. Studies with low power have a higher likelihood of missing statistical differences when they actually exist (i.e., type II error).
2. **To understand the power of a statistical test, the following aspects should be considered: the number of subjects in the study, the effect size (see subsection V, Effect Sizes), the acceptable level of type I error (usually 5%; i.e., $P \leq 0.05$), and an estimate of variability in the data.**
3. The power of statistical tests (which improve the likelihood of finding statistical differences when they exist) increases with more subjects, greater treatment effect, and lower variability among the data.
4. Researchers often design studies to maximize the potential for response to a particular treatment by using stringent inclusion and exclusion criteria and selecting a measurement device or outcome instrument that is more precise and accurate (Figure 13-6).

IV. MINIMAL CLINICALLY IMPORTANT DIFFERENCES

A. Describe the least change in a patient-oriented outcome measure that would be perceived as being beneficial to the patient or would necessitate treatment.

B. Statistical significance does not imply clinical importance.

C. Many of the patient-oriented outcome instruments that are more commonly used have research-established minimal clinically important difference values.

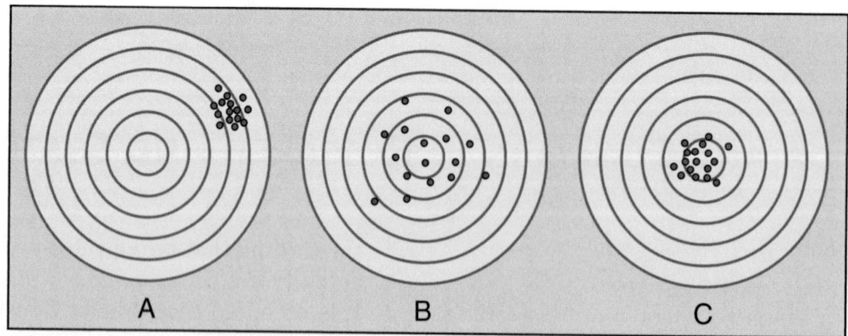

Figure 13-6 Accuracy and precision can be visually explained in the bull's-eye example. In this example, "reality" or the "truth" is at the center of the target. The analogy is used in research, because scientists are always aiming at the "truth." **A,** An example in which a cluster of data points are precise and reliable: Very similar results are seen with repeated trials. **B,** A more accurate and valid cluster than that in **A,** but precision is considerably reduced; very different results are seen with repeated trials, but they seem to cluster loosely around the center of the target. **C,** The cluster of data points is reliable and precise; the data clearly have "hit" the truth and are therefore valid and accurate. Researchers must achieve the optimal balance between accuracy and precision when selecting measurement instruments, selecting study populations, and designing research studies. (From Golish SR, et al: Design and statistics in sports medicine. In DeLee JC, et al, editors: *DeLee and Drez's orthopaedic sports medicine: principles and practice*, ed 3, Philadephia, 2009, WB Saunders, p 101, Figure 12c.)

D. Clinicians should consider whether observed differences are important enough to change practice.

V. EFFECT SIZES

A. Used to describe the magnitude of a treatment effect. An example is Cohen's d effect size.

B. Calculated as the difference between treatment groups divided by the standard deviation (typically pooled standard deviation, or the standard deviation of the reference or control group).

C. Interpretation: Effect sizes greater than 0.8 are "strong"; those less than 0.2 are "small" (between these values can be interpreted as "medium")

TESTABLE CONCEPTS

SECTION 2 COMMON RESEARCH DESIGNS AND RESEARCH TERMINOLOGY

- Observational studies can be prospective or retrospective. Common designs include case series (patients with a common injury or disease), case-control studies (similar to case series but with a defined control group, typically retrospective), cohort (defined groups of subjects to monitor over time), and cross-sectional (measurements taken on a single occasion with no retrospective or prospective review). Case reports are descriptions of a single, unique observation of a patient.
- Incidence can be calculated from prospective or longitudinal study designs because a follow-up period is required. Prevalence is calculated from cross-sectional designs to describe injury distribution at a particular time point.
- Odds ratios and relative risks can be calculated from clinical studies that are designed to determine associations among risk factor exposure and patient outcomes.
- Clinical trials are experimental studies in which a research hypothesis is tested through a specific intervention.
- The "gold standard" of experimental research designs is the randomized, blinded, and controlled clinical trial. These design types require greater time and resources; however, findings from a well-designed randomized controlled trial are considered highly influential.
- Bias is unintentional, systematic error that threatens the internal validity of a study. Randomization, matching, blinding, and using control conditions are methods to protect against the numerous forms of bias.

SECTION 3 THE LEVELS OF EVIDENCE IN ORTHOPAEDIC RESEARCH

- Findings from the best designed and most rigorous studies have the greatest influence on decision making. Such studies are of higher quality and are the most valid.
- Specific levels of evidence are assigned to published manuscripts; in level I, the highest level, results are the most valid and can best describe cause-effect relationships.
- In general, well-designed randomized and blinded clinical trials are graded as level I, prospective cohort studies as level II, case-control studies as level III, case series as level IV, and case reports or expert opinions as level V (see Figure 13-1).

SECTION 4 CONCEPTS OF EPIDEMIOLOGY

- Common epidemiologic measures of the distribution and determinants of disease include prevalence, incidence, odds ratio, and relative risk.
- Prevalence is the proportion of existing injuries or disease cases within a particular population. Incidence is the proportion of new injuries or disease cases within a specified time interval.
- Relative risk and odds ratio describe the risk and odds of a particular outcome of interest between two groups: typically a group in which subjects are treated or exposed and a reference or control group. Relative risk is calculated as the ratio between the incidence rates of an outcome in two cohorts.
- Reliability is the reproducibility of a test or measure; similarly, precision is the repeatability of the results. Validity is the ability of a measure, test, or instrument to represent truth and reality; similarly, accuracy describes the ability of a test to differentiate between correct and incorrect outcomes.
- Sensitivity is a ratio (true-positive test results divided by the number of patients with disease) that describes the proportion of patients who actually have a disease or condition and whose diagnostic test result is positive. Because highly sensitive tests (Sn) yield few false-negative results, a negative (N) result would confidently rule "OUT" the condition of interest (mnemonic: "SnNOUT").
- Specificity is a ratio (true-negative test results divided by the number of patients without disease) that describes the proportion of patients who do not have the disease or condition and whose diagnostic test result is negative. Because highly specific tests (Sp) yield few false-positives, a positive (P) test would confidently rule "IN" the condition of interest (SpPIN).
- Like specificity and sensitivity, likelihood ratios, positive predictive values, and negative predictive values are calculated from 2×2 contingency tables and can describe the accuracy of diagnostic tests.

SECTION 5 STATISTICAL METHODS FOR TESTING HYPOTHESES

- Data from research studies can be discrete (infinite possible values) or categorical (finite possible values); the latter type of data can be binary (only two options), ordered (e.g., a scale of intensity or severity), or unordered (e.g., race).
- Descriptive statistics include mean, median, mode, and standard deviation.
- Confidence intervals provide a range of values around a point estimate (e.g., mean, relative risk, odds ratio) that describe the level of confidence in the ability of the study data to accurately describe truth.
- Statistical tests can be parametric (appropriate for normally distributed continuous data) or nonparametric (appropriate for skewed data, categorical data, or small sample sizes). Each parametric test has a nonparametric equivalent.
- For comparing two groups of normally distributed data, the independent-samples *t*-test is used (paired samples if the groups are matched or measures recorded in the same individual over time). For comparisons of three or more groups, the ANOVA is used (repeated-measures ANOVA for repeated measures, ANCOVA if there is a covariate, MANOVA if there are many dependent variables). The Pearson product moment correlation coefficient is used for correlations.
- The chi-square test is used for comparing categorical data. When sample sizes are small, the Fisher exact test is used.
- For nonparametric tests, Mann-Whitney *U* test is for comparing two groups; the Wilcoxon test is for paired groups, the Friedman test is for comparisons of three or more groups, and the Spearman rho correlation coefficient is for correlations.

SECTION 6 IMPORTANT CONCEPTS IN RESEARCH AND STATISTICS

- Type I error (α error, false-positive error) is the probability that a statistical test result is *wrong* when the null hypothesis is rejected (i.e., concluding that groups are different when they actually are not). Researchers are willing to accept this error in 5% of tests.
- Type II error (β error, false-negative error) is the probability that a statistical test result is *wrong* when the test fails to reject the null hypothesis (i.e., concluding that two groups are *not* different when they actually are different).
- *P* values lower than 0.05 mean that the probability that the observed difference or relationship has occurred by chance alone, and not because of the study intervention, is less than 5%.
- Sample size estimates are used to determine the necessary number of subjects or observations needed for statistically significant results and are based on the desired statistical power (these estimates are often termed *power analyses*).
- Statistical power is the probability of finding differences among groups when differences actually exist (i.e., avoiding type II error). Higher sample sizes or highly precise measurements (lower variability) are needed in order to find small differences between study groups.
- Effect sizes are used to describe the magnitude of a treatment effect. They are calculated as the difference between treatment groups divided by the standard deviation (typically pooled standard deviation, or the standard deviation of the reference or control group).

SELECTED BIBLIOGRAPHY

The selected bibliography for this chapter can be found on www.expertconsult.com.

INDEX

Page numbers followed by "b" indicate boxes; "f" figures; "t" tables

B

C

D

E

J

K

L

M

U

V

W

X

Y

Z